Handbook of
SLEEP
DISORDERS

Handbook of
SLEEP
DISORDERS

Second Edition

Edited by
CLETE A. KUSHIDA
Stanford University School of Medicine
Stanford, California, USA

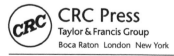

CRC Press
Taylor & Francis Group
Boca Raton London New York

CRC Press is an imprint of the
Taylor & Francis Group, an **informa** business

CRC Press
Taylor & Francis Group
6000 Broken Sound Parkway NW, Suite 300
Boca Raton, FL 33487-2742

First issued in paperback 2019

ISBN-13: 978-0-8493-7319-0 (hbk)
ISBN-13: 978-0-367-38609-2 (pbk)

Library of Congress Cataloging-in-Publication Data

Handbook of sleep disorders. — 2nd ed. / edited by Clete A. Kushida.
    p. ; cm.
  Includes bibliographical references and index.
  ISBN-13: 978-0-8493-7319-0 (hardcover : alk. paper)
  ISBN-10: 0-8493-7319-0 (hardcover : alk. paper) 1. Sleep—disorders—Handbooks, manuals, etc. I. Kushida, Clete Anthony, 1960-
  [DNLM: 1. Sleep Disorders—diagnosis. 2. Sleep Disorders—therapy. WM 188 H2363 2008]
  RC547.H36 2008
  616.8'498—dc22

                           2008035255

Visit the Taylor & Francis Web site at
http://www.taylorandfrancis.com

and the CRC Press Web site at
http://www.crcpress.com

Preface

This handbook would not exist without the excellent contributions of the talented group of international authors; their detailed and comprehensive works are greatly appreciated. I am deeply indebted to the renowned and true pioneers of the field of sleep, William Dement, Christian Guilleminault, Sonia Ancoli-Israel, Chris Gillin, and Allan Rechtschaffen, who served as my mentors through various stages of my career. In all of my endeavors, I can always count on my parents, Samiko and Hiroshi Kushida, to assist me; this book was no exception. This book is dedicated not only to my parents but also to the marvelous team of the Apnea Positive Pressure Long-Term Efficacy Study (APPLES), sponsored by the National Heart, Lung, and Blood Institute (NHLBI) of the National Institutes of Health (NIH). I have been very fortunate, along with Dr. Dement, to serve as principal investigator of APPLES; our team consists of Pamela Hyde, Deborah Nichols, Eileen Leary, Tyson Holmes, Dan Bloch, as well as NHLBI (Michael Twery and Gail Weinmann), site directors, coordinators, consultants, committee members, key Stanford site personnel (Chia-Yu Cardell, Rhonda Wong, Pete Silva, and Jennifer Blair), data and safety monitoring board (DSMB) members, and other personnel without whom this project could not have functioned in such a meticulous and efficient manner.

It is my sincere hope that the reader will strive to become an expert in the field of sleep. Although there is always room for improvement, awareness of sleep disorders by patients, physicians, and the general public is at an all-time high. However, available funding for sleep research and the number of young investigators interested in a career in basic or clinical sleep research are areas that need enhancement. The interested reader can directly contribute to the field in several ways by applying for membership in the American Academy of Sleep Medicine (www.aasmnet.org) or the Sleep Research Society (www.sleepresearchsociety.org), serving on committees in these organizations, becoming board certified in sleep medicine, submitting a sleep-related grant proposal to the NIH, and/or simply learning more about sleep and its disorders. Lastly, I'll never forget a sticker posted on the door of Mary Carskadon's former office at Stanford that contained words to live by: "Be alert. The world needs more lerts."

Clete A. Kushida

Contents

Contributors

Mohsin Ali   Department of Neurology, SUNY Upstate Medical University, Syracuse, New York, U.S.A.

Josephine Arendt   Centre for Chronobiology, School of Biomedical and Molecular Sciences, University of Surrey, Guildford, Surrey, U.K.

Najib T. Ayas   Sleep Disorders Program, University of British Columbia and Centre Clinical Epidemiology and Evaluation, Vancouver Coastal Health Research Institute, Vancouver, British Columbia, Canada

M. Safwan Badr   Division of Pulmonary, Critical Care & Sleep Medicine, Wayne State University School of Medicine, Detroit, Michigan, U.S.A.

Gang Bao   Alvarado Sleep Disorders Center and Alvarado Hospital, San Diego, California, U.S.A.

Brian Boehlecke   Division of Pulmonary and Critical Care Medicine, University of North Carolina at Chapel Hill, Chapel Hill, North Carolina, U.S.A.

Katy Borodkin   Department of Psychology, Bar Ilan University, Ramat Gan, Israel

Meredith Broderick   University Hospitals of Cleveland Case Medical Center, Cleveland, Ohio, U.S.A.

Daniel B. Brown   Greenberg Traurig, LLP, Atlanta, Georgia, U.S.A.

Theresa M. Buckley   Sleep Disorders Center, Stanford University School of Medicine, Stanford, California, U.S.A.

James B. Burch   Department of Epidemiology and Biostatistics, Norman J. Arnold School of Public Health, University of South Carolina, Dorn VA Medical Center, Columbia, South Carolina, U.S.A.

Helen J. Burgess   Biological Rhythms Research Laboratory, Department of Behavioral Sciences, Rush University Medical Center, Chicago, Illinois, U.S.A.

Erin Carlyle   Department of Psychiatry and Behavioral Sciences, Stanford University School of Medicine, Stanford, California, U.S.A.

Colleen E. Carney   Department of Psychology, Ryerson University, Toronto, Ontario, Canada

Allison Chan   Department of Psychiatry and Behavioral Sciences, Center for Narcolepsy, Stanford University School of Medicine, Stanford, California, U.S.A.

Gina H. Chen   Sleep Disorders Center, Stanford University School of Medicine, Stanford, California, U.S.A.

Yaron Dagan   Institute for Sleep Medicine, Assuta Medical Centers, and Medical Education Department, Sackler School of Medicine, Tel Aviv University, Tel Aviv, Israel

Yves Dauvilliers   Service de Neurologie, Hôpital Gui-de-Chauliac and INSERM U888, Montpellier, France

William C. Dement   Stanford University School of Medicine, Stanford, California, U.S.A.

Christopher L. Drake   Henry Ford Hospital, Sleep Disorders and Research Center, Department of Psychiatry and Behavioral Neurosciences, Wayne State College of Medicine, Detroit, Michigan, U.S.A.

Mark E. Dyken   Department of Neurology, University of Iowa College of Medicine, Iowa City; Department of Neurology Sleep Disorders Center, University of Iowa Hospitals and Clinics, Iowa City, Iowa, U.S.A.

Jack D. Edinger   Psychology Service, VA Medical Center and Department of Psychiatry and Behavioral Sciences, Duke University Medical Center, Durham, North Carolina, U.S.A.

Joan Escarrabill   UFIS Respiratòria (Chest Division) Hospital Universitari de Bellvitge, L'Hospitalet, Spain

Maria Livia Fantini   Sleep Disorders Center, Department of Clinical Neurosciences, San Raffaele Hospital-Turro, Milan, Italy

Mehran Farid   Peninsula Sleep Center, Inc., Burlingame, California, U.S.A.

Ramon Farré   Unit of Biophysics & Bioengineering, School of Medicine, University of Barcelona—IDIBAPS, Barcelona, and CIBER de Enfermedades Respiratorias (CIBERES), Bunyola, Spain

Luigi Ferini-Strambi   Sleep Disorders Center, University Vita-Salute San Raffaele, Milan, Italy

Kelleen N. Flaherty   Graduate Biomedical Writing Program, University of the Sciences in Philadelphia, Jamison, Pennsylvania, U.S.A.

Eric Frenette   Stanford University School of Medicine, Stanford, California, U.S.A.

Leah Friedman   Department of Psychiatry, Stanford University School of Medicine, Stanford, California, U.S.A.

Stephany Fulda   Max Planck Institute of Psychiatry, Munich, Germany

Anda Gershon   Department of Psychology, University of California, Berkeley, California, U.S.A.

June Gruber   Department of Psychology, University of California, Berkeley, California, U.S.A.

Christian Guilleminault   Sleep Disorders Center, Stanford University School of Medicine, Stanford, California, U.S.A.

Birgit Högl   Department of Neurology, Innsbruck Medical University, Innsbruck, Austria

Laura Haagenson   Department of Psychiatry, Stanford University School of Medicine, Stanford, California, U.S.A.

Ilana S. Hairston   Department of Psychology, University of California, Berkeley, California, U.S.A.

Allison G. Harvey   Department of Psychology, University of California, Berkeley, California, U.S.A.

Wayne A. Hening   UMDNJ-RW Johnson Medical School, New Brunswick, New Jersey, U.S.A.

Beatriz Hernandez   Department of Psychiatry, Stanford University School of Medicine, Stanford, California, U.S.A.

Aarnoud Hoekema   Department of Oral and Maxillofacial Surgery, University Medical Center Groningen, University of Groningen, Groningen, The Netherlands

Makoto Honda   Sleep Disorder Research Project, Tokyo Institute of Psychiatry, Setagaya-ku, Tokyo, Japan

Yutaka Honda   Neuropsychiatric Research Institute, Shinjuku-ku, Tokyo, Japan

Suresh Kotagal   Division of Child Neurology, Mayo Clinic, Rochester, Minnesota, U.S.A.

Clete A. Kushida   Division of Sleep Medicine, Department of Psychiatry and Behavioral Sciences, Stanford University School of Medicine, Stanford, California, U.S.A.

Scott M. Leibowitz   The Sleep Disorders Center of the Piedmont Heart Institute, Atlanta, Georgia, U.S.A.

Kenneth L. Lichstein   Department of Psychology, The University of Alabama, Tuscaloosa, Alabama, U.S.A.

Steven W. Lockley   Circadian Physiology Program, Division of Sleep Medicine, Brigham and Women's Hospital, Harvard Medical School, Boston, Massachusetts, U.S.A.

Murali Maheswaran   Center for Sleep Disorders, Skagit Valley Medical Center, Mount Vernon, Washington, U.S.A.

Rachel Manber   Department of Psychiatry and Behavioral Sciences, Stanford University School of Medicine, Stanford, California, U.S.A.

Mauro Manconi   Sleep Disorders Center, University Vita-Salute San Raffaele, Milan, Italy

Marie Marklund   Department of Orthodontics, Faculty of Medicine, Umeå University, Umeå, Sweden

Jose Mendez   Sleep Disorders Center and Division of Child Neurology, Mayo Clinic, Rochester, Minnesota, U.S.A.

Emmanuel Mignot   Department of Psychiatry and Behavioral Sciences, Center for Narcolepsy, Stanford University School of Medicine, Stanford, California, U.S.A.

Pasquale Montagna   Department of Neurological Sciences, University of Bologna, Bologna, Italy

Josep M. Montserrat   Sleep Lab, Hospital Clinic, IDIBAPS, Barcelona, and CIBER de Enfermedades Respiratorias (CIBERES), Bunyola, Spain

Alan T. Mulgrew   Sleep Disorders Program, University of British Columbia, Vancouver, British Columbia, Canada

David N. Neubauer   Sleep Disorders Center and Department of Psychiatry and Behavioral Sciences, Johns Hopkins University School of Medicine, Baltimore, Maryland, U.S.A.

Tore A. Nielsen   Centre d'Etude du Sommeil, Hôpital du Sacré-Coeur de Montréal and Département de Psychiatrie, Université de Montréal, Montréal, Québec, Canada

Seiji Nishino   Department of Psychiatry and Behavioral Sciences, Sleep and Circadian Neurobiology Laboratory & Center for Narcolepsy, Stanford University School of Medicine, Stanford, California, U.S.A.

William G. Ondo   Department of Neurology, Baylor College of Medicine, Houston, Texas, U.S.A.

Jason C. Ong Department of Psychiatry and Behavioral Sciences, Stanford University School of Medicine, Stanford, California, U.S.A.

J. F. Pagel Department of Family Practice, University of Colorado School of Medicine, Southern Colorado Residency Program, Pueblo; Sleep Disorders Center of Southern Colorado, Pueblo; and Sleepworks Sleep Laboratory, Colorado Springs, Colorado, U.S.A.

Kristen L. Payne Department of Psychology, The University of Alabama, Tuscaloosa, Alabama, U.S.A.

Dominique Petit Centre d'Etude du Sommeil, Hôpital du Sacré-Coeur de Montréal, Montréal, Québec, Canada

Tom A. Potti University of Michigan Medical School, Ann Arbor, Michigan, U.S.A.

Nelson B. Powell Department of Otolaryngology/Head and Neck Surgery, Stanford University Medical Center and Department of Behavioral Sciences, Division of Sleep Medicine, Stanford University School of Medicine, Stanford, California, U.S.A.

Mark R. Pressman Sleep Medicine Services, The Lankenau Hospital, Wynnewood; Paoli Hospital, Paoli; and Department of Medicine, Jefferson Medical College, Philadelphia, Pennsylvania, U.S.A.

Stuart F. Quan Arizona Respiratory Center, University of Arizona, Tucson, Arizona, U.S.A.

Anil N. Rama The Permanente Medical Group, San Jose, California, U.S.A.

Kathryn J. Reid Department of Neurology, Northwestern University Feinberg School of Medicine, Chicago, Illinois, U.S.A.

Robert W. Riley Department of Otolaryngology/Head and Neck Surgery, Stanford University Medical Center and Department of Behavioral Sciences, Division of Sleep Medicine, Stanford University School of Medicine, Stanford, California, U.S.A.

James A. Rowley Division of Pulmonary, Critical Care & Sleep Medicine, Wayne State University School of Medicine, Detroit, Michigan, U.S.A.

Robert L. Sack Oregon Health and Sciences University, Portland, Oregon, U.S.A.

Joan Santamaria Neurology Service and Multidisciplinary Sleep Disorders Unit, Hospital Clinic of Barcelona, University of Barcelona Medical School, Barcelona, Spain

Michael J. Sateia Section of Sleep Medicine, Dartmouth Medical School, Lebanon, New Hampshire, U.S.A.

Donald M. Sesso Department of Otolaryngology/Head and Neck Surgery, Stanford University Medical Center, Stanford, California, U.S.A.

Krista Sigurdson Sleep Disorders Program, University of British Columbia, Vancouver, British Columbia, Canada

Michael H. Silber Center for Sleep Medicine, Mayo Clinic College of Medicine, Rochester, Minnesota, U.S.A.

Debra J. Skene Centre for Chronobiology, School of Biomedical and Molecular Sciences, University of Surrey, Guildford, Surrey, U.K.

Linda Snyder Arizona Respiratory Center, University of Arizona, Tucson, Arizona, U.S.A.

James P. Soeffing   Department of Psychology, The University of Alabama, Tuscaloosa, Alabama, U.S.A.

Shannon S. Sullivan   Division of Sleep Medicine, Department of Psychiatry and Behavioral Sciences, Stanford University School of Medicine, Stanford, California, U.S.A.

Thomas C. Wetter   Max Planck Institute of Psychiatry, Munich, Germany

John Winkelman   Division of Sleep Medicine, Brigham & Women's Hospital, Harvard Medical School, Boston, Massachusetts, U.S.A.

Kenneth P. Wright, Jr.   Sleep and Chronobiology Laboratory, Department of Integrative Physiology, University of Colorado, Boulder, Colorado, U.S.A.

Thoru Yamada   Department of Neurology, University of Iowa College of Medicine, Iowa City; Division of Clinical Electrophysiology, University of Iowa Hospitals and Clinics, Iowa City, Iowa, U.S.A.

Chang-Kook Yang   Sleep Disorders Clinic, Busan Sleep Center, Busan, Korea

Shawn D. Youngstedt   Department of Exercise Science, Norman J. Arnold School of Public Health, University of South Carolina, Dorn VA Medical Center, Columbia, South Carolina, U.S.A.

1 | Perspectives

Clete A. Kushida

Division of Sleep Medicine, Department of Psychiatry and Behavioral Sciences, Stanford University School of Medicine, Stanford, California, U.S.A.

Why was this handbook written? Since the discovery of rapid eye movement (REM) sleep a little over 50 years ago, there has been a dramatic increase in the number of scientific investigations exploring sleep and its disorders. This expanding body of literature enables a clinician to learn the best practices in the diagnosis and management of sleep disorders, provided he or she knows how to access this literature. *The Handbook of Sleep Disorders* was written with the idea of providing an easy and quick way for a clinician to retrieve this information. The first edition of the *Handbook of Sleep Disorders* (1), edited by my colleague and friend, Michael J. Thorpy, M.D., of the Sleep-Wake Disorders Center at the Montefiore Medical Center in New York, was published in 1990. It consisted of 817 pages, and, at the time it was released, it was arguably the most complete reference on sleep disorders available. However, close to two decades have passed since the original handbook was published, and new clinical and basic research discoveries prompted the writing of this second edition.

What is the purpose of a handbook? The online edition of the Merriam-Webster dictionary describes a handbook as "a book capable of being conveniently carried as a ready reference"(2). It is my belief that this handbook fits this definition and serves a useful purpose. It is not intended to be a comprehensive reference about sleep or sleep medicine. Similarly, it is not intended to replace the American Academy of Sleep Medicine's International Classification of Sleep Disorders, 2nd edition (ICSD-2) (3). It is simply a reference designed to aid a clinician in the recognition and treatment of sleep disorders.

Who will benefit from this handbook? Basically, anyone who has an interest in the diagnosis and management of sleep disorders would find this handbook useful. This includes sleep specialists as well as clinicians who encounter patients with sleep disorders, such as neurologists, pulmonologists, psychiatrists, psychologists, and otolaryngologists. Given that internists, family practitioners, and pediatricians typically are at the frontline of complaints from patients about their sleep, these physicians would most likely also benefit from this handbook. Lastly, students and trainees, in particular medical students, residents, and fellows who are interested in sleep medicine would undoubtedly find the topics in this handbook informative as they progress in their training.

How will the readers use this handbook most effectively? This handbook is first and foremost a reference. The chapters are constructed so that the chapters of each section follow a specific order and structure, and the topics of each chapter also follow a particular order and structure. This enables the reader to be able to quickly access the information that he or she needs about a given sleep disorder without necessarily having to refer to the table of contents. A typical scenario for the use of this handbook would be a case in which a physician who, in the course of evaluating a patient with a sleep complaint, needs to quickly check to see if his or her diagnostic plan for the patient is reasonable and consistent with standards of care.

Enjoy, and welcome to the fascinating world of sleep disorders!

REFERENCES

1. Thorpy MJ, ed. Handbook of Sleep Disorders. New York: Informa Healthcare; 1990.
2. Merriam-Webster. Online Dictionary. Available at: http://www.merriam-webster.com/dictionary/. Accessed June 8, 2008.
3. American Academy of Sleep Medicine. ICSD-2—International classification of sleep disorders: Diagnostic and coding manual. 2nd ed. Westchester, IL: American Academy of Sleep Medicine; 2005.

2 | Description of Insomnia

Michael J. Sateia

Section of Sleep Medicine, Dartmouth Medical School, Lebanon, New Hampshire, U.S.A.

HISTORY

Background

The role and significance of sleep and sleep disturbances as important biological and psychological constructs have been the subject of human interest for millennia. Hippocrates made reference to sleep disturbance in numerous aphorisms, noting that improvement in sleep disturbance in sick individuals represents a good prognostic sign and that both insomnia and hypersomnolence are indicative of disease (1). Literature from the Old Testament to Aeschylus to Shakespeare has described insomnia and referenced the restorative and generative qualities of sleep, suggesting that sleep "brings wisdom by the awful grace of God" (2) and serves as "the balm of hurt minds." To Wordsworth, himself an insomnia sufferer, sleep was the "mother of fresh thoughts and joyous health" (3). Curiously, these literary and common sense observations regarding the importance of healthy sleep existed alongside a relatively pervasive scientific disinterest in sleep as nothing more, as Aristotle suggested, than "an inhibition of sense perception" (4) or, in Kleitman's words, a "letdown of waking activity" (5).

Theories of Etiology, Diagnosis, and Classification

Although insomnia has historically been viewed as a significant threat to physical and psychological well-being, less has been said about its causes until recent decades. For the most part, insomnia was viewed as the product of an "unquiet mind"—a consequence of conflict, stress, guilt, or depression. Hippocrates recognized insomnia as an intrinsic component of melancholia (depression). Shakespeare was especially fixated on sleep and sleep disturbance, often emphasizing vexation and treachery as the source of insomnia—"Macbeth shall sleep no more."

Early physicians and healers seem to have devoted greater attention to the potential remedies for insomnia (see below) than to descriptions or etiology of the condition. The prevailing view of sleep as a passive state "intermediate ... between wakefulness and death" likely contributed to the apparent lack of interest (6). The 19th century saw the evolution of a number of theories to explain sleep, but little consideration was devoted to the causes or consequences of insomnia. This may reflect the widespread (and still prevalent) notion that sleep disturbances are generally a function of other medical or psychological disorders, and, in that sense, of limited interest in their own right. Freud did not specifically address insomnia in great detail, although it appears as a symptom in numerous cases. Not surprisingly, his view of this symptom is largely dictated by his concept of conflict as the basis for neurosis, as in the Analysis of a Case of Sleeplessness (7).

The modern-day approach to diagnosis and classification of insomnia can be traced to publication of the initial nosology of the Association of Sleep Disorders Centers (ASDA), released in 1979 (8). This manual grouped disorders that are primarily associated with insomnia (disorders of initiating and maintaining sleep) into a single major category with eight subheadings (e.g., "psychophysiological" or "associated with ... psychiatric/substances/breathing disturbance"). In the first edition of the *International Classification of Sleep Disorders* (ICSD) (9), the major insomnia categories were clumped into intrinsic or extrinsic dyssomnias and secondary disorders. The recent publication of ICSD-2 reverted to a distinct category for major insomnia diagnoses, although it should be noted that insomnia may appear as a symptom of numerous other disorders classified under their own distinct heading (e.g., breathing or movement disorder) (10). Release of ICSD-2 was also noteworthy in that it was accompanied by a significant revision and expansion of the *International Classification of Disease* (ICD-9-CM/ICD-10) sleep diagnoses, which created far greater correspondence between systems. Finally, the *Diagnostic and Statistical Manual of Mental Disorders*, fourth edition (DSM-IV) of the American Psychiatric Association published in 1994 included a major heading for sleep disorders (11). The approach to classification paralleled ICSD, first edition in its use of dyssomnias as a major heading, though was understandably far more parsimonious in its level of detail. It seems likely that future editions of the DSM will adopt an approach that is consistent with existing ICD-10/ICSD-2 systems.

Treatment

The appearance of chemical treatments for insomnia throughout history underscores how ancient and prevalent this problem has been. It is likely that the Sumerians used opium for medicinal purposes as early as 3000 BCE. The Greek physicians employed valerian and opium as specific treatments for insomnia. The use of opioids and alcohol for relief of insomnia was taken to a new level with the 16th century development of a mixture of the two, referred to as laudanum, which remained a commonly utilized treatment for sleep problems until the 19th century.

The modern-day evolution of pharmacotherapies for insomnia began perhaps with the introduction of chloral hydrate and bromide salts in the mid-19th century. These compounds were widely used despite their potential toxicity. The discovery of barbiturates in the early 20th century further altered the face of pharmacotherapy for insomnia. Numerous congeners, most notably phenobarbital and secobarbital and barbiturate-like substances such as glutethimide, became the established treatment for insomnia through the 1950s and were undoubtedly responsible for countless addictions and a significant number of deaths during their heyday. With the serendipitous discovery of benzodiazepines (BZDs) at Hoffman-LaRoche in the late 1950s and their introduction to the market in the early 1960s, the use of barbiturates waned rapidly. Flurazepam, the first BZD approved as a hypnotic, was introduced in 1973. By the late 1970s and early 1980s, it became clear that the exceedingly long half-life of flurazepam resulted in significant daytime impairment and other adverse consequences, leading to development of several intermediate and short-acting hypnotic medications of this class (12–14). Although the more recent emergence of non-BZD compounds (zolpidem, zaleplon, eszopiclone) has significantly reduced the use of BZD hypnotics, they remain a widely used and lower-cost option in the management of insomnia.

A number of other pharmacological and herbal preparations have been administered for insomnia in recent decades. Sedating antidepressants such as amitriptyline, doxepin, and especially trazodone grew from initial application as sleep aids in patients with major depression or chronic pain to usage as hypnotic medications in varied presentations of insomnia. Melatonin emerged in the early 1990s as a potential sleep aid and, for a time, was widely touted in the lay press as a potential panacea for insomnia, despite the absence of controlled data supporting this application. Likewise, the usage of sedating antidepressant medications, particularly trazodone, grew rapidly during the 1990s because of its perceived position as a "safer" alternative (especially for longer-term use) to BZDs. As of this writing, we are witnessing a somewhat unprecedented marketing campaign for non-BZD compounds and the melatonin agonist ramelteon, a campaign that shows little sign of diminishing, as new and expensive pharmacotherapies are brought to market for this common indication.

Paralleling the developments in pharmacotherapy of the recent decades, investigation and utilization of non-pharmacological treatments, specifically cognitive-behavioral therapy for insomnia (CBT-I), have steadily increased. Numerous studies and meta-analyses have demonstrated the durable long-term efficacy of CBT-I for patients with chronic insomnia (15–18). Regrettably, its application at present remains limited by the paucity of therapists skilled in this area and lack of an effective system for referral and delivery of care.

NOMENCLATURE

An understanding of insomnia assessment and management requires familiarity with the terminology most often used in connection with this diagnosis. The most difficult challenge may be that of defining insomnia itself. Although this is a term that is widely used in common parlance, with an assumption of some common definition, closer analysis of this has proven that substantial disparities exist in operational definitions. Typically, insomnia refers to a complaint of difficulty initiating sleep (falling asleep) or maintaining sleep (mid-cycle or early morning awakening). Complaints may also include poor-quality and non-restorative sleep, which are somewhat more vaguely defined. The latter symptom is more reflective of the consequences of the sleep disturbance than the nature of the nocturnal disturbance.

To an increasing extent over the past decade, there has been emphasis, both in the clinical and research settings, on a requirement of daytime consequences as a component of insomnia. Epidemiological surveys (see below) have been confounded by variability of the precise definitions and operational assessments of insomnia (e.g., Ohayon's use of "dissatisfaction with quality of sleep" as opposed to simply "insomnia") (19). It should also be emphasized that a certain degree of confusion often arises with respect to the difference between sleep deprivation and insomnia. As the most recent edition of ICSD-2 emphasizes, insomnia represents a complaint "despite adequate opportunity and circumstance to sleep" (10). Furthermore, research demonstrates that the characteristics and sequelae of insomnia and sleep deprivation are quite different (20). Yet, in the general population and even among health care providers, this distinction often remains unclear.

The traditional diagnostic descriptions of insomnia have often included a designation as to whether the condition is "primary" or "secondary." These terms have historically been intended to indicate that insomnia is either a symptom or a function of another medical or psychiatric condition or has arisen of its own accord without subordinate relationship to another disorder. The 2005 National Institutes of Health (NIH) State of the Science Conference on Chronic Insomnia recommends that the term "comorbid insomnia" replace that of secondary insomnia (21). The principal reason for this recommendation would seem to lie in the fact that, regardless of its origins, chronic insomnia appears to be characterized by certain specific psychological and physiological characteristics that, in many cases at least, give rise to a condition that is relatively autonomous, that does not necessarily resolve with treatment of the primary medical or psychiatric condition, and that does respond effectively to therapies aimed at the more specific aspects of the insomnia process itself.

Evaluation Instruments

A variety of instruments are utilized in the comprehensive assessment of insomnia. Although a comprehensive discussion of these assessment devices is beyond the scope of this chapter (see chapt. 5), there are several basic tools with which the reader should be familiar. Complementing the clinical history, which is the most fundamental aspect of evaluation of insomnia, sleep logs represent an important component (22). These are structured instruments, completed by patients over a one- to two-week period, which document sleep-wake schedule, quality, sleep latencies, waking after sleep onset, total sleep time, and any number of other related variables of interest to the clinician. Sleep logs are sometimes referred to as sleep diaries, which may contain a more expanded set of relevant information.

Numerous questionnaires have been developed for assessment of sleep quality and insomnia. One of the most well known of these, the Pittsburgh Sleep Quality Index (PSQI), has been applied in numerous insomnia research designs (23). Others include the Insomnia Severity Scale (ISI) (24), the Dysfunctional Beliefs and Attitudes Survey (DBAS) (24), and the Sleep Disturbance Questionnaire (25), to name but a fraction. Other inventories that focus on more specific aspects of insomnia have also been developed.

Although sleep studies [polysomnography (PSG)] are not generally performed in the assessment of insomnia (26), the lower cost and portable methodology of actigraphy has been widely employed (22,27,28). An actigraph is a wrist-worn motion-sensitive device that provides quantification of sleep and wake states in a more objective manner than one-off reports or logs. Though less accurate in this respect than in-lab PSG, actigraphy is a useful adjunct in assessment of insomnia and circadian rhythm disorders.

Therapeutic Terminology

Pharmacotherapy for insomnia is reasonably straightforward with respect to terminology and includes herbal preparations and "nutritional supplements" [e.g., valerian or melatonin, which, together with other such preparations, is not subject to Food and Drug Administration (FDA) regulation], over-the-counter preparations (consisting of antihistamines marketed under a host of trade names, often in combination with analgesics), and sedating antidepressants such as trazodone, nefazodone (see FDA black box warning on hepatotoxicity), and mirtazapine. The term "hypnotic" is generally reserved for medications developed, marketed, and used primarily or exclusively for sleep. Currently, these include BZDs, other BZD-receptor agonists, and the melatonin agonist, ramelteon.

The term "non-pharmacological therapy" is widely used to describe a myriad of cognitive, behavioral, biofeedback, and common sense treatment approaches to insomnia. It is often used interchangeably with the more specific term CBT-I, although the latter is preferred when these more specific approaches are discussed. CBT-I may be further divided into its constituent components that include, among others, cognitive therapy, stimulus control, sleep restriction, biofeedback, relaxation training, paradoxical intention, and multicomponent therapies combining two or more of these. Non-pharmacological therapy also includes sleep hygiene, a perhaps unfortunate terminology employed for decades to identify healthy (and unhealthy) sleep behaviors.

KEY FEATURES AND CHARACTERISTICS

In describing the features and characteristics of patients with insomnia, it is necessary to introduce the important distinction between acute or transient insomnia and chronic insomnia. Transient insomnia is a time-limited disorder that is typically a by-product of adjustment to an acute stress, life change, illness, or time zone change. It is virtually universal, usually resolves within days or weeks, and is not generally characterized by the stigmata that accompany longer-term insomnia. Chronic insomnia problems have a number of features in common (n.b., the term "chronic insomnia" describes duration and implies a set of common characteristics, but a more specific diagnosis such as "insomnia due to mental disorder" or "psychophysio-logical insomnia" is required clinically and may have further clinical ramifications). Much of the current research has focused on primary insomnia, which has been further subdivided into psychophysiological insomnia, paradoxical insomnia (formerly known as sleep state misperception), and idiopathic (or childhood-onset) insomnia (10). Much more investigation is required to better understand the validity and clinical significance of this subdivision. The bulk of remaining insomnia disorders are comorbid with medical or psychiatric illness, or are associated with other primary sleep disorders such as movement, breathing, or circadian rhythm disorders.

Many of the characteristics of primary insomnia can be unified under the concept of *hyperarousal*. In general terms, this concept is intended to describe the overactivity and/or inappropriate timing of multiple psychological and physiological functions. Evidence for physiological hyperarousal includes increased 24-hour metabolic rate (20), heightened autonomic activity (especially in association with sleep) (29), endocrine alterations such as excessive nocturnal cortisol production (30), faster (i.e., more wake-like) sleep electroencephalo-graphic (EEG) frequencies (31), and regionally increased cerebral blood flow during sleep in comparison with controls (32). Chronic insomnia patients also tend to be cognitively hyperaroused; that is, they demonstrate heightened cognitive activity, particularly in associ-ation with efforts to sleep ("I can't turn my mind off") (33). Most of the research in this area has been accomplished in primary insomnia populations. Further investigation is necessary to extend these assessments into comorbid populations to better understand this relationship.

Features of Chronic Insomnia

The specific complaints associated with insomnia are described above. For many patients, the presentation may include more than one of these complaints. Moreover, it is quite common for complaints to evolve. For example, patients who initially present with sleep-onset difficulties may develop sleep maintenance problems over time. With respect to duration, although the minimum criterion for chronic insomnia is variously established as one to several months, the majority of patients studied demonstrate durations in the range of years to decades (34). Most of these patients have engaged in numerous self-help and self-medication (including alcohol and over-the-counter) strategies, which have proven largely unsuccessful (35). Only one in twenty chronic insomnia patients see their health care practitioner specifically for this condition, and two-thirds of them receive no medical attention at all for the problem (35). When medical attention does occur, it is typically characterized by limited or no evaluation of the problem, and when a treatment is offered at all, it is characterized by reliance on hypnotic prescription (36,37).

The subjective reports regarding sleep from insomnia patients usually overestimate the degree of disturbance when compared with objective assessment such as PSG (31,38,39). Rather than representing a deliberate distortion, it seems clear that the discrepancy is accounted for by perturbations of sleep physiology in these patients that are not well understood (see "hyperarousal" above). While this subjective-objective mismatch cuts across numerous types of chronic insomnia, it is at its most exaggerated form in patients with paradoxical insomnia, who demonstrate objectively normal sleep times but report little or no sleep at all.

Associated Conditions

Comorbid conditions are common in this population, and most clinic surveys suggest that "secondary insomnia" represents about 75% to 80% of the total (40). However, as noted above, it has become evident in recent years that conceptualizing chronic insomnia as a purely secondary symptom or condition of primary medical or psychiatric disorders does not foster an accurate understanding or therapeutic approach to the problem. Therefore, the term "comorbid" is preferred.

The presence of daytime consequences is required to establish any diagnosis of chronic insomnia. While such consequences vary from individual to individual, they typically include some form of fatigue-related complaint, often complaints of cognitive difficulties such as impaired concentration, attention or memory, psychological disturbances including dysphoric mood or irritability, and physical complaints such as headache or gastrointestinal disturbances. Clinicians should note that although it seems reasonable to include a complaint of drowsiness or sleepiness in this symptom cluster, caution must be exercised in this respect. Numerous investigations indicate that chronic insomnia patients are certainly not objectively sleepy when assessed by conventional tools (20,29,41). Therefore, patients who present with reasonably clear complaints of overwhelming drowsiness, involuntary dozing, and/or regular napping (as opposed to "fatigue," "tiredness," or "lethargy") should be assessed further for other potential causes of pathological sleepiness such as a sleep-related breathing disorder or primary hypersomnolence.

Finally, it should be noted that many chronic insomnia patients manifest a common set of psychological and behavioral characteristics that are key in the perpetuation of their disorder. These may include an excessive focus on sleep itself as well as on the consequences of not sleeping, markedly negative expectations regarding their ability to sleep, and a conditioned arousal in response to efforts to sleep. Many patients spend excessive amounts of time in bed, hoping to obtain what they perceive to be adequate quantities of sleep. In the cognitive-behavioral therapeutic approaches, these issues become key targets for effective interventions.

INCIDENCE AND PREVALENCE

Insomnia is a common condition, affecting virtually all ages and socioeconomic strata. Most epidemiological studies place the prevalence of occasional or intermittent insomnia at about 30% to 40% of the general population and that of chronic insomnia at roughly 10% to 15% (34,42–44). However, several considerations apply. It has become clear that the prevalence data are significantly influenced by the operational definition of insomnia that is employed in these studies. For example, Ohayon and Roth have pointed out that investigations utilizing only a single identifier such as "difficulty getting to sleep" or "difficulty staying asleep" as a marker for insomnia are likely to overestimate the prevalence of the disorder (45). Duration as a qualifier (greater than one month duration) has relatively little impact since most of the sample meets this criterion. However, the presence of other factors such as dissatisfaction, dread of going to bed, or the presence of hyperarousal (e.g., excessive mental activity in bed) proves critical in defining clinically relevant insomnia. In addition, earlier epidemiological studies of insomnia failed to include a criterion of daytime consequences, a factor that further narrows and defines the population. That said, the large European study that incorporated the criteria described above still demonstrated an insomnia prevalence of 11%, although only two-thirds (6.8%) received a sleep disorder diagnosis, while the remainder received mental disorder diagnoses (45). The important lesson to be derived from these data is that insomnia is a complex condition that is characterized not only by a complaint about sleep but also by an individual's assessment of and response to this complaint, as well as the consequences of the condition.

It is clear that the prevalence of insomnia is substantially higher among certain populations. Women manifest insomnia more often than men at a ratio of about 2:1 (22,46). Recent evidence suggests that this higher prevalence may not be entirely a function of higher incidence but rather of a lower remission rate, at least in the elderly (47). Certainly, higher rates of mood and anxiety disorders in women may also lead to chronic insomnia, although our current understanding raises the possibility that the converse is also true. Rates of chronic insomnia are clearly higher in clinic populations, including both psychiatric and medical clinics, and exceed 50% in some studies (44,48).

In addition to the well-recognized association between insomnia and mental disorders, including substance abuse, medical risk factors include any chronic illness or chronic pain, cancer, lung disease, and cardiovascular disease (49).

Sleep disturbance is a particular concern for the elderly, and epidemiological data are consistent with this. Depending on the definition and severity ratings, studies suggest an insomnia prevalence rate of anywhere from about 25% to over 40% (50–52). In considering this, however, it is important to recognize that much of the increased prevalence may be a function of factors that are overrepresented in the elderly population and are already known to be associated with insomnia at any age (e.g., medical/psychiatric illnesses or medications). Epidemiological studies reveal that healthy, active older adults do not demonstrate comparable increases in prevalence (52).

Insomnia is often disregarded by health care practitioners (34). The reasons for this are not clear but may represent, in part, a perception of this condition as less significant than other medical problems that may come to their attention. However, in surveys comparing health-related quality of life in a variety of chronic health conditions, insomnia sufferers demonstrate impairments that are on the same order as congestive heart failure and major depressive disorder (53–56). In assessing the significance of a chronic insomnia complaint, clinicians must also bear in mind demonstrated associations that suggest that insomnia is a significant risk factor for development of new psychiatric disorders including depression, anxiety disorders, and substance abuse (57–59). Moreover, chronic insomnia may adversely affect the course and outcome of other medical disorders, either through impaired treatment adherence, promotion of complicating psychiatric disorders, or direct impact on physiological function (e.g., lowering of pain threshold).

MODELS

Early animal studies of sleep deprivation were conducted in the late nineteenth century. De Manaceine and others demonstrated that dogs die after about one to two weeks of total sleep deprivation, although these studies lacked the controls of later investigations (60,61). The most well known of the animal sleep deprivation experiments comes from Rechtschaffen, who sleep-deprived rats using a disk over water apparatus, which forced locomotion via disk rotation every time the animal began to enter sleep (62). The study employed control animals that were similarly exposed to the apparatus and motorically active but not totally sleep deprived. The experimental animals died in 11 to 32 days, demonstrating weight loss, despite an increase in food consumption, and evidence of autonomic dysregulation. Documented human "experiments" suggest that total deprivation of up to 11 days, while resulting in significant temporary cognitive and physiological dysfunction, produced no permanent damage. Perhaps more relevant to the issue of insomnia are the studies of partial sleep deprivation by Dinges and colleagues, which reveal significant and cumulative impairments of vigilance/alertness, memory, executive function, mood, psychomotor performance, and other cognitive functions during sustained partial sleep deprivation (63).

Although the sleep loss attributed to insomnia might invite examination of this sleep deprivation literature as a potential model of insomnia and its consequences, caution must be exercised in this respect. There are numerous lines of evidence that underscore that the sleep loss associated with insomnia (which is often modest) and partial or total sleep deprivation are quite different with respect to their characteristics and consequences. Thus, while the critical importance of adequate sleep to biological and neuropsychological function in particular is not in question, the relevance of these deprivation observations to insomnia is unclear.

There are a number of models that have been put forward to further our understanding of this condition, although each addresses the issue in a limited manner, focusing primarily on a single functional perspective. Saper and colleagues have proposed animal models of insomnia on the basis of lesioning experiments and analysis of regional brain activity (64).

Lesions of the ventrolateral preoptic nucleus (VLPO) in rats result in sustained and major sleep loss over at least three months, as well as associated cognitive disturbance that correlates with degree of sleep loss. The authors note that substantial atrophy of VLPO neurons is seen in aging humans and suggests that the pattern observed in this rat model may mimic the pattern of increasing sleep disturbance associated with aging.

In unpublished data (65), Saper has also demonstrated that stress induction in this model of insomnia results in patterns of sleep disturbance similar to those observed in human stress response paradigms and is associated with patterns of central nervous system (CNS) activation that are consistent with emerging brain activation data in humans with insomnia. Other pharmacological manipulations such as recently described models of sleep-wake disturbance in hyper- and hypodopaminergic mice provide further insight into mechanisms of sleep disturbance in human disease states such as Parkinson's disease (66).

A physiological model of human insomnia, while still very incomplete, has begun to emerge over the past decade. Some of the important early work in this area was conducted by Bonnet and Arand, who demonstrated that chronic, primary insomnia was associated with heightened physiological activation as measured by 24-hour metabolic rate (20). They further demonstrated that experimental sleep deprivation that was designed to match the sleep loss of an insomnia group did not produce similar physiological activation, again underscoring key differences between sleep deprivation and insomnia. Finally, they were able to produce a model akin to the insomnia group by means of experimentally induced activation with caffeine (67). This work helped to lay the foundation for numerous investigations that have identified evidence for increased physiological activation in terms of regional CNS activation, autonomic activity, endocrine regulation, and cognition. Taken as a whole, these data constitute a theoretical *hyperarousal* model of insomnia (see above).

Complementary cognitive-behavioral models focus on the evolution and perpetuation of chronic insomnia as a result of distorted cognitions and maladaptive behaviors. These models identify factors such as excessive attention and worry regarding sleep loss and daytime consequences thereof (68), loss of "automaticity" (the routine process of sleep initiation without focus or concern) and "plasticity" (i.e., ability to adapt to normal variability of sleeping) (69), and distorted cognitions about causes of sleep disturbance as fundamental in the evolution of the disorder. Compensatory maladaptive behaviors such as spending excessive time in bed are also major contributing factors. Other models attempt to meld the physiological and cognitive perspectives by addressing the correlation of changes in EEG activity and cognitive hyperactivity that become conditioned to attempts to sleep (70).

While none of these models provides a fully unified view of this multifaceted condition, each represents a significant advancement in our understanding over the past decade.

SOCIAL AND ECONOMIC FACTORS

Although patients understandably focus on the individual suffering and impaired quality of life that are associated with chronic insomnia, it is important that as a society we also focus on the socioeconomic impact of this disorder. This impact is felt in a variety of ways, from work absenteeism and diminished productivity to substantial direct and indirect economic costs.

A recent study of absenteeism in French workers demonstrated significantly higher rates among those with insomnia compared with good sleepers. Eliminating subjects with comorbidities such as depression, anxiety, and chronic physical illness, the insomnia group had nearly double the rate of absenteeism as the control population and stayed out of work for nearly twice as long. The same investigation revealed higher rates of vehicular accidents and work errors in the insomnia group (71). The cost of absenteeism is borne largely by employers and has been estimated to be about 50% higher for the insomnia group than for controls (72). Other investigations have suggested that work performance is impaired (73). The role of insomnia in permanent work absence, that is, worker disability, has been examined in several studies. Eriksen and colleagues found that "poor sleep" predicted disability four years after initial assessment with an odds ratio of 2.16 after controlling for physical and emotional health and other factors (74). The Nord-Trøndelag Health Study (HUNT-2) of Norwegian workers, employing a prospective design with objective assessment of disability status, found that insomnia predicted subsequent permanent disability in 1.5 to 4 years with odds ratio, after adjustment for multiple health and other factors, of 1.75 (75).

Estimates of the economic costs of insomnia vary considerably, reflecting the variability in defining what constitutes direct and indirect costs, as well as the methodologies for estimating such costs. The most obvious economic burdens arise from the evaluation and treatment of the condition. This typically includes both prescription and nonprescription medication for sleep. However, at least one study also included cost estimate of alcohol used as a sleep aid, this estimate representing about 40% of the total chemical treatment costs. Direct costs of health care include doctor's visits for an insomnia complaint, other related health care visits, and sleep studies. The Walsh and Englehardt estimates of 1999 incorporated an estimate for nursing home care that was believed to be primarily a result of sleep disturbance (76). The cost attached to the latter ($10.9 billion USD) represented 78% of all direct costs. Leger and colleagues calculated the direct costs of insomnia in France, excluding alcohol use and nursing home care (77). This yielded an estimate of approximately $2.1 billion in USD. Adjusting for inflation, population and gross domestic product (GDP), the authors estimate adjusted expenses (in USD) of $6.21 billion in France and $2.38 billion in the United States. It seems likely that the significant discrepancy is more likely attributable to the problems of measurement than to this magnitude of difference in expenditure for insomnia in France and the United States.

Indirect costs are even more difficult to calculate. Such estimates factor in additional health care utilization by persons with insomnia, loss of work by absenteeism, diminished productivity, and the cost of work-related accidents and errors as well as other accidents. A 1994 estimate placed this figure at about $80 to 90 billion USD, although such figures should be regarded as gross approximations at best (78). It is clear that health care utilization is increased among insomnia populations compared with good sleepers, even when controlled for comorbidities and demographic characteristics (54,79). Both occupational and motor vehicle accidents are increased in some, though not all, studies of the impact of insomnia (54,71,79). Although there is still a great deal of work to be done in refining our understanding of the socioeconomic and professional burden of insomnia, the preliminary reports demonstrate that the burden is substantial and probably comparable to that of other chronic medical conditions.

CONCLUSIONS

Chronic insomnia is a common and complex disorder that is often overlooked in the landscape of medical care. Our current understanding suggests that it derives from a multifaceted interaction of biological and psychological factors. Although our understanding of the condition is still incomplete, emerging data have begun to shed light on important underpinnings, which can form the basis for the development of more effective therapeutic interventions. The condition has important ramifications, not only with respect to the well-being, quality of life, and psychobiological function of the affected individuals, but also with respect to socioeconomic considerations. Studies of pharmacological and non-pharmacological treatments indicate that the capability for effective intervention is already within the grasp of our health care system, but under-recognition, lack of clear treatment algorithms, and a shortage of adequately trained therapists impede our delivery of care.

REFERENCES

1. Hippocrates. Aphorisms. Available at: http://etext.library.adelaide.edu.au/mirror/classics.mit.edu/Hippocrates/aphorisms.2.ii.html. Accessed September 2006.
2. Aeschylus. Agamemnon. c.500 BCE. Available at: http://etext.library.adelaide.edu.au/mirror/classics.mit.edu/Aeschylus/agamemnon.html. Accessed September, 2006.
3. Wordsworth W. To sleep. In: Eliot C, ed. English Poetry II: From Collins to Fitzgerald. The Harvard Classics. New York: P. F. Collier and Son, 1909–1914.
4. Edelson E. Sleep. New York: Chelsea House, 1992.
5. Kleitman N. Sleep and Wakefulness. Chicago: University of Chicago Press, 1939.

6. MacNish R. The Philosophy of Sleep. New York: D. Appleton and Company, 1834.
7. Van Reterghem A. Freud and His School—New Paths of Psychopathology. Seattle: The World Wide School, 1998.
8. Association of Sleep Disorders Centers. Diagnostic classification of sleep and arousal disorders, first edition. Sleep 1979; 2(1):1–137.
9. American Sleep Disorders Association. International Classification of Sleep Disorders. Rochester, MN: American Sleep Disorders Association, 1990.
10. American Academy of Sleep Medicine. International Classification of Sleep Disorders, 2nd ed. Diagnostic and Coding Manual. Westchester, IL: American Academy of Sleep Medicine, 2005.
11. American Psychiatric Association. Diagnostic and Statistical Manual of Mental Disorders (DSM-IV). Washington DC: American Psychiatric Association, 1994.
12. Abrahamowicz M, Bartlett G, Tamblyn R, et al. Modeling cumulative dose and exposure duration provided insights regarding the associations between benzodiazepines and injuries. J Clin Epidemiol 2006; 59(4):393–403.
13. Kramer M, Schoen LS. Problems in the use of long-acting hypnotics in older patients. J Clin Psychiatry 1984; 45(4):176–177.
14. Dement WC. Objective measurements of daytime sleepiness and performance comparing quazepam with flurazepam in two adult populations using the Multiple Sleep Latency Test. J Clin Psychiatry 1991; 52(suppl):31–37.
15. Smith MT, Perlis ML, Park A, et al. Comparative meta-analysis of pharmacotherapy and behavior therapy for persistent insomnia. Am J Psychiatry 2002; 159(1):5–11.
16. Morin CM, Hauri PJ, Espie CA, et al. Nonpharmacologic treatment of chronic insomnia. An American Academy of Sleep Medicine review. Sleep 1999; 22(8):1134–1156.
17. Montgomery P, Dennis J. Cognitive behavioural interventions for sleep problems in adults aged 60+ [update of Cochrane Database Syst Rev. 2002;(2):CD003161; PMID: 12076472]. Cochrane Database Syst Rev 2003; (1):CD003161.
18. Morin CM, Culbert JP, Schwartz SM. Nonpharmacological interventions for insomnia: a meta-analysis of treatment efficacy. Am J Psychiatry 1994; 151(8):1172–1180.
19. Ohayon MM, Caulet M, Guilleminault C. How a general population perceives its sleep and how this relates to the complaint of insomnia. Sleep 1997; 20(9):715–723.
20. Bonnet MH, Arand DL. The consequences of a week of insomnia. Sleep 1996; 19(6):453–461.
21. National Institutes of Health. National Institutes of Health State of the Science Conference statement on Manifestations and Management of Chronic Insomnia in Adults, June 13–15, 2005. Sleep 2005; 28(9): 1049–1057.
22. Sateia MJ, Doghramji K, Hauri PJ, et al. Evaluation of chronic insomnia. An American Academy of Sleep Medicine review. Sleep 2000; 23(2):243–308.
23. Buysse D, Reynolds C, Monk T, et al. The Pittsburgh Sleep Quality Index: a new instrument for psychiatric practice and research. Psychiatry Res 1989; 28:193–213.
24. Morin C. Insomnia: Psychological Assessment and Management. New York: The Guilford Press, 1993.
25. Espie CA, Brooks DN, Lindsay WR. An evaluation of tailored psychological treatment of insomnia. J Behav Ther Exp Psychiatry 1989; 20(2):143–153.
26. Kushida CA, Littner MR, Morgenthaler T, et al. Practice parameters for the indications for polysomnography and related procedures: an update for 2005. Sleep 2005; 28(4):499–521.
27. Chesson A Jr., Hartse K, Anderson WM, et al. Practice parameters for the evaluation of chronic insomnia. An American Academy of Sleep Medicine report. Standards of Practice Committee of the American Academy of Sleep Medicine. Sleep 2000; 23(2):237–241.
28. Littner M, Kushida CA, Anderson WM, et al. Practice parameters for the role of actigraphy in the study of sleep and circadian rhythms: an update for 2002 [see comment]. Sleep 2003; 26(3):337–341.
29. Stepanski EJ, Glinn M, Fortier J, et al. Physiological reactivity in chronic insomnia. Sleep Res 1989; 18:306.
30. Vgontzas AN, Tsigos C, Bixler EO, et al. Chronic insomnia and activity of the stress system: a preliminary study. J Psychosom Res 1998; 45(1 spec no):21–31.
31. Perlis ML, Smith MT, Andrews PJ, et al. Beta/gamma EEG activity in patients with primary and secondary insomnia and good sleeper controls. Sleep 2001; 24(1):110–117.
32. Nofzinger EA, Buysse DJ, Germain A, et al. Functional neuroimaging evidence for hyperarousal in insomnia. Am J Psychiatry 2004; 161(11):2126–2128.
33. Regestein Q, Dambrosia J, Hallett M, et al. Daytime alertness in patients with primary insomnia. Am J Psychiatry 1993; 150:1529–1534.
34. Hohagen F, Käppler C, Schramm E, et al. Prevalence of insomnia in elderly general practice attenders and the current treatment modalities. Acta Psychiatr Scand 1994; 90(2):102–108.
35. Gallup Organization. Sleep in America. Princeton, NJ: Gallup Organization, 1995.
36. Schramm E, Hohagen F, Käppler C, et al. Mental comorbidity of chronic insomnia in general practice attenders using DSM-III-R. Acta Psychiatr Scand 1995; 91(1):10–17.

37. Hohagen F, Rink K, Käppler C, et al. Prevalence and treatment of insomnia in general practice: a longitudinal study. Eur Arch Psychiatry Clin Neurosci 1993; 242:329–336.
38. Watson NF, Kapur V, Arguelles LM, et al. Comparison of subjective and objective measures of insomnia in monozygotic twins discordant for chronic fatigue syndrome. Sleep 2003; 26(3):324–328.
39. Reynolds C, Kupfer D, Buysse D, et al. Subtyping DSM-III-R primary insomnia: a literature review by the DSM-IV work group on sleep disorders. Am J Psychiatry 1991; 148:432–438.
40. Coleman R, Roffwarg H, Kennedy S, et al. Sleep-wake disorders based on a polysomnographic diagnosis: a national cooperative study. JAMA 1982; 247:997–1003.
41. Bonnet MH, Arand DL. Physiological activation in patients with Sleep State Misperception. Psychosom Med 1997; 59(5):533–540.
42. Hatoum HT, Kania CM, Kong SX, et al. Prevalence of insomnia: a survey of the enrollees at five managed care organizations. Am J Manag Care 1998; 4(1):79–86.
43. Ohayon MM. Prevalence of DSM-IV diagnostic criteria of insomnia: distinguishing insomnia related to mental disorders from sleep disorders. J Psychiatr Res 1997; 31(3):333–346.
44. Simon GE, VonKorff M. Prevalence, burden, and treatment of insomnia in primary care. Am J Psychiatry 1997; 154(10):1417–1423.
45. Ohayon MM, Roth T. What are the contributing factors for insomnia in the general population? J Psychosom Res 2001; 51(6):745–755.
46. Foley DJ, Monjan A, Simonsick EM, et al. Incidence and remission of insomnia among elderly adults: an epidemiologic study of 6,800 persons over three years. Sleep 1999; 22(suppl 2):S366–S372.
47. Foley DJ, Monjan AA, Izmirlian G, et al. Incidence and remission of insomnia among elderly adults in a biracial cohort. Sleep 1999; 22(suppl 2):S373–S378.
48. Shochat T, Umphress J, Israel AG, et al. Insomnia in primary care patients. Sleep 1999; 22(suppl 2):S359–S365.
49. Katz DA, McHorney CA. Clinical correlates of insomnia in patients with chronic illness. Arch Intern Med 1998; 158(10):1099–1107.
50. Maggi S, Langlois JA, Minicuci N, et al. Sleep complaints in community-dwelling older persons: prevalence, associated factors, and reported causes. J Am Geriatr Soc 1998; 46(2):161–168.
51. Morgan K, Clarke D. Longitudinal trends in late-life insomnia: implications for prescribing. Age Ageing 1997; 26(3):179–184.
52. Ohayon MM, Zulley J, Guilleminault C, et al. How age and daytime activities are related to insomnia in the general population: consequences for older people. J Am Geriatr Soc 2001; 49(4):360–366.
53. Leger D, Scheuermaier K, Philip P, et al. SF-36: evaluation of quality of life in severe and mild insomniacs compared with good sleepers. Psychosom Med 2001; 63(1):49–55.
54. Hatoum HT, Kong SX, Kania CM, et al. Insomnia, health-related quality of life and healthcare resource consumption. A study of managed-care organisation enrollees. Pharmacoeconomics 1998; 14(6):629–637.
55. Idzikowski C. Impact of insomnia on health-related quality of life. Pharmacoeconomics 1996; 10(suppl 1):15–24.
56. Katz DA, McHorney CA. The relationship between insomnia and health-related quality of life in patients with chronic illness. J Fam Pract 2002; 51(3):229–235.
57. Breslau N, Roth T, Rosenthal L, et al. Sleep disturbance and psychiatric disorders: a longitudinal epidemiological study of young adults. Biol Psychiatry 1996; 39(6):411–418.
58. Weissman MM, Greenwald S, Nino-Murcia G, et al. The morbidity of insomnia uncomplicated by psychiatric disorders. Gen Hosp Psychiatry 1997; 19(4):245–250.
59. Ford D, Kamerow D. Epidemiologic study of sleep disturbances and psychiatric disorders: an opportunity for prevention? JAMA 1989; 262:1479–1484.
60. Daddi L. Sulle alterazioni del sistema nervosa centrale nella inanizione. Riv Patol Nerv Ment 1898; 3:295–300.
61. De Manaceine M. Quelques observations experimentales sur l"influence de l'insomnia absolue. Arch Ital Biol 1894; 21:322–325.
62. Rechtschaffen A, Bergmann BM, Everson CA, et al. Sleep deprivation in the rat: X. Integration and discussion of the findings, 1989. Sleep 2002; 25(1):68–87.
63. Dinges DF, Pack F, Williams K, et al. Cumulative sleepiness, mood disturbance, and psychomotor vigilance performance decrements during a week of sleep restricted to 4-5 hours per night. Sleep 1997; 20(4):267–277.
64. Lu J, Greco MA, Shiromani P, et al. Effect of lesions of the ventrolateral preoptic nucleus on NREM and REM sleep. J Neurosci 2000; 20(10):3830–3842.
65. Saper CB: Unpublished data, 2006.
66. Dzirasa K, Ribeiro S, Costa R, et al. Dopaminergic control of sleep-wake states. J Neurosci 2006; 26(41):10577–10589.
67. Bonnet MH, Arand DL. Caffeine use as a model of acute and chronic insomnia. Sleep 1992; 15(6):526–536.

68. Harvey AG. A cognitive model of insomnia. Behav Res Ther 2002; 40(8):869–893.
69. Espie CA. Insomnia: conceptual issues in the development, persistence, and treatment of sleep disorder in adults. Annu Rev Psychol 2002; 53:215–243.
70. Perlis M, Giles DE, Mendelson WB, et al. Psychophysiological insomnia: the behavioural model and a neurocognitive perspective. J Sleep Res 1997; 6:179–188.
71. Leger D, Massuel M-A, Metlaine A, et al. Professional correlates of insomnia [see comment]. Sleep 2006; 29(2):171–178.
72. Godet-Cayre V, Pelletier-Fleury N, Le Vaillant M, et al. Insomnia and absenteeism at work. Who pays the cost?[see comment]. Sleep 2006; 29(2):179–184.
73. Zammit GK, Weiner J, Damato N, et al. Quality of life in people with insomnia. Sleep 1999; 22(suppl 2): S379–S385.
74. Eriksen W, Natvig B, Bruusgaard D. Sleep problems: a predictor of long-term work disability? A four-year prospective study. Scand J Public Health 2001; 29(1):23–31.
75. Sivertsen B, Overland S, Neckelmann D, et al. The long-term effect of insomnia on work disability: the HUNT-2 historical cohort study. Am J Epidemiol 2006; 163(11):1018–1024.
76. Walsh JK, Engelhardt CL. The direct economic costs of insomnia in the United States for 1995. Sleep 1999; 22(suppl 2):S386–S393.
77. Leger D, Levy E, Paillard M. The direct costs of insomnia in France. Sleep 1999; 22(suppl 2):S394–S401.
78. Stoller MK. Economic effects of insomnia. Clin Ther 1994; 16(5):873–897; discussion 854.
79. Leger D, Guilleminault C, Bader G, et al. Medical and socio-professional impact of insomnia. Sleep 2002; 25(6):625–629.

3 | Pathophysiology, Associations, and Consequences of Insomnia

David N. Neubauer

Sleep Disorders Center and Department of Psychiatry and Behavioral Sciences, Johns Hopkins University School of Medicine, Baltimore, Maryland, U.S.A.

Kelleen N. Flaherty

Graduate Biomedical Writing Program, University of the Sciences in Philadelphia, Jamison, Pennsylvania, U.S.A.

INTRODUCTION

In a general sense, insomnia suggests inadequate sleep quality or quantity when one has an adequate opportunity to sleep. When defined as a sleep disorder, insomnia is characterized by difficulty falling asleep or remaining asleep, which may represent problems with sleep maintenance or early morning awakening despite attempts to be sleeping. Sleep disorder nosologies also may include a complaint of nonrefreshing sleep as an insomnia complaint. For a diagnosis of an insomnia disorder to be made, daytime consequences or functional impairment also should be present. These may include fatigue, inability to concentrate, or irritability. Insomnia may be characterized as primary or comorbid (1). Primary insomnia occurs independently while comorbid insomnia presumably is associated with a sleep disturbance related to another disorder. Insomnia affects approximately 30% of the general population at least occasionally and is a severe or chronic problem for about 10% of the population. Patients with co-occurring conditions have significantly increased risk for insomnia (2). People suffering with insomnia have increased healthcare costs and utilize health resources to a greater extent. They also have worse scores on quality-of-life measures. Persistent insomnia has been identified as a risk factor for the development or exacerbation of certain psychiatric and medical conditions. Overall, insomnia represents a significant socioeconomic burden both for individuals and for society. This chapter will provide an overview of current perspectives on the causes, consequences, and associations of insomnia.

ETIOLOGY, PATHOPHYSIOLOGY, AND PATHOGENESIS

The experience of insomnia may result from an extraordinary diversity of influences, including both psychologic and physiologic processes. The etiology of insomnia episodes often is multifactorial and the relative effects of different influences may vary over time. Key factors initiating an episode may no longer contribute to the persistence of insomnia as new factors exert greater influence on the maintenance on the insomnia symptoms. These conceptual relationships are very effectively delineated in Spielman's "3 Ps" model of insomnia (see section "Predisposing and Precipitating Factors") (3).

It is impossible to view insomnia as a single disease with a delineated pathogenesis that results in adverse physiologic alterations, which undermine the experience of normal sleep. An individual's vulnerabilities for developing insomnia may involve genetic and cultural factors, personality characteristics, personal history, and assorted habits and routines. Comorbid disorders and other physical conditions (e.g., pregnancy and menopause), medication and other substance use, environmental disturbances, and situational crises all may initiate insomnia episodes that then may be sustained by these elements or become complicated further by emergent perpetuating factors. Among these new processes promoting the continuance of an insomnia episode may be the evolution of a psychologically conditioned excessive arousal associated with attempts to sleep; maladaptive sleep-related behaviors, attitudes, and beliefs; and physiologic abnormalities associated with an experience of excessive arousal.

Transient insomnia episodes, typically lasting up to a few days or weeks, generally are associated with identifiable triggers. Chronic insomnia, persisting for one month or longer, is more likely to be heterogeneous in etiology. For conceptual convenience, chronic insomnia may be classed as either primary or comorbid. Primary insomnia is presumed to exist independent of other disorders, while comorbid insomnia is thought to evolve with some contribution from co-occurring conditions. However, there are no clear criteria or measures that differentiate these broad etiologic realms. Moreover, no mechanistic pathways have been delineated that would explain the association of insomnia with concurrent conditions. Insomnia patients with and without other disorders may share fundamental vulnerabilities (4).

Several theoretical models of the etiology and evolution of primary insomnia have been elaborated (5). Generally, these highlight either psychologic or physiologic underlying processes, and attempt to account for the full spectrum of nighttime and daytime insomnia symptoms. A common denominator among the recent models is an appreciation of primary insomnia not just as a nighttime sleep disturbance with daytime consequences, but rather as a 24-hour disorder that deleteriously affects the experiences of both sleep and wakefulness (6). It remains unclear whether primary insomnia is a homogeneous condition associated with shared pathophysiology or is represented by a population with similar clinical presentations but constituting numerous etiologic subsets (4).

In the broad psychologic realm, insomnia etiology models have focused on personality features, behavioral associations, and cognitive experiences. Kales and colleagues argued that persistent insomnia was more likely to occur in people who internalized psychologic disturbances and demonstrated particular Minnesota Multiphasic Personality Inventory (MMPI) patterns, including elevations on scales representing depression, psychasthenia, and conversion hysteria (7). Worry and rumination with associated emotional and physiologic arousal have been core elements in the initiation and persistence of insomnia in the cognitive models. In advocating a stimulus-control treatment for insomnia, Bootzin emphasized the role of behavioral routines in sustaining insomnia (8). The importance of arousing and conditioned psychologic processes is inherent in Spielman's model of predisposing, precipitating, and perpetuating factors influencing the development of insomnia (3).

A general cognitive model of chronic insomnia begins with an acute event associated with rumination and worry that leads to cognitive and physiologic arousal and development of the subsequent symptoms associated with insomnia (5). The focus on nighttime sleeplessness and perceived daytime consequences, along with the evolution of psychologic conditioning, reinforces and perpetuates the insomnia in a self-propagating manner. The appraisal of stressors and perceived lack of control over them are important factors contributing to insomnia (9). Harvey has proposed a cognitive model of insomnia that highlights the anxiety component and the development of selective attention and monitoring of internal and external sleep-related threat cues. This process leads to an overestimation of perceived sleep and daytime performance deficits, as well as to counterproductive safety behaviors, which may include thought control, imagery control, emotional inhibition, and difficulty in problem solving. The result of this escalating cycle may be actual deficits in sleep quality and daytime performance (10).

Perlis has proposed a neurocognitive insomnia model noting that people with chronic insomnia are not awake because they are worrying, but rather that they are worrying because they are awake (5). This neurocognitive perspective incorporates three intersecting arousal dimensions—somatic, cognitive, and cortical. The cortical arousal is associated with high-frequency electroencephalographic (EEG) activity and subsequent sleep continuity disturbance and sleep-state misperception. The insomnia experience is reinforced by enhanced long-term memory of sleep onset and non–rapid eye movement (NREM) sleep.

One hypothesis to explain the perceived waking deficits of primary insomnia subjects is increased neurophysiologic workload (11). While people with chronic insomnia may not demonstrate performance impairment relative to control populations, they may need to recruit additional cerebral resources when faced with a cognitive challenge. This may be experienced as requiring extra effort in cognitive activities.

Physiologic models of primary insomnia typically have incorporated the concept of hyperarousal, which is presumed to explain both nighttime sleep difficulty and daytime complaints, such as fatigue, tension, irritability and poor concentration (12). With this perspective, impaired wakefulness is viewed as a consequence of the hyperarousal and not the result of sleep loss. Although the primary insomnia-hyperarousal paradigm has not yet been supported with definitive pathophysiologic findings, the model has been fruitful in stimulating further research.

An early study investigating physiologic correlates of insomnia noted increased activation in poor sleepers before sleep onset and during sleep, as evidenced by increased heart rate, basal skin resistance, core body temperature, and phasic vasoconstriction (13). Bonnet and Arand have explored the relationship of sleep characteristics, indicators of hyperarousal, objective daytime sleepiness, and subjective daytime symptoms in a series of experiments. Among these have been studies with yoke-controlled normals with sleep limited to the insomnia subject patterns and investigations producing insomnia symptoms in normal sleepers given high-dose caffeine for one week (12). They have concluded that elevated arousal produces both poor sleep and related symptoms in insomnia patients.

Among the physiologic parameters studied in controlled insomnia research studies have been metabolic rate (13), heart-rate variability (14), electromyographic activity (15), hypothalamic pituitary axis (HPA) activity (16), immune function and cytokine levels (17), thermoregulation (18), and EEG patterns (19–21). Abnormalities of the stress-response system have been the focus of several hyperarousal insomnia models and have stimulated the design of numerous clinical investigations (4,22).

Vgontzas and colleagues examined the relationships of cortisol and cytokines with characteristics of sleep and waking in populations of sleep-disordered individuals, including chronic insomnia subjects (17). They found a shift of tumor necrosis factor (TNF) and interleukin (IL)-6 secretion from nighttime to daytime in the chronic insomnia group and hypothesized that this might explain daytime fatigue and performance decrements (23). Their findings of 24-hour cortisol hypersecretion in insomnia subjects could help explain nighttime difficulty falling asleep (16).

Sleep onset normally is associated with substantial thermoregulatory changes. It has been argued that insomnia may be associated with abnormalities in these processes. Thermoregulatory research has shown that subjects with sleep-onset insomnia had impaired heat loss capacity in peripheral regions in association with sleep onset (18).

EEG studies have demonstrated increased beta and gamma range activity in insomnia subjects (19). Alterations in sleep EEG microstructure as represented in cyclic alternating pattern (CAP) rate correlate with poor sleep (20). A study employing event-related potentials that indicate the processing of auditory information during sleep in insomnia subjects demonstrated an enhancement in attention and a decrease in inhibitory processes that normally facilitate sleep onset (21).

Several neuroimaging studies have explored sleep and wakefulness in people with insomnia in comparison with normal sleepers. Regional cerebral glucose metabolism was examined in a positron emission tomography (PET) study of insomnia subjects and healthy controls (24). The insomnia subjects had greater global cerebral glucose metabolism as compared with normal controls while asleep and awake, a smaller decline in wake-promoting regions in the relative metabolism from waking to sleep states, and decreased relative metabolism in the prefrontal cortex while awake. It was hypothesized that an inadequate decline in arousal mechanisms in the sleep-onset process could be associated with an inability to fall asleep and that daytime fatigue could reflect decreased activity in the prefrontal cortex. A magnetic resonance imaging (MRI) study found reduced hippocampal volumes bilaterally in insomnia subjects compared with good sleepers (25). A single photon emission computed tomography (SPECT) study found lower regional blood flow in the basal ganglia during sleep among primary insomnia subjects (26).

In summary, groups of individuals with persistent insomnia can be differentiated readily from healthy sleepers on a wide array of dimensional measures, including both psychologic and physiologic. While many of these studies support a construct of hyperarousal among insomnia subjects, the findings still must be regarded only as significant associations. It remains unclear whether hyperarousal is a cause or consequence of insomnia (4). No single underlying pathophysiologic process has been shown to represent a causal agent that would qualify for etiology status. Nevertheless, these chronic insomnia models remain powerful in stimulating further research and guiding treatment strategies.

PREDISPOSING AND PRECIPITATING FACTORS

Insomnia results from a wide range of influences, several of which have been reviewed above in the etiology discussion. Spielman developed an elegant model to highlight the factors that represent insomnia vulnerabilities and triggers. His theory posits that insomnia episodes result from the interaction of predisposing, precipitating, and perpetuating (3 Ps) factors over time. Even when they have no current sleep complaints, certain individuals are at greater risk for the development of insomnia because of underlying *predispositions*. Inherited or acquired characteristics such as female gender, advanced age, lower socioeconomic status, personality features, shift work and other irregular schedules, and comorbid illness (especially psychiatric disorders) all predispose people to the development of insomnia. Genetics, metabolism, disorders of arousal, aspects of personality, and a dysfunctional homeostatic system also serve as significant predisposing factors (4).

According to the model, predisposing factors do not initiate an insomnia episode; they simply make it more likely to occur by causing an individual to be closer to a hypothetical insomnia threshold when sleep disturbance symptoms become clinically significant. One or more *precipitating* factors must be present for one to reach this threshold. Precipitating events generally are stressful triggers and may include acute illness, loss of a job, or other financial concerns, illness or death in the family, and other situational crises. Positive stressful events (e.g., marriage, birth of a child) also may represent insomnia triggers. Insomnia sufferers may sleep better and revert to their baseline predisposition level if the crisis resolves or if they successfully adapt to it. However, it is possible for the insomnia symptoms to persist beyond the immediate influence of the initial precipitants. Once people suffer with insomnia, they may worry excessively about their sleep and the effects of not sleeping adequately. This may lead to anxiety and tension as their bedtime approaches or if they awaken during the night. Their sleep-related habits may change with irregular day and night sleeping patterns, excessive time in bed, use of alcohol or other sedating substances, and other examples of poor sleep hygiene behaviors. Conditioned hyperarousal may evolve along with dysfunctional beliefs and attitudes regarding sleep and insomnia. Together these new factors can perpetuate insomnia as it evolves into a chronic condition. The original precipitants may become irrelevant. This "3 Ps" model allows chronic insomnia to be viewed as a self-propagating condition entirely because of the perpetuating factors.

Spielman originally graphed these clusters of factors into four stacked stages in his insomnia model to suggest temporal relationships. On a vertical insomnia severity axis, predisposition represents the level of vulnerability before the onset of insomnia symptoms (preclinical) and also is the foundation at all stages. The onset of insomnia is the next stage, wherein one or more precipitating factors provide sufficient stress beyond the preclinical level to place the individual above the insomnia threshold. A short-term stage then may follow, wherein the influence of precipitating factors wane and perpetuating factors begin to accumulate and maintain the individual above the threshold. Finally, if chronic insomnia evolves, it is the perpetuating mechanisms that sustain the insomnia symptoms over time.

In an attempt to quantify trait vulnerability for insomnia, Drake and colleagues developed the Ford Insomnia Response to Stress Test (FIRST), a Likert-scale questionnaire of nine items assessing sleep disturbance in response to commonly experienced stressful situations (27). When evaluated with a population-based sample in sleep laboratory testing, individuals with higher FIRST scores had lower sleep efficiency, prolonged initial sleep onset, and elevated daytime sleep latency on the Multiple Sleep Latency Test (MSLT). The authors suggested that the results might reflect vulnerability to stress-related sleep disturbance and physiologic hyperarousal that could predispose individuals to develop chronic insomnia.

The degree to which family history represents a predisposition for developing insomnia has been examined. In a Quebec population-based sample, people with past or current insomnia were more likely to have a family history of insomnia in comparison with good sleepers (28). Drake and colleagues employed the FIRST survey with 31 sibling pairs and found a strong familial aggregation of vulnerability to stress-related sleep disturbance (29). The genetic influence on insomnia has been investigated in several twin studies (30–33). For example, a classic twin design analysis of the University of Washington Twin Registry including 1042 monozygotic and 828 dizygotic twin pairs found a heritability estimate of 57% for insomnia (33).

Epidemiologic surveys almost invariably find that insomnia occurs more frequently among women. A meta-analysis of 29 studies including over one million subjects demonstrated a risk ratio of 1.41 for females reporting insomnia compared with males (34). The greater propensity for women over men in developing insomnia increased with age.

MORBIDITY AND MORTALITY

By definition, an insomnia disorder is characterized by nighttime sleep disturbance and daytime complaints or impairment. Chronic insomnia additionally has been associated with decrements in quality of life, greater absenteeism and decreased work productivity, increased healthcare utilization and costs, higher frequency of vehicular and industrial accidents, and a significant economic burden to society. Epidemiologic studies have addressed the question of greater mortality associated with chronic insomnia. Studies demonstrating that insomnia increases the future risk of medical and psychiatric disorders are considered in the subsequent two sections of this chapter.

Impaired Daytime Functioning and General Daytime Complaints

Reports of daytime consequences and impairment among individuals with chronic insomnia are represented in multiple domains (social, physical, emotional) and may be described as fatigue, exhaustion, or malaise; attention, concentration, or memory difficulty; social or vocational dysfunction or poor school performance; mood disturbance or irritability; daytime sleepiness or excessive arousal; reduction in motivation or energy initiatives; proneness for errors or accidents at work or while driving; headache, gastrointestinal, or other physical symptoms in response to poor sleep; and concerns or worries about sleep, according to the Research Diagnostic Criteria for Insomnia Disorder developed by the American Academy of Sleep Medicine (6).

While individuals with insomnia report daytime consequences such as fatigue and sleepiness, poor performance on tasks, anxiety and dysphoria, and poor health in general, there only are replicated objective findings for impaired balance, elevated HPA activity, and sleep architecture findings associated with chronic insomnia (35). In fact, individuals with insomnia who report reduced ability to perform psychomotor tasks, memory impairment, or cognitive defects do as well as matched controls in trials. These findings suggest that these deficits are overestimated in chronic insomnia subjects. This attentional bias or sleep-related preoccupation may contribute to the development of persistent insomnia (36,37). Nevertheless, many quality-of-life indicators of chronic insomnia subjects are similar to people with other chronic illnesses (11,38–41). Subjective dysphoria, sleepiness, and fatigue have been assessed in numerous studies with validated instruments such as the Stanford Sleepiness Scale, the Profile of Mood Scales, and the Fatigue Severity Scale. Many of these studies have demonstrated significantly higher sleepiness in individuals complaining of insomnia as compared with controls (41).

Socioprofessional Impact

Insomnia has been shown to be a significant predictor of absenteeism. Two studies have shown that absenteeism was at least twice that in populations of workers with insomnia as compared with workers not complaining of insomnia (42,43). In one study, absenteeism was evaluated in a population of 1308 workers. Thirty-seven independent variables were assessed as predictors of absenteeism, with insomnia ranking as the most highly predictive. Individuals with insomnia were 2.8 times more likely to miss work than those without insomnia (43). In a study reported by Léger and colleagues, absenteeism in workers with insomnia was found to be nearly twice that of workers who were good sleepers. Further, absenteeism was higher in blue-collar jobs than white-collar jobs, and higher in men than women, although duration of absence was higher in women than men. In this same report, accidents during travel to work were assessed. Workers with insomnia were involved in more serious automobile accidents (odds ratio, OR = 1.74). More workers with insomnia reported having only one accident in the past 12 months than workers without insomnia (OR = 1.62), and three times as many workers reported having two to three accidents in the past 12 months (OR = 3.08). Twice as many workers with insomnia as those without insomnia reported that the accidents were their fault (OR = 2.03), and twice as many also reported that their accidents led to absence from work (42).

Insomnia also has been reported to impact the professional life of its sufferers through decreased productivity and efficiency, decreased job satisfaction, and reduced likelihood of career advancement (41,42). Individuals with insomnia are more prone to making serious errors than normal sleepers, have reduced self-esteem, and perceive their professional development to be reduced (i.e., received insufficient training at work) (42).

Industrial and Vehicular Accidents

Insomnia-related sleepiness, fatigue, or impaired concentration may have a negative impact on workplace safety by contributing to mistakes and accidents. In a prospective Swedish study on occupational accidents, 47,860 individuals were interviewed over a period of 20 years on issues related to work and health. One hundred and sixty six fatal occupational accidents occurred, with significant predictors being male gender, difficulties in sleeping over the past two weeks, and non-day work (44).

Vehicular accidents also are associated with insomnia. The relationship of sleep insufficiency and driving-related accidents is well established; although insomnia often is not the cause of the sleep deprivation (45). Survey data have suggested that individuals with insomnia are more likely to have driving accidents (46). An internet-based survey found a direct relationship between reported insomnia and driving accidents. An odds ratio of 1.77 was calculated for individuals reporting insomnia having three or more accidents compared with individuals with no insomnia (47).

Risk of Falls

Falls may be associated with significant immediate and long-term morbidity. Several reports have suggested that insomnia increases the risk for falls at nighttime. Balance is one of the few objective measures that differentiates chronic insomnia subjects and matched controls (41). A survey of 1526 individuals between the ages of 64 and 99 years found that 19% reported having fallen within the past year. Nighttime sleep problems were one of the independent variables significantly associated with falling (48). A database analysis of 427 Michigan nursing homes comprising 34,163 individuals aged 65 years and older found that individuals with insomnia were at greater risk for subsequent falls (49). The greatest risk among those with insomnia was in the group not treated with hypnotic medications.

Quality of Life

Several studies have investigated health-related quality-of-life features in insomnia and control subjects. Zammit and colleagues assessed 261 insomnia subjects and 101 controls without sleep complaints. Both groups completed the 36-item Short Form Health Survey of the Medical Outcomes Study (SF-36). The insomnia subjects scored significantly worse on all eight of the physical and mental quality-of-life domains, and also had greater symptomatology on surveys of depression and anxiety (46).

Léger and colleagues examined matched populations of 240 severe insomnia subjects, 422 mild insomnia subjects, and 391 good sleeper controls in a French study (50). The SF-36 quality-of-life assessment also was employed. The severe insomnia group had worse scores in all eight domains compared with the mild subjects and healthy controls. A clear correlation between the severity of the insomnia and the quality-of-life degradation was evident.

Katz and McHorney reviewed cross-sectional data from the Medical Outcomes Study, which examined health-related quality of life in 3554 patients diagnosed with one or more of five chronic conditions (hypertension, diabetes, chronic obstructive pulmonary disease, myocardial infarction, and depression) (51,52). Among these patients, 16% were categorized as having severe insomnia and 34% as having mild insomnia. It was found that insomnia was independently associated with worsened health-related quality of life to a similar extent as the patients with other chronic conditions (52). The chronic character of insomnia also was evident in the longitudinal study. The subjects were resurveyed two years after the initial evaluation. The majority of the insomnia symptoms noted at baseline persisted during the two years. Among the patients with baseline severe insomnia, 83% continued to report insomnia at the time of the follow-up survey and 59% of the mild insomnia subjects still experienced insomnia symptoms.

Economic Burden

Several studies have calculated estimates of the direct and indirect costs of insomnia in the U.S. and other selected countries (53–56). In 1995, the estimated total direct and indirect costs for insomnia ranged from $30 to $35 billion. Direct costs accounted for $13.9 billion, with $11.9 billion accounting for health care services (91% of which being nursing home costs), and $1.79 billion for medications used to treat insomnia (less than half of which being prescription medications) (54). Absenteeism, lost productivity, and accidents were estimated to account for

$80 billion in costs to society in 1994 (53). In a retrospective, observational study comparing two populations of individuals with untreated insomnia (young adults aged 18–64 and older adults 65 years of age or older) with matched individuals without insomnia, Ozminkowski and colleagues concluded that the average direct and indirect costs for younger adults with insomnia were $1253 more per six months than the matched population without insomnia, and that the direct costs for individuals in the elderly cohort were approximately $1143 more per six months than those in the matched group without insomnia (56).

Mortality

The question of whether insomnia is associated with increased mortality was examined in a large cohort of middle-aged individuals (ages 45–69 years) in the Atherosclerosis Risk in Communities Study (57). The prevalence of insomnia was 23%. Using a multivariate regression analysis and controlling for possible confounding variables, it was found that insomnia did not predict increased mortality over the study period of approximately six years. Several large-scale studies, however, have reported that both short and long sleep duration increases the risk of selected disease state and all-cause mortality (58–61). In a prospective cohort study of 10,308 white-collar British civil servants (aged 35–55 years at baseline) assessed at baseline and follow-up at 12 and 17 years, researchers in Britain looked at all-cause, cardiovascular, and noncardiovascular mortality, in addition to sleep duration. Researchers found a U-shaped association between sleep duration and mortality. After adjusting for confounders, participants who slept fewer hours than at baseline (6–8 hours) had more cardiovascular mortality (hazard ratio, HR = 2.4), but an increase in number of hours slept at baseline (>8 hours) was associated with noncardiovascular mortality (HR = 2.1) (62).

ASSOCIATIONS, COMPLICATIONS, AND CONSEQUENCES WITH CONDITIONS/DISORDERS OF ORGAN SYSTEMS

Insomnia frequently accompanies medical disorders, especially when pain or discomfort is present. Generally, most cases of insomnia are thought to be comorbid with psychiatric, medical, or other primary sleep disorders. A traditional perspective viewed insomnia as entirely secondary to the associated disorders; however, the 2005 *NIH State-of-the-Science Conference Statement on Manifestations and Management of Chronic Insomnia in Adults* argued that comorbidity should be emphasized because limited understandings of chronic insomnia mechanistic pathways prevent firm conclusions about the nature of any associations or the direction of causality (1).

Most bodily systems have been implicated with certain disorders being associated with increased prevalence of insomnia relative to the general population, although causality has not necessarily been established. Among these are the cardiovascular, pulmonary, neurologic, endocrine, urologic, rheumatologic, immunologic, gastrointestinal, dermatologic, hepatic, renal, orthopedic, hematologic, and reproductive systems. Pregnancy and menopause are associated with increased risk for insomnia. Infectious and neoplastic disease processes also may contribute to sleep disturbances. Additionally, insomnia commonly occurs in association with the following sleep disorders: circadian rhythm disorders, central or obstructive sleep-related breathing disorders, sleep-related movement disorders, restless legs syndrome, narcolepsy, and most parasomnias (63). Several studies have reported a direct relationship between the number of health problems and the likelihood of an individual reporting insomnia (64,65).

Insomnia comorbidity with medical problems was assessed in a retrospective, cross-sectional, community-based survey of 772 men and women aged 20 to 98 years (66). It was found that people with insomnia had a higher prevalence of comorbid medical problems compared with those without insomnia and, conversely, that people with chronic medical problems had a higher prevalence of insomnia compared with those without the same conditions. Insomnia subjects had higher incidences of heart disease, hypertension, neurologic disease, breathing problems, urinary problems, chronic pain, and gastrointestinal problems. Individuals reporting heart disease, cancer, hypertension, urinary problems, chronic pain, and gastrointestinal problems were more likely also to report insomnia than individuals without these health problems. The authors noted potential deleterious effects of insomnia that might complicate other health conditions and further decrease health-related quality of life. These include experimental evidence of a reduction in pain threshold and impairment in immune function.

Experimental sleep restriction (partial sleep deprivation) in healthy young adults results in glucose tolerance and immune response abnormalities, as well as enhanced sensitivity to pain (67–69). While the pathophysiology of insomnia and mechanisms of experimental sleep restriction are not necessarily the same, they do raise important questions regarding the health effects of persistent insomnia. Several epidemiologic studies have investigated specific health risks in association with insomnia.

The relationship of insomnia and hypertension was examined in a Japanese study of male workers surveyed for four years during annual health examinations (70). The hypertension incidence was significantly greater in individuals with difficulty initiating sleep and difficulty maintaining sleep. During the four years following the baseline assessment, persistent complaints of difficulty initiating and maintaining sleep were significantly associated with an increased risk of hypertension with odds ratios of 1.96 and 1.88, respectively.

The relationship of sleep habits and sleep complaints in association with the development of diabetes mellitus was examined in a Swedish study (71). In this longitudinal project, 2663 subjects were surveyed at baseline and 1244 of them were re-interviewed 12 years later. Difficulty maintaining sleep (relative risk, RR = 4.8) or the report of short sleep duration was associated with the future development of diabetes among the males. There was not a significant relationship with the women. However, a German study of 4140 men and 4129 women, followed for a mean period of 7.5 years, demonstrated a significantly increased risk for type 2 diabetes in both men and women with baseline sleep maintenance insomnia (72).

Coronary artery disease mortality was monitored prospectively in a related Swedish study during a 12-year period following an initial general population survey of adults aged 45 to 65 years (73). Difficulty initiating sleep was significantly related to coronary artery disease deaths in males with a relative risk of 3.1; however, there was not a significant relationship in females.

Prospective studies of individuals with chronic painful conditions, such as rheumatoid arthritis and fibromyalgia, have shown that insomnia is associated with an increased risk for greater clinical pain severity (74–76). Both insomnia and depression increased the risk over one year for children with regional neck pain to develop widespread pain (77).

PSYCHOLOGIC/PSYCHIATRIC ASSOCIATIONS, COMPLICATIONS, AND CONSEQUENCES

The majority of people with mood and anxiety disorders experience insomnia, and it often accompanies exacerbations of other psychiatric disorders (78). With some conditions the association is formalized in the Diagnostic and Statistical Manual of Mental Disorders, fourth edition (DSM-IV) diagnostic criteria (79). Although patients with acute episodes of mood and anxiety disorders frequently experience disturbed sleep, it has become well established that the risk of future development of these disorders increases in the context of persistent insomnia. Numerous longitudinal epidemiologic studies demonstrate that when people at the baseline evaluation have insomnia but no psychiatric disorder, they subsequently are at significantly increased risk of meeting criteria for a mood or anxiety disorder on reevaluation if the insomnia persists (80). Insomnia often is the first symptom heralding a depressive episode and symptoms of sleep disturbance may persist following improvement in mood (81,82). The relationship between insomnia and psychiatric disorders has come to be viewed as circular and synergistic. The interaction can promote a downward spiral of symptom severity and quality of life for patients, which further complicates treatment efforts.

The 1989 Ford and Kamerow publication of an analysis from the National Institute of Mental Health (NIMH) Epidemiologic Catchment Area (ECA) project documented the comorbidity of insomnia and psychiatric disorders and it was the initial key longitudinal study establishing the persistent insomnia link with future depression and anxiety (83). A general population sample of almost 8000 subjects was surveyed with standardized diagnostic interviews to identify individuals with insomnia and psychiatric disorders. Approximately

10% of the population met the relatively stringent insomnia criteria. In the insomnia group on initial evaluation, 40% of the subjects concurrently met the criteria for at least one psychiatric disorder. Among these were major depression (14.0%), dysthymia (8.5%), anxiety disorder (23.9%), alcohol abuse (7%), and other drug abuse (4.2%). The association of persistent insomnia with an increased risk for new-onset psychiatric disorders was demonstrated with a one-year follow-up survey. Those subjects with insomnia at both baseline and at follow-up interviews had a significantly increased risk (OR = 39.8) of meeting the criteria for new-onset major depression. The new-onset anxiety disorder risk also was elevated in this group (OR = 6.3). Longer-term follow-up with this ECA cohort revealed that individuals with persistent alcohol dependence had greater odds of insomnia (OR = 2.4) than those whose initial alcohol dependence had remitted (84).

A precursor analysis of the ECA database further explored the relationship of insomnia and depression (85). The age of onset and symptoms associated with the onset of major depression were examined. A significant degree of predictability was evident with the precursor-attributable risk associated with sleep disturbance identifying 47% of the new cases of major depression occurring during the following year.

Several studies have explored the prevalence of insomnia in patients with specific anxiety disorders (86). Insomnia has been shown to be especially problematic for individuals with panic disorder (87), posttraumatic stress disorder (88), generalized anxiety disorder (89), and social phobia (90). Most patients with panic disorder will experience distressing panic episodes that awaken them from sleep. Patients with posttraumatic stress disorder frequently experience poor sleep quality and vivid nightmares. The chronic anxiety of patients with generalized anxiety disorder often affects them throughout the night with resulting difficulty falling asleep and repeated awakenings. Patients with social phobia report significantly worse sleep quality and difficulty falling asleep in comparison with healthy controls.

The increased future risk of new-onset psychiatric symptoms in adult subjects with a history of insomnia was shown in a longitudinal analysis of data from over 10,000 adults in three U.S. communities where a standardized diagnostic interview was employed (91). One year following the baseline interview, 7113 of the subjects were re-interviewed. For the individuals with baseline insomnia but no previous psychiatric illness, the odds ratios for new-onset major depression, panic disorder, and alcohol abuse were 5.4, 20.3, and 2.3, respectively.

The increased risk of future mental health symptoms in people with a history of insomnia was confirmed in a study of young adults. Over 1000 members of a Michigan Health Maintenance Organization (HMO) aged 21 to 30 years were surveyed with a structured interview (92). The investigators re-interviewed 979 of the original subjects 3.5 years after the baseline survey. Those who had no psychiatric history at the baseline survey, but who previously had experienced an insomnia episode continuing for at least two weeks, were at much greater risk of having a psychiatric disorder at the time of the follow-up survey. The insomnia lifetime prevalence was 16.6% at the time of the baseline survey. A significantly increased risk for major depression, anxiety disorders, and substance abuse disorders was demonstrated in this baseline study. A gender-adjusted relative risk for new-onset major depression of 4.0 was identified.

Several studies have focused on insomnia and future psychiatric illness risk in older adults. A longitudinal United Kingdom survey of community-dwelling individuals aged 65 years and older involved a baseline semi-structured interview of 705 subjects at baseline and a reinterview of 524 of these subjects after three years (93). For the individuals with no depression at baseline, the best predictor of future depression was sleep disturbance at the time of the baseline interview. A longitudinal study in Alameda County, California assessed a 50 years and older cohort (mean age 64.9 years) (94). Baseline and one-year follow-up interviews were performed with a sample of 2370 community residents. On the baseline interview, insomnia was reported by 23.1% of the individuals. For the subjects with insomnia at both the baseline and follow-up interviews there was an odds ratio of 8.08 for the development of new-onset major depression.

The Hopkins Precursors Study demonstrated the strongest evidence for the very long-term risk of sleep disturbance contributing to future depressive symptoms (95). Over 1000 Johns Hopkins University's male medical students completed surveys while in medical school between 1948 and 1964. The questions included items about sleep characteristics. There was follow-up of these individuals for a median of 34 years with a range of 1 to 45 years. For the entire group, clinical depression was diagnosed in 101 of the subjects. Thirteen in the group committed suicide. Compared with the individuals with no sleep disturbance in medical school, the students with insomnia or with difficulty sleeping under stress had significantly greater risk of future depression with relative risks of 2.0 and 1.8, respectively. The risk of baseline insomnia and future clinical depression persisted for at least 30 years.

In a four-country European telephone structured-interview study of 14,915 subjects, insomnia with impaired daytime functioning was found in 19.1% of the general population (82). Approximately 28% of the insomnia subjects concurrently met criteria for a psychiatric diagnosis and 26% had a past psychiatric history. Data from this single-interview study suggested that insomnia often predated the onset of mood disorders, but that insomnia tended to evolve concurrently with anxiety disorders.

A large-scale Norwegian study assessed symptoms of insomnia, anxiety, and depression from general population health surveys completed by the same 25,130 individuals approximately 12 years apart (96). The study determined whether the subjects reported these symptoms on neither, both, or only on the first or second survey in an attempt to clarify whether state or trait relationships existed between insomnia and the psychiatric symptoms. Anxiety disorders on the follow-up survey were significantly associated with insomnia only on the first, only on the second, and on both surveys suggesting that insomnia may be a trait marker for subjects at risk for developing anxiety disorders. However, depression on the follow-up survey only was significantly associated with insomnia on that second survey and not with insomnia on the initial survey or both surveys. In contrast with the longitudinal studies cited above, the authors of this study suggested that there is only a state-like association between insomnia and depression.

Directionality of the association of insomnia with mood and anxiety disorders was explored in a single structured-interview study of 1014 community-based 13- to 16-year-old adolescents (97). There was a moderate lifetime association of depression and anxiety disorders with DSM-IV defined insomnia resulting in odds ratios of 3.2 to 6.8. Any previous anxiety disorder was associated with an increased risk of insomnia, but prior insomnia did not significantly increase the risk for the development of anxiety disorders. Prior insomnia did increase the risk for depression, but prior depression did not increase the risk for the onset of insomnia.

Bipolar disorder patients frequently experience insomnia during episodes of mania and depression. While some manic patients describe a decreased need for sleep, others feel distressed by an inability to sleep. Sleep loss from any cause, including jet lag and work schedules, may contribute to the onset or progression of mania in bipolar disorder patients (98,99).

Suicidal ideation and behaviors also have been shown to be more common in people with insomnia. Patients with major depression were surveyed with the Schedule for Affective Disorders and Schizophrenia (SADS), which incorporates a suicide subscale (100). Patients reporting insomnia or hypersomnia had higher suicide subscale scores and were more likely to express suicidal thoughts. In a cross-sectional study of largely tertiary-care chronic pain patients, 75% of individuals reporting sleep-onset insomnia also reported suicidal ideation. The majority of individuals without suicidal ideation reported minimal sleep-onset insomnia (101). Multivariate analyses showed that the severity of sleep-onset insomnia was a more robust correlate of suicidal ideation than depression or pain severity.

Extensive epidemiologic evidence clearly demonstrates the high degree of comorbidity between insomnia and psychiatric disorders. However, the mechanisms underlying these associations and the relationships with specific psychiatric disorders remain to be fully elucidated. Further investigations may determine the extent to which insomnia symptoms represent prodromal features, shared genetic vulnerability, or causative processes promoting related psychologic symptoms and psychiatric disorders.

SUMMARY

Insomnia is a common clinical problem that often exists as a chronic condition. Generally the etiology is multifactorial and it is frequently comorbid with psychiatric and medical disorders or in association with underlying sleep disorders. A wide spectrum of psychologic and physiologic factors has been identified as possible vulnerabilities for primary insomnia. Dominant models include psychophysiologic and hyperarousal processes. It has been argued that persistent insomnia may be associated with daytime distress and impairment, decreased quality of life, increased future risk of psychiatric illness, adverse health effects, increased falls and accidents, greater healthcare utilization, increased absenteeism, and a high societal economic burden.

REFERENCES

1. National Institutes of Health. National Institutes of Health State of the Science Conference Statement on Manifestations and Management of Chronic Insomnia in Adults, June 13–15, 2005. Sleep 2005; 28:1049–1057.
2. Stewart R, Besset A, Bebbington P, et al. Insomnia comorbidity and impact and hypnotic use by age group in a national survey population aged 16 to 74 years. Sleep 2006; 29:1391–1397.
3. Spielman AJ, Caruso LS, Glovinsky PB. A behavioral perspective on insomnia treatment. Psychiatr Clin North Am 1987; 10:541–553.
4. Drake CL, Roth T. Predisposition in the evolution of insomnia: evidence, potential mechanisms, and future directions. Sleep Medicine Clinics 2006; 1:333–349.
5. Perlis ML, Smith MT, Pigeon WR. Etiology and pathophysiology of insomnia. In: Kryger MH, Roth T, Dement WC, eds. Principles and Practice of Sleep Medicine. 4th ed. Philadelphia, PA: Elsevier, 2005:714–725.
6. Edinger JD, Bonnet MH, Bootzin RR, et al. Derivation of research diagnostic criteria for insomnia: report of an American Academy of Sleep Medicine work group. Sleep 2004; 27:1567–1596.
7. Kales A, Caldwell AB, Preston TA, et al. Personality patterns in insomnia. theoretical implications. Arch Gen Psychiatry 1976; 33:1128–1124.
8. Bootzin RR, Nicassio PM. Behavioral treatments for insomnia. In: Hersen M, Eisler RM, Miller PM, eds. Progress in Behavior Modification, Vol 6. New York: Academic Press, 1978:1–45.
9. Morin CM, Rodrigue S, Ivers H. Role of stress, arousal, and coping skills in primary insomnia. Psychosom Med 2003; 65:259–267.
10. Harvey AG. A cognitive model of insomnia. Behav Res Ther 2002; 40:869–893.
11. Orff HJ, Drummond SP, Nowakowski S, et al. Discrepancy between subjective symptomatology and objective neuropsychological performance in insomnia. Sleep 2007; 30:1205–1211.
12. Bonnet MH, Arand DL. Hyperarousal and insomnia. Sleep Med Rev 1997; 1:97–108.
13. Monroe LJ. Psychological and physiological differences between good and poor sleepers. J Abnorm Psychol 1967; 72:255–264.
14. Stepanski E, Zorick F, Roehrs T, et al. Daytime alertness in patients with chronic insomnia compared with asymptomatic control subjects. Sleep 1988; 11:54–60.
15. Haynes SN, Follingstad DR, McGowan WT. Insomnia: sleep patterns and anxiety level. J Psychosom Res 1974; 18:69–74.
16. Vgontzas AN, Bixler EO, Lin HM, et al. Chronic insomnia is associated with nyctohemeral activation of the hypothalamic-pituitary-adrenal axis: clinical implications. J Clin Endocrinol Metab 2001; 86:3787–3794.
17. Kapsimalis F, Basta M, Varouchakis G, et al. Cytokines and pathological sleep. Sleep Med 2008; 9:603–614.
18. van den Heuvel C, Ferguson S, Dawson D. Attenuated thermoregulatory response to mild thermal challenge in subjects with sleep-onset insomnia. Sleep 2006; 29:1174–1180.
19. Perlis ML, Smith MT, Andrews PJ, et al. Beta/gamma EEG activity in patients with primary and secondary insomnia and good sleeper controls. Sleep 2001; 24:110–117.
20. Parrino L, Ferrillo F, Smerieri A, et al. Is insomnia a neurophysiological disorder? The role of sleep EEG microstructure. Brain Res Bull 2004; 63:377–383.
21. Yang CM, Lo HS. ERP evidence of enhanced excitatory and reduced inhibitory processes of auditory stimuli during sleep in patients with primary insomnia. Sleep 2007; 30:585–592.
22. Richardson GS, Roth T. Future directions in the management of insomnia. J Clin Psychiatry 2001; 62 (suppl 10):39–45.
23. Vgontzas AN, Zoumakis M, Papanicolaou DA, et al. Chronic insomnia is associated with a shift of interleukin-6 and tumor necrosis factor secretion from nighttime to daytime. Metabolism 2002; 51:887–892.
24. Nofzinger EA, Buysse DJ, Germain A, et al. Functional neuroimaging evidence for hyperarousal in insomnia. Am J Psychiatry 2004; 161:2126–2128.
25. Riemann D, Voderholzer U, Spiegelhalder K, et al. Chronic insomnia and MRI-measured hippocampal volumes: a pilot study. Sleep 2007; 30:955–958.

26. Smith MT, Perlis ML, Chengazi VU, et al. Neuroimaging of NREM sleep in primary insomnia: a tc-99-HMPAO single photon emission computed tomography study. Sleep 2002; 25:325–335.
27. Drake C, Richardson G, Roehrs T, et al. Vulnerability to stress-related sleep disturbance and hyperarousal. Sleep 2004; 27:285–291.
28. Beaulieu-Bonneau S, LeBlanc M, Merette C, et al. Family history of insomnia in a population-based sample. Sleep 2007; 30:1739–1745.
29. Drake CL, Scofield H, Roth T. Vulnerability to insomnia: the role of familial aggregation. Sleep Med 2008; 9(3):297–302.
30. Heath AC, Kendler KS, Eaves LJ, et al. Evidence for genetic influences on sleep disturbance and sleep pattern in twins. Sleep 1990; 13:318–335.
31. McCarren M, Goldberg J, Ramakrishnan V, et al. Insomnia in Vietnam era veteran twins: influence of genes and combat experience. Sleep 1994; 17:456–461.
32. Partinen M, Kaprio J, Koskenvuo M, et al. Genetic and environmental determination of human sleep. Sleep 1983; 6:179–185.
33. Watson NF, Goldberg J, Arguelles L, et al. Genetic and environmental influences on insomnia, daytime sleepiness, and obesity in twins. Sleep 2006; 29:645–649.
34. Zhang B, Wing YK. Sex differences in insomnia: a meta-analysis. Sleep 2006; 29:85–93.
35. Krystal AD. Treating the health, quality of life, and functional impairments in insomnia. J Clin Sleep Med 2007; 3:63–72.
36. Taylor DJ, Lichstein KL, Durrence HH. Insomnia as a health risk factor. Behav Sleep Med 2003; 1:227–247.
37. Marchetti LM, Biello SM, Broomfield NM, et al. Who is pre-occupied with sleep? A comparison of attention bias in people with psychophysiological insomnia, delayed sleep phase syndrome and good sleepers using the induced change blindness paradigm. J Sleep Res 2006; 15:212–221.
38. Zammit GK, Weiner J, Damato N, et al. Quality of life in people with insomnia. Sleep 1999; 22(suppl 2): S379–S385.
39. Hajak G, Study of Insomnia in Europe (SINE) Study Group. Epidemiology of severe insomnia and its consequences in Germany. Eur Arch Psychiatry Clin Neurosci 2001; 251:49–56.
40. Leger D, Stal V, Guilleminault C, et al. Diurnal consequence of insomnia: impact on quality of life. Rev Neurol (Paris) 2001; 157:1270–1278.
41. Bonnet MH, Arrand DL. Consequences of insomnia. Sleep Med Clin 2006; 1:351–358.
42. Leger D, Guilleminault C, Bader G, et al. Medical and socio-professional impact of insomnia. Sleep 2002; 25:625–629.
43. Leigh JP. Employee and job attributes as predictors of absenteeism in a national sample of workers: the importance of health and dangerous working conditions. Soc Sci Med 1991; 33:127–137.
44. Akerstedt T, Fredlund P, Gillberg M, et al. A prospective study of fatal occupational accidents— relationship to sleeping difficulties and occupational factors. J Sleep Res 2002; 11:69–71.
45. Pack AI, Pack AM, Rodgman E, et al. Characteristics of crashes attributed to the driver having fallen asleep. Accid Anal Prev 1995; 27:769–775.
46. Zammit GK, Weiner J, Damato N, et al. Quality of life in people with insomnia. Sleep 1999; 22(suppl 2):S379–385.
47. Powell NB, Schechtman KB, Riley RW, et al. Sleepy driving: accidents and injury. Otolaryngol Head Neck Surg 2002; 126:217–227.
48. Brassington GS, King AC, Bliwise DL. Sleep problems as a risk factor for falls in a sample of community-dwelling adults aged 64–99 years. J Am Geriatr Soc 2000; 48:1234–1240.
49. Avidan AY, Fries BE, James ML, et al. Insomnia and hypnotic use, recorded in the minimum data set, as predictors of falls and hip fractures in Michigan nursing homes. J Am Geriatr Soc 2005; 53:955–962.
50. Leger D, Scheuermaier K, Philip P, et al. SF-36: evaluation of quality of life in severe and mild insomniacs compared with good sleepers. Psychosom Med 2001; 63:49–55.
51. Katz DA, McHorney CA. Clinical correlates of insomnia in patients with chronic illness. Arch Intern Med 1998; 158:1099–1107.
52. Katz DA, McHorney CA. The relationship between insomnia and health-related quality of life in patients with chronic illness. J Fam Pract 2002; 51:229–235.
53. Stoller MK. Economic effects of insomnia. Clin Ther 1994; 16:873–897; discussion 854.
54. Walsh JK, Engelhardt CL. The direct economic costs of insomnia in the United States for 1995. Sleep 1999; 22(suppl 2):S386–S393.
55. Chilcott LA, Shapiro CM. The socioeconomic impact of insomnia. An overview. Pharmacoeconomics 1996; 10(suppl 1):1–14.
56. Ozminkowski RJ, Wang S, Walsh JK. The direct and indirect costs of untreated insomnia in adults in the United States. Sleep 2007; 30:263–273.
57. Phillips B, Mannino DM. Does insomnia kill? Sleep 2005; 28:965–971.

58. Heslop P, Smith GD, Metcalfe C, et al. Sleep duration and mortality: the effect of short or long sleep duration on cardiovascular and all-cause mortality in working men and women. Sleep Med 2002; 3:305–314.
59. Kripke DF, Garfinkel L, Wingard DL, et al. Mortality associated with sleep duration and insomnia. Arch Gen Psychiatry 2002; 59:131–136.
60. Ayas NT, White DP, Manson JE, et al. A prospective study of sleep duration and coronary heart disease in women. Arch Intern Med 2003; 163:205–209.
61. Hublin C, Partinen M, Koskenvuo M, et al. Sleep and mortality: a population-based 22-year follow-up study. Sleep 2007; 30:1245–1253.
62. Ferrie JE, Shipley MJ, Cappuccio FP, et al. A prospective study of change in sleep duration: associations with mortality in the Whitehall II cohort. Sleep 2007; 30:1659–1666.
63. American Academy of Sleep Medicine. The International Classification of Sleep Disorders: Diagnostic & Coding Manual, ICSD-2, 2nd ed. Westchester, IL: American Academy of Sleep Medicine; 2005.
64. Foley DJ, Monjan AA, Brown SL, et al. Sleep complaints among elderly persons: an epidemiologic study of three communities. Sleep 1995; 18:425–432.
65. Mellinger GD, Balter MB, Uhlenhuth EH. Insomnia and its treatment. Prevalence and correlates. Arch Gen Psychiatry 1985; 42:225–232.
66. Taylor DJ, Mallory LJ, Lichstein KL, et al. Comorbidity of chronic insomnia with medical problems. Sleep 2007; 30:213–218.
67. Spiegel K, Leproult R, Van Cauter E. Impact of sleep debt on metabolic and endocrine function. Lancet 1999; 354:1435–1439.
68. Spiegel K, Sheridan JF, Van Cauter E. Effect of sleep deprivation on response to immunization. JAMA 2002; 288:1471–1472.
69. Roehrs T, Hyde M, Blaisdell B, et al. Sleep loss and REM sleep loss are hyperalgesic. Sleep 2006; 29:145–151.
70. Suka M, Yoshida K, Sugimori H. Persistent insomnia is a predictor of hypertension in Japanese male workers. J Occup Health 2003; 45:344–350.
71. Mallon L, Broman JE, Hetta J. High incidence of diabetes in men with sleep complaints or short sleep duration: a 12-year follow-up study of a middle-aged population. Diabetes Care 2005; 28:2762–2767.
72. Meisinger C, Heier M, Loewel H, MONICA/KORA Augsburg Cohort Study. Sleep disturbance as a predictor of type 2 diabetes mellitus in men and women from the general population. Diabetologia 2005; 48:235–241.
73. Mallon L, Broman JE, Hetta J. Sleep complaints predict coronary artery disease mortality in males: a 12-year follow-up study of a middle-aged Swedish population. J Intern Med 2002; 251:207–216.
74. Affleck G, Urrows S, Tennen H, et al. Sequential daily relations of sleep, pain intensity, and attention to pain among women with fibromyalgia. Pain 1996; 68:363–368.
75. Drewes AM, Nielsen KD, Hansen B, et al. A longitudinal study of clinical symptoms and sleep parameters in rheumatoid arthritis. Rheumatology (Oxford) 2000; 39:1287–1289.
76. Stone AA, Broderick JE, Porter LS, et al. The experience of rheumatoid arthritis pain and fatigue: examining momentary reports and correlates over one week. Arthritis Care Res 1997; 10:185–193.
77. Mikkelsson M, Sourander A, Salminen JJ, et al. Widespread pain and neck pain in schoolchildren. A prospective one-year follow-up study. Acta Paediatr 1999; 88:1119–1124.
78. Benca RM. Consequences of insomnia and its therapies. J Clin Psychiatry 2001; 62(suppl 10):33–38.
79. American Psychiatric Association. Task Force on DSM-IV. Diagnostic and Statistical Manual of Mental Disorders: DSM-IV. 4th ed. Washington, D.C: American Psychiatric Association; 1994.
80. Perlis ML, Smith LJ, Lyness JM, et al. Insomnia as a risk factor for onset of depression in the elderly. Behav Sleep Med 2006; 4:104–113.
81. Perlis ML, Giles DE, Buysse DJ, et al. Which depressive symptoms are related to which sleep electroencephalographic variables? Biol Psychiatry 1997; 42:904–913.
82. Ohayon MM, Roth T. Place of chronic insomnia in the course of depressive and anxiety disorders. J Psychiatr Res 2003; 37:9–15.
83. Ford DE, Kamerow DB. Epidemiologic study of sleep disturbances and psychiatric disorders. An opportunity for prevention? JAMA 1989; 262:1479–1484.
84. Crum RM, Ford DE, Storr CL, et al. Association of sleep disturbance with chronicity and remission of alcohol dependence: data from a population-based prospective study. Alcohol Clin Exp Res 2004; 28:1533–1540.
85. Eaton WW, Badawi M, Melton B. Prodromes and precursors: epidemiologic data for primary prevention of disorders with slow onset. Am J Psychiatry 1995; 152:967–972.
86. Mellman TA. Sleep and anxiety disorders. Psychiatr Clin North Am 2006; 29:1047–1058 (abstract x).
87. Mellman TA, Uhde TW. Patients with frequent sleep panic: clinical findings and response to medication treatment. J Clin Psychiatry 1990; 51:513–516.

88. Green B. Post-traumatic stress disorder: symptom profiles in men and women. Curr Med Res Opin 2003; 19:200–204.

89. Belanger L, Morin CM, Langlois F, et al. Insomnia and generalized anxiety disorder: effects of cognitive behavior therapy for gad on insomnia symptoms. J Anxiety Disord 2004; 18:561–571.

90. Stein MB, Kroft CD, Walker JR. Sleep impairment in patients with social phobia. Psychiatry Res 1993; 49:251–256.

91. Weissman MM, Greenwald S, Nino-Murcia G, et al. The morbidity of insomnia uncomplicated by psychiatric disorders. Gen Hosp Psychiatry 1997; 19:245–250.

92. Breslau N, Roth T, Rosenthal L, et al. Sleep disturbance and psychiatric disorders: a longitudinal epidemiological study of young adults. Biol Psychiatry 1996; 39:411–418.

93. Livingston G, Blizard B, Mann A. Does sleep disturbance predict depression in elderly people? A study in inner London. Br J Gen Pract 1993; 43:445–448.

94. Roberts RE, Shema SJ, Kaplan GA. Prospective data on sleep complaints and associated risk factors in an older cohort. Psychosom Med 1999; 61:188–196.

95. Chang PP, Ford DE, Mead LA, et al. Insomnia in young men and subsequent depression. The Johns Hopkins Precursors Study. Am J Epidemiol 1997; 146:105–114.

96. Neckelmann D, Mykletun A, Dahl AA. Chronic insomnia as a risk factor for developing anxiety and depression. Sleep 2007; 30:873–880.

97. Johnson EO, Roth T, Breslau N. The association of insomnia with anxiety disorders and depression: exploration of the direction of risk. J Psychiatr Res 2006; 40:700–708.

98. Leibenluft E, Albert PS, Rosenthal NE, et al. Relationship between sleep and mood in patients with rapid-cycling bipolar disorder. Psychiatry Res 1996; 63:161–168.

99. Young DM. Psychiatric morbidity in travelers to Honolulu, Hawaii. Compr Psychiatry 1995; 36: 224–228.

100. Agargun MY, Kara H, Solmaz M. Sleep disturbances and suicidal behavior in patients with major depression. J Clin Psychiatry 1997; 58:249–251.

101. Smith MT, Perlis ML, Haythornthwaite JA. Suicidal ideation in outpatients with chronic musculoskeletal pain: an exploratory study of the role of sleep onset insomnia and pain intensity. Clin J Pain 2004; 20:111–118.

4 | Types of Insomnia

Leah Friedman, Laura Haagenson, and Beatriz Hernandez

Department of Psychiatry, Stanford University School of Medicine, Stanford, California, U.S.A.

The term insomnia has multiple meanings–both general and specific. Over the years, a number of categorizations and definitions of insomnia have been devised for clinical and research purposes. Inconsistency in definition inevitably has led to inconsistency in the methods used to measure and to diagnose insomnia. Recently, there have been calls for greater precision and consistency in the categorizations and diagnoses of insomnia (1,2). Nosologies have varied in their approaches to improving the utility of diagnostic categories—some tend to synthesize (or lump) the various types of insomnia; others to analyze (or split) insomnia types. In this chapter, we will review some of the distinctions that have been made among types of insomnia and then present in greater detail the typology of insomnia presented in the *International Classification of Sleep Disorders*, second edition (3).

Among the several ways that insomnia has been classified, one of the more prominent distinctions has been based on the nature of the *presenting sleep complaint* or symptoms. Does the patient complain of (1) difficulty falling asleep, (2) trouble maintaining sleep, and/or (3) experiencing sleep as nonrestorative (3–5)? More recently, a complaint associated with the detrimental effects of poor nighttime sleep on the patient's daytime function has been added as an essential component of insomnia (3,6). One problem identified with classification by sleep complaint is that major sleep complaints may change over time, especially with age. Another is that presenting sleep complaints provide little information about the etiology of the complaint (7).

A second way of distinguishing insomnia types is based on the *duration* of the complaint. Accordingly, insomnia has been divided into three broad temporal categories: (*i*) transient or acute insomnia—defined as a response to an acute stressor; (*ii*) short-term insomnia—usually associated with a situational stressor that has a somewhat longer time course; and (*iii*) long-term insomnia—associated with primary insomnia or a psychiatric condition, drug or alcohol use, another medical condition or sleep disorder (prolonged time course). It has been suggested that duration of complaint as the basis for distinguishing insomnia types initially flowed out of concerns about the length of time that hypnotic medications could be safely prescribed. A challenge to this categorization is the lack of evidence demonstrating that types of insomnia based on temporal distinctions represent significantly distinct disorders (7).

A third major way of classifying insomnia distinguishes types of insomnia from a *causal perspective*. Thus, insomnia is seen either as a primary disorder or secondary to other conditions (5,8). For example, the Diagnostic and Statistical Manual of Mental Disorders (DSM-IV-TR) divides the insomnias into four groups (primary, related to another mental disorder, due to a general medical condition, and substance induced). In the case of secondary insomnia, improvement of the primary condition is frequently insufficient to treat the associated insomnia, which requires insomnia-specific treatment (7). Primary insomnias are distinguishable from each other and from secondary insomnias by differences in assumed causes, perpetuating factors, and presenting symptoms. Often, there are several causal and perpetuating factors in play, thus complicating the task of diagnosis. Although selection of a major diagnosis is preferable, when criteria for other diagnoses are met they should also be so classified (3).

Insomnias in the more precisely delineated categories of the original International Classification of Sleep Disorders (4) primarily fell under the category of dyssomnias (or disorders of either difficulty initiating or maintaining sleep or excessive sleepiness). The original ICSD separated sleep disorders into those with either extrinsic or intrinsic or circadian causes. Intrinsic dyssomnias were those thought to originate from causes internal to the body. This included primary sleep disturbances stemming from psychological or medical disorders. Extrinsic dyssomnias were thought to derive from causes external to the body. Extinction or removal of the external cause was thought to usually resolve the disorder. This distinction was explicitly eliminated in the ICSD-2 as were criteria based on severity and duration (6).

The ICSD-2 (2005) was sponsored and published by the American Academy of Sleep Medicine as a revised nosological system for sleep disorders. One of the primary goals of the revision was to make it more compatible with the larger medical diagnostic system of the International Classification of Diseases (ICD). In the ICSD-2 all the insomnias are grouped together as a distinct sleep disorder category with different variants or types. To a certain extent the various nosologies overlap each other; for example, ICSD-2 diagnoses can fit within the broader DSM-IV categories of primary and secondary insomnia. Thus, insomnia due to mental or medical disorders would logically fall under the secondary insomnia rubric while psychophysiological insomnia and adjustment or acute insomnia would be categorized as primary insomnias under the DSM-IV.

The types of insomnia presented in the ICSD-2 incorporate the several approaches described above. Eleven subtypes of insomnia are listed (two are unspecified conditions) all of which share the common complaint of insomnia. According to the ICSD-2, each of the subtypes of insomnia must meet three basic conditions: (1) adequate sleep opportunity, (2) persistent difficulty sleeping (sleep initiation, duration, consolidation, or quality), and (3) associated daytime dysfunction. Demographic and clinical features as well as the known pathophysiology of each of the various types of insomnia will be presented and discussed below and, unless otherwise noted, will be based on the contents of the ICSD-2.

ICSD-2 TYPES OF INSOMNIA

Adjustment Insomnia

Adjustment insomnia has a number of alternate names (acute insomnia, transient insomnia, short-term insomnia, stress-related insomnia, transient psychophysiological insomnia, adjustment disorder). It is by definition a transient or short-term insomnia related to an identifiable stressor. It should be noted that, although adjustment insomnia is the most commonly experienced form of insomnia (9,10), there has been little research conducted on this form of insomnia undoubtedly owing, at least in part, to its short-lived nature.

Demographics

Adjustment insomnia occurs more commonly in older adults and women. Epidemiological evidence suggests that in a given year 15% to 20% of adults experience some adjustment insomnia.

Key Symptoms and Signs

Hyperarousal has been found to play a major role in the development of acute or adjustment insomnias (11). Traditionally, the hyperarousal associated with insomnia has been conceptualized as the product of a causal chain leading from emotional arousal to physiological activation. However, it has been noted that physiological activation alone can cause insomnia (12). Although sleep disturbance is the primary symptom of adjustment insomnia, this sleep disorder is frequently associated with waking psychological symptoms of arousal such as anxiety, worry, and ruminative thoughts. Anxiety-related physical symptoms such as muscle tension, gastrointestinal upset, and headaches are also often present as well as daytime symptoms of fatigue, impaired concentration, and irritability.

Onset, Ontogeny, and Clinical Course

Adjustment insomnia is, by its short duration, the presence of a known precipitant, and absence of a learned or association component. The onset is usually acute with a less than three-month time course. The time course of the resolution of the insomnia depends on the speed at which the stressor resolves or the individual adapts to a chronic stressor. If the sleep problem lasts longer than a few months, alternate diagnoses should be considered. Chronic insomnia has been conceptualized as the product of multiple episodes of transient insomnia (13). In attempting to deal with adjustment insomnia, patients may initiate behaviors that can become factors that perpetuate their insomnia such as use of drugs or alcohol. Thus, complications frequently include the abuse of alcohol or drugs used to ameliorate the sleep disturbance associated with adjustment insomnia.

Risk Factors
A unique feature of transient insomnias is that they appear in individuals who are usually normal sleepers and whose sleep is expected to return to normal once the precipitating conditions resolve (14). On the other hand, the ICSD-2 notes a tendency for those who have a history of disturbed sleep at times of stress to be predisposed to experience insomnia at future stressful times. The individual's appraisal of stressors and the perceived lack of control over stressful events, rather than the number of events, have been found to enhance the vulnerability to insomnia. Thus, coping skills are thought to play an important mediating role between stress and sleep (11).

Psychophysiological Insomnia
Psychophysiological insomnia has a number of alternate names: primary insomnia, learned insomnia, conditioned insomnia, and chronic insomnia among others. Most research has studied patients with chronic psychophysiological insomnia (12).

Demographics
Psychophysiological insomnia is rare among children and most frequent in women. This condition is a very common form of insomnia affecting 1% to 2% of the general population and 12% to 15% of those who seek treatment at sleep centers (15).

Key Symptoms and Signs
Psychophysiological insomnia is characterized by physical and/or psychological arousal that interferes with sleep. Attention to and worry about their ability or inability to sleep are characteristic of patients with this disorder and are the primary foci for cognitive behavioral treatments for insomnia (16). Hyperarousal has been found to be a 24-hour-a-day phenomenon in patients with psychophysiological insomnia. They have been found to be more alert in the daytime than would be expected according to their sleep complaints, and they are more alert at night than asymptomatic control subjects (17). Although hyperarousal is the distinguishing feature of psychophysiological insomnia, it should be noted that heightened arousal is not exclusive to this form of insomnia (18).

Another component of psychophysiological insomnia has been conceptualized as a "learned" or "conditioned" element found to be well treated by stimulus control treatment (19). A defining characteristic of conditioned insomnia is its association with place. Stimulus control is predicated on blocking the learned association between the bed and sleeplessness.

Onset, Ontogeny, and Clinical Course
The onset of psychophysiological insomnia may be insidious or acute. In its insidious forms, adult patients often report having had symptoms in adolescence or young adulthood. As mentioned above, adjustment insomnia if unresolved can lead to psychophysiological insomnia. Psychophysiological insomnia, in turn, if not treated can be enduring. Thus, duration could be seen as a major distinction between adjustment and psychophysiological insomnia. Potential complications of psychophysiological insomnia include the appearance of a first episode or recurrence of major depression and/or the abuse of over-the-counter or prescription sleep-promoting medications.

Risk Factors
Risk factors for the development of psychophysiological insomnia include habitual light or episodic poor sleep. Anxious, overconcern about health and daytime functioning also

contribute to the risk of developing this disorder. Stressful situations such as life transitions can serve as precipitants of psychophysiological insomnia.

Paradoxical Insomnia

In this type of insomnia, subjective sleep complaints are not supported by objective findings nor is there the level of daytime impairment that would be expected given the severity of complaints (e.g., little or no sleep) about nighttime sleep. This insomnia is otherwise known as sleep state misperception, pseudo-insomnia, or sleep hypochondriasis.

Demographics

Sex distribution is unknown, but it is believed to be most common among young and middle aged adults. The prevalence of paradoxical insomnia in the general population is unknown. Among clinical populations the prevalence is less than 5%.

Key Symptoms and Signs

Overestimation of sleep latency or extreme underestimation of time spent asleep as compared with objective sleep recordings are the core characteristics of this disorder. The objective/ subjective discrepancy is greater than in other insomnias.

Onset, Ontogeny, and Clinical Course

This disorder, uncommon among children and adolescents, usually starts in young adulthood or middle age. The condition can persist for months or years without change in symptoms or presentation. Some patients' objective sleep may actually deteriorate in time to meet criteria for other insomnia disorders. If the condition persists, it may increase risk for depression, anxiety, and/or substance abuse.

There has been considerable discussion as to the nature of this complaint. Edinger and Fins (20), in a study of subjects with a broad range of insomnias, found that sleep time misperceptions ranged widely from large underestimations to large overestimations of their sleep time compared with polysomnographic results. They conclude that it is possible that the discrepancy between subjective and objective measures in this type of insomnia is due to the inability of objective measures to detect whatever is causing the individual to perceive his/her sleep as disturbed or inadequate. In discussing discrepancies between actigraphic and polysomnographic recordings, Hauri and Wisbey (21) speculate that in instances where polysomnography shows individuals as asleep while actigraphy indicates wakefulness—the actigraphy, in picking up the excessive wrist movement in these individuals, is also reflecting something about their sleep experience that they perceive as wake. Roehrs et al. (14) suggest that in such instances the problem may lie with our methods of recording sleep that do not clearly detect sleep disturbances perceived by the individual.

In fact, when Salin-Pascual et al. (22) compared subjects with paradoxical insomnia versus normals and other insomnia patients, they concluded that this type of insomnia may be a transitional state of sleep disturbance between normal and objectively classifiable insomnia. There is some argument about the value of distinguishing this type of insomnia as a distinctive type because it appears to be of relatively small prevalence. In a study comparing normal, subjective insomnia and objective insomnia subjects, Krystal et al. (23) concluded that those with subjective insomnia complaints showed distinctive physiological patterns in their non-rapid eye movement (NREM) but not their rapid eye movement (REM) electroencephalographic (EEG) recordings according to spectral analysis.

Risk Factors

Depressive traits, neuroticism, and excessive central nervous system (CNS) activation during sleep may be risk factors.

Idiopathic Insomnia

The core characteristic of idiopathic insomnia is a long-standing complaint of insomnia initiated in infancy or childhood and persisting through adulthood.

Demographics
The prevalence is approximately 0.7% of adolescents and 1% of very young adults. Among sleep clinic patients, the prevalence is less than 10%. There are no data reported regarding the sex distribution of this disorder.

Key Symptoms and Signs
The typical complaint is a lifelong difficulty with sleep. Sleep difficulties can be sleep initiation, repeated awakenings, or short sleep duration. Insomnia is persistent with few extended periods of remission. A notable feature is the absence of specific precipitants of the condition. Baseline sleep associated with this condition, however, can worsen in the presence of factors that typically precipitate insomnia such as psychosocial stressors or medical conditions.

Onset, Ontogeny, and Clinical Course
This type of insomnia is usually first evident during early childhood. After insidious onset, it is persistent throughout adulthood without the variability seen in other types of insomnia, although the type of sleep difficulty may change with time. This condition is associated with risk of major depression or substance abuse that may develop from patients' attempts to ameliorate their sleep problem.

Risk Factors
Personality has been suggested as correlated with chronic, long-term insomnia. A study of chronic insomniacs presenting for treatment at an outpatient insomnia treatment program found a cluster of personality characteristics (such as higher levels of arousal) paired with greater likelihood of a history of childhood sleep problems (24).

Some individuals with this condition had attention deficit-hyperactivity disorder (ADHD) or a history of learning disabilities during childhood. This appears to be congruent with the suggestion of an early study that insomnia with childhood onset may be more likely to be based on neurophysiological/neurochemical factors than insomnia originating in adulthood (25). A recent study suggests that children with ADHD and chronic idiopathic sleep-onset insomnia may reflect a delayed phase circadian rhythm disorder (26). These findings have been challenged as not taking into account developmental, biological, and cultural factors in defining sleep-onset insomnia in school age children (27).

Insomnia Due to a Mental Disorder
Very strong relations have been found between chronic insomnia and mental disorders (28). Insomnia due to a mental disorder is viewed as a symptom of a mental disorder when identified in the patient within a similar time frame. Thus, this type of insomnia could fall into the category of a secondary insomnia in other nosologies. In addition to the mental disorder, the insomnia itself is seen as a distinct complaint and focus of treatment. On the other hand, it has been argued that the direction of the relationship is debatable and that the insomnia may be a risk factor for certain mental disorders, for example, depression and anxiety disorders (29). A longitudinal, epidemiological study of young adults found that prior insomnia significantly predicted major depression (30). Insomnia due to a mental disorder has been associated with a variety of mood disorders, including major depressive, dysthymic, bipolar, and psychothymic disorders. Similarly anxiety and somatoform disorders have also been associated with this condition. Ohayon (31) suggested that the primacy of the symptom from the patient's perspective would distinguish an insomnia subsequent to a mental disorder from one in which the sleep complaint was dominant. Thus, for example, if a patient's insomnia followed a depressive episode, the insomnia would fall into the category of insomnia due to a mental disorder. As understanding of both insomnia and mental disorders such as depression improves, it can be expected that the causal interrelationships of these disorders will be elucidated (29).

Demographics
In sleep clinic populations, insomnia due to a mental disorder is the most common diagnosis. According to survey data, approximately 3% of the population meet criteria for this diagnosis.

This condition is more prevalent in middle age than in younger or older populations, and more common in women than in men. In a large epidemiological study, Ohayon (10) found that 5.6% of the sample had a specific sleep disorder and that insomnia due to a mental disorder was the most common diagnosis in this sample. Taylor et al. (32) found that among subjects randomly sampled from the community, African American respondents reporting insomnia had higher anxiety and depression scores than Caucasians with insomnia. In this study, there were no differences between the sexes in anxiety and depression scores among those reporting insomnia.

Key Symptoms and Signs
This insomnia is usually coincident with an associated mental disorder but insomnia complaints may be one of the first symptoms of the mental disorder. The course of the insomnia is similar to that of the associated mental condition. Difficulty in sleep initiation is typical of younger patients with anxiety disorders, while older patients, especially those with depressive disorders, have more difficulty with sleep maintenance (waking during the night and early morning awakenings). A study of 216 patients, referred for insomnia treatment, found that the presence of a psychiatric disorder was more likely to be associated with the clinicians' choice of a diagnosis of insomnia related to a mental disorder while sleep hygiene and negative conditioning were more likely to result in a primary insomnia diagnosis (33). However, the fact that 77% of patients given a primary insomnia diagnosis also had psychiatric symptoms raised questions about the validity of the distinctions upon which DSM IV insomnia diagnostic categories are chosen.

Onset, Ontogeny, and Clinical Course
As noted above, insomnia is often one of the first symptoms of a mental disorder. With prompt treatment, it may often be possible to ameliorate insomnia more quickly than the patients' underlying mental disorders. On the other hand, insomnia may persist after other symptoms of the mental disorder have improved. Indeed, even after a depressive episode has resolved, up to 44% of patients may experience residual symptoms of insomnia (34). This provides some evidence that maladaptive sleep-related behaviors may have been learned over the course of the illness episode and survived to perpetuate the individual's insomnia.

Risk Factors
The main risk factors for insomnia due to a mental disorder are those associated with the specific underlying mental disorder.

Inadequate Sleep Hygiene
Alternate names for this condition include poor sleep hygiene, sleep hygiene abuse, bad sleep habits, irregular sleep habits, excessive napping, and sleep incompatible behaviors. The essential feature of this type of insomnia is the practice of sleep behaviors inconsistent with good quality sleep and the ability to maintain alertness during the day. Sleep-incompatible behaviors can be classified into two main groups: (1) practices that increase arousal such as excessive use of caffeine and stressful and exciting activities and (2) practices, such as irregular bed and wake times, daytime napping, and excessive time in bed, that are detrimental to integrated sleep/wake patterns.

Demographics
Sex distribution is unknown for this disorder. A large sample study of university students suggested that there may be ethnic differences in both the knowledge and the practice of sleep hygiene (35). About 1% to 2% of adolescents and young adults are thought to have inadequate sleep hygiene. Older adults are believed to have similar rates of poor sleep-related behavior. This is the primary diagnosis for 5% to 10% of individuals presenting at sleep clinics. Because sleep disruptive practices are so widespread, inadequate sleep hygiene may be present as a primary or secondary diagnosis in more than 30% of sleep clinic patients.

Key Symptoms and Signs

Problems with maintaining alertness in the daytime, mood and motivational disturbance, reduced attention and concentration and daytime fatigue or sleepiness characterize this disorder, as well as a preoccupation with sleep difficulties. Many of these patients have little insight into the impact of their poor sleep practices on their sleep.

Onset, Ontogeny, and Clinical Course

This disorder may develop as early as adolescence or at any point throughout adulthood. Compensatory behaviors such as "sleeping in" late in the morning often arise as a response to insomnia but may actually exacerbate the individual's sleep problem. A complication of inadequate sleep hygiene may be alcohol or caffeine dependence that may develop as methods to compensate for poor sleep. Although good sleep practices have been found to be associated with good sleep, knowledge of good practices in and of itself does not necessarily lead to implementation of good sleep practices (36). Indeed, in one study, insomniacs had more good sleep hygiene knowledge than good sleepers, but they put this knowledge into effect less often (37). Because of this phenomenon, most nondrug treatments incorporate at least some instructions regarding basic sleep hygiene practices and encourage their use to enhance the effectiveness of the primary treatment. Although sleep hygiene instructions are commonly distributed in standardized pamphlet form, instructions often need to be tailored to the specific behaviors and needs of the individual patient (38). A recent study in a sample of older adults (60–69 years old) raised questions regarding the universal applicability of the general sleep hygiene principles since the only practice that distinguished good from poor sleepers was the frequency of napping (39).

Similarly, Harvey (2000) did not find that the sleep hygiene practices in good sleepers were better than that of subjects with sleep-onset insomnia. Schoicket and colleagues (40) found that sleep hygiene treatment produced results comparable to meditation and stimulus control but was regarded less favorably by subjects. Others have pointed out that there is insufficient evidence to demonstrate that inadequate sleep hygiene is a determinant of insomnia. Further research is needed to assess the specific mechanisms by which sleep hygiene practices play a role in insomnia (41). Lack of this information challenges the legitimacy of sleep hygiene as a separate diagnostic category.

Risk Factors

If poor sleep practices are of sufficient consequence and frequency, they may lead to insomnia or aggravate an already existing insomnia.

Behavioral Insomnia of Childhood

According to the ICSD-2, behavioral insomnia of childhood is characterized by difficulty falling asleep, staying asleep, or a combination of the two that can be attributed to a specific behavioral cause. This disorder can be subdivided into two types: sleep-onset association type or limit-setting type. In the former, the child may have difficulty with sleep onset if a specific setting (e.g., parents' bed) or object (e.g., stuffed animal) or type of stimulation (e.g., rocking) is not present. The latter subtype (limit setting) is characterized by the child stalling or refusing to go to sleep, which is viewed as a result of inadequate limit setting by the caregiver. A recent review of behavioral treatments for sleep problems in young children included another sleep-onset association type problem: nighttime waking in which the child is unable to fall back to sleep if a specific sleep association is absent (42).

Demographics

Because nocturnal sleep consolidation is not expected until three to six months, the diagnosis is usually not applied until after six months of age. Unclear understanding of normal sleep patterns in children frequently lead to sleep disturbances being underreported (43). Bedtime problems and frequent night waking in children occur at a rate of 20% to 30% in the child population, and because these problems often present together it has been difficult to come up with estimates of separate prevalence rates (42). Others have put the prevalence range of disruptive sleep at 25% to 50% (44). Interestingly, a survey of children and their parents found that the children reported experiencing significantly more sleep disturbance than their parents reported for them (45). There is not a marked difference between the rates of insomnia in girls or boys.

Key Symptoms and Signs
Sleep-onset association type symptoms include the inability to initiate sleep in the absence of certain stimuli, settings, or objects. Because sleep-onset associations are common in children, this is only seen as a disorder if the associations are highly problematic or demanding, sleep onset is significantly delayed, or caregiver intervention is required.

Onset, Ontogeny, and Clinical Course
The etiology of pediatric bedtime resistance and night waking reflects a combination of causes (biological, neurodevelopmental, or circadian) that may interact with the child's environment. Childhood insomnia, similar to insomnia in adults, involves predisposing, precipitating, and perpetuating factors (46). The onset of behavioral insomnia of childhood may occur anytime during late infancy or childhood years.

An important point about pediatric insomnia is that not only does it impact others, primarily family members, but its very existence depends on its being defined as a problem by others. Thus, the diagnosis of childhood insomnia has a large cultural component and depends on expectations of what is appropriate in a given society, subculture, or family (27). Sleep usually improves when limit-setting and negative sleep associations resolve. On the other hand, studies of the longitudinal course of childhood insomnia have shown that sleep problems beginning in infancy may persist as the child develops (46), and to be associated with somewhat higher levels of child behavior problems as well as maternal depression. This depression appears to be a result of the sleep disturbance rather than its cause (47). While success has been reported for a number of behavioral approaches to treating childhood insomnia, two behavioral interventions for childhood insomnia (extinction and parent education/prevention) have demonstrated success in controlled studies (42). Extinction (in which inappropriate behavior of the child after having been put to bed is ignored) has received the most research attention of any of the alternative behavioral treatments. The underlying operant theory, that ending the reinforcement (attention from the parent) for a behavior such as crying will over the course of time end up extinguishing the crying behavior, is relatively easy for parents to understand and for many parents to apply (48).

Risk Factors
Developmental issues such as separation anxiety may be risk factors for developing this type of insomnia.

Insomnia Due to Drug or Substance Abuse
Insomnia due to drug or substance abuse is a disruption of sleep that can be attributed to the use of a prescription medication, recreational drug, caffeine, alcohol, food, or environmental toxin. This type of insomnia can also be caused by the withdrawal of the drug or substance.

Demographics
Drug or substance abuse insomnia affects approximately 0.2% of the general population and 3.5% of clinic patients. Stimulant-related insomnia is more common in younger adults, while depressant-related insomnia is more common in older adults. High rates of both substance abuse and sleep disorders have been found among adolescents (49).

Key Symptoms and Signs
Symptoms of insomnia due to drug or substance are related to and depend on the type of drug or substance responsible for the sleep disruption. For example, the negative effects of caffeine on sleep have been well described (50). The sleeplessness caused by caffeine consumption may be accompanied by jitteriness, anxiety, and increased daytime sleepiness due to fragmented

nighttime sleep. Insomnia caused by exposure to a toxin may be accompanied by memory loss, changes in mental status, respiratory problems, cardiac symptoms, or gastrointestinal problems. Patients whose insomnia is caused by a sedative substance may have symptoms of suppressed rapid eye movement sleep, restless sleep, and daytime carryover symptoms of excessive sleepiness, sluggishness, poor coordination, reduced concentration, slurred speech, and visual-motor problems. Abrupt discontinuation of a substance may be associated with rebound insomnia characterized by a sudden worsening of sleep.

Onset, Ontogeny, and Clinical Course
This type of insomnia may arise from use of CNS stimulants (caffeine, amphetamines, cocaine) or depressants (alcohol, sedative medications). Depressants (such as alcohol) are often used as a sleep aid because they may decrease sleep-onset latency; however, they often lead to more fragmented and restless sleep and can ultimately cause insomnia. On the other hand, stimulant antidepressants [such as selective serotonin reuptake inhibitors (SSRIs)] can worsen or cause new insomnia while treating the initially presenting depression (51). Onset can occur at all ages; but it is more common for insomnia due to stimulant use to begin during adolescence or young adulthood, whereas insomnia due to depressant use usually has its onset later in adulthood. Perversely, discontinuation of a drug, for example, in alcohol recovery, can also cause insomnia that must be addressed for a therapy to be successful (52) since relapse is a real danger of insomnia associated with withdrawal in alcohol-dependent individuals (53). A further complication of chronic use of sedating medications, alcohol, or stimulants is that they can independently cause medical problems for the user (e.g., renal/hepatic failure, cardiac disorders) besides insomnia and often require intensive treatment interventions of their own.

Risk Factors
Risk factors include coexisting mood disorders and some medical disorders (e.g., chronic pain syndromes).

Insomnia Due to Medical Condition
The key feature of insomnia due to a medical condition is sleep disruption caused by a coexisting medical disorder or other physiological factor. This diagnosis is also appropriate when the insomnia itself causes significant upset or needs independent medical consideration.

Demographics
This type of insomnia has been shown by epidemiological studies to affect about 0.5% of the general population and approximately 4% of the patients seen in sleep disorders clinics. A study of a large community-based sample aged 20 to 80 years found considerable coincidence between insomnia and multiple medical conditions (54). Predictably, the occurrence of this insomnia diagnosis is most frequently noted in older adults.

Key Symptoms and Signs
Insomnia due to medical condition can be characterized by difficulty falling asleep, maintaining sleep, or concern about non-restorative sleep that is caused by any number of medical conditions that affect sleep such as arthritis, lung or breathing disorders, limited mobility, or menopausal symptoms. Similar to the symptoms of other forms of insomnia, insomnia due to medical condition often causes excessive focus on sleep, anxiety about not sleeping well, and complaints of daytime impairment. Symptoms vary as a function of the specific medical condition that is causing the insomnia.

Onset, Ontogeny, and Clinical Course
Onset of insomnia due to a medical condition may occur at any point in the life cycle but is most commonly seen during middle age or older adulthood. Results of the 2003 National Sleep Foundation Sleep in America Survey indicated that the sleep complaints reported by older adults were secondary to their comorbid illness rather than secondary to the aging process. Further, specific diseases such as heart disease, arthritis, diabetes, stroke, and lung diseases

were found to be independently associated with the experience of sleep problems (55). In a study of clinical practice patients, not only were specific chronic medical problems associated with insomnia; the insomnia itself was associated with worse health-related quality of life (56). Medications prescribed for the treatment of the underlying medical condition as well as detrimental coping strategies that patients develop may serve as perpetuating factors that may worsen an insomnia due to a medical condition. Increasingly, sleep problems are being studied in terms of specific comorbid diseases such as cancer (57) and breathing disorders (58) with methods of treatment suggested to help individuals suffering from specific medical disorders (59).

Risk Factors

Older age and, by definition, the presence of multiple medical conditions are risk factors for this form of insomnia.

Insomnia Not Due to Substance or Known Physiological Condition, Unspecified (Nonorganic Insomnia)

This insomnia diagnosis is used when a patient's insomnia appears to be related to a psychological or behavioral cause (rather than a physiological, medical or substance abuse cause), but a patient's symptoms fail to meet the diagnostic criteria for the existing categories of insomnia. This diagnosis is often used as a temporary designation while waiting for further testing.

Physiological (Organic) Insomnia, Unspecified

This diagnosis refers to insomnia that does not fit another classification but is suspected to be physiological in nature or caused by a medical condition or substance use/exposure. Similar to insomnia not due to substance of known physiological condition, it is often used as a provisional diagnosis until further testing can be conducted.

Conclusions

Concern has been voiced among insomnia experts about the paucity of research of adequate validity and reliability to support previous distinctions made among insomnia subtypes. Yet in developing current categorizations of insomnia, we have come a long way since early researchers in the field of insomnia had "...no criteria for classification of insomnia subtypes..." (60). We now have a standardized set of research criteria for the collection of reliable and valid evidence on which future typologies may be based (1). The ICSD-2 was published in 2005. With so little time elapsed, there has been little published research or clinical reports regarding either the clinical utility or the research reliability and validity of this nosology. It is hoped that the research criteria (1) for studying the types of insomnia presented in ICSD-2 will greatly facilitate and accelerate this validation process.

Some progress in such validation work was reported at the annual 2008 AASM meeting in Baltimore (61). In this work, six researchers used a multitrait method to test the validity of ICSD-2 and DSM-IV-TR diagnoses on patient volunteers. Some of the diagnostic categories of the two diagnostic systems were supported, while others were not. These findings also suggested that PSG should play a greater role in the diagnostic process than has hitherto been advised (61). Current insomnia typologies are heavily dependent on distinctions in clinical presentation. As more is learned about the underlying biological processes associated with specific sleep disorders, future categorizations could be expected to have improved clinical and research utility.

REFERENCES

1. Edinger JD, Bonnet MH, Bootzin RR, et al. Derivation of research diagnostic criteria for insomnia: report of an American Academy of Sleep Medicine work group. Sleep 2004; 27(8):1567–1596.
2. Sateia MJ, Doghramji K, Hauri PJ, et al. Evaluation of chronic insomnia. An American Academy of Sleep Medicine review. Sleep 2000; 23(2):243–308.
3. American Academy of Sleep Medicine. International Classification of Sleep Disorders, 2nd ed. Diagnostic and Coding Manual, Westchester, IL: American Academy of Sleep Medicine, 2005.

4. American Sleep Disorders Association. The International Classification of Sleep Disorders, Revised: Diagnostic and Coding Manual, Rochester, MN: American Sleep Disorders Association, 1990.
5. American Psychiatric Association. Diagnostic and Statistical Manual of Mental Disorders DSM-IV. 4th ed. Washington, DC: American Psychiatric Association, 1994.
6. Edinger JD, Means MK. Overview of insomnia: definitions, epidemiology, differential diagnosis, and assessment. In: Kryger MH, Roth T, Dement WC, ed. Principles and Practices of Sleep Medicine. Philadelphia, PA: Elsevier Saunders, 2005:702–713.
7. Krystal AD. The effect of insomnia definitions, terminology, and classifications on clinical practice. J Am Geriatr Soc 2005; 53(7 suppl):S258–S263.
8. American Psychiatric Association, Diagnostic and Statistical Manual of Mental Disorders: DSM-IV-TR. Washington, DC: American Psychiatric Association, 2000.
9. Leger D, Guilleminault C, Dreyfus JP, et al. Prevalence of insomnia in a survey of 12,778 adults in France. J Sleep Res 2000; 9:35–42.
10. Ohayon M. Epidemiological study on insomnia in the general population. Sleep 1996; 19(3 suppl): S7–S15.
11. Morin CM, Rodrigue S, Ivers H. Role of stress, arousal, and coping skills in primary insomnia. Psychosom Med 2003; 65(2):259–267.
12. Bonnet MH, Arand DL. Situational insomnia: consistency, predictors, and outcomes. Sleep 2003; 26(8): 1029–1036.
13. Borkovec TD. Insomnia. J Consult Clin Psychol 1982; 50(6):880–895.
14. Roehrs T, Zorick F, Roth T. Transient and short-term insomnias. In: Kryger MH, Roth T, Dement WC, ed. Principles and Practice of Sleep Medicine. Philadelphia, PA: Saunders, 2003:624–632.
15. Robertson JA, Broomfield NM, Espie CA. Prospective comparison of subjective arousal during the presleep period in primary sleep-onset insomnia and normal sleepers. J Sleep Res 2007; 16:230–238.
16. Morin CM. Insomnia: Psychological Assessment and Management. New York, NY: Guilford, 1993.
17. Stepanski E, Zorick F, Roehrs T, et al. Daytime alertness in patients with chronic insomnia compared with asymptomatic control subjects. Sleep 1988; 11(1):54–60.
18. Pavlova M, Berg O, Gleason R, et al. Self-reported hyperarousal traits among insomnia patients. J Psychosom Res 2001; 51(2):435–441.
19. Bootzin RR, Nicassio P. Behavioral treatments for insomnia. In: Hersen M, Eisler RM, Miller PM, eds. Progress in Behavior Modification. New York, NY: Academic Press, 1978:1–45.
20. Edinger JD, Fins AI. The distribution and clinical significance of sleep time misperceptions among insomniacs. Sleep 1995; 18(4):232–239.
21. Hauri PJ, Wisbey J. Wrist actigraphy in insomnia. Sleep 1992; 15(4):293–301.
22. Salin-Pascual RJ, Roehrs TA, Merlotti LA, et al. Long-term study of the sleep of insomnia patients with sleep state misperception and other insomnia patients. Am J Psychiatry 1992; 149(7):904–908.
23. Krystal AD, Edinger JD, Wohlgemuth WK, et al. NREM sleep EEG frequency spectral correlates of sleep complaints in primary insomnia subtypes. Sleep 2002; 25(6):626–636.
24. Edinger JD, Stout AL, Hoelscher TJ. Cluster analysis of insomniacs' MMPI profiles: relation of subtypes to sleep history and treatment outcome. Psychosom Med 1988; 50(1):77–87.
25. Hauri PJ, Olmstead E. Childhood-onset insomnia. Sleep 1980; 3(1):59–65.
26. Van der Heijden KB, Smits MG, Van Someren EJ, et al. Idiopathic chronic sleep onset insomnia in attention-deficit/hyperactivity disorder: a circadian rhythm sleep disorder. Chronobiol Int 2005; 22(3): 559–570.
27. Jenni OG. Sleep onset insomnia during childhood or poor fit between biology and culture: comment on van der Heijden et al. 'Prediction of melatonin efficacy by pre-treatment dim light melatonin onset in children with idiopathic chronic sleep onset insomnia'. J Sleep Res 2005; 14(2):195–197; discussion 197–199.
28. Schramm E, Hohagen F, Kappler C, et al. Mental comorbidity of chronic insomnia in general practice attenders using DSM-III-R. Acta Psychiatr Scand 1995; 91(1):10–17.
29. Riemann D. Insomnia and comorbid psychiatric disorders. Sleep Med 2007, 8(suppl 4):S15–S20.
30. Breslau N, Roth T, Rosenthal L, et al. Sleep disturbance and psychiatric disorders: a longitudinal epidemiological study of young adults. Biol Psychiatry 1996; 39(6):411–418.
31. Ohayon M. Prevalence of DSM-IV diagnostic criteria of insomnia: distinguishing insomnia related to mental disorders from sleep disorders. J Psychiatr Res 1997; 31(3):333–346.
32. Taylor DJ, Lichstein KL, Durrence HH, et al. Epidemiology of insomnia, depression, and anxiety. Sleep 2005; 28(11):1457–1464.
33. Nowell PD, Buysse DJ, Reynolds CF III, et al. Clinical factors contributing to the differential diagnosis of primary insomnia and insomnia related to mental disorders. Am J Psychiatry 1997; 154(10):1412–1416.
34. Nierenberg AA, Wright EC. Evolution of remission as the new standard in the treatment of depression. J Clin Psychiatry 1999; 60(suppl 22):7–11.
35. Hicks RA, Lucero-Gorman K, Bautista J, et al. Ethnicity, sleep hygiene knowledge, and sleep hygiene practices. Percept Mot Skills 1999; 88(3 pt 2):1095–1096.

36. Brown FC, Buboltz WC Jr., Soper B. Relationship of sleep hygiene awareness, sleep hygiene practices, and sleep quality in university students. Behav Med 2002; 28(1):33–38.
37. Lacks P, Rotert M. Knowledge and practice of sleep hygiene techniques in insomniacs and good sleepers. Behav Res Ther 1986; 24(3):365–368.
38. Hauri PJ. Sleep hygiene, relaxation therapy, and cognitive interventions. In: Hauri PJ, ed. Case Studies in Insomnia. New York, NY: Plenum Publishing Corp, 1991.
39. McCrae CS, Rowe MA, Dautovich ND, et al. Sleep hygiene practices in two community dwelling samples of older adults. Sleep 2006; 29(12):1551–1560.
40. Schoicket SL, Bertelson AD, Lacks P. Is sleep hygiene a sufficient treatment for sleep-maintenance insomnia? Behav Ther 1988; 19:183–190.
41. Stepanski EJ, Wyatt JK. Use of sleep hygiene in the treatment of insomnia. Sleep Med Rev 2003; 7(3): 215–225.
42. Mindell JA, Kuhn B, Lewin DS, et al. Behavioral treatment of bedtime problems and night wakings in infants and young children. Sleep 2006; 29(10):1263–1276.
43. Goetting MG, Reijonen J. Pediatric insomnia: a behavioral approach. Prim Care 2007; 34(2):427–435 (abstr x).
44. El-Sheikh M, Erath SA, Keller PS. Children's sleep and adjustment: the moderating role of vagal regulation. J Sleep Res 2007; 16(4):396–405.
45. Fricke-Oerkermann L, Pluck J, Schredl M, et al. Prevalence and course of sleep problems in childhood. Sleep 2007; 30(10):1371–1377.
46. Morgenthaler T, Kramer M, Alessi C, et al. Practice parameters for the psychological and behavioral treatment of insomnia: an update. An American Academy of Sleep Medicine report. Sleep 2006; 29(11): 1415–1419.
47. Lam P, Hiscock H, Wake M. Outcomes of infant sleep problems: a longitudinal study of sleep, behavior, and maternal well-being. Pediatrics 2003; 111(3):e203–e207.
48. Kuhn BR, Elliott AJ. Treatment efficacy in behavioral pediatric sleep medicine. J Psychosom Res 2003; 54(6):587–597.
49. Shibley HL, Malcolm RJ, Veatch LM. Adolescents with insomnia and substance abuse: consequences and comorbidities. J Psychiatr Pract 2008; 14(3):146–153.
50. Bonnet MH, Arand DL. Caffeine use as a model of acute and chronic insomnia. Sleep 1992; 15(6):526–536.
51. Kaynak H, Kaynak D, Gozukirmizi E, et al. The effects of trazodone on sleep in patients treated with stimulant antidepressants. Sleep Med 2004; 5(1):15–20.
52. Arnedt JT, Conroy DA, Brower KJ. Treatment options for sleep disturbances during alcohol recovery. J Addict Dis 2007: 26(4):41–54.
53. Brower KJ, Myra Kim H, Strobbe S, et al. A randomized double-blind pilot trial of gabapentin versus placebo to treat alcohol dependence and comorbid insomnia. Alcohol Clin Exp Res 2008; 32(8): 1429–1438.
54. Taylor DJ, Mallory LJ, Lichstein KL, et al. Comorbidity of chronic insomnia with medical problems. Sleep 2007; 30(2):213–218.
55. Foley D, Ancoli-Israel S, Britz P, et al. Sleep disturbances and chronic disease in older adults: results of the 2003 National Sleep Foundation Sleep in America survey. J Psychosom Res 2004; 56(5):497–502.
56. Katz DA, McHorney CA. The relationship between insomnia and health-related quality of life in patients with chronic illness. J Fam Pract 2002; 51(3):229–235.
57. Savard J, Simard S, Blanchet J, et al. Prevalence, clinical characteristics, and risk factors for insomnia in the context of breast cancer. Sleep 2001; 24(5):583–590.
58. Gooneratne NS, Gehrman PR, Nkwuo JE, et al. Consequences of comorbid insomnia symptoms and sleep-related breathing disorder in elderly subjects. Arch Intern Med 2006; 166(16):1732–1738.
59. Savard J, Morin CM. Insomnia in the context of cancer: a review of a neglected problem. J Clin Oncol 2001; 19(3):895–908.
60. Borkovec TD, Grayson JB, O'Brien GT, et al. Relaxation treatment of pseudoinsomnia and idiopathic insomnia: an electroencephalographic evaluation. J Appl Behav Anal 1979; 12(1):37–54.
61. Edinger JD, Wyatt JK, Olsen MK, et al. How valid are the DSM-IV-TR and ICSD-2 insomnia nosologies? Preliminary results from a multi-trait/multi-method diagnostic trial. Sleep 2008; 31 (suppl):A249.

5 | Diagnostic Tools for Insomnia

Rachel Manber, Jason C. Ong, and Erin Carlyle

Department of Psychiatry and Behavioral Sciences, Stanford University School of Medicine, Stanford, California, U.S.A.

INTRODUCTION

Insomnia has a range of clinical manifestations and involves a multitude of physical and psychological factors. In the *International Classification of Sleep Disorders*, second edition (*ICSD-2*) (1), a diagnosis of insomnia must confirm both the existence of nocturnal symptoms and a clinically significant impact during the patient's waking state. Nocturnal symptoms include difficulty initiating or maintaining sleep, early awakening, and interrupted or nonrestorative sleep. Daytime symptoms include distress about poor nocturnal sleep and impairment in any role function or other aspects of overall well-being. Researchers have traditionally used quantitative criteria to diagnose insomnia, but these criteria have not been standardized. Quantitative criteria for the frequency and duration of total wake time and/or total sleep time have been proposed (2), but these criteria have not been uniformly employed.

The assessment of insomnia begins with an initial diagnostic interview. During the initial interview the clinician must obtain sufficient information to correctly diagnose the insomnia subtype and contributing factors. Following the interview, objective measures of sleep may be used to rule out other sleep disorders when clinically indicated, laboratory tests might be ordered to rule out suspected comorbid medical conditions, and subjective self-report measures can be used to supplement information gathered in the initial interview. This chapter focuses on assessment tools and discusses assessment procedures organized by type and domain of assessment. The emphasis is on the assessment of insomnia in a clinical setting along with a discussion of additional tools most commonly used in research settings.

HISTORY AND PHYSICAL EXAMINATION

History

The ultimate goal of the initial interview is to reach a case conceptualization and formulate a treatment plan. To that end, the clinician must evaluate patients' current sleep patterns, the history of their sleeping problems, the current state of their homeostatic and circadian drives regulating normal sleep, factors that contribute to hyperarousal, and other factors that might interfere with the normal process of sleep. The latter include comorbid sleep, medical, or psychiatric disorders, substance use, current medications, and the patient's response to his or her insomnia, including behaviors originally initiated in an effort to improve sleep.

Current Sleep Pattern

A careful analysis of the patient's current sleep-wake schedule attends to a multitude of nocturnal and daytime sleep parameters. Nocturnal parameters that provide information about disturbance in sleep continuity include latency to sleep onset, wake after sleep onset, and the discrepancy between the desired and actual wake-up time. Parameters that allow evaluation of the regularity and circadian placement of sleep episodes include bedtime, lights out, final wake-up time, and time out of bed. Daytime sleep parameters include the timing, frequency, and length of naps, as well as the perceived ability to fall asleep during the day, given the opportunity. Whereas the former can assist in the evaluation of the strength of the homeostatic drive, as long naps and frequent dosing can diffuse the drive, the latter provides a behavioral index of sleep-related hyperarousal, reflecting the inability to sleep in the face of sleep deprivation. It is also important to inquire about the patient's sleep environment, including noise and comfort levels in the bedroom.

Since many patients tend to generalize their sleep problem on the basis of their worst night, it is helpful to identify a concrete time frame for discussing the sleep pattern. Usually the most recent typical week works well. It is also helpful to acknowledge the variability of sleep-wake schedules by encouraging patients to report day-to-day variability of their sleep-wake pattern. Daily sleep diaries completed prior to the initial interview can further promote the efficiency and accuracy of this portion of the interview. A detailed discussion of sleep diaries can be found later in the chapter.

History of Current and Past Episodes

Regarding the current episode, the clinician must know when the problem started; if there was an identifiable precipitating factor; how the problem progressed in terms of the frequency, severity, and the nature of the sleep symptoms; and response to past treatment. In addition, information about past episodes of insomnia should be gathered. Of particular interest is the timing of the first episode of insomnia, factors that precipitated past episodes, and the history of past treatments.

The Contribution of Circadian Rhythm Tendencies

Circadian factors are relevant to the presentation of psychophysiological insomnia (3) and are important to consider. While an absolute determination of a patient's sleep-wake rhythm is not feasible in a clinical setting, an understanding of the patient's circadian tendencies can be obtained during the interview and supplemented with sleep diaries and/or validated questionnaires (see below). The strength of the signal for optimal timing of sleep delivered by the suprachiasmatic nucleus is weakened when sleep-wake schedules change dramatically or frequently, as is the case in professions that require multiple shifts in time zones (e.g., airline industry jobs and other occupations that require frequent changes in time zones) and that involve varying shifts. Therefore, information about the patient's work schedule and travel patterns should be obtained.

Clinical indicators of a shifted sleep-wake rhythm can be gathered by relying on several core symptoms. Reports of difficulty waking up in the morning (often necessitating multiple alarms) coupled with difficulty falling asleep before very late in the night suggest a phase delay of the sleep-wake rhythm. Delayed sleep phase is often associated with prolonged time to feel fully awake after rise time and difficulty disengaging from nighttime activities. Early bedtime and involuntary evening "naps" coupled with very early wake-up times suggest a phase advance of the sleep wake rhythm. As early morning awakening is also a symptom of some psychiatric disorders, most notably depression, the assessment of these comorbidities is particularly important to fully understand the origin of this manifestation of insomnia.

Evaluating Current Treatments and Comorbidities

It is important that the initial diagnostic interview include an evaluation of comorbid conditions, whether sleep-related or more general medical or psychiatric problems. Both the conditions and their treatments can contribute to insomnia. Thus, the interview should include a review of systems most commonly associated with disturbed sleep, a physical examination, and additional laboratory tests when indicted (e.g., thyroid function and prostate-specific antigen).

Current treatments of insomnia and other conditions. Detailed information about medications and over-the-counter remedies taken to improve sleep quality is essential. A thorough assessment includes an understanding of the dose, frequency, and the time of intake of the prescribed sleep medication. It is also important to evaluate psychological factors associated with medication use—such as ambivalence or dependency—because these issues are indications of hypnotic-dependent insomnia.

A comprehensive list of a patient's medications and over-the-counter remedies for other conditions is also important. The most relevant medications to attend to in the context of assessment of insomnia are those that produce hyperarousal, such as stimulants, steroids, β-agonist medications, and some psychotropic medications. Medications in the latter class can cause insomnia or hypersomnolence and some exacerbate restless legs and periodic limb movements during sleep.

Comorbid conditions. Comorbid sleep disorders, most notably sleep-disordered breathing (SDB), can contribute to the severity of insomnia. It is imperative to evaluate clinical symptoms of SDB and follow-up with a physical examination and polysomnography when indicated. It is also important to inquire about symptoms of other comorbid sleep disorders, such as circadian rhythm disorders (discussed above), restless legs, and frequent nightmares, because they are also relevant to the presentation of insomnia and are not always spontaneously reported.

The following are the most common medical conditions associated with insomnia: hyperthyroidism, chronic pain associated with rheumatologic disorders, pulmonary diseases (most notably obstructive pulmonary disease typically treated with steroids), cardiac disorders (particularly when treated with β-agonist medications), gastrointestinal reflux, and auto-immune conditions treated with steroids. In addition, the potential impact of gender-specific factors must be considered. These include menstrual phase effects on sleep in young women, menopausal symptoms in middle-aged women, and prostate disease in older men.

Psychiatric disorders, particularly depressive disorders, account for up to 40% of cases of chronic insomnia encountered in sleep centers (4). Because depressed patients may focus on sleep complaints, most notably sleep continuity disturbances and early awakening, to the exclusion of other mood disorder symptoms, a routine evaluation of depressive disorders is important. Because anxiety disorders are associated with disturbances to the sleep system, the clinician or researcher should seek information regarding heightened general anxiety and perceived stress. Assessing comorbid psychiatric disorders and their relationship to the fluctuation in insomnia symptoms can help with differential diagnosis and treatment planning. In particular, this can aid in deciding when to refer for treatment of the comorbid psychiatric disorder.

Sleep-Related Behaviors
Several wake-time behaviors can impact sleep quality and are therefore important to assess. These include the following: (*i*) failure to unwind before bedtime, which can interfere with sleep onset and be associated with intrusive thoughts at bedtime; (*ii*) staying in bed awake for extended periods of time during the day or night, a behavior that can weaken the bed as a strong cue for sleep and thus interfere with sleep; (*iii*) patterns of substance use that can interfere with sleep, such as alcohol, caffeine, and nicotine; and (*iv*) insufficient daytime activity, as a sedentary lifestyle could hinder sleep.

Physiological and Psychological Arousal
Arousal is central to psychophysiological insomnia and is multifactorial. Research has shown increased arousal based on autonomic and cortical measures in insomniacs compared with controls. Findings of physiological arousal that have been reported include higher levels of global metabolic rates (as measured by oxygen consumption [VO_2]) and body temperature during the night and day, increased heart rate variability, and increased latency to sleep on a daytime multiple sleep latency test (5–8). Furthermore, power spectral analyses of electro-encephalography (EEG) patterns, taken as indices of cortical arousal, have found that insomniacs exhibit decreased delta activity and increased β-EEG activity compared with good sleepers (9–11). There is preliminary evidence that these EEG patterns can be improved with cognitive-behavioral therapy (CBT) for psychophysiological insomnia (12). While objective measures assessing physiological arousal are often impractical in a clinical setting, measures of cognitive arousal are practical and can be administered as part of an evaluation, particularly with candidates for CBT for insomnia. During the initial interview, the clinician needs to inquire about current life stressors and assess sleep-related cognitions, most notably sleep effort, as they often reflect cognitive arousal. While nondisturbed sleep occurs effortlessly, chronic insomnia is associated with increased sleep effort and increased preoccupation and apprehension related to sleep, which in turn hinder sleep. During the interview, the clinician should pay attention to overt and covert cognitions and behaviors that are manifestations of increased sleep effort. Attention should also be given to the coping strategies the patient uses, as many strategies actually perpetuate insomnia either directly or by increasing cognitive

arousal. Several paper and pencil scales to assess beliefs and attitudes about sleep, presleep cognition, and sleep effort exist and can be used to supplement information and clinical impression obtained during the interview. These are discussed below.

Daytime Consequences
Since a diagnosis of insomnia must include clinically significant symptoms during the day, it is important to assess whether there is significant distress regarding sleep or an impairment in function during waking hours. The *ICSD-2* indicates that at least one of the following daytime impairments must be reported in relation to sleep difficulties: (*i*) fatigue or malaise; (*ii*) attention, concentration, or memory impairment; (*iii*) social or vocational dysfunction or poor school performance; (*iv*) mood disturbance or irritability; (*v*) daytime sleepiness; (*vi*) motivation, energy, or initiative reduction; (*vii*) proneness for errors or accidents at work or while driving; (*viii*) tension, headache, or gastrointestinal symptoms; (*ix*) concerns or worries about sleep (1). Distress about poor sleep is usually expressed throughout the initial interview and is signaled by spontaneous complaints. Information about perceived impairment attributed to poor or insufficient sleep can be gathered through attention to spontaneous reporting as well as direct questioning and supplemented by the administration of self-report scales, discussed below.

Physical Examination
The clinician should carefully assess the patient for any physical conditions that may cause or contribute to difficulties initiating or maintaining sleep. Evidence of a crowded upper airway, large tongue, small mandible, large tonsils, or enlarged turbinates may indicate the presence of SDB that often results in fragmentation of sleep and contribute to sleep maintenance insomnia. Physical signs suggestive of a compressive neuropathy, such as a dermatomal distribution of sensory dysesthesia or loss and/or limb weakness, may explain limb pain or numbness that may interfere with sleep.

SUBJECTIVE ASSESSMENT TOOLS

Self-report measures can complement the initial diagnostic interview and assist in character- izing the patient's sleep complaint, associated features, and daytime distress. These measures may be given prior to the first meeting (e.g., a packet is sent out beforehand or completed in the waiting room) or after the first meeting. When given prior to the first meeting, questionnaires can provide information to guide the intake interview. When given after the first meeting, they can provide additional or more detailed information about issues discussed during the interview, as well as reveal information that was not covered during the interview. Clinicians often choose one or more of the self-report measures to use, depending on the setting of the clinic, the types of patients seen, and clinician preference. The most widely used self-report measures and their diagnostic utility are summarized in Table 1, along with references to their psychometric properties. A description of the measures and their recommended uses is given below. The measures are organized by their function (assessment of sleep, associated features, and clinical significance). We recognize that some of the measures fit more than one of the categories we formed and note this in the text when relevant.

Subjective Tools for Characterizing Nocturnal Symptoms
Prospective and retrospective tools for characterizing the patterns, frequency, and severity of the nocturnal symptoms of insomnia can be used to determine the current state of the problem and to monitor change with treatment. The sleep diary (or sleep log) is the primary tool for providing prospective data on a night-to-night basis. In addition to characterizing the frequency and severity of the nighttime problem, the sleep diary can provide useful information on the variability of the patient's sleep-wake habit, circadian tendencies, patterns of medication use, and nap behaviors. While sleep diaries provide prospective data on the sleep problem, questionnaires provide retrospective data on global indices of insomnia severity and take into account both nocturnal and daytime symptoms. Of the many sleep questionnaires that provide retrospective data on global indices of insomnia severity, we describe

Table 1 Table of Subjective Measures

Measure	Domain	Diagnostic utility	Original citation
Insomnia Severity Index (ISI)	Global severity	Insomnia severity	13,20
Pittsburgh Sleep Quality Index (PSQI)	Global severity	Insomnia severity	21
Presleep Arousal Scale (PSAS)	Hyperarousal	Assess arousal related to psychophysiological insomnia	26
Hyperarousal Scale	Hyperarousal	Assess arousal related to psychophysiological insomnia	29
Arousal Predisposition Scale	Hyperarousal	Assess arousal related to psychophysiological insomnia	28
Dysfunctional Beliefs and Attitudes about Sleep (DBAS)	Sleep-related cognitions	Assess cognitions related to psychophysiological arousal	30,34,35
Thought Control Questionnaire for Insomnia (TCQ-I)	Sleep-related cognitions	Assess strategies for controlling sleep-related cognitions	36
Glasgow Content of Thoughts Inventory (GCTI)	Sleep-related cognitions	Assess content of presleep thoughts	37
Glasgow Sleep Effort Scale (GSES)	Sleep-related cognitions	Assess sleep effort to arousal	38
Horne-Östberg Morningness-Eveningness scale	Circadian tendencies	Assess circadian factors, rule out circadian rhythm sleep disorders CRSD	39
Morningness-Eveningness Composite Scale (MECS)	Circadian tendencies	Assess circadian factors, rule out CRSD	40
Epworth Sleepiness Scale (ESS)	Sleepiness	Assess daytime sleepiness in different situations	14,45
Fatigue Severity Scale (FSS)	Fatigue	Assess daytime fatigue	46
Beck Depression Inventory (BDI)	Depression	Assess depressive symptoms, rule out mood disorder	15,48
Inventory of Depressive Symptoms (IDS)	Depression	Assess severity of depressive symptoms	49,50
State Trait Anxiety Inventory (STAI)	Anxiety	Assess anxiety symptoms, rule out anxiety disorder	51
Profile of Mood States (POMS)	General mood	Assess mood states and changes	53
SF-36	General psychological well-being	Assesses overall quality of life	55
Symptoms Checklist-90 (SCL-90)	General psychological symptoms	Assesses psychological symptoms across several domains	56
Brief Symptoms Inventory (BSI)	General psychological symptoms	Short form derived from SCL-90	57

the following two: the Insomnia Severity Index (ISI) and the Pittsburgh Sleep Quality Index (PSQI). Both are well validated, easy to administer and often used in research as well as clinic settings.

Sleep Diaries
Sleep diaries are considered the standard of practice for the subjective assessment of insomnia (16), with a duration of two weeks of diaries recommended for a baseline assessment of the sleep problem (17). Sleep diaries typically include the items necessary for deriving the following sleep parameters: sleep onset latency (SOL), the total amount of time awake during the night after sleep onset (WASO), terminal wakefulness (TWAK), the number of awakenings during the night (NWAK), the total time in bed (TIB), the total amount of sleep (TST), and sleep efficiency (SE). In addition, estimates of number of naps and medication use, as well as

ratings of sleep quality, daytime sleepiness, and daytime fatigue and tiredness are frequently included in a sleep diary. A section for notes or comments provides patients the space to elaborate on specific problems and unusual circumstances.

Sleep diaries provide detailed quantitative raw data from which the severity and frequency of different aspects of the problem across the recorded period can be derived. In addition, a review of diary data with the patient can be helpful for testing the accuracy of the relationship between the sleep symptoms and other factors, such as perceived daytime consequences (e.g., sleepiness, fatigue, mood), consumption of alcohol and caffeine, and use of sleep medications. Completion of the sleep diary can alert clinicians to areas that should be addressed and might not otherwise be disclosed. For example, when patients report precise times (e.g., nocturnal awakening at 3:21 a.m.) the clinician is alerted to the presence of excessive clock monitoring, a behavior that is likely to interfere with sleep. The timing and regularity of bedtimes and wake-up times (e.g., weekday versus weekend) can assist in the assessment of circadian rhythm factors that might be relevant to the patient's presentation. Baseline sleep diaries are particularly important for the initial TIB prescription for a sleep restriction protocol, a component of CBT. While initial sleep diaries are helpful for assessment and diagnosis, continued completion of a sleep diary during treatment provides information about compliance and progress. These continued data are the basis for adjustments to the treatment.

Although sleep diaries are considered the primary tool for assessing insomnia, they can be problematic and difficult to implement. Given the subjective nature of the data, issues with missing or inaccurate data lead to problems in calculating sleep parameters. Clear instructions, corrective feedback, and methods to ensure daily completion need to be implemented in order to increase accuracy. In addition, for some patients compliance can be challenging, and thus researchers have used several methods to enhance data collection. These include having patients leave a voice message each morning into an answering machine that has a time stamp, or using electronic devices, such as personal data assistants (PDAs). In some cases, completion of sleep diaries may heighten anxiety and exacerbate insomnia. Also, subjective estimates of sleep may not accurately reflect objectively measured sleep, as insomniacs tend to overestimate wakefulness and underestimate total sleep time during the night (17,18). Finally, although most sleep diaries contain items on the essential aspects of nocturnal sleep, there is no consensus on the exact language of the diary items, the sequence of items, and the format (e.g., table versus graphical). When developed, a standardized set of core questions to be included in sleep diaries will permit a more meaningful comparison of results from different studies on insomnia than is presently possible.

Despite these limitations, sleep diaries may provide a more representative sample of an individual's sleep than retrospective questionnaires or polysomnographic (PSG) studies (18). Moreover, the practicality and cost-effectiveness of a sleep diary versus objective sleep measures support its status as the primary self-report tool for assessing insomnia.

Insomnia Severity Index

The ISI (19,20) is a seven-item scale that measures the degree of severity on three nighttime symptoms (difficulty falling asleep, difficulty staying asleep, problem waking too early) and daytime consequences, distress, and dissatisfaction. Each item is rated on a five-point scale and the total score provides an index of severity of the insomnia. The instruction is to "rate the current (i.e., last 2 weeks) severity of your insomnia problem(s)." Guidelines for interpreting the total score are as follows: 0–7 (no significant insomnia), 8–14 (subthreshold insomnia), 15–21 (moderate insomnia), 22–28 (severe insomnia) (19). In addition, a score > 14 has been found to be the optimum cutoff for insomnia as a disorder (19). Given its brevity, face validity, sensitivity to detect change with treatment, and its direct relevance for assessing insomnia as a disorder, the ISI can be easily added to a clinic questionnaire or research protocol. However, the ISI is exclusively focused on insomnia symptoms and does not provide information on sleep pattern and frequency of disturbed sleep, nor does it assess for the use of sleep medication.

Pittsburgh Sleep Quality Index

The PSQI is a 19-item scale that measures general sleep disturbances over a one-month interval (21). Although it was developed as a measure of disturbed sleep in general (including symptoms of other sleep disturbances such as apnea) rather than a pure measure of insomnia severity, it has been used in several insomnia studies (22,23). Unlike the ISI, which instructs the patient to rate the severity of insomnia symptoms, the PSQI provides a global severity of sleep disturbance based on questions about sleep patterns, frequency of sleep onset, and maintenance difficulties, as well frequency of a range of other sleep disturbances (e.g., snoring, feeling too hot or too cold, dreams, and pain), medication use, and a range of daytime consequences. Each item is ranked on a 0–3 scale. Scoring the PSQI consists of deriving scores for the following seven components: subjective sleep quality, sleep latency, sleep duration, sleep efficiency, sleep disturbance, use of sleep medication, and daytime dysfunction, from which a global score is derived. A score >5 represents clinically meaningful insomnia. More specifically, this cutoff score indicates moderate sleep problems in at least three sleep components or severe sleep problems in at least two areas. A 3-factor scoring of the PSQI has been proposed using factor analytic methods on a large data set obtained from older adults. The three subscales are sleep efficiency, perceived sleep quality, and daily disturbance (24). Similar to the ISI, the PSQI is easy to administer in a clinical setting. The retrospective time frame for the PSQI is the last month, making it somewhat less sensitive than the ISI for detecting change with brief treatments, but it has been used with a reference period as little as one week (25).

Subjective Tools for Characterizing Factors or Features Associated with Nocturnal Symptoms

Assessment of potential contributing factors and associated features (e.g., hyperarousal, circadian rhythm tendencies, and increased sleep effort) can help establish the subtype of insomnia and identify factors that may be perpetuating the insomnia disorder. We discuss below a few such measures, organized by domain assessed (see also Table 1).

Hyperarousal

Diagnosing psychophysiological insomnia requires evidence of heightened or conditioned arousal (or hyperarousal) regarding sleep (e.g., anxiety about sleep, physical tension or difficulty relaxing, and intrusive thoughts at bedtime). Research has revealed evidence of higher levels of presleep rumination (26) and a more negative tone of sleep-related cognitions when insomniacs are compared to good sleepers (27). Several measures of arousal have been developed, of which the following three are discussed: the Presleep Arousal Scale (PSAS) (26), the Arousal Predisposition Scale (APS) (28), and the Hyperarousal Scale (HAS) (29).

The PSAS is a 16-item questionnaire with two subscales (cognitive and somatic arousal). Patients are asked to rate a variety of symptoms related to hyperarousal in the period preceding sleep on a five-point Likert scale. Typically, patients are asked to complete the PSAS daily (for example, with the sleep diary). The APS has 12 items. It was originally designed to measure cognitive arousability as a trait or predisposition. Similar to the PSAS, items are rated on a five-point Likert scale. The HAS is another measure of trait-like hyperarousal. Patients are asked to rate 26 self-descriptive items on a four-point Likert scale.

These three self-report tools can provide quantitative information on levels of arousal in people with insomnia, who in general score higher than good sleepers. However, there are no known cutoff scores for quantifying pathological levels of hyperarousal. To the best of our knowledge, these measures have not yet been employed in published treatment studies and it is not known how much change in arousal occurs with treatment. It is also not known whether these measures prime the responder to self-monitor these symptoms more closely, potentially leading to increased arousal. Further research is needed to refine measures of arousal and to understand their role in clinical and research settings focused on the assessment and treatment of insomnia.

Sleep-Related Cognitions

Individuals with insomnia exhibit more distorted sleep-related cognitions than good sleepers (20,30,31). Moreover, treatment with CBT-I is associated with decreased distortions (31–33). Whereas the causal relationship between insomnia and distorted beliefs and attitude about sleep has yet to be clarified, it is agreed that these beliefs play a role in the perpetuation of insomnia (20).

The most widely used scale for measuring cognitions in treatment studies is the Dysfunctional Beliefs and Attitudes About Sleep (DBAS). Morin and colleagues (30) originally developed the DBAS as a 30-item scale. Subsequently, two 10-item short forms have been extracted using factor analytic techniques (34,35). The short forms reduce the time required to complete the scale without sacrificing the psychometric properties. Other scales for measuring cognitive processes have been developed to elucidate the cognitive factors associated with insomnia. These include the Thought Control Questionnaire for Insomnia (TCQ-I) (36) and the Glasgow Content of Thoughts Inventory (37). Both require further evaluation for use in clinical samples. Another validated scale of sleep-related cognition is the Glasgow Sleep Effort Scale (GSES) (38). The GSES is an eight-item scale focused on sleep-related effort, which represents the need to control sleep.

Circadian Factors

To assess the potential contribution of circadian factors to insomnia, the clinician typically uses behavioral correlates of the circadian rhythms, either during the interview (described earlier) or through self-report questionnaires measuring morning and evening tendencies. These questionnaires inquire about preferences for various activities and ease with which a person rises in the morning. The Horne-Östberg (Owl-Lark) scale (39) and a later derivative, the Morningness-Eveningness Composite Scale (MECS) (40), are of note here. The Horne-Östberg is a 19-item questionnaire whose score correlates with markers of the circadian pacemaker. It has been adapted to several languages [e.g., Dutch (41) and Portuguese (42)] and age groups [e.g., young adults and middle-aged adults (43)]. Normative values for young and middle-aged adults have been developed (39,43). The MECS (40) is a 13-item scale based upon 9 items from the Horne-Östberg scale and 4 items from the Torsvall and Åkerstedt scale (44). Data from these questionnaires provide information on patients' preferred sleep schedules independent of social and occupational commitments. The combination of questionnaire data and information about current sleep schedule allows the clinician to identify instances when changes to the amount of the time spent in bed are indicated.

Subjective Tools for Characterizing Waking Correlates

The assessment of daytime sequelae of poor sleep provides the context for evaluating the clinical significance of poor sleep. In a clinical setting, the impact of nocturnal symptoms on daytime activities can be assessed during the diagnostic interview by asking about the patient's inference regarding the relationship between poor sleep and daytime correlates. In a research setting, quantification of daytime consequences of poor sleep (waking correlates) is recommended (18). Of the range of waking correlates mentioned in the *ICSD-2*, self-report questionnaires commonly used by behavioral sleep medicine specialists and insomnia researchers are briefly discussed. Domains assessed by these measures are sleepiness, fatigue, depression, and anxiety. It is important to keep in mind that questionnaires quantify daytime impairment but do not inform the relationship between nighttime symptoms and the reported daytime impairments.

Sleepiness can be assessed using the Epworth Sleepiness Scale (ESS) (45), a brief eight-item questionnaire with a score above 10 suggesting excessive daytime sleepiness, though insomniacs tend to score below this cutoff. Fatigue can be assessed using the Fatigue Severity Scale (FSS) (46), a nine-item measure scored on a 1–7 scale. The FSS can detect changes in self-reported fatigue following insomnia treatments. Coadministration of the ESS and the FSS can help the clinician distinguish between sleepiness and fatigue, two constructs that are often confused by insomniacs. Several depression symptom inventories exist. The reader is referred elsewhere (47) for an extensive review of empirically based measures of depression. The two most widely used in the United States are the Beck Depression Inventory (BDI) (48), a 21-item scale that measures depression symptom severity and the Inventory of Depressive Symptoms (IDS), a validated 30-item scale (49) from which a shorter 16-item scale has been derived and validated (50). These measures can also be used to screen for the presence of a coexisting depressive disorder. Among the anxiety scales, a well-validated scale used frequently in insomnia research is the State-Trait Anxiety Inventory (STAI) (51), a 20-item questionnaire with two versions measuring state and trait anxiety, respectively. The reader is referred elsewhere (52) for an extensive review of other empirically based anxiety measures. Other subjective measures that can be used to assess a broader range of symptoms include the Profile of Mood States (POMS) (53), which assesses mood disturbance and mood changes, the SF-36 (54,55), which indexes quality of life (54), and the Symptom Checklist-90 (SCL-90) (56) and its shorter derivative, the Brief Symptoms Inventory (BSI) (57), both of which assess several domains of psychopathology.

Choosing among these subjective tools often depends on clinician preference, patient burden, and the need for further assessment beyond the interview. At a minimum, in a clinical setting it is helpful to include one questionnaire in each of the following three areas: (*i*) a measure of circadian rhythm tendency, as this tendency can guide the prescription of time in bed for sleep restriction; (*ii*) a measure of depression symptom severity, as such symptoms are common among insomniacs and can aid in deciding when to refer for the treatment of depression; and (*iii*) a measure of behaviors and cognitions that interfere with sleep quality so that they can be addressed during treatment.

OBJECTIVE ASSESSMENT TOOLS

In clinical settings, objective measures of sleep are used for differential diagnosis of other sleep disorders and when paradoxical insomnia is suspected. In addition to PSG, which remains the gold standard objective measure of sleep, other less expensive objective measures of sleep are also useful. These devices provide objective information on sleep-wake states by relying on physiological data other than EEG, and some can even provide a distinction between REM and non-REM sleep. However, these devices are typically unattended and are often battery operated—two attributes that could be associated with technical failure or power loss and subsequently with loss of data. Finally, a few behavioral-based devices have been developed and are briefly discussed below.

Polysomnography
Polysomnography is routinely used for the diagnosis of several sleep disorders, but it is not routinely indicated for the diagnosis of insomnia (58,59). Nevertheless, PSG can help rule out SDB when clinical symptoms are present and could be useful when insomnia does not respond to an adequate course of treatment. Night-to-night variability and the "first-night" effect (i.e., poor sleep associated with adapting to the laboratory setting and recording equipment) are greater for measures of sleep continuity relevant to insomnia than for indices of SDB and periodic leg movements. Contemporary home-based PSG studies, which are typically unattended, allow the collection of a full montage of sleep data. Unlike laboratory PSG studies, the first-night effect of home-based PSG is generally absent, suggesting that home PSG provides more reliable data on sleep continuity of insomniacs (60). Home PSG is gaining prominence as an objective measure of sleep in insomnia treatment outcome studies.

Actigraphy
Actigraphs are wristwatch-sized devices containing a motion sensor that records and stores information on gross motor activity. Typical epoch length for insomnia studies is one minute, and most devices also include an event marker that can indicate events of interest, such as the onset and offset of the intended sleep period. Some models have additional features, such as light sensors or programmable alarm prompts, so that the user may mark subjective ratings of interest.

Unlike PSG, which evaluates sleep based on multiple channels of information [EEG, EMG (electromyography) and EOG (electrooculography)], actigraphy determines sleep-wake states based solely on wrist movement. Consequently, sleep and wake states during the intended sleep period can be estimated but actigraphs do not provide information about sleep stages. Although the agreement between actigraphy-derived estimates of sleep parameters and PSG is not perfect, it is within a range that has been acceptable for other medical and psychological tests (61). Correlations between actigraphy and PSG-derived sleep parameters vary depending on the specific actigraphy model and specific scoring algorithm. These typically exceed 0.5 for both laboratory PSG (62,63) and home-based PSG (64). Although the validity of the method might vary according to the device and the scoring algorithm (65), when used in primary insomnia actigraphy appears to have acceptable agreement with PSG on measures such as number of awakenings, total time spent awake after sleep onset, total sleep time, and sleep efficiency, but not latency to sleep onset (66). Actigraphy can also be reliably used to detect change in sleep following treatment (62,63,66,67). Nevertheless, compared with PSG, actigraphy tends to underestimate total sleep time and sleep efficiency and overestimate total wake time in primary insomnia (63) and in hypnotic-dependent insomnia (66).

The main advantage of actigraphy is its suitability for recording sleep-wake data continuously for long periods of time in the patient's habitual sleep environment. It can reliably assess circadian patterns in sleep-wake organization over time (68) and can therefore assess circadian influences on sleep. Though actigraphy is not indicated for the routine diagnosis of insomnia, it can serve as an adjunct to routine clinical evaluation of specific aspects of insomnia (68). For instance, it is useful for evaluation of sleep when paradoxical insomnia is suspected (69) and whenever clinically derived information is deemed unreliable.

It is recommended that actigraphs be used along with sleep diaries to confirm timing of lights out and the end of the sleep period and to allow rejecting of artifacts. It is also recommended that actigraphs be used for at least three consecutive 24-hour periods (68).

NEW DIAGNOSTIC TOOLS

Nightcap and REMview

Nightcap and its later derived FDA-approved REMview are home-based sleep monitoring systems that can differentiate between wakefulness, non-REM, and REM sleep based on eyelid and body movements. The device works by distinguishing between slow and rapid eye movements (70,71). The validity of this device for determination of sleep parameters as compared with PSG is not uniform across sleep variables. Edinger and colleagues (72) found that it performed worse on sleep onset latency and time awake after sleep onset, yet concluded that it is valid for measuring sleep onset latency (73). Though the device is able to differentiate between poor and good sleepers, its main utility for assessing insomnia is in research, rather than clinical settings.

Other sleep devices rely on monitoring physiological and behavioral changes that occur during the transition to sleep onset. These changes include the sleeper's response to a probe, as is the case with the sleep-assessment device (74), change in respiration (75), or change in muscle tone (76,77). These devices provide an accurate measure of latency to sleep onset when compared with laboratory PSG, but are either less accurate than actigraphy or unable to evaluate total sleep time or other sleep variables after sleep onset (77). These devices are used in research but not in clinical settings.

CONCLUSIONS

An initial diagnostic interview is critical for the clinician to accurately diagnose insomnia and contributing factors. Subjective assessment tools can be used to characterize nocturnal symptoms, identify factors contributing to insomnia, assess baseline sleep patterns and sleep-related habits, measure insomnia severity and sleep quality, identify features associated with poor sleep, such as cognitive hyperarousal, and assess waking correlates of poor sleep. Objective measures of sleep could assist in ruling out other sleep disorders (e.g., polysomnogram), and in confirming a diagnosis of paradoxical insomnia (e.g., actigraphs or PSG).

REFERENCES

1. American Academy of Sleep Medicine. The International Classification of Sleep Disorders: Diagnostic and Coding Manual. 2nd ed. Westchester: American Academy of Sleep Medicine, 2005.
2. Lichstein KL, Durrence HH, Taylor DJ, et al. Quantitative criteria for insomnia. Behav Res Ther 2003; 41(4):427–445.

3. Lack L, Bootzin R. Circadian rhythm factors in insomnia and their treatment. In: Perlis ML, Lichstein K, eds. Treating Sleep Disorders: Principles and Practice of Behavioral Sleep Medicine. Hoboken, NJ: John Wiley & Son, Inc., 2003:305–344.
4. Buysse DJ, Reynolds CF, Hauri PJ. Diagnostic concordance for DSM-IV sleep disorders: A report from the APA/NIMH DSM-IV field trial. Am J Psychiatry 1994; 151:1351–1360.
5. Adam K, Tomeny M, Oswald I. Physiological and psychological differences between good and poor sleepers. J Psychiatr Res 1986; 20(4):301–316.
6. Bonnet MH, Arand DL. Twenty-four hour metabolic rate in insomniacs and matched normal sleepers. Sleep 1995; 18:581–588.
7. Bonnet MH, Arand DL. Heart rate variability in insomniacs and matched normal sleepers. Psychosom Med 1998; 60:610–615.
8. Stepanski E, Zorick F, Roehrs T, et al. Daytime alertness in patients with chronic insomnia compared with asymptomatic control subjects. Sleep 1988; 11:54–60.
9. Hall M, Buysse DJ, Nowell PD, et al. Symptoms of stress and depression as correlates of sleep in primary insomnia. Psychosom Med 2000; 62(2):227–230.
10. Perlis ML, Merica H, Smith MT, et al. Beta EEG in insomnia. Sleep Med Rev 2001; 5:363–374.
11. Merica H, Blois R, Gaillard JM. Spectral characteristics of sleep EEG in chronic insomnia. Eur J Neurosci 1998; 10(5):1826–1834.
12. Cervena K, Dauvilliers Y, Espa F, et al. Effect of cognitive behavioural therapy for insomnia on sleep architecture and sleep EEG power spectra in psychophysiological insomnia. J Sleep Res 2004; 13(4): 385–393.
13. Bastien CH, Vallieres A, Morin CM. Validation of the Insomnia Severity Index as an outcome measure for insomnia research. Sleep Med 2001; 2(4):297–307.
14. Johns MW. Reliability and factor analysis of the Epworth Sleepiness Scale. Sleep 1992; 15(4):376–381.
15. Beck AT, Steer RA, Garbin MG. Psychometric properties of the beck depression inventory: twenty-five years of evaluation. Clin Psychol Rev 1988; 8:77–100.
16. Smith LJ, Nowakowski S, Soeffing JP, et al. The measurement of sleep. In: Perlis ML, Lichstein KL, eds. Treating Sleep Disorders: Principles and Practice of Behavioral Sleep Medicine. Hoboken, NJ: John Wiley & Sons, Inc, 2003:29–73.
17. Sateia MJ, Doghramji K, Hauri PJ, et al. Evaluation of chronic insomnia. An American Academy of Sleep Medicine review. Sleep 2000; 23(2):243–308.
18. Buysse D, Ancoli-Israel S, Edinger JD, et al. Recommendations for a Standard Research Assessment of Insomnia. Sleep 2006; 29(9):1155–1173.
19. Bastien CH, Vallieres A, Morin CM. Validation of the Insomnia Severity Index as an outcome measure for insomnia research. Sleep Med 2001; 2(4):297–307.
20. Morin C. Insomnia. New York: Guilford Press, 1993.
21. Buysse DJ, Reynolds CF, Monk TH, et al. The Pittsburgh sleep quality index: a new instrument for psychiatric practice and research. Psychiatry Res 1989; 28(2):193–213.
22. Backhaus J, Junghanns K, Broocks A, et al. Test-retest reliability and validity of the Pittsburgh Sleep Quality Index in primary insomnia. J Psychosom Res 2002; 53(3):737–740.
23. Carpenter JS, Andrykowski MA. Psychometric evaluation of the Pittsburgh Sleep Quality Index. J Psychosom Res 1998; 45(1 Spec No):5–13.
24. Cole JC, Motivala SJ, Buysse DJ, et al. Validation of a 3-factor scoring model for the Pittsburgh sleep quality index in older adults. Sleep 2006; 29(1):112–116.
25. Carter PA. A brief behavioral sleep intervention for family caregivers of persons with cancer. Cancer Nurs 2006; 29(2):95–103.
26. Nicassio PM, Mendlowitz DR, Fussell JJ, et al. The phenomenology of the pre-sleep state: the development of the pre-sleep arousal scale. Behav Res Ther 1985; 23(3):263–271.
27. Kuisk LA, Bertelson AD, Walsh JK. Presleep cognitive hyperarousal and affect as factors in objective and subjective insomnia. Percept Mot Skills 1989; 69(3 pt 2):1219–1225.
28. Coren S. Prediction of insomnia from arousability predisposition scores: scale development and cross-validation. Behav Res Ther 1988; 26(5):415–420.
29. Pavlova M, Berg O, Gleason R, et al. Self-reported hyperarousal traits among insomnia patients. J Psychosom Res 2001; 51(2):435–441.
30. Morin CM, Stone J, Trinkle D, et al. Dysfunctional beliefs and attitudes about sleep among older adults with and without insomnia complaints. Psychol Aging 1993; 8:463–467.
31. Carney CE, Edinger JD. Identifying critical beliefs about sleep in primary insomnia. Sleep 2006; 29(4):444–453.
32. Morin CM, Blais F, Savard J. Are changes in beliefs and attitudes about sleep related to sleep improvements in the treatment of insomnia? Behav Res Ther 2002; 40(7):741–752.
33. Edinger JD, Wohlgemuth WK, Radtke RA, et al. Cognitive behavioral therapy for treatment of chronic primary insomnia: a randomized controlled trial. JAMA 2001; 285:1856–1864.

34. Espie CA, Inglis SJ, Harvey L, et al. Insomniacs' attributions: psychometric properties of the Dysfunctional Beliefs and Attitudes about Sleep Scale and the Sleep Disturbance Questionnaire. J Psychosom Res 2000; 48(2):141–148.

35. Edinger JD, Wohlgemuth WK. Psychometric comparisons of the standard and abbreviated DBAS-10 versions of the dysfunctional beliefs and attitudes about sleep questionnaire. Sleep Med 2001; 2(6):493–500.

36. Ree MJ, Harvey AG, Blake R, et al. Attempts to control unwanted thoughts in the night: development of the thought control questionnaire-insomnia revised (TCQI-R). Behav Res Ther 2005; 43(8):985–998.

37. Harvey KJ, Espie CA. Development and preliminary validation of the Glasgow Content of Thoughts Inventory (GCTI): a new measure for the assessment of pre-sleep cognitive activity. Br J Clin Psychol 2004; 43(pt 4):409–420.

38. Broomfield NM, Espie CA. Towards a valid, reliable measure of sleep effort. J Sleep Res 2005; 14(4):401–407.

39. Horne JA, Ostberg O. A self-assessment questionnaire to determine morningness-eveningness in human circadian rhythms. Int J Chronobiol 1976; 4(2):97–110.

40. Smith C, Reilly C, Midkiff K. Evaluation of three circadian rhythm questionnaires with suggestions for an improved measure of morningness. J Appl Psychol 1989; 74:728–738.

41. Zavada A, Gordijn MC, Beersma DG, et al. Comparison of the Munich Chronotype Questionnaire with the Horne-Ostberg's Morningness-Eveningness Score. Chronobiol Int 2005; 22(2):267–278.

42. Benedito-Silva AA, Menna-Barreto L, Marques N, et al. A self-assessment questionnaire for the determination of morningness-eveningness types in Brazil. Prog Clin Biol Res 1990; 341B:89–98.

43. Taillard J, Philip P, Chastang JF, et al. Validation of Horne and Ostberg morningness-eveningness questionnaire in a middle-aged population of French workers. J Biol Rhythms 2004; 19:76–86.

44. Torsvall L, Akerstedt T. A diurnal type scale. Construction, consistency and validation in shift work. Scand J Work Environ Health 1980; 6(4):283–290.

45. Johns MW. A new method for measuring daytime sleepiness: the Epworth sleepiness scale. Sleep 1991; 14(6):540–545.

46. Krupp LB, LaRocca NG, Muir-Nash J, et al. The fatigue severity scale. Application to patients with multiple sclerosis and systemic lupus erythematosus. Arch Neurol 1989; 46(10):1121–1123.

47. Nezu AM, Ronan GF, Meadows EA, et al. Practitioner's Guide to Empirically Based Measures of Depression. New York: Kluwer Academic/Plenum Publishers, 2000.

48. Beck AT, Ward CH, Mendelson M, et al. An inventory for measuring depression. Arch Gen Psychiatry 1961; 4:561–571.

49. Rush AJ, Gullion CM, Basco MR, et al. The Inventory of Depressive Symptomatology (IDS) Psychometric properties. Psychol Med 1996; 26:477–486.

50. Rush AJ, Trivedi M, Ibrahim HM, et al. The 16-Item Quick Inventory of Depressive Symptomatology (QIDS), clinician rating (QIDS-C), and self-report (QIDS-SR): a psychometric evaluation in patients with chronic major depression. Biol Psychiatry 2003; 54(5):573–583.

51. O'Neil HFJ, Spielberger CD, Hansen DN. Effects of state anxiety and task difficulty on computer-assisted learning. J Educ Psychol 1969; 60(5 pt 1):343–350.

52. Antony MM, Orsillo SM, Roemer L. Practitioner's Guide to Empirically Based Measures of Anxiety. New York: Kluwer Academic/Plenum Publishers, 2001.

53. Norcross JC, Guadagnoli E, Prochaska JO. Factor structure of the profile of mood states (POMS): two partial replications. J Clin Psychol 1984; 40(5):1270–1277.

54. McHorney CA, Ware JE Jr., Raczek AE. The MOS 36-Item Short-Form Health Survey (SF-36): II. Psychometric and clinical tests of validity in measuring physical and mental health constructs. Med Care 1993; 31(3):247–263.

55. Ware J, Snow K, Kosinski M, et al. SF-36® Health Survey Manual and Interpretation Guide. Boston, MA: New England Medical Center, The Health Institute, 1993.

56. Derogatis LR, Lipman RS, Covi L. SCL-90: an outpatient psychiatric rating scale—preliminary report. Psychopharmacol Bull 1973; 9(1):13–28.

57. Derogatis LR, Melisaratos N. The Brief Symptom Inventory: an introductory report. Psychol Med 1983; 13(3):595–605.

58. Kushida CA, Littner MR, Morgenthaler T, et al. Practice parameters for the indications for polysomnography and related procedures: an update for 2005. Sleep 2005; 28(4):499–521.

59. Chesson AL Jr., Ferber RA, Fry JM, et al. The indications for polysomnography and related procedures. Sleep 1997; 20(6):423–487.

60. Edinger JD, Fins AI, Sullivan RJ Jr., et al. Sleep in the laboratory and sleep at home: comparisons of older insomniacs and normal sleepers. Sleep 1997; 20(12):1119–1126.

61. Tryon WW. Issues of validity in actigraphic sleep assessment. Sleep 2004; 27(1):158–165.

62. Friedman L, Benson K, Noda A, et al. An actigraphic comparison of sleep restriction and sleep hygiene treatments for insomnia in older adults. J Geriatr Psychiatry Neurol 2000; 13(1):17–27.

63. Vallieres A, Morin CM. Actigraphy in the assessment of insomnia. Sleep 2003; 26(7):902–906.

64. Gehrman P, Edinger J, Means M, et al. Measurement of sleep in young insomniacs: a multi-trait, multi-method approach. Sleep 2003; 26(suppl):A310–A311 (abstr).
65. Jean-Louis G, Zizi F, von Gizycki H, et al. Actigraphic assessment of sleep in insomnia: application of the Actigraph Data Analysis Software (ADAS). Physiol Behav 1999; 65(4–5):659–663.
66. Lichstein KL, Stone KC, Donaldson J, et al. Actigraphy validation with insomnia. Sleep 2006; 29(2): 232–239.
67. Edinger JD, Wohlgemuth WK, Krystal AD, et al. Behavioral insomnia therapy for fibromyalgia patients: a randomized clinical trial. Arch Intern Med 2005; 165(21):2527–2535.
68. Littner M, Kushida CA, Anderson WM, et al. Practice parameters for the role of actigraphy in the study of sleep and circadian rhythms: an update for 2002. Sleep 2003; 26(3):337–341.
69. Hauri PJ, Wisbey J. Wrist actigraphy in insomnia. Sleep 1992; 15(4):293–301.
70. Ajilore O, Stickgold R, Rittenhouse CD, et al. Nightcap: laboratory and home-based evaluation of a portable sleep monitor. Psychophysiology 1995; 32(1):92–98.
71. Mamelak A, Hobson JA. Nightcap: a home-based sleep monitoring system. Sleep 1989; 12(2):157–166.
72. Edinger JD, Means MK, Stechuchak KM, et al. A pilot study of inexpensive sleep-assessment devices. Behav Sleep Med 2004; 2(1):41–49.
73. Cantero JL, Atienza M, Stickgold R, et al. Nightcap: a reliable system for determining sleep onset latency. Sleep 2002; 25(2):238–245.
74. Lichstein KL, Nickel R, Hoelscher TJ, et al. Clinical validation of a sleep assessment device. Behav Res Ther 1982; 20(3):292–297.
75. Naifeh KH, Kamiya J. The nature of respiratory changes associated with sleep onset. Sleep 1981; 4(1):49–59.
76. Viens M, De Koninck J, Van den Bergen H, et al. A refined switch-activated time monitor for the measurement of sleep-onset latency. Behav Res Ther 1988; 26(3):271–273.
77. Hauri PJ. Evaluation of a sleep switch device. Sleep 1999; 22(8):1110–1117.

6 | Diagnostic Algorithm for Insomnia

Anil N. Rama
The Permanente Medical Group, San Jose, California, U.S.A.

Tom A. Potti
University of Michigan Medical School, Ann Arbor, Michigan, U.S.A.

CLINICAL VIGNETTE

Frances is a 76-year-old woman who had difficulties initiating and maintaining sleep. She often experienced "electric shock"-like sensations in her legs at night, which were relieved by walking. Frances complained of being fatigued and sleepy during the day. She typically obtained five to six hours of sleep each night. Frances reported that her father also suffered from similar symptoms.

Frances had been diagnosed with angina, hypertension, and depression. She takes clopidogrel, atenolol, lisinopril, zolpidem, and mirtazapine on a regular basis. Frances is married with three grown children. She drinks one to two glasses of wine with dinner and smokes one pack of cigarettes a day.

Frances meets the clinical criteria for restless legs syndrome (RLS), which includes an urge to move the legs in the evening after lying down, with movement attenuating the symptoms, and a positive family history (1). Her neurological examination was normal, and measurement of her nerve conduction velocities revealed no evidence of a peripheral neuropathy. Iron, ferritin, creatinine, hematocrit, and other serological tests were normal. A sleep study revealed severe periodic limb movement disorder (PLMD), with more than eight hundred periodic limb movements of sleep (PLMS) detected during her sleep. Approximately one-third of the PLMS were associated with electroencephalographic cortical arousals. There was no evidence of significant respiratory disturbances.

Frances was diagnosed with insomnia secondary to RLS, PLMD, poor sleep hygiene, and hypnotic dependence by her internist. Dopamine agonists such as ropinirole or pramipexole are considered first-line agents in the treatment of RLS by most sleep specialists. A secondary etiology for RLS was not detected (i.e., iron deficiency, peripheral neuropathy, or renal insufficiency). Antidepressants such as mirtazapine are sedating and can worsen RLS (2). Frances was asked to switch to a different antidepressant, such as bupropion, that does not worsen RLS. Lifestyle choices such as smoking or drinking might also exacerbate RLS and insomnia. Therefore, smoking cessation and alcohol abstinence were also encouraged (3,4). Zolpidem use can lead to tolerance and dependence, while cessation may lead to rebound insomnia, and it was recommended that she taper use of this medication.

Frances followed the various recommendations. She improved her sleep hygiene, made the necessary medication changes, started a dopamine agonist, and achieved adequate control of her RLS and PLMD. Her long-standing difficulties with sleep initiation and maintenance difficulties resolved, and she was able to gradually discontinue use of zolpidem.

KEY STEPS IN THE DIAGNOSIS OF INSOMNIA

First Step: Clinical History

Obtaining a complete clinical history from the patient, bed partner, parent, or caregiver is the first and most important step in the diagnosis of insomnia. The onset, duration, and type of insomnia (i.e., sleep-onset insomnia, sleep maintenance insomnia, sleep-offset insomnia, or non-restorative sleep) with special attention paid to temporal events in the patient's life surrounding the insomnia should be elicited. Nighttime symptoms such as snoring, apneas, leg jerks, dream-enacting behaviors, somnambulism, diaphoresis, enuresis, and bruxism should be elicited. Daytime symptoms such as fatigue, sleepiness, poor concentration, restless legs, depression, and anxiety should also be explored. Reviewing the patient's past medical, family, and social history along with current medications and allergies may also unmask an underlying cause of the insomnia for which a specific therapy can be implemented.

Second Step: Physical Examination

A general physical examination is necessary but often overlooked by many physicians treating insomnia. The examination should include an evaluation of the mental status. For instance, is the patient alert, demented, depressed, or anxious? The upper airway should be carefully assessed for evidence of sleep-related breathing disorders. Specifically, is the nasal septum deviated, are the nasal turbinates enlarged, are the nasal valves collapsing, is the hard palate high and arched, is the soft palate low, is the tongue large, or is the mandible recessed? A cardiovascular and pulmonary examination should be conducted. For example, is there evidence of congestive heart failure, pulmonary hypertension, or restrictive or obstructive lung disease? A brief neurological examination should also be performed. In particular, is there a peripheral neuropathy or a neurodegenerative disorder such as Parkinson's disease or Alzheimer's dementia? A comprehensive physical examination can often elicit clues to the underlying etiology of the patient's insomnia.

Third Step: Sleep Log, Scales, Actigraphy, and Polysomnogram

Sleep testing for insomnia should be considered, but ordered only after obtaining a comprehensive clinical history and performing a meticulous physical examination. Sleep logs are important to characterize the nature and pattern of the sleep problem and to assess the effectiveness of treatment intervention. Self-report rating scales such as the Pittsburg Sleep Quality Index, Insomnia Severity Index, and Women's Health Initiative Insomnia Rating Scale can be used as screening tools or to assess the severity of insomnia or response to treatment. Actigraphy involves wearing a motion-sensing device on the wrist that may help define sleep patterns and circadian rhythm disorders as well as response to treatment. Polysomnography should be used to rule out specific sleep disorders such as obstructive sleep apnea (OSA) and PLMS that may result in fragmentation of sleep and sleep maintenance difficulties.

IMPORTANT DIAGNOSTIC FEATURES AND CRITERIA TO DISTINGUISH INSOMNIA TYPES

The following categories used to classify insomnia are derived from the *International Classification of Sleep Disorders*, second edition (*ICSD-2*) (5). In general, insomnia is characterized by a complaint of difficulty with the initiation or maintenance of sleep, early morning awakening, or chronically non-restorative or poor-quality sleep, despite adequate opportunity and circumstances for sleep (5). In addition, at least one of the following forms of daytime impairment related to the nighttime sleep difficulty should be reported by the patient: fatigue or malaise; attention, concentration, or memory impairment; social or vocational dysfunction or poor school performance; mood disturbance or irritability; daytime sleepiness; motivation, energy, or initiative reduction; proneness for errors or accidents at work or while driving; tension, headaches, or gastrointestinal symptoms in response to sleep loss; and/or concerns or worries about sleep (5).

Adjustment Insomnia

Adjustment insomnia refers to insomnia with daytime impairment that develops in reaction to one or more identifiable stressors. The insomnia typically resolves in less than three months with resolution of or acclimation to the stressor (5).

Psychophysiological Insomnia

Psychophysiological insomnia involves insomnia lasting over one month perpetuated by two maladaptive behaviors: heightened arousal and learned sleep-preventing behaviors. Specifically, the patient may have increased anxiety primarily about sleep, difficulty falling asleep when desired, mental arousal, and somatic tension. Interestingly, the patient often sleeps better away from his or her own bedroom.

Paradoxical Insomnia
Paradoxical insomnia refers to a patient's complaint of arousal for at least one month in the absence of any objective evidence of a sleep disturbance.

Idiopathic Insomnia
Idiopathic insomnia refers to lifelong sleeplessness with no defined etiology.

Insomnia Due to Mental Disorder
In this condition, the symptom of insomnia is present for more than one month and correlates with a mental disorder such as depression or anxiety.

Inadequate Sleep Hygiene
Inadequate sleep hygiene refers to insomnia lasting at least one month due to routine activities that are non-conducive to promoting good sleep. Smoking, drinking, excessive napping, exercising near bedtime, exposure to bright lights prior to bedtime, intense mental activity prior to bedtime, and using the bed for activities other than sleeping are a few examples of behaviors that may contribute to this disorder.

Behavioral Insomnia of Childhood
There are two types of behavioral insomnia of childhood. One type involves difficulty with sleep onset without the presence of special or routine conditions such as falling asleep while sucking on a bottle or having a parent read to the child in bed. The other type involves improper limit setting in which the caregiver fails to enforce bedtimes for the child.

Insomnia Due to Drug or Substance
This category of insomnia lasts at least one month and is directly due to the use, abuse, or withdrawal from a drug or substance known to disrupt sleep.

Insomnia Due to Medical Condition
Insomnia lasting at least one month that is directly due to a medical condition known to disrupt sleep.

Insomnia Due to Substance or Known Physiological Condition, Unspecified
This diagnosis is used when a patient fails to meet the diagnostic criteria for the categories above but a substance or psychological condition is felt to be contributing to the patient's insomnia.

Physiological (Organic) Insomnia, Unspecified
This diagnosis is used when a patient fails to meet the criteria for the categories above but a physiological condition is felt to be contributing to the patient's insomnia.

DIFFERENTIAL DIAGNOSIS

Insomnia is not a disease but a symptom of other conditions. A physician's approach to insomnia should be similar to how he or she would approach any symptom: A differential diagnosis should be constructed, and various disease states need to be ruled in or out, and one of the goals of this chapter is to present a straightforward differential diagnosis for the patient complaining of insomnia. By methodically evaluating each potential etiology in the context of the patient's medical history and physical examination, it is our belief that a cause for the vast majority of cases of insomnia can be determined. Disease-specific treatments can then be employed, and unnecessary use of hypnotics can hopefully be avoided.

Insomnia can be characterized as either difficulty initiating sleep, difficulty maintaining sleep, an early morning awakening with the inability to return to sleep, or non-restorative sleep. When evaluating a patient with insomnia, various categories of disease states should be considered. These include behavioral, psychiatric, neurological, circadian rhythm, movement, and respiratory disorders. They also include various medication effects, environmental factors, paradoxical insomnia, and miscellaneous medical conditions. Idiopathic insomnia is a rare entity that should also be considered.

Table 1 Insomnia: Differential Diagnosis

- Behavioral disorders
- Psychiatric disorders
- Circadian rhythm disorders
- Movement disorders
- Respiratory disorders
- Neurological disorders
- Miscellaneous medical conditions
- Medications
- Idiopathic

Table 2 Behavioral Disorders Associated with Insomnia

- Adjustment insomnia
- Psychophysiological insomnia
- Inadequate sleep hygiene
- Behavioral insomnia of childhood
- Paradoxical insomnia

By formulating a differential diagnosis in the context of the patient's medical history and physical examination, one or more etiologies for the patient's insomnia can be determined. The remainder of the chapter will review in detail the various categories comprising the differential diagnosis of insomnia. Table 1 contains a general list of disorders that lead to the formation of insomnia.

Behavioral Disorders

Behavioral disorders occur because of stressful circumstances in the daily life of the patient. An identifiable stressor or habitual activities near bedtime may result in insomnia. Behavioral disorders are not severely debilitating, but the presence of insomnia can cause patients to become irritable and hinder their ability to function in the daytime. Table 2 lists common behavioral disorders that lead to insomnia.

Adjustment insomnia is temporally associated with an identifiable stressor that is psychological, environmental, or physical in nature. The insomnia resolves over a period of a few weeks when the specific stressor resolves or when the patient adapts to the stress. Negative stressors, such as bereavement or unexpected medical illness, and positive stressors, such as anticipating a vacation or securing a job promotion, can result in this type of insomnia.

Like adjustment insomnia, psychophysiological insomnia is associated with a specific life stressor. However, psychophysiological insomnia persists long after the resolution of the stressor. The persistence of the insomnia results from heightened physiological and mental arousal and learned sleep-preventing associations. The patient is anxious about sleep but not by other aspects of his or her life (which helps to distinguish this condition from a generalized anxiety disorder). Because of chronic sleep difficulties, the patient inappropriately develops negative associations to sleep in his or her usual sleeping environment (6). Therefore, the individual may report sleeping better in a new environment where no negative associations have been developed.

Inadequate sleep hygiene refers to insomnia that develops as a result of daily or nightly activities that prevent good quality sleep and full daytime alertness. Behaviors that produce increased arousal can result in this type of insomnia (7). These behaviors can include using alcohol, nicotine, tobacco, and caffeine, engaging in intense mental or physical activity near bedtime, or using the bed for activities other than sleep. In addition, behaviors that interfere with the regular timing and duration of sleep such as engaging in variable bedtimes or rise times and taking long daytime naps could also lead to this condition (8).

Behavioral insomnia of childhood develops as a result of inappropriate sleep associations or inadequate limit setting. The child is unable to fall asleep without a specific stimulation (e.g., rocking, watching television), object (e.g., bottle, teddy bear), or setting (e.g., lighted room, parents' bed). Behavioral insomnia of childhood can also develop when the child stalls or refuses to go to sleep. Fortunately, when the parent enforces limits to these situations, the insomnia quickly resolves (9).

Paradoxical insomnia, also referred to as sleep state misperception, is a unique condition in which the patient complains of insomnia, however, objective evidence (i.e., polysomnograms, actigraphy, etc.) indicates normal sleep patterns. The patient typically overestimates time spent awake and underestimates time spent sleeping. Some believe that paradoxical insomnia may be a milder version or precursor of psychophysiological insomnia (10).

Psychiatric Disorders

Psychiatric disorders involve disruptions in thinking, perception, or mood. Mood disorders, anxiety disorders, panic disorders, alcohol and drug dependency, and psychosis are associated with long-term insomnia. Table 3 lists common psychiatric disorders that lead to insomnia.

Mood disorders include, but are not limited to, major depressive disorder, dysthymia, and bipolar disorder. It is estimated that up to 90% of patients with depression complain of sleep quality (11). Patients with major depressive disorder have a high frequency of awakenings consistent with their level of depression (12). Patients with dysthymia have insomnia symptoms that are more enduring, in accordance with the longer period of depression. Insomnia in patients with bipolar disorder during a depressive episode is similar to that of insomnia in patients with major depressive disorder. Insomnia in patients with bipolar disorder during a manic episode is characterized by reduced amounts of sleep (13). In depressed patients, insomnia tends to persist only as long as the depressive symptoms are present. In general, the objective and subjective measures of sleep in depressed patients improves during three to four weeks of effective antidepressant treatment.

Anxiety disorders include panic disorder, posttraumatic stress disorder, and acute stress disorder. Anxiety disorders can result in difficulties initiating and maintaining sleep (14). Panic attacks occurring during sleep may lead to insomnia (15). Patients report awakening with rapid alertness in a sudden state of fear. A panic attack is associated with rapid eye movement (REM) sleep, differentiating it from sleep terrors, which occur during non–rapid eye movement (NREM) stage N3 (formerly NREM stage 3 and 4 sleep) (16). After an attack, the patient may become anxious about returning to sleep, which contributes to the insomnia. If panic attacks occur only during sleep and not during the day, then the diagnosis of panic disorder should be questioned and an alternative diagnosis (e.g., OSA) should be considered. Insomnia in posttraumatic stress disorder is most often a result of reoccurring nightmares due to a traumatic stressor experienced by the patient. Insomnia in patients with acute stress disorder is similar to that found in patients with posttraumatic stress disorder, but the insomnia is not as long lasting.

Drugs or substances can disrupt sleep if used inappropriately. The most common forms of drug and substance used include alcohol, sedative-hypnotic medications, and stimulants such as caffeine and nicotine. Alcohol can help initiate sleep and increase slow-wave sleep in the first half of the night but can lead to restless sleep or awakenings in the second half of the night when the alcohol wears off. Routine use of alcohol or sedative-hypnotic medications leads to tolerance and dependence. Abrupt discontinuation of these agents can result in rebound insomnia characterized by a sudden drop in sleep quality. In addition, alcohol and certain sedative-hypnotic medications can worsen coexisting sleep disorders such as OSA. Use and withdrawal of illicit drugs such as cocaine and methamphetamine are associated with insomnia (17,18). Nicotine use near bedtime causes insomnia by increasing the patient's alertness (19). Heavy smokers may experience insomnia from nightly withdrawal or possibly from respiratory disturbances. If a patient is trying to quit smoking, the ensuing withdrawal syndrome leads to significantly increased chances of insomnia (20). Sleep disturbances (e.g., nightmares, fragmented sleep, early morning arousals) induced by nicotine replacement aids may make it more difficult for smokers to quit smoking (21).

Table 3 Psychiatric Disorders Associated with Insomnia

- Mood disorders
- Anxiety disorders
- Panic disorder
- Alcohol or drug dependency
- Psychoses

Table 4 Neurological Disorders Associated with Insomnia

- Narcolepsy
- Parkinson's disease
- Sleep-related epilepsy
- Degenerative brain disorders
- Stroke
- Fatal familial insomnia

Patients with psychoses display disordered thinking and perception. Schizophrenia is the most common disorder manifested by psychosis. Sleep may be disrupted in schizophrenic patients as a result of inadequate sleep hygiene or by a dysfunctional sleep-wake schedule. Abuse of alcohol, illicit drugs, or prescription drugs used by the schizophrenic population may also lead to decreased amounts of sleep. Although insomnia is not the primary complaint of schizophrenics, sleep-onset and maintenance difficulties are characteristic features, as well as reduced REM and slow-wave sleep (22).

Neurological Disorders

Neurological disorders can impair the central, peripheral, and autonomic nervous systems. Disorders of the nervous system present with a wide variety of somatic symptoms, including insomnia. Table 4 lists important neurological disorders that are associated with insomnia.

Narcolepsy is characterized by excessive daytime sleepiness, cataplexy, automatic behaviors, sleep paralysis, hypnagogic or hypnopompic hallucinations, and fragmented sleep (23). Although patients with narcolepsy have excessive daytime sleepiness, approximately 50% of narcoleptics complain of sleep disturbances at night. Nighttime awakenings occur because of rapid transitions from REM sleep to a conscious state (24).

Parkinson's disease is characterized by a mask-like face, stooped posture, shuffling gait, bradykinesia, resting tremor, and cogwheel rigidity. Sleep disorders occur in approximately 94% of Parkinson's disease patients (25). Insomnia may be due to the disease process itself or coexisting RLS, PLMS, or OSA (26). Insomnia can also occur because of the dose-related side effects of dopaminergic agents (e.g., nightmares) used to treat the disease.

Individuals with sleep-related epilepsy frequently complain of insomnia or excessive daytime sleepiness (27). In these patients, epileptic activity is enhanced during sleep, particularly during sleep onset or awakenings (28). Epileptiform discharges provoke sleep disruption and can lead to severe sleep deprivation in patients (29). Stress, sleep deprivation, irregular sleep-wake patterns, and use of stimulants may exacerbate the condition.

Patients with degenerative brain disorders may experience a variety of sleep disorders including insomnia (30–32). Examples of common degenerative brain disorders include Alzheimer's disease, Huntington's disease, and multiple sclerosis. The severity and location of the underlying neuropathology correlates to the intensity of sleep disturbances experienced by the patient. Coexisting depression, sleep-disordered breathing, and sleep-related movement disorders may also contribute to insomnia in patients with degenerative brain disorders (33).

Over half of stroke patients develop insomnia (34). Insomnia is associated with the location of the stroke, especially if it involves the thalamus or brain stem. Over 50% of stroke patients have sleep-disordered breathing, mostly in the form of OSA, which can also result in insomnia (35).

Fatal familial insomnia is an untreatable lethal prion disease. Familial and sporadic fatal insomnia produces disrupted sleep (i.e., insomnia, reduced slow-wave sleep, alterations in circadian rhythm), and motor abnormalities (i.e., muscle twitches, difficulty swallowing, difficulty speaking, or ataxia) (36,37). Research indicates that neuronal apoptosis may be responsible for the disrupted sleep and insomnia (38).

Circadian Rhythm Disorders

The circadian system is the foundation of the sleep-wake cycle. Circadian rhythm sleep disorders are associated with dysfunctions or insufficiencies in the circadian system (39). The misalignment between the internal circadian timing system and the external environment is typically due to either an alteration in the functioning of the circadian timing system [e.g., circadian rhythm sleep disorder, delayed or advanced sleep phase type (ASP)] or changes in the external environment (e.g., jet lag or shift work). When both insomnia and excessive

Table 5 Circadian Rhythm Disorder Types Associated with Insomnia

- Jet lag
- Shift work
- Delayed sleep phase
- Advanced sleep phase
- Free running
- Irregular sleep-wake
- Short sleeper

daytime sleepiness coexist, a circadian rhythm sleep disorder may be present (40,41). Table 5 lists the types of circadian rhythm disorders that are associated with insomnia.

Jet lag disorder is a short-lived impairment manifested by insomnia or excessive daytime sleepiness in those who cross several time zones by air travel (42,43). The severity of the disorder is affected by the number of time zones traversed, the direction in which travel occurs, and the age of the traveler (44). Those crossing multiple time zones, traveling east (due to the advancement of bedtime), and the elderly may require additional time for recovery. Although jet lag symptoms may mimic those seen in circadian rhythm sleep disorder, delayed sleep phase type (DSP), and ASP, the symptoms in jet lag are relatively short lived.

Shift work disorder is characterized by insomnia and daytime fatigue due to a persistent work schedule that overlaps with a patient's typical sleep time (45). Shift work disorder can lead to a reduction in the total number of hours a patient sleeps in a given day. As such, the patient may complain of a reduction in sleep quality, alertness, and reduced cognitive efficiency (46,47). Additional problems can arise if the patient remains active during periods that he or she should be resting. Daylight will usually have an adverse effect on the patient's ability to adapt to a new sleep-wake cycle.

DSP typically affects adolescents and young adults and is characterized by a sleep-wake cycle that is delayed relative to social norms (48). These patients are often referred to as "night owls." A DSP patient will naturally choose a sleep time past 1 a.m. and will typically awaken in the late morning or early afternoon. Consequently, the patient often fails to meet various morning social obligations (e.g., school, work). Increased sleep latency and insomnia may occur when these patients attempt to retire at a more socially accepted bedtime (49). Patients with DSP typically display abnormalities such as increased anxiety, depression, and lack of control of emotional expression (50).

ASP typically affects the elderly and is characterized by a sleep-wake cycle that is advanced relative to social norms (51,52). Patients with ASP may naturally choose a sleep time between 6 p.m. and 9 p.m. and will typically awaken between 2 a.m. and 5 a.m. Consequently, the patient often fails to meet various evening social obligations (e.g., parties, dinners). Insomnia may occur when these patients attempt to remain asleep after awakening in the early morning.

Circadian rhythm sleep disorder, free-running type, also known as non-24-hour sleep-wake syndrome, involves the endogenous circadian clock not being able to use external cues to calibrate the sleep-wake cycle. Although the normal sleep-wake cycle is slightly longer than 24 hours, individuals use light and other external cues to maintain synchrony to the 24-hour day. A patient suffering from this free-running disorder has a sleep-wake cycle that is significantly longer than the 24-hour day and is unable to use external cues to adjust his or her sleep-wake cycle (53). Consequently, the patient's sleep cycle tends to delay further relative to the normal sleep schedule with each passing day. This disorder is typically seen in blind individuals because they lack the ability to perceive light-dark cycles, but rare cases occur in sighted individuals (54). The patient may experience insomnia and excessive sleepiness when attempting to sleep at regular times.

Irregular sleep-wake rhythm is characterized by a sleep-wake cycle that is highly variable during a 24-hour period because of a random circadian timing system. There is day-to-day variability in sleep onset and sleep duration (55). Although total sleep time is normal, patients may take frequent naps at variable times during the day and night. Because the sleep-wake cycle does not adjust to environmental cues, insomnia and excessive daytime sleepiness develop when attempting to adhere to a regular sleep-wake schedule. This condition can occur at any age.

A short sleeper is an individual with no apparent reduction in alertness or impairment in functioning after receiving less than five hours of sleep per night (56). The patient does not have difficulties initiating and maintaining sleep. Short sleepers may only complain of insomnia if they attempt to sleep longer than their natural sleep-wake cycle.

Movement Disorders

Sleep-related movement disorders involve physical movements that may result in insomnia (57). The movements are irresistible or involuntary, occur during sleep or periods of rest, and frequently result in insomnia and daytime fatigue. Table 6 lists the types of movement disorders that are associated with insomnia.

RLS is a common sensorimotor disorder characterized by unpleasant sensations deep inside the legs. These sensations primarily occur when the patient is sedentary during rest periods and can become more pronounced during bedtime (58,59). The paresthesias are accompanied by an irresistible urge to move the limb, which results in a temporary relief of symptoms. Approximately 80% of patients with RLS have PLMS. RLS can result in sleep-onset insomnia as well as difficulties in returning to sleep following nocturnal awakenings (60). Patients often complain of excessive daytime sleepiness and fatigue (61).

PLMD is a condition in which frequent and involuntary muscle spasms occur only during sleep. These are stereotyped, periodic, jerking movements typically consisting of flexion of the ankle, knee, and hip. PLMS are regularly accompanied by an awakening resulting in sleep fragmentation and subsequent excessive daytime sleepiness, although this is controversial (62,63). In virtually all patients with RLS, PLMS are observed, however, patients with PLMD do not necessarily experience RLS. There is some evidence that certain antidepressants, such as venlafaxine or selective serotonin reuptake inhibitor (SSRI) groups, may worsen PLMS (64).

Sleep starts, also referred to as hypnic jerks, are spontaneous muscle twitches of various body parts that occur throughout the night, typically during sleep onset (65). Sleep starts arising in the relaxation and drowsiness period preceding sleep onset have been reported to cause severe sleep-onset insomnia (66). The patient often complains of a feeling of falling or other sensory hallucination during the occurrence (67). Sleep starts are differentiated from RLS and PLMS because the movements tend to be more rapid, short lived, and erratic in pattern. Furthermore, sleep starts are not associated with unpleasant sensations or an irresistible urge to move the legs at night.

Sleep-related leg cramps are painful muscle contractions, which occur during sleep. Leg cramps are common occurrences among the elderly (68). The spasms are involuntary and begin abruptly at irregular times throughout the night. The painful experiences may delay sleep onset or trigger arousals from sleep. Unlike the discomfort felt in RLS, the pain from leg cramps does not subside with continued activity of the legs. Instead, relief is only achieved through stretching of the muscle, massage, or heat.

Respiratory Disorders

Disordered respiration during sleep due to OSA, central sleep apnea (CSA), sleep-related hypoventilation/hypoxemia, and chronic lung diseases may lead to sleep fragmentation. Table 7 lists the types of respiratory disorders that are associated with insomnia.

Table 6   Movement Disorders Associated with Insomnia

- Restless legs syndrome
- Periodic limb movement disorder
- Sleep starts
- Sleep-related leg cramps

Table 7   Respiratory Disorders Associated with Insomnia

- Obstructive sleep apnea
- Central sleep apnea
- Cheyne–Stokes breathing pattern
- High-altitude periodic breathing
- Sleep-related hypoventilation syndromes
- Chronic lung diseases

OSA is characterized by repetitive partial (i.e., hypopneas) or total (i.e., apneas) obstruction of the upper airway with subsequent increased ventilatory effort (e.g., snoring, gasping, choking) resulting in cortical arousals and/or oxygen desaturations. The fragmentation of sleep may lead to excessive daytime sleepiness as well as insomnia. If untreated, OSA may lead to hypertension, stroke, and cardiovascular morbidity (69–71). OSA should be considered in those with excess body weight but also in thin individuals or children with abnormal anatomical features (72,73).

CSA is characterized by cessation of respiration due to repetitive lapses in ventilatory effort resulting in sleep fragmentation (74). Unlike OSA, patients with CSA commonly complain of awakening during sleep and insomnia, but less commonly of daytime sleepiness (75,76). An increased ventilatory response to carbon dioxide is a predisposing factor to the development of CSA. Patients with CSA sometimes have a lower than normal carbon dioxide level (i.e., hypocapnia) due to hyperventilation, and a small increase in carbon dioxide levels may result in cessation of ventilation. CSA is often idiopathic (i.e., primary CSA), but can be triggered by drug use (i.e., opioids) or dysfunctions in the cardiac, renal, or central nervous systems (77).

Cheyne–Stokes breathing pattern is a specific CSA syndrome in which the recurring apneic episodes involve a gradually increasing tidal volume followed by a gradually decreasing tidal volume (78). This is distinguishable from OSA and other types of CSA in which the respiration changes are more rapid. Cheyne–Stokes breathing pattern may develop secondary to congestive heart failure, stroke, or renal failure (79). The sleep-disordered breathing pattern generally arises during the sleep-wake transition and may result in difficulties with sleep maintenance and excessive daytime sleepiness.

High-altitude periodic breathing is a specific CSA syndrome manifested by headaches, loss of appetite, nausea, dizziness, and insomnia, which become present after a rapid ascent (i.e., greater than 300 m/day to an altitude above 4000 m) (80). The occurrence of the disorder involves a periodic cycle between apneic and hyperpneic episodes, and, similar to other types of CSA, there is no forced ventilatory effort with the apnea (81). The sleep disturbances may involve frequent arousals at night and an increase in sleep onset latency during initial adaptation (82). High-altitude periodic breathing is thought to occur after hyperventilation with associated hypocapnic alkalosis. This occurs at high altitude when hyperventilation is induced by hypoxia. This suggests that the $PaCO_2$ may be the primary stimulus to ventilation during sleep, and loss of this drive, as occurs with hypocapnia, could produce dysthymic breathing. The condition is usually self limited and benign but may progress to cerebral edema and end in coma. A second, less common type of high-altitude illness presents with symptoms of pulmonary edema such as fatigue, chest tightness, dyspnea, cough, and hemoptysis.

Patients with sleep-related hypoventilation/hypoxemia syndromes suffer from nocturnal hypoxia and may develop similar complications as patients with CSA and OSA. Hypoventilation syndromes are characterized by an elevation of the arterial carbon dioxide tension to above 45 mmHg due to an imbalance between the metabolic production, circulation, and elimination of carbon dioxide through exhaled gas (83). Sleep-related hypoventilation syndromes most commonly stem from pulmonary parenchymal or vascular pathologies, lower airway obstructions, or neuromuscular and chest wall disorders (84). The disorders often predispose patients to developing insomnia and daytime sleepiness and may coexist with other forms of sleep-disordered breathing (85). Hypoventilation/hypoxemia disorders are generally distinguishable from OSA and CSA because the oxygen desaturation level is consistent and sustained throughout the nocturnal period; whereas in CSA and OSA, the oxygen desaturation level may fluctuate in accordance with altered airflow during the apneic episodes.

Insomnia is common in patients with chronic lung diseases such as chronic obstructive pulmonary disease (COPD), cystic fibrosis, and asthma (86,87). These relatively common disorders can lead to the development of sleep-related hypoventilation/hypoxemia syndrome and other problems that can disrupt sleep (88). For example, patients with COPD may have disrupted sleep due to cough, excess mucous production, arousals from sleep due to hypercapnia, and secondary to medications used to manage the lung disease (89,90).

Miscellaneous Medical Conditions

Insomnia may result from medical conditions that do not fit under the previous categories. Table 8 lists common miscellaneous medical conditions that are associated with insomnia.

Table 8 Miscellaneous Medical Conditions Associated with Insomnia

- Gastroesophageal reflux
- Hyperthyroidism
- Fibromyalgia
- Pregnancy
- Menopause
- Sleep-related headaches

Approximately three quarters of individuals who suffer from gastroesophageal reflux disease (GERD) experience its symptoms at night, when stomach contents are regurgitated into the esophagus, causing pain or discomfort. The nighttime symptoms (e.g., sour taste in mouth, heartburn, coughing, or choking) may disturb sleep and cause insomnia (91). Sleep-related GERD affects between 21% and 56% of individuals (92,93). In addition, nighttime gastro-esophageal reflux is common in individuals with respiratory disorders such as sleep apnea and asthma, and may affect the severity of these disorders (94).

Disorders of the endocrine system such as hyperthyroidism, hypothyroidism, and hyperparathyroidism may lead to sleep disturbances. Insomnia, irritability, and anxiety are the most common psychiatric complaints of hyperthyroid patients (95). Patients with hypo-thyroidism are at increased risk for developing OSA, which in turn may fragment sleep and lead to insomnia (96). Insomnia is highly prevalent in patients with symptomatic secondary hyperparathyroidism. The mitigation of sleep disturbances after parathyroidectomy demon-strates a link between the thyroid gland and insomnia (97). Parathyroidectomy can relieve symptoms such as skin itching, bone pain, and general weakness, which may be responsible for the improvement in sleep and reduction in insomnia.

Insomnia is common and debilitating in patients with fibromyalgia (98). Fibromyalgia causes widespread pain in the body. Fibromyalgia patients frequently complain of inadequate sleep, fatigue, dizziness, cognitive impairments, anxiety, and depression. The disease is more prevalent in women, especially after menopause, than men (99). Patients with fibromyalgia may have an increased number of arousals during the night. The severity of the patient's disease relates to the quality of their sleep (100).

Women can be prone to insomnia during certain points in the menstrual cycle, pregnancy, and menopause (101). The increased prevalence of insomnia and daytime sleepiness in pregnancy may be associated with RLS, sleep-disordered breathing, as well as the physical discomfort of pregnancy (102,103). Pregnancy is associated with the narrowing of the upper airway, which may lead to OSA (104,105). In addition, the large fluctuations in hormone levels during pregnancy and after childbirth may lead to physiological changes, which can cause sleep disturbances. Sleep disturbances can also occur in pregnant women who have experienced a previous pregnancy loss, as these women may have increased anxiety associated with pregnancy (106).

Hot flashes, mood disorders, and increased sleep-disordered breathing can lead to insomnia during the menopausal transition (107,108). Partial upper airway obstructions, vasomotor symptoms, and depression tend to be the primary causes for sleep disturbances in women undergoing menopause (109,110). There is a possibility that during menopause the circadian rhythm is altered by a change in melatonin expression (111).

Sleep-related headaches may affect sleep onset and maintenance (112). Headaches are caused by numerous factors, from physical to environmental, and vary in severity and extent. Common headache syndromes include migraines, cluster headaches, chronic paroxysmal hemicrania, and hypnic headaches. Migraines are recurring unilateral headaches ranging from moderate to severe intensity and can trigger insomnia in over 50% of patients (113). Migraines have an equal chance of occurring during the day or night. Cluster headaches are severe headaches characterized by unilateral paroxysmal attacks of severe pain, which occur during REM sleep (114). The headaches have a much shorter duration than migraines, but may occur multiple times a day over a period of one to two months in a year. Chronic paroxysmal hemicrania resembles cluster headaches, but are of even shorter duration (i.e., less than an hour) and occur more frequently in a day. Like cluster headaches, these headaches appear mostly during REM sleep (115). Hypnic headaches only occur during sleep and awaken the patient from sleep multiple times a night (116). Patients often complain that the headaches appear at approximately the same time each night. Unlike the previously described headache syndromes, hypnic headaches are bilateral and are typically less severe.

Medication Classes

Prescription drugs and substances can have adverse effects on sleep and wakefulness and aggravate preexisting sleep disorders (117). Table 9 lists medications that are associated with insomnia.

Antidepressants can cause or exacerbate insomnia (118). Most antidepressants, particularly SSRIs, monoamine oxidase inhibitors, and tricyclic antidepressants, decrease REM sleep (119). Antidepressants, with the exception of bupropion, can also worsen RLS, PLMS, and REM sleep behavior disorder (120). Sleep initiation and maintenance are affected by antidepressants, but the effects are less consistent between drugs. Some antidepressants, such as clomipramine and the SSRIs (in particular fluoxetine), are sleep disturbing early in treatment, and others such as amitriptyline and the serotonin 5-HT2-receptor antagonists are sleep promoting. However, these effects are short lived, and there are very few significant differences between drugs after a few weeks of treatment (121).

Antihypertensives are commonly used to reduce blood pressure. Nearly 20% of patients using antihypertensives will suffer from side effects including insomnia, tiredness, and depression (122).

Antiepileptic drugs, also known as anticonvulsants, are used to prevent the occurrence of epileptic seizures. Patients using antiepilectic drugs such as levetiracetam have frequent arousals and stage shifts, which can lead to daytime sleepiness and insomnia (123).

Antihistamines alleviate allergic reactions caused by histamine release. First-generation H1-antihistamines are associated with adverse reactions such as sedation, dizziness, tremor, anxiety, and insomnia (124,125). These drugs may also exacerbate RLS. First-generation antihistamines are inexpensive and widely available. As such, they may be inappropriately used by patients with insomnia for their hypnotic effects. Repetitive use may lead to tolerance and rebound insomnia upon discontinuation.

Decongestants are a broad class of medications used to treat nasal congestion. Decongestants can have stimulatory effects and produce insomnia (126,127). Pseudoephedrine, a common ingredient used in decongestant drugs, can lead to insomnia and dry mouth in patients (128).

Bronchodilators function to improve bronchial airflow and are effective in treating diseases such as asthma, emphysema, pneumonia, and bronchitis. These medications often have stimulant properties, which can lead to insomnia.

Thyroid supplements are used to treat hypothyroidism. Because the thyroid has a necessary function in the control of circadian rhythms, any medication that alters the levels of thyroid-stimulating hormone (TSH) or thyroxin may, in effect, change sleeping patterns in the patient (129). This could possibly lead to the development of insomnia in the patient.

Oral contraceptives can increase the severity and frequency of migraines among women (130). As described previously, headaches contribute to insomnia. Oral contraceptives may also induce sleep disturbances by reducing REM latency and slow-wave sleep (131).

High doses of stimulants such as methylphenidate and dextroamphetamine used to treat conditions such as narcolepsy, hypersomnia, attention deficit hyperactivity disorder (ADHD),

Table 9 Medication Classes Associated with Insomnia

- Antidepressants
- Antihypertensives
- Antiepileptics
- Antihistamines
- Decongestants
- Bronchodilators
- Thyroid supplements
- Oral contraceptives
- Stimulants
- Steroids
- Theophylline

and depression may lead to substance abuse and psychosis in patients (132). Use or withdrawal of such drugs may result in insomnia. Modafinil can cause insomnia because of its half-life of approximately 15 hours (133). Caffeine and illicit drugs with stimulant activity are also capable of causing insomnia in patients.

Steroid use is associated with insomnia (134). Dexamethasone, a drug commonly used for various medical problems (e.g., cerebral edema, inflammation), leads to a prolonged sleep latency (135).

Theophylline has been used as a treatment for asthma, COPD, and CSA (136). Theophylline can contribute to insomnia by delaying nocturnal sleep onset, increasing wakefulness after sleep onset, and decreasing slow-wave sleep (137,138).

Idiopathic Insomnia

Idiopathic insomnia is lifelong and occurs without a known etiology. Studies have indicated that a hyperactive awakening system or a hypoactive sleep system could be the basis for insomnia (139). Although a dysfunctional sleep-wake center in the brain seems likely, the true cause of this disorder is not fully known.

CONCLUSIONS

Insomnia is not a disease; it is a symptom associated with various medical or psychiatric conditions causing insufficient or poor quality sleep. A physician should approach insomnia as he or she would approach any symptom. A differential diagnosis should be formulated and systematically evaluated in the context of the patient's medical history and physical examination, given the multitude of behavioral, psychiatric, neurological, circadian rhythm, movement, respiratory, and other disorders or conditions that may contribute to the symptoms of insomnia. The etiology of the patient's insomnia can then be elucidated, and relevant treatment can be instituted, thereby avoiding the unnecessary use of hypnotic medication.

REFERENCES

1. Allen RP, Pacchietti D, Hening WA, et al. Restless legs syndrome: diagnostic criteria, special considerations, and epidemiology. A report from the restless legs syndrome diagnosis and epidemiology workshop at the National Institutes of Health. Sleep Med 2003; 4:101–119.
2. Agargun MY, Kara H, Ozbek H, et al. Restless legs syndrome induced by mirtazapine. J Clin Psychiatry 2002; 63(12):1179.
3. Mountifield JA. Restless legs syndrome relieved by cessation of smoking. CMAJ 1985; 133(5):426–427.
4. Aldrich MS, Shipley JE. Alcohol use and PLMS. Alcohol Clin Exp Res 1993; 17:192–196.
5. American Academy of Sleep Medicine. International classification of sleep disorders. 2nd ed. Diagnostic and coding manual. Illinois: American Academy of Sleep Medicine, 2005.
6. de Carvalho LB, Lopes EA, Silva L, et al. Personality features in a sample of psychophysiological insomnia patients. Arq Neuropsiquiatr 2003; 61(3A):588–590.
7. Jefferson CD, Drake CL, Scofield HM, et al. Sleep hygiene practices in a population-based sample of insomniacs. Sleep 2005; 28(5):611–615.
8. Jefferson CD, Drake CL, Scofield HM, et al. Sleep hygiene practices in a population-based sample of insomniacs. Sleep 2005; 28(5):611–615.
9. Ferber RA. Behavioral "insomnia" in the child. Psychiatr Clin North Am 1987; 10(4):641–653.
10. Bonnet MH, Arand DL. Physiological activation in patients with Sleep State Misperception. Psychosom Med 1997; 59(5):533–540.
11. Tsuno N, Besset A, Ritchie K. Sleep and depression. J Clin Psychiatr 2005; 66(10):1254–1269.
12. Taylor DJ, Lichstein KL, Durrence HH, et al. Epidemiology of insomnia, depression, and anxiety. Sleep 2005; 28(11):1362–1363.
13. Harvey AG, Schmidt DA, Scarna A, et al. Sleep-related functioning in euthymic patients with bipolar disorder, patients with insomnia, and subjects without sleep problems. Am J Psychiatry 2005; 162(1):50–57.
14. Tiepkema M. Insomnia. Health Rep 2005; 17(1):9–25.
15. Agargun MY, Kara H. Recurrent sleep panic, insomnia, and suicidal behavior in patients with panic disorder. Compr Psychiatry 1998; 39(3):149–151.

16. Craske MG, Tsao JC. Assessment and treatment of nocturnal panic attacks. Sleep Med Rev 2005; 9(3): 173–184.
17. Sofuoglu M, Dudish-Poulsen S, Poling J, et al. The effect of individual cocaine withdrawal symptoms on outcomes in cocaine users. Addict Behav 2005; 30(6):1125–1134.
18. Nakatani Y, Hara T. Disturbance of consciousness due to methamphetamine abuse. A study of 2 patients. Psychopathology 1998; 31(3):131–137.
19. Underner M, Paquereau J, Meurice J. [Cigarette smoking and sleep disturbance] Rev Mal Respir 2006; 23(3 suppl):6S67–6S77.
20. Cummings KM, Giovino G, Jaen CR, et al. Reports of smoking withdrawal symptoms over a 21 day period of abstinence. Addict Behav 1985; 10(4):373–381.
21. Wetter DW, Fiore MC, Baker TB, et al. Tobacco withdrawal and nicotine replacement influence objective measures of sleep. J Consult Clin Psychol 1995; 63(4):658–667.
22. Monti JM, Monti D. Sleep disturbance in schizophrenia. Intl Rev Psychiatry 2005; 17(4):247–253.
23. Bittencourt LR, Silva RS, Santos RF, et al. Excessive daytime sleepiness. Rev Bras Psiquiatr 2005; 27(suppl 1):16–21.
24. Saper CB, Cano G, Scammell TE. Homeostatic, circadian, and emotional regulation of sleep. J Comp Neurol 2005; 493(1):92–98.
25. Lauterbach EC. The neuropsychiatry of Parkinson's disease. Minerva Med 2005; 96(3):155–173.
26. Boczarska-Jedynak M, Opala G. Sleep disturbances in Parkinson's disease. Neurol Neurochir Pol 2005; 39(5):380–388.
27. Eisensehr I, Schmidt D. Epilepsy and sleep disorders. MMW Fortschr Med 2005; 147(spec no 2):54–57.
28. Foldvary-Schaefer N, Grigg-Damberger M. Sleep and epilepsy: what we know, don't know, and need to know. J Clin Neurophysiol 2006; 23(1):4–20.
29. Vaughn BV, D'Cruz OF. Sleep and epilepsy. Semin Neurol 2004; 24(3):301–313.
30. McCurry SM, Gibbons LE, Logsdon RG, et al. Anxiety and nighttime behavioral disturbances. Awakenings in patients with Alzheimer's disease. J Gerontol Nurs 2004; 30(1):12–20.
31. Fleming WE, Pollak CP. Sleep disorders in multiple sclerosis. Semin Neurol 2005; 25(1):64–68.
32. Ohadinia S, Noroozian M, Shahsavand S, et al. Evaluation of insomnia and daytime napping in Iranian Alzheimer disease patients: relationship with severity of dementia and comparison with normal adults. Am J Geriatr Psychiatry 2004; 12(5):517–522.
33. Fleming WE, Pollak CP. Sleep disorders in multiple sclerosis. Semin Neurol 2005; 25(1):64–68.
34. Leppavuori A, Pohjasvaara T, Vataja R, et al. Insomnia in ischemic stroke patients. Cerebrovasc Dis 2002; 14(2):90–97.
35. Bassetti CL. Sleep and stroke. Semin Neurol 2005; 25(1):19–32.
36. Montagna P. Fatal familial insomnia: a model disease in sleep physiopathology. Sleep Med Rev 2005; 9(5):339–352.
37. Montagna P, Gambetti P, Cortelli P, et al. Familial and sporadic fatal insomnia. Lancet Neurol 2003; 2 (3):167–176.
38. Delisle MB, Uro-Coste E, Gray F, et al. Fatal familial insomnia. Clin Exp Pathol 1999; 47(3–4):176–180.
39. Richardson GS. The human circadian system in normal and disordered sleep. J Clin Psychiatry 2005; 66(suppl 9):3–9; quiz 42–43.
40. Doghramji K. Assessment of excessive sleepiness and insomnia as they relate to circadian rhythm sleep disorders. J Clin Psychiatry 2004; 65(suppl 16):17–22.
41. Reid KJ, Zee PC. Circadian rhythm disorders. Semin Neurol 2004; 24(3):315–325.
42. Waterhouse J, Nevill A, Finnegan J, et al. Further assessments of the relationship between jet lag and some of its symptoms. Chronobiol Int 2005; 22(1):121–136.
43. Katz G, Durst R, Zislin Y, et al. Psychiatric aspects of jet lag: review and hypothesis. Med Hypotheses 2001; 56(1):20–23.
44. Lagarde D, Doireau P. Jet lag. Med Trop (Mars) 1997; 57(4 bis):489–492.
45. Santhi N, Duffy JF, Horowitz TS, et al. Scheduling of sleep/darkness affects the circadian phase of night shift workers. Neurosci Lett 2005; 384(3):316–320.
46. Rouch I, Wild P, Ansiau D, et al. Shiftwork experience, age and cognitive performance. Ergonomics 2005; 48(10):1282–1293.
47. Boivin DB, James FO. Light treatment and circadian adaptation to shift work. Ind Health 2005; 43(1): 34–48.
48. Wyatt JK. Delayed sleep phase syndrome: pathophysiology and treatment options. Sleep 2004; 27(6): 1195–1203.
49. Watanabe T, Kajimura N, Kato M, et al. Sleep and circadian rhythm disturbances in patients with delayed sleep phase syndrome. Sleep 2003; 26(6):657–661.
50. Shirayama M, Shirayama Y, Iida H, et al. The psychological aspects of patients with delayed sleep phase syndrome (DSPS). Sleep Med 2003; 4(5):427–433.
51. Ondze B, Espa F, Ming LC, et al. Advanced sleep phase syndrome. Rev Neurol (Paris) 2001; 157(11 pt 2): S130–S134.

52. Avidan AY. Sleep in the geriatric patient population. Semin Neurol 2005; 25(1):52–63.
53. Kohsaka M. Non-24-hour sleep-wake syndrome. Nippon Rinsho 1998; 56(2):410–415.
54. Klein T, Martens H, Dijk DJ, et al. Circadian sleep regulation in the absence of light perception: chronic non-24-hour circadian rhythm sleep disorder in a blind man with a regular 24-hour sleep-wake schedule. Sleep 1993; 16(4):333–343.
55. Doljansky JT, Kannety H, Dagan Y. Working under daylight intensity lamp: an occupational risk for developing circadian rhythm sleep disorder? Chronobiol Int 2005; 22(3):597–605.
56. Aeschbach D, Sher L, Postolache TT, et al. A longer biological night in long sleepers than in short sleepers. J Clin Endocrinol Metab 2003; 88(1):26–30.
57. Barriere G, Cazalets JR, Bioulac B, et al. The restless legs syndrome. Prog Neurobiol 2005; 77(3):139–165.
58. Phillips B, Hening W, Britz P, et al. Prevalence and correlates of restless legs syndrome: results from the 2005 National Sleep Foundation Poll. Chest 2006; 129(1):76–80.
59. Sonka K, Kemlink D. Restless legs syndrome in 2004. Prague Med Rep 2004; 105(4):337–356.
60. Montplaisir J. Abnormal motor behavior during sleep. Sleep Med 2004; 5(suppl 1):S31–S34.
61. Gerhard R, Bosse A, Uzun D, et al. Quality of life in restless legs syndrome. Influence of daytime sleepiness and fatigue. Med Klin (Munich) 2005; 100(11):704–709.
62. Nozawa T. Periodic limb movement disorder. Nipon Rinsho 1998; 56(2):389–395.
63. Lesage S, Hening WA. The restless legs syndrome and periodic limb movement disorder: a review of management. Semin Neurol 2004; 24(3):249–259.
64. Yang C, White DP, Winkelman JW. Antidepressants and periodic leg movements of sleep. Biol Psychiatry 2005; 58(6):510–514.
65. Fusco L, Pachatz C, Cusmai R, et al. Repetitive sleep starts in neurologically impaired children: an unusual non-epileptic manifestation in otherwise epileptic subjects. Epileptic Disord 1999; 1(1):63–67.
66. Montagna P, Provini F, Plazzi G, et al. Propriospinal myoclonus upon relaxation and drowsiness: a cause of severe insomnia. Mov Disord 1997; 12(1):66–72.
67. Sander HW, Geisse H, Quinto C, et al. Sensory sleep starts. J Neurol Neurosurg Psychiatry 1998; 64(5):690.
68. Kanaan N, Sawaya R. Nocturnal leg cramps. Clinically mysterious and painful–but manageable. Geriatrics 2001; 56(6):34, 39–42.
69. Caples SM, Kara T, Somers VK. Cardiopulmonary consequences of obstructive sleep apnea. Semin Respir Crit Care Med 2005; 26(1):25–32.
70. Baguet JP, Narkiewicz K, Mallion JM. Update on hypertension management: obstructive sleep apnea and hypertension. J Hypertens 2006; 24(1):205–208.
71. Collop NA. Obstructive sleep apnea: what does the cardiovascular physician need to know? Am J Cardiovasc Drugs 2005; 5(2):71–81.
72. Ryan CM, Bradley TD. Pathogenesis of obstructive sleep apnea. J Appl Physiol 2005; 99(6):2440–2450.
73. Deane S, Thomson A. Obesity and the pulmonologist. Arch Dis Child 2006; 91(2):188–191.
74. White DP. Pathogenesis of obstructive and central sleep apnea. Am J Respir Crit Care Med 2005; 172(11):1363–1370.
75. White DP. Central sleep apnea. Med Clin North Am 1985; 69(6):1205–1219.
76. Wisskirchen T, Teschler H. Central sleep apnea syndrome and Cheyne-Stokes respiration. Ther Umsch 2000; 57(7):458–462.
77. Caples SM, Wolk R, Somers VK. Influence of cardiac function and failure on sleep-disordered breathing: evidence for a causative role. J Appl Physiol 2005; 99(6):2433–2439.
78. Ingbir M, Freimark D, Adler Y. Cheyne-Stokes breathing disorder in patients with congestive heart failure: incidence, pathophysiology, treatment and prognosis. Harefuah 2001; 140(12):1209–1212, 1227.
79. Cherniack NS, Longobardo G, Evangelista CJ. Causes of Cheyne-Stokes respiration. Neurocrit Care 2005; 3(3):271–279.
80. Maggiorini M. Mountaineering and altitude sickness. Ther Umsch 2001; 58(6):387–393.
81. Przybylowski T, Ashirbaev A, Le Roux J, et al. Sleep and breathing at altitude of 3800 m–the acclimatization effect. Pneumonol Alergol Pol 2003; 71(5–6):213–220.
82. Mizuno K, Asano K, Inoue Y, et al. Consecutive monitoring of sleep disturbance for four nights at the top of Mt Fuji (3776 m). Psychiatry Clin Neurosci 2005; 59(2):223–225.
83. Krachman S, Criner GJ. Hypoventilation syndromes. Clin Chest Med 1998; 19(1):139–155.
84. Annane D, Chevrolet JC, Chevret S, et al. Nocturnal mechanical ventilation for chronic hypoventilation in patients with neuromuscular and chest wall disorders. Cochrane Database Syst Rev 2000; (2): CD001941.
85. Perrin C, D'Ambrosio C, White A, et al. Sleep in restrictive and neuromuscular respiratory disorders. Semin Respir Crit Care Med 2005; 26(1):117–130.
86. Kutty K. Sleep and chronic obstructive pulmonary disease. Curr Opin Pulm Med 2004; 10(2):104–112.
87. Henry Benitez M, Morera Fumero AL, Gonzalez Martin IJ, et al. Insomnia in asthmatic patients. Spanish. Actas Luso Esp Neurol Psiquiatr Cienc Afines 1994; 22(4):164–170.
88. McNicholas WT. Impact of sleep in COPD. Chest 2000; 117(2 suppl):48S–53S.

89. George CF. Perspectives on the management of insomnia in patients with chronic respiratory disorders. Sleep 2000; 23(suppl 1):S31–S35; discussion S36–S38.
90. Weitzenblum E, Chaouat A. Sleep and chronic obstructive pulmonary disease. Sleep Med Rev 2004; 8(4):281–294.
91. Johnson DA, Orr WC, Crawley JA, et al. Effect of esomeprazole on nighttime heartburn and sleep quality in patients with GERD: a randomized, placebo-controlled trial. Am J Gastroenterol 2005; 100 (9):1914–1922.
92. de Oliveira SS, dos Santos Ida S, da Silva JF, et al. Gastroesophageal reflux disease: prevalence and associated factors. Arq Gastroenterol 2005; 42(2):116–121.
93. Fass R, Ouan SF, O'Connor GT, et al. Predictors of heartburn during sleep in a large prospective cohort study. Chest 2005; 127(5):1658–1666.
94. Orr WC. Therapeutic options in the treatment of nighttime gastroesophageal reflux. Digestion 2005; 72(4):229–238.
95. Lu CL, Yee YC, Tsai SJ, et al. Psychiatric disturbances associated with hyperthyroidism: an analysis report of 30 cases. Zhonghua Yi Xue Za Zhi (Taipei) 1995; 56(6):393–398.
96. Kittle WM, Chaudhary BA. Sleep apnea and hypothyroidism. South Med J 1988; 81(11):1421–1425.
97. Chou FF, Lee CH, Chen JB, et al. Sleep disturbances before and after parathyroidectomy for secondary hyperparathyroidism. Surgery 2005; 137(4):426–430.
98. Edinger JD, Wohlgemuth WK, Krystal AD, et al. Behavioral insomnia therapy for fibromyalgia patients: a randomized clinical trial. Arch Intern Med 2005; 165(21):2527–2535.
99. Polanska B. Fibromyalgia syndrome—pathogenesis, diagnosis, and treatment problems. Pol Merkur Lekarski 2004; 16(91):93–96.
100. Rizzi M, Sarzi-Puttini P, Atzeni F, et al. Cyclic alternating pattern: a new marker of sleep alteration in patients with fibromyalgia? J Rheumatol 2004; 31(6):1193–1199.
101. Dzaja A, Arber S, Hislop J, et al. Women's sleep in health and disease. J Psychiatr Res 2005; 39(1):55–76.
102. Manconi M, Govoni V, De Vito A, et al. Restless legs syndrome and pregnancy. Neurology 2004; 63(6):1065–1069.
103. Pien GW, Schwab RJ. Sleep disorders during pregnancy. Sleep 2004; 27(7):1405–1417.
104. Izci B, Vennelle M, Liston WA, et al. Sleep-disordered breathing and upper airway size in pregnancy and post-partum. Eur Respir J 2006; 27(2):321–327.
105. Izci B, Riha RL, Martin SE, et al. The upper airway in pregnancy and pre-eclampsia. Am J Respir Crit Care Med 2003; 167(2):137–140.
106. Van P, Cage T, Shannon M. Big dreams, little sleep: dreams during pregnancy after prior pregnancy loss. Holist Nurs Pract 2004; 18(6):284–292.
107. Landis CA, Moe KE. Sleep and menopause. Nurs Clin North Am 2004; 39(1):97–115.
108. Moline ML, Broch L, Zak R, et al. Sleep in women across the life cycle from adulthood through menopause. Sleep Med Rev 2003; 7(2):155–177.
109. Miller EH. Women and insomnia. Clin Cornerstone 2004; 6(suppl 1B):S8–S18.
110. Polo-Kantola P, Rauhala E, Helenius H, et al. Breathing during sleep in menopause: a randomized, controlled, crossover trial with estrogen therapy. Obstet Gynecol 2003; 102(1):68–75.
111. Walters JF, Hampton SM, Ferns GA, et al. Effect of menopause on melatonin and alertness rhythms investigated in constant routine conditions. Chronobiol Int 2005; 22(5):859–872.
112. Jennum P, Jensen R. Sleep and headache. Sleep Med Rev 2002; 6(6):471–479.
113. Kelman L, Rains JC. Headache and sleep: examination of sleep patterns and complaints in a large clinical sample of migraineurs. Headache 2005; 45(7):904–910.
114. Weintraub JR. Cluster headaches and sleep disorders. Curr Pain Headache Rep 2003; 7(2):150–156.
115. Cohen AS, Kaube H. Rare nocturnal headaches. Curr Opin Neurol 2004; 17(3):295–299.
116. Manni R, Sances G, Terzaghi M, et al. Hypnic headache: PSG evidence of both REM- and NREM-related attacks. Neurology 2004; 62(8):1411–1413.
117. Obermeyer WH, Benca RM. Effects of drugs on sleep. Neurol Clin 1996; 14(4):827–840.
118. Lam RW. Sleep disturbances and depression: a challenge for antidepressants. Int Clin Psychopharmacol 2006; 21(1):S25–S29.
119. Mayers AG, Baldwin DS. Antidepressants and their effect on sleep. Hum Psychopharmacol 2005; 20(8):533–559.
120. Yang C, White DP, Winkelman JW. Antidepressants and periodic leg movements of sleep. Biol Psychiatry 2005; 58(6):510–514.
121. Wilson S, Argyropoulos S. Antidepressants and sleep: a qualitative review of the literature. Drugs 2005; 65(7):927–947.
122. Bardage C, Isacson DG. Self-reported side-effects of antihypertensive drugs: an epidemiological study on prevalence and impact on health-state utility. Blood Press 2000; 9(6):328–334.
123. Cicolin A, Magliola U, Giordano A, et al. Effects of levetiracetam on nocturnal sleep and daytime vigilance in healthy volunteers. Epilepsia 2006; 47(1):82–85.

124. Welch MJ, Meltzer EO, Simons FE, et al. H1-antihistamines and the central nervous system. Clin Allergy Immunol 2002; 17:337–388.

125. Haydon RC 3rd. Are second-generation antihistamines appropriate for most children and adults? Arch Otolaryngol Head Neck Surg 2001; 127(12):1510–1513.

126. Meltzer EO. Antihistamine- and decongestant-induced performance decrements. J Occup Med 1990; 32(4):327–334.

127. Ferguson BJ. Influences of allergic rhinitis on sleep. Otolaryngol Head Neck Surg 2004; 130(5):617–629.

128. Storms WW, Bodman SF, Nathan RA, et al. SCH 434: a new antihistamine/decongestant for seasonal allergic rhinitis. J Allergy Clin Immunol 1989; 83(6):1083–1090.

129. Steiger A. Thyroid gland and sleep. Acta Med Austriaca 1999; 26(4):132–133.

130. No authors listed. Headache, migraine and oral contraceptives. Contracept Rep 1998; 8(6):12–14, 16.

131. Burdick RS, Hoffmann R, Armitage R. Short note: oral contraceptives and sleep in depressed and healthy women. Sleep 2002; 25(3):347–349.

132. Auger RR, Goodman SH, Silber MH, et al. Risks of high-dose stimulants in the treatment of disorders of excessive somnolence: a case-control study. Sleep 2005; 28(6):667–672.

133. Becker PM, Schwartz JR, Feldman NT, et al. Effect of modafinil on fatigue, mood, and health-related quality of life in patients with narcolepsy. Psychopharmacology 2004; 171(2):133–139.

134. Hall RC, Popkin MK, Stickney SK, et al. Presentation of the steroid psychoses. J Nerv Ment Dis 1979; 167(4):229–236.

135. Meixner R, Gerhardstein R, Day R, et al. The alerting effects of dexamethasone. Psychophysiology 2003; 40(2):254–259.

136. Hansel TT, Tennant RC, Tan AJ, et al. Theophylline: mechanism of action and use in asthma and chronic obstructive pulmonary disease. Drugs Today (Barc) 2004; 40(1):55–69.

137. Richardt D, Driver HS. An evaluative study of the short-term effects of once-daily, sustained-release theophylline on sleep in nocturnal asthmatics. S Afr Med J 1996; 86(7):803–804.

138. Sacco C, Braghiroli A, Grossi E, et al. The effects of doxofylline versus theophylline on sleep architecture in COPD patients. Monaldi Arch Chest Dis 1995; 50(2):98–103.

139. Sano H, Itoh H. Idiopathic insomnia. Nippon Rinsho 1998; 56(2):361–364.

7 | Behavioral Treatment of Insomnia

Jack D. Edinger
Psychology Service, VA Medical Center and Department of Psychiatry and Behavioral Sciences, Duke University Medical Center, Durham, North Carolina, U.S.A.

Colleen E. Carney
Department of Psychology, Ryerson University, Toronto, Ontario, Canada

INTRODUCTION AND TREATMENT RATIONALE

Insomnia is a prevalent disorder characterized by difficulty initiating or maintaining sleep or by chronically poor sleep quality. Accompanying nocturnal sleep disruption are daytime complaints (e.g., fatigue, poor concentration, lowered social functioning, etc.) that can significantly compromise daily functioning, health status, and quality of life (1–5). Sleep difficulties may arise from a variety of conditions or circumstances, such as stress, environmental factors, changes to the sleep-wake cycle, medical or psychiatric illnesses, or ingestion of sleep-disrupting substances. Regardless of the precipitating factors, insomnia may assume a chronic course perpetuated by psychological, emotional, and behavioral anomalies that persist over time and cause continual sleep disruption (6–8). Included among these are dysfunctional beliefs and attitudes that may contribute to sleep-related performance anxiety and lead to sleep-disruptive bedtime arousal (6,9). In addition, patient's misconceptions about sleep-promoting practices may give way to a variety of compensatory strategies that only further disrupt sleep. For example, daytime napping or spending extra time in bed in pursuit of elusive, unpredictable sleep may only serve to interfere with normal homeostatic mechanisms designed to operate automatically in the face of sleep debt. Alternately, the habit of remaining in bed well beyond the normal rising time, following a poor night's sleep, may disrupt circadian mechanisms and make subsequent sleep more difficult. Additionally, failure to discontinue mentally demanding work and allot sufficient *wind-down time* before bed may serve as a significant sleep inhibitor during the subsequent sleeping period. Over time, these cognitive and behavioral anomalies may result in the repeated association of the bed and bedroom with unsuccessful sleep attempts and lead to the development of sleep-disruptive conditioned arousal in response to the home sleeping environment.

Given the important perpetuating roles various cognitive and behavioral factors may play in insomnia, behavior therapy is often appropriate as a primary or adjunctive treatment for managing this condition. In the current chapter we describe the nature and treatment focus of each of the more commonly employed behavioral insomnia therapies. We also review results from applications of these treatments with various subtypes of insomnia and consider both the relative and combined efficacy of behavioral and pharmacologic insomnia therapies. In addition, we discuss various issues related to treatment implementation such as cost-effectiveness, methods of delivery, treatment durability, treatment adherence, and predictors of long-term treatment response. We conclude our discussion by outlining the current limitations in the cognitive-behavioral therapy (CBT) insomnia literature and suggesting directions for future research.

DESCRIPTION OF THE BEHAVIORAL INSOMNIA THERAPIES

To date, a variety of behavior therapies have been developed to treat chronic insomnia. Although the nature and focus of these treatments varies considerably, they all are designed to reestablish normal functioning of the human biological sleep system via eradicating behavioral and conditioning factors that serve to perpetuate insomnia. The following text provides more detailed descriptions and general evaluations of each of these treatments.

Relaxation Therapies

Relaxation therapies were among the earliest behavioral strategies used to treat insomnia with case studies describing such approaches first appearing in the late 1950s. Since that time, a host of formal relaxation therapies including progressive muscle relaxation training, autogenic training, imagery training, biofeedback, and hypnosis have been used to treat insomnia (10–13). Common to these approaches is their focus on sleep-related performance anxiety and bedtime arousal, which often perpetuate sleep difficulties. Regardless of the specific relaxation strategy used, treatment entails teaching the insomnia patients formal exercises designed to reduce anxiety and arousal at bedtime so that sleep initiation is facilitated. For example, progressive muscle relaxation training (14) involves teaching these patients to alternately tense then relax each of 16 major skeletal muscle groups so as to help them discriminate between somatic tension and relaxation and to enhance their ability to develop a relaxation response to sleep-disruptive bedtime arousal. Whereas the specific training exercises vary from one form of relaxation to the next, most forms of this therapy require multiple treatment sessions with additional intersession home practice to achieve optimal result. The goal of this training is to assist the patient in achieving sufficient relaxation skills so that insomnia resulting from sleep-related performance anxiety and bedtime arousal can be minimized or eliminated.

Relaxation therapies have been used with relative frequency in addressing various insomnia subtypes. Available evidence suggests that the relaxation therapies are moderately effective in managing insomnia symptoms, particularly sleep onset complaints. A recent evidence-based review (15), in fact, supports the efficacy of relaxation therapy for insomnia and suggests that it can be considered a well-established and recommended treatment for this condition. Currently the various forms of this treatment are considered equally effective as evidence suggesting that the superiority of one relaxation technique over another for treating insomnia is currently lacking.

Stimulus Control

This approach, developed by Bootzin (16), is based on the assumption that both the timing (bedtime) and setting (bed/bedroom) associated with repeated unsuccessful sleep attempts, over time, become conditioned cues that perpetuate insomnia. Given this assumption, the goal of this treatment is that of reassociating the bed and bedroom with successful sleep efforts. To achieve this endpoint, patients are encouraged to follow a structured regimen designed to curtail sleep-incompatible activities in the bed and bedroom and to establish a consistent sleep-wake schedule. In practice, stimulus control requires instructing the insomnia patient to (*i*) go to bed only when sleepy; (*ii*) establish a standard wake-up time; (*iii*) get out of bed whenever awake for more than15 to 20 minutes; (*iv*) avoid reading, watching TV, eating, worrying and other sleep-incompatible behaviors in the bed and bedroom; and (*v*) refrain from daytime napping. From a theoretical perspective, it is probable that strict adherence to this regimen not only eliminates sleep-disruptive conditioned arousal but also reestablishes a normal sleep drive and sleep-wake rhythm. From a practical viewpoint, this treatment is easily understood and usually can be administered in one visit. However, follow-up visits are usually conducted to assure treatment adherence and achieve optimal success.

Both the straightforward nature of the stimulus control regimen and extensive research with this technique have made this treatment one of the most popular and widely used behavioral insomnia therapies. Current evidence (17–19) suggests that stimulus control is more efficacious than most other stand-alone behavioral insomnia therapies in the management of sleep onset and sleep maintenance difficulties. As a consequence it is currently regarded as a well-established and recommended therapy (15) for the management of chronic insomnia complaints.

Sleep Restriction

All too commonly, insomnia patients spend excessively long periods in bed at night to offset their extended periods of wakefulness by providing them ample additional opportunity to get the sleep they feel they need. Unfortunately, insomnia patients may experience excessive time awake each night simply *because* they are allotting far too much time for sleep. Given this observation, Spielman and colleagues (20) developed the behavioral intervention, sleep restriction therapy (SRT) to correct this sleep-disruptive habit. In practice, SRT entails instructing the patient to restrict time allotted for sleep each night so that the time spent in bed closely matches the patient's actual sleep requirement. Typically this treatment begins by having the patient maintain a sleep diary (a record of each night's sleep) for two to three weeks. Subsequently, the patient's average total sleep time (ATST) is calculated from the diary.

An initial time-in-bed (TIB) prescription may be set either at the ATST or at a value equal to the ATST plus an amount of time that is deemed to represent normal nocturnal wakefulness for the patient's particular age group (21). However, unless persuasive evidence suggests the patient has an unusually low sleep requirement, the initial TIB prescription is seldom set below 5 hours per night. On subsequent visits, the TIB prescription is increased by 15- to 20-minute increments following weeks the patient is sleeping more than 85% or 90% of the TIB, on average, and continues to report daytime sleepiness. Conversely, TIB is usually reduced by similar amounts following weeks wherein the individual, on average, sleeps less that 80% of the time spent in bed. Since TIB adjustments are usually necessary, SRT typically entails an initial visit to introduce treatment instructions and follow-up visits to alter TIB prescriptions.

Like stimulus control therapy, SRT is a straightforward and simple-to-implement approach. Moreover, current evidence suggests that its efficacy is well established (15) and it is among the most effective stand-alone behavioral insomnia therapies (17–19). Nonetheless, for a subset of insomnia patients, SRT enhances sleep-related performance anxiety because they interpret reduced TIB as a reduced opportunity to sleep. Such patients often have difficulty adhering to SRT due to their heightened sleep-related anxiety. For these patients, gradual rather than precipitous TIB reductions have been suggested (22,23) to improve patient adherence and enhance treatment outcome.

Paradoxical Intention

Designed mainly to address patients' sleep-disruptive performance anxiety and exaggerated efforts to sleep, paradoxical intention involves instructing the insomnia patient to remain awake as long as possible after retiring to bed (24). The patient is instructed to purposefully engage in the feared activity (staying awake) in order to reduce performance anxiety and conscious intent to sleep that confound associated goal-directed behavior (falling asleep). This method alleviates both the patient's excessive focus on sleep and anxiety over not sleeping; as a result, sleep becomes less difficult to initiate. Treatment implementation typically involves an initial visit to provide treatment instructions and follow-up sessions to support the patient and assess treatment enactment. Although less widely used than the above-described approaches, paradoxical intention is currently regarded as a well-established and efficacious behavioral insomnia therapy (15). However, some authors (25,26) have noted rather mixed results across patients with this approach.

Sleep Hygiene

Sleep hygiene connotes a loosely defined set of recommendations targeting lifestyle and environmental problems that may disrupt sleep. Sleep hygiene therapy typically consists of education about healthy sleep behaviors and sleep-conducive environmental conditions (27). For example, insomnia patients may be encouraged to exercise daily; eliminate the use of caffeine, alcohol, and nicotine; eat a light bedtime snack that includes food items (e.g., milk products, peanut butter) rich in the sleep-promoting amino acid, L-tryptophan; and ensure that the sleeping environment is quiet, dark, and comfortable. Whereas such commonsense advice is often useful in the overall management of insomnia, sleep hygiene therapy is among the lesser effective behavioral interventions when used in isolation (15). Thus, sleep hygiene is seldom used as a primary intervention, but is often combined with other behavioral therapies.

Cognitive Therapies

Underlying and supporting performance anxiety and sleep-disruptive habits of insomnia sufferers is a host of cognitive/psychological factors that serve to perpetuate sleep disturbance. Among these are dysfunctional beliefs and attitudes about sleep (9,28) that heighten sleep-related anxiety and promote sleep-interfering habits. For example, beliefs that sleep is unpredictable and uncontrollable or that one must obtain 8 hours of sleep at night to function each day can add to anxiety about sleep and, in turn, interfere with the sleep process. Furthermore, insufficient knowledge about how one should respond to a night of poor sleep may lead to practices such as daytime napping or "sleeping in," which disrupt the ensuing night's sleep. Given increasing recognition of these types of sleep-related misconceptions, therapeutic strategies that specifically target and correct these dysfunctional beliefs have increasingly been used in insomnia treatment. Most often this form of cognitive therapy entails formalized patient education modules or cognitive restructuring methods similar to those commonly used in cognitive therapy with clinically depressed individuals (29).

In addition to dysfunctional sleep-related beliefs, cognitive arousal arising from sleep-disruptive practices such as engagement in mentally stimulating activities immediately prior to bedtime or the habit of *taking ones worries to bed* is a fairly common sleep disruptor among insomnia patients. As such, encouraging patients to avoid mentally stimulating activities in the hour or so before bedtime and schedule an early-evening structured problem-solving time to address daily worries (30) are additional cognitive therapy approaches that may be employed to reduce mental arousal during the sleep period. Whereas these and the above-mentioned cognitive strategies are generally regarded as useful for the overall management of insomnia, no studies have examined the efficacy of such approaches used in isolation to treat insomnia patients.

Cognitive-Behavioral Therapy

This treatment strategy might best be regarded as a *second-generation*, multicomponent behavioral insomnia treatment that evolved from the above-described strategies. CBT typically consists of one or more of the cognitive therapy strategies used in combination with both stimulus control and sleep-restriction therapies (6,7,15). Often sleep hygiene and some type of relaxation therapy are included in the CBT protocol. One presumed advantage of this multicomponent treatment is that it includes strategies for addressing the range of cognitive and behavioral anomalies that perpetuate insomnia. As a result, this treatment should be more universally effective across insomnia sufferers regardless of their presenting complaint (i.e., sleep onset complaints vs. sleep maintenance difficulty). Although CBT is a multicomponent and seemingly more complex treatment than those previously described, in practice, this intervention usually requires no more therapist or patient treatment time than do the first-generation treatments reviewed above. The cognitive therapy and behavioral instructions are typically provided in two to eight sessions; however, most CBT clinicians employ multiple treatment sessions to provide sufficient support and follow-up. Over recent years, CBT has become an increasingly popular form of insomnia therapy and arguably now represents the treatment of choice among the available behavioral insomnia therapies. Moreover, there is ample evidence that this multicomponent treatment, with or without the addition of a form of relaxation therapy, is an effective intervention (15,31,32). As such, much of the discussion in the ensuing sections considers the utility and effectiveness of CBT for various types of insomnia patients.

Applications to Primary Insomnia

CBT for insomnia developed out of a translational research tradition. Translational research bridges between the development or modification of treatments and psychopathology/risk factor research. Research on the factors thought to purport insomnia thus informs interventions designed to address such factors. This approach would be of most value to clinical researchers in insomnia if evidence supported that the intervention (*i*) improved sleep and related outcome measures such as quality of life or mood and (*ii*) improved the factors that CBT is targeting (i.e., excessive TIB). For example, research suggests that some insomnia patients catastrophize about the effects of sleep loss. An ideal outcome for such a patient would be a reduction in catastrophizing about sleep loss, in addition to a decreased amount of time spent awake in bed, thus addressing the sleep complaint and the risk factor. In the ensuing sections, we will review the evidence that CBT produces improvements in sleep outcomes, and has a positive effect on the sleep-interfering factors thought to be mechanistically important in insomnia.

The effect of CBT on sleep and other outcomes. Early single-subject studies supported the efficacy of CBT in significantly reducing the time spent awake after sleep onset (33,34). These studies also suggested the effects of CBT are durable, as treatment gains are maintained into the three- to six-month follow-up period (33,34). Large-scale randomized clinical trials (RCTs) have also supported the use of CBT with primary insomnia patients. In an early RCT (35), CBT produced a 53% reduction in the time spent awake after sleep onset on a subjective measure (i.e., daily monitoring of sleep via sleep diary). Equally as impressive, this study showed patients achieved a 51% reduction on wakefulness after sleep onset (WASO) measured by polysomnography. Furthermore, meta-analytic studies suggest that behavioral insomnia therapies produce large mean treatment effects on subjective sleep estimates of sleep onset latency (SOL), WASO, number of awakenings (NWAK), total sleep time (TST), and sleep quality ratings (17–19).

In addition to examining changes from pre- to posttreatment and the associated effect sizes for continuous sleep variables, it is also useful to evaluate sleep change on a criterion variable. One RCT (31) found that greater proportions of those treated with CBT (64%) met clinical improvement criteria (i.e., a 50% pre- to posttreatment reduction in wake time after sleep onset) relative to those treated with relaxation (12%) or placebo control (8%). In a study of abbreviated two-session CBT, 60% of CBT patients achieved at least a 50% pre- to posttreatment reduction in wake time after sleep onset as compared to 0% of a group treated solely with sleep hygiene therapy. Similarly, 56% of the CBT group had posttreatment scores in the normal range on an Insomnia Symptom Questionnaire (20), as compared with none of the sleep hygiene group members. In a meta-analytic look at clinical effectiveness, at least 50% of those treated with CBT or other validated behavioral insomnia treatment experienced at least a 33% reduction in sleep diary SOL as well as a posttreatment SOL of 35 minutes or less (18).

Along with the large number of efficacy trials, there have been a number of clinical effectiveness studies designed to test CBT with these types of patients seen in day-to-day clinic settings (36,37). One such study (37) evaluated an abbreviated CBT developed for a primary care setting against a wait-list control group. CBT produced a mean reduction in SOL of 33 minutes, as compared to a mean reduction of 4 minutes for the control condition (37). Of those in the CBT group using sleep medications at baseline, 76% were medication-free at the end of treatment and 80% were medication-free at one-year posttreatment. The results of this effectiveness study are thus commensurate with efficacy study findings. That is, CBT is not just effective in highly selected/screened study patients; it is also an effective treatment in the types of primary insomnia sufferers seen in typical clinical venues.

Does CBT address the perpetuating mechanisms it targets? There are several hypothesized cognitive and behavioral factors that purportedly perpetuate or maintain insomnias. Of the perpetuating cognitive factors, maladaptive sleep-related beliefs are among the most commonly implicated. Thus, a belief-targeted treatment such as CBT would be expected to modify maladaptive beliefs, and such a decline in these beliefs should relate to sleep improvement. As expected, CBT trials have demonstrated significant pre- to posttreatment reduction in the beliefs thought to perpetuate insomnia, and such belief modification relates to clinical indices of sleep improvement (31,32,38,39). Another cognitive factor implicated in insomnia relates to a reduced sense of self-efficacy or confidence in the ability to produce sleep (26,40). Thus, one would predict that sleep-related self-efficacy should improve as treated patients implement the behavioral strategies and gain more experience with improved sleep. Studies have supported that clinical improvement on sleep indices in CBT-treated groups are related to significant increases in sleep-related self-efficacy at follow-up assessments (31,36,41).

Lastly, the most common cognitive factor cited by patients as perpetuating insomnia is "cognitive arousal" (42,43). "Cognitive arousal" is an umbrella term that has been used to describe mental processes in bed (i.e., excessive mentation, worry, environmental monitoring, racing thoughts, rumination, and problem solving). Thus, it is expected that CBT would reduce cognitive arousal in successfully treated patients. Although there are many studies documenting the sleep-interfering effects of cognitive arousal (44–46) there are few studies wherein the effect of CBT on the arousal is reported (47). Some studies using progressive muscle relaxation (PMR) have reported decreased cognitive intrusions (48). Other studies have combined elements of CBT, such as paradoxical intention or PMR, with cognitive techniques, such as thought stopping, and generally, these interventions have resulted in decreased cognitive arousal as well as sleep improvements (49–51). Most studies however report on isolated cognitive-specific strategies to target the arousal. Such studies have demonstrated both improved sleep and improved presleep cognitive arousal (30,52–54). It should be noted that many of these strategies have not been tested in clinical trials with treatment-seeking people with insomnia; thus, more work is needed to assess their utility in a clinical setting. The preponderance of studies documenting that this is a problem for patients

(30,42,43) and that presleep mental activity has sleep-interfering effects (44–46) suggests that this is an important area for future research.

In addition to cognitive factors, a number of behavioral factors in insomnia have been identified. One such maintaining factor is spending an "excessive" amount of time in bed. Remaining in bed for a longer period than the hours of sleep reliably produced results in an increased time spent awake in bed. One would predict that clinical improvement on sleep variables would be associated with a decrease in the amount of time in bed. Studies suggest that behavioral interventions successfully address excessive time in bed and reductions are associated with sleep improvement (20). The reductions in TIB are not associated with decreased TST, thus matching TIB to sleep need. Lastly, variability in bedtime and rise time has been implicated in disturbed sleep (8,16,40,55). A number of studies have suggested that regulating bedtime and rise time is associated with sleep improvement (16,32,33,35–37,56–58). Thus, clinical trials have generally supported that CBT produces an improvement in sleep indices, and also improves many of the cognitive and behavioral factors thought to be important in insomnia.

Pharmacological, Behavioral, and Combined Treatments

Both cognitive-behavioral insomnia treatments and pharmacotherapy with benzodiazepine receptor agonists (BZRAs) have well-proven efficacy (15,32,59,60), but studies designed as head-to-head comparisons of these two forms of treatment have been surprisingly absent from the literature. One notable exception to this trend is the study by Waters et al. (61) that compared behavioral treatments consisting of sleep hygiene alone, relaxation treatment combined with a cognitive distraction technique, and a combined stimulus control/sleep restriction intervention with a medication treatment consisting of 15 mg of the BZRA, flurazepam, administered nightly at bedtime. Pre- to posttreatment comparisons conducted over a two-week treatment phase suggested that the medication therapy was more effective in reducing subjective sleep onset and maintenance difficulties than were the three behavioral treatments. Furthermore, treatment adherence to medication therapy was somewhat better than it was for the behavioral treatments. Unfortunately, a relatively small sample size ($N = 53$) and lack of long-term follow-up data limit this study's generalizability and obviate conclusions about the durability of treatments over time.

Despite the general lack of direct comparisons of cognitive-behavioral and pharmacological therapies for insomnia, several meta-analytic reviews of behavioral and pharmacological treatment studies have provided some insights into the relative efficacy of these treatment approaches. These meta-analyses reviewed and extracted treatment outcome data reported for various behavioral insomnia therapies (17,18), BZRAs (60), or both types of treatment (19) in order to derive estimates of their treatment effect sizes on subjective indices of SOL, sleep maintenance difficulty, and sleep quality. Figure 1 shows the averaged treatment effect sizes for the behavioral and pharmacological insomnia therapies derived from these meta-analyses. This figure shows that both the behavioral and pharmacological therapies have medium to large effect sizes for improving the sleep measures considered. The behavioral therapies appear to have an advantage over pharmacotherapy in reducing SOL and improving subjective sleep quality, whereas pharmacotherapy is relatively more effective than the behavioral treatments in reducing the frequency of arousals and increasing total sleep time. Overall, these findings suggest that behavioral insomnia therapies perform relatively well and compare favorably to the BZRAs for treating insomnia.

Of course, each of these treatment approaches has its relative advantages and disadvantages. BZRA therapy usually results in immediate improvement in sleep once treatment is initiated. However, concerns have been raised about the long-term efficacy of various BZRA agents and the potential for psychological dependence on such medications (62). In contrast, treatment effects are more delayed with CBT and other behavioral treatments although such therapies tend to produce improvements that endure over extended time periods (15,63). In view of these considerations, some investigators have explored the utility of combining pharmacological and behavioral insomnia therapies to take advantage of each approach's relative advantages and overcome their individual limitations. In the short term, a combined treatment would be expected to result in rapid sleep improvements due to the quick action of sleep medication, whereas in the long term, improvements should endure after

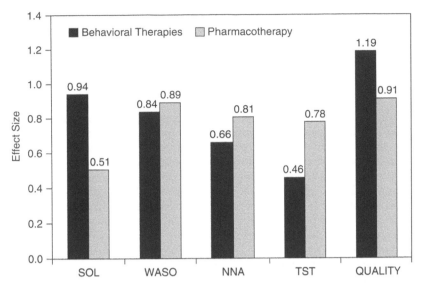

Figure 1 Relative treatment effect sizes for behavioral and pharmacological insomnia therapies. This figure was provided to the authors for use in this chapter by Charles M. Morin, Ph.D., and we wish to thank him for his willingness to share this figure. Information presented in the figure was drawn from meta-analyses conducted by Morin et al. (17), Murtagh and Greenwood (18), and Smith et al. (19) concerning the efficacy of behavioral insomnia treatments, and by Nowell et al. (60) concerning the efficacy of benzodiazepine hypnotics and zolpidem for treating insomnia. As employed in these meta-analyses, the term, *treatment effect size,* reflects the average amount of difference (expressed as a fraction of the pooled standard deviation) observed between treated and untreated subjects. Hence, an effect size of 0.5 would indicate that treated subjects, on average, showed one-half standard deviation greater improvement than did control subjects. In clinical treatment studies, effect sizes in the 0.2 range typically are considered *small,* those in the 0.5 range are considered *medium,* and those ≥ 0.8 are considered *large* (147). *Abbreviations*: SOL, sleep onset latency; WASO, wake time after sleep onset; NNA, number of nocturnal awakenings; TST, total sleep time; Quality, subjective sleep quality ratings.

medication withdrawal as a function of the behavioral therapy included in the combined intervention.

However, clinical trials conducted to test such combined treatments have provided rather mixed results. A number of studies (32,64–66) have suggested that combined behavioral/pharmacological insomnia treatments produce greater short-term improvements (e.g., via pre- vs. posttreatment comparisons) than do either forms of treatment used alone. In contrast, one study (67) showed the short-term treatment results from a BZRA medication used alone to be superior to combined medication/behavioral treatment, whereas another study (68) found CBT to be superior to a therapy wherein medication was used in combination with CBT for the initial three weeks of a six-week treatment. Furthermore, two (32,64) of the studies supporting the relative short-term benefits of combined therapies also showed better long-term results at one- to two-year follow-ups in those treated with behavioral insomnia therapy alone. However, a small ($N = 17$) clinical trial (69) showed that a treatment sequence of five weeks of combined medication/CBT treatment followed by five weeks of CBT alone was superior to the reverse sequence or to CBT alone when both short- and long-term benefits of treatment were considered. These latter results suggest that proper treatment sequencing may be needed to optimize therapy outcomes. Nonetheless, it appears most accurate to conclude that an optimum model for combining behavioral and pharmacological treatments has yet to be determined; hence, more studies designed to test combined treatment models are definitely merited.

Using CBT to Aid Hypnotic Discontinuation

Although sleep medications have demonstrated efficacy, their long-term use may become problematic for many insomnia patients. For example, some BZRA medications have a risk of tolerance and reduced efficacy over time. Such medications also have risks for increased falls and decreased cognitive functioning particularly among the disproportionate number of older adults who use such medications. In addition, there is some suggestion that tapering benzodiazepine (BZD) medications in many long-term users does not result in any sleep changes relative to those who remain on their medications (70). Discontinuing BZD medication may also result in cognitive functioning improvements. Given these considerations and the ongoing cost of pharmacotherapy, many long-term users of sleep medications may eventually desire to discontinue their use of these agents.

However, many with this desire encounter the problem of insomnia rebound upon discontinuation either due to physiological dependence, or owing more commonly to their psychological dependence. Indeed, within the diagnostic nomenclature is an insomnia diagnosis characterized by an insomnia that is "hypnotic induced." As noted by Lichstein et al. (71) the threat of withdrawal symptoms and rebound insomnia can discourage those wanting to stop their medications from doing so. To address this phenomenon, there has been a growing interest in using psychological and behavioral insomnia therapies to assist patients in their hypnotic discontinuation. Kirmil-Gray et al. (72), for example, tested the effectiveness of a stress-management skill training program in helping women discontinue their sleep medications. In this study, stress management training resulted in reductions in sleep medicine use and greater improvement in sleep and mood measures relative to supportive therapy.

Since the time of this early study, there have been five large studies investigating the efficacy of behavioral interventions to aid hypnotic discontinuation (71,73–76). In a study of 209 chronic hypnotic users (74), CBT improved subjective sleep quality and reduced hypnotic use through a six-month follow-up relative to care as usual. The proportion of patients reducing their hypnotic use by at least 50% from baseline was less than half in the usual care group (11%) relative to those treated with CBT (39%). In a comparison study of physician-supervised taper, supervised taper plus CBT, and CBT alone, all three interventions produced large reductions in the amount (90%) and frequency (80%) of medication use (75). Compared to the single component treatments, there were more patients in the supervised taper plus CBT (85%) group that were medication-free at the end of treatment. The medication-free rates for the supervised taper alone and CBT alone were far more modest than those for the combined approach (48% and 54%, respectively). Both CBT groups reported greater sleep improvements than the supervised taper alone. In addition, there was no evidence of rebound insomnia or increased anxiety. In fact, there were notable reductions in insomnia symptom severity, as well as anxious and depressive mood-related symptoms. Whereas the use of CBT without a supervised taper produced the highest rate of relapse, those receiving the supervised taper alone were much less likely to become medication-free at posttreatment.

In addition, Lichstein and colleagues have conducted two studies showing that relaxation therapy may be a useful adjunct to supervised medication tapering (71,73). Both studies revealed that the therapy was helpful in reducing hypnotic use. Moreover, in a more recent study, those receiving relaxation training in addition to supervised taper reported greater improvement in sleep efficiency and subjective sleep quality (77). In a similar study comparing supervised taper with or without stimulus control (78), stimulus control produced greater sleep improvements by follow-up. Collectively, these studies suggest that CBT and other behavioral insomnia therapies may benefit long-term hypnotic users who wish to discontinue their sleep medication use.

Applications to Comorbid Insomnia

As noted in the National Institutes of Health State of the Science Conference Statement (59), most presentations of insomnia occur coincident to or comorbid with other conditions (79,80). As a result, there has been a call for increased clinical research in the treatment of sleep complaints in comorbid patient populations (59). Although the mechanisms are poorly understood, insomnia is believed to contribute to or complicate the comorbid condition. In cases wherein a medical condition may have initially caused insomnia, behavioral factors can set the stage for insomnia to remain after the condition resolves (81). This situation can also occur in psychiatric disorders, which may explain the high rate of residual insomnia after remission from the comorbid psychiatric disorder (82,83). In some cases of comorbid insomnia, the assumption that insomnia will remit when the comorbid condition remits is not always true, and treatment of the insomnia is necessary.

In ascertaining what represents optimal sleep therapy for comorbid patients, it is useful to consider the factors that sustain some sleep difficulties. Although the onset of insomnia comorbid to medical or psychiatric conditions may relate to endogenous physiological changes or acute stress reactions to the onset of illness, a host of cognitive and behavioral factors have been implicated in sustaining insomnia in these individuals over time (84). Even among individuals whose sleep disturbance initially represented an absolute secondary symptom of the comorbid condition, the nightly experience of unsuccessful sleep attempts could result in conditioned arousal and subsequent attempts to make up for lost sleep by spending excessive time in bed each night or napping during the day (20,40,85). These practices are associated with prolonged sleep difficulties because of the deleterious effects on homeostatic and circadian mechanisms that control the normal sleep-wake rhythm (20,40,85). Thus, sleep-disruptive cognitions and habits may play important roles in perpetuating insomnia in comorbid patients and merit-specific treatment attention (84).

Given these considerations, CBT appears a particularly viable treatment for insomnia comorbid to medical and psychiatric conditions since it addresses the myriad cognitive and behavioral mechanisms presumed to sustain chronic insomnia in many patient subtypes (32,33,35,36,38,86–90). Thus far, there have been a limited number of studies investigating the efficacy of CBT in patients with insomnia and comorbid mixed medical and/or psychiatric conditions (89,91–93). Results of these studies have suggested that CBT is efficacious in reducing sleep problems in these mixed patient groups. There have also been studies evaluating the efficacy of CBT in treating insomnia of specific medical patient groups. For example, CBT has shown promising results for several patient groups with cancer (94–98). This is particularly promising given that insomnia often remains long after remission from cancer (99,100).

In addition to these applications, there has been a series of studies highlighting the applicability of CBT in patients with chronic pain syndromes. Those with chronic pain tend to have the same maladaptive beliefs about sleep and sleep-disruptive behaviors known to perpetuate insomnia in those with primary insomnia. In addition, sleep may be an important factor in etiological models of pain syndromes. For example, analog studies have shown that experimenter-induced disruption of deep, slow-wave sleep elicits symptoms such as fatigue, myalgias, and mood disturbance among initially noncomplaining normal individuals (101). In addition, studies of clinical fibromyalgia patients have shown that a worsening of sleep enhances subsequent daytime distress and myalgias, and exacerbations of daytime pain and/or psychosocial distress often are followed by increased nocturnal sleep disruption (102–104). Given such findings, it seems reasonable to postulate that symptoms of some pain syndromes may be modulated by the reciprocal interaction of nocturnal sleep disturbance and cardinal daytime symptoms (pain, myalgia, fatigue, distress). Thus, therapy to correct sleep disturbance in such patients may interrupt the vicious sleep/distress/fatigue feedback cycle and lead to overall symptom improvement. Studies testing CBT for insomnia in those with chronic pain have shown promising results for both sleep and pain symptoms (41,88). Likewise, CBT for insomnia in fibromyalgia patients has support for improving both insomnia and fibromyalgia symptoms (105).

Given the efficacy of behavioral therapies for insomnia comorbid to medical conditions, there has been growing interest (84) in testing these treatments among those with comorbid mental disorders such as major depressive disorder (MDD). There are several possible reasons for this interest. One relates to the enormous cost and prevalence of this often recurrent disorder (1,106–109). Another reason relates to the high incidence of insomnia within this patient group. Coincident MDD and insomnia is particularly common in clinical settings inasmuch as up to 90% of those with MDD have sleep problems (110,111). Likewise, patients with insomnia and concurrent psychiatric disorders represent the largest group of insomnia sufferers that present to sleep clinics (112). Those patients who present with coincident insomnia and MDD comprise a particularly challenging group who warrant separate recognition and special treatment attention. Insomnia may predate and predict initial MDD onset, exacerbate MDD symptoms, and remain as a clinically significant condition long after the associated MDD episode remits (113,114). Although conditioned arousal and poor sleep habits could play a significant role in the insomnia co-occurring with MDD, this possibility tends to be ignored by clinicians. Indeed, insomnia in the context of MDD has traditionally been regarded as merely a product of the larger MDD disease process that fails to merit separate diagnostic or treatment attention (59,115).

Thus far, there have been a limited number of studies suggesting the applicability and potential efficacy of CBT with MDD patients. Some studies, for example, have shown that those with MDD and insomnia manifest the type of treatment targets for which CBT has been designed. Specifically, patients with insomnia and MDD exhibit more dysfunctional beliefs about sleep (116,117), sleep-disruptive behaviors, and sleep effort than those with primary insomnia alone (117). Furthermore, preliminary treatment studies have suggested CBT for insomnia may benefit the sleep and mood of depressed patients. In this regard, Morawetz (118) found that the vast majority of insomnia patients with MDD treated with a self-help form of CBT reported both marked sleep and mood improvements as a function of treatment. Finally, Morin and colleagues (119) showed CBT resulted in an improvement in sleep, and an associated mood improvement among a series of cases with comorbid insomnia and MDD. Given these various results, it appears that sleep-targeted therapies should play an important role in the acute management and long-term course of patients suffering from insomnia comorbid to MDD. For these patients, CBT seems particularly promising since it targets cognitive-behavioral mechanisms thought to sustain chronic insomnia, and the studies mentioned here suggest its applicability and likely efficacy with MDD patients. Moreover the apparent durability of CBT's posttreatment effects enhances its appeal for this patient group.

There is evidence for the use of CBT for insomnia in other mental disorders such as post-traumatic stress disorder (PTSD) (120) or alcohol dependence (41), but much more clinical trials are needed in this area. In some populations, components are added to CBT for insomnia to address disorder-specific problems. For example, in a treatment study of those with PTSD, combined behavioral insomnia treatment with a component called "dream rehearsal" to improve the incidence of nightmares resulted in improved sleep (120). Although treatment studies of patients with comorbid medical and psychiatric illnesses would suggest that the insomnia of these patients can be treated as effectively with CBT as primary insomnia (PI) patients (121), future research will likely explore whether disorder-specific modifications to CBT produce superior results to the CBT delivered to PI patients.

Considerations for Treatment Implementation

The discussion thus far supports the efficacy of behavioral insomnia therapies in general and CBT interventions specifically for treating patients with primary insomnia, comorbid insomnia, and hypnotic dependence. However, a number of factors related to treatment implementation may help determine the general utility of these therapies and influence the eventual treatment outcomes obtained. The following sections review several of these factors including the methods of treatment delivery, patients' treatment adherence, predictors of treatment response, and the accessibility and costs of treatment.

Methods of delivery. Behavioral insomnia treatments were initially designed for delivery via individual therapy sessions. In efforts to improve cost-effectiveness and increase accessibility, a number of alternative delivery methods have been developed. By far the most common alternative delivery format is group therapy. Although a previous meta-analytic review (17) suggested a slight superiority of individually administered treatments over group therapy, several controlled evaluations have shown that group CBT models involving six to eight sessions produce significant improvements in subjective/objective sleep patterns, general mood status, and dysfunctional beliefs about sleep (9,37,122,123). Although group CBT is a popular approach, studies directly comparing the relative benefits of individual versus group formats have been extremely limited. One study (124) did show comparable outcomes for insomnia patients assigned to either group or individualized CBT therapy, but clearly more studies are needed to further explore this issue.

To further enhance the cost-effectiveness of behavioral insomnia therapies, several investigators have developed and tested treatment protocols that can be self-administered outside of the clinic setting. Mimeault and Morin (125), for example, tested a self-help, CBT bibliotherapy with and without supportive phone consultations against a wait-list control group. Compared to the control condition, those treated with the bibliotherapy showed substantially greater sleep improvements than control patients, and these improvements were maintained at a three-month follow-up. The addition of phone consultations with a therapist conferred some advantage over bibliotherapy alone at posttreatment, but these benefits disappeared by follow-up. Strom et al. (126) tested a five-week self-help interactive CBT program delivered to insomnia patients via the Internet. Although those receiving this treatment demonstrated many sleep improvements, individuals randomized to a wait-list control group also showed similarly improved sleep. The treated group did show significantly greater reductions in dysfunctional sleep-related beliefs than did untreated patients, but treatment and control groups otherwise did not differ on study outcome measures. Considered collectively, these findings imply that some therapist involvement, even if provided via phone consultation, seems advantageous to behavioral treatment outcomes with insomnia sufferers.

In efforts to facilitate dissemination of behavioral insomnia treatments, some investigators have tested treatment delivery models suitable for common medical practice settings or the general public at large. Given that insomnia sufferers typically present first in primary care settings, it seems reasonable to consider training nonspecialist healthcare professionals (e.g., nurses, general practitioners) to provide behavioral interventions. Two studies designed to test the efficacy of such an approach have demonstrated that both family physicians (127) and office-practice nurses (37) can effectively administer these treatments in general medical practice settings. In contrast, Oosterhuis and Klip (128) reported promising results from a novel study wherein behavioral insomnia therapy was provided via a series of eight, 15-minute educational programs broadcast on radio and television in the Netherlands. Over 23,000 people ordered the accompanying course material, and data from a random subset of these showed sleep improvements; reductions in hypnotic use, medical visits, and physical complaints were achieved among those who took part in this educational program. Thus, it appears that behavioral insomnia treatments can be effectively delivered by various providers and delivery of such treatment, even via mass media outlets, may provide benefits to some insomnia sufferers. Of course, the relative efficacy of these alternate treatment delivery methods vis-à-vis traditional individual or group therapy has yet to be established.

Treatment acceptance and adherence. The success of behavioral insomnia therapy is dependent on a patient's acceptance of treatment and subsequent consistent adherence to the particular strategies prescribed. In a sense, acceptance and adherence are related processes in that patients' pretreatment preferences affect their subsequent willingness to enact and adhere to treatment recommendations (129) Studies of patients' preferences have shown that most insomnia sufferers rate behavioral insomnia therapies as more acceptable than long-term pharmacotherapy for their sleep problems (129,130). Furthermore, one study (1999) (32) showed patients were more satisfied with behavioral insomnia therapy and rated it as more effective than sleep medication. Findings from another study (130) suggested that individuals with chronic insomnia not only prefer a behavioral insomnia therapy such as CBT to pharmacotherapy, but also expect CBT to produce greater improvements in daytime functioning, better long-term effects, and fewer negative side effects. Collectively, these data suggest that insomnia patients regard behavioral insomnia therapy as a viable and acceptable treatment for their sleep difficulties.

Whereas patients' adherence to behavioral insomnia treatment is important in assuring their overall success, currently no standardized methodology for measuring adherence exists. Some investigators (32,131,132) have solicited treatment adherence/compliance ratings from the patients themselves, their significant others, or their therapists. Results of such ratings suggest moderate to high patient adherence to treatment strategies, but adherence ratings are highly subjective and likely subject to an overly favorable reporting bias, particularly when solicited from patients themselves. As an alternative to adherence ratings, some researchers have used indices derived from sleep diaries completed by patients throughout the course of treatment. Bouchard et al. (133), for example, employed seven indices taken from patients sleep diaries to assess daily adherence to stimulus control and sleep-restriction therapy recommendations. Overall, patients showed a high level of adherence by virtue of meeting 6 of the 7 adherence indices on average each day. Furthermore, perceptions of sleep-related self-efficacy were positively related to adherence, suggesting that self-efficacy may play an important role in promoting adherence behaviors. More recently, Carney et al. (116) tested the utility of actigraphy for measuring adherence to behavioral sleep schedule prescriptions in a sample of normal sleepers. Results of this analog study showed that actigraphy identified adherence violations not revealed by coincident sleep diary monitoring. Hence, methods such as actigraphy may ultimately be needed to obtain an appraisal of insomnia patients' actual adherence to behavioral treatment recommendations.

Despite their limitations, studies employing subjective ratings or sleep diary indices of treatment adherence have shown the importance of treatment enactment to eventual treatment outcome. One study (132), for example, showed that patients rated as highly adherent by their therapists had higher sleep quality, fewer sleep-related dysfunctional beliefs, and less sleep-related impairment at posttreatment than did those with poorer adherence. In another study (134), a sleep diary measure of sleep schedule consistency predicted sleep improvements at a posttreatment assessment. In still another study (131), adherence to sleep restriction and stimulus-control components was found to be the strongest predictor of clinical sleep improvements in sleep latency and nighttime wakefulness. Adherence to cognitive therapy strategies also predicted reductions in wakefulness, but use of sleep hygiene strategies was unrelated to sleep outcome. Interestingly, Vincent and Lionberg (129) found that sleep hygiene was the most liked whereas the more consistently effective treatment, sleep restriction, was the least liked form of behavioral treatment. Nonetheless, both the previously cited efficacy studies and the research specifically focused on adherence suggest that a substantial proportion of patients receiving behavioral insomnia therapies manifest sufficient treatment adherence to achieve clinically significant sleep improvements.

Economic considerations. The relative cost-effectiveness of behavioral and pharmacological insomnia therapies is an important consideration, given current capitation and managed care models of healthcare delivery. As compared to sedative hypnotic therapy, behavioral insomnia treatments are rather time-consuming and initially expensive to administer. Hence, for those patients with acute insomnia, pharmacotherapy may be far more cost-effective. However, in the treatment of chronic insomnia, this may not be the case. Patients provided ongoing pharmacotherapy for chronic insomnia incur the costs of medications in addition to repeat physician visits for medication prescriptions. Since behavioral insomnia therapies are designed to eradicate the cognitive and behavioral anomalies that sustain insomnia, they often produce durable improvements that persist long after the treatment course is completed (7,15). As such, behavioral insomnia therapies may represent the more cost-effective treatment when long-term outcomes are considered. Unfortunately both comparisons of the long-term treatment outcomes and the relative cost-effectiveness/cost-benefits of behavioral and pharmacological insomnia therapies are currently lacking (7,19).

Thus, additional research is needed to establish relative economic merits of these treatments.

Another important economic consideration is the reduction in healthcare costs and utilization associated with insomnia treatment. Various studies (4,135–137) have shown that insomnia enhances healthcare costs and utilization among affected individuals. Since behavioral insomnia treatments produce long-term sleep improvements, they may reduce healthcare utilization. Whereas currently there are limited data to support this speculation, one uncontrolled case series study (138) showed a marked reduction in healthcare utilization (e.g., outpatient clinic visits) among patients who underwent behavioral group therapy for their insomnia. Nonetheless, additional clinical trials with adequate control groups are needed to cross-validate these preliminary findings and confirm the positive effects behavioral therapies may have on the healthcare utilization patterns of insomnia patients.

Treatment accessibility. Despite the proven efficacy and potential advantages that behavioral insomnia therapies may hold for many insomnia patients, a number of treatment barriers currently limit accessibility to such treatments. Most individuals who do seek treatment for insomnia typically do so in primary care settings (139,140) wherein provider time constraints and general lack of knowledge about behavioral treatment options obviate the delivery of such interventions. Furthermore, there are currently a very limited number of sleep specialists and other healthcare providers who have expertise in behavioral insomnia therapies (141). Hence, even when insomnia patients present to sleep specialty centers or otherwise specifically seek behavioral interventions, they often have difficulty finding trained professionals who can administer such treatments. Moreover, many health insurance plans decline to cover the costs of these therapies (141). As a result, those patients who are successful in locating a behavioral insomnia therapist may be dissuaded from pursuing such treatment due to financial considerations. Given these various barriers, insomnia patients currently have relatively limited access to behavioral treatments for their sleep difficulties. This state of affairs is unfortunate since such treatment may be preferred or even optimal for many insomnia sufferers. Thus, efforts to reduce these barriers and make such treatments more widely accessible seem warranted.

Predictors of treatment outcome. As noted earlier, behavioral insomnia therapies have proven efficacy with various patient types, yet not all insomnia sufferers benefit equally from these treatments. In order to understand who may and may not respond to such treatments, various investigators have attempted to identify factors that predict patients' responses to these therapies. Studies of various demographic variables have shown that factors such as gender, marital status, education, and occupational status are not significant predictors of treatment outcome (17,37,142). Thus, for the most part, demographic characteristics seem to have little bearing on behavioral insomnia treatment outcomes.

It might be expected that factors such as a history of hypnotic use as well as the duration and severity of insomnia may influence treatment response. Research (37) that has examined the influence of sleep medication use has shown that those who use such medications do about as well as medication-free patients during CBT treatment. In contrast, findings regarding the influence of insomnia severity and duration have been mixed. One study (37) showed that those with more severe pretreatment levels of insomnia showed greater overall treatment-related improvement, yet they were less likely to achieve normative treatment endpoints than were those with milder insomnia. Another study (142) however found that those with the marked pretreatment insomnia severity had lower posttreatment sleep efficiencies on polysomnography than did those who entered treatment with milder insomnia. Likewise, studies to date have not shown a consistent relationship between insomnia duration and the treatment outcomes resulting from behavioral insomnia therapies (37,38,142). Overall, these studies suggest that patients should not be excluded from behavioral insomnia therapies purely on the basis of their insomnia severity/duration or prior medication use. Nonetheless, more research concerning the influence of these factors on eventual treatment outcome would be useful.

FUTURE RESEARCH

Over the past three and half decades, behavioral insomnia therapies have proven their value to the sleep medicine community such that current-day CBT are widely accepted as viable, frontline treatments for chronic insomnia (59). Despite the proven efficacy of such treatments, much more basic and clinical research is needed to provide a better understanding of such interventions and maximize their effectiveness with the array of insomnia patients encountered in day-to-day clinical practice. In this regard, it seems useful to outline several specific lines of research that warrant consideration.

As noted previously, there is currently rather limited knowledge concerning the mechanisms whereby such treatments produce their effects. To date, studies of treatment mechanisms have focused primarily on sleep-related beliefs or observable sleep habits and shown that interventions such as CBT effectively reduce dysfunctional beliefs about sleep and correct certain sleep-disruptive habits (e.g., spending excessive time in bed, maintaining an erratic sleep-wake schedule) purported to perpetuate insomnia. However, little is known about the effects of behavioral insomnia therapies on arousal mechanisms thought to play important perpetuating roles in chronic sleep difficulties. Although many insomnia patients report pre-sleep cognitive arousal as the most important factor in their insomnia (43), it is striking that our efficacy and effectiveness trials have not measured whether cognitive arousal is reduced after CBT. This may be due in part to the current vagueness of the cognitive arousal construct. Thus, future studies designed to better define this construct and assess whether cognitive arousal is effectively ameliorated by behavioral insomnia therapies appear warranted.

There are also many questions that remain concerning the general and relative efficacy of cognitive-behavioral insomnia treatments. It seems noteworthy that not all patients respond to these treatments and a notable portion or treatment responders fail to become good sleepers

(15,123). Hence, it appears that research focused on enhancing the efficacy of these treatments would be useful. Moreover, despite the voluminous published clinical trials concerning both behavioral and pharmacological treatments for insomnia, head-to-head comparisons of these two types of interventions have been absent from the insomnia treatment literature (59). As a result, the relative short- and long-term benefits of these two forms of treatment remain unknown. It seems possible, if not probable, that different insomnia patient subtypes may respond differently to these forms of treatment such that some patient types benefit more from behavioral treatments, whereas others respond best to pharmacological therapies. Thus, studies designed to investigate these issues would be useful.

Our literature review also suggests that cognitive-behavioral insomnia therapies are a useful component of the treatment regimen employed to assist patients wishing to discontinue their use of hypnotic medications. The studies in the area have been limited in number and focus. The few studies concerning hypnotic discontinuation have considered patients with long-term BZRA usage. However, medications other than BZRAs (e.g., sedating antidepressants) are often prescribed for insomnia by frontline providers (143,144). Hence, future research in this area should examine whether behavioral insomnia therapies are useful in aiding discontinuation from other non-BZD medications commonly used to treat insomnia.

It is clear from much of the previous discussion that behavioral treatments are effective with both primary and comorbid forms of chronic insomnia. Nonetheless, to date, no studies have been conducted to evaluate the relative efficacy of cognitive-behavioral insomnia treatments with such distinctive insomnia subtypes. As such, it remains unclear whether these treatments, in their current forms, perform equally well in both primary and comorbid insomnia patients. Patients with comorbid disorders often have symptoms (e.g., pain, lethargy, anxiety, etc.) that may add to or confound sleep. Since existing cognitive-behavioral insomnia treatments do not typically include strategies to address such symptoms, it is possible that those with comorbid insomnia may respond less well to these insomnia treatment strategies. Of course, a corollary of this speculation is that cognitive-behavioral insomnia treatments may benefit from special tailoring or augmentation (84) to address sleep-disruptive symptoms of the comorbid disorder as well as the more common cognitive-behavioral anomalies (dysfunctional beliefs, sleep-disruptive compensatory strategies) that emerge in many forms of insomnia. Hopefully, future research will address these questions and speculations.

A final area that appears ripe for research concerns the issue of treatment dissemination. Currently, the population of insomnia patients who might benefit from behavioral insomnia therapies far outstrips the limited number of behavioral sleep medicine specialists with established expertise in such interventions (59). Consequently, many patients who might prefer and benefit from such therapies may have difficulty accessing such treatments. The challenge to the sleep medicine community, both currently and in the foreseeable future, is that of determining effective methods for accomplishing the widest and most cost-effective dissemination of these behavioral interventions. Training more qualified behavioral therapists in these techniques clearly is one option, but this approach is fairly narrow in scope and will require an extended period of time before enough trained providers are available to make a significant impact on treatment accessibility. Hence, this strategy, at best, represents only a small portion of the overall strategy required to address this challenge.

From the literature reviewed herein, many behavioral insomnia treatment resources are currently available to allow the sleep medicine community to take a broader public health perspective toward insomnia and test a stepped care (145,146) model for the treatment of the insomnia population. Figure 2 presents a schematic of how this model might be enacted. Given some recent research (128) concerning the use of mass media to address insomnia, efforts to disseminate basic behavioral treatment principles through such media should be explored. Whereas this level of *intervention* may not prove effective for many insomnia patients, media-based treatments have the advantage of very extensive dissemination; hence, it is likely that a notable number of insomnia patients could be effectively "treated" by this intervention alone. Those not benefited by mass media education could step up to more structured albeit relatively accessible interventions such as the self-help (125) or Internet-based (126) programs. Such treatments can also reach a sizable proportion of the insomnia population and likely will be helpful to a proportion of those not helped by media education alone. Of course, many insomnia patients may prefer to seek treatment from their primary care providers. For those

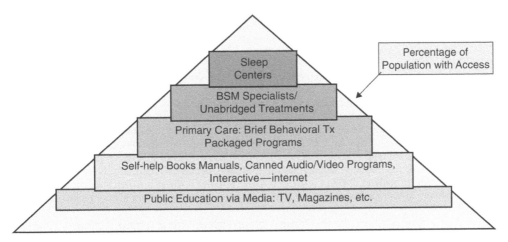

Figure 2 Taking a broader public health perspective—stepped care model to behavioral insomnia treatment. *Abbreviations*: BSM, behavioral sleep medicine; Tx, treatment.

who step up to this level of care, basic behavioral treatments could be provided either by physicians themselves (127) or by their office nurses (37), although admittedly many such providers would first need training to administer such interventions. Assuming such training can be accomplished, it is likely that a portion that fails to respond to the lower level interventions would respond to this level of intervention. Those patients requiring more intensive treatment, of course, could be referred to behavioral insomnia treatment specialists, and it is likely that some of the more complex cases in this cohort will eventually be referred to full-service sleep centers for more comprehensive evaluation and treatment.

Admittedly many of our speculations regarding the functioning of this stepped care model remain hypothetical and require extensive testing before they can be confirmed. Moreover, much additional provider training will need to be accomplished at the upper "steps" in this model to assure adequate dissemination of the behavioral insomnia therapies. Nonetheless, inasmuch as 10% of the population suffers from chronic insomnia, this stepped care model has significant heuristic appeal for assuring the broadest dissemination of the behavioral insomnia treatments. Therefore, research designed to test various individual steps in this model as well as the model as a whole would seem useful.

CONCLUSIONS

Chronic insomnia is a fairly prevalent and significant health concern that often is perpetuated by dysfunctional beliefs about sleep, heightened anxiety, and a host of sleep-disruptive compensatory practices. Whereas pharmacotherapy is often prescribed for this condition, such treatment may be encumbered with side effects and usually fails to address the psychological and behavioral anomalies sustaining the sleep problems. In contrast, the behavioral insomnia therapies are specifically designed to address one or more of these perpetuating mechanisms. Research has shown that the range of cognitive-behavioral insomnia therapies are moderately to highly effective, particularly for ameliorating sleep difficulties in a range of patients including those with primary insomnia, those with insomnia comorbid to mental or medical conditions, and those trying to overcome dependence on sleep medications. As a function of this research, such treatments are now regarded as the treatments of choice for chronic insomnia sufferers. The evolution of behavioral insomnia therapies over the last several decades has been impressive. Nonetheless, further development is needed to maximize the efficacy, clinical utility, and availability of these interventions. Hopefully, future studies will focus on maximizing the effectiveness and dissemination of these treatments to the patients whom might benefit from them.

REFERENCES

1. Ford D, Kamerow D. Epidemiologic study of sleep disturbances in psychiatric disorders. JAMA 1989; 262:1479–1484.
2. Ohayon MM. Epidemiology of insomnia: what we know and what we still need to learn. Sleep Med Rev 2002; 6:97–111.
3. Katz DA, McHorney CA. Clinical correlates of insomnia in patients with chronic illness. Arch Intern Med 1998; 158:1099–1107.
4. Hajak G, SINE Study Group. Study of Insomnia in Europe. Epidemiology of severe insomnia and its consequences in Germany. Euro Arch Psychiatry Clin Neurosci 2001; 251:49–56.
5. Zammit GK, Weiner J, Damato N et al. Quality of life in people with insomnia. Sleep 1999; 22:S379–S385.
6. Morin CM, Espie CA. Insomnia: A Clinical Guide to Assessment and Treatment. New York: Kluwer Academic/Plenum Publishers, 2003.
7. Edinger JD, Means MK. Cognitive-behavioral therapy for primary insomnia. Clin Psychol Rev 2005; 29:539–558.
8. Spielman AJ, Caruso LS, Glovinsky PB. A behavioral perspective on insomnia treatment. Psychiatr Clin N Am 1987; 10:541–553.
9. Morin CM, Stone J, Trinkle D, et al. Dysfunctional beliefs and attitudes about sleep among older adults with and without insomnia complaints. Psychol Aging 1993; 8:463–467.
10. Schultz JH, Luthe W. Augenic Training. New York: Grune & Stratton, 1959.
11. Jacobson E. Anxiety and Tension Control. Philadelphia: Lippincott, 1964.
12. Borkovec TD, Fowles DC. Controlled investigation of the effects of progressive relaxation and hypnotic relaxation on insomnia. J Abnorm Psychol 1973; 82:153–158.
13. Nicassio P, Bootzin RR. A comparison of progressive relaxation and autogenic training as treatments for insomnia. J Abnorm Psychol 1974; 83:253–260.
14. Bernstein D, Borkovec TD. Progressive relaxation training. Champaign, Ill: Research Press, 1973.
15. Morin CM, Bootzin R, Buysse DJ, et al. Psychological and behavioral treatment of insomnia: update of the recent evidence (1998–2004). Sleep 2006; 29(11):1398–1414.
16. Bootzin RR. Stimulus control treatment for insomnia. Proceedings of the 80th Annual Meeting of the American Psychological Association, Honolulu, HI, 1972; 7:395–396.
17. Morin CM, Culbert JP, Schwartz SM. Nonpharmacological interventions for insomnia: a meta-analysis of treatment efficacy. Am J Psychiatry 1994; 151:1172–1180.
18. Murtagh DR, Greenwood KM. Identifying effective psychological treatments for insomnia: a meta-analysis. J Consult Clin Psychol 1995; 63:79–89.
19. Smith MT, Perlis ML, Park A, et al. Comparative meta-analysis of pharmacotherapy and behavior therapy for persistent insomnia. Am J Psychiatry 2002; 159:5–11.
20. Spielman AJ, Saskin P, Thorpy MJ. Treatment of chronic insomnia by restriction of time in bed. Sleep 1987; 10:45–55.
21. Wohlgemuth WK, Edinger JD. Sleep restriction therapy. In: Lichstein KL, Morin CM, eds. Treatment of Late-life Insomnia. Thousand Oaks, CA: Sage, 2000:147–184.
22. Lichstein KL. Sleep compression treatment of an insomnoid. Behav Ther 1988; 19:625–632.
23. Glovinsky P, Spielman A. The Insomnia Answer: A Personalized Program for Identifying and Overcoming the Three Types of Insomnia. New York: Penguin Group, 2006.
24. Turner RM, Ascher LM. Controlled comparison of progressive relaxation, stimulus control, and paradoxical intention therapies for insomnia. J Consult Clin Psychol 1979; 47:500–508.
25. Espie CA, Lindsay WR. Paradoxical intention in the treatment of chronic insomnia: six case studies illustrating variability in therapeutic response. Behav Res Ther 1985; 23:703–709.
26. Lacks P. Behavioral treatment for persistent insomnia. New York: Pergamon Press, 1987.
27. Hauri PJ. Sleep Hygiene, Relaxation Therapy, and Cognitive Interventions. New York: Plenum Publishing, 1991:65–84.
28. Carney CE, Edinger JD. Identifying critical dysfunctional beliefs about sleep in primary insomnia. Sleep 2006; 29:325–333.
29. Beck AT, Rush AJ, Shaw BF, et al. Cognitive Therapy of Depression. New York: Guilford Press, 1979.
30. Carney CE, Waters WF. Effects of a Structured Problem-Solving Procedure on Pre-Sleep Cognitive Arousal in College Students with Insomnia. Behav Sleep Med 2006; 4:13–28.
31. Edinger JD, Wohlgemuth WK, Radtke RA, et al. Cognitive behavioral therapy for treatment of chronic primary insomnia: a randomized, controlled trial. JAMA 2001; 285:1856–1864.
32. Morin CM, Colecchi C, Stone J, et al. Behavioral and pharmacological therapies for late-life insomnia: a randomized controlled trial. JAMA 1999; 281:991–999.
33. Edinger JD, Hoelscher TJ, Marsh GR, et al. A cognitive-behavioral therapy for sleep-maintenance insomnia in older adults. Psychol Aging 1992; 7(2):282–289.
34. Hoelscher T, Edinger JD. Treatment of sleep-maintenance insomnia in older adults: sleep period reduction, sleep education and modified stimulus control. Psychol Aging 1988; 3:258–263.

35. Morin CM, Kowatch RA, Barry T, et al. Cognitive-behavior therapy for late-life insomnia. J Consult Clin Psychol 1993; 61:137–147.
36. Edinger JD, Sampson WS. A primary care "friendly" cognitive behavioral insomnia therapy. Sleep 2003; 26:177–182.
37. Espie CA, Inglis SJ, Tessier S, et al. The clinical effectiveness of cognitive behaviour therapy for chronic insomnia: implementation and evaluation of a sleep clinic in general medical practice. Behav Res Ther 2001; 39:45–60.
38. Espie CA, Inglis SJ, Harvey L, et al. Insomniacs' attributions: psychometric properties of the dysfunctional beliefs about sleep scale and the sleep disturbance questionnaire. J Psychosom Res 2000; 48:141–148.
39. Morin CM, Blais F, Savard J. Are changes in beliefs and attitudes related to sleep improvements in the treatment of insomnia? Behav Res Ther 2002; 40(7):741–752.
40. Morin CM. Insomnia: psychological assessment and management. New York: Guilford Press, 1993.
41. Currie SR, Wilson KG, Pontefract AJ, et al. Cognitive-behavioral treatment of insomnia secondary to chronic pain. J Consult Clin Psychol 2000; 68:407–416.
42. Broman JE, Hetta J. Perceived pre-sleep arousal in patients with persistent psychophysiological and psychiatric insomnia. Nord J Psychiatry 1994; 48:203–207.
43. Lichstein KL, Rosenthal TL. Insomniacs' perceptions of cognitive versus somatic determinants of sleep disturbance. J Abnorm Psychol 1980; 89:105–107.
44. Gross R, Borkovec T. Effects of cognitive intrusion manipulation on the sleep onset latency of good sleepers. Behav Ther 1982; 13:112–116.
45. Haynes SN, Adams A, Franzen M. The effects of pre-sleep stress on sleep-onset insomnia. J Abnorm Psychol 1981; 90:601–606.
46. Hauri P. Effects of evening activity on early night sleep. Psychophysiology 1969; 4:267–276.
47. Backhaus J, Junghanns K, Broocks A, et al. Test-retest reliability of the Pittsburgh Sleep Quality Index in primary insomnia. J Psychosom Res 2002; 53:737–740.
48. Borkovec T, Hennings BL. The role of physiological attention-focusing in the relaxation treatment of sleep disturbance, general tension, and specific stress reaction. Behav Res Ther 1978; 16:7–19.
49. Mitchell KR. Behavioral treatment of pre-sleep tension and intrusive cognitions in patients with severe predormital insomnia. J Behav Med 1978; 2:57–69.
50. Mitchell KR, White RG. Self-management of severe pre-dormital insomnia. J Behav Ther Exp Psychol 1977; 8:57–63.
51. Sanavio E. Pre-sleep cognitive intrusions and treatment of onset-insomnia. Behav Res Ther 1988; 26:451–459.
52. Espie CA, Lindsay WR. Cognitive strategies for the management of severe sleep maintenance insomnia: a preliminary investigation. Behav Psychother 1987; 15:388–395.
53. Harvey AG, Farrell C. The efficacy of a Pennebaker-like writing intervention for poor sleepers. Behav Sleep Med 2003; 1:115–123.
54. Levey AB, Aldaz JA, Watts FN, et al. Articulatory suppression and the treatment of insomnia. Behav Res Ther 1991; 29:85–89.
55. Carney CE, Edinger JD, Meyer B, et al. Daily activities and sleep quality in college students. Chronobiol Int 2006; 23(3):623–637.
56. Monk TH, Petrie SR, Hayes AJ, et al. Regularity of daily life in relation to personality, age, gender, sleep quality and circadian rhythms. J Sleep Res 1994, 3:196–205.
57. Edinger JD, Wohlgemuth WK, Radtke RA, et al. Cognitive behavioral therapy for treatment of chronic Primary Insomnia: a randomized controlled trial. JAMA 2001; 285:1856–1864.
58. Monk TH, Reynolds CF III, Buysse DJ, et al. The relationship between lifestyle regularity and subjective sleep quality. Chronobiol Int 2003; 20:97–107.
59. National Institutes of Health. National Institutes of Health State of the Science Conference statement on manifestations and management of chronic insomnia in adults. Sleep 2005; 28:1049–1057.
60. Nowell PD, Mazumdar S, Buysse DJ, et al. Benzodiazepines and zolpidem for chronic insomnia: a meta-analysis of treatment efficacy. JAMA 1997; 278:2170–2177.
61. Waters WF, Hurry MJ, Binks PG, et al. Behavioral and hypnotic treatments of insomnia subtypes. Behav Sleep Med 2003; 1:81–101.
62. Greenblatt DJ. Pharmacology of benzodiazepine hypnotics. J Clin Psychiatry 1992; 53(suppl):7–13.
63. Morin CM, Belanger L, Bastien CH, et al. Long-term outcome after discontinuation of benzodiazepines for insomnia: a survival analysis of relapse. Behav Res Ther 2005; 43:1–14.
64. Hauri PJ. Can we mix behavioral therapy with hypnotics when treating insomniacs? Sleep 1997; 20:1111–1118.
65. Milby JB, Williams V, Hall JN, et al. Effectiveness of combined triazolam-behavioral therapy for primary insomnia. Am J Psychiatry 1993; 150:1259–1260.
66. Rosen RC, Lewin DS, Goldberg RL, et al. Psychophysiological insomnia combined effects of pharmacotherapy and relaxation-based treatments. Sleep Med 2000; 1:279–288.

67. Lewin DS, Rosen RC, Goldberg L, et al. Drug and non-drug interactions in psychophysiologic insomnia: preliminary findings. Paper presented at: Association for Advancement of Behavioral Therapy, San Diego, 1994.
68. Jacobs GD, Pace-Schott EF, Stickgold R, et al. Cognitive behavior therapy and pharmacotherapy for insomnia: a randomized controlled trial and direct comparison. Arch Intern Med 2004; 164:1888–1896.
69. Vallieres A, Morin CM, Guay B. Sequential combinations of drug and cognitive behavioral therapy for chronic insomnia: an exploratory study. Behav Res Ther 2005; 43:1611–1630.
70. Curran HV, Collins R, Fletcher S, et al. Older adults and withdrawal from benzodiazepine hypnotics in general practice: effects on cognitive function, sleep, mood and quality of life. Psychol Med 2003; 33:1223–1237.
71. Lichstein KL, Peterson BA, Riedel BW, et al. Relaxation to assist sleep medication withdrawal. Behav Modif 1999; 23:379–402.
72. Kirmil-Gray K, Eagleston JR, Thoresen CE, et al. Brief consultation and stress management treatments for drug-dependent insomnia: effects on sleep quality, self-efficacy, and daytime stress. J Behav Med 1985; 8:79–99.
73. Lichstein KL, Johnson RS. Relaxation for insomnia and hypnotic medication use in older women. Psychol Aging 1993; 8:103–111.
74. Morgan K, Dixon S, Mathers N, et al. Psychological treatment for insomnia in the management of long-term hypnotic drug use: a pragmatic randomized controlled trial. Br J Gen Pract 2003; 53:923–928.
75. Morin CM, Bastien CH, Guay B, et al. Randomized clinical trial of supervised tapering and cognitive-behavior therapy to facilitate benzodiazepine discontinuation in older adults with chronic insomnia. Am J Psychiatry 2004; 161:332–342.
76. Reidel BW, Lichstein KL, Peterson BA, et al. A comparison of the efficacy of stimulus control for medicated and non-medicated insomniacs. Behav Modif 1998; 22:3–28.
77. Lichstein KL, Peterson BA, Riedel BW, et al. Relaxation to assist sleep medication withdrawal. Behav Modif 1999; 23:379–402.
78. Riedel B, Lichstein KL, Peterson BA, et al. A comparison of the efficacy of stimulus control for medicated and non-medicated insomniacs. Behav Modif 1998; 22:3–28.
79. Lichstein KL, Wilson NM, Johnson CT. Psychological treatment of secondary insomnia. Psychol Aging 2000; 15:232–240.
80. Ohayon MM, Roberts RE. Comparability of sleep disorders diagnoses using DSM-IV and ICSD classifications with adolescents. Sleep 2001; 24:920–925.
81. Katz DA, McHorney CA. The relationship between insomnia and health-related quality of life in patients with chronic illness. J Fam Pract 2002; 51:229–235.
82. Zayfert C, DeViva JC. Residual insomnia following cognitive behavioral therapy for PTSD. J Trauma Stress 2004; 17:69–73.
83. Nierenberg AA, Keefe BR, Leslie VC, et al. Residual symptoms in depressed patients who respond acutely to fluoxetine. J Clin Psychiatry 1999; 60:221–225.
84. Smith MT, Huang MI, Manber R. Cognitive behavior therapy for chronic insomnia occurring within the context of medical and psychiatric disorders. Clin Psychol Rev 2005; 25:559–592.
85. Edinger JD, Wohlgemuth WK. The significance and management of persistent primary insomnia. Sleep Med Rev 1999; 3:101–118.
86. Edinger JD, Wohlgemuth WK, Radtke RA, et al. Dose response effects of cognitive-behavioral insomnia therapy: a randomized clinical trial. Sleep 2007; 30(2):203–212.
87. Edinger JD, Fins AI, Sullivan RJ, et al. Comparison of cognitive-behavioral therapy and clonazepam for treating periodic limb movement disorder. Sleep 1996; 19:442–444.
88. Morin CM, Kowatch RA, Wade JB. Behavioral management of sleep disturbances secondary to chronic pain. J Behav Ther Exp Psychiatry 1989; 20:295–302.
89. Morin CM, Stone J, McDonald K, et al. Psychological management of insomnia: a clinical replication series with 100 patients. Behav Ther 1994; 25:291–309.
90. Perlis M, Aloia M, Millikan A, et al. Behavioral treatment of insomnia: a clinical case series study. J Behav Med 2000; 23:149–161.
91. Lichstein KL, Wilson NM, Johnson CT. Psychological treatment of secondary insomnia. Psychol Aging 2000; 15:232–240.
92. Perlis ML, Sharpe MC, Smith MT, et al. Behavioral treatment of insomnia: treatment outcome and the relevance of medical and psychiatric morbidity. J Behav Med 2001; 24:281–296.
93. Rybarczyk B, Lopez M, Benson R, et al. Efficacy of two behavioral treatment programs for comorbid geriatric insomnia. Psychol Aging 2002; 17:288–298.
94. Cannici J, Malcolm R, Peek LA. Treatment of insomnia in cancer patients using muscle relaxation training. J Behav Ther Exp Psychiatry 1983; 14:251–256.
95. Davidson JR, Waisberg JL, Brundage MD, et al. Nonpharmacologic group treatment of insomnia: a preliminary study with cancer survivors. Psychooncology 2001; 10:389–397.

96. Savard J, Simard S, Ivers H, et al. Randomized study on the efficacy of cognitive-behavioral therapy for insomnia secondary to breast cancer. Part I: Sleep and psychological effects. J Clin Oncol 2005; 23:6083–6096.
97. Simeit R, Deck R, Conta-Marx B. Sleep management training for cancer patients with insomnia. Support Care Cancer 2004; 12:176–183.
98. Quesnel C, Savard J, Simard S, et al. Efficacy of cognitive-behavioral therapy for insomnia in women treated for nonmetastatic breast cancer. J Consult Clin Psychol 2003; 71:189–200.
99. Couzi RJ, Helzlsouer KJ, Fetting JH. Prevalence of menopausal symptoms among women with a history of breast cancer and attitudes toward estrogen replacement therapy. J Clin Oncol 1995; 13:2737–2744.
100. Lindley C, Vasa S, Sawyer WT, et al. Quality of life and preferences for treatment following systemic adjuvant therapy for early-stage breast cancer. J Clin Oncol 1998; 16:1380–1387.
101. Moldofsky H, Scarisbrick P, England R, et al. Musculoskeletal symptoms and non-REM sleep disturbance in patients with 'Fibrositis Syndrome' and healthy subjects. Psychosom Med 1975; 37:341–351.
102. Goldenberg DL. Treatment of fibromyalgia syndrome. Rheum Dis Clin N Am 1989; 15:61–71.
103. Pilowsky I, Crettenden I, Townley M. Sleep disturbance in pain clinic patients. Pain 1985; 23:27–33.
104. Smythe HA. Does modification of sleep patterns cure fibromyalgia? Br J Rheumatol 1988; 27:449.
105. Edinger JD. Behavioral insomnia therapy for fibromyalgia patients: a randomized clinical trial, Arch Intern Med 2005; 165:1–9.
106. Goldman LS, Nielsen NH, Champion HC. Awareness, diagnosis, and treatment of depression. J Gen Intern Med 1999; 14:569–580.
107. Pearson SD, Katzelnick D, Simon G, et al. Depression among high utilizers of medical care. J Gen Intern Med 1999; 14:461–468.
108. Murray CJL, Lopez AD. The global burden of disease: a comprehensive assessment of mortality, injuries and risk factors in 1990 and projected to 2000. Cambridge: MA, Harvard School of Public Health and the World Health Organization, 1998.
109. Keller MB, Lavori PW, Mueller TI, et al. Time to recovery, chronicity and levels of psychotherapy in major depression. Arch Gen Psychiatry 1992; 49:809–816.
110. Kupfer DJ, Reynolds CF III, Ulrich RF, et al. EEG sleep, depression and aging. Neurobiol Aging 1982; 3(4):351–360.
111. Reynolds CF, Kupfer D. Sleep research in affective illness: state of the art circa 1987. Sleep 1987; 10:199–215.
112. Edinger JD, Hoelscher TJ, Webb MD, et al. Polysomnographic assessment of DIMS: empirical evaluation of its diagnostic value. Sleep 1989; 12:315–322.
113. Judd LL, Akiskal HS, Maser JD, et al. A prospective 12-year study of subsyndromal and syndromal depressive symptoms in unipolar major depressive disorders. Arch Gen Psychiatry 1998; 55:994–700.
114. Perlis M, Giles DE, Buysse DJ, et al. Self-reported sleep disturbance as a prodromal symptom in recurrent depression. J Affect Disord 1997; 42:209–212.
115. Lichstein KL. Secondary insomnia. In: Lichstein KL, Morin CM, eds. Treatment of Late-life Insomnia. Thousand Oaks, CA: Sage, 2000:297–319.
116. Carney CE, Edinger JD, Segal ZV. Those with depression report different beliefs about sleep than those with primary insomnia or good sleepers. Sleep 2005; 28(suppl):A313(abstr).
117. Kohn L, Espie CA. Sensitivity and specificity of measures of the insomnia experience: a comparative study of psychophysiologic insomnia, insomnia associated with mental disorder and good sleepers. Sleep 2005; 29:104–112.
118. Morawetz D. Depression and insomnia: What comes first? Aust J Couns Psychol 2001; 3:19–24.
119. Vallieres A, Bastien CH, Ouellet MC, et al. Cognitive-behavior therapy for insomnia associated with anxiety or depression. Sleep 2000; 23(suppl):A311.
120. Krakow B, Johnston L, Melendrez D, et al. An open-label trial of evidence-based cognitive behavior therapy for nightmares and insomnia in crime victims with PTSD. Am J Psychiatry 2001; 158:2043–2047.
121. Verbeek I, Schreuder K, Declerck G. Evaluation of short-term nonpharmacological treatment of insomnia in a clinical setting. J Psychosom Res 1999; 47:369–383.
122. Backhaus J, Hohagen F, Voderholzer U, et al. Long-term effectiveness of a short-term cognitive-behavioral group treatment for primary insomnia. Eur Arch Psychiatry Clin Neurosci 2001; 251:35–41.
123. Morin CM, Hauri PJ, Espie CA, et al. Nonpharmacologic treatment of chronic insomnia. an American Academy of Sleep Medicine review. Sleep 1999; 22:1134–1156.
124. Morin CM, Bastien C, Savard J. Current status of cognitive-behavior therapy for insomnia: evidence for treatment effectiveness and feasibility. In: Perlis ML, Lichstein KL, eds. Treating Sleep Disorders: Principles and Practice of Behavioral Sleep Medicine. New York: Wiley & Sons, 2003:262–285.
125. Mimeault V, Morin CM. Self-help treatment for insomnia: bibliotherapy with and without professional guidance. J Consult Clin Psychol 1999; 67:511–519.

126. Strom L, Pettersson R, Andersson G. Internet-based treatment for insomnia: a controlled evaluation. J Consult Clin Psychol 2004; 72:113–120.

127. Baillargeon L, Demers M, Ladouceur R. Stimulus-control: nonpharmacologic treatment for insomnia. Can Fam Physician 1998; 44:73–79.

128. Oosterhuis A, Klip EC. The treatment of insomnia through mass media, the results of a televised behavioral training programme. Soc Sci Med 1997; 45:1223–1229.

129. Vincent N, Lionberg C. Treatment preference and patient satisfaction in chronic insomnia. Sleep 2001; 24:411–417.

130. Morin CM, Gaulier B, Barry T, et al. Patients' acceptance of psychological and pharmacological therapies for insomnia. Sleep 1992; 15:302–305.

131. Harvey L, Inglis SJ, Espie CA. Insomniacs' reported use of CBT components and relationship to long-term clinical outcome. Behav Res Ther 2002; 40:75–83.

132. Vincent NK, Hameed H. Relation between adherence and outcome in the group treatment of insomnia. Behav Sleep Med 2003; 1:125–139.

133. Morin CM, Vallieres A, Ivers H, et al. Dysfunctional beliefs and attitudes and sleep (DBAS): validation of a briefer version (DBAS-16). Sleep 2003; 26:A294.

134. Riedel BW, Lichstein KL. Strategies for evaluating adherence to sleep restriction treatment for insomnia. Behav Res Ther 2001; 39:2001–2212.

135. Simon GE, VonKorff M. Prevalence, burden, and treatment of insomnia in primary care. Am J Psychiatry 1997; 154:1417–1423.

136. Weissman MM, Greenwald S, Nino-Murcia G, et al. The morbidity of insomnia uncomplicated by psychiatric disorders. Gen Hosp Psychiatry 1997; 19:245–250.

137. Dement WC, Pelayo R. Public health impact and treatment of insomnia. Eur Psychiatry 1997; 12:31s–39s.

138. Bourne LS, Edinger JD, Carpenter K, et al. Does behavioral insomnia therapy reduce health care utilization? Sleep 2001; 24:A75.

139. Ancoli-Israel S, Roth T. Characteristics of insomnia in the United States: results of the 1991 National Sleep Foundation Survey I. Sleep 1999; 2(suppl):S347–S353.

140. Hajak G. Insomnia in primary care. Sleep 2000; 23:S54–S63.

141. Perlis ML, Smith MT, Cacialli DO, et al. On the comparability of pharmacotherapy and behavior therapy for chronic insomnia. Commentary and implications. J Psychosom Res 2003; 54:51–59.

142. Gagne A, Morin CM. Predicting treatment response in older adults with insomnia. J Clin Geropsychol 2001; 7:131–143.

143. Walsh JK, Engelhardt CL. Trends in the pharmacologic treatment of insomnia. J Clin Psychiatry 1992; 53:10–17.

144. Walsh JK, Roehrs T, Roth T. Pharmacologic treatment of primary insomnia. In: Kryger MH, Roth T, Dement WC, eds. Principles and Practice of Sleep Medicine. Philadelphia, PA: Elsevier-Saunders, 2005:749–760.

145. Newman MG. Recommendations for a cost-offset model of psychotherapy allocation using generalized anxiety disorder as an example. J Consult Clin Psychol 2000; 68:549–555.

146. Wilson GT, Vitousek KM, Loeb KL. Stepped care treatment of eating disorders. J Consult Clin Psychol 2000; 68:564–572.

147. Cohen J. Statistical power analyses for the behavioral sciences. San Diego: Academic Press, 1977.

8 | Pharmacologic Treatment of Insomnia

Clete A. Kushida

Division of Sleep Medicine, Department of Psychiatry and Behavioral Sciences, Stanford University School of Medicine, Stanford, California, U.S.A.

INTRODUCTION

The treatment of insomnia since antiquity to the 1960s has included substances and medications such as alcohol, laudanum, bromides, chloral hydrate, paraldehyde, urethane, and barbiturates. Benzodiazepines have been used to treat insomnia, but problems such as dependence, daytime drowsiness, and prevention of the transition from N2 to N3 sleep have resulted in providers prescribing this class of medications less frequently to their patients. Similarly, antidepressants with sedating properties such as trazodone are commonly prescribed to insomnia sufferers, despite considerable adverse effects such as tolerance, constipation, orthostatic hypotension, blurred vision, and priapism. Atypical antipsychotics such as olanzapine and quetiapine are also prescribed to patients with insomnia and also are associated with adverse effects that are not minor, such as dizziness, anticholinergic effects, and weight gain. Newer treatment options, which will be the focus of this chapter, include medications acting on the α-1 subunit of the benzodiazepine receptor complex and a novel MT1/MT2 receptor agonist, have rapidly become the first-line therapy for patients with insomnia, in conjunction with behavioral therapy.

Z-HYPNOTICS

Benzodiazepines (e.g., clonazepam, lorazepam, estazolam) act on the benzodiazepine receptor complex in the brain to facilitate γ-aminobutyric acid (GABA) and serve to decrease sleep latency and increase total sleep time. The newer "Z"-hypnotics, which include zolpidem, zaleplon, and eszopiclone, have increased selectivity for the α-1 subunit of the benzodiazepine receptor complex and have less of an effect on sleep architecture and a more rapid onset of action compared to benzodiazepines. This selectivity translates to less dependence and tolerance compared with benzodiazepines and nonsignificant anxiolytic, anticonvulsant, and muscle relaxant activity at doses prescribed for insomnia. Although Z-hypnotics have less adverse effects compared with benzodiazepines, gastrointestinal problems such as diarrhea and stomach upset may occur in some patients, and in the case of eszopiclone, a transient metallic or unpleasant taste on awakening in the morning has been reported. In addition, perceptual difficulties, memory problems, confusion, and rarely sleepwalking have been observed in patients using Z-hypnotics. The specific use of these medications often is tailored to their half-lives; patients who suffer from sleep-initiation insomnia (i.e., difficulty falling asleep) are more likely to benefit from a Z-hypnotic with a short half-life of less than two hours such as zaleplon (1) as opposed to those who suffer mainly from a sleep-maintenance insomnia (i.e., difficulty staying asleep). In the latter case, these patients are more likely to benefit from a medication such as eszopiclone (2), which has a longer half-life.

MT1/MT2 RECEPTOR AGONIST

Ramelteon binds to the MT1/MT2 receptor and has a rapid onset of action and a short half-life of less than three hours (half-life of its active metabolite is 2–5 hours) (3). Similar to other hypnotics, this medication results in a reduced sleep latency and increased total sleep time, but due to its short half-life, may not be effective in maintaining sleep throughout the night. Although difficulty concentrating and decreased alertness are reported dose-related adverse effects, no abuse potential has been reported for ramelteon.

BENZODIAZEPINES

Some benzodiazepines such as triazolam and temazepam have been shown to reduce sleep latency and wake after sleep onset and increase total sleep time. However, tolerance, adverse effects such as memory impairment, and the longer half-lives of these medications with resultant daytime drowsiness compared with Z-hypnotics limit their utility as first-line hypnotics. In addition, triazolam has also been associated with rebound insomnia, in which the insomnia following discontinuation of the drug's use may be worsened. Flurazepam is not usually considered due to its prolonged half-life, and other benzodiazepines such as clonazepam or lorazepam may be considered for off-label use in some restricted circumstances.

ANTIDEPRESSANTS

Sedating low-dose antidepressants (e.g., trazodone, mirtazapine, amitriptyline, doxepin) may be considered as a pharmacologic treatment for insomnia; however, since they are antidepressants, they should be considered in patients who have comorbid depression. As described earlier, this class of medication is not without adverse effects, and there are specific adverse effects associated with certain antidepressants (e.g., mirtazapine is associated with weight gain).

ATYPICAL ANTIPSYCHOTICS

Olanzapine and quetiapine have been prescribed for patients with insomnia, but adverse effects such as dizziness, weight gain, hyperglycemia, and anticholinergic effects limit their use. These medications should be prescribed only in patients with psychosis who have concomitant insomnia.

OTHER PRESCRIPTION DRUGS

There are other medications that have been prescribed for insomnia, although their indications may be for other diseases (e.g., epilepsy). Such medications include gabapentin and tiagabine. However, given their potential for adverse effects and limited data on efficacy, off-label use of these medications as a treatment for insomnia is rarely considered. Lastly, chloral hydrate has been used in the past in patients with insomnia. However, it is associated with significant adverse effects, such as gastrointestinal upset, and rapid tolerance to this drug limits its utility in these patients.

NON-PRESCRIPTION DRUGS AND SUBSTANCES

Compounds such as diphenhydramine, melatonin, kava-kava, and valerian have been used as over-the-counter remedies for insomnia. Unfortunately, limited evidence support their use, and potentially life-threatening adverse effects (e.g., hepatic impairment with kava-kava) should be considered in any patient with insomnia who is considering taking these drugs or substances. Since these compounds are not approved by the national Food and Drug Administration (FDA), their safety is untested and the strengths of the active ingredient may vary from one preparation to another. In addition, the occurrence of daytime drowsiness and cognitive impairment may be present the day following use of these drugs or substances. Melatonin is secreted by the pineal gland and affects the suprachiasmatic nucleus, the brain's circadian pacemaker. It has been used in the treatment of jet lag, but its efficacy in improving sleep initiation and/or maintenance difficulties in patients with insomnia is questionable. However, some studies have shown that early-evening administration of this compound improved sleep latency and sleep duration in healthy individuals (4–6), and the adverse effect profile is mild, with nausea, fatigue, and dizziness reported in some individuals.

CONCLUSIONS

There are various medications, substances, and preparations that may be used to treat insomnia. Physicians and patients should be aware of the indications, onsets of action, half-lives, and adverse effects of these treatments, in order to ensure appropriate efficacy, decreased tolerance, and minimal safety-related issues. This is especially true when a patient with insomnia is considering use of a non-FDA-approved drug or substance for his or her condition.

REFERENCES

1. Drover DR. Comparative pharmacokinetics and pharmacodynamics of short-acting hypnosedatives. Clin Pharmacokinet 2004; 43:227–238.
2. Krystal AD, Walsh JK, Laska E, et al. Sustained efficacy of eszopiclone over 6 months of nightly treatment: results of a randomized, double-blind, placebo-controlled study in adults with chronic insomnia. Sleep 2003; 26:793–799.
3. Morin CM, Hauri PJ, Espie CA, et al. Nonpharmacologic treatment of chronic insomnia. An American Academy of Sleep Medicine review. Sleep 1999; 22:1134–1156.
4. Turek FW, Gillette MU. Melatonin, sleep, and circadian rhythms: rationale for development of specific melatonin agonists. Sleep Med 2004; 5:523–532.
5. Wagner J, Wagner ML, Hening WA. Beyond benzodiazepines: alternative pharmacologic agents for the treatment of insomnia. Ann Pharmacother 1998; 32:680–691.
6. Brzezinski A, Vangel MG, Wurtman RJ, et al. Effects of exogenous melatonin on sleep: a meta-analysis. Sleep Med Rev 2005; 9:41–50.

9 | Adjunctive and Alternative Treatment of Insomnia

Kristen L. Payne, James P. Soeffing, and Kenneth L. Lichstein

Department of Psychology, The University of Alabama, Tuscaloosa, Alabama, U.S.A.

INTRODUCTION

Numerous contributing factors may play a role in chronic insomnia, but there is no definitive model that establishes how these factors combine and interact to initiate and perpetuate the condition. With so many factors potentially playing a role, it makes sense for clinicians to be as inclusive as possible when considering treatment options for the diverse array of persons suffering with insomnia. Interventions such as prescription hypnotics and cognitive-behavioral therapy offer some heavily researched options for persons seeking treatment, but these conventional interventions do not address every potential contributing factor in every individual. They also may not be optimal in all situations because of associated costs and side effects. For example, patients may avoid cognitive-behavioral interventions because of their relatively high upfront costs and benzodiazepines because of dependence potential.

Alternative therapies may appeal to those concerned about some of the negative side effects or costs of traditional insomnia therapies. These alternative treatments range from bright light therapy to herbal medications to biofeedback treatment. Approximately 25% to 50% of people in industrialized nations use some sort of alternative treatment (1). Thirty percent of respondents in another survey reported using alternative or complementary treatments for insomnia (2). With so many individuals utilizing alternative treatments, more information needs to be disseminated to practitioners and patients. This chapter will examine the available research for each of the alternative treatments and will pay special attention to the quality of the research studies in an attempt to help clinicians make informed decisions about each therapy.

LIMITATIONS OF THE EVIDENCE FOR ALTERNATIVE THERAPIES

To evaluate the existent literature appropriately, one must be aware that there are some inherent difficulties when describing research in the area of alternative therapies. First, studies are typically funded based on what sponsors deem interesting or important at the time. Alternative medicine is typically given less weight than traditional Western medicine and may be less likely to be funded. This translates into the possibility that alternative treatments are effective for certain disorders, but we lack the scientific evidence to support it.

Second, some alternative treatments originated in areas other than the United States and are more often practiced in these areas. For example, acupuncture is a prevalent practice in China, and thus many of the articles published are written in Chinese. This review is limited to articles published in English.

Third, the methodology of many studies evaluating alternative treatments is often criticized by researchers trained in Western science. This may be because researchers in alternative medicine are using a different theoretical model than those trained in traditional Western science. The biomedical model focuses on disease with the underlying assumption that some agent(s) leads to this disease (3).

On the other hand, complementary medicine focuses on a more holistic approach to illness and is concerned with several factors that may be multidimensional in nature and are difficult to study independently. Relatedly, the nature of some alternative therapies makes controlled study difficult. For example, acupuncture cannot be simulated without sham needle insertion. Whether this is a valid placebo condition is often questioned (4,5). The reader should keep these issues in mind when evaluating the findings presented in the current chapter.

VITAMINS/HERBAL/HORMONAL SUPPLEMENTS

Vitamins

Approximately 33% of Americans take at least one vitamin supplement daily (6). However, very little is known about how vitamins impact sleep. A study by our group (7) showed that people taking vitamins (either multivitamins or multiple vitamins) tended to have more awake time during the night than those who did not take vitamins. It should be noted that this study used secondary data analysis to explore the topic, and future studies would benefit from a more prospective research design. This is the first attempt to examine the association between vitamins and sleep. There has been more published information on specific medicinal herbs and nutritional supplements used to treat insomnia, and this discussion follows.

Valerian

In some studies, valerian has been shown to improve sleep compared with placebo based on physician and self-rating forms, increase slow-wave sleep and decrease stage 1 sleep, improve quality and decrease sleep latency compared to placebo, and sedate for a shorter duration as compared with traditional benzodiazepines (8). Several controlled trials have found positive effects on sleep (9,10) such that participants report significantly better sleep, specifically with reductions in sleep-onset latency (SOL) (11).

A systematic review of valerian was also conducted (12) by examining only randomized controlled trials (9 studies). The authors concluded that there was contradictory evidence in the literature. For example, some of the studies reported decreases in SOL, whereas others did not find any differences between those taking valerian and those in the control condition. The authors do mention that the methodologies in the studies were different, which could have contributed to the contradictions. Some studies used subjective measures of sleep variables and others used polysomnographic (PSG) data. The overall conclusion that the authors made was that more rigorous studies needed to be conducted in this area before any firm conclusions could be reached about the efficacy of valerian. Valerian appears to be fairly safe, with few adverse side effects reported (11). The side effects of valerian include dizziness, headache, and nausea.

In a study on the efficacy of a valerian-hops combination treatment for insomnia, researchers found that there were modest improvements in SOL, sleep efficiency (SE), and total sleep time (TST) (13), although the changes in SE and TST were not statistically significant. According to the authors, this combination treatment may be a helpful adjunctive therapy for insomnia.

In conclusion, valerian's efficacy to treat insomnia needs to be examined more closely and rigorously. The studies that have been published offer contradictory results and have used different methodologies, which makes firm conclusions difficult.

Melatonin

Melatonin is a hormone secreted by the pineal gland, which plays a significant role in sleep regulation and onset. Several randomized placebo-controlled trials have been conducted (14–16) to evaluate melatonin's effects on sleep. In one study, a significant number of patients who were taking melatonin and were also taking benzodiazepines (8 out of 13) were able to reduce or discontinue their use of the benzodiazepines (17). These findings are especially important for populations that are prone to experiencing negative side effects from benzodiazepines (e.g., older adults).

A meta-analysis (18) was used to examine 12 studies on melatonin's effects on sleep. The major findings were that SOL was reduced by an average of 7.5 minutes, SE was increased by 2.2%, and TST increased by 12.8 minutes for those taking melatonin. In another meta-analysis focused on the safety of melatonin (19), few adverse side effects were reported. The most common side effects included nausea, headaches, dizziness, and drowsiness. There were no differences in side effects reported between those receiving placebo as compared with those receiving melatonin. Interestingly, some authors point out that acupuncture, yoga, and meditation can naturally increase the secretion of melatonin, which may explain some of these treatments' ability to improve sleep (20,21).

Dosing and time of administration of melatonin plays a role in its therapeutic effect. Melatonin given from mid-day to early evening can have beneficial effects on sleep (22,23). A randomized, double-blinded controlled study with older adults found that 2 mg of continued-release melatonin was effective for helping to maintain sleep, after just one week of administration (24). In this same study a one-week treatment of 2 mg fast-release melatonin was effective in improving SOL. Maintenance on 1-mg continued-release melatonin over the course of two months improved both maintenance and initiation of sleep. Some researchers have demonstrated that low doses of melatonin ranging from 0.3 to 1 mg do not improve SOL (25), while others have found that doses between 3 and 6 mg given approximately 30 to 120 minutes before sleep are effective in reducing SOL (26). At this time, optimal dosing is unclear (27).

Overall, melatonin appears to improve sleep, but only modestly by effecting SOL, SE, and TST. There is some evidence that melatonin can be used as a substitute for benzodiazepines for patients who are wary of taking or who are unable to tolerate such medication. However, dosing and time of administration plays an important role in the therapeutic outcome of this drug and should be considered carefully. Unfortunately, at this time firm recommendations about dosing are not available.

Sleep-Aid Tea

Little research has been published on the effects of sleep-aid tea for the treatment of insomnia. Sleep-Aid Tea is a tea consisting of substances from natural fruits and plants that are thought to have sleep-inducing effects (28). Studies have been conducted using this tea, mostly on animal subjects, and the results have been positive in comparison with placebo (29). Specifically, the tea has increased TST in these animals.

Research with human participants is still in its preliminary phase. In one study, 40 insomniacs were asked to take the tea and perform self-assessment measures of their sleep quality (SQ) (28). In this sample, TST was enhanced by an average of 1.5 hours. However, no control group was used in this study, and details about the participants are vaguely reported. Details about the makeup of the tea used with the human participants were also not reported.

Kava

Kava, a plant that grows on the South Sea Islands, can produce depressant effects in the central nervous system (CNS) of animals (30). It has been used to treat anxiety disorders and to improve sleep (31). Many more studies have been conducted with kava as a treatment for anxiety than for sleep. The few studies that have evaluated its effects on sleep have found favorable results. For instance, it has been shown to increase subjective ratings of SQ, as well as decrease in SOL and wake time after sleep onset (WASO) (31). However, there are few studies evaluating kava specifically for insomnia, so caution should be taken until more controlled studies have been conducted for this particular population. Logically, it seems that kava might be helpful with those insomniacs who have trouble sleeping due to anxiety problems, but direct testing of this hypothesis is needed.

In conclusion, positive results have been shown for treating insomnia with melatonin and valerian. Although some of the findings in meta-analyses for valerian are contradictory, both valerian (32) and melatonin (33) are widely cited in alternative therapy handbooks (3,34), are used frequently for sleep problems, and are gaining more visibility in scientific literature. Less is known about Sleep-Aid Tea and kava, and no definitive statement can be made about their effects on sleep.

BIOFEEDBACK

Biofeedback involves monitoring physiological signals and learning to influence them through conscious effort. Proponents of biofeedback treatments suggest that the control of these signals can help relieve symptoms related to a variety of physical and mental health problems (35). In a typical biofeedback treatment session, sensors or electrodes are attached to different parts of the body and used to detect physiological measures such as muscle tension, heart rate, temperature, perspiration, or brain waves. Special hardware and software is then used to amplify and process these bodily signals in such a way that audio or visual feedback can be given to the patient. Patients can then monitor the feedback and use a variety of techniques such as relaxation exercises to alter their physiology. Essentially then, biofeedback is designed to help patients gain voluntary control of involuntary functions.

Two types of biofeedback have been used for the treatment of insomnia: electromyographic (EMG) and electroencephalographic (EEG). EMG biofeedback involves the measurement and control of somatic arousal in the form of muscle tension. With the help of biofeedback instrumentation, patients are taught how to recognize and control the tension in a specific muscle group through special relaxation exercises. In this way, biofeedback can be considered closely related to relaxation treatments for insomnia. Auditory or visual feedback communicates information about the level of tension and offers cues to the patient's level of physiological arousal. Thus, when the auditory or visual cues show a reduction in muscle tension, the patients know that they are successfully administering the relaxation exercise. Over time, the goal is to have the patients be able to utilize their relaxation skills without the biofeedback paraphernalia and to reduce physiological arousal at bedtime.

Several reports suggest that EMG biofeedback is effective for improving measures of sleep continuity. The sleep variable most commonly associated with improvement has been SOL. Several studies using EMG biofeedback have indicated statistically significant reductions in SOL for persons with insomnia (36–41). Research has also shown significant improvements in WASO (40) and TST (39). Despite these encouraging results, EMG biofeedback consistently fails to perform better than other relaxation treatments (36–38,42) or placebo biofeedback (38,41,42).

EEG biofeedback involves training to manipulate brain waves and includes two main subtypes: theta and sigma. Theta waves range from 3 to 7 Hz and are a dominant waveform in stage N1 and N2 sleep. The rationale for using theta biofeedback is to help patients produce brain waves that are compatible with sleep to encourage sleep onset and increase the patient's ability to maintain sleep. Although not formally considered a relaxation therapy, theta biofeedback does involve attempts to move toward a low arousal state. The research literature regarding theta biofeedback is rather sparse relative to that for EMG biofeedback. A case study by Bell (43) described improvements in SOL and TST at posttreatment and three-month follow-up for a 42-year-old woman with a complaint of sleep-onset insomnia. Other work (44) indicated improvements in SOL and TST at posttreatment and follow-up for persons treated with theta biofeedback. However, the lack of control groups and statistical analyses should be considered in evaluation of this treatment literature.

The other subtype of EEG biofeedback, sigma, is also called sensorimotor rhythm (SMR) biofeedback and involves the strengthening of 12 to 14 Hz EEG activity that characterizes healthy non–rapid eye movement (NREM) sleep. Research has suggested that this type of brain activity is less prominent during wakefulness in persons with insomnia relative to healthy sleepers (45). Thus, increasing this 12 to 14 Hz activity may be a useful treatment approach for insomnia. An early study using SMR biofeedback (46) produced a reduction in SOL and movement time during sleep. Further research by Hauri (47) and Hauri and colleagues (44) also revealed improvement in SOL from pre- to posttreatment and pre- to follow-up analyses. However, these improvements were not statistically significant in either study, and improvements in the SMR biofeedback group were not significantly different from a control group (47). Despite these findings, the two studies by Hauri and colleagues revealed an interesting relationship between the type of biofeedback and the type of insomnia. Persons with insomnia who were either muscularly or psychologically tense at baseline appeared to benefit more from the interventions designed to lower arousal (EMG and theta), while initially less tense participants benefited more from the SMR biofeedback.

In conclusion, biofeedback has shown some efficacy in the treatment of insomnia. Persons with insomnia fairly consistently show improvements in SOL after being treated with a variety of biofeedback subtypes. Unfortunately, biofeedback treatments also consistently fail to outperform other behavioral treatments and placebo control groups. If biofeedback treatment is to be used, assessing baseline somatic and psychological tension levels and delivering a biofeedback type consistent with these levels may be one way to maximize treatment outcome for persons with insomnia. Despite this interesting possibility, the dearth of biofeedback for insomnia research in the past 20 years suggests a loss of interest in this potential treatment option.

LOW-ENERGY EMISSION THERAPY

Low-energy emission therapy (LEET) consists of delivering low levels of amplitude-modulated radio frequency electromagnetic fields through an electrically conductive mouthpiece. The mouthpiece must have direct contact with the mucus in the mouth. The electricity is passed through the mouthpiece and to the patient's brain (48). The therapy is usually conducted in 15-minute intervals with a 42.7-Hz amplitude modulation of 27.12 MHz (48). It has been shown that the administration of LEET modulates calcium release in animal cortexes (49,50).

Several studies have been conducted to assess the efficacy of the LEET device in treating insomnia (48,51,52) and the long-term side effects of the treatment (53). A placebo-controlled trial (52) showed that those receiving active treatment had an increase in TST after treatment, whereas the placebo group did not show this increase, even after controlling for baseline TST. In addition, those receiving active treatment had a significant decrease in SOL and an increase in SE. The inactive treatment group did not show a significant increase in SOL; however, this group did show an increase in SE, although this increase was much smaller than in the active treatment group.

Safety of the LEET device and treatment has been assessed in a retrospective manner (53). The side effects reported most often were pleasant dreaming (7% of 807) and increased dreaming (5%). Two participants reported a diagnosis of cancer after receiving the LEET treatment; however, the authors of the study concluded it was likely not due to the treatment. The electromagnetic fields given off during LEET treatment are far less than that of a cell phone. The authors of the study called for prospective and more rigorous research to be conducted to help establish the safety of this treatment. Overall, this treatment appears to be promising and is currently used frequently in Europe for the treatment of insomnia.

BRIGHT LIGHT

Research has suggested that environmental light is the most potent tool for synchronizing and stabilizing human circadian rhythms (54). Emerging evidence also suggests that a circadian rhythm that is out of synch with the day-night cycle can produce and contribute to the symptoms of insomnia (55). Considering these conclusions, it makes sense to consider the use of bright light exposure as a treatment for certain types of insomnia.

Two types of persons with insomnia appear to be best suited to bright light interventions: (*i*) those who have a delayed circadian rhythm that causes them to fall asleep later and wake up later than what is considered normal and (*ii*) those who have an advanced circadian rhythm that causes them to fall asleep earlier and wake up earlier than is considered normal.

Two studies have reported success in treating sleep-onset insomnia in younger patients by administering bright-light treatment during the morning hours (56,57). Other studies have successfully used bright-light therapy administered in the evening to improve sleep maintenance and delay early morning awakenings in older adults with advanced circadian rhythms (58–60). On the basis of results, clinicians may want to consider bright-light therapy for patients whose insomnia appears to be related to either an advanced or delayed circadian rhythm.

RELAXATION-TYPE TREATMENT

Relaxation is a treatment often used in behavioral management of insomnia (61). "Relaxation" refers to several related methods with common procedures including conducting relaxation in a quiet environment; concentrating on a repetitive, calming stimulus; maintaining a peaceful attitude; and resting in a comfortable position (62). There are several types of relaxation used to treat insomnia. The techniques that have been studied the most include progressive and passive muscle relaxation and imagery (chap. 7). However, there are other types of relaxation therapy that are used to combat insomnia but are less visible in the scientific literature. We will now examine these treatments in detail.

Yoga

Yoga is a system of breathing techniques and postures used to help improve breathing and flexibility as well as a spiritual rejuvenation. Yoga has been recommended as a system that promotes relaxation and may be suitable for those people experiencing insomnia, especially insomnia associated with psychological distress. However, there is little research in this area. What does exist suggests that yoga can improve subjective sleep measures, including TST,

WASO, and SOL (63), and feelings of being rested in older adults (64). It should be noted that only the study with older adults contained a controlled condition. Few other studies have been done in a controlled manner, although some complementary medicine books tout this as an effective treatment for insomnia (34). It should be stressed that research in the area is young, and more controlled research trials would benefit practitioners and patients alike by shedding more light on yoga's effects on sleep.

Meditation

A component of many Eastern relaxation techniques, including yoga, is a focus on meditation, which involves concentrating on a specific object (concentrative meditation) or a broader field (mindfulness meditation) (65). One of the goals of meditation is an altered state of consciousness, and this has been found to reduce excitation of the nervous system and cortex. For people who have insomnia and complain of physiological arousal, meditation may be a helpful treatment.

The data on meditation and insomnia are not abundant but some do exist. Woolfolk and colleagues (66) compared meditation to relaxation training and a waitlist control group. They found that those in both the relaxation and meditation treatments had less SOL and lower subjective ratings on difficulty falling asleep as compared with the waitlist control treatment. What is especially interesting is that the relaxation and meditation groups did not differ from each other on any variable. Thus, this treatment may be comparable to traditional relaxation techniques.

A study on transcendental meditation examined the sleep of 10 insomniacs and found a significant reduction in SOL (67). The reduction in SOL was maintained at one-year follow-up.

Aromatherapy

Aromatherapy oils are absorbed either through the skin or through inhalation. Common aromatherapy oils used for sleep include lavender and chamomile.

Lavender has been shown to have anticonvulsant effects in laboratory studies involving mice (68). Repeat dosing of lavender oil seems to increase TST and decrease SOL in animals (69). Some clinical trials have been conducted to assess the efficacy of using lavender to promote sleep in humans (70). These studies found depressant effects on CNS and improved TST. One issue to consider when using lavender is that it tends to increase the potential of other drugs that have sleep-promoting effects (71).

There are studies that name other essential oils as sleep promoting, including sour orange (*Citrus aurantium* L.) (72) and chamomile (73). The preliminary reports on sour orange and chamomile are encouraging although sour orange has only been tested in animals at this stage. Chamomile, typically taken as a tea, has been shown to induce sleep in 10 cardiac patients (73).

While the verdict is still out on the soporific effect of most essential oils, lavender has had some encouraging results and looks promising as an aid to promote sleep. However, randomized placebo-controlled trails would help make the case stronger for lavender. Special care should be taken to assess the possibility of drug interactions with lavender.

Music Therapy

Few studies have been conducted to assess the effect that music has on sleep (74–76). The earlier studies tended to use mixed samples including several different age groups, lacked random assignment to groups, and did not assess possible confounding variables such as depression.

Lai and Good (74) conducted a randomized controlled trail and assigned participants to the music or control group. Music was played for 45 minutes before bedtime in this sample of older adults suffering from difficulty sleeping. However, these participants did not necessarily meet the criteria for insomnia. The participants chose a music style that they preferred from a list of songs with similar tempos. Experimenters arrived at the participants' home, played the tape for them, and observed physical reactions to the tape. Experimenters instructed the participants on how to relax, if needed. Those in the music therapy group had better global sleep quality, SOL, SE, and less daytime impairment (as measured by the Pittsburgh Sleep Quality Index). One obvious question is whether the relaxation techniques or the music itself (or both) were responsible for the effects that were seen. Although from preliminary studies music looks like a possible treatment for insomnia, further research should look into the role of music in relaxation as separate from a training exercise in relaxation techniques.

In summary, most relaxation-type therapies show some promise in treating insomnia. However, at this stage, meditation and lavender appear to have the most support. There is some support for music therapy and yoga, but not enough to establish their efficacy.

ACUPUNCTURE

Acupuncture has been used to treat insomnia by the Chinese for a long period of time (3). However, it is difficult to evaluate acupuncture's efficacy in treating insomnia for a couple of reasons. First, the research that exists on the efficacy of acupuncture in treating insomnia is complicated by the use of chronic pain patients as research participants. Second, most articles in this area are not published in English.

Several PSG studies have been conducted to assess the efficacy of acupuncture (77,78) but are published in other languages. Other reviews of existing literature are also available in other languages (79). One study published in English found a decrease in SOL and an increase in TST, SE, and SQ from baseline to posttreatment (21).

A systematic review of the effect of acupuncture on insomnia examined studies that used an experimental design, were written in English, and were published between 1975 and 2002 (80). Eleven articles met these criteria. The authors of this review reported that acupuncture's rate of success was greater than 80%, meaning that most participants in the studies perceived effectiveness of acupuncture or had a longer duration of sleep. However, the authors also note that there was quite a bit of variability between the studies in the definitions of insomnia.

The basic mechanism by which acupuncture aids in effecting sleep is largely unknown. However, the information available on the neurobiology of acupuncture shows that the CNS sites that react to acupuncture are also indicated in the regulation of the sleep-wake cycle (81). Other research has shown that acupuncture increases the level of melatonin that the body produces, thereby possibly aiding in sleep (21).

In summary, acupuncture is used frequently in other countries to treat insomnia. From the research available in English, it appears that acupuncture needs to have more controlled trials conducted before the efficacy of its use as an insomnia treatment can be assessed. The Western literature would benefit from a review of the literature in other languages.

WHITE NOISE

There is no definitive definition of white noise as it is used in the pursuit of better sleep, but it can be described as a constant, low-intensity, mixed frequency sound. A good example of white noise from common experience would be the constant hum of a cooling fan or air conditioning unit. Another commonly used sound that people often use in place of truer forms of white noise is a recording of the ocean lapping against the shore. There has been little published research exploring the soporific impact of white noise, but the few published reports that exist are encouraging.

Spencer and colleagues (82) explored the effect of white noise on neonates ranging in age from two to seven days. The authors found that 80% of neonates exposed to white noise fell asleep within five minutes, while only 25% in a no-noise control group did the same. This study hints at the possibility that white noise can actually facilitate the process of falling asleep, but the results have not been replicated in studies with adults. Other research suggests that white noise can be a helpful tool to maintain sleep in environments where sudden noise leads to frequent arousals from sleep.

Stanchina and colleagues (83) exposed sleeping participants to the recorded noise of an intensive care unit (ICU) under two conditions where white noise was also either present or absent. They found that participants had more consolidated sleep and fewer arousals in the white noise condition. Another interesting outcome of the study was that the peak noise level in the white noise condition was higher than in the ICU noise only condition. On the basis of this information, the authors concluded that the sleep-enhancing effects of white noise are due to its ability to reduce the difference between background noise and peak noise.

It is not clear what intensity of white noise is optimal for promoting sleep, but some research suggests that very loud white noise can affect the architecture of sleep in unexpected ways. Scott (84) exposed college students to 93 db of continuous white noise across eight consecutive nights and found that the amount of time spent in rapid eye movement (REM) sleep decreased significantly and was replaced by increases in stage N1 and stage N2 sleep.

In conclusion, white noise has shown some efficacy in improving sleep. The evidence suggesting that white noise improves SOL is sparse. However, it does appear that white noise can facilitate the continuation and quality of sleep in situations where there are frequent intrusive noises. This effect appears to be due to the ability of white noise to reduce the difference between environmental background noise and peak noise. Those who choose to use white noise to promote sleep should be aware that very loud white noise might have a potentially negative impact on sleep architecture. Further research is needed to assess whether white noise can actually help people fall asleep faster.

CHIROPRACTIC TREATMENT

Anecdotal evidence is often reported in support of chiropractic treatment for insomnia (85) since no experimentally controlled studies have been published. One pilot study was conducted to assess patients' expectations, experience with chiropractic treatment, and sleep after treatment (85).

In patients who had received chiropractic treatment, approximately two-thirds reported no change in their sleep difficulties. Those who did report change in sleeping, most often reported sleeping more soundly. The prospective part of the study examining sleep patterns of patients with insomnia showed that three-fourths of participants recorded sleep improvement in the first days after chiropractic adjustment.

The precise mechanism of action for which chiropractic treatment can affect sleep is not known. One possibility is that it relieves pain, which may be an underlying contributor to insomnia (85). Research in this area is very preliminary, and more is needed to establish if chiropractic treatment is helpful to treat insomnia.

EXERCISE

It is a commonly held belief that exercise improves sleep, and this belief has been supported by survey-based epidemiologic research. For example, epidemiological studies have shown a positive correlation between exercise and sleep (86–88). Conclusions drawn from these types of studies are limited due to alternative explanations for the relationship between exercise and sleep.

A review of the applicable literature by Youngstedt (89) highlights some of these alternative explanations that are not controlled for in epidemiologic studies. Alternative explanations include (1) better sleep may be associated with a greater willingness to exercise (2), better sleep and ability or willingness to exercise are related to better overall health and less stress (3), people who exercise also tend to engage in other healthy behaviors such as avoidance of excessive alcohol, caffeine, and tobacco, and (4) outdoor exercise may be associated with more exposure to bright light, which in turn could have a positive impact on sleep.

Experimental research examining the impact of acute exercise offers a second avenue of exploration to clarify the relationship between exercise and sleep. A majority of experimental studies in this area compared groups that took part in acute active daily exercise with sedentary control groups, and compared their sleep on the evening after the day the exercise occurred. A meta-analysis by Youngstedt et al. (90) synthesized the extant research and reached the following conclusions: (1) SOL and WASO are nearly unaffected by exercise (2), exercise leads to a small increase in TST, and (3) slow-wave sleep slightly increases after exercise and REM sleep slightly decreases. Although these results are somewhat disappointing, one aspect of these studies may help explain the modest results. The participants in these studies were almost entirely good sleepers who were likely limited in their ability to improve because their current sleep was already good.

Some researchers (90) have identified variables that moderate the effects of exercise on sleep. These authors concluded that (*i*) exercise has the most positive impact on sleep if it occurs four to eight hours before bedtime; (*ii*) exercise durations of one to two hours appears to have the greatest positive effect on sleep; and (*iii*) light, moderate, and vigorous exercise elicit similar outcomes.

Another area of interest is chronic exercise, which refers to long-term exercise regimens. Three studies examining chronic exercise compared older adults engaging in chronic exercise with a control group and found no significant differences between groups on sleep variables such as SOL, WASO, and TST (91–93). Unfortunately, like the research on acute exercise, these studies used healthy sleepers as participants, again creating a ceiling effect.

One study that actually used participants who met the criteria for a diagnosis of primary insomnia had more encouraging results. King and colleagues (94) found that a sample of predominantly older adults randomized into a moderate exercise treatment group self-reported significantly larger improvements in SOL and TST relative to a waitlist control group at posttreatment.

In conclusion, the majority of research exploring the influence of exercise on sleep has been conducted with healthy older sleepers and was found to have minimal improvement on sleep. Research on participants meeting criteria for insomnia has shown more promise, but only with self-report measures. Further research with both subjective and objective measures is needed to clarify the efficacy of exercise for improving sleep in persons with insomnia. Clinical applications of exercise to aid in sleep should include strategies to maximize outcomes by using optimal duration of exercise and time of exercise relative to bedtime.

CONCLUSIONS

The majority of alternative and adjunctive treatments are difficult to evaluate as treatments for insomnia because of a lack of controlled research, poor sampling procedures, or lack of information about the specific treatment. Many complementary and alternative therapy handbooks include a list of helpful treatments for insomnia, yet conservative scientific support for their efficacy is lacking. The area of complementary medicine would benefit from having more information and efficacy trials as well as information about safety for these treatments.

LEET and meditation are somewhat helpful for treating insomnia; however, these therapies would benefit from a more thorough examination of the safety of each treatment and other variables that may affect the outcomes (i.e., type of insomnia). Several of the treatments included in this chapter have some evidence that supports its use for insomnia, yet each treatment's success seems to be dependent on the type of insomnia present. Treatments falling into this category include kava, biofeedback, bright light, and chiropractic treatment. Melatonin appears to be marginally helpful for decreasing sleep, but its therapeutic effects depend on the time of administration and dosage. Other treatments such as yoga, aromatherapy, acupuncture, and music therapy simply lack the rigorous research needed for any firm conclusions to be reached. The research on Sleep-Aid Tea does not give enough information about the contents of the tea to be fully evaluated, and the research on exercise has been conducted almost exclusively with older normal sleepers, making conclusions about its effects on the sleep of insomniacs virtually impossible. White noise does seem to be a helpful remedy for sleep disturbances if one is in an environment that contains sleep-disrupting noises. Contradictory evidence exists for valerian, and thus conclusions about its effects on sleep are difficult.

To add to the difficulty in evaluating some complementary and alternative treatments' effects on sleep is the fact that they are not regulated by the U.S. Food and Drug Administration (FDA), and thus purity of ingredients and accuracy of labeled dosing can be variable. This is particularly true for supplements and aromatherapy treatment.

Overall, it appears that research in the area of complementary and alternative treatment for insomnia has a long but promising road ahead in the treatment of insomnia. Although proponents of these alternative treatments state the difficulties in measuring these treatments' effects, empirical evidence would help physicians and patients make informed decisions about treatment options. There are negative side effects associated with traditional treatments for insomnia (especially with benzodiazepines), and finding other effective tools to combat insomnia may help those with sleeping difficulties achieve a better quality of life.

REFERENCES

1. Mamtani R, Cimino A. A primer of complementary and alternative medicine and its relevance in the treatment of mental health problems. Psychiatr Q 2002; 73:367–381.
2. Brown RP, Gerbarg PL. Herbs and nutrients in the treatment of depression, anxiety, insomnia, migraine, and obesity. J Psychiatr Pract 2001; 7:75–91.
3. Spencer JW, Jacobs JJ. Complementary/Alternative Medicine: An Evidence-Based Approach. New York: Mosby, 1999.
4. Ballegaard S, Meyer CN, Trojaborg W. Acupuncture in angina pectoral: does acupuncture have a specific effect? J Intern Med 1991; 229:357–362.
5. Zaslawski C, Rogers C, Garvey M, et al. Strategies to maintain the credibility of sham acupuncture used as a control treatment in clinical trials. J Altern Complement Med 1997; 3:257–266.
6. Millen AE, Dodd KW, Subar AF. Use of vitamin, mineral, nonvitamin, and nonmineral supplements in the United States: the 1987, 1992, and 2000 National Health Interview Survey results. J Am Diet Assoc 2004; 104:942–950.
7. Lichstein KL, Payne KL, Soeffing JP, et al. Vitamins and sleep: an exploratory study. Sleep Med 2007; 9(1):27–32.
8. Gyllenhaal C, Merritt SL, Peterson SD, et al. Efficacy and safety of herbal stimulants and sedatives in sleep disorder. Sleep Med Rev 2000; 4:229–251.
9. Lindahl O, Lindwall L. Double blind study of valerian preparation. Pharmacol Biochem Behav 1989; 32:1065–1066.
10. Ziegler G, Ploch M, Miettinen-Baumann A, et al. Efficacy and tolerability of valerian extract LI 156 compared with oxazepam in the treatment of non-organic insomnia—a randomized, double-blind, comparative clinical study. Eur J Med Res 2002; 25:480–486.
11. Hadley S, Petry JJ. Valerian. Am Fam Physician 2003; 67:1755–1758.
12. Stevinson C, Ernst E. Valerian for insomnia: a systematic review of randomized clinical trials. Sleep Med 2000; 1:91–99.
13. Morin CM, Koetter U, Bastien C, et al. Valerian-Hops combination and diphenhydramine for treating insomnia: a randomized placebo-controlled clinical trial. Sleep 2005; 28:1465–1471.
14. Hughes RJ, Badia P. Sleep promoting and hypothermic effects of daytime melatonin administration in humans. Sleep 1997; 20:124–131.
15. Singer C, Tractenberg RE, Kaye J, et al. A multicenter, placebo-controlled trial of melatonin for sleep disturbance in Alzheimer's disease. Sleep 2002; 26:893–901.
16. Stone BM, Turner C, Mills SL, et al. Hypnotic activity of melatonin. Sleep 2000; 23:1–7.
17. Fainstein I, Bonetto AJ, Brusco LI, et al. Effects of melatonin in elderly patients with sleep disturbance: a pilot study. Curr Ther Res 1997; 58:990–1000.
18. Brzezinski A, Vangel MG, Wurtman RJ, et al. Effects of exogenous melatonin on sleep: a meta-analysis. Sleep Med Rev 2005; 9:41–50.
19. Buscemi N, Vandermeer B, Hooton N, et al. The efficacy and safety of exogenous melatonin for primary sleep disorders. J Gen Intern Med 2005; 20:1151–1158.
20. Harinath K, Malhorta AS, Pal K, et al. Effects of Hatha yoga and Omkar meditation on cardiorespiratory performance, psychologic profile, and melatonin secretion. J Altern Complement Med 2004; 10:261–268.
21. Spence DW, Kayumov L, Chen A, et al. Acupuncture increases nocturnal melatonin secretion and reduces insomnia and anxiety: a preliminary report. J Neuropsychiatry Clin Neurosci 2004; 16:19–28.
22. Vollrath L, Semm P, Gammel G. Sleep induction by intranasal application of melatonin. In: Birau N, Schloot W, eds. Melatonin: Current Status and Perspectives. Advances in Biosciences. Vol 29. London: Pergamon Press, 1981:327–329.
23. Zhdanova IV, Wurtman RJ, Lynch HJ, et al. Sleep-inducing effects of low melatonin doses. Sleep Res 1995; 24:66.
24. Haimov I, Lavie P, Laudon M, et al. Melatonin replacement therapy of elderly insomniacs. Sleep 1995; 18:598–603.
25. Attenburrow MEJ, Cowen PJ, Sharpley AL. Low dose melatonin improves sleep in healthy middle-aged subjects. Psychopharmacology 1996; 126:179–181.
26. Nave R, Peled R, Lavie P. Melatonin improves evening napping. Eur J Pharmacol 1995; 275:213–216.
27. Attele AS, Xie JT, Yuan CS. Treatment of insomnia: an alternative approach. Altern Med Rev 2000; 5:249–259.
28. Liu SY. Some basic features of the new sleep-aid tea (SAT) for the treatment of insomnia. Sleep Res Online 2000; 3:49–52.
29. Liu SY, Zhang WY, Zhang Y, et al. Somnogenic effects of isomeric oxidized glutathione (IGSSG) and oxidized glutathione (GSSG). Isolated from roots of *Panax ginseng* (PG-R). In: Du TC, Tam JP, Zhang YS, eds. Peptides-Biology and Chemistry. Leiden: ESCOM, 1993:101–102.
30. Schultz V, Hansel R, Tyler VE. Rational Phototherapy. Berlin: Springer, 1998.

31. Kieser M. Efficacy of kava-kava in the treatment of non-psychotic anxiety, following pretreatment with benzodiazepines. Psychopharmacology 2001; 157:277–283.
32. Kuhn MA. Complementary Therapies for Health Care Providers. New York: Lippincott Williams & Wilkins, 1999:91–93.
33. Kuhn MA. Complementary Therapies for Health Care Providers. New York: Lippincott Williams & Wilkins, 1999:134–136.
34. Novey DW. A Physician's Complete Reference to Complementary and Alternative Medicine. St. Louis: Mosby, 2000.
35. Gatchel RJ, Price KP. Clinical Applications of Biofeedback: Appraisal and Status. New York: Pergamon Press, 1979.
36. Freedman RF, Papsdorf JD. Biofeedback and progressive relaxation treatment of sleep-onset insomnia. Biofeedback Self Regul 1976; 1:253–271.
37. Haynes SN, Sides H, Lockwood G. Relaxation instructions and frontalis electromyographic feedback intervention with sleep-onset insomnia. Behav Ther 1977; 8:644–652.
38. Nicassio PM, Boylan MB, McCabe TG. Progressive relaxation, EMG biofeedback and biofeedback placebo in the treatment of sleep-onset insomnia. Br J Med Psychol 1982; 55:159–166.
39. Sanavio E. Pre-sleep cognitive intrusions and treatment of onset-insomnia. Behav Res Ther 1988; 26:451–459.
40. Sanavio E, Vidotto G, Bettinardi O, et al. Behaviour therapy for DIMS: comparison of three treatment procedures with follow-up. Behav Psychother 1990; 18:151–167.
41. VanderPlate C, Eno EN. Electromyograph biofeedback and sleep-onset insomnia: comparison of treatment and placebo. Behav Eng 1983; 8:146–153.
42. Hughes RC, Hughes HH. Insomnia: effects of EMG biofeedback, relaxation training, and stimulus control. Behav Eng 1978; 5:67–72.
43. Bell JS. The use of EEG theta biofeedback in the treatment of a patient with sleep onset insomnia. Biofeedback Self Regul 1979; 4:229–236.
44. Hauri PJ, Percy L, Hellekson C, et al. The treatment of psychophysiologic insomnia with biofeedback: a replication study. Biofeedback Self Regul 1982; 7:223–235.
45. Jordan JB, Hauri P, Phelps PJ. The sensorimotor rhythm (SMR) in insomnia. In: Chase MH, Mitler MM, Walter PL, eds. Sleep Research. University of California, Los Angeles: Brain Information Services/Brain Research Institute, 1976.
46. Feinstein B, Sterman MB, Macdonald LR. Effects of sensorimotor rhythm training on sleep. Sleep Res 1974 3:134.
47. Hauri PJ. Treating psychophysiologic insomnia with biofeedback. Arch Gen Psychiatry 1981; 38:752–758.
48. Reite M, Higgs L, Lebet JP, et al. Sleep inducing effect of low energy emission therapy. Bioelectromagnetics 1994; 15:67–75.
49. Bawin SM, Kaczmarek LK, Adey WR. Effects of modulated VHF fields on the central nervous system. Ann N Y Acad Sci 1975; 247:74–91.
50. Blackman CF, Elder JA, Weil CM, et al. Induction of calcium ion efflux from brain tissue by radiofrequency radiation. Radio Sci 1979; 14:93–98.
51. Lebet JP, Barbault A, Rossel C, et al. Electroencephalographic changes following low energy emission therapy. Ann Biomed Eng 1996; 24:424–429.
52. Pasche B, Erman M, Hayduk R, et al. Effects of low energy emission therapy in chronic psychophysiological insomnia. Sleep 1996; 19:327–336.
53. Amato D, Pasche B. An evaluation of the safety of low energy emission therapy. Compr Ther 1993; 19:242–247.
54. Duffy JF, Kronauer RE, Czeisler CA. Phase shifting human circadian rhythms: influence of sleep timing, social contact and light exposure. J Physiol 1996; 495:289–297.
55. Bootzin RR, Lack L, Wright H. Efficacy of bright light and stimulus control instruction for sleep onset insomnia. Sleep 1998; 22:1328–1333.
56. Rosenthal NE, Joseph-Vanderpool JR, Levendosky AA, et al. Phase-shifting effects of bright morning light as treatment for delayed sleep phase syndrome. Sleep 1990; 13:354–361.
57. Lack L, Wright H, Paynter D. The treatment of sleep onset insomnia with morning bright light. Sleep Res 1995; 24A:338.
58. Campbell SS, Dawson D, Anderson MW. Alleviation of sleep maintenance insomnia with timed exposure to bright light. J Am Geriatr Soc 1993; 41:829–836.
59. Cooke KM, Kreydatus MA. The effect of evening light exposure on the sleep of elderly women expressing sleep complaints. J Behav Med 1998; 21:103–114.
60. Lack L, Wright H. The effect of evening bright light in delaying the circadian rhythms and lengthening the sleep of early morning awakening insomniacs. Sleep 1993; 16:436–443.
61. Morin CM, Culbert JP, Schwartz SM. Nonpharmacological interventions for insomnia: a meta-analysis of treatment sleep efficacy. Am J Psychiatry 1994; 151:1172–1178.
62. Benson HB. The Relaxation Response. New York: William Morrow, 1975.

63. Khalsa, SBS. Treatment of chronic insomnia with yoga: a preliminary study with sleep-wake diaries. Appl Psychophysiol Biofeedback 2004; 29:269–278.

64. Manjunath NK, Telles S. Influence of yoga and Ayurveda on self-rated sleep in a geriatric population. Indian J of Med Res 2005; 121:683–690.

65. Delmonte MM. The relevance of meditation to clinical practice: an overview. Appl Psychol: Int Rev 1999; 39:331–354.

66. Woolfolk RL, Carr-Kaffashan, McNulty TF. Meditation training as a treatment for insomnia. Behav Ther 1976; 7:359–365.

67. Miskiman DE. The treatment of insomnia by the Trancendental Meditation program in the treatment of insomnia. In: Orme-Johnson DW, Farrow JT, eds. Scientific Research on the Trancendental Meditation Program: Collected Papers. Vol 1, 2nd ed. Livingston Manor, NY: Maharishi European Research University Press, 1977:296–298.

68. Lis-Balchin M, Hart S. Studies on the mode of action of the essential oil of lavender (*Lavandula angustifolia* P. Miller). Phytother Res 1999; 13:540–542.

69. Wheatley D. Medicinal plants for insomnia: a review of their pharmacology, efficacy and tolerability. J Psychopharmacol 2005; 19:414–421.

70. Schultz V, Hubner WD, Ploch, M. Clinical trials with photo-psychopharmacological agents. Phytomedicine 1997; 4:379–387.

71. Atanassove-Shopova S, Roussinov KS. On certain central neurotropic effects of lavender essential oil. Bull Inst Physiol 1970; 5:349–354.

72. Carvalho-Freitas MI, Costa M. Anxiolytic and sedative effects of extracts and essential oil from *Citrus aurantium* L. Biol Pharm Bull 2002; 25:1629–33.

73. Gould L, Reddy CVR, Comprecht RF. Cardiac effect of chamomile tea. J Clin Pharmacol 1973; 13:475–479.

74. Lai HL, Good M. Music improves sleep quality in older adults. J Adv Nurs 2005; 49:234–244.

75. Mornhinweg GC, Voignier RR. Music for sleep disturbance on the elderly. J Holist Nurs 1995; 13:248–254.

76. Zimmerman L, Nieveen J, Barnason S, et al. The effects of music interventions on postoperative pain and sleep in coronary artery bypass graft (CABG) patients. Sch Inq Nurs Pract 1996; 10:153–170.

77. Buguet A, Satre M, LeKerneau J. Continuous nocturnal automassage of an acupuncture point modifies sleep in healthy subjects. Neurophysiol Clin 1995; 25:78–83.

78. Montakab H, Langel G. The effect of acupuncture in the treatment of insomnia. Clinical study of subjective and objective evaluation. Schweiz Med Wochenschr Suppl 1994; 62:49–54.

79. Li N, Wu B, Wang C-W, et al. A systematic evaluation of randomized controlled trials for acupuncture and moxibustion treatment of insomnia. Zhongguo Zhen Jiu 2005; 25(1):7–10.

80. Sok SR, Erlen JA, Kim KB. Effects of acupuncture therapy on insomnia. J Adv Nurs 2003; 44:375–384.

81. Lin Y. Acupuncture treatment for insomnia and acupuncture analgesia. Psychiatry Clin Neurosci 1995; 29:199–200.

82. Spencer JA, Moran DJ, Lee A, et al. White noise and sleep induction. Arch Dis Child 1990; 65:135–137.

83. Stanchina ML, Abu-Hijleh M, Chaudhry BK, et al. The influence of white noise on sleep in subjects exposed to ICU noise. Sleep Med 2004; 6:423–428.

84. Scott TD. The effects of continuous, high intensity, white noise on the human sleep cycle. Psychophysiology 1972; 9:227–232.

85. Jamison JR. Insomnia: does chiropractic help? J Manipulative Physiol Ther 2005; 28:179–186.

86. Kim K, Uchiyama M, Okawa M, et al. An epidemiological study of insomnia among the Japanese general population. Sleep 2000; 23:41–47.

87. Morgan K. Daytime activity and risk factors for lat-life insomnia. J Sleep Res 2003; 12:231–238.

88. Sherrill DL, Kotchou K, Quan SF. Association of physical activity and human sleep disorders. Arch Intern Med 1998; 158:1894–1898.

89. Youngstedt SD. Effects of exercise on sleep. Clin Sports Med 2005; 24:355–365.

90. Youngstedt SD, O'Connor PJ, Dishman RK. The effects of acute exercise on sleep: a quantitative synthesis. Sleep 1997; 20:203–214.

91. Naylor E, Penev PD, Orberta L, et al. Daily social and physical activity increases slow-wave sleep and daytime neuropsychological performance in the elderly. Sleep 2000; 23:87–95.

92. Tworoger SS, Yasui Y, Vitiello MV, et al. Effects of a yearlong moderate-intensity exercise and a stretching intervention on sleep quality in postmenopausal women. Sleep 2003; 26:830–836.

93. Vitiello MV, Prinz PN, Schwartz RS. Slow wave sleep but not over-all sleep quality of healthy older men and women is improved by increased aerobic fitness. Sleep Res 1994; 23:149.

94. King AC, Oman RF, Brassington GS, et al. Moderate-intensity exercise and self-rated quality of sleep in older adults. A randomized controlled trial. J Am Med Assoc 1997; 277:32–37.

10 | Special Considerations for Treatment of Insomnia

Allison G. Harvey, Ilana S. Hairston, Anda Gershon, and June Gruber

Department of Psychology, University of California, Berkeley, California, U.S.A.

SPECIAL CONSIDERATIONS FOR TREATMENT OF INSOMNIA

Several of the preceding chapters have already raised important issues that require consideration when treating patients with insomnia. The aim of this chapter is to address a number of additional special considerations including side effects, gender, age, comorbidity, reasons insomnia may be treatment resistant (e.g., presence of unhelpful beliefs or worry, daytime distress), and legal issues.

SIDE EFFECTS OF TREATMENT

Aside from some sleep deprivation in the first one to two weeks of stimulus control and sleep restriction, cognitive behavior therapy for insomnia (CBT-I) has no known side effects.

The side effects associated with medication treatments for insomnia depend on the half-life, target receptor, and specificity to that receptor site. For example, benzodiazepines (such as temazepam and flurazepam) have the most side effects and are associated with tolerance and rebound (1), as they have the longest half-life and the least specificity (targeting the $GABA_A$ receptor complex broadly). The newer non-benzodiazepine hypnotics (such as zolpidem and zalelpon) have a shorter half-life and specific targets within the $GABA_A$ receptor site. Hence, they have fewer associated side effects relative to the benzodiazepines (2,3). Although much less researched Ramelteon, a newer medication targeting the melatonin receptors, appears to be associated with relatively few side effects (4). Research investigating other receptor targets (such as orexin, leptin, and serotonin) is ongoing in the hope of developing additional medications with low side effect profiles.

GENDER EFFECTS OF TREATMENT

Gender Differences in Rates of Insomnia

It is well documented that women meet diagnostic criteria for insomnia at higher rate than men. A meta-analysis investigating these sex differences reported that insomnia is approximately 1.4 times more prevalent among women than among men (95% confidence interval: 1.28–1.55) (5). This female-to-male ratio has been shown to increase slightly after the age of 45 (6). Before examining possible implications of this gender difference for treatment, we first briefly review two possible explanations for the difference.

Biological Sex Differences in Sleep Patterns

While a large number of studies have assessed gender (or sex) differences in sleep patterns, a reliable pattern is yet to emerge. This may relate to the cyclic nature of the female hormonal profile as well as the interaction of gender with age-related changes. For example, an examination of gender differences comparing patients diagnosed with insomnia ($n = 86$) and good sleepers ($n = 86$) found no evidence of gender-related differences in objective measures of sleep continuity and amounts of rapid eye movement (REM) or non-REM (NREM) sleep. The authors concluded that the increased prevalence of insomnia among women compared to men is not due to sex-related differences in sleep parameters (6). By contrast, Carrier et al. (7) assessed the spectral signature of different NREM sleep stages in 100 healthy men and women between 20 to 60 years of age. The authors reported higher power density in the lower frequency range of the electroencephalogram (EEG) in women compared to men, suggesting that differences in sleep quality between women and men go beyond behavioral measures of sleep (e.g., sleep efficiency, sleep onset latency, etc.). They also found a gender-independent decline in lower frequency, with an increase in higher frequency bands with age.

Hormonal events or changes that occur throughout the life course, including menstruation, pregnancy, and menopause, have been suggested to be important contributors to the disruption of sleep in women.

Menstruation

Both gonadal steroid hormones (e.g., estrogen, progesterone, testosterone) and core body temperature, two factors that vary considerably across the menstrual cycle, can significantly impact sleep patterns (8). However, although subjective changes in sleep are common in premenstrual syndrome, dysmenorrhea, and premenstrual dysphoric disorder, no reliable differences in objective sleep measures have been reported (8).

Pregnancy

Pregnancy is linked with disturbed sleep and daytime sleepiness (9). Sleep disturbances are associated with hormonal changes in the early months of the pregnancy, and fetus size and motion in later months. Studies using both polysomnographic and subjective sleep measures have documented decreased slow wave sleep (SWS), decreased sleep efficiency, increased wake after sleep onset and decreased REM sleep among pregnant women (9). Sleep often continues to be disturbed after delivery due to frequent awakenings to attend to the newborn as well as hormonal changes (10). Interestingly, a study of women in their ninth month of pregnancy showed that severity of sleep disruption predicted the duration and difficulty of labor and the likelihood of having a cesarean delivery (11). These results raise the possibility that interventions to improve sleep quality in late pregnancy may reduce difficulty during labor and its associated risks.

Menopause

Menopause is also associated with increased occurrence of impaired sleep quality, although the direct effects of menopause on objective sleep measures have failed to yield reliable results. That said, between 50% and 70% of post-menopausal women report suffering from insomnia and 70% to 85% report vasomotor symptoms ("hot flashes"), which interfere with sleep quality (for review see Ref. 8).

To sum up, the role of biological sex differences on objective and subjective parameters of sleep quality is not well understood in the human population. Clearly, steroidal hormones can play a significant role in regulating parameters that affect sleep, such as core body temperature or mood, suggesting that hormonal status needs to be taken into account when assessing a sleep complaint and determining the treatment approach.

Comorbidity with Anxiety and Depression

Another possible explanation of the gender difference is that insomnia is frequently comorbid with depression and anxiety disorders (12) that are themselves more prevalent among women than men. Because of this comorbidity between insomnia, depression, and anxiety disorders, it has been proposed that the increased prevalence of insomnia observed among women relative to men may be due to the increased prevalence of depression and anxiety disorders among women relative to men (13). It is possible that these disorders share a similar underlying causal mechanism (14).

Gender Differences in the Treatment of Insomnia

Other than age, most demographic variables such as gender, marital status, education, and occupational status are not predictors of treatment outcome following CBT-I (15,16). On the other hand, there is some evidence for gender differences in the use of medications. Some studies have reported that women use tranquilizers two to three times more frequently than men (17,18). However, more recently accrued evidence indicate that the gender difference that emerged in previous studies has markedly decreased (19).

There is mixed evidence regarding whether physicians prescribe medication differently for male and female insomnia patients. Walsh and Schweitzer (19) have reported that women diagnosed with insomnia are more likely to receive a prescription for a hypnotic than men. By contrast, Brownlee and colleagues (20) found no gender difference in the rate at which zopiclone, benzodiazepines, antidepressants, or antihistamines were prescribed to female versus male insomnia patients.

AGE EFFECTS OF TREATMENT: TREATING INSOMNIA ACROSS THE LIFE SPAN

As reviewed in chapters 7 and 8, there is evidence for the efficacy and effectiveness of CBT-I and medication for both adults and older adults. However, the efficacy of interventions in adolescence and children is not as well documented. This is of critical concern because sleep quantity and patterns vary substantially with age, such that the application of treatments for insomnia developed and tested for adults are unlikely to be directly transportable to younger age groups. To emphasize this point, the challenges to sleep across development are reviewed in the following section.

Newborns average a total of 16 to 20 hours of sleep and lack diurnal organization. Circadian organization of sleep emerges in infancy and consolidation of sleep gradually increases to full night around the age of 6, with a concomitant decline in daytime naps. The total amount of sleep gradually declines through adolescence, such that by young adulthood average nighttime sleep varies between seven and nine hours and in the middle adult years between six and eight hours (21,22).

The polysomnographic and EEG markers of sleep also differ between infancy and later developmental stages. Thus, in newborns REM and NREM phases are termed "active" and "quiet" sleep, respectively (21). There are also alterations in sleep architecture over the course of development. Newborn infants may enter sleep with a REM (or active sleep) episode, and their REM-NREM cycle lasts about 50 to 60 minutes, compared with about 90 minutes in adults (22,23). Whereas at birth approximately 50% of sleep is spent in active sleep, once a child is two years of age this percentage is reduced to 20% to 30% of total sleep time, similar to adult levels. Amount of stages 3 and 4 sleep decreases and stage 2 sleep increases during adolescence and the second decade of life sleep (22). Finally, during adolescence there is a delay in circadian phase and a corresponding delay in sleep onset, often shifting past midnight to the early morning hours (24,25). This has been attributable to a number of influences, including a tendency toward increasing autonomy in deciding what time to go to bed, which coincides with both a natural biological delay in the circadian cycle plus irregularity in the sleep schedule associated with psychosocial stress and activities (21,24).

Given these considerable changes in sleep across development, defining, assessing, and devising appropriate treatment regimens for children and adolescents suffering from a sleep disorder provides considerable challenge. Although the prevalence of insomnia in children and adolescents is not yet well quantified, studies highlight high rates of sleep problems. For example, prevalence of sleep disorders in children aged 2 to 13.9 was assessed in a large sample ($n = 1038$) by questionnaires administered to parents (26). The authors found that 20% of the children had two to four insomnia symptoms and 41.1% had one symptom. The prevalence of daytime sleepiness was 15.4%. Similarly, a telephone survey of 1125 adolescents aged 15 to 18, across several European countries, found that approximately 20% were sleepy during the day, 25% had insomnia symptoms, and 4% met clinical diagnostic criteria for insomnia. Given the importance of sleep in brain development and learning (27), impaired sleep quality in youth is likely to have a critical long-term impact.

A key consideration is how to adapt existing treatments or develop new treatments for sleep disturbance in younger individuals. Unfortunately, this is an under-researched domain. However, there is a small evidence-based reporting on the effectiveness of some of the interventions with children and adolescents who suffer from sleep disturbance (28,29). As will become evident, the approaches described vary in their suitability for younger children (for specialist coverage of the treatment for younger children see Ref. 29, for older children see Ref. 28, and for adolescents see Ref. 30). The core strategies fall into four broad categories.

Bedtime Routine

A presleep routine that helps children and adolescents reduce their arousal, regulate their mood and prepare for sleep is recommended, as is maintaining consistent bed and wake times. The latter has the dual advantage of ensuring the child is ready for bed at bedtime while also promoting stability in the circadian rhythm (21).

Bedtime Resistance

This difficulty can be a source of sleeplessness and stress for the entire family. The intervention is based on the assumption that difficulty going to sleep is, at least in part, maintained by parental attention. The aim is to reduce bedtime behaviors that are inconsistent with getting to sleep by reducing parental attention to them. Owens et al. (29) describe several modifications to an extinction procedure, the goal of which is to increase acceptance of the intervention by the parents. First, there is "parental presence" to reduce separation anxiety in the child during the first week of the program. During the next week the parent sleeps in the child's bedroom but in a separate bed but without interacting with the child during the night. For the third week, the parent moves to a separate room. A second approach is "graduated extinction and fading" in which the parents reduce their response slowly over time either in the form of increasing the latency to respond or decreasing the length of the response. Third, parents can provide "minimal brief checks," at regular intervals of 5 to 20 minutes, whilst crying persists.

In older children, this intervention needs to be altered by facilitating enforcement of bedtime by the parent and maintenance of regular bed and wake times with age appropriate incentives.

Insomnia

Insomnia in children and adolescents is addressed with similar treatments as for adults, particularly stimulus control (see chap. 7 for a full description). There is preliminary data that a multi-component treatment featuring stimulus control is helpful for a subgroup of adolescents with insomnia; namely, those who have had substance-related difficulties (31). However, the field awaits a full evaluation of this treatment approach in adolescents who suffer from insomnia without psychiatric comorbidity and those with insomnia that is comorbid with psychiatric comorbidity, such as the anxiety and mood disorders. As already described in chapter 7, stimulus control involves asking the insomnia sufferer to go to bed *only* when he or she is tired, to limit the activities in bed to sleep, to get up at the same time every morning, and when sleep-onset does not occur within 10 to 20 minutes, to get up and go to another room. The underlying rationale of this treatment is that insomnia is the result of maladaptive conditioning between the environment (bed/bedroom) and sleep incompatible behaviors (e.g., worry/frustration at not being able to sleep). The intervention developed by Bootzin (32) aims to reverse this association by limiting the sleep incompatible behaviors that may be engaged in by the patient with this disorder.

Phase Delay

As we have already described, a key feature of sleep leading up to and during the adolescent years is the delay in circadian phase, such that sleep onset does not occur until the early hours of the morning (33). Although the literature for treating delayed phase is small, the interventions tested include exposure to bright light, although the optimal timing and dose of the exposure remains to be established for children and adolescents (21). More simply, such procedures as gradual advances in bedtime and wakeup times (say by 15 minutes a day), avoiding daytime napping and maintaining consistency on the weekend are recommended. Or, when the bedtime is very late, it may be easier to institute successive delays in bedtime. The reason that moving in this direction may be favorable is that the circadian cycle naturally runs over 24 hours. Hence, delays that capitalize on the natural tendency for the circadian system to run over 24 hours may be more easily achieved than advances in bedtime (30).

COMORBIDITY

Insomnia can occur as the sole presenting problem or as a condition that is comorbid with another psychiatric or medical disorder (12). There has been a tendency in the past to assume that insomnia is secondary to a so-called "primary disorder" (e.g., depression, anxiety). However, it is now widely agreed that perceiving of the insomnia as merely epiphenomenal to the comorbid disorder is unwise. Prominent among the reasons are the following. First, the evidence indicates that insomnia is a risk factor for, and can be causal in, the development or maintenance of the comorbid disorder (34,35). Second, substantial evidence is accruing to suggest that insomnia that is comorbid with another psychiatric or medical disorder does not necessarily remit with the treatment of the so-called "primary disorder" (36). Third, there is convincing evidence of a bi-directional relationship between daytime mood and symptoms and nighttime sleep (37,38) whereby a vicious cycle of symptoms and mood disturbance interfere with sleep and the effects of sleep deprivation at night exacerbates daytime symptoms and mood. For reviews of this evidence see Smith et al. (36) who discuss a range of psychiatric disorders, and Dahl and Lewin (38) who focus on adolescents, and Harvey et al. who focused on bipolar disorder (39) and the anxiety disorders (40).

PATIENT PREFERENCE

Assessing the acceptability of a treatment to a patient population is of high importance. If a treatment is unacceptable, patients will decline it, withdraw during the treatment, or not comply with the treatment. Several studies indicate that patients with insomnia rate pharmacological interventions to be a significantly less acceptable form of treatment compared to psychological interventions. Vincent and Lionberg (41) asked patients with chronic insomnia to rate their acceptance and perceived efficacy of CBT-I versus pharmacotherapy. The results suggest that individuals with chronic insomnia preferred CBT-I. The authors speculated that this preference may be accounted for by the perceived benefits of CBT to daytime function combined with the negative aversive side effects the patients' associate with pharmacological treatments. Similarly, Morin and colleagues (42) evaluated the acceptability of psychological treatments, as compared to pharmacotherapy in patients with chronic insomnia and good sleepers. They asked participants to read brief descriptions of CBT-I and pharmacotherapy and to rate the two treatment modalities according to preference, acceptance, and suitability. The results suggested that both patients with chronic insomnia and good sleepers rated CBT-I as more preferable, acceptable, and suitable compared to pharmacotherapy.

UNHELPFUL BELIEFS ABOUT SLEEP

Following the pioneering work of Morin and colleagues (43), the evidence that patients with insomnia hold more unhelpful and inaccurate beliefs about sleep, relative to individuals without insomnia, continues to accrue. Also, the finding that reduced unhelpful beliefs about sleep is associated with better treatment outcome (44,45) highlights their importance to the treatment of insomnia.

In CBT-I unhelpful beliefs about sleep are typically corrected through education about sleep. When unhelpful beliefs are resistant to education, we suggest devising an individualized behavioral experiment (46,47). Behavioral experiments are "planned experiential activities, based on experimentation or observation, which are undertaken by patients in or between ... therapy sessions. Their design is derived directly from a ... formulation of the problem, and their primary purpose is to obtain new information which ... [includes]. Contributing to the development and verification of the cognitive formulation" (p. 8, 48). To give one example, for patients who continue to believe that "even one night of poor sleep substantially impairs my daytime functioning," an individualized behavioral experiment is collaboratively devised and conducted toward the end of treatment. We do it toward the end because this is when the patients feel they have developed an ability to manage the daytime consequences of a poor night[a] and we time it so that no activities known to be adversely affected by sleepiness (like driving) are to be engaged in the day following. This experiment involves actually choosing to have one "poor night" of sleep (e.g., choosing to sleep 6.5 hours for a patient who believes he/she needs 8 hours). It has typically been done by the patient by accident on several occasions (i.e., those sessions when a patient has come in and said "you know I only slept 6 hours last night and I actually feel OK today"). However, these experiences still haven't always fundamentally changed the belief that "I need 8 hours of sleep every single night in order to cope" and may even have been dismissed as a fluke or attributed to some other occurrence (e.g., "I coped because I drank a lot of coffee"). So by actually choosing to sleep less, for just one night, the patient has the opportunity to learn that getting less than the ideal amount of sleep on one night is not necessarily devastating to next day performance and actually often leads to improvement the following night. Before attempting this experiment, the patient decides whether they wish to go to bed later, set the alarm earlier, or some combination of both. We plan interesting and engaging activities to do during this time to keep awake and ensure the experiment is memorable. For example, those who choose to wake earlier in the morning might decide to have a leisurely breakfast in bed or take more time reading the morning newspaper. Care should be exercised to NOT choose a night prior to a day when the patient is driving or would be at risk if he or she is sleepy and we only attempt this experiment when the patient feels he or she has developed an ability to manage the daytime consequences of a poor night of sleep. With a careful rationale, planning and support (e.g., phone calls), most patients will give this experiment a try and the results provide a compelling and memorable refutation of the belief that "even one night of poor sleep substantially impairs my daytime functioning." Perhaps paradoxically, by reducing fear of poor sleep, the potential to obtain more sleep of better quality can be markedly increased.

THE WORRIED PATIENT

It is well documented that people with insomnia lie in bed worrying about a range of topics, including not being able to get to sleep (49,50). Cognitive models of insomnia suggest that worry activates the sympathetic nervous system (the so-called "fight or flight response") thereby triggering physiological arousal and distress. This combination of worry, arousal, and distress spirals the individual into a state of heightened anxiety that is antithetical to falling asleep and staying asleep (51,52). In support, there is convergent empirical evidence suggesting that worry, while trying to get to sleep, serves to maintain insomnia (53,54). A new topic, just starting to attract research attention, relates to the finding that some thought control strategies, like thought suppression, are important contributors to the maintenance of worry in insomnia patients (55–57). Accordingly, some insomnia patients may benefit from an intervention to reduce worry and establish helpful strategies for managing unwanted thoughts. These are two features of insomnia that are not always included in CBT-I. It is certainly possible that components within CBT-I may indirectly target worry. For example, although a behavioral theory underpins the stimulus control and relaxation components of CBT-I, it has been suggested that these components may operate via a cognitive mechanism in that stimulus control may prevent people lying in bed worrying about not sleeping (59) and relaxation may function by calming presleep cognitive activity (60), reducing concern about the sleep disturbance, and fostering a more positive outlook (61). However, on the basis (a) that directly and explicitly targeting worry in CBT for insomnia may improve outcome and (b) of our clinical experience that worry can be an important residual symptom after treatment with CBT-I, we have been developing an intervention that explicitly targets worry (62). We begin the intervention for worry by defining negative automatic thoughts (NATs) and then teaching the patient to monitor for, catch, and evaluate their NATs (63). Patients are asked to pick sleep-related NATs as examples to work on, although we suggest to the patient that the procedure for worrisome thoughts is helpfully applied to any topic. Themes that emerge from the patient observing and recording their NATs are then used to detect unhelpful beliefs that serve to

---

[a] Methods used to manage the daytime consequences of poor sleep are addressed below under the heading "Daytime Distress and Impairment."

maintain the insomnia. These can then be tested with an individualized behavioral experiment (46). This procedure alone is rarely sufficient for managing worry among patients with insomnia. Hence, several other approaches are required, three of which will now be briefly described (for a fuller description see Ref. 64).

1. Assess how the patient attempts to manage his/her worry as he/she is trying to get to sleep. Typically he or she will report trying to stop worrying by "blanking my mind" or "trying to stop all thought" (for a questionnaire that assesses thought management strategies see Ref. 56). For these patients it can be helpful to conduct a behavioral experiment within the session to demonstrate the adverse consequences of thought suppression. We do Wegner's (65) white bear experiment in the session. The patient is asked to close his or her eyes and try to suppress *all* of his or her thoughts relating to white bears (the therapist does this too). After a couple of minutes, the patient is asked to stop and share how successful his or her suppression attempts were (or more typically, were not!). This provides a stunning demonstration of the counterproductive nature of thought control and is a springboard to discussing alternative thought management strategies like letting the thoughts come (i.e., the opposite of suppression) or gently redirecting attention to interesting and engaging imagery. Then, for homework during the subsequent week, one or more individualized behavioral experiments are devised in which the client tries out the various alternative thought control strategies (including imagery approaches (55,66).

2. On the basis of a paper by Watkins and Baracaia (67), we listen to patients asking themselves "why questions" (e.g., Why am I not sleepy? Why are my thoughts racing? Why do I always feel so sleepy?). These often become evident either (*i*) during the initial case formulation when the thoughts the patient has as he or she is trying to get to sleep are elicited or (*ii*) when the content of worry episodes is unpacked. "Why questions" rarely have definite answers. Hence, asking them tends to lead to *more* distress. For example, if a person were to ask "why can't I control my sleep?" the chances are that he or she would not find a simple, definite answer, and would end up feeling as if there was no solution to the problem, heightening anxiety and distress.

3. We also assess whether the patient holds positive beliefs about worrying in bed. The importance of positive beliefs about worry is drawn from the generalized anxiety disorder literature which suggests that pathological worry may be, at least partly, maintained because the individual believes that worry will lead to positive consequences (68). To help identify positive beliefs we ask our patients to complete a questionnaire that lists a range of positive and negative beliefs about worry (69). Examples of the positive beliefs included in this questionnaire are: "worrying while trying to get to sleep helps me get things sorted out in my mind and is a way to distract myself from worrying about even more emotional things, things that I don't want to think about." If we discover that patients hold these beliefs we use Socratic questioning and experiments to examine and test their validity.

DRIVING RISK AND MEDICOLEGAL ASPECTS

Excessive sleepiness and sleep-inducing drugs are a significant public health concern because they represent a risk factor for driving fatalities. According to epidemiological studies of road accidents in the United States and Europe, sleep-related accidents constitute 10% to 20% of accidents (70,71). Moreover, Connor and colleagues (70) identified sleepiness at the wheel, sleeping less than 5 hours in the 24 hours before an accident, and driving between the hours of 2 a.m. and 5 a.m. as major risk factors for driving accidents [odds ratio (OR) = 8.2, OR = 2.7, and OR = 5.6, respectively]. Other studies suggest relevance to insomnia patients. For example, Ohayon et al. reported that patients with insomnia have twice the risk of accident relative to individuals without insomnia (72). Furthermore, there are a handful of studies suggesting increased risk for driving accidents among insomnia patients taking benzodiazepines. For example, Hemmelgarn et al. (73) showed that among older patients, the use of the long-acting benzodiazepines was positively associated with increased driving accidents. Similarly, in a large community sample Neutel (74) assessed the risk of hospitalization due to injuries from driving accidents among individuals who filled a first prescription for benzodiazepine anxiolytics, benzodiazepine hypnotics and controls. The findings indicated that individuals prescribed either benzodiazepine hypnotics or benzodiazepine anxiolytics were at an increased risk for hospitalization due to driving accidents within four weeks of the prescription being filled (OR = 3.9 and OR = 2.5, respectively). These findings underscore the potential danger of insomnia and sleep-inducing pills on driving accidents.

Although several countries have restrictions on commercial drivers' hours and shifts, to date, only the State of New Jersey has specifically criminalized fatigued driving in the general population (75). There are at least two difficulties in criminalizing fatigued driving: defining sleepiness and the structure of the law. Criminalizing drunk driving required the ability to objectively determine dangerous levels of alcohol. An equivalent measure for sleepiness does not yet exist. Moreover, unlike alcohol, the consumption of which is a recreational choice, sleep curtailment can be due to factors over which the individual has less control such as care giving, work requirements, or a sleep disorder. From the legal perspective, in order to prosecute an individual for committing a crime, it is necessary to prove culpability. This is typically determined by assessing two main elements of the crime—voluntary act (*actus reus*) and intent (*mens rea*). Falling asleep while driving is typically perceived as lacking these two elements, raising the question of whether the decision to drive while fatigued (i.e., the prior action) is the criminal act.

A good example of this issue can be found in the case of *State v. Olsen* in which a woman fell asleep while driving and killed a child playing on the sidewalk; she was convicted of involuntary manslaughter (76). The Supreme Court of Utah reasoned that an individual could be held accountable for allowing oneself to become unconscious (i.e., fall asleep). In other words, the court held that knowing that falling asleep while performing a hazardous activity (e.g., driving) results in harm to others, the question of criminal culpability depends on prior conduct of the defendant. To the best of our knowledge, however, there are no cases of an insomnia-related conviction yet documented.

To sum up, insomnia patients may be at risk for driving accidents, particularly if taking sleep-inducing medications, such as benzodiazepines. In treating insomnia patients, health care providers should inform patients of the risk for driving accidents due to excessive sleepiness at the wheel. Providers may also wish to evaluate the patient's ability to safely drive throughout the course of treatment.

DAYTIME DISTRESS AND IMPAIRMENT

The vast majority of the research, theory, and treatment for chronic insomnia focus on nighttime symptoms and processes (77). This is surprising given that there are well-established daytime consequences of chronic insomnia. Specifically, during the day people with insomnia report decreased ability to accomplish daily tasks and more sleepiness, tiredness, and difficulty functioning socially. They also report impaired concentration and memory problems. In addition, work absenteeism, increased use of medical services, and self-medication with either over-the-counter medications or alcohol are common among individuals with insomnia (78). Other studies have reported the daytime consequences of insomnia to include increased anxiety and depression, poor self-esteem, and social withdrawal (79). These impairments adversely affect interpersonal, social, and occupational functioning (80). Moreover, there is empirical evidence that daytime processes may be independent of nighttime processes (81).

Despite the reliable and durable changes reported on several sleep parameters following treatment for insomnia, to date, there is very limited evidence that treatment improves daytime functioning (82). This is because few trials have included measures of daytime functioning as outcome measures. Accordingly, some patients may require a specific intervention for daytime distress. The seeds of this approach are in the process of being developed and tested (46,64), such as "energy generating" experiments and conducting surveys of friends and family to normalize that some daytime tiredness and lapses in attention and memory during the day are experienced by everyone, even good sleepers. In an open trial, this approach was associated with marked improvement in daytime impairment (83).

CONCLUSIONS

Building on the special considerations for treating insomnia highlighted in chapters 7 and 8, we have aimed to address a range of additional considerations; namely, gender differences, legal issues, driving risk, sleep changes across development, comorbidity, patient preference, unhelpful beliefs about sleep, the worried patient, and daytime distress and impairment. These considerations highlight the complexity involved in understanding, assessing and treating patients with insomnia.

REFERENCES

1. Fleming JAE, Kushida CA. Medications, drugs of abuse and alcohol. In: Kushida CA, ed. Sleep Deprivation, in press.
2. Patat A, Paty I, Hindmarch I. Pharmacodynamic profile of Zaleplon, a new non-benzodiazepine hypnotic agent. Hum Psychopharmacol 2001; 16(5):369–392.
3. Blin O, Micallef J, Audebert C, et al. A double-blind, placebo- and flurazepam-controlled investigation of the residual psychomotor and cognitive effects of modified release zolpidem in young healthy volunteers. J Clin Psychopharmacol 2006; 26(3):284–289.
4. Johnson MW, Suess PE, Griffiths RR. Ramelteon: a novel hypnotic lacking abuse liability and sedative adverse effects. Arch Gen Psychiatry 2006; 63(10):1149–1157.
5. Zhang B, Wing YK. Sex differences in insomnia: a meta-analysis. Sleep 2006; 29(1):85–93.
6. Voderholzer U, Al-Shajlawi A, Weske G, et al. Are there gender differences in objective and subjective sleep measures? A study of insomniacs and healthy controls. Depress Anxiety 2003; 17:162–172.
7. Carrier J, Land S, Buysse DJ, et al. The effects of age and gender on sleep EEG power spectral density in the middle years of life (ages 20–60 years old). Psychophysiology 2001; 38(2):232–242.
8. Manber R, Armitage R. Sex, steroids, and sleep: a review. Sleep 1999; 22(5):540–555.
9. Santiago JR, Nolledo MS, Kinzler W, et al. Sleep and sleep disorders in pregnancy. Ann Intern Med 2001; 134:396–408.
10. Lee KA, Zaffke ME. Longitudinal changes in fatigue and energy during pregnancy and the postpartum period. J Obstet Gynecol Neonatal Nurs 1999; 28(2):183–191.
11. Lee KA, Gay CL. Sleep in late pregnancy predicts length of labor and type of delivery. Am J Obstet Gynecol 2004; 191(6):2041–2046.
12. Benca RM, Obermeyer WH, Thisted RA, et al. Sleep and psychiatric disorders: a meta-analysis. Arch Gen Psychiatry 1992; 49:651–668.
13. Kornstein SG. Gender differences in depression: implications for treatment. J Clin Psychiatry 1997; 58 suppl 15:12–18.
14. Harvey AG, Watkins E, Mansell W, et al. Cognitive Behavioural Processes Across Psychological Disorders: A Transdiagnostic Approach to Research and Treatment. Oxford: Oxford University Press, 2004.
15. Edinger JE, Means MK. Cognitive-behavioral therapy for primary insomnia. Clin Psychol Rev 2005; 25:539–558.
16. Espie CA, Inglis SJ, Harvey L. Predicting clinically significant response to cognitive behavior therapy for chronic insomnia in general medical practice: analyses of outcome data at 12 months posttreatment. J Consult Clin Psychol 2001; 69:58–66.
17. Ashton H, Goldin JF. Tranquillisers: prevalence, predictors and possible consequences. Data from a large United Kingdom survey. Br J Addict 1989; 84:541–546.
18. Taggart LAP, McCammon SL, Allred LJ, et al. Effect of patient and physician gender on prescriptions for psychotropic drugs. J Womens Health 1993; 2:353–357.
19. Walsh JK, Schweitzer PK. Ten-year trends in the pharmacological treatment of insomnia. Sleep 1999; 22:371–375.
20. Brownlee K, Devins GM, Flanigan M, et al. Are there gender differences in the prescribing of hypnotic medications for insomnia? Hum Psychopharmacol 2003; 18:69–73.
21. Hoban TF. Sleep and its disorders in children. Semin Neurol 2004; 24:327–340.
22. Carskadon MA, Dement WC. Normal human sleep: an overview. In: Kryger MH, Roth T, Dement WC, eds. Principles and Practice of Sleep Medicine. 4th ed. Philadelphia: Elsevier, 2005.
23. Carskadon MA. Sleep and circadian rhythms in children and adolescents: relevance for athletic performance of young people. Clin Sports Med 2005; 24:319–328.
24. Carskadon MA. Factors influencing sleep patterns of adolescents. In: Carskadon MA, eds. Adolescent Sleep Patterns: Biological, Social, and Psychological Influences. New York, NY: Cambridge University Press, 2002:4–26.

25. Tate BA, Richardson GS, Carskadon MA. Maturational changes in sleep-wake timing: longitudinal studies of the circadian activity rhythm of a diurnal rodent. In: Carskadon MA, ed. Adolescent Sleep Patterns: Biological, Social, and Psychological Influences. New York, NY: Cambridge University Press, 2002:40–49.

26. Archbold KH, Pituch KJ, Panahi P, et al. Symptoms of sleep disturbances among children at two general pediatric clinics. J Pediatr 2002; 140(1):97–102.

27. Dahl RE. Adolescent development and the regulation of behavior and emotion: introduction to part VIII. Ann N Y Acad Sci 2004; 1021:294–295.

28. Sadeh A. Cognitive-behavioral treatment for childhood sleep disorders. Clin Psychol Rev 2005; 25:612–628.

29. Owens JL, France KG, Wiggs L. Behavioural and cognitive-behavioural interventions for sleep disorders in infants and children: a review. Sleep Med Rev 1999; 3:281–302.

30. Dahl R. Child and adolescent sleep disorders. In: Kaufmann D, ed. Child and Adolescent Neurology for the Psychiatrist. Baltimore, MD: Williams & Wilkins, 1992:169–194.

31. Bootzin RR, Stevens SJ. Adolescents, substance abuse, and the treatment of insomnia and daytime sleepiness. Clin Psychol Rev 2005; 25:629–644.

32. Bootzin RR. Stimulus control treatment for insomnia. Proc Am Psychol Assoc 1972; 7:395–396.

33. Carskadon MA. Patterns of sleep and sleepiness in adolescents. Pediatrician 1990; 17:5–12.

34. Harvey AG. Insomnia: symptom or diagnosis? Clin Psychol Rev 2001; 21:1037–1059.

35. McCrae CS, Lichstein KL. Secondary insomnia: diagnostic challenges and intervention opportunities. Sleep Med Rev 2001; 5:47–61.

36. Smith MT, Huang MI, Manber R. Cognitive behavior therapy for chronic insomnia occurring within the context of medical and psychiatric disorders. Clin Psychol Rev 2005; 25:559–592.

37. Dahl RE. The regulation of sleep and arousal: development and psychopathology. Dev Psychopathol 1996; 8:3–27.

38. Dahl RE, Lewin DS. Pathways to adolescent health sleep regulation and behavior. J Adolesc Health 2002; 31(6 suppl):175–184.

39. Harvey AG, Mullin BC, Hinshaw SP. Sleep and circadian rhythms in children and adolescents with bipolar disorder. Dev Psychopathol 2006; 18(4):1147–1168 (review).

40. Harvey AG, Hairston IS, Gruber J, et al. Anxiety and Sleep. In: Antony MM, Stein MB, eds. Handbook of Anxiety and the Anxiety Disorders. New York: Oxford University Press, 2006.

41. Vincent N, Lionberg C. Treatment preference and patient satisfaction in chronic insomnia. Sleep 2001; 24:411–417.

42. Morin CM, Gaulier B, Barry T, et al. Patients' acceptance of psychological and pharmacological therapies for insomnia. Sleep 1992; 15:302–305.

43. Morin CM, Stone J, Trinkle D, et al. Dysfunctional beliefs and attitudes about sleep among older adults with and without insomnia complaints. Psychol Aging 1993; 8:463–467.

44. Edinger JD, Wohlgemuth WK, Radtke RA, et al. Does cognitive-behavioral insomnia therapy alter dysfunctional beliefs about sleep? Sleep 2001; 24:591–599.

45. Morin CM, Blais F, Savard J. Are changes in beliefs and attitudes about sleep related to sleep improvements in the treatment of insomnia? Behav Res Ther 2002; 40:741–752.

46. Ree M, Harvey AG. Insomnia. In: Bennett-Levy J, Butler G, Fennell M, eds. Oxford Guide to Behavioural Experiments in Cognitive Therapy. Oxford: Oxford University Press, 2004:287–305.

47. Tang NK, Anne Schmidt D, Harvey AG. Sleeping with the enemy: clock monitoring in the maintenance of insomnia. J Behav Ther Exp Psychiatry 2007; 38(1):40–55 [Epub Jun 21, 2006].

48. Bennett-Levy J, Butler G, Fennell MJV, et al. The Oxford Handbook of Behavioural Experiments. Oxford: Oxford University Press, 2004.

49. Harvey AG. Pre-sleep cognitive activity: a comparison of sleep-onset insomniacs and good sleepers. Br J Clin Psychol 2000; 39:275–286.

50. Wicklow A, Espie CA. Intrusive thoughts and their relationship to actigraphic measurement of sleep: towards a cognitive model of insomnia. Behav Res Ther 2000; 38:679–693.

51. Harvey AG. A cognitive model of insomnia. Behav Res Ther 2002; 40:869–894.

52. Espie CA. Insomnia: conceptual issues in the development, persistence, and treatment of sleep disorder in adults. Annu Rev Psychol 2002; 53:215–243.

53. Harvey AG. Trouble in bed: the role of pre-sleep worry and intrusions in the maintenance of insomnia. J Cogn Psychother 2002; 16:161–177.

54. Harvey AG. What about patients who can't sleep? Case formulation for insomnia. In: Tarrier N, ed. Case Formulation in Cognitive Behaviour Therapy: The Treatment of Challenging and Complex Clinical Cases. London: Brunner-Routledge, in press.

55. Harvey AG, Payne S. The management of unwanted pre-sleep thoughts in insomnia: distraction with imagery versus general distraction. Behav Res Ther 2002; 40:267–277.

56. Ree MJ, Harvey AG, Blake R, et al. Attempts to control unwanted thoughts in the night: development of the thought control questionnaire-insomnia revised (TCQI-R). Behav Res Ther 2005; 43:985–989.

57. Bélanger L, Morin CM, Gendron L, et al. Presleep cognitive activity and thought control strategies in insomnia. J Cogn Psychother 2005; 19:17–27.
58. Harvey AG. The attempted suppression of presleep cognitive activity in insomnia. Cognit Ther Res 2003; 27:593–602.
59. Lichstein KL, Fisher SM. Insomnia. In: Hersen M, Bellack AD, eds. Handbook of Clinical Behavior Therapy with Adults. New York: Plenum Press, 1985:319–352.
60. Borkovec TD. Insomnia. J Consult Clin Psychol 1982; 50:880–895.
61. Espie CA, Lindsay WR, Brooks DN, et al. A controlled comparative investigation of psychological treatments for chronic sleep-onset insomnia. Behav Res Ther 1989; 27:79–88.
62. Harvey AG. Unwanted intrusive thoughts in insomnia. In: Clark DA, ed. Intrusive thoughts in clinical disorders: theory, research, and treatment. New York: Guilford Press, 2005:86–118.
63. Beck J. Cognitive Therapy: Basics and Beyond. New York: Guilford, 1995.
64. Harvey AG. A cognitive theory of and therapy for chronic insomnia. J Cogn Psychother 2005; 19:41–60.
65. Wegner DM, Schneider DJ. Mental control: the war of the ghosts in the machine. In: Uleman JS, Bargh JA, eds. Unintended Thought. New York, NY: Guilford Press, 1989:287–305.
66. Nelson J, Harvey AG. An exploration of pre-sleep cognitive activity in insomnia: imagery and verbal thought. Br J Clin Psychol 2003; 42:271–288.
67. Watkins E, Baracaia S. Why do people ruminate in dysphoric moods? Pers Individ Dif 2001; 30:723–734.
68. Wells A. Meta-cognition and worry: a cognitive model of generalized anxiety disorder. Behav Cogn Psychother 1995; 23:301–320.
69. Harvey AG. Beliefs about the utility of presleep worry: an investigation of individuals with insomnia and good sleepers. Cognit Ther Res 2003; 27:403–414.
70. Connor J, Norton R, Ameratunga S, et al. Driver sleepiness and risk of serious injury to car occupants: population based case control study. BMJ 2002; 324:1125.
71. Horne JA, Reyner LA. Sleep related vehicle accidents. BMJ 1995; 310:565–567.
72. Ohayon MM, Caulet M, Philip P, et al. How sleep and mental disorders are related to complaints of daytime sleepiness. Arch Intern Med 1997; 157:2645–2652.
73. Hemmelgarn B, Suissa S, Huang A, et al. Benzodiazepine use and the risk of motor vehicle crash in the elderly. JAMA 1997; 278:27–31.
74. Neutel CI. Risk of traffic accident injury after a prescription for a benzodiazepine. Ann Epidemiol 1995; 5:239–244.
75. Jones CB, Dorrian J, Rajaratnam SMW. Fatigue and the criminal law. Ind Health 2005; 43:63–70.
76. Shuman D, Smith AM, Pritzlaff CJ. Legal implications. In: Kushida CA, ed. Sleep deprivation: clinical issues, pharmacology, and sleep loss effects. New York: Marcel Dekker, 2005:363–385.
77. Riedel BW, Lichstein KL. Insomnia and daytime functioning. Sleep Med Rev 2000; 4:277–298.
78. Roth T, Ancoli-Israel S. Daytime consequences and correlates of insomnia in the United States: results of the 1991 National Sleep Foundation Survey. II. Sleep 1999; 22:S354–S358.
79. Alapin I, Fichten CS, Libman E, et al. How is good and poor sleep in older adults and college students related to daytime sleepiness, fatigue, and ability to concentrate? J Psychosom Res 2000; 49:381–390.
80. Rombaut N, Maillard F, Kelly F, et al. The quality of life insomniacs questionnaire. Med Sci Res 1990; 18:845–847.
81. Neitzert Semler C, Harvey AG. Misperception of sleep can adversely affect daytime functioning in insomnia. Behav Res Ther 2005; 43:843–856.
82. Means MK, Lichstein KL, Epperson MT, et al. Relaxation therapy for insomnia: nighttime and daytime effects. Behav Res Ther 2000; 38:665–678.
83. Harvey AG, Sharpley A, Ree MJ, et al. An open trial of cognitive therapy for chronic insomnia. Behav Res Ther 2007; 45:2491–2501.

11 | Description of Circadian Rhythm Sleep Disorders

Shannon S. Sullivan

Division of Sleep Medicine, Department of Psychiatry and Behavioral Sciences, Stanford University School of Medicine, Stanford, California, U.S.A.

HISTORY AND NOMENCLATURE

Circadian rhythm sleep disorders (CRSDs) are a family of disorders that include problems with the timing of sleep and resultant daytime or nighttime symptoms. The term "circadian rhythm" refers to the endogenous rhythm of slightly greater than 24 hours, which has an important influence over many biological and physiological processes. Circadian variation has been recognized and recorded in living things since ancient times. Though endogenously generated, it may be modified or entrained by external environmental cues. Human circadian rhythms, including sleep-wake cycles, are driven by the suprachiasmatic nucleus (SCN) of the anterior hypothalamus. The SCN responds to light and non-light cues to synchronize the body's internal rhythms with the external world. The near–24 hour rhythm of the SCN is normally entrained to the 24-hour light-dark cycle of the earth's rotation around the sun (1). Melatonin secretion from the pineal gland, which is driven by the SCN, peaks after dark onset and is linked to sleep propensity (1). Light in the evening causes a rapid suppression of melatonin concentrations (2,3).

KEY FEATURES AND CHARACTERISTICS OF CRSD

The timing of sleep is optimal when one's circadian sleep/wake rhythms are well aligned with the actual sleep schedule. Misalignment between the endogenous circadian timing and the exogenous social and physical environment, or alterations in the circadian timekeeping of sleep, can lead to persistent or recurrent sleep disturbances known as CRSDs. According to criteria established by the *International Classification of Sleep Disorders* (ICSD), second edition, such disturbances must (*i*) lead to insomnia, excessive daytime sleepiness, or both; and (*ii*) affect social, occupational, or other types of functioning (4). A careful history, actigraphy, and sleep diaries may be useful to investigate and document CRSDs.

Incidence and Prevalence

CRSD, delayed sleep phase type (DSP), characterized by habitually delayed (late) sleep and wake times, and *CRSD, advanced sleep phase type* (ASP), characterized by habitually advanced (early) sleep and wake times, have unknown prevalences in the general population. DSP has a mean age of onset of 20 years, and prevalence is higher in adolescents and young adults, at 7% to 16%. Family history is positive in an estimated 40% of DSP patients. It is also estimated that 10% of chronic insomnia patients in sleep clinic have DSP (4). On the other hand, ASP has about a 1% prevalence in middle-aged and older adults, and increases with age. Both sexes are affected equally by ASP (4).

CRSD, irregular sleep-wake type, characterized by a lack of clearly defined circadian rhythm of the sleep and wake cycle, has unknown incidence and prevalence. Onset can occur at any age. *CRSD, free-running type,* is characterized by an abnormal synchronization between the 24-hour light-dark cycle and the endogenous circadian rhythm. The disorder occurs equally in males and females, is associated with a variable, "non-entrained" sleep pattern, and occurs in completely blind individuals more than 50% of the time; however, about 70% of blind individuals complain of sleep disturbances, and 40% have chronic cyclic sleep disturbances (4).

Environmentally induced CRSDs, such as *jet lag type*, which occurs as travelers cross multiple time zones, can affect all age groups, though the elderly have more pronounced symptoms and a prolonged rate of recovery. In *shift work type*, prevalence depends on the prevalence of shift wok in the population; in industrialized countries an estimated 20% of workers are shift workers, and prevalence of shift work disorder is 2% to 5% (4). There are no known sex differences. Finally, *CRSD due to a medical condition* has an unknown prevalence overall and varies with both underlying condition and exposure to light, structured physical and social activities. Two other disorders are described in the *ICSD*, second edition, *other circadian rhythm disorder and other circadian rhythm disorder due to a drug or substance*; while these fit the general requirements for CRSDs, they do not meet criteria for other specific types of CRSDs. Prevalence and incidence data are unknown.

Phylogeny and Animal Models

Internal circadian clocks are found in all eukaryotic and some prokaryotic organisms (5). From algae to humans, external environmental stimuli entrain the non-24-hour intrinsic cycle to a 24-hour rhythm (1). However, humans are unique in that they are routinely awake when their internal clock is signaling for sleep, and often want to sleep when the intrinsic rhythm is signaling for wake (6).

To explain how humans are able to consolidate approximately eight hours of sleep at night, Borbely proposed a two-process model of sleep regulation in which a homeostatic process (i.e., sleep drive), which builds as the day progresses, interacts with a circadian process (7). In 1993, Edgar et al. proposed an extension of this model, the "opponent process" model (8). This model incorporates the circadian pacemaker in the SCN as an active facilitator of wakefulness and opponent of homeostatic sleep tendency during the day. This model was derived from the observation that squirrel monkeys (*Saimiri sciureus*) demonstrated a profoundly increased daily sleep time, loss of sleep-wake consolidation, and short sleep latencies (at lights-out) following lesions of the SCN (9). There is evidence to support both a wake- and sleep-promoting role for the SCN in sleep-wake regulation (9).

In addition, the interrelationship between circadian and homeostatic processes has been investigated using circadian clock gene mutant or recombinant mouse models. Such models are used to understand the regulation of sleep in the absence of usual circadian control. Among the first studied was the circadian Clock mutant mouse, which demonstrated a two-hour decrease in total daily sleep (in both light-dark and constant-dark conditions) that was largely attributable to a decrease in nocturnal non–rapid eye movement (NREM) sleep, without a corresponding decrease in sleep intensity (as assessed by NREM delta power) (10). Now many genes with circadian influence have been studied in rodent models. Evidence suggests that circadian genes functionally influence both circadian and homeostatic components of sleep-wake regulation.

Social and Economic Factors

Shift work is expected to increase as second jobs, overtime work, and expanded service hours increase (11). Workers in around-the-clock occupations report obtaining less sleep and experiencing sleepiness on the job (12). There is abundant documentation that this is the case: National Aeronautics and Space Administration (NASA) studies of commercial airline pilots (13) demonstrated that, overall, 85% of pilots studied accumulated sleep debt across their trip schedules. Truck drivers, train engineers, air traffic controllers, public safety workers, and health care providers have all been studied and have been shown to have acute sleep deprivation and accumulation of sleep debt (12). Overall, 60% to 70% of shift workers report difficulty with work, sleepiness on the job, or actually falling asleep at work (14).

Consequences of sleepiness on the job are significant. For example, in one study, 41% of medical trainees report fatigue-related errors (15). In another report, extended work hours were associated with a three-fold increase in on-the-job injuries (16). Acute sleep loss increases sleepiness more than ethanol and had effects comparable to ethanol in blunting psychomotor performance (17), and sleepiness has been suggested to pose as great a risk to driving safety as alcohol (18,19). Drowsy work-related driving has been demonstrated to have alarming consequences, with a reported 39% of health care workers and 30% of police officers reporting an accident or near miss due to being tired (12).

Both sleep deprivation and circadian changes in chemoreceptor responsiveness and control of breathing (20) may also contribute to other coexisting sleep disorders such as obstructive sleep apnea. This will increase symptom burden, daytime sleepiness, and risk of adverse outcomes.

The personal burden and overall societal cost of CRSD is unknown but thought to be extensive. Accidents, lapses in public safety, lost work days, and decreased efficiency at work are just some of the consequences of CSRD, and a full accounting of these costs has yet to be estimated.

CONCLUSIONS

CRSDs refer to a family of disorders that include problems with the timing of sleep and resultant daytime or nighttime symptoms. These disorders lead to insomnia, excessive daytime sleepiness, or both, and impact social, occupational, or other types of functioning. The incidence and prevalence of these disorders vary depending on type, age, and gender; in some populations, such as those who are completely blind, CRSD can occur more than 50% of the time. Species, such as squirrel monkeys and rodents, have been used to study sleep-wake regulation. The social and economic impact of CRSDs should not be underestimated, particularly in light of consequent sleepiness leading to industrial and motor vehicle accidents.

REFERENCES

1. Sheer F, Cajochen C, Turek F, et al. Melatonin in the regulation of sleep and circadian rhythms. In: Kryger M, Roth T, Dement W, eds. Principles and Pratice of Sleep Medicine. 4th ed. Philadelphia: Elsevier Health Sciences, 2005:395–399.
2. Lewy AJ, Wehr TA, Goodwin FK, et al. Light suppresses melatonin secretion in humans. Science 1980; 210:1267–1269.
3. Zeitzer JM, Dijk DJ, Kronauer R, et al. Sensitivity of the human circadian pacemaker to nocturnal light: melatonin phase resetting and suppression. J Physiol 2000; 526(pt 3):695–702.
4. International Classification of Sleep Disorders: Diagnostic and Coding Manual. Illinois: American Academy of Sleep Disorders, 2005:117–131.
5. Takahashi JS, Turek FW, Moore RY, eds. Handbook of Behavioral Neurobiology. New York: Kluwer Academic/Plenum, 2001.
6. Turek F. Introduction: disorders of chronobiology. In: Kryger M, Roth T, Dement W, eds. Principles and Practice of Sleep Medicine. 4th ed. Philadelphia: Elsevier, 2005:657–658.
7. Borbély AA. Sleep regulation: Circadian rhythm and homeostasis. In: Ganten D, Pfaff D, eds. Current Topics in Neuroendocrinology. vol 1. Sleep: Clinical and Experimental Aspects. Berlin: Springer, 1982: 83–103.
8. Edgar DM, Dement WC, Fuller CA. Effect of SCN lesions on sleep in squirrel monkeys: evidence for opponent processes in sleep-wake regulation. J Neurosci 1993; 13:1065–1079.
9. Fuller PM, Gooley JJ, Saper CB. Neurobiology of the sleep-wake cycle: sleep architecture, circadian regulation, and regulatory feedback. J Biol Rhythms 2006; 21:482–493.
10. Naylor E, Bergmann BM, Krauski K, et al. The circadian clock mutation alters sleep homeostasis in the mouse. J Neurosci 2000; 20:8138–8143.
11. Biological Rhythms: Implications for the Worker. Office of Technology Assessment, U.S. Congress. Washington, D.C.: U.S. Government Printing Office, 1991:OTA-BA-463.
12. Rosekind M. Managing work schedules: an alertness and safety perspective. In: Kryger M, Roth T, Dement W, ed. Principles and Practice of Sleep Medicine. Philadelphia: Elsevier Saunders, 2005:680–690.
13. NASA-Ames Research Center. Crew factors in flight operations: the initial NASA-Ames field studies on fatigue. Aviat Space Envion Med 1998; 69:B1–60.
14. Akerstedt T, Torsvall L. Shift work. Shift-dependent well-being and individual differences. Ergonomics 1981; 24:265–273.
15. Gaba DM, Howard SK, Jump B. Production pressure in the work environment. California anesthesiologists' attitudes and experiences. Anesthesiology 1994; 81:488–500.
16. Akerstedt T. Work injuries and time of day—national data. In: Proceedings of a Consensus Development Symposium on Work Hours, Sleepiness, and Accidents. Stockholm, Sweden, September 8–10, 1994:106.
17. Roehrs T, Burduvali E, Bonahoom A, et al. Ethanol and sleep loss: a "dose" comparison of impairing effects. Sleep 2003; 26:981–985.
18. Roehrs T, Beare D, Zorick F, et al. Sleepiness and ethanol effects on simulated driving. Alcohol Clin Exp Res 1994; 18:154–158.
19. Dawson D, Reid K. Fatigue, alcohol and performance impairment. Nature 1997; 388:235.
20. Stephenson R. Circadian rhythms and sleep-related breathing disorders. Sleep Med 2007; 8:681–687.

12 | Pathophysiology, Associations, and Consequences of Circadian Rhythm Sleep Disorders

Shawn D. Youngstedt
Department of Exercise Science, Norman J. Arnold School of Public Health, University of South Carolina, Dorn VA Medical Center, Columbia, South Carolina, U.S.A.

James B. Burch
Department of Epidemiology and Biostatistics, Norman J. Arnold School of Public Health, University of South Carolina, Dorn VA Medical Center, Columbia, South Carolina, U.S.A.

INTRODUCTION

Circadian rhythm sleep disorders (CRSDs) are a family of sleep disorders affecting the timing of sleep. They result from a mismatch between the body's endogenous clock and external timing cues provided by an individual's 24-hour schedule. People with CRSDs typically cannot sleep or wake at the times required for work, school, or other social routines, but can generally get enough sleep if allowed to sleep and wake at preferred times. CRSDs diagnoses include delayed sleep phase type (DSPT), advanced sleep phase type (ASPT), irregular sleep-wake type, free-running type, jet lag type, shift work type, and CRSD due to medical conditions. This chapter will briefly describe each disorder, its etiology, pathophysiology, and pathogenesis; predisposing and precipitating factors; associated morbidity and mortality; and associations, complications, and consequences.

DELAYED SLEEP PHASE TYPE

CRSD of DSPT is characterized by inability to fall asleep before 2:00 a.m. (often later) and extreme difficulty awakening at a "normal" time in the morning, that is, before 10:00 a.m. (1,2). A delayed phase in individuals with CRSD of DSPT has been noted in multiple circadian markers, including the rhythms of core body temperature (3), and dim light melatonin onset (DLMO) (4).

If given the opportunity on weekends or holidays, or through special arrangements of school/work and social schedules, individuals with CRSD of DSPT will often wake up at times between 10:00 a.m. and 1:00 p.m., and they demonstrate normal sleep quantity and quality (5). However, most people with CRSD of DSPT face chronic sleep deprivation, with all of its consequences. When attempting to wake at more normal times, they exhibit severe sleep inertia and even "sleep drunkenness."

Etiology, Pathophysiology, and Pathogenesis

Sleep and wakefulness are regulated by two processes, a circadian process, which promotes sleep during the night and wakefulness during the day, and a homeostatic process, which promotes sleep as a function of duration of wakefulness (6). These processes interact to promote consolidated bouts of sleep and wakefulness (7). There is evidence that the interaction between circadian and homeostatic processes is altered in CRSD of DSPT (8,9). Specifically, compared with normal controls, individuals with CRSD of DSPT display a longer interval between circadian phase markers (e.g., body core temperature nadir) and wake time (8,9). Difficulty arising in these patients probably stems not only from a delay in the circadian system but also from this altered interaction between circadian and homeostatic processes.

It has been hypothesized that CRSD of DSPT might be attributed to a longer circadian period, which would lead to a tendency for circadian phase to gradually drift to later times (1,2). However, to our knowledge there is no compelling empirical support for this hypothesis.

Sleep deprivation studies have shown that, compared with normal sleepers, individuals with CRSD of DSPT have reduced ability to sleep in the evening and early night (10,11), which might be attributed to reduced homeostatic pressure for sleep with prolonged wakefulness. This could explain a tendency for these individuals to delay bedtime compared with normal sleepers.

Staying up late and waking up late, even over just a few days, can delay the circadian system (12); chronic maintenance of such a schedule probably results in further phase delays. These delays can be attributed to several interacting factors, including exposure to phase-delaying effects of both nighttime light and later timing of sleep, as well as decreased exposure to morning light, which advances the circadian system (13).

Predisposing and Precipitating Factors

Predisposing and precipitating factors that mediate CRSD of DSPT include a biological tendency for circadian delay coupled with behavior that exacerbates this tendency. A familial pedigree for CRSD of DSPT has been demonstrated (14), and CRSD of DSPT has been linked to polymorphisms in circadian clock genes, *hPer3*, arylakylamine *N*-acetyltransferase, HLA, and *Clock* (15–17). The usual onset of CRSD of DSPT occurs in adolescence or young adulthood, which is associated with a delay in the circadian system (18).

Another precipitating biological factor for CRSD of DSPT might be increased sensitivity to the phase-delaying effects of evening light (2). Consistent with this hypothesis is evidence that evening bright light elicits exaggerated suppression of melatonin in CRSD of DSPT patients compared with controls (19).

A biological delay in the circadian system undoubtedly contributes to voluntarily staying up and waking up later, resulting in increased exposure to the phase-delaying effects of evening light and decreasing exposure to the phase-advancing effects of morning light. Likewise, anecdotes suggest that long-term night work can precipitate CRSD of DSPT (1), though there is likely significant self-selection of night work by people with delayed body clocks.

Similar delay in circadian timing can be precipitated by medical, psychiatric, or substance abuse disorders. However, the diagnosis of CRSD of DSPT requires that the pattern cannot be primarily attributed to these other causes (1).

Morbidity and Mortality

CRSD of DSPT does not cause much sleep loss so long as an individual is permitted to sleep until 10:00 a.m. to 12:00 noon. However, this is often not possible, particularly at its typical onset during adolescence and early adulthood (18). Thus, individuals with CRSD of DSPT are typically chronically sleep deprived.

Psychological/Psychiatric Associations, Complications, and Consequences

A relatively high prevalence of depression has been found in individuals with CRSD of DSPT (20,21). Moreover, winter depression (aka seasonal affective disorder) has been associated with a delayed circadian system (22,23), and remission from winter depression is associated with a normalization of circadian phase (23). A causal association between delayed phase and depression has also been suggested by some evidence that antidepressant effects of bright light treatment for winter depression are correlated with the phase-advancing effects of morning light (23,24). However, other studies have found that phase-advancing and antidepressant effects of light treatment are not necessarily correlated (25,26). Nevertheless, having a delayed wake time can result in low levels of exposure to environmental bright light (27), which has been associated with nonseasonal depression, as well as winter depression.

A variety of psychosocial problems arise for many individuals with CRSD of DSPT, who are often assumed to be lazy and unmotivated (21). Awakening at normal and, especially, earlier than normal times can be extremely difficult for individuals with CRSD of DSPT. Work tardiness and absenteeism are relatively common in individuals with CRSD of DSPT compared with normal sleepers (21). In an extreme example, a Marine with CRSD of DSPT was court-martialed for these offenses (28).

ADVANCED SLEEP PHASE TYPE

CRSD of ASPT is characterized by sleep ($\sim$6–9 p.m.) and wake ($\sim$2–5 a.m.) times that are $\geq$3 hours earlier than societal norms (1,2). Advanced circadian phase in other markers [e.g., of DLMO (29)] is also evident in individuals with CRSD of ASPT, though the advance in these markers is typically not as profound as the advance in sleep phase (2). When sleep is scheduled for these advanced times, CRSD of ASPT patients demonstrate normal age-related sleep duration and architecture (1,2).

Etiology, Pathophysiology, and Pathogenesis

The precise pathophysiology of CRSD of ASPT is not clear. A short circadian period has been noted in a family with CRSD of ASPT (30). It has been hypothesized that CRSD of ASPT might be attributed to reduced ability of the circadian system to delay and/or a relatively larger window of time of sensitivity to the phase-advancing effects of light (1,2).

Predisposing and Precipitating Factors

Family pedigrees of CRSD of ASPT have been documented with an autosomal dominant mode of inheritance (29,30). Mutations in the circadian clock *hPer2* and *CK1 δ* genes have been linked with inheritance of CRSD of ASPT (31).

The prevalence of CRSD of ASPT increases with age (32), as does a general trend toward earlier circadian phase (33,34). Research is mixed regarding whether aging is associated with a shortening of the circadian period (33), which could explain the phase advance. Some research has indicated remarkably low levels of exposure to evening light in older adults (35). Inadequate exposure to the phase-delaying effect of evening light could contribute to the relatively high prevalence of CRSD of ASPT among older adults. Conversely, exposure to high levels of morning light could precipitate or exacerbate CRSD of ASPT. Anecdotal accounts suggest that work schedules requiring chronic very early awakening can lead to subsequent CRSD of ASPT (1,2).

Morbidity and Mortality

As with CRSD of DSPT, CRSD of ASPT does not cause health problems so long as individuals are able to maintain schedules that accommodate their abnormal circadian phases. Individuals with CRSD of ASPT generally have less difficulty maintaining such schedules than individuals with CRSD of DSPT since most people have fewer professional obligations in the evening than in the morning (2). Excessive late-afternoon sleepiness is common in CRSD of ASPT and could contribute to decreased work productivity and increased risk of accidents (2). Fulfilling various evening obligations, which are contrary to an advanced circadian system, can lead to chronically insufficient sleep and associated health problems.

Psychological/Psychiatric Associations, Complications, and Consequences

Earlier speculation had been that major depression might be associated with a phase advance of the strong oscillator relative to the sleep-wake cycle, as evidenced by shortened rapid eye movement (REM) onset latency. However, data generally do not support that CRSD of ASPT is a cause of depression, or vice versa, and depression and CRSD of ASPT are characterized by different sleep and circadian profiles (36). For example, unlike CRSD of ASPT, extreme late-afternoon sleepiness, early bedtimes, and advancement in other markers of circadian phase (such as melatonin and body temperature) are generally not found in depressed individuals (36).

Adherence to very early bedtimes can lead to some strain in social and work relations, and many individuals with CRSD of ASPT would prefer to stay up late (37,38). Moreover, extreme early morning awakening is often a source of frustration and loneliness (38).

FREE-RUNNING TYPE (NON-24-HOUR SLEEP-WAKE SYNDROME)

CSRD of free-running type is characterized by periodic, recurring sleep symptoms of difficulty initiating asleep, maintaining sleep, and arising, depending on the current phase of the circadian system, which regulates sleep propensity and alertness (1,2). When the circadian system is in synchrony with the sleep-wake schedule, individuals with free-running rhythms sleep normally. However, when the circadian system gradually drifts out of phase with the sleep-wake cycle, sleep problems appear. It is more difficult to recognize and diagnose CSRD of free-running type compared with other CRSDs. There is typically not a dramatic abnormality in behavior; rather, individuals with free-running circadian rhythms generally attempt to maintain a consistent, normal sleep-wake schedule (1,39).

Etiology, Pathophysiology, and Pathogenesis

Under normal circumstances in sighted individuals, the circadian system is entrained to precisely 24 hours via daily exposure to zeitgebers ("time givers") (40), particularly light exposure, which shifts the clock via a direct retinohypothalamic pathway (41). However, under experimental conditions in which these zeitgebers are removed (or distributed equally across the 24-hour day), such as in the constant routine (42) or the ultrashort sleep-wake cycle (43), the circadian system oscillates at its endogenous frequency. In humans, the endogenous period is ~24.2 to 24.5 hours (44,45), as evidenced by a progressive phase delay under these experimental conditions.

In real-world conditions, CSRD of free-running type is usually observed in blind people (46), and can be attributed to a lack of photic input to the suprachiasmatic nuclei. Nonetheless, many blind people remain normally or partly entrained (46), and this can be explained by the existence of separate photoreceptors in the retina, which are responsive to light, independent of visual perception (47,48). Not surprisingly, an important predictor of free running in blind individuals is whether their eyes have been enucleated. Blind individuals probably also remain entrained via regular exposure to other zeitgebers, such as exercise, social interaction, and daily melatonin treatment.

CSRD of free-running type in sighted individuals has often been preceded by psychiatric disorders, especially depression (49). The pathophysiology of this association is not clear. It has been hypothesized that depressed individuals might have a relative absence of exposure to social zeitgebers (50). Reduced sensitivity to light could plausibly explain the etiology of both depression and free-running rhythms (50). One case of CSRD of free-running type in a mentally retarded individual with very low melatonin excretion prompted speculation that the disorder might be due to a congenital deficiency in melatonin production (51). Another case in which onset occurred following a car accident led to speculation that CSRD of free-running type might also be attributed to "microscopic damage in the vicinity of the suprachiasmatic nucleus (SCN) or its output pathways" (52).

Predisposing and Precipitating Factors

As discussed, blindness is the most common precipitating factor for free-running rhythms. Sighted individuals with free-running rhythms have reported that night shift work, unemployment, and voluntary lifestyle habits of extreme eveningness are common precipitating factors (53).

IRREGULAR SLEEP-WAKE TYPE

CSRD of irregular sleep-wake type is characterized by the absence of a clear circadian pattern of sleep and wakefulness (1,2). Rather, patients demonstrate a sporadic pattern of sleep episodes (≥3) over a 24-hour period, though the total amount of sleep obtained over a 24-hour period is generally normal for one's age (54,55).

Etiology, Pathophysiology, and Pathogenesis

CSRD of irregular sleep-wake type has been most often associated with dementia (55–57), but it has also been associated with mental retardation and head injury. These associations might be attributed to anatomical or functional abnormalities in the SCN or pineal gland, which have been associated with aging in general, and particularly with dementia (58). Similar sleep-wake patterns have been noted in animals following ablation of the SCN (59). Neurological diseases and mental retardation have been linked to CSRD of irregular sleep-wake type.

Having a poorly entrained environment, such as insufficient light exposure in the day, excessive nighttime light exposure, and continuous inactivity, have also been associated with irregular sleep-wake cycle patterns in nursing home and hospital patients (60,61). Indeed, even young, healthy individuals display a similar sleep pattern when subjected to continuous bed rest (62).

JET LAG TYPE

Rapid transmeridian travel elicits a host of symptoms, particularly insomnia during the nighttime and reduced alertness during the daytime. Although CRSD of jet lag type is the most transitory of the CRSDs, it can nonetheless have profound negative effects on physical and mental health.

Etiology, Pathophysiology, and Pathogenesis
CRSD of jet lag type is elicited by rapid transmeridian travel, which causes a desynchronization between the circadian system and the environmental schedule (1,2,63). Moreover, symptoms might be partly attributed to internal desynchronization between various biological rhythms (64). Following air travel, rhythms can re-entrain to the new time zones at different rates, and even in opposite directions of phase shifts, for example, either advancing 9 hours or delaying 15 hours (63). Symptoms of jet lag become progressively worse with the number of time zones crossed, and persist until the circadian system is resynchronized to the new time zone (63).

Resynchronization takes an average of approximately one day per time zone crossed, but there are considerable individual differences in rate of adjustment. Readjustment is generally more difficult following eastward than westward travel, and this can be attributed partly to the fact that the endogenous period length is greater than 24 hours, making delays more natural. Similarly, people generally find it easier to adjust to the end (fall back) than the beginning of daylight savings (spring forward). Depending on the number of time zones crossed, daytime light exposure following travel is more likely to counteract adjustment to eastward than westward travel. For example, since maximal phase-delaying effects of light occur zero to six hours before the body temperature nadir (on average, ~11:00 p.m.–5:00 a.m., in one's home time zone), the traveler who has flown ≥7 time zones east should initially avoid light exposure until after 11:00 a.m.

Predisposing and Precipitating Factors
Considerable individual differences exist in the rate of resynchronization and the degree of symptoms associated with jet lag (63). Anecdotal accounts suggest that some individuals do not experience jet lag. These individual differences are not well understood, but might be explained by differences in the flexibility of the circadian system and differences in the ability to sleep at an abnormal circadian phase (65,66).

There is some evidence that older age is associated with slower resynchronization and worse symptoms of jet lag (67). Although slower adjustment might be expected with age because of decrements in eye function, laboratory studies have failed to reveal differences in phase responses to light exposure in humans (68). Theoretically, "morning types" and "evening types" might have relatively more difficulty traveling westward and eastward, respectively.

Behavior during the days preceding travel as well as following travel can delay the time for complete resynchronization and/or exacerbate symptoms of jet lag (69). Whereas late bedtimes and excessive evening light exposure prior to travel can slow complete adjustment to eastward travel, early rise times and morning light prior to travel can slow adjustment following westward travel (69). Light exposure following travel can also facilitate or impair resynchronization according to the phase response curve for light. Sleep deprivation before and after travel can also exacerbate other symptoms.

Morbidity and Mortality
The most common symptoms associated with jet lag disorder are insomnia, low alertness during the daytime, general malaise, gastrointestinal distress, and urination and defecation at abnormal, inconvenient times of day (70). Chronic repeated exposure to transmeridian air travel in airline crews has been associated with cardiovascular disease (71), cognitive deficits (72,73), and temporal lobe atrophy (73). Chronic air travel in female flight attendants has been associated with menstrual cycle dysfunction (74). To our knowledge, there is no compelling

evidence that chronic exposure to jet lag influences mortality in humans. However, there is compelling evidence from animal studies that chronic exposure to simulated jet lag can increase mortality (75,76) and the rate of cancer progression (77–79).

Psychological/Psychiatric Associations, Complications, and Consequences

Severe impairments in mood have been documented following acute air travel with validated questionnaires such as the Profile of Mood States (POMS). Moreover, there is evidence that acute air travel can exacerbate and possibly precipitate the onset of major affective disorders (80). Chronic exposure to jet lag in flight crews has been associated with dementia.

SHIFT WORK TYPE

Shift work refers both to rotating work hours as well as permanent work at unusual times, such as the all-night (graveyard) shift. Approximately 20% of the work force are shift workers, and this number is expected to grow (81). The fastest growing job sector in western societies is the service sector, which often requires 24-hour operation (81). Like jet lag, CRSD of shift work type arises as people attempt to function at times that are contrary to their circadian systems. However, unlike jet lag, CRSD of shift work type is typically chronic, essentially persisting as long as the individual is required to maintain one of these debilitating schedules.

Etiology, Pathophysiology, and Pathogenesis

Shift work varies considerably in work hours, frequency, and direction of shift, etc. The all-night ("graveyard") schedule results in the greatest sleep loss, which arises from a desynchronization between the work schedule and the workers' circadian rhythms. Shift workers almost never completely synchronize their body clocks to these schedules (82). Resistance to synchronization can be attributed to exposure to light and other zeitgebers at inappropriate times for shifting the clock to a shift work schedule (e.g., morning light exposure on the drive home from work), and social commitments, which tend to keep one entrained to a diurnal schedule (81,82). Indeed, most shift workers revert back to a normal diurnal schedule on weekends (81). Lack of resynchronization results in reduced alertness during work hours, chronically insufficient sleep duration and quality, and increased risk of accidents (69,83,84). Eating meals during shift work hours could result in abnormally timed pancreatic and metabolic responses, which might increase the risk of diabetes and heart disease (63,85).

Epidemiological studies have suggested an association of melatonin suppression with cancer in night workers (86–88). Several lines of evidence indicate that melatonin has antiproliferative, immune-enhancing, and antioxidant properties, and, conversely, that blocking or suppressing melatonin can increase the risk of cancer onset and progression (89). Melatonin synthesis, which normally occurs at night, is suppressed by light exposure, which is unavoidable for many night workers. On the other hand, light exposure is helpful for increasing alertness during night work, and this effect is mediated partly by melatonin suppression. Further experiments are needed to clarify the potential benefits and risks of melatonin suppression for shift workers (63).

The association of shift work with cancer could also be explained by disrupted clock protein function. The molecular clock responsible for circadian rhythms both in supra-chiasmatic nuclei and in peripheral tissues consists of at least nine core clock genes whose expression coordinates DNA repair, cell proliferation, and apoptosis, processes that are all critical to carcinogenesis (90–93). Mutation or disregulation of specific clock genes (e.g., *Per*) has been associated with functional disruption of circadian rhythms (94), and with increased tumor development and cancer mortality (92,94,95).

Predisposing and Precipitating Factors

Numerous factors have been associated with tolerance of shift work, many of which relate to a greater ability to obtain sleep on shift work schedules. Older age (>50 years) is associated with less tolerance of shift work, and this has been observed even in individuals who had previously been highly tolerant (96). The age-related decline in shift work tolerance might be partly attributed to a general phase advance of the circadian system with age, and decreased "flexibility" of sleep timing, that is, ability to sleep at odd hours (65,66).

"Night owls" (individuals high in "eveningness") are clearly more tolerant of all-night work schedules than "morning larks" (individuals high in "morningness") (96), and this greater tolerance has been linked with a delay in the circadian system and greater sleep flexibility following night work.

Having other preexisting sleep disorders, health and psychiatric morbidities, and history of alcohol or drug abuse are all associated with greater risk of developing CRSD of shift work sleep type. Employers would be well advised to screen for these characteristics.

Both cross-sectional and experimental evidence indicate that aerobic exercise can enhance tolerance to shift work (97–100), perhaps by improving sleep and promoting alertness and energy levels during work hours. Moreover, regular exercise can attenuate numerous morbidities associated with shift work (101).

Varying levels of family and social obligations influence sleep and tolerance to shift work. Workers who must sacrifice sleep to care for family, performing errands, etc. tend to have worse tolerance and greater levels of marital and family strife (81).

Morbidity and Mortality

Shift work has been associated with an increased risk of multiple morbidities, including psychiatric disturbance (see below), cancer (86,102), cardiovascular disease (101,103), gastrointestinal distress (104), and menstrual cycle dysfunction. Higher mortality rates have also been demonstrated in workers with long durations of shift work exposure (105). It is clear that the risk of accidents increase during the night (69,83). Indeed, many of the world's most notorious catastrophes, such as Chernobyl and Bhopal, have been attributed to shift work.

Psychological/Psychiatric Associations, Complications, and Consequences

Self-selection of individuals able to cope with shift work probably results in an underestimation of its negative impact on psychological/psychiatric disorders. Nonetheless, compared with day workers, shift workers have a higher prevalence of psychiatric disorders, and worse mood levels on standardized questionnaires (106). A night of sleep deprivation can precipitate or exacerbate mania in predisposed individuals (107).

Common methods to self-treat insomnia associated with shift work include drug and alcohol use, which can lead to abuse and dependence (1). Conversely, excessive use of caffeine or other stimulants for combating sleepiness on the job can exacerbate insomnia and anxiety disorders (1).

CONCLUSIONS

CRSDs are associated with significant physiological consequences, ranging from sleep inertia to more serious medical conditions, such as cardiovascular disease and dementia. The interaction between homeostatic and circadian processes is believed to be altered in individuals with these circadian disorders. Genetic mechanisms have been identified in some of these disorders, such as CRSDs of delayed and advanced sleep types. Shift work has been associated with an increased risk of multiple morbidities, and a higher mortality rate has been demonstrated in workers with prolonged shift work exposure.

ACKNOWLEDGMENTS

This work was supported by HL71560 as well as VA (VISN-7) Career Development Awards (SDY, JBB).

REFERENCES

1. Zee P, Ancoli-Israel S, Carskadon M, et al. Circadian rhythm sleep disorders. In: Sateia MJ, ed. The International Classification of Sleep Disorders. 2nd ed. Westchester: American Academy of Sleep Medicine, 2005:117–141.
2. Reid KJ, Zee PC. Circadian disorders of the sleep-wake cycle. In: Kryger MH, Roth T, Dement WC, eds. Principles and Practice of Sleep Medicine. 4th ed. Philadelphia: Elsevier Saunders, 2007:691–701.

3. Vignau J, Dahlitz M, Arendt J, et al. Biological rhythms and sleep disorders in man: the delayed sleep phase syndrome. In: Wetterberg L, ed. Light and Biological Rhythms in Man. 1st ed. Stockholm: Pergamon Press, 1993:261–271.

4. Shibui K, Uchiyama M, Okawa M. Melatonin rhythms in delayed sleep phase syndrome. J Biol Rhythms 2000; 14:72–76.

5. Wyatt JK. Delayed sleep phase syndrome: pathophysiology and treatment options. Sleep 2007; 27:1195–1203.

6. Borb'ely AA. A two-process model of sleep regulation. Hum Neurobiol 1982; 1:195–204.

7. Dijk DJ, Czeisler CA. Paradoxical timing of the circadian rhythm of sleep propensity serves to consolidate sleep and wakefulness in humans. Neurosci Lett 1994; 166:63–68.

8. Ozaki S, Uchiyama M, Shirakawa S, et al. Prolonged interval from body temperature nadir to sleep offset in patients with delayed sleep phase syndrome. Sleep 1996; 19(1):36–40.

9. Uchiyama M, Okawa M, Shibui K, et al. Altered phase relation between sleep timing and core body temperature rhythm in delayed sleep phase syndrome and non-24-hour sleep-wake syndrome in humans. Neurosci Lett 2000; 294(2):101–104.

10. Uchiyama M, Okawa M, Shibui K, et al. Poor recovery sleep after sleep deprivation in delayed sleep phase syndrome. Psychiatry Clin Neurosci 1900; 53:195–197.

11. Uchiyama M, Okawa M, Shibui K, et al. Poor compensatory function for sleep loss as a pathogenic factor in patients with delayed sleep phase syndrome. Sleep 2000; 23(4):553–558.

12. Burgess HJ, Eastman CI. A late wake time phase delays the human dim light melatonin rhythm. Neurosci Lett 2006; 395(3):191–195.

13. Crowley SJ, Lee C, Tseng CY, et al. Combinations of bright light, scheduled dark, sunglasses, and melatonin to facilitate circadian entrainment to night shift work. J Biol Rhythms 2003; 18(6):513–523.

14. Ancoli-Israel S, Schnierow B, Kelsoe J, et al. A pedigree of one family with delayed sleep phase syndrome. Chronobiol Int 2001; 18(5):831–840.

15. Iwase T, Kajimura N, Uchiyama M, et al. Mutation screening of the human *Clock* gene in circadian rhythm sleep disorders. Psychiatry Res 2002; 109:121–128.

16. Archer SN, Robilliard DL, Skene DJ, et al. A length polymorphism in the circadian clock gene per3 is linked to delayed sleep phase syndrome and extreme diurnal preference. Sleep 2003; 26(4):413–415.

17. Hohjoh H, Takasu M, Shishikura K, et al. Significant association of the arylalkylamine N-acetyltransferase (AA-NAT) gene with delayed sleep phase syndrome. Neurogenetics 2003; 4: 151–153.

18. Crowley SJ, Acebo C, Carskadon MA. Sleep, circadian rhythms, and delayed phase in adolescence. Sleep Med 2007; 8(6):602–612.

19. Aoki H, Ozeki Y, Yamada N. Hypersensitivity of melatonin suppression in response to light in patients with delayed sleep phase syndrome. Chronobiol Int 2001; 18(2):263–271.

20. Weiner P. Can chronotherapy of chronic obstructive pulmonary disorder improve treatment? J Intern Med 2000; 246:422.

21. Regenstein QR, Monk TH. Delayed sleep phase syndrome: a review of its clinical aspects. Am J Psychiatry 1995; 152:602–608.

22. Dahl K, Avery DH, Lewy AJ, et al. Dim light melatonin onset and circadian temperature during a constant routine in hypersomnic winter depression. Acta Psychiatr Scand 1993; 88:60.

23. Lewy AJ, Sack RL, Singer CM, et al. Winter depression and the phase-shift hypothesis for bright light's therapeutic effects: history, theory, and experimental evidence. J Biol Rhythms 1988; 3(2): 121–134.

24. Lewy AJ, Leflur BJ, Emens JS, et al. The circadian basis of winter depression. Proc Natl Acad Sci 2006; 103(19):7414–7419.

25. Eastman CI, Gallo LC, Lahmeyer HW, et al. The circadian rhythm of temperature during light treatment for winter depression. Biol Psychiatry 1993; 34:210–220.

26. Murray G, Michalak EE, Levitt AJ, et al. Therapeutic mechanism in seasonal affective disorder: do fluoxetine and light operate through advancing circadian phase? Chronobiol Int 2005; 22(5):937–943.

27. Goulet G, Mongrain V, Desrosiers C, et al. Daily light exposure in morning-type and evening-type individuals. J Biol Rhythms 2007; 22(151):158.

28. deBeck TW. Delayed sleep phase syndrome-Criminal offense in the military? Mil Med 1990; 155(1): 14–15.

29. Reid KJ, Chang A-M, Dubocovich ML, et al. Familial advanced sleep phase syndrome. Arch Neurol 2001; 58:1089–1094.

30. Jones CR, Campbell SS, Zone SE, et al. Familial advanced sleep-phase syndrome: a short-period circadian rhythm variant in humans. Nat Med 1999; 5(9):1062–1065.

31. Toh KL, Jones CR, He Y, et al. An hPer2 phosphorylation site mutation in familial advanced sleep-phase syndrome. Science 2001; 291:1040–1043.

32. Ando K, Kripke DF, Ancoli-Israel S. Estimated prevalence of delayed and advanced sleep phase syndromes. Sleep Res 1995; 24:509.

33. Monk TH. Aging human circadian rhythms: conventional wisdom may not always be right. J Biol Rhythms 2007; 20(4):366–374.
34. Duffy JF, Czeisler CA. Age-related change in the relationship between circadian period, circadian phase, and diurnal preference in humans. Neurosci Lett 2002; 318:117–120.
35. Youngstedt SD, Kripke DF, Elliott JA, et al. Light exposure, sleep quality, and depression in older adults. In: Holick MF, Jung EG, eds. Biologic Effects of Light 1998. 5th ed. Boston: Kluwer Academic Publishers, 1999:427–435.
36. Benca RM. Mood Disorders. In: Kryger MH, Roth T, Dement WC, eds. Principles and Practice of Sleep Medicine. 4th ed. Philadelphia: Elsevier Saunders, 2007:1311–1326.
37. Ishihara K, Miyake S, Miyasita A, et al. Morningness-eveningness preference and sleep habits in Japanese office workers of different ages. Chronobiologia 1992; 19:9.
38. Ancoli-Israel S, Cooke JR. Prevalence and comorbidity of insomnia and effect on functioning in elderly populations. J Am Geriatr Soc 2007; 53(S7):S264–S271.
39. Klein T, Martens H, Dijk DJ, et al. Circadian sleep regulation in the absence of light perception: chronic non-24-hour circadian rhythm sleep disorder in a blind man with a regular 24-hour sleep-wake schedule. Sleep 1993; 16(4):333–343.
40. Johnson CH, Elliott JA, Foster R. Entrainment of circadian programs. Chronobiol Int 2003; 20(5):741–774.
41. Moore RY. Retinohypothalamic projection in mammals: a comparative study. Brain Res 1972; 49: 403–409.
42. Duffy JF, Dijk D-J. Getting through to circadian oscillators: why use constant routines? J Biol Rhythms 2002; 17(1):4–13.
43. Lavie P, Segal S. Twenty-four-hour structure of sleepiness in morning and evening persons investigated by ultrashort sleep-wake cycle. Sleep 1989; 12(6):522–528.
44. Czeisler CA, Duffy JF, Shanahan TL, et al. Stability, precision, and near-24-hour period of the human circadian pacemaker. Science 1999; 284:2177–2181.
45. Lewy AJ, Hasler BP, Emens JS, et al. Pretreatment circadian period in free-running blind people may predict the phase angle of entrainment to melatonin. Neurosci Lett 2001; 313:158–160.
46. Sack RL, Lewy AJ, Blood ML, et al. Circadian rhythm abnormalities in totally blind people: incidence and clinical significance. J Clin Endocrinol Metab 1992; 75(1):127–134.
47. Lucas RJ, Freedman MS, Munoz M, et al. Regulation of the mammalian pineal by non-rod, non-cone, ocular photoreceptors. Science 1999; 284:505–508.
48. Brainard GC, Hanifin JP, Greeson JM, et al. Action spectrum for melatonin regulation in humans: evidence for a novel circadian photoreceptor. J Neurosci 2001; 21(16):6405–6412.
49. Hayakawa T, Uchiyama M, Kamei Y, et al. Clinical analyses of sighted patients with non-24-hour sleep-wake syndrome: a study of 57 consecutively diagnosed cases. Sleep 2005; 28(8):945–952.
50. McArthur AJ, Lewy AJ, Sack RL. Non-24-hour sleep-wake syndrome in a sighted man: circadian rhythm studies and efficacy of melatonin treatment. Sleep 1996; 19(7):544–553.
51. Akaboshi S, Inoue Y, Kubota N, et al. Case of a mentally retarded child with non-24 hour sleep-wake syndrome caused by deficiency of melatonin secretion. Psychiatry Clin Neurosci 2000; 54(3):379–380.
52. Boivin DB, James FO, Santo JB, et al. Non-24-hour sleep-wake syndrome following a car accident. Neurobiology 2003; 60(11):1841–1843.
53. Uchiyama M, Shibui K, Hayakawa T, et al. Larger phase angle between sleep propensity and melatonin rhythms in sighted humans with non-24-hour sleep-wake syndrome. Sleep 2002; 25(1): 83–88.
54. Okawa M, Mishima K, Hishikawa Y, et al. Circadian rhythm disorders in sleep-waking and body temperature in elderly patients with dementia and their treatment. Sleep 1991; 14(6):478–485.
55. Witting W, Kwa IH, Eikelenboom P, et al. Alterations in the circadian rest-activity rhythm in aging and Alzheimer's disease. Biol Psychiatry 1990; 27:563–572.
56. Mirmiran M, Witting W, Swaab DF, et al. Sleep and circadian rhythm changes in Alzheimer's disease. In: Smirne S, Franceschi M, Ferini-Strambi L, eds. Sleep and Ageing. Milano, Italy: Masson Press, 1991:57–64.
57. Van Someren EJW. Circadian and sleep disturbances in the elderly. Exp Gerontol 2000; 35(9–10): 1229–1237.
58. Wu YH, Swaab DF. Disturbance and strategies for reactivation of the circadian rhythm system in aging and Alzheimer's disease. Sleep Med 2007; 8(6):623–636.
59. Rusak B. Neural mechanisms for entrainment and generation of mammalian circadian rhythms. Fed Proc 1979; 38(12):2589–2595.
60. Ancoli-Israel S, Martin JL, Kripke DF, et al. Effect of light treatment on sleep and circadian rhythms in demented nursing home patients. J Am Geriatr Soc 2002; 50(2):282–289.
61. van Someren E, Kessler A, Mirmiran M, et al. Indirect bright light improves circadian rest-Activity rhythm disturbances in demented patients. Biol Psychiatry 1997; 41:955–963.
62. Campbell SS. Duration and placement of sleep in a "disentrained" environment. Psychophysiology 1984; 21(1):106–113.

63. Arendt J, Stone B, Skene DJ. Sleep disruption in jet lag and other circadian rhythm-related disorders. In: Kryger MH, Roth T, Dement WC, eds. Principles and Practice of Sleep Medicine. 4th ed. Philadelphia: Elsevier Saunders, 2005:659–672.

64. Wever RA. The Circadian System of Man: Results of Experiments Under Temporal Isolation. New York: Springer-Verlag, 1979.

65. Ashkenazi IE, Reinberg AE, Motohashi Y. Interindividual differences in the flexibility of human temporal organization: pertinence to jet lag and shiftwork. Chronobiol Int 1997; 14(2):99–113.

66. Costa G, Lievore F, Casaletti G, et al. Circadian characteristics influencing interindividual differences in tolerance and adjustment to shiftwork. Ergonomics 1989; 32(4):373–385.

67. Monk TH, Buysse DJ, Carrier J, et al. Inducing jet-lag in older people: directional asymmetry. J Sleep Res 2000; 9:101–116.

68. Benloucif S, Green K, L'Hermite-Balériaux M, et al. Responsiveness of the aging circadian clock to light. Neurobiol Aging 2006; 27(12):1870–1879.

69. Revell VL, Eastman CI. How to trick mother nature into letting you fly around or stay up all night. J Biol Rhythms 2005; 20(4):353–365.

70. Spitzer RL, Terman M, Williams JBW, et al. Jet lag: clinical features, validation of a new syndrome-specific scale, and lack of response to melatonin in a randomized, double-blind trial. Am J Psychiatry 1999; 156(9):1392–1396.

71. Ekstrand K, Bostrom PA, Arborelius M, et al. Cardiovascular risk factors in commercial flight aircrew officers compared with those in the general population. Angiology 1996; 47(11):1089–1094.

72. Cho K, Ennaceur A, Cole JC, et al. Chronic jet lag produces cognitive deficits. J Neurosci 2000; 20(6): RC66.

73. Cho K. Chronic 'jet lag' produces temporal lobe atrophy and spatial cognitive deficits. Nat Neruosci 2007; 4(6):567–568.

74. Lauria L, Ballard TJ, Caldora M, et al. Reproductive disorders and pregnancy outcomes among flight attendants. Aviat Space Environ Med 2006; 77(5):533–539.

75. Davidson AJ, Sellix MT, Daniel J, et al. Chronic jet-lag increases mortality in aged mice. Curr Biol 2006; 16(21):R914–R916.

76. Penev PD, Kolker DE, Zee PC, et al. Chronic circadian desynchronization decreases the survival of animals with cardiomyopathic heart disease. Am J Physiol Heart Circ Physiol 1998; 275(44): H2334–H2337.

77. Filipski E, Delaunay F, King VM, et al. Effects of chronic jet lag on tumor progression in mice. Cancer Res 2004; 64:7879–7885.

78. Filipski E, King VM, Li XM, et al. Disruption of circadian coordination accelerates malignant growth in mice. Pathol Biol 2003; 51:216–219.

79. Filipski E, Innominato PF, Wu M, et al. Effects of light and food schedules on liver and tumor molecular clocks in mice. J Natl Cancer Inst 2005; 97(7):507–517.

80. Katz G, Knobler HY, Laibel Z, et al. Time zone change and major psychiatric morbidity: the results of a 6-year study in Jerusalem. Compr Psychiatry 2002; 43(1):37–40.

81. Monk TH. Shift work: basic principles. In: Kryger MH, Roth T, Dement WC, eds. Principles and Practice of Sleep Medicine. 4th ed. Philadelphia: Elsevier Saunders, 2005:673–679.

82. Eastman CI, Boulos Z, Terman M, et al. Light treatment for sleep disorders: consensus report. VI. shiftwork. J Biol Rhythms 1995; 10(2):157–164.

83. Folkard S, Akerstedt T. Trends in the risk of accidents and injuries and their implications for models of fatigue and performance. Aviat Space Environ Med 2007; 75(suppl 3):A161–A167.

84. Akerstedt T. Shift work and disturbed sleep/wakefulness. Occup Med 2003; 53(2):89–94.

85. Ha M, Park J. Shiftwork and metabolic risk factors of cardiovascular disease. J Occup Health 2005; 47 (2):89–95.

86. Schernhammer ES, Kroenke CH, Laden F, et al. Night work and risk of breast cancer. Epidemiology 2006; 17(1):108–111.

87. Burch JB, Yost MG, Johnson W. Melatonin, sleep and shift work adaptation. J Occup Environ Med 2005; 47(9):893–901.

88. Schernhammer ES, Kroenke CH, Dowsett M, et al. Urinary 6-sulphatoxymelatonin levels and their correlations with lifestyle factors and steroid hormone levels. J Pineal Res 2006; 40(2):116–124.

89. Blask DE, Sauer LA, Dauchy RT, et al. New insights into melatonin regulation of cancer growth. In: Olcese J, ed. Melatonin After Four Decades: an Assessment of Its Potential. New York: Kluwer Academic/Plenum Publishers, 1999:337–343.

90. Fu L, Lee CC. The circadian clock: pacemaker and tumor suppressor. Nat Rev Cancer 2003; 3:350–361.

91. Matsuo T, Yamaguchi S, Mitsui S, et al. Control mechanism of the circadian clock for timing of cell division in vivo. Science 2003; 302:255–259.

92. Reddy AB, Wong GK, O'Neill J, et al. Circadian clocks: neural and peripheral pacemakers that impact upon the cell division cycle. Mutat Res 2005; 574(1–2):76–91.

93. Collis SJ, Boulton SJ. Emerging links between the biological clock and the DNA damage response. Chromosoma 2007; 116:331–339.
94. Albrecht U, Zheng B, Larkin D, et al. Mper1 and mper2 are essential for normal resetting of the circadian clock. J Biol Rhythms 2001; 16:100–104.
95. Lee CC. Tumor suppression by the mammalian period genes. Cancer Causes Control 2006; 17:525–530.
96. Harma M, Kandolin I. Shiftwork, age and well-being: recent developments and future perspectives. J Hum Ergol (Tokyo) 2001; 30(1–2):287–293.
97. Harma M. Ageing, physical fitness and shiftwork tolerance. Appl Ergon 1996; 27(1):25–29.
98. Harma M. Sleepiness and shiftwork: individual differences. J Sleep Res 1995; 4(S2):57–61.
99. Harma M, Ilmarinen J, Knauth P. Physical fitness and other individual factors relating to the shiftwork tolerance of women. Chronobiol Int 1988; 5:417.
100. Harma MI, Ilmarinen J, Knauth P, et al. Physical training intervention in female shift workers: II. The effects of intervention on the circadian rhythms of alertness, short-term memory, and body temperature. Ergonomics 1988; 31(1):51–63.
101. Tenkanen L, Sjoblom T, Harma M. Joint effect of shift work and adverse lifestyle factors on the risk of coronary heart disease. Scand J Work Environ Health 1998; 24(5):351–357.
102. Davis S, Mirick DK, Stevens RG. Night shift work, light at night, and risk of breast cancer 2001; 93(20):1557–1562.
103. Knutsson A, Boggild H. Shiftwork and cardiovascular disease: review of disease mechanisms. Rev Environ Health 2000; 15(4):359–372.
104. Costa G, Apostoli P, d'Andrea G, et al. Gastrointestinal and neurotic disorders in textile shift workers. In: Reinberg A, Vieux N, Andlauer P, eds. Night and Shift Work: Biological and Social Aspects. Oxford: Pergamon Press, 1981:215–221.
105. Karlsson B, Alfredsson L, Knutsson A, et al. Total mortality and cause-specific mortality of Swedish shift and dayworkers in the pulp and paper industry in 1952–2001. Scand J Work Environ Health 2007; 31(1):30–35.
106. Drake CL, Roehrs T, Richardson G, et al. Shift work sleep disorder: prevalence and consequences beyond that of symptomatic day workers. Sleep 2004; 27(8):1453–1462.
107. Wehr TA, Sack DA, Rosenthal NE. Sleep reduction as a final common pathway in the genesis of mania. Am J Psychiatry 1987; 144:201–204.

13 | Types of Circadian Rhythm Sleep Disorders

Helen J. Burgess

Biological Rhythms Research Laboratory, Department of Behavioral Sciences, Rush University Medical Center, Chicago, Illinois, U.S.A.

Kathryn J. Reid

Department of Neurology, Northwestern University Feinberg School of Medicine, Chicago, Illinois, U.S.A.

INTRODUCTION

There are six types of circadian rhythm sleep disorders described in the *International Classification of Sleep Disorders*, second edition (*ICSD-2*) (1): delayed sleep phase type, advanced sleep phase type, irregular sleep-wake type, free-running type, jet lag type, and shift work type. Details of the demographics; key symptoms and signs; onset, ontogeny, and clinical course; and risk factors for these six circadian rhythm sleep disorders will be discussed in this chapter. Circadian rhythm sleep disorders due to medical condition, as well as other circadian rhythm sleep disorders due to drug or substance use, are not covered in this chapter since they are due to extrinsic causes.

The general criteria for a circadian rhythm sleep disorder includes a persistent or recurrent pattern of sleep disturbance resulting from either an alteration to the circadian system or misalignment between the endogenous circadian clock and exogenous factors that influence the timing and duration of sleep. As a result of this sleep disturbance, individuals complain of insomnia and/or excessive daytime sleepiness that leads to impaired waking function (1).

DELAYED SLEEP PHASE TYPE

Demographics

The exact prevalence of delayed sleep phase type in the general population is not known. There are a few studies reporting prevalence in different populations. A single epidemiological study from Norway reported a prevalence of 0.17% (2). The prevalence in adolescents and young adults is considerably higher at approximately 7% (3). There is a tendency for circadian sleep-wake cycles to be delayed in adolescents and young adults and as such delayed sleep phase type is typically more commonly seen in this age group. In middle age the prevalence is considerably less at 0.7% (4). The prevalence in patients attending sleep clinics with a complaint of primary insomnia has been reported to be between 6.7% and 16% (5,6). There is no known gender or ethnic associations with delayed sleep phase type (2).

Key Symptoms and Signs

The *ICSD-2* outlines the following criteria for the diagnosis of delayed sleep phase type (1). It is characterized by a stable habitual delay in the sleep-wake schedule of two or more hours compared to the conventional sleep times. Individuals with delayed sleep phase type typically report difficulty falling asleep at a socially acceptable or desired time, but once they are asleep, sleep is usually normal for age. Attempts to fall asleep earlier are typically unsuccessful. They also report difficulty waking at a desired or conventional wake time. When social or work responsibilities require earlier than desired wake times, morning sleepiness is usually reported. Sleep logs or activity monitoring (i.e., actigraphy in conjunction with a sleep log) for at least seven days displays a stable delay of the sleep-wake period (Fig. 1). The sleep complaints should not be better explained by another current sleep, mental, neurological, and medical or substance use disorder.

Individuals with delayed sleep phase type may occasionally exhibit periods where their sleep-wake schedule is progressively delayed by an hour or so a day similar to that seen in free-running type (see section on free-running type below). In such cases, a longer (a month or

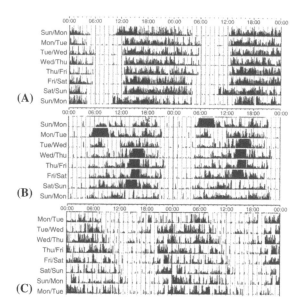

Figure 1 Examples of eight days of rest-activity cycles in patients with circadian rhythm sleep disorders recorded with wrist activity monitoring. Actograms are double plotted in clock hours. (**A**) Delayed sleep phase type has a sleep time of approximately 4 to 6 a.m. and a wake time of approximately 12 p.m. (**B**) Advanced sleep phase type has a sleep time of approximately 8 to 9 p.m. and a wake time of 4 to 5 a.m. (there is a short period on Tuesday between 9 a.m. and 12 p.m. in which the subject removed the activity monitor). (**C**) Free-running type has a rest-activity cycle that typically progressively delays each day with the rest period during the daytime.

more) assessment of sleep-wake cycles and detailed sleep-wake history may be required to differentiate between delayed sleep phase type and free-running type.

Onset, Ontogeny, and Clinical Course
The mean age of onset of delayed sleep phase type is 20 years of age (1–7). However, onset has been reported in early childhood too (8,9). Delayed sleep phase type is a chronic disorder that, if left untreated, may continue into old age; however, with increasing age there tends to be an advance in the timing of the sleep-wake cycle and, as such, the delay may be reduced. Self-medication with alcohol and hypnotics to induce sleep and stimulants to combat daytime sleepiness may lead to substance abuse. Treatment of this disorder can alleviate some symptoms but the underlying tendency and preference to be delayed typically remains; therefore, continual treatment is usually required. It is important to distinguish delayed sleep phase type from individuals who just have a delayed sleep-wake schedule ("night owls") but no impaired functioning.

Risk Factors
Behavioral factors may play a role in predisposing or precipitating delayed sleep phase type. However, delayed sleep phase type is a multifactorial condition due to a combination of lifestyle, mood, personality, and genetic factors (8). Due to the delayed sleep-wake episode, individuals with delayed sleep phase type may have a reduction in light exposure during the phase-advance portion of the light phase response curve (PRC) and/or exposure to bright light during the phase delay portion, which may result in maintaining or further delaying the sleep-wake episode. This phenomenon has been demonstrated in normal subjects (10). It has also been suggested that there may be an alteration to the light PRC, such that individuals with delayed sleep phase type may have a smaller advance region of the light PRC (11).

Genetics may also predispose some individuals to delayed sleep phase type. Polymorphisms in the following circadian rhythm genes have been identified in individuals with delayed sleep phase type: *CKIepsilon*, *hPer3*, arylalkylamine *N*-acetyltransferase, HLA genes, and *Clock* (12–18). There is also one reported case of familial delayed sleep phase type; however, this family has yet to be genetically characterized (19).

ADVANCED SLEEP PHASE TYPE

Demographics
The prevalence of advanced sleep phase type in the general population is unknown but believed to be rare (2). The prevalence in middle-aged adults has been reported to be approximately 1% (4). There is a tendency for circadian sleep-wake cycles to advance with age,

and as such, advanced sleep phase type is typically more commonly seen in the elderly. Several familial cases of advanced sleep phase type have been reported in affected individuals as young as 11 years of age (20–22). The reduction in the reported numbers of advanced sleep phase type is most likely due to the resulting degree of impairment. Unless the advanced sleep phase is extreme, it probably does not hinder daily functioning to the same degree as a delayed sleep phase because the advanced phase conforms more to societal schedules and norms. There is no known gender or ethnic associations with advanced sleep phase type.

Key Symptoms and Signs

The *ICSD-2* outlines the following criteria for a diagnosis of advanced sleep phase type (1). It is characterized by a stable advance in the habitual sleep-wake schedule of several hours compared to conventional sleep times. There is an inability to stay awake till the desired or conventional bedtime and an inability to remain asleep till desired or conventional wake times. Individuals with advanced sleep phase type report afternoon and early evening sleepiness and early morning awakening. When they are able to sleep at their preferred times, sleep is normal for age. Sleep logs or activity monitoring (i.e., actigraphy in conjunction with a sleep log) for at least seven days displays a stable advance of the sleep-wake period (Fig. 1). The sleep complaints cannot be better explained by another current sleep, mental, neurological, and medical or substance use disorder.

Onset, Ontogeny, and Clinical Course

The onset of advanced sleep phase type is typically in middle age (1), although it has been reported in children (20). Advanced sleep phase type is a chronic disorder that, if left untreated, may be lifelong. Self-medication with alcohol and hypnotics to induce sleep and stimulants to combat daytime sleepiness may lead to substance abuse. Treatment of this disorder can alleviate some symptoms but the underlying tendency and preference to be advanced typically remains; therefore, continual treatment is usually required. It is important to distinguish advanced sleep phase type from individuals who just have an advanced sleep-wake schedule ("early birds") but have no impaired functioning.

Risk Factors

Genetics may predispose some individuals to advanced sleep phase type. Several familial cases of the advanced sleep phase type have been reported (20–22). Polymorphisms in circadian rhythm genes (*hPer2* and *CKIdelta*) have been identified, which alter the phosphorylation of proteins within the molecular circadian clock system (21–23).

A shorter circadian period would also explain an advance in circadian phase and has been reported in one familial case of advanced sleep phase type (24). In addition, behavioral factors such as increased light exposure in the morning hours due to early morning awakening may exacerbate and perpetuate the advanced sleep phase. It has also been suggested that there may be an alteration in the light PRC, such that individuals with advanced sleep phase type may have a dominant phase-advance portion of the light PRC (25).

IRREGULAR SLEEP-WAKE TYPE

Demographics

There is less known about the demographics of irregular sleep-wake type but it is believed to be rare (7). Irregular sleep-wake type has been most commonly reported in association with neurological disorders such as dementia (26–28), following brain injury and in children with mental retardation (29). There are no known gender or ethnic associations with irregular sleep-wake type.

Key Symptoms and Signs

The *ICSD-2* outlines the following criteria for a diagnosis of irregular sleep-wake type (1). Irregular sleep-wake type is characterized by the lack of a circadian rhythm of sleep-wake activity. Individuals with irregular sleep-wake type complain of insomnia and/or excessive daytime sleepiness. Sleep logs or activity monitoring (i.e., actigraphy in conjunction with a sleep log) for at least 7 days displays at least three irregular sleep bouts in a 24-hour period.

Total sleep time during the 24-hour period should be normal for age. The sleep complaints cannot be better explained by another current sleep, mental, neurological, and medical or substance use disorder.

Onset, Ontogeny, and Clinical Course

The onset of irregular sleep-wake type can occur at any age. There is very limited information available about the clinical course of irregular sleep-wake type (1). If irregular sleep-wake type is the result of an endogenous dysfunction of the circadian clock, it is likely that, if untreated, the disorder will be lifelong.

Risk Factors

Irregular sleep-wake type is most commonly seen in individuals who have an alteration to the circadian clock due to brain injury or dementia or in those who have reduced exposure or ability to process circadian time cues because of dementia and mental retardation. Institutionalized elderly with dementia may be at particular risk for irregular sleep-wake disorder resulting from a reduction in exposure to circadian time cues such as light and activity (30–32). Several cases of irregular sleep-wake type have been reported in children with psychomotor retardation (29). It has been suggested that disruption of the melatonin rhythm due to irregular or reduced light/dark exposure may play a role in such cases (29). More recently, there have been single cases reporting that nighttime exposure to bright light (33) or prolactin-secreting pituitary microadenoma (34) resulted in the development of irregular sleep-wake type. An understanding of whether the sleep disturbance results from alterations to the endogenous circadian clock or altered exposure to time cues is important in the development of treatment strategies for patients with irregular sleep-wake type.

FREE-RUNNING TYPE

Demographics

Free-running type is most commonly seen in totally blind people with no conscious light perception (35–38), particularly in those who are enucleated (37–39); sometimes it can occur in sighted individuals (40–54). It is estimated that 18% to 40% of totally blind individuals experience chronic cyclical sleep disturbances suggestive of free running (36,37,55,56). In sighted individuals, free-running type may constitute 12% to 23% of circadian rhythm sleep disorder cases (57,58), and may be more commonly seen in men (57). There are no known ethnic associations.

Key Symptoms and Signs

The *ICSD-2* outlines the following criteria for a diagnosis of free-running type (1). First, there must be a complaint of insomnia or excessive sleepiness related to an abnormal synchronization between the 24-hour light/dark cycle and the endogenous circadian rhythm of sleep and wake propensity. Second, a week of completed sleep diaries either with or without actigraphy monitoring demonstrates a pattern of sleep and wake times that typically delay, or shift later in time each day with a period longer than 24 hours (Fig. 1). Third, the sleep disturbance is not better explained by another current sleep disorder, medical or neurological disorder, mental disorder, or drug or substance use disorder.

"Free running" refers to the phenomenon when the internal circadian clock oscillates at its own endogenous circadian period ("tau"), independent of the external environment. Most typically, a person's tau is greater than 24 hours, and thus the patient typically shows progressively later and later bedtimes and wake times, with a delay between 1 and 2 hr/day (35,40,52). When sleeping at appropriate circadian times, sleep and daytime function will be normal, but the individual will periodically sleep outside of conventional sleep times (45,59). When individuals with free-running type attempt to maintain conventional sleep and wake times within the 24-hour day, they can experience insomnia and daytime sleepiness as they cycle through periods of circadian misalignment (39,41,43,59,60). The increased daytime sleepiness can be expressed as an increased incidence of daytime naps (60). Patients will likely report negative repercussions in their social life (51,59) and in their employment if they are required to work fixed regular hours (41,55). A detailed sleep-wake history may be required to differentiate between delayed sleep phase type and free-running type.

Onset, Ontogeny, and Clinical Course

The onset of free-running type can occur at any age in blind individuals, and thus can be present in congenitally blind children at birth (35,36,61,62). Free-running type can be a lifelong condition in the blind unless treated. In sighted individuals, the majority of patients report that the onset of symptoms occurs during their teenage years (51). Alcohol, hypnotics, and stimulants are sometimes used by individuals with free-running type (whether sighted or blind) to combat the cyclical occurrence of excessive daytime sleepiness and insomnia (36,44,55,59), and thus substance abuse is possible.

In some cases of sighted individuals, free-running type is likely a severe form of delayed sleep phase type, where exposure to light prior to sleep causes the circadian clock to phase delay, leading to the progressive phase delays in the sleep-wake schedule characteristic of free-running type (44,46,48). Indeed this is likely the cause of nonentrainment in sighted individuals who spontaneously remit (41), or who are able to maintain stable sleep times after a series of fixed forced awakenings at conventional times (42) or after regular exposure to light (44,48,54,63,64).

Risk Factors

Totally blind individuals are most at risk for free-running type (35–38), especially those with both eyes enucleated, (37–39), as this completely prohibits the light/dark cycle from entraining the circadian clock to the 24-hour day. Sighted individuals are at increased risk for developing free-running type when they are isolated from an external light/dark cycle, such as during Antarctic winters, and do not maintain set sleep times (65).

Patients with delayed sleep phase type may be at greater risk for developing free-running type, if their exposure to evening light progressively occurs later in time (delays) in association with their sleep-wake schedule (44,51). Additionally, chronotherapy, a possible treatment for delayed sleep phase type, where sleep is timed three hours later each day (5), has led to some cases of delayed sleep phase type to develop into free-running type (45,66).

There is an increased incidence of psychiatric and personality disorders in free-running type, including depressive symptoms and mood disorders (45,51,52). In sighted individuals these can precede the development of free-running type (51); they may result from the social and occupational difficulties associated with free-running type (41,51), and may also exacerbate the condition by further reducing exposure to social time cues (41,45,51).

Occasionally, free-running type is associated with head injury (67), mental retardation (42), or dementia (68), perhaps due to neurological damage and/or a reduced ability to process 24-hour social cues that may otherwise help entrain the clock (69).

JET LAG TYPE

Demographics

In 2004, approximately 27.4 million U.S. residents jet traveled to overseas destinations (excluding commercial flight crew and military/government flights) (70). Of these, 66% crossed a significant number of time zones to reach Europe, Asia, Oceania, the Middle East, or Africa; the great majority of travelers visited only one country (81%). Almost all of the travelers were adults (93%) who had traveled overseas before (89%), having taken an average of 2.8 overseas trips in the past 12 months. On average they spent 16.2 nights outside the United States, and most were traveling for a vacation or to visit friends and/or relatives (71%). The majority of the travelers were male (57%) and, on average, 45 years old. Little is known about the ethnic and racial characteristics of these travelers, but due to the expense of international travel, it is not surprising that the average household income of these travelers was $110,100 (70).

Key Symptoms and Signs

The *ICSD-2* outlines the following criteria for a diagnosis of jet lag (1). First, there must be a complaint of insomnia or excessive daytime sleepiness associated with transmeridian jet travel across at least two time zones. Second, there is an additional associated impairment of daytime function, general malaise, or somatic symptoms such as gastrointestinal disturbance within one to two days of travel. Third, the sleep disturbance is not better explained by another current sleep disorder, medical or neurological disorder, mental disorder, or medication or substance use disorder.

Survey data collected from over 500 business people illustrate the relative prevalence of the different symptoms associated with jet lag (71). The primary complaint of jet travelers was disturbed sleep (78%), followed by daytime fatigue (49%), decreased mental performance (26%), gastrointestinal problems (24%), and increased irritability (18%). Disruption of menstrual cycles is also relatively common in female travelers, especially frequent travelers such as flight attendants (72).

Onset, Ontogeny, and Clinical Course

Theoretically, jet lag will occur in any entrained individual who via jet travel finds himself or herself in a distinctly altered time zone. Thus, jet lag could conceivably begin in the first few months after birth, which is when humans are typically first entrained by the light/dark cycle to the 24-hour day (73).

Jet lag will usually be felt in the first day or two after travel. If substantial sleep deprivation has occurred during travel resulting in significant sleep pressure, then the first night of sleep in the new time zone may not be greatly disturbed. However, subsequent sleep episodes are likely to be disturbed by the circadian misalignment. Flying east usually results in difficulty initiating sleep, whereas flying west results in early morning awakenings (74). Daytime alertness and function will be immediately impaired, even if sleep and/or alertness are enhanced by pharmacological means, due to the underlying circadian misalignment (75).

Jet lag is a temporary condition, and typically, the symptoms subside as there is an increase in the number of days in the new time zone. A rough estimate is one day of jet lag for every hour of difference between the home and destination time zone (1), although this will vary depending on the light exposure received on arrival, which determines the direction in which the circadian clock shifts (76). Eastward jet travel typically results in worse jet lag than westward jet travel (71) because the circadian phase advances required for eastward travel are slower than the circadian phase delays required for westward travel (77–79). Eastward travel can also increase the chances of receiving light at an inappropriate time, causing the circadian clock to shift in the opposite direction to the desired sleep time ("antidromic reentrainment"), thereby further exacerbating the circadian misalignment that causes jet lag (76). Occasionally the sleep disturbance due to jet lag will precipitate the development of a psychophysiological insomnia (1,80), in which case the "jet lag" can continue beyond 2 weeks. In such cases, referral to a sleep specialist is warranted (80,81).

Risk Factors

As we age we are at greater risk for jet lag because while circadian clocks in older people can adjust as quickly as in younger people (82,83), tolerance to the circadian misalignment resulting from jet travel is reduced with increasing age, resulting in more lost sleep and worse daytime functioning (84,85). Thus, as we age we may experience worse jet lag and for a longer period of time.

Circadian theory suggests that an individual traveler's circadian phase may affect their jet lag. Morning types (early birds) typically have earlier circadian phases (86), and thus are likely to find traveling east a little easier because the resulting circadian misalignment may be less than when they travel west. Conversely, evening types (night owls) who have later circadian phases (86) may find traveling west a little easier.

A history of short sleep episodes could theoretically worsen jet lag, as experimental studies in humans have shown that two weeks of short six-hour sleep episodes significantly reduces the response of the circadian clock to light (87,88). This reduction in the response of the circadian clock to light could be due to significant sleep deprivation, although to date this has only been found in nonhuman animal studies (89,90).

Greater experience with jet travel per se is not associated with a lower likelihood or reduced severity of jet lag (91), as jet lag is a normal physiological response to a rapidly shifted time zone. Frequent fliers such as flight attendants can jet travel so frequently that their circadian clocks do not have enough time to adjust to the new time zone (92), resulting in chronic jet lag. Chronic jet lag has been associated with cognitive deficits (93). Flight attendants are also at increased risk for cancer, however, further work is required to determine the relative contributions of increased exposure to circadian misalignment and ionizing radiation to this increased risk (94).

SHIFT WORK TYPE

Demographics
The most recent data on the prevalence of shift work in the United States comes from a survey conducted by the Bureau of Labor Statistics (95). The results from this survey suggest that in 2004 approximately 15% of full-time American workers were employed in jobs that required them to work nonstandard hours: 4.7% worked evening shifts, 3.2% worked night shifts, 3.1% worked irregular schedules, 2.5% worked rotating shifts, and 1.2% worked split shifts or "other" shifts (95). Morning shifts were not considered shift work in this survey because work between 6 a.m. and 6 p.m. was considered a "daytime schedule." The age distribution of the surveyed shift workers was as follows: 42% were 16 to 34 years old, 47% were 35 to 54 years old, and 11% were 55 years or older. Men were more likely to work an alternative shift (17% of male full-time workers) than women (12% of female full-time workers). Blacks or African-Americans were more likely than Whites, Latinos, or Asians to work alternative shifts. The majority of shift workers (55%) reported working alternative hours because it was "the nature of the job" (95).

Sleep disturbance and sleepiness are normal physiological responses to shift work. However, it is estimated that 1% to 5% of the population, or up to a third of all shift workers suffer symptoms significant enough to meet the criteria for shift work "disorder," as defined below (1,96).

Key Symptoms and Signs
The *ICSD-2* outlines the following criteria for a diagnosis of shift work disorder (1). First, there must be a complaint of insomnia or excessive sleepiness that is temporally associated with a recurring work schedule that occurs during the usual sleep period. Second, the symptoms are associated with the shift work schedule for at least one month. Third, a week of completed sleep diaries either with or without actigraphy monitoring demonstrates circadian and sleep misalignment. Fourth, the sleep disturbance is not better explained by another current sleep disorder, medical or neurological disorder, mental disorder, or medication or substance use disorder.

The insomnia and excessive sleepiness described above often lead to shift workers experiencing reduced alertness, impaired mental performance, worsening mood, increased accidents, and absenteeism (96). This in turn can raise safety concerns, particularly in workers whose mistakes can have significant public health and safety consequences, such as nuclear power plant operators, health care workers, and train and truck drivers (97).

Onset, Ontogeny, and Clinical Course
The negative symptoms associated with shift work will likely begin shortly after the onset of shift work and, in most cases, will resolve once the shift work schedule ends (1). The sleep disturbance due to shift work could precipitate the development of a psychophysiological insomnia (1) and thus continue well beyond the shift work schedule.

In general, shift workers are at greater risk for gastrointestinal, cardiovascular and reproductive disturbance, and cancer (98). There are likely several contributing factors to this increased risk, including the psychosocial stress of shift work (1,96,99), the type and timing of food intake (100), circadian misalignment (101), potentially suppressed melatonin in those workers exposed to light at night (102), and the physiological effects of the sleep loss associated with shift work that include negative alterations in insulin sensitivity, glucose tolerance, thyrotropin concentrations (103), and suppressed immune activity (104). Shift workers are also at greater risk of sleepiness-related car accidents (96). Drug and alcohol dependence may also result from attempts to improve sleep quality and quantity (1).

Risk Factors

The type of shift is a significant determinant of shift work disorder. Shift work that contains night shifts and/or early morning shifts are most likely to cause shift work disorder (1) because these work schedules produce the most circadian misalignment. Night shift workers typically struggle to stay awake at night and sleep poorly during the day. Self-reported average sleep length per day for permanent night workers is only 6.6 hours, but this decreases to 5.9 hours if the night shifts occur during rotating shift work (105). Early morning shift workers often have difficulty initiating sleep earlier in the evening and waking in the early morning. Morning shifts as part of a rotating schedule reduce sleep to only 6.6 hours (105). Rapid rotating shifts (≤4 days on each shift) reduce average sleep lengths to 6.5 hours (105). Notably, even this short sleep period in many shift workers is likely to be disturbed (1). By contrast, slowly rotating shift workers (>4 days on each shift) report obtaining 6.9 hours of sleep and permanent evening shift workers report obtaining 7.6 hours (105) more sleep than the average daytime worker (7.4 hours) (106).

A shift worker's morningness–eveningness propensity and age can also affect their adjustment to shift work. Morning types (early birds) typically have earlier circadian phases (86), and thus may not find great difficulty working early morning shifts, but struggle to work the night shift. Conversely, evening types (night owls) who have later circadian phases (86) may find it easier to work at night but are likely to have great difficulty working early morning shifts. As people age they tend to sleep and wake at earlier times (107), in part because of an earlier circadian phase (84), thereby reducing their suitability for night shifts. Older individuals also have a reduced tolerance to circadian misalignment, and thus shift work in these individuals can result in worse sleep and daytime functioning (84,85). Thus, some shift workers who had previously coped well can find themselves struggling to cope with shift work as they get older, particularly after the age of 50 years (99). Naturally long sleepers could be at greater risk of shift work disorder, as they will likely lose more sleep than naturally short sleepers, potentially leading to greater impairment than naturally short sleepers.

The geographical location of the workplace and season can also affect adjustment to shift work. Problems with shift work are often reduced when workers are not exposed to bright outdoor light, which contributes to the circadian misalignment, which underlies the insomnia and sleepiness often associated with shift work. For example, night workers in extreme northern (North Sea offshore oilrigs) or extreme southern locations (Antarctic stations), are often not exposed to bright outdoor light, particularly in winter, and consequently do not show the circadian misalignment typical of most night workers (108,109). Similarly, some night workers who commute home in winter before sunrise can show some circadian adjustment to night work (110–112).

CONCLUSIONS

Circadian rhythm sleep disorders result from either a disturbance to the circadian system or misalignment between the internal body clock and external factors that affect sleep timing and duration.

Genetics may play a role in the delayed and advanced sleep phase types, and irregular sleep-wake disorder has been associated with neurological diseases. The free-running disorder is most commonly seen in those who are totally blind, has an association with psychiatric and personality disorders, and may be a lifelong condition unless treated. Jet lag is affected by direction of travel, age, and circadian phase; however, more frequent travel is not associated with a less frequent or reduced severity of the condition. Lastly, shift work disorder may affect as many as a third of all shift workers, and a given individual's adjustment to shift work is influenced by the type of shift, morningness-eveningness tendency, age, geographical location, and season.

ACKNOWLEDGMENTS

This work was supported by Grants HL69988, HL072408, and NR07677 from the National Institutes of Health and Grant OH003954, from the Centers for Disease Control and Prevention.

REFERENCES

1. Sateia M, ed. International Classification of Sleep Disorders: Diagnostic and Coding Manual. 2nd ed. Westchester, IL: American Academy of Sleep Medicine, 2005.
2. Schrader H, Bovim G, Sand T. The prevalence of delayed and advanced sleep phase syndromes. J Sleep Res 1993; 2:51–55.
3. Pelayo RP, Thorpy MJ, Glovinsky P. Prevalence of delayed sleep phase syndrome among adolescents. Sleep Res 1988; 17:391.
4. Ando K, Kripke DF, Ancoli-Israel S. Estimated prevalence of delayed and advanced sleep phase syndromes. Sleep Res 1995; 24:509.
5. Czeisler CA, Richardson GS, Coleman RM, et al. Chronotherapy: resetting the circadian clocks of patients with delayed sleep phase insomnia. Sleep 1981; 4(1):1–21.
6. Regestein QR, Monk TH. Delayed sleep phase syndrome: a review of its clinical aspects. Am J Psychiatry 1995; 152:602–608.
7. Yamadera H, Takahashi K, Okawa M. A multicenter study of sleep-wake rhythm disorders: clinical feature of sleep-wake rhythm disorders. Psychiatry Clin Neurosci 1996; 50:195–201.
8. Alvarez B, Dahlitz MJ, Vignau J, et al. The delayed sleep phase syndrome: clinical and investigative findings in 14 subjects. J Neurol Neurosurg Psychiatry 1992; 55:665–670.
9. Garcia J, Rosen G, Mahowald M. Circadian rhythms and circadian rhythm disorders in children and adolescents. Semin Pediatr Neurol 2001; 8(4):229–240.
10. Burgess HJ, Eastman CI. A late wake time phase delays the human dim light melatonin rhythm. Neurosci Lett 2006; 395:191–195.
11. Weitzman ED, Czeisler CA, Coleman RM, et al. Delayed sleep phase syndrome. Arch Gen Psychiatry 1981; 38(7):737–746.
12. Takahashi Y, Hohjjoh H, Matsuura K. Predisposing factors in delayed sleep phase syndrome. Psychiatry Clin Neurosci 2000; 54:356–358.
13. Archer SN, Robilliard DL, Skene DJ, et al. A length polymorphism in the circadian clock gene per3 is linked to delayed sleep phase syndrome and extreme diurnal preference. Sleep 2003; 26:413–415.
14. Iwase T, Kajimura N, Uchiyama M, et al. Mutation screening of the human Clock gene in circadian rhythm sleep disorders. Psychiatry Res 2002; 109:121–128.
15. Hohjoh H, Takasu M, Shishikura K, et al. Significant association of the arylalkylamine N-acetyltransferase (AA-NAT) gene with delayed sleep phase syndrome. Neurogenetics 2003; 4:151–153.
16. Ebisawa T, Uchiyama M, Kajimura N, et al. Association of structural polymorphisms in the human period3 gene with delayed sleep phase syndrome. EMBO Rep 2001; 2:342–346.
17. Takano A, Uchiyama M, Kajimura N, et al. A missense variation in human casein kinase I epsilon gene that induces functional alteration and shows an inverse association with circadian rhythm sleep disorders. Neuropsychopharmacology 2004; 29(10):1901–1909.
18. Pereira DS, Tufik S, Louzada FM, et al. Association of the length polymorphism in the human Per3 gene with the delayed sleep-phase syndrome: does latitude have an influence upon it? Sleep 2005; 28:29–32.
19. Ancoli-Israel S, Schnierow B, Kelsoe J, et al. A pedigree of one family with delayed sleep phase syndrome. Chronobiol Int 2001; 18:831–840.
20. Reid KJ, Chang AM, Dubocovich ML, et al. Familial advanced sleep phase syndrome. Arch Neurol 2001; 58:1089–1094.
21. Toh KL, Jones CR, He Y, et al. An hper2 phosphorylation site mutation in familial advanced sleep phase syndrome. Science 2001; 291:1040–1043.
22. Satoh K, Mishima K, Inoue Y, et al. Two pedigrees of familial advanced sleep phase syndrome in Japan. Sleep 2003; 26:416–417.
23. Xu Y, Padiath QS, Shapiro RE, et al. Functional consequences of a CKIdelta mutation causing familial advanced sleep phase syndrome. Nature 2005; 434:640–644.
24. Jones CR, Campbell SS, Zone SE, et al. Familial advanced sleep-phase syndrome: a short-period circadian rhythm variant in humans. Nat Med 1999; 5:1062–1065.
25. Reid KJ, Zee PC. Circadian disorders of the sleep-wake cycle. In: Kryger MH, Roth T, Dement WC, eds. Principles and Practice of Sleep Medicine. Philadelphia: Elsevier, 2005:691–701.
26. Hoogendijk WJ, van Someren EJ, Mirmiran M, et al. Circadian rhythm-related behavioral disturbances and structural hypothalamic changes in Alzheimer's disease. Int Psychogeriatr 1996; 8:245–252.
27. Witting W, Kwa IH, Eikelenboom P, et al. Alterations in the circadian rest-activity rhythm in aging and Alzheimer's disease. Biol Psychiatry 1990; 27(6):563–572.
28. Okawa M, Mishima K, Hishikawa Y, et al. Circadian rhythm disorders in sleep-waking and body temperature in elderly patients with dementia and their treatment. Sleep 1991; 14(6):478–485.
29. Pillar G, Shahar E, Peled N, et al. Melatonin improves sleep-wake patterns in psychomotor retarded children. Pediatr Neurol 2000; 23:225–228.

30. van Someren EJ, Hagebeuk EE, Lijzenga C, et al. Circadian rest-activity rhythm disturbances in Alzheimer's disease. Biol Psychiatry 1996; 40(4):259–270.
31. Pollak CP, Stokes PE. Circadian rest-activity rhythms in demented and nondemented older community residents and their caregivers. J Am Geriatr Soc 1997; 45(4):446–452.
32. Ancoli-Israel S, Klauber MR, Jones DW, et al. Variations in circadian rhythms of activity, sleep, and light exposure related to dementia in nursing-home patients. Sleep 1997; 20:18–23.
33. Doljansky JT, Kannety H, Dagan Y. Working under daylight intensity lamp: an occupational risk for developing circadian rhythm sleep disorder? Chronobiol Int 2005; 22:597–605.
34. Borodkin K, Ayalon L, Kanety H, et al. Dysregulation of circadian rhythms following prolactin-secreting pituitary microadenoma. Chronobiol Int 2005; 22(1):145–156.
35. Okawa M, Nanami T, Wada S, et al. Four congenitally blind children with circadian sleep-wake rhythm disorder. Sleep 1987; 10(2):101–110.
36. Leger D, Guilleminault C, Defrance R, et al. Prevalence of sleep/wake disorders in persons with blindness. Clin Sci 1999; 97:193–199.
37. Sack RL, Lewy AJ, Blood ML, et al. Circadian rhythm abnormalities in totally blind people: incidence and clinical significance. J Clin Endocrinol Metab 1992; 75:127–134.
38. Lockley SW, Skene DJ, Arendt J, et al. Relationship between melatonin rhythms and visual loss in the blind. J Clin Endocrinol Metab 1997; 82:3763–3770.
39. Czeisler CA, Shanahan TL, Klerman EB, et al. Suppression of melatonin secretion in some blind patients by exposure to bright light. N Engl J Med 1995; 332:6–11.
40. Elliott AL, Mills JN, Waterhouse JM. A man with too long a day. J Physiol 1971; 212:30–31.
41. Kokkoris CP, Weitzman ED, Pollak CP, et al. Long-term ambulatory temperature monitoring in a subject with a hypernychthemeral sleep-wake cycle disturbance. Sleep 1978; 1(2):177–190.
42. Okawa M, Nakajima S, Sasaki H, et al. A case with free-running of the sleep-waking rhythm and successful non-drug treatment by forced awakening. Sleep Res 1980; 9:215.
43. Weber AL, Cary MS, Connor N, et al. Human non-24-hour sleep-wake cycles in an everyday environment. Sleep 1980; 2(3):347–354.
44. Kamgar-Parsi B, Wehr TA, Gillin JC. Successful treatment of human non-24-hour sleep-wake syndrome. Sleep 1983; 6(3):257–264.
45. McArthur AJ, Lewy AJ, Sack RL. Non-24-hour sleep-wake syndrome in a sighted man: circadian rhythm studies and efficacy of melatonin treatment. Sleep 1996; 19:544–553.
46. Uchiyama M, Okawa M, Ozaki S, et al. Delayed phase jumps of sleep onset in a patient with non-24-hour sleep-wake syndrome. Sleep 1996; 19:637–640.
47. Eastman CI, Anagnopoulos CA, Cartwright RD. Can bright light entrain a free-runner? Sleep Res 1988; 17:372.
48. Hoban TM, Sack RL, Lewy AJ, et al. Entrainment of a free-running human with bright light? Chronobiol Int 1989; 6(4):347–353.
49. Tomoda A, Miike T, Uezono K, et al. A school refusal case with biological rhythm disturbance and melatonin therapy. Brain Dev 1994; 16:71–76.
50. Zallek SN. A teenager with insomnia and fatigue; habit or hard wiring? J Clin Sleep Med 2006; 2:92–93.
51. Hayakawa T, Uchiyama M, Kamei Y, et al. Clinical analyses of sighted patients with non-24-hour sleep-wake syndrome: a study of 57 consecutively diagnosed cases. Sleep 2005; 28:945–952.
52. Dagan Y, Ayalon L. Case study: psychiatric misdiagnosis of non-24-hours sleep-wake schedule disorder resolved by melatonin. J Am Acad Child Adolesc Psychiatry 2005; 44:1271–1275.
53. Akaboshi S, Inoue Y, Kubota N, et al. Case of a mentally retarded child with non-24 hour sleep-wake syndrome caused by deficiency of melatonin secretion. Psychiatry Clin Neurosci 2000; 54(3):379–380.
54. Sugita Y, Ishikawa H, Mikami A, et al. Successful treatment for a patient with hypernychthemeral syndrome. Sleep Res 1987; 16:642.
55. Miles LE, Wilson MA. High incidence of cyclic sleep/wake disorders in the blind. Sleep Res 1977; 6:192.
56. Martens H, Endlich H, Hildebrandt G, et al. Sleep/wake distribution in blind subjects with and without sleep complaints. Sleep Res 1990; 19:398.
57. Kamei Y, Urata J, Uchiyaya M, et al. Clinical characteristics of circadian rhythm sleep disorders. Psychiatry Clin Neurosci 1998; 52:234–235.
58. Dagan Y, Eisenstein M. Circadian rhythm sleep disorders: toward a more precise definition and diagnosis. Chronobiol Int 1999; 16:213–222.
59. Miles LEM, Raynal DM, Wilson MA. Blind man living in normal society has circadian rhythms of 24.9 hours. Science 1977; 198:421–423.
60. Lockley SW, Skene DJ, Butler LJ, et al. Sleep and activity rhythms are related to circadian phase in the blind. Sleep 1999; 22:616–623.
61. Martens H, Endlich H, Hildebrandt G, et al. Sleep/wake distribution in blind subjects with and without sleep complaints. Sleep Res 1990; 19:398.

62. Lapierre O, Dumont M. Melatonin treatment of a non-24-hour sleep-wake cycle in a blind retarded child. Biol Psychiatry 1995; 38:119–122.

63. Shibui K, Uchiyama M, Iwama H, et al. Periodic fatigue symptoms due to desynchronization in a patient with non-24-h sleep-wake syndrome. Psychiatry Clin Neurosci 1998; 52:477–481.

64. Watanabe T, Kajimura N, Kato M, et al. Case of a non-24 h sleep-wake syndrome patient improved by phototherapy. Psychiatry Clin Neurosci 2000; 54:369–370.

65. Kennaway DJ, Van Dorp CF. Free-running rhythms of melatonin, cortisol, electrolytes, and sleep in humans in Antarctica. Am J Physiol 1991; 260:R1137–R1144.

66. Oren DA, Wehr TA. Hypernyctohemeral syndrome after chronotherapy for delayed sleep phase syndrome. N Engl J Med 1992; 327:1762.

67. Boivin DB, James FO, Santo JB, et al. Non-24-hour sleep-wake syndrome following a car accident. Neurology 2003; 60:1841–1843.

68. Mikami A, Sugita Y, Teshima Y, et al. A 48-hour sleep-wake cycle in a patient with Parkinsonism. Sleep 1987; 10:625.

69. Palm L, Blennow G, Wetterberg L. Correction of non-24-hour sleep/wake cycle by melatonin in a blind retarded boy. Ann Neurol 1991; 29:336–339.

70. U.S. Department of Commerce, Office of Travel and Tourism Industries. 2004 profile of U.S. resident traveler visiting overseas destinations reported from: survey of international air travelers. Available at: www.tinet.ita.doc.gov/view/f-2004-101-001/index.html, 2005.

71. Leger D, Badet D, de La Giclais B. The prevalence of jet-lag among 507 traveling businessmen. Sleep Res 1993; 22:409.

72. Iglesias R, Terres A, Chavarria A. Disorders of the menstrual cycle in airline stewardesses. Aviat Space Environ Med 1980; 51:518–520.

73. Rivkees SA. Emergence and influences of circadian rhythmicity in infants. Clin Perinatol 2004; 31 (2):217–228.

74. Boulos Z, Campbell SS, Lewy AJ, et al. Light treatment for sleep disorders: consensus report. VII. Jet lag. J Biol Rhythms 1995; 10:167–176.

75. Walsh JK, Muehlbach MJ, Schweitzer PK. Hypnotics and caffeine as countermeasures for shiftwork-related sleepiness and sleep disturbance. J Sleep Res 1995; 4:80–83.

76. Burgess HJ, Crowley SJ, Gazda CJ, et al. Preflight adjustment to eastward travel: 3 days of advancing sleep with and without morning bright light. J Biol Rhythms 2003; 18:318–328.

77. Aschoff J, Hoffmann K, Pohl H, et al. Re-entrainment of circadian rhythms after phase shifts of the zeitgeber. Chronobiologia 1975; 2:23–78.

78. Eastman CI, Martin SK. How to use light and dark to produce circadian adaptation to night shift work. Ann Med 1999; 31:87–98.

79. Shanahan TL, Kronauer RE, Duffy JF, et al. Melatonin rhythm observed throughout a three-cycle bright-light stimulus designed to reset the human circadian pacemaker. J Biol Rhythms 1999; 14:237–253.

80. Reid KJ, Burgess HJ. Circadian rhythm sleep disorders. Prim Care 2005; 32:449–473.

81. Burgess HJ, Eastman CI. Prevention of jet lag. Physicians' Information and Education Resource (PIER). American College of Physicians. Available at: http://Pier.acponline.org, 2003.

82. Campbell SS. Effects of timed bright-light exposure on shift-work adaptation in middle-aged subjects. Sleep 1995; 18:408–416.

83. Benloucif S, Green K, L'hermite-Baleriaux M, et al. Responsiveness of the aging circadian clock to light. Neurobiol Aging 2006; 27:1870–1879.

84. Moline ML, Pollak CP, Monk TH, et al. Age-related differences in recovery from simulated jet lag. Sleep 1992; 15:28–40.

85. Dijk DJ, Duffy JF, Riel E, et al. Ageing and the circadian and homeostatic regulation of human sleep during forced desynchrony of rest, melatonin and temperature rhythms. J Physiol 1999; 516.2:611–627.

86. Baehr EK, Revelle W, Eastman CI. Individual differences in the phase and amplitude of the human circadian temperature rhythm: with an emphasis on morningness-eveningness. J Sleep Res 2000; 9:117–127.

87. Burgess HJ, Eastman CI. Short nights attenuate light-induced circadian phase advances in humans. J Clin Endocrinol Metab 2005; 90:4437–4440.

88. Burgess HJ, Eastman CI. Short nights reduce light-induced circadian phase delays in humans. Sleep 2006; 29(1):25–30.

89. Mistlberger RE, Landry GL, Marchant EG. Sleep deprivation can attenuate light-induced phase shifts of circadian rhythms in hamsters. Neurosci Lett 1997; 238:5–8.

90. Challet E, Turek FW, Laute M, et al. Sleep deprivation decreases phase-shift responses of circadian rhythms to light in the mouse: role of serotonergic and metabolic signals. Brain Res 2001; 909:81–91.

91. Flower DJ, Irvine D, Folkard S. Perception and predictability of travel fatigue after long-haul flights: a retrospective study. Aviat Space Environ Med 2003; 74:173–179.

92. Harma M, Laitinen J, Partinen M, et al. The effect of four-day round trip flights over 10 time zones on the circadian variation of salivary melatonin and cortisol in airline flight attendants. Ergonomics 1993; 37:1479–1489.

93. Cho K. Chronic 'jet lag' produces temporal lobe atrophy and spatial cognitive deficits. Nat Neurosci 2001; 4:567–568.

94. Buja A, Mastrangelo G, Perissinotto E, et al. Cancer incidence among female flight attendants: a meta-analysis of published data. J Womens Health (Larchmt) 2006; 15(1):98–105.

95. Beers TM. Workers on flexible and shift schedules in May 2004. United States Department of Labor, Bureau of Labor Statistics, July 1, 2005:1–14. Available at: http://www.bls.gov/news.release/flex.toc.htm. Retrieved January 19, 2006.

96. Drake CL, Roehrs T, Richardson G, et al. Shift work sleep disorder: prevalence and consequences beyond that of symptomatic day workers. Sleep 2004; 27:1453–1462.

97. Rosekind MR. Managing work schedules: an alertness and safety perspective, In: Kryger MH, Roth T, Dement WC, eds. Principles and Practice of Sleep Medicine. Philadelphia: Elsevier, 2005:680–690.

98. Knutsson A. Health disorders of shift workers. Occup Med 2003; 53:103–108.

99. Monk TH. Shift work: basic principles. In: Kryger MH, Roth T, Dement WC, eds. Principles and Practice of Sleep Medicine. Philadelphia: Elsevier, 2005:673–679.

100. Ribeiro DC, Hampton SM, Morgan L, et al. Altered postprandial hormone and metabolic responses in a simulated shift work environment. J Endocrinol 1998; 158:305–310.

101. Penev PD, Kolker DE, Zee PC, et al. Chronic circadian desynchronization decreases the survival of animals with cardiomyopathic heart disease. Am J Physiol 1998; 275:H2334–H2337.

102. Schernhammer ES, Schulmeister K. Melatonin and cancer risk: does light at night compromise physiologic cancer protection by lowering serum melatonin levels? Br J Cancer 2004; 90:941–943.

103. Spiegel K, Leproult R, Van Cauter E. Impact of sleep debt on metabolic and endocrine function. Lancet 1999; 354:1435–1439.

104. Spiegel K, Sheridan JF, Van Cauter E. Effect of sleep deprivation on response to immunization. JAMA 2002; 288:1471–1472.

105. Pilcher JJ, Lambert BJ, Huffcutt AI. Differential effects of permanent and rotating shifts on self-report sleep length: a meta-analytic review. Sleep 2000; 23:155–163.

106. National Sleep Foundation. Less fun, less sleep, more work an American portrait. A National Sleep Foundation Poll. Available at: www.sleepfoundation.org, 2001.

107. National Sleep Foundation. 2003 Sleep in America poll. A National Sleep Foundation Poll. Available at: www.sleepfoundation.org.

108. Barnes RG, Deacon SJ, Forbes MJ, et al. Adaptation of the 6-sulphatoxymelatonin rhythm in shiftworkers on offshore oil installations during a 2-week 12-h night shift. Neurosci Lett 1998; 241:9–12.

109. Midwinter MJ, Arendt J. Adaptation of the melatonin rhythm in human subjects following night-shift work in Antarctica. Neurosci Lett 1991; 122:195–198.

110. Dumont M, Benhaberou-Brun D, Paquet J. Profile of 24-h light exposure and circadian phase of melatonin secretion in night workers. J Biol Rhythms 2001; 16:502–511.

111. Weibel L, Spiegel K, Gronfier C, et al. Twenty-four-hour melatonin and core body temperature rhythms: their adaptation in night workers. Am J Physiol 1997; 272:R948–R954.

112. Sack RL, Blood ML, Lewy AJ. Melatonin rhythms in night shift workers. Sleep 1992; 15:434–441.

14 | Diagnostic Tools for Circadian Rhythm Sleep Disorders

Kenneth P. Wright, Jr.

Sleep and Chronobiology Laboratory, Department of Integrative Physiology, University of Colorado, Boulder, Colorado, U.S.A.

Christopher L. Drake

Henry Ford Hospital, Sleep Disorders and Research Center, Department of Psychiatry and Behavioral Neurosciences, Wayne State College of Medicine, Detroit, Michigan, U.S.A.

Steven W. Lockley

Circadian Physiology Program, Division of Sleep Medicine, Brigham and Women's Hospital, Harvard Medical School, Boston, Massachusetts, U.S.A.

INTRODUCTION

Disorders of the circadian timekeeping system are a specialized class of sleep disorders generally characterized by inappropriate phase relationships between internal biological time and the light-dark or desired wakefulness-sleep cycle. Both sleep disruption and reduced ability to sustain wakefulness can result from these inappropriate phase relationships. These disorders are caused by both biological (e.g., changes in circadian and sleep neurobiology) and environmental (e.g., light exposure) factors (see American Academy of Sleep Medicine Task Force reviews) (1,2). This chapter will discuss the tools used to help diagnose circadian rhythm sleep disorders (CRSDs). The general use of diagnostic tools for CRSDs is discussed followed by their application to each specific CRSD disorder.

The clinical utility of sleep and circadian diagnostic tools depends on the ability of the tools to provide reliable and accurate information regarding the status of the sleep-wake and circadian systems. Acceptable, practical and cost-effective tools are required to assist the clinician in assessing and tracking circadian phase and sleep. The recognition of these methods as essential diagnostic tools of sleep medicine by practitioners and insurance providers is important for ensuring accurate diagnosis and effective treatment. Recommended use of diagnostic tools outlined in this chapter is based on evidence from the scientific literature.

HISTORY AND PHYSICAL EXAMINATION

A detailed medical and sleep history as well as physical examination should be included in the evaluation and diagnosis of CRSDs. A sleep history should include questions about the patient's sleep patterns (e.g., duration, timing, and quality), signs, and symptoms of primary sleep disorders including snoring, excessive sleepiness, medical comorbidities and related safety and performance concerns (e.g., drowsy driving, falling asleep at work or in school). This history should be used to determine whether a patient's sleep and/or sleepiness problem may be the result of a primary sleep disorder or is associated with a medical or psychiatric disorder. Use of drugs (prescription or non-prescription), caffeine, nicotine, and alcohol should be assessed. CRSDs can have negative family and social consequences, since sleep often occurs at non-standard times and thus queries should be made regarding these issues.

It is also helpful to determine whether the presenting symptoms existed prior to changes in sleep-wake scheduling (e.g., before shift work began), as major schedule changes can exacerbate an already existing condition. Finally, it is important to distinguish general fatigue from excessive sleepiness due to circadian rhythm disruption as these represent different constructs and require different treatment approaches. Sleepiness caused by CRSDs should exhibit a particular pattern, related to the phase of the circadian system, whereas general fatigue may not. The differentiation of these symptoms is complicated by the fact that patients with excessive sleepiness typically present with complaints of fatigue rather than "sleepiness." When differentiating these underlying problems, it is helpful to understand that sleepiness is exacerbated or "unmasked" by sedentary activity (e.g., watching TV, reading) while fatigue may improve following rest.

Non-Entrained Type (Non-24-Hour Sleep-Wake Syndrome, Free-Running Type)

Individuals with non-entrained or free-running CRSDs complain of periodic sleep-wake problems characterized by alternating episodes of good sleep followed by episodes of poor nighttime sleep and excessive daytime sleepiness as the desired sleep pattern cycles in and out of synchrony with the internal non-24-hour body clock phase (Fig. 1B vs. A). Each episode can last for up to several months and during a bad sleep phase, may be misdiagnosed as chronic insomnia and/or excessive sleepiness. Longitudinal assessment of the cyclical nature of the sleep disorder is therefore key, along with the observation that the sleep disorder remits spontaneously every so often.

Reports of non-24-hour sleep-wake disorders are rare in sighted individuals (4–6) but can sometimes occur in association with psychiatric (e.g., schizophrenia) (7) or other behavioral disorders. In these cases, the patient's self-selected light-dark exposure likely induces temporary non-24-hour sleep-wake patterns due to repeated daily light-induced phase delays (8). Restoration of a stable 24-hour light-dark cycle may alleviate the disorder in these cases.

Non-entrained CRSDs are common in totally blind patients due to the lack of a light signal from the eyes reaching the circadian pacemaker in the hypothalamus (9–11). Patients without eyes, whether through bilateral enucleation, trauma, or developmental disorders (e.g., anophthalmia, microphthalmia), have a very high incidence of non-entrained CRSDs, and totally blind individuals who have eyes but lack any conscious light perception are also likely to have this disorder. Such patients will complain of cyclic sleep-wake problems as described above, and during the bad phase of the cycle will usually exhibit short nighttime sleep duration and excessive daytime napping or extreme sleepiness, the timing of which gradually gets later and later (if their internal circadian clock period is >24 hours) or earlier and earlier (if their circadian period is <24 hours) (12,13). The duration of each episode of poor sleep will depend on the individuals' circadian period (see Circadian Period Assessment below). For example, a patient with a period of 24.7 hours will take ~35 days to complete one cycle of good and bad sleep, with poor sleep for about half that time. A patient with a period of 24.2 hours, however, will take ~121 days to complete a full cycle with respect to their 24-hour social day and will therefore experience sleep problems for ~2 months of each cycle. Estimation of the individual's circadian period is the key to managing expectations in relation to the sleep disorder and may be important for treating the disorder. Onset of the sleep disorder will often coincide with or occur shortly after loss of light perception in those with progressive visual disorders or those who lost their light perception rapidly (e.g., eye trauma). Patients with visual acuity of light perception or better, and who report sleep-wake disturbances are unlikely to suffer from non-entrained CRSDs (11,14) and should be evaluated for non-circadian sleep disorders.

Prolonged episodes of poor nighttime sleep and excessive daytime napping may be misperceived as narcolepsy. The cyclic nature and severity of the disorder may be less apparent in young individuals, who may be able to withstand higher levels of sleep pressure during episodes associated with significant sleep disruption.

Delayed Sleep Phase Type (Delayed Sleep Phase Syndrome)

Delayed sleep phase type (DSPT) is characterized by bed and wake times that are typically hours later than desired and/or are required by work/school (Fig. 2). Therefore, patients may present with difficulty falling asleep and/or difficulty awakening in the morning. DSPT is more common in adolescents and young adults, and in some cases may correlate with a psychopathological condition that differs from insomnia in that the primary sleep complaint is difficulty with sleep onset whereas sleep maintenance problems are rare (15,16). The disorder may also be induced behaviorally by repeated late-night light exposure that causes a phase delay of the circadian system. Patients with DSPT would not exhibit sleep disruption or difficulty awakening if bed and wake times were permitted on a delayed schedule. DSPT

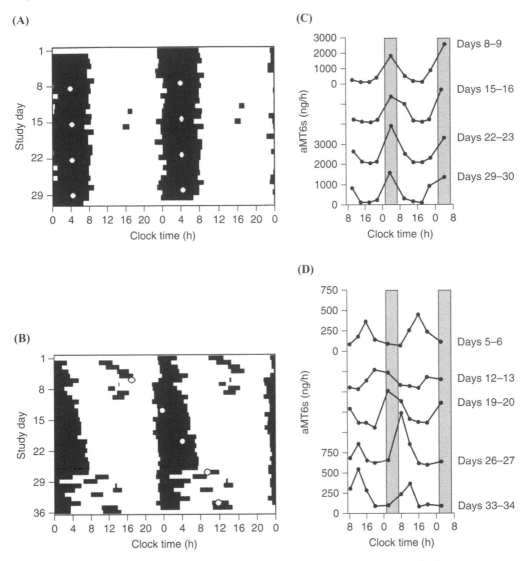

Figure 1 Circadian rhythms of sleep and melatonin in two visually impaired subjects. (**A**, **B**) Subjects completed daily sleep and nap diaries for four to five weeks and their sleep times (■) are double-plotted according to the time of day (abscissa) and study day (ordinate). Subjects also collected sequential 4 to 8 hourly urine samples for 48 hours per week, and the peak time of urinary 6-sulfatoxymelatonin (aMT6s) production each week (○) are plotted. (**C**, **D**) The weekly rhythms of urinary aMT6s production (●) that correspond to the peak times shown, and the gray bars represent the normal range of peak production for aMT6s (1:00–7:00 hours). (**A**, **C**) Data from a visually impaired female aged 35 years with a visual acuity to detect "hand movements only." Both the sleep-wake cycle and aMT6s rhythm remain entrained to 24 hours (**A**) with normal nighttime production of melatonin (**C**) and such rhythms would be typical of most normally sighted subjects. Note that her visual impairment, while severely disrupting the visual system, does not affect the circadian photoreception system, illustrating the functional separation of the visual and circadian photoreceptor systems. The subject in **B** and **D** is a 66-year old totally blind man with one eye and no conscious light perception. He exhibits a sleep-wake cycle and melatonin rhythm that are not entrained to 24 hours (**B**). The aMT6s rhythm exhibits a non-24-hour period ($\tau = 24.68$ hour), which clearly delays from week-to-week and is not entrained to the night (**D**). Closer observation of the sleep patterns show a cyclic sleep disorder in this subject where sleep occurs normally at night with no daytime naps when the endogenous aMT6s rhythm coincides with the night but becomes very disturbed at night and is accompanied by many daytime naps when the aMT6s rhythm does not occur at night. The timing of the naps follows the timing of the aMT6s rhythm, which represents the internal "biological" night and the time when the circadian system promotes sleep. The subject tries to remain on a normal social day, that is, sleeping at night and remaining awake in the day, but cannot sleep well when the circadian system in not entrained to the light-dark cycle. This example of a non-24-hour sleep-wake disorder is typical of most totally blind subjects and highlights the disturbance caused by a failure of light-dark information to reach the hypothalamic circadian pacemaker on our ability to sleep and wake on a 24-hour pattern. *Source*: Reproduced with permission from Ref. 3.

Delayed Sleep Phase Syndrome

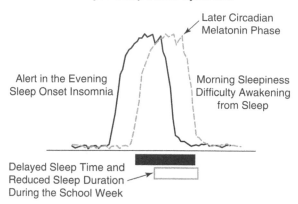

Figure 2 Delayed sleep phase syndrome or delayed sleep phase type (DSPT). DSPT is the most common circadian sleep disorder in adolescents. Patients report difficulty falling asleep and difficulty awakening at the times required by school/work schedules. When responsibilities no longer dictate an early sleeping schedule (e.g., summer vacation), the patient has no difficulty sleeping or awakening when the timing of the major sleep episode is delayed, and the patient is allowed to sleep late. The drive to go to bed later and sleep late in the morning is related to a shift in circadian phase, as represented by the delayed timing of the melatonin rhythm (*dashed line*). This delay in circadian timing is associated with sleep-onset insomnia and may be its primary cause (i.e., patients attempt to go to sleep at a circadian time when the biological clock is promoting wakefulness) and morning sleepiness (i.e., patients awaken at a circadian time when the biological clock is promoting sleep). The phase delay in circadian timing may be related to biological (circadian physiology) and behavioral changes (e.g., social activities, increased light exposure in the evening, earlier school start times) that occur during adolescence. A goal of treatment should be to advance circadian phase so that melatonin onset and sleep time occur earlier. The shift in circadian phase and the sleep-wake cycle may not be equal, potentially exacerbating decrements in waking function when the patient is awake at an inappropriate circadian phase.

combined with early school start times is thought to contribute to poor school performance and reduced sleep during the week. Inadequate sleep associated with DSPT in adolescents may contribute to increased risk of automobile accidents and increased use of caffeine, nicotine, and alcohol. Adults with DSPT report difficulty conforming to conventional work schedules or other social demands. Nearly 50% of patients report a family history of DSPT (17). Primary insomnia and stimulant use as potential causes of sleep onset insomnia at the required bedtime should be excluded by verifying that insomnia is not present when bedtime is sufficiently delayed and that stimulant use is reduced or avoided all together. It is also important to consider an underlying psychiatric disorder (e.g., obsessive compulsive disorder) in the differential diagnosis of DSPT.

Advanced Sleep Phase Type (Advanced Sleep Wake Syndrome)
Advanced sleep phase type (ASPT) is characterized by late afternoon/early evening sleepiness and early morning terminal awakening, which result in bedtimes and wake times being hours earlier than desired (Fig. 3). ASPT is more common in middle age and in old age compared to young adults. Early sleep patterns associated with ASPT often result in fewer social and work conflicts than DSPT. Repeated early-morning light exposure may also induce an advanced phase. As major depression may present with frequent early morning awakenings, it is important to consider an underlying psychiatric disorder in the differential diagnosis of ASPT. Assessment of the temporal relationship between the onset of sleep and mood symptoms can sometimes provide important information in this regard. A family history of ASPT has been reported (18–20).

Irregular Sleep-Wake Type
Irregular sleep-wake type (ISWT) is characterized by an erratic pattern of sleep episodes that occur across day and night. ISWT is more common in patients with developmental and degenerative neurological disorders (e.g., mental retardation, autism, and dementia). Total daily sleep duration may be in the normal range, but the timing of sleep is altered such that sleep may occur in multiple, fragmented, shorter than normal episodes over the 24-hour day. Circadian phase markers may indicate a normal phase in these cases (21), suggesting a

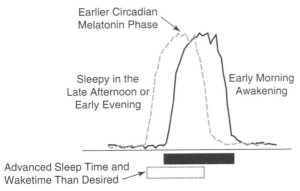

Advanced Sleep Phase Syndrome

Earlier Circadian
Melatonin Phase

Sleepy in the
Late Afternoon or
Early Evening

Early Morning
Awakening

Advanced Sleep Time and
Waketime Than Desired

Figure 3 Advanced sleep phase syndrome or advanced sleep phase type (ASPT). ASPT is the most common circadian sleep disorder in older adults. Patients report sleepiness in the late afternoon and early evening hours and early morning awakenings. The drive to go to bed and awaken earlier is related to a shift in circadian phase, as represented by the advanced timing of the melatonin rhythm (*dashed line*). This advance in circadian timing is associated with late afternoon/early evening sleepiness, and sleep maintenance insomnia may be an important contributor to this phenomenon. The phase advance in circadian timing may be related to biological (sleep and circadian physiology) and behavioral factors (e.g., increased light exposure in the early morning hours). A goal of treatment may be to delay circadian phase so that melatonin and sleep time occur later. As for DSPT, the shift in circadian phase and the sleep-wake cycle may not be equal, potentially exacerbating decrements in waking function when the patient is awake at an inappropriate circadian phase.

disorder of the output of the circadian system to other brain areas rather than an intrinsic disorder of the central circadian pacemaker itself.

Time Zone Change Type

Time zone change type (jet lag) is characterized by desynchronization between the circadian system and the light-dark cycle due to the rapid change in the light-dark cycle experienced following travel across multiple time zones. As with shift work type (see below), the circadian system cannot adapt to the rapid change in light-dark schedule and symptoms may persist upward of 12 days depending on the number of time zones crossed. Symptoms of jet lag include sleep difficulty and daytime sleepiness directly associated with a change in time zones usually ≥2 hours. Complaints of initiating sleep (especially following eastward travel), maintaining sleep (eastward and westward travel), excessive daytime sleepiness, fatigue, headache, and gastrointestinal disturbance are common. Daytime sleepiness may impair work performance and increase the risk of accidents (e.g., drowsy driving). Symptoms typically subside after a few days following arrival in the new time zone and circadian adaptation is generally ~1 day per time zone traveled (22,23).

Shift Work Type (Shift Work Sleep Disorder/Shift Work Disorder)

Shift work type (SWT) is thought to be primarily caused by desynchronization between the shift-work schedule and the light-dark cycle. Shift workers schedules' (and therefore light-dark cycle) often change more rapidly than the circadian system can adapt to, resulting in wake (work) and sleep occurring at an inappropriate circadian phase. Consequently, the characteristic symptoms of SWT are excessive sleepiness and/or insomnia that result in disruption of social, occupational, or other areas of function. Early morning shift workers may have shortened sleep schedules at night associated with their early morning shift start times and may exhibit excessive sleepiness as well. Gastrointestinal disturbance such as ulcers and gastrointestinal reflux disease, sleepiness-related accidents, absenteeism, depression, and missed family and social activities are also common in patients with SWT (24). Meals are also taken at inappropriate internal circadian phases causing elevation of postprandial insulin, glucose, and fats (25–28) potentially increasing the long-term risk of heart disease and diabetes (29). Long-term shift workers are also reported to have a higher incidence of some types of cancers compared to non-shift workers, particularly breast cancer in female shift workers (30,31). The mechanism of increased risk is unknown but may be related to change in hormone levels due to light exposure at night (32) and/or repeated circadian disruption (33,34).

SUBJECTIVE ASSESSMENT TOOLS

General Use
Sleep-Wakefulness Diaries
Sleep diaries have a long history of use in assessing sleep disorders (35,36). Prospective sleep diaries have been reported to be reliable and valid measures of sleep patterns, whereas retrospective diaries are subject to recall errors and bias. In general, for diaries to be useful they need to be completed on a daily basis. Importantly, when using sleep diaries for CRSD assessment, one must take into account the timing and duration of naps and self-assessment of waking function/sleepiness. Diaries should be collected for a minimum of one week and at least should assess bed times, wake times, sleep latency, sleep duration, and sleep quality. In many but not all CRSDs, the timing of sleep is most important in the clinical diagnosis. Electronic diaries [e.g., use of a personal digital assistant (PDA)] are an option to traditional paper diaries. A number of validated diaries have been published and a useful diary incorporating many of the components above can be downloaded free from the National Sleep Foundation website (www.sleepfoundation.org).

Sleepiness Scales
The Epworth Sleepiness Scale (ESS) is commonly used to document excessive daytime sleepiness in primary sleep disorders. Scores ≥ 10 are indicative of potential excessive daytime sleepiness (37). Although the ESS may be used to help document excessive sleepiness associated with CRSDs, it has not been specifically validated in CRSDs. The ESS may be particularly useful in tracking treatment progress. However, more frequent measurements that determine the timing of sleepiness across the waking day (e.g., 2-hourly assessments of sleepiness) with the Karolinska Sleepiness Scale (KSS) (38), Stanford Sleepiness Scale (39) (SSS), or visual analog scales (40) may provide more insight into the pattern of circadian-driven sleepiness. For example, two-hourly assessments using the KSS for two days when awake per week shows that the daily profile, but not average sleepiness, is indicative of advanced/ delayed phase in morning and evening types (41).

Morningness-Eveningness Assessment
Morningness-eveningness questionnaires can be used to assess morning versus evening behavioral patterns and preferences. The Horne-Üstberg Morningness-Eveningness Questionnaire (42) is the most widely used tool to assess morningness-eveningness. The questionnaire contains 19 items and possible scores range from 16 to 86. High scores between 69 and 86 indicate morning types and low scores between 16 and 41 indicate evening types. The Munich Chronotype Questionnaire is a more recent assessment tool for behavioral preferences with a version specific for shift workers (43). Extreme scores on these questionnaires may be associated with certain CRSDs.

Non-Entrained Type
Sleep-Wakefulness Diaries
Recommended. Diaries can be used to document episodes of poor sleep, naps, and excessive sleepiness. Complaints of poor nighttime sleep include prolonged sleep latency, reduced sleep duration, frequent and long duration awakenings, and poor sleep quality. There is also a high prevalence of naps and excessive daytime sleepiness in a repetitive cycle (12,13) (Fig. 1B). In most cases (those with a circadian period > 24 hours), sleep onset and offset times will become progressively delayed, although a minority of patients may have a period <24 hours (10,44) and report progressively earlier sleep times. Both good and poor sleep episodes can last for several weeks up to six months, although in the latter case the cyclic nature of the disorder may not be recognized and without prolonged evaluation may be perceived as intermittent insomnia. Therefore in patients who do not readily describe a cyclic disorder, at least 2 months of sleep diaries may be required to detect a non-24-hour pattern.

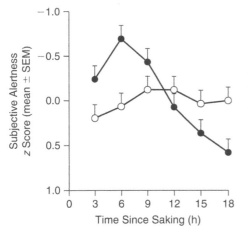

Figure 4 Average alertness (least squares mean z score $\pm$ SEM) is plotted in relation to time elapsed since waking from nighttime sleep episodes for abnormally advanced (•) and abnormally delayed blind (○). Changes in the circadian phase at which waking occurred had a dramatic effect on waking function. Advanced subjects, despite waking at an earlier clock time, wake at a later phase of their circadian cycle (Fig. 5A) and exhibit advanced alertness and performance profiles with an earlier peak and a prolonged decline. Delayed subjects show an opposite tendency in that although they wake at a later clock time, sleep occurs at a relatively earlier phase in the circadian cycle (Fig. 5A) and waking function remains relatively stable throughout the day, and is generally higher at the end of the day than advanced subjects. The internal phase relationship between sleep-wake behavior and the circadian system therefore contributes to the daily profile of alertness, mood, and performance in a predictable manner. *Source*: Adapted with permission from Ref. 45.

Sleepiness Scales
Average daytime sleepiness tends to depend on whether the patient's circadian phase is aligned with the sleep-wakefulness schedule. Assessment of sleepiness every two hours for two days when awake shows that the daily profile, but not average sleepiness, is indicative of advance/delay and the phase of non-entrained blind subjects (Fig. 4).

Morningness-Eveningness Assessment
Given the cyclical nature of the sleep disorders, Morningness-Eveningness Assessments may be hypothesized to vary depending on the circadian phase at which they are done. Multiple assessments over weeks or months may illustrate the cyclical pattern of sleep preferences, and may differentiate from permanently advanced- or delayed-sleep phase types although this has not been tested.

Delayed Sleep Phase Type
Sleep-Wakefulness Diaries
Recommended. Diaries can be used to document delayed sleep and/or wake times. DSPT is associated with evening alertness that results in bedtimes and wake times much later than desired (Fig. 5). However, wake time may be in the normal range due to work/school schedule requirements and in this case delayed sleep onset accompanied by short sleep duration may be observed. Patients may adopt a delayed sleep-wake schedule with adequate sleep duration during weekends and vacations.

Sleepiness Scales
May be helpful to document daytime sleepiness. Based on data from evening types without DSPT, it would be hypothesized that assessment of sleepiness every two hours using the KSS for two days when awake may show a daily profile consisting of morning sleepiness and evening alertness in patients with DSPT (Fig. 4).

Morningness-Eveningness Assessment
DSPT patients would be expected to score as evening types (16) suggesting physiological and behavioral tendencies to have delayed circadian rhythms. Evening types with DSPT have been hypothesized to be particularly difficult to phase advance, which may impact treatment considerations, however, the latter has not been demonstrated (16).

Advanced Sleep Phase Type
Sleep-Wakefulness Diaries
Recommended. Diaries can be used to document advanced sleep and wake times. ASPT is associated with late afternoon/early evening sleepiness that results in bedtimes and wake times much earlier than desired (Fig. 5).

(A)   **(B)**

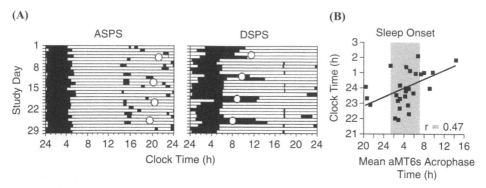

Figure 5 Relationship between sleep timing and circadian phase in entrained blind subjects. **(A)** Subjective sleep (■) and urinary aMT6s rhythm (○) timing over four weeks (study day on ordinate axis, clock time on abscissa) in two blind subjects, one with advanced sleep phase syndrome (ASPS) and one with delayed sleep phase syndrome (DSPS). In the ASPS subject, the advanced aMT6s peak (~20:00 hours, 8 hours earlier than normal) is associated with many daytime naps in the late afternoon and early evening, as the circadian system attempts to initiate sleep during the biological day, and an early wake-time from the main sleep episode. The DSPS subject exhibits a relatively delayed sleep onset time on most days but shows a particularly delayed sleep pattern during weekends when not having to set the alarm for work, as on other days. **(B)** The correlation between the timing of the aMT6s peak (abscissa) and sleep onset time (ordinate) in visually impaired entrained subjects, illustrating the change in sleep timing associated with altered circadian phase. *Source*: Adapted with permission from Ref. 13.

Sleepiness Scales
May be helpful to document daytime sleepiness. Based on data from morning types without ASPT, it would be hypothesized that assessment of sleepiness every two hours using the KSS for two days when awake may show a daily profile consisting of morning alertness and evening sleepiness in patients with ASPT (Fig. 4).

Morningness-Eveningness Assessment
Clinical use has been limited. ASPT patients will commonly score as morning types (19,20) suggesting physiological and behavioral tendencies to have advanced circadian rhythms.

Time Zone Change Type
Sleep-Wakefulness Diaries
Estimates of habitual bed and wake times in the home time zone are helpful when designing treatment interventions. Diaries can be used to help document impaired sleep in the new time zone.

Sleepiness Scales
May be helpful to document daytime sleepiness in the new time zone.

Morningness-Eveningness Assessment
Clinical use has been limited. It would be hypothesized that morning types would adapt easier to eastward travel and evening types would adapt easier to westward travel. However, there is no experimental evidence in the literature to support such hypotheses.

Other Assessments
The Columbian Jet Lag Scale (46) and the Liverpool Jet Lag Questionnaire (47,48) have been used as tools to rate symptoms associated with jet lag.

Irregular Sleep-Wake Type
Sleep-Wakefulness Diaries
Recommended. Diaries can be used to document irregular sleep patterns. Sleep will often be distributed in short episodes across the 24-hour day. Caregivers might need to complete diaries, as many individuals with ISWT have dementia and developmental disorders.

Sleepiness Scales
May be helpful to document daytime sleepiness. This scale may need to be completed by a caregiver. Note that caregivers of patients with ISWT are reported to show high levels of excessive daytime sleepiness because of sleep disruption associated with the care of the patient with ISWT (49).

Morningness-Eveningness Assessment
Clinical use has been limited.

Shift Work Type
Sleep-Wakefulness Diaries
Recommended. Diaries can be used to document insomnia during daytime sleep episodes and improved sleep on days off. Queries about sleepiness on the drive to and from work as well as sleepiness during the work schedule can help document clinical significance/disruption in waking function. Shift workers report average sleep durations of ~6.4 hours per day across the week, which is shorter than that of the general adult population. Patients with SWT often report even shorter average daily sleep durations of ~5.5 hours (24). In addition, sleep diaries can be used to help to document increased sleep duration on days off/vacation when sleep occurs at night and can help rule out primary insomnia.

Sleepiness Scales
The ESS may be helpful to document excessive sleepiness associated with shift work. On average, shift workers do not appear to have higher ESS scores than non-shift workers (50–52). However, a large subset of shift workers experience excessive sleepiness throughout the 24-hour day. Thus, it becomes important to use appropriate screening methods to identify this subset with standardized measures such as the ESS. Clinically, ESS scores ≥ 10 are typically used to identify individuals with excessive sleepiness. However, a more conservative criterion of >13 (consistent with one standard deviation above the population mean) has been used in some research settings. In terms of screening in clinical settings, the standard cutoff of ≥ 10 may provide a more useful measure to identify at risk individuals. Sleepiness scales such as the KSS and the SSS can be used to help to document excessive sleepiness on the night shift (53). These scales are useful because they rate sleepiness at the time of testing, not retrospectively or situational.

Morningness-Eveningness Assessment
Morning types reportedly do not cope as well with night work as do evening types (54,55), and/or morning types have more altered sleep patterns (56).

OBJECTIVE ASSESSMENT TOOLS

General Use
Polysomnography
Clinical polysomnography (PSG) in a sleep center is rarely used in the diagnosis of CRSDs, except to rule out primary sleep disorders such as apnea, narcolepsy, and or periodic limb disorder movements, all of which may be the cause of and/or contribute to excessive sleepiness. PSG to rule out primary sleep disorders should be scheduled at the patient's habitual sleep time in order to obtain an accurate assessment of sleep quality and pattern.

Actigraphy
Actigraphy is recommended to document irregular sleep patterns in patients with CRSDs. An actigraphy monitor capable of assessing light exposure may also help to determine whether inappropriate light exposure may contribute to the problem. Some actigraphy monitors also can measure subjective sleepiness during the day. Sleep timing and duration derived from actigraphy generally correlate well with PSG (57–60) and with sleep logs (61); however, quiet

wakefulness (e.g., watching a movie) is often difficult to differentiate from sleep via actigraphy. Actigraphy is particularly helpful in documenting the timing of sleep episodes, including naps in CRSD patients (60,62,63). The monitor should be worn for a minimum of one week and ideally accompanied by a sleep log. Actigraphy may be particularly useful in populations who cannot maintain a sleep log (e.g., children, the elderly, and in patients with neurological, psychiatric, or developmental disorders).

Multiple Sleep Latency Test
Multiple sleep latency test (MSLT) scores may be helpful in documenting excessive sleepiness and ruling out other sleep disorders such as narcolepsy.

Cognitive Function
Assessment of cognitive function may be helpful in documenting the negative impact of CRSDs on waking function, especially since objective measurements of sleepiness such as the MSLT and maintenance of wakefulness test (MWT) do not always correlate with cognitive capabilities (64–66). A number of standardized cognitive function tests have been used as research tools in the literature to better understand cognitive impairments associated with CRSDs and improvement in performance following treatment (e.g., psychomotor vigilance, digit symbol substitution, mathematical addition, and executive function). The sensitivity of many of these tasks to sleepiness and countermeasures as well as test-retest reliability is well documented. However, population norms are not currently available for most tasks and implementation of these tasks requires training. Improvements within a patient from before to after treatment may be helpful in documenting improvement in daytime function. However, it should be noted that many tasks have large learning curves, and improvement in some scores may be due to learning the task and not representative of improved cognitive function following treatment per se. Any sign or complaint of cognitive impairment may warrant further evaluation.

Laboratory Tests
There are no established laboratory tests specific for CRSDs.

Non-Entrained Type
Polysomnography
Typically not performed. Sleep quality on a given night will depend on the phase relationship between internal biological time and sleep.

Actigraphy
Recommended. Actigraphy can be effectively used to document cyclic sleep-wake patterns (Fig. 6B), including poor nighttime sleep and the occurrence of daytime naps across several weeks or months. Patients often present with consolidated sleep with no naps for several weeks and may then report several weeks of disrupted sleep and an increase in daytime naps. Therefore, assessment of one to two months or longer with actigraphy is recommended for the non-entrained type.

Multiple Sleep Latency Test
Typically not performed. MSLT scores on a given day will depend on the phase relationship between internal biological time and sleep.

Cognitive Function
Typically not performed. Cognitive function scores on a given day will depend on the phase relationship between internal biological time and sleep.

Laboratory Tests
Typically not performed. If one is considering removing a blind patient's eyes for cosmetic rather than medical reasons, a melatonin suppression test (68,69) may be useful to determine

(A)

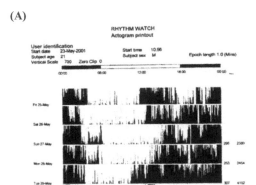

Delayed Sleep Phase Syndrome.

(B)

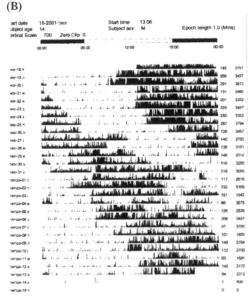

Non-24-Hour Sleep Wake syndrome.

(C)

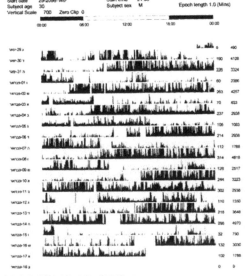

Irregular (or Disorganized) Sleep Wake Pattern.

Figure 6 Example of actigraphy recording from patients with delayed sleep phase type, free-running type, and irregular sleep-wake type. Black spikes represent activity. Clock hour is shown at the top of the figures. (**A**) Sleep (inactivity) occurs in the delayed sleep phase patient between 0300 and 0600 hours and wake time occurs between 1030 and 1400 hours depending on the day of the week. Also, note that bedtime and wake time are later on the weekend. (**B**) An example of actigraphy in a patient with non-24-hour type whose sleep-wakefulness schedule is not maintained on a 24-hour day. The timing of sleep and wakefulness occurs progressively later across days, consistent with a longer than 24-hour period of the circadian clock for this individual. Note that many patients may show stable timing of the primary sleep episode and yet their circadian clock may not be entrained to the 24-hour day (Fig. 1B). (**C**) An example of activity for a patient with irregular sleep-wake type. Wakefulness and sleep are irregular occurring at all times of day and night. *Source*: Adapted with permission from Ref. 67.

whether photic information is reaching the circadian clock. If this test is positive, the eyes should not be removed unless clinically necessary, as the development of non-entrained CRSDs is virtually certain in bilaterally enucleated cases.

Delayed Sleep Phase Type

Polysomnography
Typically not performed. If PSG is performed to rule out other sleep disorders, it should be done at the patient's delayed/preferred sleep time in order to obtain adequate sleep duration. The impact of inadequate sleep in this condition may also need to be assessed, since patients with DSPT reportedly sleep more than controls (70). Comparison of PSG sleep on the patient's preferred schedule versus that imposed by work/school requirements may verify disturbed sleep on the imposed schedule (71); however, such sleep disturbances are likely to last as long as the imposed schedule is followed.

Actigraphy
Recommended. Actigraphy can be effectively used to document delayed sleep and wake times (Fig. 6A) and/or shortened sleep duration. Actigraphy with light exposure recordings can document a pattern of evening light exposure that reinforces the delay in the patient's circadian phase and sleep schedule.

Multiple Sleep Latency Test
Typically not performed.

Cognitive Function
Typically not performed. Cognitive function would be expected to be worst in the morning and improve later in the day. Students may have difficulties with school performance due to delayed circadian phase and inadequate sleep.

Laboratory Tests
None.

Advanced Sleep Phase Type

Polysomnography
Typically not performed. If PSG is performed to rule out other sleep disorders, it should be done at the patient's early/preferred sleep time in order to obtain adequate sleep duration.

Actigraphy
Recommended. Actigraphy can be effectively used to document early sleep and wake times. Actigraphy with light exposure recordings can document a pattern of early morning light exposure that reinforces the advance in the patient's circadian phase and sleep schedule.

Multiple Sleep Latency Test
Typically not performed.

Cognitive Function
Typically not performed although cognitive function would be expected to be best in the morning and deteriorate later in the day.

Laboratory Tests
None.

Time Zone Change Type

Polysomnography
Typically not performed.

Actigraphy
Typically not performed. Actigraphy can be used to help document impaired sleep in the new time zone relative to the home time zone.

Multiple Sleep Latency Test
Typically not performed.

Cognitive Function
Typically not performed.

Laboratory Tests
None.

Irregular Sleep-Wake Type

Polysomnography
Typically not performed.

Actigraphy
Recommended. Actigraphy can be effectively used to document irregular sleep-wakefulness patterns (Fig. 6C) and in fact may be particularly useful in this population, since patients may have difficulty completing sleep diaries. A minimum of two weeks recording is suggested.

Multiple Sleep Latency Test
Typically not performed.

Cognitive Function
A complete neuropsychological examination should be considered if the patient shows signs of severe cognitive impairment, a developmental disorder, or neurodegenerative disease.

Laboratory Tests
Brain imaging may be considered if the patient shows signs of neurodegenerative disease.

Shift Work Type

Polysomnography
Typically not performed. If PSG is performed to rule out primary sleep disorders, it should be scheduled during a time consistent with the patient's ability to sleep well (e.g., at night) so that an adequate sample of sleep can be obtained. In general, shift workers exhibit a shorter latency to sleep, reduced non–rapid eye movement (NREM) stage N2 and rapid eye movement (REM) sleep, and more wake after sleep onset (WASO) when sleep occurs during the day. No study to date has compared PSG sleep of shift workers with and without SWT.

Actigraphy
Actigraphy may be helpful in documenting daytime insomnia. If circadian adaptation is the goal of treatment, generally when a patient is on a stable night work schedule, assessment of light exposure patterns may also be useful (e.g., early morning exposure to bright sunlight is thought to maintain the patient's circadian phase such that his or her clock is promoting sleep at night while he or she is working) (72,73).

Multiple Sleep Latency Test
If an MSLT is performed, it should be done at night during the patient's habitual work hours. An MSLT may help document excessive sleepiness on the night shift when the patient is typically active and reduced sleepiness with treatment. Findings from studies of SWT patients

indicate MSLT latencies on average <3 minutes (53). Findings from studies of simulated shift work indicate that this degree of sleepiness is not necessarily caused by being awake at night when the circadian clock is promoting sleep (74); however, the available data indicate that nighttime MSLTs may not reach the normal daytime range of 10 to 20 minutes even in healthy volunteers.

Cognitive Function
Standardized cognitive function testing may help document impaired behavioral alertness on the night shift and improved cognitive function with treatment.

Laboratory Tests
None.

OTHER CLINICAL TOOLS TO MEASURE CIRCADIAN PHASE/INTERNAL BIOLOGICAL TIME

General Principles
Circadian rhythms of melatonin, core body temperature, and cortisol are considered markers of the phase (75–77), amplitude, (76) and period (8,78) of the master circadian clock in the suprachiasmatic nucleus (SCN) of the hypothalamus (Fig. 7). In humans, the circadian timekeeping system approximates the ∼24-hour solar light dark cycle and is designed to promote sleep and its associated functions during the solar darkness (79,80). Assessment of the status of the circadian timekeeping system has proved helpful in understanding the nature of circadian sleep disorders and for testing the effectiveness of new treatment strategies.

Shipping Biological Specimens
The U.S. Centers for Disease Control and Prevention (CDC) guidelines for transport of biological specimens within the United States (USPS 18 USC 1716) should be strictly followed. Also refer to U.S. Department of Transportation (DOT) and International Air Transporters Association (IATA) regulations.

Circadian Phase Assessment
Circadian phase (ϕ) is defined as the time within the circadian cycle, at which a particular event occurs (e.g., the onset/rise of the melatonin rhythm, the minimum of the temperature rhythm, the maximum of the cortisol rhythm). Circadian phase angle (Ψ) is defined as the time within the circadian cycle relative to other events (biological or environmental), at which a particular circadian phase occurs (e.g., melatonin onset occurs on average ∼2 hours prior to habitual bedtime) (81). Most people sleep at night and therefore show high body temperatures during the daytime and low temperatures at night, with the minimum occurring several hours before habitual wake time (82,83). Cortisol levels decrease across the day, are lowest near the end of the day and increase across the night, reaching peak values near habitual wake time (75). Melatonin levels typically rise several hours before habitual bedtime, are high during the nocturnal sleep period, peak in the middle of the night, decline thereafter and are low during the daytime. High melatonin, low body temperature, and rising cortisol levels are representative of the internal biological night. Sleep is optimal when initiated during a relatively narrow window during the biological night when melatonin levels are high and temperature levels are low, whereas wakefulness is optimal during the biological day when melatonin levels are low and temperature levels are high.

Due to the masking effects of activity, posture, and sleep on temperature levels, and the frequent sampling rate required when assessing the pulsatile release of the hormone cortisol, the melatonin rhythm is the easiest circadian phase marker assessed to help diagnose and treat CRSDs. Melatonin can be reliably measured in blood and saliva, and its metabolite 6-sulfatoxy-melatonin (aMT6s) can easily be assessed in urine. Accurate assessment of circadian phase using melatonin requires that sighted patients are studied in dim room light (<25 lux, e.g., between

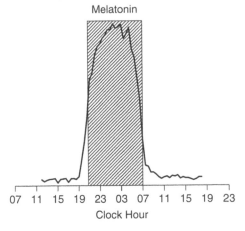

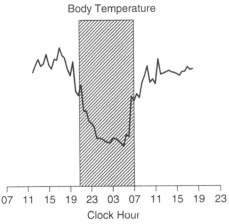

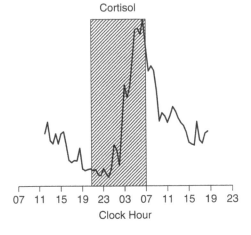

Figure 7 Markers of internal biological time relative to sleep under entrained conditions. High melatonin levels define the biological night, and low melatonin levels define the biological day with the onset of melatonin occurring on average ~2 hours prior to habitual bedtime. Body temperature levels are high during the biological day and low during the biological night, with the minimum temperature occurring ~2.5 hours before habitual wake time. Cortisol levels decrease across the biological day, are lowest near habitual bedtime, rise across the biological night, and peak near habitual wake time.

candle light and a reading light) because light exposure can acutely reduce melatonin levels (76,84,85). The influence of behavior, diet, and drugs should also be controlled when possible (see below).

The most often used marker of melatonin phase in a laboratory setting is the dim light melatonin onset (DLMO). The DLMO is most commonly defined as the point where melatonin levels increase over 10 pg/mL in plasma (86), although a lower absolute threshold or methods based on relative melatonin levels (e.g., 25% of the peak-to-trough range) may be more appropriate for low producers or older patients (81,87). Melatonin content in saliva is ~30% to 50% of plasma levels (88,89); therefore, a range of 3 to 5 pg/mL has been used as a threshold criterion for DLMO in saliva (53,90–92). Alternative methods of defining DLMO and other melatonin circadian phase markers have been reviewed (93). Under field conditions, for repeated longitudinal assessments, and for assessing relative changes in circadian phase, urinary measures are preferred. The acrophase or cosinor-derived fitted peak time of aMT6s production is generally used and its utility has been shown in assessment of adaptation rates of shift workers (94–96), circadian phase disorders in the blind (11), and when combined with urinary cortisol measures efficacy of ongoing melatonin treatment for non-24-hour disorder in the blind (97,98). One advantage of 24 to 48 hours urinary assessments is that the entire circadian rhythm is assessed, minimizing the risk of "missing" the DLMO which can occur when the correct timing of the collection of saliva and plasma samples is difficult to predict. Moreover this technique, compared to saliva or plasma measures, would likely be least affected by environmental light as collecting integrated urine samples may "wash out" the acute suppression of melatonin if bright light is relatively transient, although this remains to be tested systematically.

Protocol for Assessing Melatonin Phase in Saliva

In the home, instruct the patient to dim the lights. If the sun has not set, the windows should be covered with drapes or shades. Saliva samples can easily be collected using commercially available devices. This involves placing a piece of cotton in the mouth between the cheek and gum. Patients should be provided with 10 saliva sample collection devices numbered 1 to 10.

Instructions to the patient. The patient should be instructed to refrain from eating or drinking within 30 minutes of a subsequent saliva sample. Patients should avoid caffeine (99,100), alcohol (101–103), marijuana (104), non-steroidal anti-inflammatory drugs (NSAIDS) (105), and high carbohydrate meals (106) on the day of saliva collection. They should participate in sedentary activities during the test (e.g., reading, no exercise except light stretching) (107,108). A DLMO is not recommended for patients taking medications that may impact melatonin levels [e.g., beta blockers, selective serotonin-reuptake inhibitors (SSRIs), and monoamine oxidase inhibitors (MAOIs)] unless a sufficient washout period without medication is clinically feasible prior to assessment (109). Exogenous melatonin in pill form on the day of the test should be avoided as it may induce supraphysiological levels on the test. Patients should be instructed to drink only water during the test. If food is consumed between samples, patients should be instructed to rinse their mouth with water at least 30 minutes before providing a saliva sample. If gums bleed and a saliva sample contains blood, this should be noted on the collection sheet as salivary melatonin levels will be high because of blood contamination. Instruct the patient to place the cotton swab between cheek and gum for 5 minutes. The saliva soaked cotton swab should be placed in the collection device with the teeth and pushed into the tube with the tongue. Instruct the patient to refrain from handling the cotton swab with their fingers, as the sample may become contaminated. The samples should be placed in a freezer bag and kept frozen until they are returned to the physician's office. It is often helpful to provide patients with a timer with an auditory alarm to prompt them when to collect each sample. Instruct the patient to collect the sample at the time scheduled and note any deviations. Saliva should be collected every 60 minutes beginning ~6 to 7 hours prior to habitual bedtime, and saliva collection should end ~2 hours past habitual bedtime (Table 1). Clinicians can contact melatonin assay kit providers for the names of laboratories that perform melatonin assays.

After receiving the melatonin results, the following procedures can be used to determine DLMO time. Note that clock hour should be converted to military time and a value of 24 should be added to times after 2400 hours (e.g., 0100 should be 2500). Furthermore, minutes should be converted to decimal time (e.g., 21:36 should be 21.60; to convert minutes to decimal time, divide minutes by 60, e.g., $36/60 = 0.6$) (Table 2). Data should be plotted to review the rhythm profile. If melatonin values are unstable (Fig. 8), sampling time errors may have occurred.

Select the sample times and values immediately before and after melatonin levels rise above 3 pg/mL and enter those columns into the following formula in Microsoft Excel: =TREND (enter the time associated with the sample immediately below 3 pg/mL:enter the time associated with the sample immediately above 3 pg/mL, enter the sample value immediately below 3 pg/mL:enter the sample value immediately above 3 pg/mL, enter 3). In the above example, enter "=TREND(C6:C7,D6:D7,3)" and the resulting DLMO time will be

Table 1 Sample Saliva Collection Sheet

Sample number	Sample time (note that actual times will depend on the patient's habitual bedtime)	Comments (e.g., bleeding gums)
1	6:30 p.m.	
2	7:30 p.m.	
3	8:30 p.m.	
4	9:30 p.m.	
5	10:30 p.m.	
6	11:30 p.m.	
7	12:30 a.m.	
8	1:30 a.m. (habitual bedtime)	
9	2:30 a.m.	
10	3:30 a.m.	

Table 2 Sample Calculation of DLMO

A	B	C	D
Sample/row number	Sample time (clock hour)	Sample decimal time	Sample value (pg/mL)
1	6:30 p.m.	18.50	1.16
2	7:30 p.m.	19.50	1.52
3	8:35 p.m.	20.58	1.29
4	9:30 p.m.	21.50	1.58
5	10:30 p.m.	22.50	1.36
6	11:40 p.m.	23.67	2.52
7	12:30 a.m.	24.50	8.02
8	1:30 a.m. (habitual bedtime)	25.50	8.49
9	2:30 a.m.	26.60	9.75
10	3:30 a.m.	27.50	12.35

23.74 hour or 11:44 p.m. [to convert decimal time back to minutes multiply the numbers after the decimal by 60 (e.g., 0.74 × 60 = 44 minutes)]. If melatonin in saliva samples does not rise above the 3 pg/mL threshold, then the patient's circadian phase is likely outside the sampling interval. If all values are above 5 pg/mL, then the onset of the melatonin rhythm may have been missed and a 24-hour urine assessment may be necessary (see below). Note that patients with suspected DSPT may require samples to be taken at later times to ensure that DLMO is sampled, and patients with suspected non-entrained type disorders should be assessed multiple times over several weeks to assess whether DLMO changes over time. In such cases, sampling saliva every hour across the waking day may be useful to assess the drift in melatonin phase observed in non-entrained type patients.

Protocol for Assessing Melatonin Phase in Urine
See dietary, medication, and activity instructions above. In addition, use of diuretics should be noted, as should any liver or kidney disorder that may affect the metabolism or excretion of melatonin. Approximately 90% of melatonin is converted to urinary aMT6s; and while it is possible to measure melatonin in urine, measurement of aMT6s provides a more robust assay signal and is utilized more widely. Urinary aMT6s levels correlate highly with circulating plasma levels, although the peak occurs approximately two hours later and this lag should be taken into account when assessing aMT6s phase (110). Urinary cortisol can also be used if the patient is taking drugs that affect melatonin (97,111), and although the pulsatile nature of cortisol production is less apparent in urine sampling, phase estimates can be more variable using this method (111). Urine voids should be collected for at least 48 hours and depending on the suspected disorder, on multiple occasions. All urine produced during this time should be collected approximately every four hours during wakefulness plus an eight-hour overnight collection. More frequent collection times are acceptable. Sample times and total urine volume should be noted as outlined below.

(A)

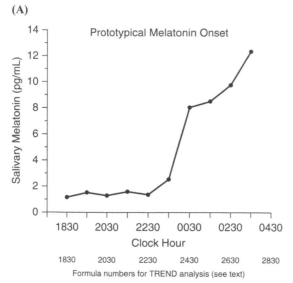

Formula numbers for TREND analysis (see text)

(B)

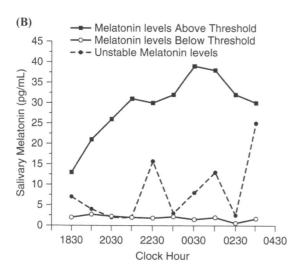

Figure 8 Examples of salivary melatonin data. (**A**) Example of a prototypical melatonin onset with a habitual bedtime near 0200 hours. Data show an example of salivary melatonin onset with an increase in melatonin levels between 2400 (0000 hours) and 0030 hours, and subsequent levels remain above the 3 pg/mL threshold. Note that the clock hour of melatonin onset will vary among patients. (**B**) Examples of salivary melatonin data consistently above (*closed squares*) and below (*open circles*) 3 pg/mL threshold and of unstable melatonin levels that rise above and go below the 3 pg/mL threshold (*dashed line, closed circles*). Melatonin onset cannot be accurately determined with these salivary assessments. Melatonin onset already occurred in the data showing melatonin levels above threshold, although it is clear that melatonin peaks during the nighttime hours. Melatonin phase cannot be determined in the example where melatonin levels are below threshold. It is also possible that melatonin amplitude is flattened in this example; assessment of additional salivary time points or 48-hour urine assessment is required to distinguish among these possibilities. Unstable melatonin onset could be a result of sampling error (e.g., incorrect order of sampling tubes, exposure to light prior to sampling, assay error). Repeated melatonin assessment is required.

Instructions to the patient The patient should collect all the urine they produce at four- to eight-hour intervals. Collection time and total urine volume (mL) for each collection should also be measured. For visually impaired patients or those unable to use a measuring cylinder, urine weight (g) can be used instead of volume, and a speaking kitchen scale can be provided for this purpose. The patient should be given the following equipment for each 48-hour collection: 2 × 1 L urine collection bottles or containers (male- and female-appropriate), 10 small urine vials (5–10 mL) labeled and Provided in order of use (e.g., ordered left to right) in a Styrofoam container, 10 disposable plastic Pasteur pipettes, 10 small grip-seal bags large enough for one urine sample vial, several larger grip-seal bags for double-bagging the samples, disposable gloves, a measuring cylinder or speaking kitchen scale, a Styrofoam container for returning samples or federally-approved container, and pre-paid addressed packaging for returning samples by mail.

The collection procedure for each 48-hour sampling episode is as follows: upon waking on day 1, empty your bladder but do not collect any urine. All urine produced from then on should be collected at four- to eight-hour intervals. For example, if you wake at 7:00 a.m. on Saturday, empty your bladder then and do not collect it. All urine you produce between 7:00 and 11:00 a.m. should be collected in the same large sample bottle. At 11:00 a.m., measure the total volume and record the collection times using military time (e.g., 07:00–11:00, 450 mL).

Then transfer a 5-mL sample from the large collection bottle to the first urine vial in the sequence using a disposable pipette. Only fill the small bottle about two-thirds full, not to the top, as the volume will expand when frozen and if the bottle is too full, the top will be pushed off. Put the filled urine vial in a small bag, seal it, and then place it in a larger grip-seal bag in the freezer. Throw away the remaining urine and wash the large collection bottle with warm water only (do not use bleach or other chemicals); then begin collecting all urine produced for the next 4 hours (e.g., 11:00–15:00). At 15:00, repeat the procedure, then collect all urine produced between 15:00 and 19:00 and then from 19:00 until bedtime, remembering to record the exact time and volume of each collection before saving the sample. The fifth collection of the day is the overnight collection and any urine produced during the night plus the first void upon waking should be collected in the same large bottle (e.g., 07:00 on Sunday morning). The first morning void belongs to the overnight sample, as the urine will collect in the bladder overnight and will therefore reflect nighttime melatonin production. Times and volumes should be measured as before, and a small sample saved. Repeat the sequence on the second day and make the final urine collection on the third morning (e.g., collect on Sunday 07:00–11:00, 11:00–15:00, 15:00–19:00, 19:00-bedtime, bedtime-wake time on Monday morning). At the end of each 48-hour collection, the patient will have 10 small frozen urine vials, each contained in its own sealed bag (to prevent cross-contamination and save the samples if they thaw while being returned) and 10 sets of times and volumes/weights. If the samples cannot be frozen, then refrigeration is preferred to room temperature. Samples should be returned frozen if possible, but aMT6s is stable at room temperature for four days (112), allowing samples to be sent by next-day or two-day delivery if they cannot be returned in person. If the patient forgets to record the times and volumes, they should try to estimate the data; if this is not possible, some information about the peak timing may still be redeemed from the uncorrected aMT6s amount (see below). If the patient throws away the urine without collecting a sample, they should try to retrieve any remaining sample in the bottle, as volumes as small as 2 µL can be used in some assays (e.g., radioimmunoassay, Stockgrand Ltd., University of Surrey, U.K.). The times and durations indicated above are only guidelines; actual times and durations can vary to fit the patients' schedule as long as there are five collections per day and the actual times are recorded. If the patient cannot do 48 hours, at least 30 hours will still provide enough information to assess the phase and the rhythm profiles, although having two cycles makes interpretation of the results easier.

Assay results (e.g., ng/mL) should be converted into hourly rates for each collection episode as follows: (ng/mL × total sample volume)/total sample hours. This rate should be plotted versus the midpoint collection time (Fig. 1). Normality of phase can be assessed either from the observed peak time of the plotted data (Fig. 1) or after being fit to a simple cosine function (11). If the patient habitually sleeps at night, the aMT6s peak should occur between ~1:30 and 6:30 a.m. (mean ± 2 SD = 4.2 ± 2.4, Arendt and English, unpublished results) (111). Earlier or later stable peak times would indicate a relatively advanced or delayed phase, respectively (Fig. 5). Peak times that occur progressively later or earlier would indicate a non-24-hour period (see below and Fig. 1).

Circadian Amplitude Assessment

Although melatonin and body temperature rhythms have been used as markers of the amplitude of the circadian timekeeping system (76,87,113,114), the role of circadian amplitude in CRSDs is not well understood. However, increased circadian amplitude has been hypothesized to be important for treatment of older adults, especially those with dementia (115).

Circadian Period Assessment

Circadian period (τ) refers to the time it takes to complete a circadian cycle (i.e., the time between the circadian phase on one day and the same circadian phase on the following day). Under typical conditions, the intrinsic near-24-hour period of the circadian clock in humans is adjusted daily by environmental time cues to be equal to the ~24.0-hour light-dark cycle (116). Some individuals have an intrinsic circadian period shorter than 24 hours and thus require a daily lengthening/phase delay of their circadian clock to be synchronized to the 24-hour day, whereas individuals with a longer than 24-hour intrinsic period require a daily shortening/phase advance of their circadian clock to remain synchronized (116). Circadian period has been reported to regulate the timing of melatonin onset relative to sleep time in sighted humans such that those with shorter circadian periods have an earlier onset of melatonin relative to habitual sleep time (81,117), and thus the biological night starts and ends earlier than in patients with longer circadian periods (80). Circadian period has also been associated with morningness-eveningness preferences (118), such that evening types are more likely to have circadian periods longer than 24 hours, whereas morning types are more likely to have circadian periods near or shorter than 24 hours.

Repeated assessment of melatonin, temperature, and cortisol rhythms across weeks has been used to estimate the period of the human circadian clock. Studies of sighted humans using the "forced desynchrony" protocol (8,79,80,91,117,119–121) or a constant dim light protocol (78) have reported period estimates close to but on average a little longer than 24 hours in sighted humans. Using the "free running protocol," where sleep-wake behavior (and therefore light-dark exposure) is left up to the patient, circadian periods tend to be overestimated and much closer to 25 hours (8).

Non-Entrained Type

Circadian Phase Assessment
Recommended but typically not done. Repeated assessment of circadian phase should be performed in order to document instability of circadian timing (see period assessment above) and confirm whether the sleep-wake disorder is accompanied by a non-24-hour period of the circadian clock or is the result of a behavioral disorder not related to a circadian phase abnormality. Multiple phase assessments using 48-hour urine collections are recommended in this population. Patients with non-entrained type disorders often demonstrate a circadian phase whose angle is constantly changing with respect to the external time of day/sleep-wakefulness schedule. The most common pattern observed is that the individual maintains a normal 24-hour sleep-wake schedule with the sleep episode scheduled at night, but their internal clock oscillates at a period longer than 24 hours. When internal biological time matches the socially imposed sleep schedule, sleep at night and daytime alertness are normal; however, when the clock is out of phase with the normal schedule, sleep at night occurs during the biological day, resulting in disturbed sleep and subsequent wakefulness. Wakefulness and sleep are impaired when sleep and wakefulness occur at an inappropriate circadian phase. Another manifestation of this disorder involves individuals who no longer maintain a normal 24-hour schedule and instead go to sleep and awaken according to internal biological time, typically later and later each day. Assessment of circadian phase may be useful in determining when to begin melatonin treatment (97).

Circadian Amplitude Assessment
Not recommended for clinical treatment.

Circadian Period Assessment
Recommended but typically not done. In field studies of blind patients with non-entrained type disorders, weekly or bimonthly melatonin phase estimates from urine collections across many months have been used to assess the circadian period. Patients with non-entrained type disorders, especially blind individuals who lack photic input to their circadian clock (9–11,122), will often exhibit circadian periods longer than 24 hours; however, patients with circadian periods shorter than 24 hours have been observed (10,44). There is disagreement over whether assessment of circadian period is useful clinically for the ultimate treatment of non-entrained type disorders (123), although the time to successful treatment may be decreased with accurate low-dose (0.5 mg) melatonin treatment timing based on circadian phase and period (98,124). In these patients, 4 × 48-hour collections spaced every 1 or 2 weeks, again accompanied by sleep diaries and/or actigraphy are recommended in order to ensure sufficient time to observe a change in circadian phase (Fig. 1).

Delayed Sleep Phase Type

Circadian Phase Assessment
Assessment of circadian phase may be useful in documenting that a late circadian phase underlies the delayed sleep-wake pattern and establishing the proper timing of treatment interventions

designed to phase shift the circadian clock. Salivary or urinary melatonin assessment is recommended in this population. The phase angle between circadian phase and sleep has been reported to be altered in some (125,126) but not all studies (127) of DSPT patients.

Circadian Amplitude Assessment
Not recommended for clinical treatment.

Circadian Period Assessment
Not recommended for clinical treatment. It could be hypothesized that patients with DSPT may have longer circadian periods. However, to date, circadian period has not been assessed in this patient population.

Advanced Sleep Phase Type

Circadian Phase Assessment
Assessment of circadian phase may be useful in documenting that an early circadian phase underlies the advanced sleep-wake pattern. Salivary or urinary melatonin assessment is recommended in this population. The phase angle of entrainment has not been reported in ASPT patients. The timing of melatonin onset is reportedly earlier in ASPT patients (18,128).

Circadian Amplitude Assessment
Not recommended for clinical treatment.

Circadian Period Assessment
Not recommended for clinical treatment. The circadian period of one individual with ASPT was reported to be shorter than 24 hours, consistent with a biological drive from the circadian clock to go to bed early at night (18).

Time Zone Change Type

Circadian Phase Assessment
Not recommended for clinical treatment. Transient misalignment between circadian phase and environmental time is observed during jet lag.

Circadian Amplitude Assessment
Not recommended for clinical treatment.

Circadian Period Assessment
Not recommended for clinical treatment. It could be hypothesized that patients with shorter than 24-hour circadian periods would adapt more easily to eastward travel while patients with longer than 24-hour circadian periods would adapt more easily to westward travel. The finding that most individuals studied to date show circadian periods longer than 24 hours is consistent with the general notion that it is easier to adapt to westward travel. However, whether circadian period is associated with ease of adjustment to jet travel has not been studied.

Irregular Sleep-Wake Type

Circadian Phase Assessment
Not recommended for clinical treatment.

Circadian Amplitude Assessment
Not recommended for clinical treatment. Circadian amplitude may be reduced in patients with ISWT and amplitude may be increased with treatment (115,129).

Circadian Period Assessment
Not recommended for clinical treatment. Whether circadian period is altered in ISWT is unknown.

Shift Work Sleep Type
Circadian Phase Assessment
Failure to adapt the patient's circadian phase to the wakefulness-sleep schedule is observed in many shift workers who attempt to sleep during the day and work at night (96,130,131). Assessment of circadian phase may be helpful in order to ascertain the degree of circadian adjustment to the shift work schedule and to inform treatment strategies. Melatonin assessment across the 24-hour day may be useful in this population if circadian adaptation is a goal of treatment.

Circadian Amplitude Assessment
Not recommended for clinical treatment. Whether circadian amplitude is altered in patients with SWT is unknown.

Circadian Period Assessment
Not recommended for clinical treatment. Whether circadian period contributes to SWT symptoms is unknown. It would be hypothesized that direction of shift in internal circadian phase is influenced by intrinsic circadian period and that patients with shorter circadian periods may have more difficulty with night work because, as noted, a shorter circadian period is associated with a behavioral morning preference.

FUTURE DIAGNOSTIC TOOLS

Genetic Markers
Evidence for a genetic mutation being involved in a familial form of ASPT (18) and for human Per3 gene and hClock gene mutations in DSPT (132) have been reported. However, use of genetic markers in these populations has not been applied in clinical practice.

CONCLUSIONS

As with any sleep assessment, a detailed clinical history is necessary to rule out other primary sleep disorders and/or other concomitant medical conditions. As patients with CRSDs typically present with symptoms of fatigue, mood disturbance, and/or insomnia it is important to explore potential psychiatric comorbidity as a primary cause of the underlying symptoms. Standardized assessments such as the Beck Depression Inventory or Hamilton Depression Rating Scale can be useful in this regard. Sleep diaries and actigraphy recordings with light exposure assessment are perhaps the most effective tools to assess CRSD and improvements with treatment. PSG is typically not recommended unless the goal is to rule out other primary sleep disorders. Assessment of circadian phase using salivary and urinary melatonin measures are helpful yet underutilized tools to determine whether the circadian timekeeping system is aligned appropriately with the desired sleep-wakefulness schedule. Circadian phase assessment may also be helpful to verify an appropriate change in circadian phase with treatment. Assessment of circadian phase is particularly useful for CRSDs, especially in patients who do not respond to treatment. Health care insurers are strongly encouraged to reimburse the costs of assessing circadian phase and actigraphy, as these clinical procedures are crucial for proper diagnosis and treatment of CRSDs. Use of these procedures will improve the effectiveness of treatment, which will reduce economic costs associated with the health and safety consequences of CRSDs.

REFERENCES

1. Sack RL, Auckley D, Auger R, et al. Circadian rhythm sleep disorders, Part I: Basic principles, shift work and jet lag disorders. An American Academy of Sleep Medicine review. Sleep 2007; 30(11): 1456–1479.

2. Sack RL, Auckley D, Auger R, et al. Circadian rhythm sleep disorders, Part II: Advanced sleep phase disorder, delayed sleep phase disorder, free-running disorder, and irregular sleep-wake rhythm. An American Academy of Sleep Medicine review. Sleep 2007; 30(11):1480–1497.

3. Lockley SW. Human circadian rhythms: circadian rhythms: influence of light in humans. In: Squire LR, ed. New Encyclopedia of Neuroscience. Oxford, UK: Elsevier, 2008, in press.

4. Kokkoris CP, Weitzman ED, Pollak CP, et al. Long-term ambulatory temperature monitoring in a subject with a hypernychthemeral sleep-wake cycle disturbance. Sleep 1978; 1(2):177–190.

5. McArthur AJ, Lewy AJ, Sack RL. Non-24-hour sleep-wake syndrome in a sighted man, circadian rhythm studies and efficacy of melatonin treatment. Sleep 1996; 19(7):544–553.

6. Hayakawa T, Uchiyama M, Kamei Y, et al. Clinical analyses of sighted patients with non-24-hour sleep-wake syndrome, a study of 57 consecutively diagnosed cases. Sleep 2005; 28(8):945–952.

7. Wulff K, Joyce E, Middleton B, et al. The suitability of actigraphy, diary data, and urinary melatonin profiles for quantitative assessment of sleep disturbances in schizophrenia, a case report. Chronobiol Int 2006; 23(1–2):485–495.

8. Czeisler CA, Duffy JF, Shanahan TL, et al. Stability, precision, and near-24-hour period of the human circadian pacemaker. Science 1999; 284(5423):2177–2181.

9. Lewy AJ, Newsome DA. Different types of melatonin circadian secretory rhythms in some blind subjects. J Clin Endocrinol Metab 1983; 56(6):1103–1107.

10. Sack RL, Lewy AJ, Blood ML, et al. Circadian rhythm abnormalities in totally blind people, incidence and clinical significance. J Clin Endocrinol Metab 1992; 75(1):127–134.

11. Lockley SW, Skene DJ, Arendt J, et al. Relationship between melatonin rhythms and visual loss in the blind. J Clin Endocrinol Metab 1997; 82(11):3763–3770.

12. Lockley SW, Skene DJ, Tabandeh H, et al. Relationship between napping and melatonin in the blind. J Biol Rhythms 1997; 12(1):16–25.

13. Lockley SW, Skene DJ, Butler LJ, et al. Sleep and activity rhythms are related to circadian phase in the blind. Sleep 1999; 22(5)616–623.

14. Tabandeh H, Lockley SW, Buttery R, et al. Disturbance of sleep in blindness. J Ophthalmol 1998; 126(5): 707–712.

15. Dagan Y, Eisenstein M. Circadian rhythm sleep disorders, toward a more precise definition and diagnosis. Chronobiol Int 1999; 16(2):213–222.

16. Wyatt JK. Delayed sleep phase syndrome, pathophysiology and treatment options. Sleep 2004; 27(6): 1195–1203.

17. Ancoli-Israel S, Schnierow B, Kelsoe J, et al. A pedigree of one family with delayed sleep phase syndrome. Chronobiol Int 2001; 18(5):831–840.

18. Jones CR, Campbell SS, Zone SE, et al. Familial advanced sleep-phase syndrome: a short-period circadian rhythm variant in humans. Nat Med 1999; 5(9): 1062–1065.

19. Reid KJ, Chang AM, Dubocovich ML, et al. Familial advanced sleep phase syndrome. Arch Neurol 2001; 58(7):1089–1094.

20. Satoh K, Mishima K, Inoue Y, et al. Two pedigrees of familial advanced sleep phase syndrome in Japan. Sleep 2003; 26(4):416–417.

21. Hatfield CF, Herbert J, Van Someren EJ, et al. Disrupted daily activity/rest cycles in relation to daily cortisol rhythms of home-dwelling patients with early Alzheimer's dementia. Brain 2004; 127(5): 1061–1074.

22. Takahashi T, Sasaki M, Itoh H, et al. Re-entrainment of the circadian rhythms of plasma melatonin in an 11-h eastward bound flight. Psychiatry Clin Neurosci 2001; 55(3):275–276.

23. Takahashi T, Sasaki M, Itoh H, et al. Re-entrainment of circadian rhythm of plasma melatonin on an 8-h eastward flight. Psychiatry Clin Neurosci 1999; 53(2):257–260.

24. Drake CL, Roehrs T, Richardson G, et al. Shift work sleep disorder, prevalence and consequences beyond that of symptomatic day workers. Sleep 2004; 27(8):1453–1462.

25. Ribeiro DC, Hampton SM, Morgan L, et al. Altered postprandial hormone and metabolic responses in a simulated shift work environment. J Endocrinol 1998; 158(3):305–310.

26. Hampton SM, Morgan LM, Lawrence N, et al. Postprandial hormone and metabolic responses in simulated shift work. J Endocrinol 1996; 151(2):259–267.

27. Lund J, Arendt J, Hampton SM, et al. Postprandial hormone and metabolic responses amongst shift workers in Antarctica. J Endocrinol 2001; 171(3):557–564.

28. Sopowski MJ, Hampton SM, Ribeiro DC, et al. Postprandial triacylglycerol responses in simulated night and day shift, gender differences. J Biol Rhythms 2001; 16(3):272–276.

29. Knutsson A. Health disorders of shift workers. Occup Med (Lond) 2003; 53(2):103–108.

30. Davis S, Mirick DK, Stevens RG. Night shift work, light at night, and risk of breast cancer. J Natl Cancer Inst 2001; 93(20):1557–1562.

31. Schernhammer ES, Laden F, Speizer FE, et al. Rotating night shifts and risk of breast cancer in women participating in the nurses' health study. J Natl Cancer Inst 2001; 93(20):1563–1568.

32. Stevens RG, Blask DE, Brainard GC, et al. Meeting report, the role of environmental lighting and circadian disruption in cancer and other diseases. Environ Health Perspect 2007; 115(9):1357–1362.

33. Filipski E, Delaunay F, King VM, et al. Effects of chronic jet lag on tumor progression in mice. Cancer Res 2004; 64(21):7879–7885.

34. Filipski E, King VM, Li X, et al. Disruption of circadian coordination accelerates malignant growth in mice. Pathol Biol (Paris) 2003; 51(4):216–219.

35. Manber R, Blasey C, Arnow B, et al. Assessing insomnia severity in depression, comparison of depression rating scales and sleep diaries. J Psychiatr Res 2005; 39(5):481–488.

36. Perlis ML, Smith M, Jungquist C, et al., eds. The Cognitive-Behavioral Treatment of Insomnia: A Session by Session Guide. New York: Springer Publishing, 2005.

37. Johns MW. Reliability and factor-analysis of the Epworth Sleepiness Scale. Sleep 1992; 15(4):376–381.

38. Akerstedt T, Gillberg M. Subjective and objective sleepiness in the active individual. Int J Neurosci 1990; 52(1–2):29–37.

39. Hoddes E, Zarcone V, Smythe H, et al. Quantification of sleepiness, a new approach. Psychophysiology 1973; 10(4):431–436.

40. Hull JT, Wright KP, Czeisler CA. The influence of subjective alertness and motivation on human performance independent of circadian and homeostatic regulation. J Biol Rhythms 2003; 18(4):329–338.

41. Kerkhof GA, Van Dongen HP. Morning-type and evening-type individuals differ in the phase position of their endogenous circadian oscillator. Neurosci Lett 1996; 218(3):153–156.

42. Horne JA, Ostberg O. A self-assessment questionnaire to determine morningness-eveningness in human circadian rhythms. Int J Chronobiol 1976; 4(2):97–110.

43. Zavada A, Gordijn MC, Beersma DG, et al. Comparison of the Munich Chronotype Questionnaire with the Horne-Ostberg's Morningness-Eveningness Score. Chronobiol Int 2005; 22(2):267–278.

44. Lewy AJ, Emens J, Jackman A, Yuhas K. Circadian uses of melatonin in humans. Chronobiol Int 2006; 23(1–2):403–412.

45. Lockley SW, Dijk D-J, Kosti O, et al. Alertness, mood and performance rhythm disturbances associated with circadian sleep disorders in the blind. J Sleep Res 2008; 17(2):207–216.

46. Spitzer RL, Terman M, Williams JB, et al. Jet lag, clinical features, validation of a new syndrome-specific scale, and lack of response to melatonin in a randomized, double-blind trial. Am J Psychiatry 1999; 156(9):1392–1396.

47. Waterhouse J, Edwards B, Nevill A, et al. Do subjective symptoms predict our perception of jet-lag? Ergonomics 2000; 43(10):1514–1527.

48. Waterhouse J, Reilly T, Atkinson G, et al. Jet lag: trends and coping strategies. Lancet 2007; 369(9567):1117–1129.

49. Lee D, Morgan K, Lindesay J. Effect of institutional respite care on the sleep of people with dementia and their primary caregivers. J Am Geriatr Soc 2007; 55(2):252–258.

50. Shen J, Botly LC, Chung SA, et al. Fatigue and shift work. J Sleep Res 2006; 15(1):1–5.

51. Garbarino S, De Carli F, Nobili L, et al. Sleepiness and sleep disorders in shift workers: a study on a group of Italian police officers. Sleep 2002; 25(6):648–653.

52. Sanford SD, Lichstein KL, Durrence HH, et al. The influence of age, gender, ethnicity, and insomnia on Epworth sleepiness scores: a normative US population. Sleep Med 2006; 7(4):319–326.

53. Czeisler CA, Walsh JK, Roth T, et al. Modafinil for excessive sleepiness associated with shift-work sleep disorder. N Engl J Med 2005; 353(5):476–486.

54. Akerstedt T. Psychological and psychophysiological effects of shift work. Scand J Work Environ Health 1990; 16(suppl 1):67–73.

55. Hilliker NA, Muehlbach MJ, Schweitzer PK, et al. Sleepiness/alertness on a simulated night shift schedule and morningness-eveningness tendency. Sleep 1992; 15(5):430–433.

56. Costa G, Lievore F, Casaletti G, et al. Circadian characteristics influencing interindividual differences in tolerance and adjustment to shiftwork. Ergonomics 1989; 32(4):373–385.

57. Kushida CA, Chang A, Gadkary C, et al. Comparison of actigraphic, polysomnographic, and subjective assessment of sleep parameters in sleep-disordered patients. Sleep Med 2001; 2(5):389–396.

58. Lichstein KL, Stone KC, Donaldson J, et al. Actigraphy validation with insomnia. Sleep 2006; 29(2): 232–239.

59. de Souza L, Benedito-Silva AA, Pires ML, et al. Further validation of actigraphy for sleep studies. Sleep 2003; 26(1):81–85.

60. Morgenthaler T, Alessi C, Friedman L, et al. Practice parameters for the use of actigraphy in the assessment of sleep and sleep disorders: an update for 2007. Sleep 2007; 30(4):519–529.

61. Lockley SW, Skene DJ, Arendt J. Comparison between subjective and actigraphic measurement of sleep and sleep rhythms. J Sleep Res 1999; 8(3):175–183.

62. Ancoli-Israel S, Cole R, Alessi C, et al. The role of actigraphy in the study of sleep and circadian rhythms. Sleep 2003; 26(3):342–392.

63. Littner M, Kushida CA, Anderson WM, et al. Practice parameters for the role of actigraphy in the study of sleep and circadian rhythms: an update for 2002. Sleep 2003; 26(3):337–341.

64. Frey DJ, Badia P, Wright Jr. KP. Inter- and intra-individual variability in performance near the circadian nadir during sleep deprivation. J Sleep Res 2004; 13(4):305–315.
65. Bliwise DL, Carskadon MA, Seidel WF, et al. MSLT-defined sleepiness and neuropsychological test performance do not correlate in the elderly. Neurobiol Aging 1991; 12(5):463–468.
66. Kraemer S, Danker-Hopfe H, Dorn H, et al. Time-of-day variations of indicators of attention, performance, physiologic parameters, and self-assessment of sleepiness. Biol Psychiatry 2000; 48 (11):1069–1080.
67. Dagan Y. Circadian rhythm sleep disorders (CRSD). Sleep Med Rev 2002; 6(1):45–54.
68. Czeisler CA, Shanahan TL, Klerman EB et al. Suppression of melatonin secretion in some blind patients by exposure to bright light. N Engl J Med 1995; 332(1):6–11.
69. Klerman EB, Shanahan TL, Brotman DJ, et al. Photic resetting of the human circadian pacemaker in the absence of conscious vision. J Biol Rhythms 2002; 17(6):548–555.
70. Uchiyama M, Okawa M, Shibui K, et al. Poor compensatory function for sleep loss as a pathogenic factor in patients with delayed sleep phase syndrome. Sleep 2000; 23(4):553–558.
71. Thorpy MJ, Korman E, Spielman AJ, Glovinsky PB. Delayed sleep phase syndrome in adolescents. J Adolesc Health Care 1988; 9(1):22–27.
72. Eastman CI, Stewart KT, Mahoney MP, et al. *Shiftwork*, dark goggles and bright light improve circadian rhythm adaptation to night-shift work. Sleep 1994; 17(6):535–543.
73. Eastman CI, Martin SK. How to use light and dark to produce circadian adaptation to night shift work. Ann Med 1999; 31(2):87–98.
74. Muehlbach MJ, Walsh JK. The effects of caffeine on simulated night-shift work and subsequent daytime sleep. Sleep 1995; 18(1):22–29.
75. Van Cauter E, Sturis J, Byrne MM, et al. Demonstration of rapid light-induced advances and delays of the human circadian clock using hormonal phase markers. Am J Physiol 1994; 266(6 pt 1):E953–E963.
76. Czeisler CA, Wright Jr. KP. Influence of light on circadian rhythmicity in humans. In: Turek FW, Zee PC, eds. Regulation of Sleep and Circadian Rhythms. New York: Marcel Dekker, Inc., 1999:149–180.
77. Lewy AJ, Cutler NL, Sack RL. The endogenous melatonin profile as a marker for circadian phase position. J Biol Rhythms 1999; 14(3):227–236.
78. Middleton B, Arendt J, Stone BM. Human circadian rhythms in constant dim light (8 lux) with knowledge of clock time. J Sleep Res 1996; 5(2):69–76.
79. Wyatt JK, Ritz-De Cecco A, Czeisler CA, et al. Circadian temperature and melatonin rhythms, sleep, and neurobehavioral function in humans living on a 20-h day. Am J Physiol 1999; 277(4): R1152–R1163.
80. Wright KP Jr., Hull JT, Hughes RJ, et al. Sleep and wakefulness out of phase with internal biological time impairs learning in humans. J Cogn Neurosci 2006; 18(4):508–521.
81. Wright KP Jr., Gronfier C, Duffy JE, et al. Intrinsic period and light intensity determine the phase relationship between melatonin and sleep in humans. J Biol Rhythms 2005; 20(2):168–177.
82. Duffy JF, Dijk D-J, Klerman EB, et al. Later endogenous circadian temperature nadir relative to an earlier wake time in older people. Am J Physiol 1998; 275(5):R1478–R1487.
83. Mongrain V, Lavoie S, Selmaoui B, et al. Phase relationships between sleep-wake cycle and underlying circadian rhythms in morningness-eveningness. J Biol Rhythms 2004; 19(3):248–257.
84. Lewy AJ, Wehr TA, Goodwin FK, et al. Light suppresses melatonin secretion in humans. Science 1980; 210(4475):1267–1269.
85. Zeitzer JM, Dijk D-J, Kronauer RE, et al. Sensitivity of the human circadian pacemaker to nocturnal light: melatonin phase resetting and suppression. J Physiol (Lond) 2000; 526(3):695–702.
86. Lewy AJ, Sack RL. The dim light melatonin onset as a marker for circadian phase position. Chronobiol Int 1989; 6(1):93–102.
87. Hughes RJ, Sack RL, Lewy AJ. The role of melatonin and circadian phase in age-related sleep-maintenance insomnia: assessment in a clinical trial of melatonin replacement. Sleep 1998; 21(1):52–68.
88. Pang SF, Lee PPN, Chan YS, et al. Melatonin secretion and its rhythms in biological fluids. In: Yu HS, Reiter RJ, eds. Melatonin, Biosynthesis, Physiological Effects, and Clinical Applications. Boca Raton, CRC Press, 1993:129–153.
89. Voultsios A, Kennaway DJ, Dawson D. Salivary melatonin as a circadian phase marker, validation and comparison to plasma melatonin. J Biol Rhythms 1997; 12(5):457–466.
90. Weber JM, Schwander JC, Unger I, et al. A direct ultrasensitive RIA for the determination of melatonin in human saliva, comparison with serum levels. Sleep Res 1997; 26:757.
91. Carskadon MA, Labyak SE, Acebo C, et al. Intrinsic circadian period of adolescent humans measured in conditions of forced desynchrony. Neurosci Lett 1999; 260(2):129–132.
92. Wirz-Justice A, Werth E, Renz C, et al. No evidence for a phase delay in human circadian rhythms after a single morning melatonin administration. J Pineal Res 2002; 32(1):1–5.
93. Wright KP Jr., Rogers NL. Endogenous versus exogenous effects of melatonin. In: Pandi-Perumal SR, Cardinali DP, eds. Melatonin, from Molecules to Therapy. New York: Nova Science Publishers, 2007:547–569.

94. Barnes RG, Deacon SJ, Forbes MJ, et al. Adaptation of the 6-sulphatoxymelatonin rhythm in shiftworkers on offshore oil installations during a 2-week 12-h night shift. Neurosci Lett 1998; 241(1): 9–12.

95. Barnes RG, Forbes MJ, Arendt J. Shift type and season affect adaptation of the 6-sulphatoxymelatonin rhythm in offshore oil rig workers. Neurosci Lett 1998; 252(3):179–182.

96. Dumont M, Benhaberou-Brun D, Paquet J. Profile of 24-h light exposure and circadian phase of melatonin secretion in night workers. J Biol Rhythms 2001; 16(5):502–511.

97. Lockley SW, Skene DJ, James K, et al. Melatonin administration can entrain the free-running circadian system of blind subjects. J Endocrinol 2000; 164(1):R1–R6.

98. Hack LM, Lockley SW, Arendt J, et al. The effects of low-dose 0.5-mg melatonin on the free-running circadian rhythms of blind subjects. J Biol Rhythms 2003; 18(5):420–429.

99. Wright KP Jr., Badia P, Myers BL, et al. Caffeine and light effects on nighttime melatonin and temperature levels in sleep-deprived humans. Brain Res 1997; 747(1):78–84.

100. Wright KP Jr., Myers BL, Plenzler SC, et al. Acute effects of bright light and caffeine on nighttime melatonin and temperature levels in women taking and not taking oral contraceptives. Brain Res 2000; 873(2):310–317.

101. Badia P, Murphy PJ, Myers BL, et al. Alcohol ingestion and nighttime melatonin levels. Sleep Res 1994; 32:477.

102. Ekman AC, Leppaluoto J, Huttunen P, et al. Ethanol inhibits melatonin secretion in healthy volunteers in a dose-dependent randomized double blind cross-over study. J Clin Endocrinol Metab 1993; 77(3):780–783.

103. Rojdmark S, Wikner J, Adner N, et al. Inhibition of melatonin secretion by ethanol in man. Metabolism 1993; 42(8):1047–1051.

104. Lissoni P, Resentini M, Mauri R, et al. Effects of tetrahydrocannabinol on melatonin secretion in man. Horm Metab Res 1986; 18(1):77–78.

105. Murphy PJ, Myers BL, Badia P. Nonsteroidal anti-inflammatory drugs alter body temperature and suppress melatonin in humans. Physiol Behav 1996; 59(1):133–139.

106. Krauchi K, Cajochen C, Werth E, et al. Alteration of internal circadian phase relationships after morning versus evening carbohydrate-rich meals in humans. J Biol Rhythms 2002; 17(4):364–376.

107. Deacon S, Arendt J. Posture influences melatonin concentrations in plasma and saliva in humans. Neurosci Lett 1994; 167:191–194.

108. Shanahan TL, Czeisler CA. Melatonin rhythm observed during forced desynchrony: circadian and forced components. Sleep Res 1995; 24A:544.

109. Skene DJ, Bojkowski CJ, Arendt J. Comparison of the effects of acute fluvoxamine and desipramine administration on melatonin and cortisol production in humans. Br J Clin Pharmacol 1994; 37(2): 181–186.

110. Arendt J. Melatonin and the Mammalian Pineal Gland. London: Chapman and Hall, 1995.

111. Skene DJ, Lockley SW, James K, et al. Correlation between urinary cortisol and 6-sulphatoxymelatonin rhythms in field studies of blind subjects. Clin Endocrinol (Oxf) 1999; 50(6):715–719.

112. Bojkowski CJ, Arendt J, Shih MC, et al. Melatonin secretion in humans assessed by measuring its metabolite, 6-sulfatoxymelatonin. Clin Chem 1987; 33(8):1343–1348.

113. Jewett ME, Kronauer RE, Czeisler CA. Light-induced suppression of endogenous circadian amplitude in humans. Nature 1991; 350(6313):59–62.

114. Zeitzer JM, Daniels JE, Duffy JF, et al. Do plasma melatonin concentrations decline with age? Am J Med 1999; 107(5):432–436.

115. Van Someren EJW, Raymann RJEM, Scherder EJA, et al. Circadian and age-related modulation of thermoreception and temperature regulation, mechanisms and functional implications. Ageing Res Rev 2002; 1(4):721–778.

116. Duffy JF, Wright Jr. KP. Entrainment of the human circadian system by light. J Biol Rhythms 2005; 28 (4):326–338.

117. Gronfier C, Wright KP Jr., Kronauer RE, et al. Entrainment of the human circadian pacemaker to longer-than-24-h days. Proc Natl Acad Sci U S A 2007; 104(21):9081–9086.

118. Duffy JF, Rimmer DW, Czeisler CA. Association of intrinsic circadian period with morningness-eveningness, usual wake time, and circadian phase. Behav Neurosci 2001; 115(4):895–899.

119. Hiddinga AE, Beersma DGM, van den Hoofdakker RH. Endogenous and exogenous components in the circadian variation of core body temperature in humans. J Sleep Res 1997; 6(3):156–163.

120. Wright KP Jr., Hughes RJ, Kronauer RE, et al. Intrinsic near-24-h pacemaker period determines limits of circadian entrainment to a weak synchronizer in humans. Proc Natl Acad Sci U S A 2001; 98(24): 14027–14032.

121. Scheer FA, Wright KP Jr., Kronauer RE, et al. Plasticity of the intrinsic period of the human circadian timing system. PLoS ONE 2007; 2(1):e721.

122. Miles LEM, Raynal DM, Wilson MA. Blind man living in normal society has circadian rhythms of 24.9 hours. Science 1977; 198(4315):421–423.

123. Lockley SW, Arendt J, Skene DJ. Visual impairment and circadian rhythm disorders. Dialog Clin Neurosci 2007; 9(3):301–314.
124. Lewy AJ, Emens JS, Bernert RA, et al. Eventual entrainment of the human circadian pacemaker by melatonin is independent of the circadian phase of treatment initiation: clinical implications. J Biol Rhythms 2004; 19(1):68–75.
125. Shibui K, Uchiyama M, Okawa M. Melatonin rhythms in delayed sleep phase syndrome. J Biol Rhythms 1999; 14(1):72–76.
126. Uchiyama M, Okawa M, Shibui K, et al. Altered phase relation between sleep timing and core body temperature rhythm in delayed sleep phase syndrome and non-24-hour sleep-wake syndrome in humans. Neurosci Lett 2000; 294(2):101–104.
127. Wyatt JK, Stepanski EJ, Kirkby J. Circadian phase in delayed sleep phase syndrome, predictors and temporal stability across multiple assessments. Sleep 2006; 29(8):1075–1080.
128. Terman M, Lewy AJ, Dijk DJ, et al. Light treatment for sleep disorders: consensus report. IV. Sleep phase and duration disturbances. J Biol Rhythms 1995; 10(2):135–147.
129. Van Someren EJ. Circadian rhythms and sleep in human aging. Chronobiol Int 2000; 17(3):233–243.
130. Czeisler CA, Dijk DJ. Use of bright light to treat maladaptation to night shift work and circadian rhythm sleep disorders. J Sleep Res 1995; 4(S2):70–73.
131. Sack RL, Blood ML, Lewy AJ. Melatonin rhythms in night shift workers. Sleep 1992; 15(5):434–441.
132. Archer SN, Robilliard DL, Skene DJ, et al. A length polymorphism in the circadian clock gene Per3 is linked to delayed sleep phase syndrome and extreme diurnal preference. Sleep 2003; 26(4):413–415.

15 | Diagnostic Algorithm for Circadian Rhythm Sleep Disorders

Yaron Dagan

Institute for Sleep Medicine, Assuta Medical Centers, and Medical Education Department, Sackler School of Medicine, Tel Aviv University, Tel Aviv, Israel

Katy Borodkin

Department of Psychology, Bar Ilan University, Ramat Gan, Israel

INTRODUCTION

This chapter provides recommendations for the clinical diagnosis of circadian rhythm sleep disorders (CRSDs). The *International Classification of Sleep Disorders*, second edition (*ICSD-2*) (1) lists nine types of CRSDs, all of which meet the following general criteria: (*i*) the sleep disturbance is primarily due to a mismatch between the internal biological clock and the environment; (*ii*) the disorder involves complaints of insomnia, excessive daytime sleepiness, or both; and (*iii*) the sleep disruption is associated with impaired daytime functioning in multiple areas, such as academic, occupational, social, and family performance.

The various types of CRSDs can be classified to three categories according to their etiology. Primary CRSDs arise from an abnormality of the intrinsic biological clock. This group consists of four disorders: CRSD of delayed sleep phase type (DSPT), in which the habitual timing of sleep episode is delayed relative to conventional or socially accepted time; CRSD of advanced sleep phase type (ASPT), in which the habitual sleep onset and wake-up times are advanced relative to conventional or socially accepted times; CRSD of free-running type, which is usually characterized by steady, gradual daily delay of several hours in sleep onset and wake-up times; and CRSD of irregular sleep-wake type, in which sleep and wake periods occur at variable times throughout the 24-hour period.

The second group of CRSDs includes disorders that emerge when the activity of the normal intrinsic biological clock is disrupted by external factors. These are CRSD of shift work type, which is consequent to work hours scheduled during the habitual sleep period, and CRSD of jet lag type, in which the sleep-wake cycle is out of phase with the environment as a result of changing time zones. Secondary CRSDs, the third group, are diagnosed if the CRSD is due to an underlying medical or neurological condition, or the CRSD is a side effect of a drug or substance. The last disorder is CRSD, not otherwise specified (NOS), which is defined as CRSD that does not meet criteria for other CRSDs.

The diagnosis of CRSDs can be established by means of three diagnostic procedures: clinical interview, monitoring of sleep-wake cycle, and assessment of biological markers of the internal circadian rhythmicity. This chapter describes the specific features of each procedure for the various types of CRSDs.

The clinical interview includes questions about sleep onset and offset times, sleep-related symptomatology, hunger and preferred cognitive activity hours, hereditary trends, presence of other diseases, and use of medications. It should be noted that in most types of these disorders, clinical interview is helpful in establishing the general diagnosis of CRSD, but the particular type is usually defined by monitoring of the sleep-wake patterns.

The monitoring of sleep-wake cycle is performed for several days (7–10 days are recommended) using actigraphy or sleep log. Actigraph is a watch-sized device sampling hand motion that is worn on the nondominant wrist. The output of this device is an actogram, in which sleep episodes are represented by white areas and wake episodes by black areas. The 24-hour period can be double-plotted in a raster format (e.g., Figs. 1–4). Visual screening of an actogram is usually sufficient to recognize the sleep-wake pattern. Actigraphy also produces quantitative data that allows for a more precise evaluation of such sleep variables as sleep onset and offset, sleep duration, number of awakenings, number of limb movements, and sleep efficiency.

For clinical purposes, sleep logs can be applied where actigraphic devices are not available. Patients are required to record bedtime and waking up time for several days. Such records were found to correlate well with actigraphic data (2). Since at least several days are required to assess sleep-wake patterns, actigraphy or sleep log, rather than polysomnography, is the preferred objective tool for diagnosis of CRSDs. All actograms shown in this chapter demonstrate rest-activity patterns recorded in unconstrained conditions, in which the patient is free to choose bedtime and wake-up hours. This feature of actigraphic/sleep log monitoring for diagnosis of CRSD is highly important because sleep-wake schedule obtained under forced conditions can mask the true pattern of the schedule thus misleading the diagnosis.

The third diagnostic procedure is assessment of biological markers of the internal biological clock, as captured by melatonin and body temperature circadian rhythms. This procedure is not mandatory, but can be helpful in complicated cases, especially when CRSD of free-running type or irregular sleep-wake type is suspected. Although melatonin can be measured in urine or blood, melatonin collected in saliva is also reliable and a more practical method for clinical purposes. Similarly, body temperature can be assessed rectally or orally. Less inconvenience is caused to a patient by the latter technique.

In clinical practice, salivary melatonin and oral temperature samplings can be made simultaneously every 2 hours for 36 hours during wakefulness. The acrophase (time of rhythm's maximal values) of melatonin rhythm and the nadir of temperature rhythm (time of rhythm's minimal values) are the most straightforward chronobiological markers to establish the phase of the rhythm. The period of each rhythm and phase relationships between the rhythms are also useful in defining the abnormality of the intrinsic biological clock.

CIRCADIAN RHYTHM SLEEP DISORDER, DELAYED SLEEP PHASE TYPE

Clinical Vignette

The patient, a 15-year-old boy at referral had difficulties falling asleep and awakening since early childhood. On school days, he usually went to bed around midnight; however, the actual sleep onset occurred at about 02:00. This timing of sleep episode led to chronic sleep deprivation during weekdays, since the boy obtained around five hours of nocturnal sleep. As a result, he felt sleepy throughout the day. He reported being unable to stay concentrated and alert at school and dozing off in class. The patient lacked appetite in the morning and preferred to have the main meal of the day in the evening. Female relatives on his mother's side of the family (mother, aunt, and grandmother) were all described by his mother as "owls." Other than the sleep disturbances, he was healthy and free of drugs.

During 10 days of actigraphic monitoring, sleep onset occurred between 05:00 to 07:30 and awakenings were between 13:30 and 18:00 (Fig. 1A). His mother has also undergone actigraphic study, which demonstrated a similar pattern of delayed sleep-wake cycle (sleep episode during 6 days of the study usually started at 04:00 and ended at 12:00, as shown in Fig. 1B). The boy and his mother both received diagnosis of CRSD of DSPT and were recommended for treatment with oral melatonin.

Key Steps in the Diagnosis of the Disorder
Clinical Interview
The interview should refer to the patient's sleep-wake patterns and sleep-related complaints. Typical patients with CRSD of DSPT have difficulty initiating sleep until 02:00 to 06:00. Waking up at the desired or necessary time in the morning to fulfill social or occupational duties often presents a true challenge for these patients. Most of them also experience profound daytime sleepiness. Attempts to deliberately advance sleep onset by early bedtime or by hypnotic medication may promote prolonged periods of time in bed awake.

Monitoring of Sleep-Wake Cycle
Actigraphy/sleep log shows delay in sleep onset and offset times (Fig. 1A,B). Timing of sleep episode is relatively stable throughout the tested days.

Assessment of Biological Markers
Melatonin and temperature samples show clear circadian rhythmicity marked by a phase delay. It was shown that whereas plasma melatonin in patients with CRSD of DSPT peaked at around 08:00, in healthy controls this occurred at around 04:00 (3). Similar gap in the

(A) **(B)**

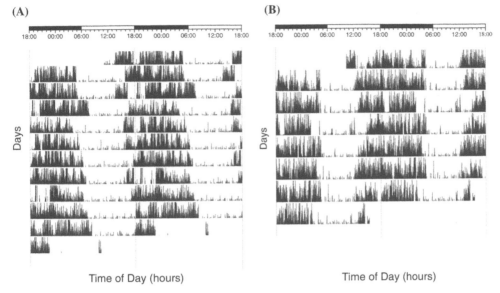

Figure 1   Actogram of a boy (**A**) and his mother (**B**) suffering from circadian rhythm sleep disorder of delayed sleep phase type (CRSD, DSPT).

timing of rectal temperature nadir between CRSD of DSPT (07:30) and control (05:00) group was reported in another study (4). Since the only abnormality in the biological rhythms of patients with CRSD of DSPT is phase delay, both melatonin and temperature rhythms exhibit 24-hour periodicity. If the rhythms are measured simultaneously, the overall rise of melatonin rhythm and fall of temperature rhythm will occur in the time window of sleep episode. In addition, temperature and melatonin rhythms are synchronized with each other, which can be seen in the approximate co-occurrence of the melatonin peak and temperature nadir on the time axis.

Important Diagnostic Features and Criteria to Distinguish Types
Patients with CRSD of DSPT often experience severe difficulties in daytime functioning, which can lead to an inability to keep up with school requirements in adolescence and maintain a steady job in adulthood. Additional clinical features of CRSD of DSPT that are useful in establishing the diagnosis are as follows (5): (*i*) preference of late evening and night hours as hours of highest alertness and functioning; (*ii*) lack of appetite in the morning and increased hunger in the late evening or night hours; (*iii*) family history of delayed sleep onset and offset (6); (*iv*) onset of the delay in sleep-wake schedule in childhood or early adolescence; (*v*) the sleep disturbance, which is a chronic, lifelong condition, unless treated.

Another interesting characteristic of patients with CRSD of DSPT is their poor ability to compensate for sleep loss. It was demonstrated that these patients were able to compensate for previous sleep loss mainly throughout their subjective night (between 06:00 and 12:00), whereas healthy controls compensated for previous sleep loss at almost all times throughout the 24-hour period (7). Our clinical experience supports this laboratory finding in that many patients with CRSD of DSPT report that if they did not obtain enough sleep on the previous night they would feel sleepier in the morning than in the evening of the next day, a pattern that is the reverse of the expected for healthy individuals. Further, despite the sleep loss, they would fall asleep at their habitual time on the following night, even if attempts were made to go to bed earlier.

Lastly, CRSD of DSPT tends to co-occur with personality disorders (5,8,9) and learning disabilities (5,10).

Differential Diagnosis
CRSD of DSPT should be distinguished from "normal" sleep patterns. Some individuals tend to delay sleep onset voluntarily, as a consequence of occupational, academic, and social activities in the late evening hours. These individuals differ from patients with CRSD of DSPT

mainly in the flexibility of their biological clock. Thus, an individual with intact biological clock who is used to falling asleep later than accepted is able to adjust his or her sleep-wake schedule to environmental changes (such as vacations, new working hours, etc). Patients with CRSD of DSPT seem to be unable to phase shift sleep episodes by motivation or education.

Due to complaints of difficulties falling asleep, CRSD of DSPT symptoms can sometimes be confused with sleep-onset insomnia. Patients suffering from sleep-onset insomnia feel sleepy at the desired bedtime but are unable to fall asleep. Sleep-onset difficulties do not persist on a daily basis. By comparison, in patients with CRSD of DSPT who attempt to advance their sleep-wake cycle by earlier bedtime, the inability to fall asleep is not accompanied by sleepiness. Further, sleep-onset difficulties continue as long as the patient keeps his bedtime out of phase with his endogenous sleep-wake rhythm. When allowed to maintain the preferred schedule, sleep initiation is normal.

CRSD of DSPT should be differentiated from sleep disorders that involve excessive daytime sleepiness complaint (such as idiopathic hypersomnia, sleep apnea, and narcolepsy). Patients with CRSD of DSPT are not sleepy if allowed to follow their intrinsic sleep-wake cycle.

Some individuals with free-running sleep-wake schedule might show CRSD of DSPT-like symptoms, such as difficulty falling asleep, daytime sleepiness, and delayed sleep onset. To establish the diagnosis, actigraphic monitoring is required. In unconstrained conditions, rest-activity pattern of a patient with CRSD of DSPT shows relative stability in sleep onset and offset, whereas sleep episodes of a patient with a free-running sleep-wake schedule is progressively delayed to later hours from day to day. If the actogram is inconclusive, as it might occur in atypical cases, assessment of melatonin/temperature circadian rhythm is helpful (see sect. "Differential Diagnosis" of CRSD of free-running type). Primary CRSD of DSPT should also be distinguished from delayed sleep-wake cycle that is secondary to a drug or an underlying medical condition. A thorough patient interview and physical examination may help to establish the etiology of CRSD of DSPT in such cases.

CIRCADIAN RHYTHM SLEEP DISORDER, ADVANCED SLEEP PHASE TYPE

Clinical Vignette
The patient, a 57-year-old man at referral, complained of early-morning awakening from which he suffered for as long as he could remember. He used to wake up between 03:00 and 05:00. At around 20:00 to 21:00, he typically felt extremely sleepy and experienced an inability to maintain alertness, but nevertheless delayed bedtime to 23:00 in attempts to delay his wake time. Throughout the day, he felt sleepy, which interrupted his daily routines. He remembered that during his university years, he had a strong preference for early morning hours as the best hours for studying. He underwent previous sleep studies at another institute and was diagnosed as having depression, for which he was treated with escitalopram [an antidepressant that acts as a selective serotonin reuptake inhibitor (SSRI)]. Shortly after treatment initiation, it was discontinued due to ineffectiveness and multiple side effects.

Actigraphic monitoring showed an advanced sleep-wake pattern that confirmed the patient's report (Fig. 2). During 10 days of the study, awakening occurred between 03:30 and 05:30. Decreased activity (which can be interpreted as napping) appeared at as early as 19:00 to 20:00, whereas the actual rest episode began at around 23:00. The patient was diagnosed with CRSD of ASPT. Two therapeutic options were suggested: administration of 4-mg slow-release oral melatonin before bedtime, 3-mg melatonin at awakening or, alternatively, one hour exposure to bright light at 19:00.

Key Steps in the Diagnosis of the Disorder
Clinical Interview
Patients with CRSD of ASPT often complain of early-morning insomnia, excessive evening sleepiness, and early sleep onset. A typical patient reports that he or she falls asleep between 18:00 and 21:00 and wakes up at 02:00 to 05:00.

Monitoring of Sleep-Wake Cycle
Sleep onset and offset are advanced (Fig. 2). However, timing of the sleep episode is relatively stable throughout the tested days.

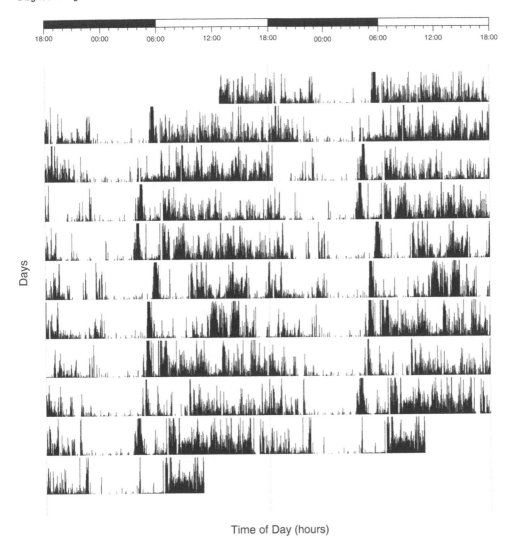

Figure 2 Actogram of a patient with circadian rhythm sleep disorder of advanced sleep phase type (CRSD, ASPT).

Assessment of Biological Markers

Both melatonin and temperature rhythms in CRSD of ASPT have a statistically significant 24-hour periodicity. The phase of these rhythms, on the other hand, is advanced, which can be seen in the melatonin peak and temperature nadir. If both rhythms are measured simultaneously, their phases are synchronized with each other.

Important Diagnostic Features and Criteria to Distinguish Types

When the patients are allowed to follow an advanced sleep-wake schedule, sleep is normal for age. In order to adjust to the conventional timetable, these patients might attempt to delay sleep onset. Since early awakening still occurs regardless of the sleep onset time, the patients might experience sleep loss. CRSD of ASPT is associated with functional difficulties, especially during late afternoon and early evening hours. These are usually less severe than in CRSD of DSPT and other types of CRSDs, which might partially explain the low prevalence known for this disorder (11).

Additional features useful in the diagnosis of CRSD of ASPT are as follows (5): (*i*) preference of early morning hours as hours of highest alertness; (*ii*) presence of other family members who can be described as "larks" (12,13); (*iii*) onset of the condition at early childhood; and (*iv*) the sleep disturbance, which is a chronic, lifelong condition, unless treated.

Differential Diagnosis

CRSD of ASPT should be differentiated from normal sleep-wake patterns, especially in the elderly. Whereas normal advancement in the phase of sleep-wake cycle tends to occur with growing age, CRSD of ASPT is a chronic condition that appears as early as childhood. CRSD of ASPT should also be distinguished from early-morning insomnia due to depression. As opposed to patients with CRSD of ASPT, patients with depression feel sleepy when they wake up in the early morning hours. They do not go to sleep at the early evening hours, as patients with CRSD of ASPT do. Lastly, sleep disturbances in depression occur once in a while, when there is a depressive episode, whereas symptoms of CRSD of ASPT are present on a daily basis throughout the life, unless treated. CRSD of ASPT should be differentiated from hypersomnias based on the dependency of occurrence of sleepiness on the sleep-wake schedule: whereas in CRSD of ASPT sleepiness appears only while on an imposed schedule, in hypersomnias it is present regardless of sleep-wake timetable.

CIRCADIAN RHYTHM SLEEP DISORDER, FREE-RUNNING TYPE

Clinical Vignette

Since the age of 12 years, the patient experienced sleep difficulties that became particularly severe about 3 years later. He complained of difficulty falling asleep, long sleep duration, and tiredness at awakening. He also described his sleep onset time as irregular. He remembered repeatedly nodding off at daytime whenever the situation did not require his active involvement. The patient did not eat in the morning and felt more alert at night.

The real crisis occurred when he was recruited to compulsory army service at the age of 18. He was unable to adjust to the requirements of military service, and even attempted suicide. Three months after recruitment, he was found unfit for military service and discharged. Following his suicidal attempt, he was seen for psychiatric evaluation and received a diagnosis of a personality disorder. Neurological examination that preceded referral was normal.

The patient's actogram (Fig. 3) indicated that his sleep onset was progressively delayed by two to four hours each day during the first seven days of the actigraphic monitoring. During this week, the sleep episode occurred during the light hours of the day. Throughout the last five days of the study, day-to-day variability in sleep onset timing was more considerable, and no clear pattern of consistent delay in sleep onset could be detected. During these days, sleep episode tended to occur during the darkness hours of the 24-hour period.

The patient was diagnosed with CRSD of free-running type and received treatment with 5-mg oral melatonin to be taken at 20:00. At follow-up visit, three weeks after treatment initiation, he reported that with melatonin, he typically fell asleep shortly after the ingestion and woke up at 06:00. His sleep-wake schedule was more stable, and sleep-related symptoms were reduced.

Key Steps in the Diagnosis of the Disorder

Clinical Interview

Clinical symptoms of CRSD of free-running type are often difficult to distinguish from those of CRSD of DSPT. When forced to follow an imposed sleep-wake schedule that is incompatible with their intrinsic circadian rhythms, patients with CRSD of free-running type also complain of daytime sleepiness and difficulties falling asleep and awakening. They typically are not aware of the gradual delay in their sleep onset. Rather, they might report that their habitual bedtime is either later than desired or irregular. Many of the patients feel that typically, their sleep duration is very long, although objective assessment is not always consistent with the subjective report (see sect. "Clinical Vignette" and Fig. 3).

Monitoring of Sleep-Wake Cycle

Figure 3 demonstrates a relatively common pattern in these patients consisting of two distinct periods. One period (the first 7 days in Fig. 3) is marked by consistent delay in the timing of sleep episode that extends to later hours each day. Following the first period, an episode of

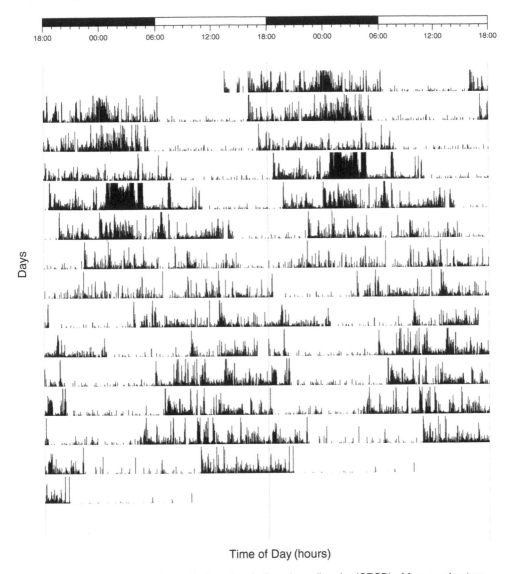

Figure 3 Actogram of a patient with circadian rhythm sleep disorder (CRSD) of free-running type.

greater variability in sleep onset time (the last 5 days in Fig. 3) occurs as if during these days, the internal clock resets itself to begin the next cycle of gradual delays in sleep onset.

Assessment of Biological Markers
Measuring melatonin/temperature circadian rhythm is especially useful for patients whose actogram can be interpreted either as evidence of CRSD of DSPT, irregular sleep-wake type, or free-running type. In the latter condition, both melatonin and temperature rhythms might have longer than a 24-hour period (14–17). If temperature, melatonin, and sleep-wake rhythms are measured simultaneously, they might show desynchronization with each other (14–17).

Important Diagnostic Features and Criteria to Distinguish Types
Similar to patients with CRSD of DSPT, some of the patients with CRSD of free-running type lack appetite in the morning and prefer night hours for activities involving concentration and attention. Daytime functional difficulties associated with CRSD, free-running type condition might be even more severe than those of patients with CRSD of DSPT. Like the latter condition, CRSD of free-running type is frequently comorbid to personality disorders (8). Contrary to CRSD of DSPT, familial patterns are unknown in this condition. In sighted individuals, the

disorder usually emerges first during childhood or early adolescence and lasts throughout the entire life, unless treated (5).

The description above highlights the importance of clinical interview in revealing clinical features of CRSD of free-running type that are consistent with the diagnosis of CRSD. To finalize the diagnosis and to identify the disorder as CRSD of free-running type, actigraphic monitoring of rest-activity patterns is obligatory.

Differential Diagnosis

The clinical features of CRSD of free-running type are at times similar to those seen in CRSD of DSPT. Patients with CRSD of DSPT might delay sleep onset toward later hours each day for several days, which might further complicate the diagnosis. Evaluation of melatonin/temperature circadian rhythms is helpful in distinguishing between the types. In CRSD of DSPT, both rhythms have a clear 24-hour periodicity whereas in CRSD of free-running type, the period is usually longer than 24 hours. Further, if both melatonin and temperature rhythms are measured simultaneously, their phases will be desynchronized with each other only in the case of CRSD of free-running type. CRSD of free-running type should also be differentiated from insomnias and hypersomnias.

CIRCADIAN RHYTHM SLEEP DISORDER, IRREGULAR SLEEP-WAKE TYPE

Clinical Vignette

The patient was a 17-year-old high school student when he first attended the Institute for Fatigue and Sleep Medicine. He complained of insomnia and daytime sleepiness. He described his sleep as occurring at irregular times, which caused severe disturbance in his daily routines. He could not attend school at the required schedule, and thus had troubles accomplishing school tasks and obtaining a matriculation certificate. The patient's second visit to the Institute took place when he was a soldier in compulsory service. As a result of his disorganized sleep-wake cycle, he was unable to fulfill his duties at the required schedule, for which he was repeatedly punished and charged.

At his first visit at the age of 17, the patient underwent assessment of rest-activity patterns for 11 days, which revealed that his sleep episodes were of variable length and unstable timing. For example, on some nights the patient fell asleep at around 01:00, whereas on others at 05:00 or 06:00. Further, the rest period could last for 4 as well as for 12 hours. Daytime napping was noted on days with short nocturnal sleep duration, probably to compensate for sleep loss (actogram illustrating rest-activity patterns of a patient with irregular sleep-wake cycle is shown in Fig. 4).

Based on the actigraphy and the clinical findings, the patient was diagnosed with irregular sleep-wake rhythm. The patient was unsuccessfully treated with melatonin, and therefore rehabilitative treatment approach was recommended (18).

Key Steps in the Diagnosis of the Disorder

Clinical Interview

A typical patient with CRSD of irregular sleep-wake type is unable to reliably describe his or her sleep onset as irregular. The patients complain of daytime sleepiness and insomnia, which usually arises from attempts to fall asleep when feeling alert. Complaint of long sleep hours is also common in this condition.

Monitoring of Sleep-Wake Cycle

An actogram/sleep log shows that rest and activity episodes occur at inconsistent and unpredictable times throughout the 24-hour period. Some days may include more than one sleep episode. Another important feature of this condition is the day-to-day variability in sleep duration (Fig. 4).

Assessment of Biological Markers

Melatonin/temperature rhythms may show loss of clear circadian rhythmicity and desynchrony between the rhythms, if measured simultaneously.

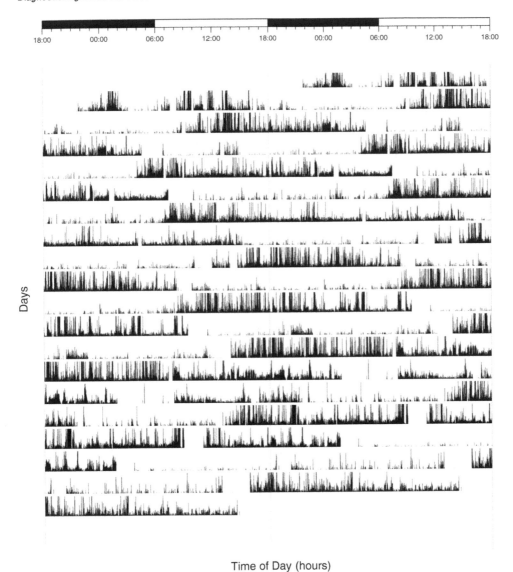

Figure 4 Actogram of a patient with circadian rhythm sleep disorder (CRSD) due to a drug, who displayed irregular rest-activity patterns.

Important Diagnostic Features and Criteria to Distinguish Types

The disorganization in sleep-wake cycle can result in particular difficulty to follow an imposed timetable. There are no known circadian features distinctive for this disorder (such as hunger and alertness hours). Familial patterns are also unknown. The condition first appears in childhood or early adolescence and can last throughout the entire life.

Differential Diagnosis

CRSD of irregular sleep-wake type is extremely rare as a primary disorder. In the majority of cases, this condition emerges as a result of a medical or neurological disorder and therefore should be classified as CRSD due to medical condition. To define CRSD of irregular sleep-wake type as primary disease, particular efforts should be made to rule out other causes for sleep disruption.

CIRCADIAN RHYTHM SLEEP DISORDER, SHIFT WORK TYPE

Clinical Vignette
The patient suffered from difficulty falling asleep, frequent nocturnal arousals, and excessive daytime sleepiness. These symptoms lasted for three years. For the last five years before the admission, she has been working early morning and night shifts at a bakery. Following a night shift, she usually fell asleep at 10:00 and woke up at 13:00, thus obtaining a total of three hours of sleep. On the night following a morning shift, her bedtime was 23:00 and the sleep episode ended after two to three hours. Based on these data, the patient was diagnosed with CRSD of shift work type and recommended to explore employment options that will not require shift work.

Key Steps in the Diagnosis of the Disorder
Clinical Interview
Patients suffering from CRSD of shift work type usually complain of insomnia and daytime sleepiness that occur as a result of working hours scheduled during the habitual sleep hours.

Monitoring of Sleep-Wake Cycle
In many cases the disorder can be diagnosed based solely on patient interview. Actigraphy can be used if the etiology of the sleep disturbance is unclear. If the patient undergoes actigraphic assessment in unconstrained conditions, a few days of prolonged sleep episode is expected as a compensation for sleep deprivation during shift work. Following these, the patient is expected to return to normal sleep-wake patterns, which are synchronized with the environment. Normal patterns are likely to be seen since the disorder is due to an externally imposed schedule that does not match the light-dark cycle, and as soon as this schedule is removed, the person is able to regain his internal sleep-wake cycle.

Important Diagnostic Features and Criteria to Distinguish Types
The total sleep time of these individuals is shorter than they need, especially in night and early morning workers. Sleep is regarded as insufficient. The sleep disturbances are accompanied by cognitive deficits, mood disturbances, and disruptions of social and family life. The condition may last as long as the person continues working in shifts. In some cases, though, it may persist beyond the duration of shift work.

Differential Diagnosis
Complaints of excessive daytime sleepiness present in CRSD of shift work type can sometimes be misinterpreted as a symptom of other primary sleep disorders, such as sleep apnea. If another primary sleep disorder is suspected, polysomnographic study of nocturnal sleep is recommended following two weeks in which the patient's sleep-wake cycle is not restricted by the timetable of shift work. The combination of symptoms of daytime sleepiness and insomnia might suggest other primary CRSDs. CRSD of shift work type can be distinguished from primary CRSDs by collecting the relevant information on work hours schedule during the patient interview.

CIRCADIAN RHYTHM SLEEP DISORDER, JET LAG TYPE

Clinical Vignette
The patient, a 38-year-old man, was admitted to the Institute for Fatigue and Sleep Medicine with complaints of sleepiness, insomnia, and decreased cognitive functioning following frequent and short visits to the United States and Japan. He traveled to these destinations for business negotiations as president of an Israeli high-tech company. As a hobby, he used to test his cognitive abilities by playing mathematical computer games. He noticed that, while abroad, his performance on these games as well as his ability to negotiate was significantly reduced. He was diagnosed with CRSD of jet lag type. To improve his functioning following a transmeridian flight, he was recommended to adjust meal hours to the local time while abroad

and to take 5-mg melatonin two to three hours before midnight when traveling eastward or before bedtime (earlier than midnight) when traveling westward.

Key Steps in the Diagnosis of the Disorder
Clinical Interview
Patients suffering from CRSD of jet lag type complain of sleep disturbances, insomnia, daytime sleepiness, decreased alertness, difficulties in daytime functioning, general malaise, and sometimes, gastrointestinal disturbance.

Important Diagnostic Features and Criteria to Distinguish Types
The symptoms arise following a transmeridian flight across at least two time zones and begin within one to two days following the air travel. The severity and duration of the symptoms usually depend on the number of time zones crossed and the direction of the flight. Traveling eastward, which requires advancement of the internal biological clock with the new environmental light-dark cycle, is usually more difficult to adjust than traveling westward.

Differential Diagnosis
Other mental, physical, or sleep disorders should be ruled out through patient history.

CIRCADIAN RHYTHM SLEEP DISORDER DUE TO MEDICAL CONDITION

Clinical Vignette
At age 20, the patient was involved in a car accident that resulted in minor head trauma without loss of consciousness. Following the accident, he started feeling excessive daytime sleepiness. He also noticed that the timing of sleep onset and offset became irregular.

To establish the diagnosis, polysomnography was performed that revealed no sleep disorder. Actigraphic monitoring of 15 days indicated that the patient had an irregular sleep-wake cycle. Statistical analyses revealed a significant 24-hour periodicity in salivary melatonin, whereas no significant circadian pattern could be found for temperature rhythm. Visual screening of the best-fit models indicated that the rhythms were uncoupled (Fig. 5).

The patient was diagnosed with CRSD due to medical condition and treated with 5-mg melatonin administered at 21:00 for a month. Since he did not respond to the treatment, we recommended the rehabilitative approach to be adopted. According to this approach, the patient is encouraged to accept his disorder and its functional outcomes as permanent and is guided to overcome the deficits by organizing his life routines to fit wakefulness hours (18).

Key Steps in the Diagnosis of the Disorder
The CRSD of this type is diagnosed when it is secondary to an underlying neurological or medical condition, among which are brain tumors (19,20), head trauma (21–24), dementia (25), and Parkinson's disease (26).

Important Diagnostic Features and Criteria to Distinguish Types
The sleep-wake pattern can be similar to any of the four primary intrinsic types (CRSD of DSPT, ASPT, free-running, or irregular sleep-wake type). For example, minor head trauma was previously reported to be associated with delayed (21,23,24), free-running (22), and irregular (21) sleep-wake cycle. The patients may present with a variety of symptoms, including insomnia and daytime sleepiness. The condition is chronic and may arise at any age.

Depending on the type of the particular sleep-wake abnormality, the diagnostic criteria are similar to those described for the primary disorders. The diagnosis of CRSD due to medical condition is made if an underlying medical or neurological condition accounts for the CRSD.

Differential Diagnosis
CRSD due to medical condition should be differentiated from primary intrinsic CRSDs. Additional criteria for differential diagnosis can be seen in "Differential Diagnosis" sections of other specific CRSDs.

(A)

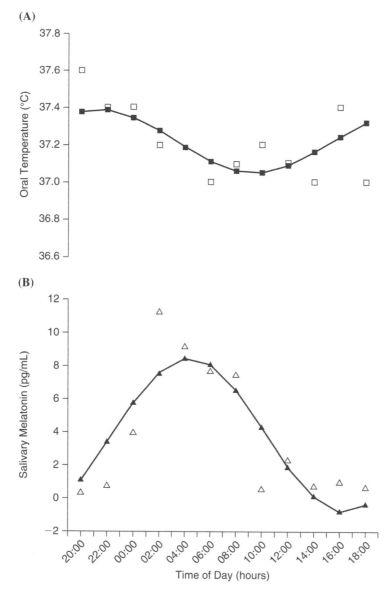

(B)

Figure 5 Raw data and best-fit cosine curve of 24 hours of (**A**) oral temperature and (**B**) salivary melatonin of a patient suffering from circadian rhythm sleep disorder (CRSD) due to medical condition. The patient displayed irregular sleep-wake patterns. □, Raw data of oral temperature; —■—, best-fit curve of oral temperature; △, raw data of salivary melatonin; —▲—, best-fit curve of salivary melatonin.

CIRCADIAN RHYTHM SLEEP DISORDER DUE TO DRUG OR SUBSTANCE

Clinical Vignette

When he was 16, the patient was diagnosed with Gilles de la Tourette syndrome, for which he was successfully treated with haloperidol (10 mg/day). Two years after commencing the treatment his sleep onset and offset became irregular. His inability to maintain a stable sleep-wake schedule severely disrupted his daily life routines, and he was unable to hold a job on a regular basis. Being a talented computer systems analyst, he began working at home during his waking hours.

The patient was referred to the Institute for Fatigue and Sleep Medicine by his psychiatrist with complaints of severe insomnia. Actigraphic monitoring of rest-activity patterns for 18 days revealed an irregular and disorganized sleep-wake pattern (Fig. 4). The timing and length of sleep episodes varied from day to day considerably. Since the patient reported that prior to treatment with haloperidol his sleep was normal, we considered the abnormality of the sleep-wake schedule as secondary to haloperidol, rather than to the illness itself. Therefore, the patient was diagnosed with CRSD due to medication or substance. To treat his condition, haloperidol was replaced with atypical neuroleptic risperidone. When oral melatonin (5 mg at 21:00) was added as a secondary therapy, normal sleep-wake cycle was fully restored (30).

Key Steps in the Diagnosis of the Disorder
The CRSD of this type is diagnosed when it emerges as a side effect of drug use. Typical neuroleptics, such as haloperidol and flupentixol, were observed to trigger CRSDs in patients with schizophrenia (27,28), Alzheimer's disease (29), and Gilles de la Tourette syndrome (30). CRSDs can also emerge as an iatrogenic effect of specific SSRIs. Delayed sleep-wake rhythm as a side effect of this class of drugs was previously described in 10 patients with obsessive-compulsive disorder who received treatment with fluvoxamine (31).

Important Diagnostic Features and Criteria to Distinguish Types
Any of the four patterns of sleep-wake abnormalities described for primary intrinsic types (CRSD of DSP, ASP, free-running, and irregular sleep-wake type) can emerge following administration of psychoactive medications. The CRSD of this type may occur at any age. In many cases, it will last for as long as the medication that alters the circadian rhythm of sleep-wake cycle is administered (27,29,31). The diagnosis of this condition is made in accordance with the steps described for the primary types and after determining that the CRSD is secondary to drug or substance.

Differential Diagnosis
Sleep-related complaints of patients treated with psychoactive drugs are often regarded as drug-induced insomnia or daytime somnolence. As the findings demonstrate, in some cases these could be symptoms of iatrogenic CRSD. This condition should also be differentiated from primary intrinsic CRSDs. Additional criteria for differential diagnosis can be seen in "Differential Diagnosis" sections of other specific CRSDs.

CIRCADIAN RHYTHM SLEEP DISORDER, NOT OTHERWISE SPECIFIED

Clinical Vignette
The patient, a 47-year-old man, admitted to the Institute for Fatigue and Sleep Medicine complaining of severe fatigue, daytime sleepiness, and an inability to maintain a regular sleep schedule. This condition severely impaired his well-being and ability to maintain normal daily functioning. The sleep-related disturbances lasted for as long as 20 years, since he started to work in the diamond industry. As a diamond grader, the patient owned a professional high-intensity (8000 lux) daylight lamp, which he regularly used in his work at different times of the day, including at night. During the years, he was diagnosed with depression and chronic fatigue syndrome (CFS). Antidepressant and hypnotic drugs failed to improve his condition.

Actigraphic assessment of sleep-wake cycle for 14 days demonstrated that the patient had an irregular sleep-wake rhythm. Oral temperature and saliva melatonin circadian rhythms also showed abnormal patterns, with salivary melatonin peak at 11:28 and oral temperature nadir at 13:55 (Fig. 6).

We assumed that the disorganization of the patient's circadian rhythms resulted from chronic exposure to the professional bright light lamp and therefore diagnosed it as CRSD, NOS. To treat his condition, we recommended to (*i*) cease using the lamp in the nighttime, (*ii*) take 5-mg melatonin in the evening, and, as a complementary treatment, (*iii*) sit under the bright light lamp (8000 lux) for one hour every morning to increase his daytime alertness. Two months after initiation of the treatment, sleep-wake and oral temperature circadian rhythms were reassessed and found to be stabilized (32).

Key Steps in the Diagnosis of the Disorder
CRSD, NOS is diagnosed when the disorder is a CRSD, but does not meet criteria for any of the eight types of CRSDs. The patient described in the clinical vignette suffered from an irregular

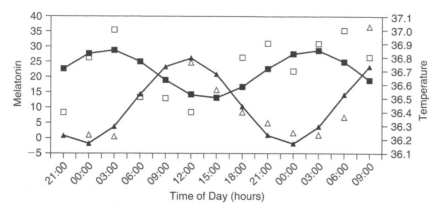

Figure 6 Raw data and best-fit cosine curve of 24 hours of oral temperature and salivary melatonin of a patient suffering from circadian rhythm sleep disorder not otherwise specified (CRSD, NOS). The patient displayed irregular sleep-wake patterns. □, Raw data of oral temperature; —■—, best-fit curve of oral temperature; △, raw data of salivary melatonin; —▲—, best-fit curve of salivary melatonin.

sleep-wake cycle that was neither intrinsic (and thus could not be categorized as CRSD of irregular sleep-wake type), nor due to medical condition or drug/substance. Rather, it was most likely caused by external factors (but not those that can account for shift work or jet lag disorder), that is, exposure to bright light at times inconsistent with the environmental light-dark cycle.

Important Diagnostic Features and Criteria to Distinguish Types

CRSD, NOS is also diagnosed in cases where the primary source of CRSD is difficult to establish. For example, in cases of patients with neurological/ developmental disorders it is not always possible to unambiguously define the CRSD as primary or secondary disorder. Likewise, there are patients with psychiatric disorders whose CRSD could either be primary or secondary to psychotic states or drug use.

Sleep complaints and sleep-wake patterns might be similar to those described for each of the primary types of CRSDs. The patient interview, actigraphy/sleep log, and melatonin/ temperature daily rhythm assessment (if required) aims to recognize that a patient has a CRSD and to rule out all other types of CRSDs described above.

Differential Diagnosis

CRSD, NOS should be distinguished from all other types of CRSDs. Additional criteria for differential diagnosis can be seen in "Differential Diagnosis" sections of other specific CRSDs.

CONCLUSIONS

CRSDs are diagnosed when the sleep disturbance is due to a mismatch between the internal clock and the environment, the patient complains of insomnia and/or excessive daytime sleepiness, and the sleep disruption is associated with impaired daytime functioning in multiple areas of the patient's life. The CRSDs can be classified into three categories according to their etiology, which are primary CRSDs arising from an abnormality of the intrinsic clock (DSPT, ASPT, free-running type, and irregular sleep-wake type); disorders that emerge when the activity of the normal intrinsic clock is disrupted by external factors (shift work type and jet lag type); and secondary CRSDs (due to an underlying medical or neurological condition, side effect of a drug or substance, or not otherwise specified). A clinical interview with a thorough review of the patient's history is often sufficient in establishing the diagnosis of a CRSD, but monitoring of sleep-wake cycle and assessment of biological markers of the internal circadian rhythmicity are frequently useful in confirming the diagnosis of the disorder and differentiating it from other similar disorders.

REFERENCES

1. American Academy of Sleep Medicine, . International Classification of Sleep Disorders: Diagnostic and Coding Manual. 2nd ed. Westchester, IL: American Academy of Sleep Medicine, 2005.
2. Lockley SW, Skene DJ, Arendt J. Comparison between subjective and actigraphic measurement of sleep and sleep rhythms. J Sleep Res 1999; 8(3):175–183.
3. Shibui K, Uchiyama M, Okawa M. Melatonin rhythms in delayed sleep phase syndrome. J Biol Rhythms 1999; 14(1):72–76.
4. Ozaki S, Uchiyama M, Shirakawa S, et al. Prolonged interval from body temperature nadir to sleep offset in patients with delayed sleep phase syndrome. Sleep 1996; 19(1):36–40.
5. Dagan Y, Eisenstein M. Circadian rhythm sleep disorders: toward a more precise definition and diagnosis. Chronobiol Int 1999; 16(2):213–222.
6. Ebisawa T, Uchiyama M, Kajimura N, et al. Association of structural polymorphisms in the human period3 gene with delayed sleep phase syndrome. EMBO Rep 2001; 2(4):342–346.
7. Uchiyama M, Okawa M, Shibui K, et al. Poor compensatory function for sleep loss as a pathogenic factor in patients with delayed sleep phase syndrome. Sleep 2000; 23(4):553–558.
8. Dagan Y, Sela H, Omer H, et al. High prevalence of personality disorders among circadian rhythm sleep disorders (CRSD) patients. J Psychosom Res 1996; 41(4):357–363.
9. Dagan Y, Stein D, Steinbock M, et al. Frequency of delayed sleep phase syndrome among hospitalized adolescent psychiatric patients. J Psychosom Res 1998; 45(1 spec no.):15–20.
10. Szeinberg A, Borodkin K, Dagan Y. Treatment with melatonin for adolescents with delayed sleep phase syndrome. Clin Pediatr (Phila) 2006; 45(9):809–818.
11. Ando K, Kripke DF, Ancoli-Israel S. Estimated prevalence of delayed and advanced sleep phase syndromes. Sleep Res 1995; 24:509.
12. Toh KL, Jones CR, He Y, et al. An hPer2 phosphorylation site mutation in familial advanced sleep phase syndrome. Science 2001; 291(5506):1040–1043.
13. Ancoli-Israel S, Schnierow B, Kelsoe J, et al. A pedigree of one family with delayed sleep phase syndrome. Chronobiol Int 2001; 18(5):831–840.
14. Masubuchi S, Hashimoto S, Endo T, et al. Amplitude reduction of plasma melatonin rhythm in association with an internal desynchronization in a subject with non-24-hour sleep–wake syndrome. Psychiatry Clin Neurosci 1999; 53(2):249–251.
15. McArthur AJ, Lewy AJ, Sack RL. Non-24-hour sleep–wake syndrome in a sighted man: circadian rhythm studies and efficacy of melatonin treatment. Sleep 1996; 19(7):544–553.
16. Kokkoris CP, Weitzman ED, Pollak CP, et al. Long-term ambulatory temperature monitoring in a subject with a hypernychthemeral sleep–wake cycle disturbance. Sleep 1978; 1(2):177–190.
17. Dagan Y, Ayalon L. Case study: psychiatric misdiagnosis of non-24-hours sleep–wake schedule disorder resolved by melatonin. J Am Acad Child Adolesc Psychiatry 2005; 44(12):1271–1275.
18. Dagan Y, Abadi J. Sleep–wake schedule disorder disability: a lifelong untreatable pathology of the circadian time structure. Chronobiol Int 2001; 18(6):1019–1027.
19. Cohen RA, Albers HE. Disruption of human circadian and cognitive regulation following a discrete hypothalamic lesion: a case study. Neurology 1991; 41(5):726–729.
20. Borodkin K, Ayalon L, Kanety H, et al. Dysregulation of circadian rhythms following prolactin-secreting pituitary microadenoma. Chronobiol Int 2005; 22(1):145–156.
21. Ayalon L, Borodkin K, Dishon L, et al. Circadian rhythm sleep disorders following mild traumatic brain injury. Neurology 2007; 68(14):1136–1140.
22. Boivin DB, James FO, Santo JB, et al. Non-24-hour sleep-wake syndrome following a car accident. Neurology 2003; 60(11):1841–1843.
23. Nagtegaal JE, Kerkhof GA, Smits MG, et al. Traumatic brain injury-associated delayed sleep phase syndrome. Funct Neurol 1997; 12(6):345–348.
24. Quinto C, Gellido C, Chokroverty S, et al. Posttraumatic delayed sleep phase syndrome. Neurology 2000; 54(1):250–252.
25. Witting W, Kwa IH, Eikelenboom P, et al. Alterations in the circadian rest-activity rhythm in aging and Alzheimer's disease. Biol Psychiatry 1990; 27(6):563–572.
26. Bliwise DL, Watts RL, Watts N, et al. Disruptive nocturnal behavior in Parkinson's disease and Alzheimer's disease. J Geriatr Psychiatry Neurol 1995; 8(2):107–110.
27. Wirz-Justice A, Cajochen C, Nussbaum P. A schizophrenic patient with an arrhythmic circadian rest-activity cycle. Psychiatry Res 1997; 73(1–2):83–90.
28. Wirz-Justice A, Haug HJ, Cajochen C. Disturbed circadian rest-activity cycles in schizophrenia patients: an effect of drugs? Schizophr Bull 2001; 27(3):497–502.
29. Wirz-Justice A, Werth E, Savaskan E, et al. Haloperidol disrupts, clozapine reinstates the circadian rest-activity cycle in a patient with early-onset Alzheimer disease. Alzheimer Dis Assoc Disord 2000; 14(4):212–215.

30. Ayalon L, Hermesh H, Dagan Y. Case study of circadian rhythm sleep disorder following haloperidol treatment: reversal by risperidone and melatonin. Chronobiol Int 2002; 19(5):947–959.
31. Hermesh H, Lemberg H, Abadi J, et al. Circadian rhythm sleep disorders as a possible side effect of fluvoxamine. CNS Spectr 2001; 6(6):511–513.
32. Doljansky JT, Kannety H, Dagan Y. Working under daylight intensity lamp: an occupational risk for developing circadian rhythm sleep disorder? Chronobiol Int 2005; 22(3):597–605.

16 | Treatment of Circadian Rhythm Sleep Disorders

Robert L. Sack
Oregon Health and Sciences University, Portland, Oregon, U.S.A.

The thesis of this chapter is that a rational treatment approach to circadian rhythm sleep disorders (CRSDs) can be based on an understanding of the biology of the human circadian system. With this viewpoint in mind, the chapter will begin with a discussion of circadian misalignment—the pathophysiological mechanism that is thought to underlie most of the CRSDs. This will be followed by an overview of the circadian timing mechanisms that can be recruited to correct this misalignment. Finally, some specific recommendations will be made for treatment of each of the disorders, drawn from research in which the principles of circadian rhythm biology have been applied to the currently recognized CRSDs.

CIRCADIAN MISALIGNMENT: THE UNDERLYING PATHOPHYSIOLOGY OF CIRCADIAN RHYTHMS SLEEP DISORDERS

A description of the currently recognized CRSDs has been presented in an earlier chapter. Most of these disorders share a common element; namely, a misalignment of endogenous circadian rhythms, generated by the body clock, with the desired (or required) time for sleep. Both endogenous and exogenous factors can contribute to this circadian misalignment. For example, the vulnerability of teenagers and young adults to delayed sleep phase disorder (DSPD) could be due to both a lengthening of the intrinsic circadian period (perhaps related to hormonal influences) as well as socially reinforced behavior patterns, such as staying up late and "sleeping in."

The consequences of circadian misalignment can be satisfactorily explained by current theories of sleep regulation such as the opponent process model as formulated by Edgar et al. (1). This model postulates that the homeostatic and circadian mechanisms that control the sleep-wake cycle are normally synchronized with each other and with the 24-hour solar day-night cycle. During the day, the circadian system generates an alerting signal that counteracts (opposes) the expression of the homeostatic sleep drive. At night, the circadian alerting signal is withdrawn, and sleep commences and discharges the accumulated sleep drive through the night (Fig. 1).

When the homeostatic and circadian processes are out of alignment, sleep is undermined by an inappropriately timed circadian alerting signal. Moreover, the circadian alerting signal is absent when it is needed to counteract the expression of an accumulation of homeostatic sleep drive during wakefulness (Fig. 2). In addition to the disrupted timing of endogenous processes, attempted sleep at nonstandard times can be interrupted by exogenous factors such as ambient noise and light, as well as pressing social obligations. Furthermore, there is an unavoidable burden of sleep deprivation associated with sudden transitions in the timing of sleep. For example, the night worker who stays awake for 36 hours on the first tour of duty is acutely sleep deprived. The various consequences of circadian misalignment are illustrated in Figure 2 and discussed in the accompanying legend.

PRINCIPLES OF TREATMENT

Given that CRSDs involve a mismatch between the endogenous circadian rhythm and the desired (or required) time for sleep, there are three different treatment strategies that can be logically adopted: (1) circadian phase shifting ("resetting the body clock" to a more favorable

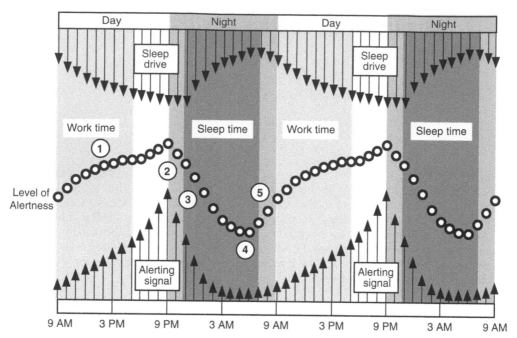

Figure 1   The opponent process model of sleep-wake regulation for a person on a conventional schedule [as proposed by Edgar et al. (1)] is presented in a double-plotted hypothetical diagram. According to the model, the level of alertness (*filled circles*) results from of the opposing forces of sleep drive (which accumulates in proportion to the duration of waking), and an alerting process, which is generated by the circadian pacemaker. (1) During the day, sleep drive accumulates, but is counteracted by the opposing alerting signal. (2) In the late afternoon or early evening, the alerting signal peaks, and there is a "forbidden zone" for sleep. (3) The alerting signal then recedes, and sleep commences and is sustained during the night. (4) The low point for alertness is coincident with the nadir of core body temperature. (5) At the time of final awakening, alertness and body temperature are rising and sleep drive has dissipated.

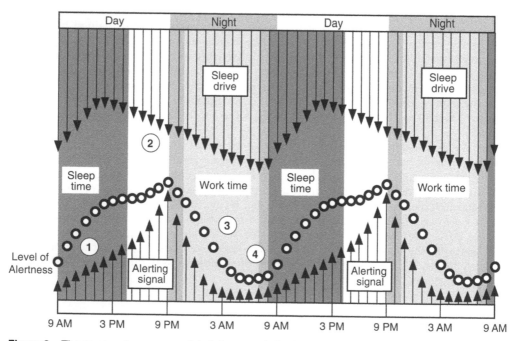

Figure 2   The opponent process model of sleep regulation in a night shift worker. This diagram assumes that a night shift worker has made no adaptation. (1) Sleep during the day is coincident with the circadian alerting process, and consequently sleep is shortened. (2) Overall sleep drive is increased because of relative sleep deprivation. (3) Work is coincident with a recession of the alerting process and in the context of accumulated sleep drive. (4) At the alertness minimum, sleep may be impossible to resist.

alignment), (2) prescribed sleep scheduling, based on circadian principles, that aims to minimize the consequences of circadian misalignment, and (3) pharmacotherapy aimed at counteracting the symptoms of sleepiness and insomnia generated by circadian misalignment. The principles for these interventions are described below.

Circadian Phase Shifting

Timed Light Exposure

It is well documented that mammalian circadian rhythms are primarily generated within the neurons of the suprachiasmatic nucleus (SCN) of the hypothalamus, and that in most humans, the intrinsic period of this rhythm is different from 24 hours—usually slightly longer [reviewed by Dijk and Lockley (2)]. Consequently, synchronization of the body clock with the 24-hour solar day (called *entrainment*) is a dynamic, ongoing process that depends on recurrent timing adjustments (phase resetting) of the body clock via exposure to the relevant environmental time cues (*zeitgebers*)—most importantly, the solar light-dark cycle. In the absence of these critical environmental timing signals (e.g., temporal isolation or total blindness), circadian rhythms will typically "free-run" on a non-24-hour cycle, expressing the intrinsic period of the circadian pacemaker.

Although it is now well established that the solar light-dark cycle is the primary cue for synchronizing the circadian system of most living organisms (both plant and animal), it was once thought that the human species, with more developed cognitive and social capacities, might be an exception; indeed, many patients implicitly hold the belief that these sleep disorders can be overcome with effort and willpower. However, the demonstration that light exposure could suppress melatonin secretion in humans, as it did in other species (if the light were sufficiently bright) (3), led to discoveries regarding the phase-resetting effects of light on the human circadian system (4,5). These discoveries were critical because they demonstrated the continuity between human and other mammalian circadian systems and gave rise to the clinical use of timed light exposure as a treatment for CRSDs.

Non-photic time cues such as the timing of sleep and exercise may have some influence on the body clock, but the potency of these cues in humans, compared with light exposure, appears to be relatively weak. Because people ordinarily sleep at night, in a dark space, with eyes closed, the timing of sleep inevitably gates the exposure to the light-dark cycle, and in this way, an individual's sleep schedule can significantly influence circadian rhythms by structuring the timing of light exposure.

The clock-resetting effects of light are critically dependent on the timing of exposure. In normally entrained individuals, light exposure in the morning resets the body clock to an earlier time (causes a phase advance), whereas light exposure in the evening resets the body clock to a later time (causes a phase delay). These timing-dependent effects of environmental cues on the circadian system can be plotted as a phase response curve (PRC) as shown in Figure 3. This *push-pull* effect of light helps to maintain the stability of the circadian system, but other factors may be involved as well. The magnitude of the phase shifts is greatest around the inflection point of the PRC (around 5 a.m. in normally entrained individuals) and is least (but not absent) with light exposure in midday [reviewed by Duffy and Wright (6)]. Thus, in the treatment of CRSDs, the timing of an intervention (e.g., prescribed bright light exposure) is often more important than the intensity (dose).

Recently, specialized photoreceptors (non-rod, non-cone) associated with the ganglion cells of the retina have been shown to be important for the phase-resetting effects of light on the circadian system (7)). These photoreceptors are maximally sensitive to blue-green light.

Although bright light exposure (3000–10,000 lux) has been shown to produce robust phase shifts, it has been shown that even modest intensities (100–550 lux) can produce substantial phase shifts if the light is presented to subjects who have been living in a constant dim light environment (8). Also, recent studies have shown that intermittent bright light exposure can produce almost as much phase shifting as continuous exposure (9). Thus, in addition to absolute intensity, both light exposure history and the contrast of the light exposure with the background intensity appear to be important for chronobiological effects. An experiment that reported phase-shifting effects of light exposure to the skin has not been replicated (10,11).

Questions have been raised about the safety of bright light exposure for humans, especially the possibility of phototoxic effects on the lens and/or the retina. To mimic sunlight,

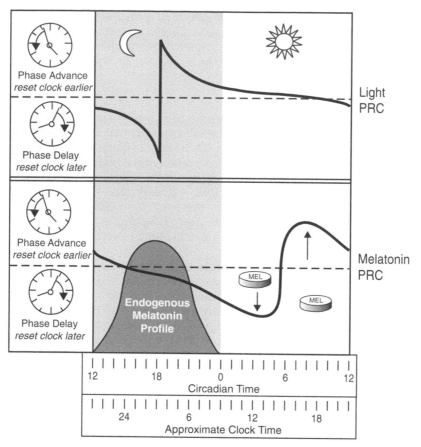

Figure 3 Schematic phase response curves (PRCs) for light and melatonin administration. The effects of light and melatonin are dependent on the timing of administration. The relationship can be plotted as a phase response curve. In summary, light exposure late in the day or melatonin administration in the morning will cause the circadian clock to shift later (a phase delay), while light exposure in the morning or melatonin administration late in the day will cause the circadian clock to shift earlier (a phase advance). Both PRCs have an inflection point, the crossover time between advances and delays. According to convention, circadian time 0 is the beginning of the light phase (daytime) and circadian time 12 is the beginning of the dark phase (nighttime).

some early experiments involved "full spectrum" light sources that included ultraviolet (UV) radiation, but there is now a consensus that UV wavelengths are unnecessary for the phase-shifting effect of light and should be avoided (12). A diffuser panel placed over the light sources effectively filters UV radiation. Because most light sources used for treatment are no brighter than ordinary sunlight, they would seem to be as safe. However, caution is in order for patients with ocular pathology (e.g., lenticular cataracts or retinal degeneration).

In summary, the chronobiological effects of light are dependent on intensity, timing, wavelength, pattern (intermittent or continuous), duration, exposure history, and the level of contrast with background light exposure. The exact importance of each of these parameters remains to be worked out. It is customary in clinical practice to employ light exposure from a commercially available light source that generates diffuse illumination with an intensity of 3000 to 10,000 lux for 30 to 60 minutes. The light exposure should be integrated into some other activity (e.g., eating, watching television, reading) if it is to be carried out on a regular basis. The light can be indirect (patients do not need to stare at the light box). Used in this way, timed bright light exposure appears to be safe within the parameters that have been tested. An artificial light source may be unnecessary if appropriately timed exposure to ordinary daylight is an option.

If the goal is to synchronize the circadian system to the desired (or required) sleep schedule, timed light exposure should, in principle, be a helpful intervention for almost all of the CRSDs, although it may be impractical or even impossible to carry out in some circumstances. In addition to timed light exposure, eliminating (or reducing) the unwanted effects of light on the circadian system (e.g., wearing goggles to prevent light-induced phase shifting) has been proven effective in several simulated shift work studies (13,14).

Timed Melatonin Administration

Melatonin administration to both animals and humans has been shown to shift circadian rhythms and to entrain free-running rhythms. As with light exposure, the effects of melatonin administration are dependent on the timing (phase) of administration. For normally entrained individuals, melatonin administration in the morning shifts rhythms later while melatonin administration in the evening shifts rhythms earlier (Fig. 3). In other words, the melatonin PRC is about 180 degrees out of phase with the light PRC, and therefore, melatonin can be thought of as a "darkness signal." It is tempting to speculate that endogenous melatonin secretion at night may have a role in promoting the stability of the circadian system, but this remains to be clearly demonstrated.

A variety of doses of melatonin have been used for phase shifting, and it appears that the shape of a dose response curve for this effect is rather flat; that is, there is not much difference in effect between lower and higher doses. Recent studies suggest that timing is more important than dose. In fact, one study indicated that a high dose was less effective than a low dose for entrainment of a blind person with free-running rhythms, possibly because the high dose interacted with both the advance and delay portions of the melatonin PRC (15). Melatonin probably has some direct soporific effects, especially at higher doses and when administered at times when endogenous melatonin is not being secreted (16). Appropriately timed melatonin and light exposure may be synergistic, but it is less clear that melatonin can overcome the effect of light exposure on the circadian system, if light and melatonin are promoting shifts in opposite directions.

Although melatonin has not been approved by the Food and Drug Administration (FDA) as a drug, it is widely available in the United States as a "nutritional supplement." Concerns have been raised about the purity of the available preparations as well as the reliability of stated doses. Labels that feature a GMP seal, which stands for *Good Manufacturing Practice*, provide some assurance of the purity and accuracy of stated doses.

Generally available formulations of 3 mg produce blood levels that are at least 10-fold higher than physiological concentrations; however, no serious adverse reactions have been attributed to these supraphysiological doses. Recently, a melatonin agonist ramelteon has been licensed as a hypnotic in the United States, and other agonists are in development. Animal studies suggest that ramelteon has phase-shifting effects that are analogous to melatonin (17), but at this time, no studies have been reported in humans.

Other Phase-Shifting Treatments

Timed vigorous exercise has been tested for its phase-shifting effects, but the results are not robust. In some experiments, animals have been entrained to the time of feeding, but this time cue has not been demonstrated to be effective in humans.

Prescribed Sleep Scheduling

The term *chronotherapy* was originally coined to describe a prescribed sleep schedule treatment of DSPD. It was based on the discovery that the human circadian period is usually longer than 24 hours (18) and might be exceptionally long in patients with DSPD. This could explain the great difficulty these patients have in shifting their circadian pacemaker and sleep schedule to an earlier time. With chronotherapy, the timing of sleep is *intentionally delayed* several hours per day until it is aligned to a targeted bedtime. After this goal is achieved, patients are advised to scrupulously maintain a regular sleep-wake schedule. If relapse occurs, the procedure is repeated.

Certain recommendations for rotating night work can be thought of as sleep schedule prescriptions based on similar circadian considerations; that is, emphasizing delays rather than advances. For example, it has been suggested that rotating shifts should be scheduled in a clockwise direction. Another, more refined, proposed schedule for shift workers involves gradual delays in the timing of sleep that are consistent with an understanding that the circadian pacemaker can only be reset an hour or two per day (19).

Symptomatic Treatment: Counteracting Insomnia

As discussed above, the circadian pacemaker generates an alerting signal during the day (in diurnal species) that counteracts the expression of accumulated homeostatic sleep drive (1). During the normal time for sleep at night, this alerting signal is withdrawn. In CRSDs, there is a mismatch so that the circadian alerting signal occurs during the desired (or required) time for sleep, potentially generating insomnia, usually manifested as foreshortened sleep. Hypnotic drugs or other treatments for insomnia can be justified to counteract the unwelcome clock-dependent alerting in patients with CRSDs.

Symptomatic Treatment: Counteracting Excessive Sleepiness

The symptom of excessive sleepiness in CRSD can be explained in two ways: (*i*) because circadian misalignment causes foreshortened or inefficient sleep, there is an accumulation of sleep drive; and (*ii*) because of circadian misalignment, clock-dependent alerting does not occur when the person is awake.

Caffeine is the most widely used alerting agent in our culture and is effective in counteracting sleepiness from almost any cause. Amphetamine-related drugs are more potent than caffeine and may be indicated in some patients with CRSDs. However, modafinil is the only drug that has been approved by the FDA for a CRSD; namely, night shift sleep disorder.

TREATMENT SUGGESTIONS FOR SPECIFIC CIRCADIAN RHYTHM SLEEP DISORDERS

Having discussed some of the overarching principles, we now turn to the therapy of specific CRSDs. Treatment needs to be preceded by a careful history to rule out other primary sleep disorders and to characterize behavior patterns (e.g., ill-timed recreational or social activities) or other factors (e.g., chronic illness, medication side effects, caffeine intake) that may be exacerbating the problem. Also, it is very important to set realistic goals for treatment that the patient is clearly motivated to accomplish. If the problem is impacting the family, they should be involved in the treatment as well.

Treatment of Delayed Sleep Phase Type

Delayed sleep phase disorder (DSPD), first described by Weitzman et al. (20), is characterized by a stable sleep schedule that is at least two hours later than the conventional or desired time. Patients with DSPD consult sleep specialists because they are unable to conform to conventional work schedules or other social demands. A tendency for a delayed sleep schedule is very common in adolescence and can lead to academic failure. Weitzman originally proposed that a significant number of patients diagnosed with sleep-onset insomnia may have underlying DSPD—a tantalizing but unproven hypothesis.

It is often suggested that patients with DSPD have an intrinsic circadian period that is longer than average and that is why they have such difficulty advancing their body clock. However, other mechanisms such as a sub-sensitivity to the phase-advancing effects of light, could explain the disorder (for a detailed review, see Ref. 21).

Clock Resetting with Light

In an early study, Rosenthal et al. (22) treated 20 DSPD patients for two weeks with two hours of bright light exposure (2500 lux) in the morning (between 6 and 9 a.m.) using an artificial source ("light box"), combined with restricted light exposure in the evening. The active treatment was compared with two hours of ordinary morning light exposure (300 lux) in a crossover design. The bright light treatment produced an increase in morning alertness as measured with the multiple sleep latency test (MSLT) as well as significant phase advances of the core body temperature rhythm.

In clinical practice, an artificial light source may be unnecessary if the wake-up time occurs after sunrise; going outside into sunlight for 20 to 30 minutes upon awakening may provide sufficient exposure. On the other hand, patients with DSPD often have considerable morning sleep inertia, and getting them out of bed on time for either natural or artificial light exposure can be challenging and may require help from the family. The optimal duration for morning bright light exposure is unknown, and practical adjustments and arrangements need to be negotiated with the patient. We aim for at least 30 minutes, integrated with other morning activities such as eating breakfast or applying makeup.

Clock Resetting with Melatonin
Using a crossover design, Dahlitz et al. gave eight patients DSPD melatonin (5 mg) or placebo at 10 p.m., five hours before the average time of sleep onset as determined by pretrial sleep logs (23). With melatonin treatment, sleep onset times were shifted earlier (mean 82 minutes) as were wake times (mean 117 minutes). Similar results were obtained by Nagtegaal et al. who also showed a 1.5 hour advance of the endogenous melatonin onset (24).

Treatment with melatonin is most effective if the dose is administered at the optimal time point of the melatonin PRC for advancing rhythms. Until the dim light melatonin onset (DLMO) (25), or some other circadian marker, becomes clinically available, appropriate timing has to be estimated. In our clinic, we provide the patient with a schedule that initiates treatment (0.5 or 3 mg) about three hours prior to habitual bedtime and then gradually shifts the timing earlier over a period of several weeks. When the targeted sleep schedule has been achieved, the timing of light exposure and melatonin administration can remain constant.

Prescribed Sleep Schedule
The use of chronotherapy (systematically delaying sleep times by about three hours per day around the clock) has been discussed above. Although it requires a high level of patient compliance, it is rational and can be quite effective, but there are no controlled studies of its safety and efficacy. In our clinic, we more commonly prescribe a sleep schedule that slowly advances bedtimes in conjunction with treatments that promote circadian phase advances (see combination treatment below).

Symptom Control
Hypnotic medications have not been systematically tested for DSPD and are not recommended as monotherapy, but can be a reasonable adjunctive measure for those nights when the patient's sleep latency extends 30 minutes beyond the prescribed bedtime (see below).

Combination Treatment
In our clinic, evening melatonin and morning bright light are often prescribed in tandem utilizing a schedule [provided by a computer-generated worksheet (Table 1)] that gradually advances the timing of attempted sleep and the timing of both treatments by 15 to 30 minutes every few days. These gradual shifts in schedule are based on the presumption that large circadian "phase jumps" are difficult to achieve, especially phase advances, and therefore, attempting to shift sleep times too quickly may lead to failure and the abandonment of treatment. Once the desired schedule is accomplished, maintenance treatment with light and melatonin can be continued on a stable, fixed schedule.

Many patients with DSPD have a strong personal preference for being awake late at night (e.g., they may enjoy the solitude at this time of day), and unless there is a serious consequence such as failing in school or losing a job, they may not want to change their sleep schedule. Consequently, cultivating patient motivation is important for the success of any treatment for DSPD. With adolescents, a great deal of tension has often developed with their parents regarding sleep schedules. To reduce unproductive blaming, we spend considerable time and effort educating patients and their parents about the factors that regulate circadian rhythms and sleep, attempting to frame the problem in a more dispassionate way.

Treatment of Advanced Sleep Phase Disorder
Advanced sleep phase disorder (ASPD) is characterized by a sleep schedule that is persistently several hours earlier than the conventional or desired time. ASPD is thought to be much less common than DSPD, but because an early sleep pattern results in fewer social conflicts (people are not usually punished for getting to work too early), the incidence of ASPD may be underestimated. A familial form has been described to be associated with a specific clock

Table 1 Proposed Sleep, Light Exposure, and Medication Schedule for Delayed Sleep Phase Disorder

| Date | Wake up | Bright light exposure | | Melatonin (3 mg) | Targeted bedtime | Sleeping pill, if needed |
		Start	Stop			
1/2/2007	11:00 a.m.	11:00 a.m.	12:00 p.m.	1:00 a.m.	3:00 a.m.	3:30 a.m.
1/3/2007	11:00 a.m.	11:00 a.m.	12:00 p.m.	1:00 a.m.	3:00 a.m.	3:30 a.m.
1/4/2007	11:00 a.m.	11:00 a.m.	12:00 p.m.	1:00 a.m.	3:00 a.m.	3:30 a.m.
1/5/2007	10:30 a.m.	10:30 a.m.	11:30 a.m.	12:30 a.m.	2:30 a.m.	3:00 a.m.
1/6/2007	10:30 a.m.	10:30 a.m.	11:30 a.m.	12:30 a.m.	2:30 a.m.	3:00 a.m.
1/7/2007	10:30 a.m.	10:30 a.m.	11:30 a.m.	12:30 a.m.	2:30 a.m.	3:00 a.m.
1/8/2007	10:00 a.m.	10:00 a.m.	11:00 a.m.	12:00 a.m.	2:00 a.m.	2:30 a.m.
1/9/2007	10:00 a.m.	10:00 a.m.	11:00 a.m.	12:00 a.m.	2:00 a.m.	2:30 a.m.
1/10/2007	10:00 a.m.	10:00 a.m.	11:00 a.m.	12:00 a.m.	2:00 a.m.	2:30 a.m.
1/11/2007	9:30 a.m.	9:30 a.m.	10:30 a.m.	11:30 p.m.	1:30 a.m.	2:00 a.m.
1/12/2007	9:30 a.m.	9:30 a.m.	10:30 a.m.	11:30 p.m.	1:30 a.m.	2:00 a.m.
1/13/2007	9:30 a.m.	9:30 a.m.	10:30 a.m.	11:30 p.m.	1:30 a.m.	2:00 a.m.
1/14/2007	9:00 a.m.	9:00 a.m.	10:00 a.m.	11:00 p.m.	1:00 a.m.	1:30 a.m.
1/15/2007	9:00 a.m.	9:00 a.m.	10:00 a.m.	11:00 p.m.	1:00 a.m.	1:30 a.m.
1/16/2007	9:00 a.m.	9:00 a.m.	10:00 a.m.	11:00 p.m.	1:00 a.m.	1:30 a.m.
1/17/2007	8:30 a.m.	8:30 a.m.	9:30 a.m.	10:30 p.m.	12:30 a.m.	1:00 a.m.
1/18/2007	8:30 a.m.	8:30 a.m.	9:30 a.m.	10:30 p.m.	12:30 a.m.	1:00 a.m.
1/19/2007	8:30 a.m.	8:30 a.m.	9:30 a.m.	10:30 p.m.	12:30 a.m.	1:00 a.m.
1/20/2007	8:00 a.m.	8:00 a.m.	9:00 a.m.	10:00 p.m.	12:00 a.m.	12:30 a.m.
1/21/2007	8:00 a.m.	8:00 a.m.	9:00 a.m.	10:00 p.m.	12:00 a.m.	12:30 a.m.
1/22/2007	8:00 a.m.	8:00 a.m.	9:00 a.m.	10:00 p.m.	12:00 a.m.	12:30 a.m.
1/23/2007	7:30 a.m.	7:30 a.m.	8:30 a.m.	9:30 p.m.	11:30 p.m.	12:00 a.m.
1/24/2007	7:30 a.m.	7:30 a.m.	8:30 a.m.	9:30 p.m.	11:30 p.m.	12:00 a.m.
1/25/2007	7:30 a.m.	7:30 a.m.	8:30 a.m.	9:30 p.m.	11:30 p.m.	12:00 a.m.
1/26/2007	7:00 a.m.	7:00 a.m.	8:00 a.m.	9:00 p.m.	11:00 p.m.	11:30 p.m.

Current average wake-up time is 11.00 a.m.
This table was generated by a spreadsheet incorporating the premise that treatment of DSPD can be accomplished by gradual phase advances (30 minutes every three days) augmented by morning light exposure, evening melatonin, and sleeping medication, when necessary. The rate of phase advancement can be altered depending on the needs and progress of the patient.

gene mutation, and a shortening of circadian period was demonstrated in one of the family members; however, other mechanisms may be involved. As normal people age, bedtimes, wake times, and circadian markers often shift earlier (26,27). Older patients may be diagnosed with ASPD, although the etiology might be different from younger people; for example, it might be related to a decrease in homeostatic sleep drive (28) that results in early morning awakening and light exposure that secondarily causes an advance in the circadian pacemaker.

Clock Resetting with Light
According to circadian principles, light exposure in the evening or melatonin administration in the morning should counteract the tendency for phase-advanced rhythms. Most of the research has been focused on older people with advanced sleep schedules and sleep maintenance insomnia who may not meet the full criteria for ASPD. Although light-induced phase delays have been reported (29), the treatment was not well tolerated and was not continued after the experimental period. In summary, evening light exposure can be tried as a method for delaying rhythms, but clinical research on ASPD has been quite limited.

Clock Resetting with Melatonin
Although there are no systematic reports of melatonin administration for ASPD, low doses of melatonin (e.g., 0.5 mg), upon early awakening, can be tried as a method to promote phase delays. Higher doses might cause some daytime drowsiness.

Prescribed Sleep Schedules
Chronotherapy (systematic sleep scheduling), shifting sleep around the clock in an advance direction, was found to be effective in one case of ASPD (30).

Symptom Control
Because patients with ASPD are unable to stay up late enough to enjoy social or cultural activities, the intermittent use of a low-dose, short-acting stimulant (e.g., ritalin 5 mg) to counteract evening sleepiness may be useful. A short-acting hypnotic such as zaleplon could be used as a middle-of-the-night sleeping aid.

Combination Treatment
A combination of the treatments described above could be tried as there are no known adverse interactions.

Treatment of Shift Work Type CRSD
Shift work is a term that applies to a broad spectrum on nonstandard work schedules including permanent night shifts, rotating shifts, and random work schedules. It can also apply to schedules demanding an early awakening from nocturnal sleep. About one in five workers in the United States do some form of shift work, women almost as frequently as men (31). Rapidly rotating shifts clearly do not allow sufficient time for circadian adaptation, and even permanent night workers compromise adaptation by adopting a conventional schedule on their days off. In addition to circadian misalignment, the burdens of shift work involve social conflicts as well as sleep deprivation from interruptions during nonstandard sleep times.

There is presumably a subset of shift workers who, for a variety of reasons, fail to adapt to their required work and sleep schedule and meet criteria for a formal diagnosis of shift work sleep disorder (32). However, the boundary between a non-pathological, normally expected response to an unnatural situation and a diagnosable disorder is not easy to determine. Most of the interventional research studies on shift work have been done in a laboratory setting, employing a simulated shift work protocol; far fewer have been carried out in the field.

The prevailing belief is that most shift workers do not shift their circadian rhythms to match their nonstandard sleep schedules. However, some field studies, using standard circadian phase makers, have documented phase resetting—at least in some people—indicating that it is possible. On the other hand, even if phase shifting can be accomplished, many night workers would find it undesirable because they would be out of phase on their days off.

Clock Resetting with Timed Light Exposure
Experimental protocols, in which subjects are placed in a controlled environment on a sleep-wake schedule that simulates shift work, have amply demonstrated that appropriately timed bright light exposure can facilitate adaptive phase shifts (33). Furthermore, Eastman et al. have shown that wearing dark goggles on the morning commute home, to minimize phase advances, can facilitate adaptive phase delays (14).

Field studies have provided some confidence that this strategy can be used in the "real world." For example, Boivin and James (34) treated 10 night duty nurses for the first six hours of their shift with intermittent bright light exposure administered when the subjects were working at their nurse's station. The bright light treatment was combined with morning light avoidance by wearing goggles on the commute home. Circadian phase shifts in the treated group were significantly greater than in nine untreated workers on the same schedule. Treatment normalized the phase angle with daytime sleep and lengthened the duration of daytime sleep. Despite these kinds of encouraging results, bright light treatment has not been adopted widely as a treatment for shift work disorder, presumably because of the expense and difficulty in incorporating it into the work environment.

Clock Resetting with Melatonin
As with light treatment, melatonin administration can facilitate phase shifts in simulated shift work experiments (33). However, a field study done by our group (35) illustrates both the efficacy and the complexity of melatonin treatment. Permanent night nurses ($N = 24$) who

worked seven consecutive shifts alternating with seven days off (a "7–70 schedule") were treated with melatonin (0.5 mg) or placebo at bedtime for four weeks in a crossover design. Nine of the subjects shifted equally well on placebo or melatonin, and eight failed to shift with either treatment. Seven were specific melatonin responders; that is, they failed to shift with placebo but shifted with melatonin treatment. Melatonin given just prior to daytime sleep may produce a hypnotic effect (perhaps by counteracting the unwelcome daytime circadian alerting signal) as well as promote phase resetting. In summary, some night workers do not need treatment, others fail melatonin treatment, and some respond specifically to melatonin treatment.

Symptom Control: Promoting Sleep
Hypnotic medications have been used to promote daytime sleep, both in simulated shift work studies and in field studies (36,37). However, the increase of time asleep with hypnotic use does not necessarily counteract the circadian-mediated dip in nighttime alertness. The usual misgivings about hypnotics apply, but in some cases, regular treatment can be quite appropriate.

Symptom Control: Promoting Alertness
In the largest ($N = 209$), double-blind, placebo-controlled study of shift workers to date, Czeisler et al. (38) tested modafinil (300 mg) as a treatment to counteract excessive sleepiness during night work. At baseline, and then on three occasions, one month apart, MSLTs, clinical symptom ratings, and simple reaction time performance testing were performed. Modafinil produced a modest, but statistically significant, lengthening of nighttime sleep latency (1.7 ± 0.4 vs. 0.3 ± 0.3 minutes; $p = 0.002$). Self-rated symptom improvement occurred in 74% of those treated versus 36% on placebo. There were concomitant improvements in performance measures. Although modafinil counteracted nighttime sleepiness, it did not restore alertness to a daytime level. It is unknown whether a higher dose would have produced a more robust effect.

In several studies, caffeine has been shown to be an effective countermeasure for sleepiness during night work or experimentally induced sleep deprivation (39,40).

Combination Treatment
Although good treatments are available, shift workers who are having problems with their sleep and alertness do not often seek help from sleep clinics but rather assume that their sleep and alertness burdens are unavoidable and untreatable. Given the wide variety of shift work schedules and the various desires of patients, treatment should be tailored to meet the needs of the individual workers. For an occasional overnight duty (e.g., 24-hour duty in the emergency room), phase resetting would not be possible or desirable. A stimulant medication to maintain alertness during the shift and perhaps a hypnotic for daytime sleep might be indicated. For workers on a steady night shift (who maintain a relative nocturnal orientation on their days off), promoting phase resetting with light exposure or melatonin would be more logical. For a worker who is at risk for costly mistakes (e.g., a nuclear power plant supervisor), more aggressive treatment may be required. Some people are very intolerant of shift work and may need a medical authorization to be excused.

Treatment of Jet Lag
The circadian misalignment associated with jet lag sleep disorder is the inevitable consequence of crossing time zones too rapidly for the circadian system to keep pace. Depending on the number and direction of time zones crossed, it may take days or even weeks for the circadian system to resynchronize. The intensity and duration of the jet lag symptoms are related to (*i*) the number of time zones crossed, (*ii*) the direction of travel (*iii*), the ability to sleep while traveling, (*iv*) the availability and intensity of local circadian time cues upon arrival, and (*v*) individual differences in tolerance to circadian misalignment. Long-distance jet travel can also be associated with sleep deprivation caused by sitting in a cramped seat all night and drinking too much coffee or alcohol. Jet lag is generally benign and self limited, but travel time is precious, and therefore, treatment, if safe and effective, is warranted.

There are two potential targets for treatment. The first involves accelerating the rate of resynchronization (re-entrainment) using timed light exposure or melatonin. The second involves alleviating the symptoms of jet lag, particularly insomnia, with hypnotic medications and, possibly, daytime sleepiness with alerting agents. The gastrointestinal dysfunction associated with jet lag can be targeted as well. Our patient recommendations for jet lag are summarized in Table 2.

Clock Resetting with Melatonin
Melatonin has been found to be helpful for jet lag in a number of well-controlled trials (for a systematic, evidence-based review, see Ref. 41). It is of interest that most studies have tested it

Table 2 Recommendations for Counteracting Jet Lag

	Traveling Westward	Traveling Eastward
	Getting ready to travel	
Light exposure	Go to bed later and get up later for a few days before your trip. Get plenty of bright light exposure in the evening.	Go to bed earlier and get up earlier for a few days before your trip. Get plenty of bright light exposure in the morning.
Sleep	Don't leave packing, etc. to the last minute. Get a good night's sleep the night before your flight. If possible, schedule your flight at a time that won't cut your prior sleep time short.	
Melatonin	Take 0.5 mg (low dose) at 6 a.m. on the day of departure.	Take 0.5 to 3 mg at 3 p.m. on the day of departure.
	In flight	
Comfort	Go first class if you can afford it.	
Food and drink	Stay hydrated (drink lots of water). No coffee if you expect to sleep. Go easy on the alcohol—don't drink if you intend to use a sleeping pill.	
Sleep	If you can, get some sleep during the flight, but don't expect your usual amount. When attempting to sleep, use an eye mask, ear plugs and a pillow.	
Sleeping medication	A very short acting sleeping pill (e.g., zaleplon) can help you sleep during the flight. (A longer acting one could leave you feeling groggy upon arrival).	
Avoid blood clots (deep vein thrombosis)	Sitting for a long time can increase the risk of getting a blood clot in your leg. Change position and walk around when you can. Taking an aspirin can help to prevent blood clots.	
	Upon arrival	
Sleep	Expect trouble *staying* asleep.	Expect trouble *getting* to sleep.
Napping	Take a nap if you are tired, but keep it as short as possible (you don't want to undermine your nighttime sleep).	
Sleeping medication	Take a longer acting sleeping medication (zolpidem, iszopiclone) at bedtime (if needed) until you have adjusted to local time.	
Melatonin	Take 0.5 mg (low dose) if you wake up too early (it will extend your night).	Take 0.5 to 3 mg at bedtime on the first night. Then 1 hour earlier each night until you feel adapted to local time.
Light exposure	Get bright light exposure in the evening.	Bright light exposure in the morning.
Light exposure if your travel is over 8 time zones	For the first 2 days after arrival, avoid bright light for 2–3 hours before going to bed for; then get bright light exposure in the evening.	For the first 2 days after arrival, avoid bright light for the first 2–3 hours after getting up. Then get bright light exposure in the morning.

for eastward flight, when a bedtime dose might have hypnotic effects as well as promote phase advance clock resetting. With westward flight, melatonin taken at bedtime could (in theory) inhibit clock resetting in the desired delay direction. Timing is therefore as important as dose (studies have tested doses ranging from 0.5 to 10 mg for up to three days prior to departure and up to five days upon arrival at the destination).

Clock Resetting with Timed Light Exposure
A number of studies of simulated jet lag have demonstrated accelerated re-entrainment using appropriately timed light exposure; however, there are almost no field trials. In most cases, natural daylight at the destination would be expected to facilitate circadian adaptation to local time. However, as Daan and Lewy pointed out (42), travel over about eight time zones will result in light hitting on the "wrong" part of the light PRC. Avoiding bright light after long flights (greater than eight time zones) for the first few hours in the morning after eastward travel or a few hours in the evening after westward travel should help to minimize this problem. After a few days, the light PRC will have presumably shifted enough so that light avoidance will not be needed. Eastman et al. demonstrated that almost complete circadian adaptation can be accomplished with planned light exposure for the week prior to travel (43), but this requires more effort than most people want to invest.

Symptom Control: Promoting Sleep
As jet lag–induced insomnia is self limited, a short course of hypnotic pharmacological treatment can be readily justified, and a number of field trials have demonstrated a benefit. On the other hand, adverse effects have been reported; for example, triazolam was implicated in several dramatic cases of global amnesia following its use to promote sleep during jet travel (44); concurrent consumption of alcohol may have been a contributing factor in these adverse events. The immobility associated with hypnotic use might increase the risk for deep vein thrombosis, known to be a risk of jet travel.

Symptom Control: Promoting Alertness
Increased coffee consumption is the first countermeasure most travelers use to combat wake time sleepiness, but elevated caffeine levels may exacerbate jet lag–induced insomnia. Modafinil has been shown to improve alertness in phase-shifting experiments that simulate jet lag, but there have been no field studies to date.

Treatment of Non-24-Hour Sleep Disorder (Sighted)
Clock Resetting with Timed Light Exposure
Non-24-hour (free-running) CRSD is uncommon in sighted people, so almost all we know about the disorder has come from a few case reports. For reasons that remain obscure, the timing of sleep persistently delays, expressing a free-running period of greater than 24 hours, presumably reflecting the intrinsic rhythm of the pacemaker (as if the person were in temporal isolation). Bright light exposure was found to successfully entrain circadian rhythms in several case reports; however, no placebo-controlled trials have been conducted.

Clock Resetting with Melatonin
A few case reports have also reported successful treatment with melatonin administered around the time of the desired bedtime, or when it would be predicted to cause a phase advance. The most common dose was 3 mg, and the duration of treatment ranged from one month to six years.

Prescribed Sleep Scheduling
Almost by definition, patients with this diagnosis are unable to adapt to a prescribed sleep schedule.

Combination Treatment

Non-24-hour CRSD may be an extreme form of DSPD, and similar treatment strategies can be tried; for example, morning light exposure, evening melatonin, and intermittent hypnotics (as described above).

Treatment of Non-24-Hour Sleep Disorder (Blind)

Although non-24-hour CRSD is very rare in normally sighted people, about half of the totally blind, who have no access to the entraining effects of light, have free-running circadian rhythms. For some, recurrent symptoms of daytime sleepiness and nighttime insomnia, when their rhythms are out of phase, are very burdensome.

Entrainment with Melatonin

Daily melatonin administration has been shown to entrain free-running rhythms in totally blind subjects (45,46) and appears to be the current treatment of choice. In a study by our group (46), six out of seven subjects entrained to 10 mg given at the usual bedtime for three to nine weeks. Subsequently, treatment was repeated in three subjects, starting with a 10-mg dose that was gradually stepped down every other week to 0.5 mg. Entrainment was maintained, even at the lowest dose, and free-running rhythms recurred after the cessation of treatment. Later, these same subjects were successfully entrained with 0.5 mg de novo (47). Furthermore, the blind subject who failed to entrain in the initial trial to 10 mg was subsequently entrained with a 0.5-mg dose (15). The effectiveness of the lower dose was attributed to its selective activity on the advance zone of the melatonin PRC with no "spillover" to the delay zone. In a recent trial by another group (48), a 0.5-mg dose entrained 6 out of 10 subjects. In summary, the evidence is compelling that melatonin can entrain the majority of totally blind patients with non-24-hour CRSD. A *physiological* dose (0.5 mg) appears to be as effective as a *pharmacological* dose (5 to 10 mg), and in some cases, more effective.

Treatment of Irregular CRSD

In this disorder, sleep and wake times tend to be randomly distributed over the night and day. The diagnosis is uncommon in healthy adults and is usually associated with dementia, retardation, or brain injury. Patients with irregular CRSD cause their caretakers to lose sleep, and consequently, it is the caretakers who often bring them to medical attention. Rarely, the pattern is seen in otherwise normal individuals with either very poor sleep hygiene or no apparent etiology.

The goal of therapy is to consolidate sleep, as much as possible, into a major nighttime bout. Bright light exposure during the day (sometimes combined with more intense social activity) has been used with some success in institutional settings. In brain-injured children with mental retardation, moderately high-dose bedtime melatonin has been used with some success. The usual sedative/hypnotic drugs can be justified in difficult cases, but may make matters worse if they cause confusion and disorientation. Stimulant medications during the day have not been tested but might be justified in some individuals.

CONCLUSIONS

The first priority in the treatment of CRSDs is to educate patients about circadian rhythms, sleep, and the consequences of circadian misalignment, the probable underlying cause for their symptoms. Furthermore, successful treatment requires a therapeutic alliance based on a good understanding of what the patient hopes to obtain from treatment. The delineation of the PRCs for light exposure and melatonin administration has provided the clinician with at least two strategies for resetting of the body clock to match the desired (or required) sleep schedule, thereby addressing circadian misalignment. When clock resetting is impractical, unsuccessful, or undesirable, the symptoms of sleepiness and insomnia (however unconventional the sleep-wake schedule) can be counteracted with stimulant or hypnotic medications.

REFERENCES

1. Edgar DM, Dement WC, Fuller CA. Effect of SCN lesions on sleep in squirrel monkeys: evidence for opponent processes in sleep-wake regulation. J Neurosci 1993; 13(3):1065–1079.
2. Dijk DJ, Lockley SW. Integration of human sleep-wake regulation and circadian rhythmicity. J Appl Physiol 2002; 92(2):852–862.
3. Lewy AJ, Wehr TA, Goodwin FK, et al. Light suppresses melatonin secretion in humans. Science 1980; 210(4475):1267–1269.
4. Czeisler CA, Allan JS, Strogatz SH, et al. Bright light resets the human circadian pacemaker independent of the timing of the sleep-wake cycle. Science 1986; 233(4764):667–671.
5. Lewy AJ, Sack RL, Miller LS, et al. Antidepressant and circadian phase-shifting effects of light. Science 1987; 235(4786):352–354.
6. Duffy JF, Wright KP Jr. Entrainment of the human circadian system by light. J Biol Rhythms 2005; 20(4):326–338.
7. Rollag MD, Berson DM, Provencio I. Melanopsin, ganglion-cell photoreceptors, and mammalian photoentrainment. J Biol Rhythms 2003; 18(3):227–234.
8. Zeitzer JM, Dijk DJ, Kronauer R, et al. Sensitivity of the human circadian pacemaker to nocturnal light: melatonin phase resetting and suppression. J Physiol 2000; 526 pt 3:695–702.
9. Gronfier C, Wright KP Jr., Kronauer RE, et al. Efficacy of a single sequence of intermittent bright light pulses for delaying circadian phase in humans. Am J Physiol Endocrinol Metab 2004; 287(1):E174–E181.
10. Eastman CI, Martin SK, Hebert M. Failure of extraocular light to facilitate circadian rhythm reentrainment in humans. Chronobiol Int 2000; 17(6):807–826.
11. Wright KP Jr., Czeisler CA. Absence of circadian phase resetting in response to bright light behind the knees. Science 2002; 297(5581):571.
12. Reme CE, Rol P, Grothmann K, et al. Bright light therapy in focus: lamp emission spectra and ocular safety. Technol Health Care 1996; 4(4):403–413.
13. Crowley SJ, Lee C, Tseng CY, et al. Combinations of bright light, scheduled dark, sunglasses, and melatonin to facilitate circadian entrainment to night shift work. J Biol Rhythms 2003; 18(6):513–523.
14. Eastman CI, Stewart KT, Mahoney MP, et al. Dark goggles and bright light improve circadian rhythm adaptation to night-shift work. Sleep 1994; 17(6):535–543.
15. Lewy AJ, Emens JS, Sack RL, et al. Low, but not high, doses of melatonin entrained a free-running blind person with a long circadian period. Chronobiol Int 2002; 19(3):649–658.
16. Wyatt JK, Dijk DJ, Ritz-de Cecco A, et al. Sleep-facilitating effect of exogenous melatonin in healthy young men and women is circadian-phase dependent. Sleep 2006; 29(5):609–618.
17. Hirai K, Kita M, Ohta H, et al. Ramelteon (TAK-375) accelerates reentrainment of circadian rhythm after a phase advance of the light-dark cycle in rats. J Biol Rhythms 2005; 20(1):27–37.
18. Czeisler CA, Richardson GS, Coleman RM, et al. Chronotherapy: resetting the circadian clocks of patients with delayed sleep phase insomnia. Sleep 1981; 4(1):1–21.
19. Eastman CI. Squashing versus nudging circadian rhythms with artificial bright light: solutions for shift work? Perspect Biol Med 1991; 34(2):181–195.
20. Weitzman ED, Czeisler CA, Coleman RM, et al. Delayed sleep phase syndrome. A chronobiological disorder with sleep-onset insomnia. Arch Gen Psychiatry 1981; 38(7):737–746.
21. Wyatt JK. Delayed sleep phase syndrome: pathophysiology and treatment options. Sleep 2004; 27(6): 1195–1203.
22. Rosenthal NE, Joseph-Vanderpool JR, Levendosky AA, et al. Phase-shifting effects of bright morning light as treatment for delayed sleep phase syndrome. Sleep 1990; 13(4):354–361.
23. Dahlitz M, Alvarez B, Vignau J, et al. Delayed sleep phase syndrome response to melatonin. Lancet 1991; 337(8750):1121–1124.
24. Nagtegaal JE, Kerkhof GA, Smits MG, et al. Delayed sleep phase syndrome: a placebo-controlled cross-over study on the effects of melatonin administered five hours before the individual dim light melatonin onset. J Sleep Res 1998; 7(2):135–143.
25. Lewy AJ, Sack RL, Miller LS, et al. The use of plasma melatonin levels and light in the assessment and treatment of chronobiologic sleep and mood disorders. J Neural Transm Suppl 1986; 21:311–322.
26. Dijk DJ, Duffy JF. Circadian regulation of human sleep and age-related changes in its timing, consolidation and EEG characteristics. Ann Med 1999; 31(2):130–140.
27. Carrier J, Paquet J, Morettini J, et al. Phase advance of sleep and temperature circadian rhythms in the middle years of life in humans. Neurosci Lett 2002; 320(1–2):1–4.
28. Duffy JF, Czeisler CA. Age-related change in the relationship between circadian period, circadian phase, and diurnal preference in humans. Neurosci Lett 2002; 318(3):117–120.
29. Campbell SS, Dawson D, Anderson MW. Alleviation of sleep maintenance insomnia with timed exposure to bright light. J Am Geriatr Soc 1993; 41(8):829–836.
30. Moldofsky H, Musisi S, Phillipson EA. Treatment of a case of advanced sleep phase syndrome by phase advance chronotherapy. Sleep 1986; 9(1):61–65.

31. Presser HB. Toward a 24-hour economy. Science 1999; 284:1778–1779.
32. Ohayon MM, Lemoine P, Arnaud-Briant V, et al. Prevalence and consequences of sleep disorders in a shift worker population. J Psychosom Res 2002; 53(1):577–583.
33. Burgess HJ, Sharkey KM, Eastman CI. Bright light, dark and melatonin can promote circadian adaptation in night shift workers. Sleep Med Rev 2002; 6(5):407–420.
34. Boivin DB, James FO. Circadian adaptation to night-shift work by judicious light and darkness exposure. J Biol Rhythms 2002; 17(6):556–567.
35. Sack RL, Lewy AJ. Melatonin as a chronobiotic: treatment of circadian desynchrony in night workers and the blind. J Biol Rhythms 1997; 12(6):595–603.
36. Hart CL, Ward AS, Haney M, et al. Zolpidem-related effects on performance and mood during simulated night-shift work. Exp Clin Psychopharmacol 2003; 11(4):259–268.
37. Monchesky TC, Billings BJ, Phillips R, et al. Zopiclone in insomniac shiftworkers. Evaluation of its hypnotic properties and its effects on mood and work performance. Int Arch Occup Environ Health 1989; 61(4):255–259.
38. Czeisler CA, Walsh JK, Roth T, et al. Modafinil for excessive sleepiness associated with shift-work sleep disorder [see comment]. N Engl J Med 2005; 353(5):476–486.
39. McLellan TM, Bell DG, Kamimori GH. Caffeine improves physical performance during 24 h of active wakefulness. Aviat Space Environ Med 2004; 75(8):666–672.
40. Wyatt JK, Cajochen C, Ritz-De Cecco A, et al. Low-dose repeated caffeine administration for circadian-phase-dependent performance degradation during extended wakefulness. Sleep 2004; 27(3): 374–381.
41. Herxheimer A, Petrie KJ. Melatonin for the prevention and treatment of jet lag. Cochrane Database Syst Rev 2002; (2):CD001520.
42. Daan S, Lewy AJ. Scheduled exposure to daylight: a potential strategy to reduce "jet lag" following transmeridian flight. Psychopharmacol Bull 1984; 20(3):566–568.
43. Eastman CI, Gazda CJ, Burgess HJ, et al. Advancing circadian rhythms before eastward flight: a strategy to prevent or reduce jet lag. Sleep 2005; 28(1):33–44.
44. Morris HH 3rd, Estes ML. Traveler's amnesia. Transient global amnesia secondary to triazolam. JAMA 1987; 258(7):945–946.
45. Lockley SW, Skene DJ, James K, et al. Melatonin administration can entrain the free-running circadian system of blind subjects. J Endocrinol 2000; 164(1):R1–R6.
46. Sack RL, Brandes RW, Kendall AR, et al. Entrainment of free-running circadian rhythms by melatonin in blind people. N Engl J Med 2000; 343(15):1070–1077.
47. Lewy AJ, Bauer VK, Hasler BP, et al. Capturing the circadian rhythms of free-running blind people with 0.5 mg melatonin. Brain Res 2001; 918(1–2):96–100.
48. Hack LM, Lockley SW, Arendt J, et al. The effects of low-dose 0.5-mg melatonin on the free-running circadian rhythms of blind subjects. J Biol Rhythms 2003; 18(5):420–429.

17 | Special Considerations for Treatment of Circadian Rhythm Sleep Disorders

Josephine Arendt and Debra J. Skene

Centre for Chronobiology, School of Biomedical and Molecular Sciences, University of Surrey, Guildford, Surrey, U.K.

INTRODUCTION

The characteristics, diagnosis, and treatment of circadian rhythm sleep disorder (CRSD) are described in this section. These are briefly summarized here to introduce the specific applications and problems of treatments that shift the timing of rhythms (chronobiotics, exposure to light, and other time cues).

CRSD occurs when the timing of internal rhythms is at odds with desired or imposed sleep time. The most common manifestation of CRSD is found in persons working night shifts (approximately 15–20% of the population in developed countries). In this case inappropriate timing of internal rhythms with respect to the external environment is a transitory but recurrent condition and is referred to as "external desynchronization." The situation arises because the circadian system adapts slowly to abrupt changes of time cues. The symptoms of jet lag have the same origin (1). Abnormal timing of internal rhythms with respect to each other has also been reported (internal desynchronization), and both external and internal desynchrony may occur together. Extreme variants of internal periodicity (the inherent frequency of an individuals circadian clock) leading to abnormal timing of the circadian system also come into the category of CRSD but are less common. Lack of sufficiently strong time cues in everyday life is associated with (usually) delayed circadian rhythms relative to sleep time. In the polar winter with no natural daylight and in rare cases of sighted people this may lead to complete desynchronization from the 24-hour day or "free-run." Blind people with no perception of light frequently show free-running circadian rhythms. In a small number of people with no eyes studied to date, all manifested this phenomenon (2).

SHIFT WORK

Most night shift workers, even working permanent night shifts, never adapt fully to their imposed work schedule. Thus they work during the time of maximum sleepiness, minimum alertness, lowest performance, and least efficient metabolism (3) (Fig. 1). Sleep is short and of poor quality when taken during the day, out of phase with the circadian peak of sleep propensity, the minimum of core body temperature, and the peak of melatonin secretion.

Full adaptation to night shift is accompanied by normalization of sleep and other functions. It only occurs naturally in unusual situations when people are not subject to conflicting time cues, in particular, natural bright light and social obligations. For example, certain night work schedules on offshore oil rigs, or in winter in polar regions, lead to complete circadian adaptation within a few days (4,5). In these conditions there is every reason to use strategies to hasten adaptation. Sleep and other problems then arise when returning to day work and can be addressed in theory (but efficacy is not yet fully demonstrated in practice) by use of similar strategies to those advised when adapting to night work (see later).

The most numerically important shift work conditions, at least in the United Kingdom, are irregular night shifts (sometimes night and sometimes days) and rotating schedules in a "normal" environment (information from the Office of National Statistics). Examples of rotations include two to three days early shift (e.g., 06-14 hours), three days late shift (e.g., 14-22 hours), three days night shift (e.g., 22-06 hours), rest days. Neither of these schedules allows the internal

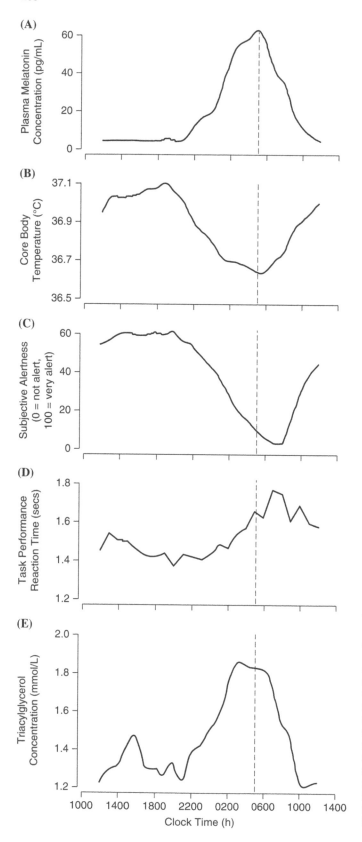

Figure 1 Diagrammatic representation of the circadian rhythms of plasma melatonin, core body temperature, subjective alertness, task performance (reaction time, in seconds), and triacylglycerol, from human beings held in constant routine conditions (i.e., controlled light, posture, activity, and meals). The peak in the melatonin rhythm (**A**), shown by the dotted line, and the low point of the temperature rhythm (**B**) are within one hour of each other. The low- point of the alertness and performance rhythms (**C** and **D**, respectively) is shortly after the melatonin peak, and the peak in triacylglycerol (**E**) coincides with the melatonin peak. *Source*: From Ref. 3.

clock to adapt to nights, since there is substantial inertia in the circadian system, and exposure to morning light (travel home window) counters any tendency to adapt.

The answers to this problem are not simple. However, for very short periods of night shift (one to three days) interspersed with longer periods of day work or leisure, it is advisable not to try and adapt the circadian clock to nights, but to counter poor nighttime alertness and daytime sleep with measures that have minimal phase shifting actions. This approach preserves the normal alignment of rhythms with the predominant day schedule. Increasing light intensity in the work environment, toward the latter part of the night during and after the core body temperature minimum, will in principle improve alertness and performance and should counter circadian adaptation (6–8). A nap taken prior to night work may be beneficial and administration of the pineal hormone melatonin can, in controlled studies, enhance the ability to sleep in late afternoon/evening during the "wake maintenance zone" (9). There are few data to attest to the success, or otherwise, of this approach in real life situations. Melatonin has also been used to help daytime sleep in shift workers, with inconsistent results (10) (http://www.ahrq.gov/news/press/pr2004/melatnpr.htm). The drug modafinil is able to increase nighttime alertness apparently without compromising daytime sleep, however, there is little information on practical applications to date (11,12).

For longer periods of night shift, particularly if subjects show partial circadian adaptation, there is reason to hasten adaptation using timed exposure to light and/or chronobiotic treatment, however, the problem of readaptation to daywork then occurs. Timed exposure to increased light intensity with or without concomitant melatonin treatment appears to be quite effective in limited field data (13–16).

JET LAG

Jet lag might be considered a minor problem of long-haul holidays, however for a substantial proportion of long-distance travelers (approx. 50%), the first few days after crossing a large number of time zones can be very unpleasant. For the business traveler the ability to function correctly is critical. Like the unadapted night shift worker she/he will be desynchronized from the external environment, sleep deprived, and at a low point of alertness and performance. However, after crossing time zones, eventually everyone adapts the circadian clock if they stay long enough in the new time zone. On average, without interventions, the circadian clock takes a day to adapt for each time zone crossed. However, greater shifts are seen initially and substantial differences in response are seen between eastward and westward transitions (17,18). For a sufficient length of stay in the new time zone, treatment strategies to hasten adaptation are clearly to be recommended. For short stopovers the problem is different and the best advice is to return home as soon as possible, to travel over daytime as far as is possible, to schedule work for the predicted time of maximum alertness in the departure time zone, and to conserve sleep by whatever means. For short stopovers followed by a second, third and, in the case of long-haul pilots, more long-haul flights, conservation of sleep is again the priority. Attempting to shift the circadian clock appropriately in these conditions is extremely difficult (19).

ABNORMAL TIMING OF INTERNAL RHYTHMS WITH RESPECT TO EACH OTHER (INTERNAL DESYNCHRONY)

Abnormal timing of internal rhythms with respect to each other has been reported in conditions such as jet lag (20). "Re-entrainment by partition" refers to different internal rhythms shifting at different rates, and also in different directions (by advance or by delay) after abrupt change of time zone or work schedule. Most of this information comes from early data and may not have been gathered in appropriately controlled conditions. However, recent evaluation of genetic function following phase shifts in animals suggests strongly that different peripheral organs adapt at different rates to each other and to the central clock in the suprachiasmatic nucleus (SCN) (21). Rhythms timed "directly" by the SCN such as melatonin, cortisol, and core body temperature normally shift together. Even here, however, there is evidence for differential downstream control leading to internal desynchrony (22). The rare condition of Smith–Magenis Syndrome is accompanied by daytime melatonin secretion but with normally timed cortisol secretion: daytime sleepiness and poor nighttime sleep are present (23).

EXTERNAL AND INTERNAL DESYNCHRONY

Clearly, in view of the above sections, both external and internal desynchrony can be present simultaneously after abrupt change of time zones or work schedules.

EXTREME VARIANTS OF INTERNAL PERIODICITY

Extreme variants of internal periodicity are reflected in extreme diurnal preference and appear to be genetically determined. Most attention has been paid to familial advanced sleep phase syndrome (FASPS), which is a rare condition associated with a mutation in the clock gene per 2 (24). There is some evidence that delayed sleep phase type (DSPT) is associated with polymorphisms in the clock gene per 3 (25), particularly a length polymorphism (26) that is in turn associated with diurnal preference. However there is as yet no evidence that DSPT patients have abnormal periodicity. Seasonal affective disorder (SAD), which may be accompanied by hypersomnia, is often associated with phase changes of the circadian system, more commonly delays (27). However the delay may not be of such magnitude that it differs from delayed phase in winter in people who do not suffer this condition. There is no evidence as yet for abnormal periodicity in SAD.

INSUFFICIENT TIME CUES

Environment

The circadian system is maintained on a 24-hour period and optimally phased by time cues (zeitgebers), the most important of which is alternation of light and darkness. The most obvious situation deficient in bright light is during winter in high latitudes and polar regions of the earth. Here delayed timing of the internal clock is evident in winter and can lead to suboptimal phase relationships between sleep and the internal clock (28). "Midwinter insomnia" has been reported from northern high latitudes associated with delayed circadian phase (29).

Urban humans are rarely exposed to bright natural sunlight especially in winter (30). It seems likely that some incidence of DSPT may be due to this problem. In institutional situations, such as residential homes for the elderly, artificial ambient light levels may be unacceptably low (31,32). Yellowing of the lens with aging leads to less exposure to the short wavelengths of light implicated as the most powerful acting on the circadian system. Circadian photoreception is demonstrably less sensitive in the elderly (33). In addition poor mobility, loss of appetite, and insufficient social interactions further reduce the time cues that maintain optimal synchrony. These factors undoubtedly contribute to poor sleep in older people. However, curiously, phase advance of the circadian system and sleep (together with an altered, earlier phase relationship of sleep to the melatonin rhythm) (34), rather than phase delay, is reported in the elderly.

Blindness

People with no perception of light have a major risk of non-24-hour sleep-wake disorder. All subjects with no eyes show this phenomenon, and these findings underpin the importance of light as the principal time cue maintaining our rhythms in synchrony with the 24-hour day (2). In the absence of the light-dark time cue, people desynchronize from 24 hours and "free-run" at their own endogenous periodicity. Circadian period is an individual trait linked to clock gene characteristics. In our experience, on average in the blind it is approximately 24.5 hours, slightly longer than that found in sighted subjects (35). Living on a non-24-hour day means that the circadian system is regularly out of synchrony with the external environment: effectively people suffer "intermittent jet lag" as described by one of our subjects. It is a lifetime problem leading to poor sleep, alertness, performance, and no doubt other problems related to circadian desynchrony during each out of phase period. It is often misdiagnosed and inappropriately treated (at least anecdotally).

Free-Running Sighted Subjects

A few reports exist of sighted people living in a "normal environment" who desynchronize from the 24-hour day and suffer the same problems as blind free-runners (36). The reasons for this are obscure. They may be behavioral (e.g., willed avoidance of light), extreme long or short internal periodicity, which cannot synchronize to 24 hours, or possibly defective perception of light by the circadian clock in the SCN.

PSYCHIATRIC DISORDERS

Abnormal rhythmicity has frequently been reported in psychiatry, particularly bipolar disorder, depression, and schizophrenia, as well as SAD (37,38). Sleep disturbance accompanies these conditions and may be either a consequence or a cause of abnormal rhythms.

TREATMENT STRATEGIES: CHRONOBIOLOGICAL APPROACHES

Recognition of circadian rhythm disorders has led to development of a new class of treatment: chronobiotics, the precursor of which is the pineal hormone melatonin. Melatonin can change the timing of the circadian clock, reinforce internal phase relationships and increase the amplitude of the circadian system (39,40). It is of course preferable to use a non-pharmacological approach, if possible, and to this end the use of light, the major time cue of the circadian system, has been prominent. Correct treatment with pharmacological and non-pharmacological interventions ideally requires knowledge of the timing of the internal clock in each patient. Both phase advances and phase delays, as well as (less commonly) rhythm suppression/increased amplitude, can be obtained by chronobiological strategies, depending on the timing of treatment relative to the individuals' internal clock.

LIGHT

Timed application of bright light of suitable intensity and spectral composition can in principle re-phase, synchronize, and reinforce the amplitude of circadian rhythms. Thus for all conditions, except those with defective light perception or retinal pathology, light is the treatment of choice.

Delayed circadian phase can be adjusted by light treatment in the subjective early morning (Fig. 2—melatonin profile defines biological (subjective) night) and this has been employed with some success in DSPT (41), in SAD (38), and in environments with insufficient time cues (40). Successful treatment usually depends on knowledge of circadian phase, since light shifts rhythms according to a phase-response curve (PRC). Light timed to delay will evidently exacerbate the problem. Circadian phase in DSPS and other conditions can be evaluated using the melatonin rhythm and to a certain extent inferred using sleep timing (42). In theory, abnormally advanced circadian phase can be treated by light treatment in the first half of the subjective night but little data exist to substantiate the theory (43).

Sufficiently bright light at night will hasten adaptation to simulated and real night shift work, and back to dayshift work with consequent improvement in sleep and other problems (14,44,45). Similarly, timed light treatment together with avoidance of light at the right time can in theory hasten adaptation to time zone change (19,46). Application of light at the "wrong" time will, however, drive the circadian system to adapt in the "wrong" direction. For example, instead of adapting to an 8-hour phase shift by advancing 8 hours, the system may delay by 16 hours. Avoidance of light at the wrong time is possibly more important than the light

---

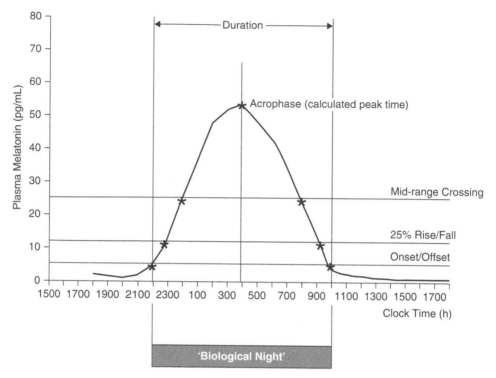

Figure 2 Diagram to illustrate the normal profile of melatonin secretion (plasma) defining "biological night." The features of this profile and that of salivary melatonin and urinary 6-sulphatoxymelatonin (aMT6s) (acrophase, duration, mid-range crossing, 25% rise and fall, onset and offset of secretion), used to characterize the timing of the circadian clock, are indicated. Melatonin treatment timing is ideally based on "circadian time" (CT) where by convention CT 14 is melatonin onset. aMT6s acrophase is approximately two hours after the plasma melatonin acrophase. *Source*: From Ref. 40.

treatment itself (44). For example, traveling eastwards overnight across eight time zones, natural morning light exposure on arrival will drive the system to delay unless it is avoided. Computer programs exist to predict optimal light exposure and avoidance (47).

In environments deficient in time cues, light has been successfully employed to restore correct circadian phase. Either "skeleton" photoperiod (two one-hour bright-light pulses daily, morning and evening), light exposure in the subjective morning, or a full photoperiod (whole day) of bright light has been employed (28,48–50). SAD is successfully treated with light, notably given in the morning (30 minutes, 10,000 lux), with restoration of normal sleep and mood (38). Most recently it appears that a similar light treatment can be used as an adjunct to conventional antidepressants in major depression to address both the cognitive and sleep dysfunction (37). However, this approach is in its infancy. To what extent light acts by correcting circadian phase and/or amplitude and/or optimizing internal phase relationships remains unclear.

SIDE EFFECTS OF LIGHT

The vast bulk of data associated with light treatment of circadian dysfunction concerns the use of broad spectrum white light from 2000–10,000 lux and 30 minutes to 3 hours exposure. It has been reported that exposure to some commercial equipment causes excessive visual glare such as exposure to naked bulbs, direct intense illumination from below the eyes, and intentionally augmented UV radiation (38). Suggested criteria for choosing lamps are listed on the suppliers page of the nonprofit Center for Environmental Therapeutics Web site (http://www.cet.org). In a recent comprehensive review, primarily concerned with SAD,

Terman and Terman (38) report that there is very little evidence for side effects of light treatment such as retinal damage. Mild visual complaints have included blurred vision, eyestrain, and photophobia. One study evaluated 83 patients with SAD for 88 potential side effects of 30 minutes, 10,000 lux, broad spectrum white light, and found a frequency of 6% to 16% complaints, including nausea, headache, jumpiness/jitteriness, and eye irritation. Ophthalmological evaluations of untreated patients with normal oculoretinal status have shown no obvious acute light-induced pathology or long-term sequelae. According to Terman and Terman, there are no definite contraindications for bright-light treatment other than for the retinopathies. Interactions of light treatment with photosensitizing medication are evident and avoidable. It should also be noted that concomitant treatment with a number of drugs, notably antidepressant medication, may lead to both desirable (possibly enhanced action of some antidepressants) and undesirable effects (37,38).

Recently it has become clear that the most effective wavelengths with regard to circadian function are in the blue region of the spectrum (460–480 nm) (51–53). Very little clinical data has emerged yet using short-wavelength light. At present it is important to consider the safety aspects of blue-light treatment. The reader is referred to reviews by Reme (54,55). However avoidance of short-wavelength light may yet be a solution for increasing light at night in shiftwork without undesirable phase shifts and without compromising performance etc. (56).

There is another possible down side to the use of light treatment during biological darkness in humans. A hypothesis has been proposed to the effect that the increased risk of cancer (particularly breast and colorectal cancer) in shift workers is due to light experienced at night and the presumed suppression of melatonin that occurs (57). This hypothesis is based on accumulating evidence for anticancer effects of melatonin in animals and humans, and some preliminary evidence for anticancer effects in humans in combination chemotherapy (58–61). The hypothesis as stated is generating a considerable amount of research. Blind subjects (with no light perception at all) may have a decreased incidence of cancer, which has been attributed to lack of melatonin suppression (62); however, some confounding factors cannot be eliminated.

Sparse and inconsistent evidence exists for a decline in melatonin during night shift work, but it is probable that this can occur (63). In a light-induced forced nine-hour phase shift using approximately 1000 lux white light, a clear decline in 6-sulphatoxymelatonin (aMT6s) production was noted (64). In real shift workers adaptation to night shift may be accompanied by a significant decline on returning to daywork (65). Actual light exposure at night needs to be evaluated carefully in field studies. Moreover light at night has numerous effects. The mere fact of frequent disruption of all circadian rhythms, not just melatonin, is effectively a physiological insult. Most importantly, perhaps, light directly influences the expression of the clock gene feedback loops involving both central and peripheral circadian oscillators. Disruption of clock gene function by simulated phase shifts is associated with increased risk of cancer in recent animal studies (66,67).

These possible associations of major disease risk with light exposure during subjective nighttime await further research to confirm the correlations and determine any causality.

MELATONIN

Clearly light cannot be used for circadian adjustment in subjects with no light perception. In this case the chronobiotic melatonin is the treatment of choice (40,68).

Low (0.05–10 mg) doses of melatonin during the "biological day," i.e., when endogenous melatonin levels are low, can induce transient sleepiness or sleep, and lower core body temperature, in suitably controlled circumstances (posture is important, the greatest effects are seen with recumbent subjects in very dim light) (68). These effects are opposite to the acute effects of bright light given at night. The effects of melatonin on sleep have been extensively reviewed recently (69).

In the same dose range (0.05–10 mg) it is able to shift circadian timing to both later and earlier times when administration is appropriately timed. Phase advances (and possibly phase delays) are dose dependent using a single dose in the range 0.05 to 5 mg. As for light, appropriate timing of treatment to delay or advance according to a PRC requires knowledge of

(A)   (B)

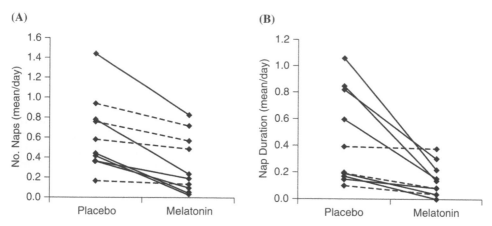

Figure 3 Reduction in the number and duration of naps in 10 free-running totally blind subjects treated daily with 0.5 mg melatonin (fast release) for a complete circadian "beat" cycle. *Source*: From Ref. 71.

internal circadian timing. The reported phase-response curves to melatonin are approximately the reverse of that to light (40).

Timed melatonin administration (0.5–5 mg at 24-hour intervals, usually at desired bedtime) can fully entrain (or synchronize) the free-running circadian rhythms of most blind subjects, with a consequent improvement in sleep (70–72) (Fig. 3) and daytime alertness (even without entrainment, sleep is improved).

Two recent meta-analyses with regard to the effects of melatonin on jet lag have different conclusions. One considers that existing evidence shows a robust positive effect (73). The other (reporting on the use of nutritional supplements, for a variety of conditions including shiftwork) found little evidence for a consistent effect on sleep after time zone change (10) but confirmed the efficacy of melatonin in DSPT (Agency for Healthcare Research and Quality (http://www.ahrq.gov/news/press/pr2004/melatnpr.htm). This latter analysis discarded very large numbers of jet lag studies for reasons that were not apparent (74). With regard to shift work the data are indeed inconsistent. Exceptions are studies where careful treatment timing was used in the field or in simulation laboratory studies (45). As for light, timing is critical to avoid precipitating phase shifts in the "wrong" direction. Preflight treatment with melatonin and/or light can be timed to initiate a shift in the right direction (but has rarely been used) (75,76). In field studies individual variability in rate and direction of adaptation of the circadian clock is large (Fig. 4) and exposure to conflicting natural bright light is always a problem [although one simulation study has shown that melatonin can partially counter conflicting light (77)].

Results from DSPT have also been consistently good—and here timing of treatment is relatively easy to predict. Patients are entrained, albeit with a delay, and it is evident that afternoon/early evening melatonin will induce shifts in the right direction. To the authors knowledge there is little information on the treatment of ASPT by melatonin. Hack (78) successfully delayed a blind subject with ASPT by stepwise shifting of melatonin treatment to later times.

The use of melatonin for elderly sleep disorder has given somewhat inconsistent results according to a limited meta-analysis (79). A recent large scale study in demented elderly using light, melatonin and a combination of both treatments has provided evidence for clinically relevant improvements in sleep and cognitive functioning (80). It is likely that melatonin is most effective if the sleep problem is related to rhythm disorder. A "melatonin deficiency" syndrome has been invoked whereby melatonin treatment of the elderly replaces a deficiency in endogenous melatonin (81). However, while a decline of melatonin in the elderly has frequently been reported, this does not necessarily relate to sleep problems.

There has been considerable success treating sleep and behavioral problems in multiply disabled children, usually with neurological disorders. However, to what extent this involves changes in circadian rhythms remains unclear (82,83).

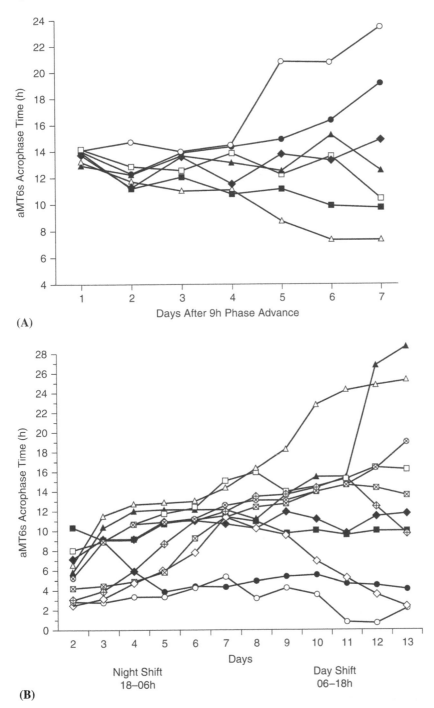

(A)

(B)

Night Shift
18–06h

Day Shift
06–18h

Figure 4 Timing chronobiotic treatment in jet lag and shift work situations is a challenge, since individuals shift their circadian rhythms at different speeds and in different directions after an abrupt change of time cues. (**A**) Simulated jet lag with a forced nine hour phase advance, timing of the 6-sulphatoxymelatonin (aMT6s) rhythm in seven subjects in the days following phase shift. (**B**) Real shift work on an offshore oil rig, timing of the aMT6s rhythm in eleven subjects working seven nights followed by seven days. Ideally treatment should start before the phase change to specify the most appropriate direction of shift. *Source*: From Ref. 19.

Melatonin Agonists and Antagonists

Several agonists and antagonists have been described, for example, in references 84 and 85. One, ramelteon, has recently been licensed. It is too soon to evaluate their effectiveness compared with melatonin, and their short- and long-term side effects.

SIDE EFFECTS OF MELATONIN

There are remarkably few reported side effects of melatonin and it is considered to be safe in healthy adults in the dose range quoted here (0.05–10 mg fast or slow release) (10,73,86,87), (http://www.ahrq.gov/news/press/pr2004/melatnpr.htm). Numerous publications attest to its beneficial effects in conditions not (as yet) related to rhythm disorder (primarily in animals) (88). However, its physiological function as an internal time cue or "zeitgeber" provided the initial rationale for treatment of CRSD.

It has very low toxicity in reported animal and human data (review Arendt, 1997). Since it has the effects of lowering alertness, performance, core body temperature, and increasing sleepiness when taken during subjective daytime (and which might be considered side effects), the usual advice is to take it prior to a period of desired sleep. It is most effective at increasing sleep propensity when taken during the afternoon/early evening (89). However, it is possible to advance circadian rhythms at this time using a low dose, which does not have major sleepiness inducing effects (76,90).

Probably the most efficient use of melatonin (and no doubt other chronobiotic treatments) with regard to sleep and circadian timing is to combine it with other time cues. Thus taken daily at 1600 hours (in normally phased individuals) followed by a period of dim light and recumbency, it is highly efficacious at advancing all measured rhythms (9,91). Few data exist to specify the best conditions in which to generate a delay in circadian timing with melatonin (suppression of melatonin enhances light-induced delays (92)).

Safety in Clinical Studies

A large number of clinical studies using melatonin now exist in the published literature. The majority concern healthy volunteers. One early report concerning subjects taking part in field studies of jet lag found the following incidence of side effects reported more than once (melatonin %, N = 474, placebo %, N = 112): sleepiness (8.3%, 1.8%), headache (1.7%, 2.7%), nausea (0.8%, 0.9%), fuzziness/giddiness (0.6%, 0%) and lightheadedness (0.8%, 0%) (86). This review reported treatment of a blind man since 1988 with 5 mg melatonin daily, with no side effects, and a single case (healthy female) of melatonin self-administration (2–5 mg daily) since 1981. These individuals continue to take melatonin in the same dose range with no problems.

A recent safety evaluation of the literature provided the following information: Considering the dose range from 3 mg, (which is a low pharmacological dose in terms of plasma concentrations), to 1600 mg, the reported incidence of side effects in 5607 adults was 3.87% over the period 1984–2001 (references available on request). The duration of treatment varied from a single dose to 18 months. Side effects included depression, increased anger or psychosis; increased anxiety, loss of sleep or weight; transitory sedation and occasional flushing; drowsiness, sleepiness, or fatigue; hangover effect; headache; slight "fuzziness;" odd taste in mouth; thrombocytopenia; intentional overdose; bad mood; instability in sleep-wake cycle; suspected suppression of endogenous melatonin secretion; lack of motivation; increased nighttime hypotension; "rocking" sensation; weakness; heavy head; insomnia; palpitations; vomiting; delusions and hallucinations; diarrhea; asthenia; leukopenia; thrombocytopenia and anemia. As for the 1997 report, the most common were drowsiness/sleepiness/ fatigue (to be expected) and headache.

Over the same period and considering doses less than 3 mg (lowest was 200 µg) an incidence of 0.99% adverse events was found in 3342 adults, with the treatment period ranging from one day to six months (references available on request). These included poor mood during the early part of the evening; pruritus; possible autoimmune hepatitis; bad dreams; headache; recurrent migraine, heartburn, tremor, anxiety, and somnolence; vivid dreams; mild faintness on standing up; sleepiness, alopecia; gastric intolerance, increased body weight, insomnia, and constipation.

In 545 pediatric patients with various conditions, 1.5% adverse events were reported, the most common being moodiness and mild headache. The dose range was 0.14–10 mg, and the duration of treatment from one day to six years (references available on request).

However, by no means all papers report adverse events, many do not distinguish between side effects of placebo and melatonin, and some do not give exact numbers of occurrences.

One interesting report described the use of melatonin for sleep disturbance in psychiatric patients where one subject was unable to remain synchronized to 24 hours after withdrawal from melatonin treatment (93). This single observation may suggest that in vulnerable subjects "addiction" to melatonin is possible. There is no other evidence for tolerance/addiction however.

Since melatonin has powerful physiological effects in photoperiodic species, and humans show residual photoperiodism (39,94) it behoves us to be certain of its uses and limitations and long-term safety needs to be assessed.

AGE AND GENDER EFFECTS OF TREATMENT WITH LIGHT OR MELATONIN

It is likely that a greater light intensity will be necessary in the elderly compared with the young, to achieve restoration of abnormal circadian function (see above) although little data addresses this as yet. Since metabolic function changes with age, dose response studies for the use of melatonin in the very elderly are required, indeed more dose response studies are required for all its uses.

There are no reports of gender effects with regard to the ability of light to phase shift the circadian clock to the authors' knowledge.

The bioavailability of oral melatonin (250 μg) is reported to be three-fold higher in women than in men, with no differences in clearance when corrected for body weight (95). However there are as yet no reported gender differences in the effects of melatonin administration to the author's knowledge.

DRIVING RISK

Anyone taking melatonin should be advised not to drive for seven to eight hours after the dose in view of potential decrements in alertness and performance, although this advice will perhaps be modified in future for very low doses. One study (96) has evaluated the driving risk of 5 mg melatonin at 16-30 hours. The overall result of a computer test battery showed no objective adverse impact of melatonin on driving performance. However, caution was advised in view of increased sleepiness. One study is not sufficient for firm conclusions to be drawn.

Shift workers have been advised to avoid light (by wearing sunglasses) in the "going home window" after night shift if adaptation is desired. Unfortunately this can lead to lowered alertness and visual acuity and increase potential accident risk (already large at this time). Recently sunglasses (blue blockers) which selectively remove the wavelengths of light which most affect the circadian system, but preserve vision, have been developed and initial reports are encouraging (56,97). Further information is required before recommendations can be made.

GENERAL PROBLEMS

Light as a non-pharmacological treatment does not require registration. The Society for Light Treatment and Biological Rhythms website (http://www.sltbr.org) provides much useful information on the use of light, its attributes, and problems. Melatonin however is not a registered medication in many countries. Development to registration is underway, and one formulation has recently been approved by the European authorities. It is available via the internet and over the counter notably in the United States where it is classified as a food supplement. The quality of these over the counter products may be questionable and the advice is always to obtain a registered product from a licensed manufacturer. There are insufficient comparative dose-response and formulation trials of melatonin for any indication as yet. It should be noted that oral contraceptives (and a number of other common drugs, for example, nonsteroidal antiinflammatories, beta adrenergic receptor antagonists) can modify endogenous melatonin secretion (68). Thus potential drug interactions are many.

The application/avoidance of light, melatonin, or other treatment according to chronobiological principles is a challenge in terms of advice to clinicians and individuals who self-medicate, particularly in occupational health, with regard to timing the treatment. It is likely that "side effects" are observed primarily with inappropriate timing. Results from controlled laboratory studies are hard to extrapolate to real life situations in view of the individual variability in response to phase shift (Fig. 4). It is possible that assessment of individual chronotype (morningness-eveningness) and habitual sleep times will help to predict appropriate timing of light and chronobiotic treatments in the future. Should a rapid, simple, objective method of ascertaining internal clock timing become available, no doubt its use will maximize the efficacy of the treatment of CRSD.

STANDARD CAUTIONS WITH REGARD TO SELF-TREATMENT WITH MELATONIN (19)

Melatonin can induce sleepiness and lowered alertness. You are advised not to drive, operate heavy or dangerous machinery, or do equivalent tasks requiring alertness for seven to eight hours after taking your pill.

We do not advise to use melatonin if (i) you are a long-haul pilot, air crew, or shift worker (this is due to potential difficulties with timing the dose.), (ii) you or a close blood relative suffers from a psychiatric condition, migraine, or an auto-immune disease, (iii) you are less than 18 years old or know (or suspect) that you are pregnant, (iv) you are taking any medication other than minor analgesics or oral contraceptives, and (v) you are breastfeeding.

CONCLUSIONS

Timed light and melatonin treatments have proved successful in specific cases of CRSD. In controlled conditions both are effective at optimizing circadian timing, however, in real life situations of shift work and jet lag, the results are as yet inconsistent, probably due to conflicting environmental and behavioral time cues. Both light and melatonin are considered safe provided suitable precautions are taken as outlined above. There is insufficient information to evaluate recently registered chronobiotic medications, however, they will be subject to the same problems of treatment timing as light and melatonin. Non-pharmacological interventions such as timed exercise and meals have no associated side effects as yet.

ACKNOWLEDGMENTS

This Chapter was written during the tenure of grants from the U.K. Health and Safety Executive, the Energy Institute, the Antarctic Funding Initiative, the European Union, EU Marie Curie RTN grant (MCRTN-CT-2004-512362) and EU FP6 EUCLOCK (no.018741) and with support from Stockgrand Ltd., University of Surrey, Guildford, Surrey, U.K. We would like to thank Alliance Pharmaceuticals Ltd., Chippenham, Wiltshire, U.K., for providing their unpublished evaluation of the safety of melatonin in clinical reports.

REFERENCES

1. Dunlap JC, Loros J, Decoursey PJ, eds. Chronobiology: Biological Timekeeping. Sunderland, MA: Sinauer Associates Inc., 2004.
2. Lockley SW, Skene DJ, Arendt J, et al. Relationship between melatonin rhythms and visual loss in the blind. J Clin Endocrinol Metab 1997; 82(11):3763–3770.
3. Rajaratnam SM, Arendt J. Health in a 24-h society. Lancet 2001, 358(9286), 999–1005.
4. Barnes RG, Forbes MJ, Arendt J, Shift type and season affect adaptation of the 6-sulphatoxymelatonin rhythm in offshore oil rig workers. Neurosci Lett 1998; 252(3):179–182.
5. Ross JK, Arendt J, Horne J, et al. Night-shift work in Antarctica: sleep characteristics and bright light treatment. Physiol Behav 1995; 57(6):1169–1174.
6. Revell VL, Arendt J, Terman M, et al. Short-wavelength sensitivity of the human circadian system to phase-advancing light. J Biol Rhythms 2005; 20(3):270–272.
7. Revell VL, Arendt J, Fogg LF, et al. Alerting effects of light are sensitive to very short wavelengths. Neurosci Lett 2006; 399(1–2):96–100.

8. Khalsa SB, Jewett ME, Cajochen C, et al. A phase response curve to single bright light pulses in human subjects. J Physiol 2003; 549(pt 3):945–952.
9. Rajaratnam SM, Middleton B, Stone BM, et al. Melatonin advances the circadian timing of EEG sleep and directly facilitates sleep without altering its duration in extended sleep opportunities in humans. J Physiol 2004; 561(pt 1):339–351.
10. Buscemi N, Vandermeer B, Hooton N, et al. Efficacy and safety of exogenous melatonin for secondary sleep disorders and sleep disorders accompanying sleep restriction: meta-analysis. BMJ 2006; 332 (7538):385–393.
11. Czeisler C, Wenes K. Armodafinil improves memory and attention in patients with excessive sleepiness associated with shift work sleep disorder. Proceedings of the Association of Professional Sleep Societies Conference, Salt Lake City, Utah, 17–22 June 2006. Sleep 2006; 29(suppl):93 (abstr).
12. Czeisler CA, Walsh JK, Roth T, et al. Modafinil for excessive sleepiness associated with shift-work sleep disorder. N Engl J Med 2005; 353(5):476–486.
13. Bjorvatn B, Stangenes K, Oyane N, et al. Effects of bright light and melatonin on adaptation to night work. A randomised placebo-controlled field study at an oil rig. Proceedings of the Association of Professional Sleep Societies Conference, Salt Lake City, Utah, 17–22 June 2006. Sleep 2006, 29 (suppl):92 (abstr).
14. Bjorvatn B, Kecklund G, Akerstedt T. Bright light treatment used for adaptation to night work and re-adaptation back to day life. A field study at an oil platform in the North Sea. J Sleep Res 1999; 8(2):105–112.
15. Boivin DB, James FO. Light treatment and circadian adaptation to shift work. Ind Health 2005; 43(1): 34–48.
16. Bjorvatn B, Stangenes K, Oyane N, et al. Randomized placebo-controlled field study of the effects of bright light and melatonin in adaptation to night work. Scand J Work Environ Health 2007; 33(3): 204–214.
17. Gundel A, Wegmann HM. Resynchronization of the circadian system following a 9-hr advance or a delay zeitgeber shift: real flights and simulations by a Van-der-Pol oscillator. Prog Clin Biol Res 1987; 227B:391–401.
18. Reddy AB, Field MD, Maywood ES, et al. Differential resynchronisation of circadian clock gene expression within the suprachiasmatic nuclei of mice subjected to experimental jet lag. J Neurosci 2002; 22(17):7326–7330.
19. Arendt J, Stone B, Skene D. Sleep disruption in jet lag and other circadian rhythm disturbances. In: Kryger M, Roth T, Dement W, eds. Principles and Practice of Sleep Medicine. Philadelphia: WB Saunders, 2005:659–672.
20. Wegmann HM, Gundel A, Naumann M, et al., Sleep, sleepiness, and circadian rhythmicity in aircrews operating on transatlantic routes. Aviat Space Environ Med 1986; 57(12 pt 2):B53–B64.
21. Stokkan KA, Yamazaki S, Tei H, et al. Entrainment of the circadian clock in the liver by feeding. Science 2001; 291(5503):490–493.
22. Gordijn MC, Beersma DG, Korte HJ, et al. Effects of light exposure and sleep displacement on dim light melatonin onset. Journal of Sleep Research, 1999, 8, 163–174.
23. De Leersnyder H, Claustrat B, Munnich A, et al. Circadian rhythm disorder in a rare disease: Smith-Magenis syndrome. Mol Cell Endocrinol 2006; 252(1–2):88–91.
24. Toh KL, Jones CR, He Y, et al. An hPer2 phosphorylation site mutation in familial advanced sleep phase syndrome. Science 2001; 291(5506):1040–1043.
25. Ebisawa T, Uchiyama M, Kajimura N, et al. Association of structural polymorphisms in the human period3 gene with delayed sleep phase syndrome. EMBO Rep 2001;2(4):342–346.
26. Archer SN, Robilliard DL, Skene DJ, et al. A length polymorphism in the circadian clock gene Per3 is linked to delayed sleep phase syndrome and extreme diurnal preference. Sleep 2003; 26(4):413–415.
27. Lewy AJ, Lefler BJ, Emens JS, et al. The circadian basis of winter depression. Proc Natl Acad Sci U S A 2006; 103(19):7414–7419.
28. Broadway J, Arendt J, Folkard S. Bright light phase shifts the human melatonin rhythm during the Antarctic winter. Neurosci Lett 1987; 79(1–2):185–189.
29. Hansen T, Bratlid T, Lingjarde O, et al. Midwinter insomnia in the subarctic region: evening levels of serum melatonin and cortisol before and after treatment with bright artificial light. Acta Psychiatr Scand 1987;75(4):428–434.
30. Okudaira N, Kripke DF, Webster JB. Naturalistic studies of human light exposure. Am J Physiol 1983; 245(4):R613–R615.
31. Ancoli-Israel S, Gehrman P, Martin JL, et al., Increased light exposure consolidates sleep and strengthens circadian rhythms in severe Alzheimer's disease patients. Behav Sleep Med 2003; 1(1):22–36.
32. Van Someren EJ, Riemersma RF, Swaab DF. Functional plasticity of the circadian timing system in old age: light exposure. Prog Brain Res 2002; 138:205–231.
33. Herljevic M, Middleton B, Thapan K, et al. Light-induced melatonin suppression: age-related reduction in response to short wavelength light. Exp Gerontol 2005; 40(3):237–242.

34. Duffy JF, Zeitzer JM, Rimmer DW, et al. Peak of circadian melatonin rhythm occurs later within the sleep of older subjects. Am J Physiol Endocrinol Metab 2002; 282(2):E297–E303.
35. Skene DJ, Lockley SW, Thapan K, et al. Effects of light on human circadian rhythms. Reprod Nutr Dev 1999; 39(3):295–304.
36. McArthur AJ, Lewy AJ, Sack RL. Non-24-hour sleep-wake syndrome in a sighted man: circadian rhythm studies and efficacy of melatonin treatment. Sleep 1996; 19(7):544–553.
37. Wirz-Justice A. Biological rhythm disturbances in mood disorders. Int Clin Psychopharmacol 2006; 21 (suppl 1):S11–S15.
38. Terman M, Terman JS. Light therapy for seasonal and nonseasonal depression: efficacy, protocol, safety, and side effects. CNS Spectr 2005; 10(8):647–663;quiz 672.
39. Arendt J. Melatonin and the Mammalian Pineal Gland. London: Chapman Hall, 1995.
40. Arendt J, Skene DJ. Melatonin as a chronobiotic. Sleep Med Rev 2005; 9(1):25–39.
41. Campbell SS, Murphy PJ, van den Heuvel CJ, et al. Etiology and treatment of intrinsic circadian rhythm sleep disorders. Sleep Med Rev 1999; 3(3):179–200.
42. Wyatt JK. Delayed sleep phase syndrome: pathophysiology and treatment options. Sleep 2004; 27(6): 1195–1203.
43. Palmer CR, Kripke DF, Savage HC, Jr., et al. Efficacy of enhanced evening light for advanced sleep phase syndrome. Behav Sleep Med 2003; 1(4):213–226.
44. Boivin DB, James FO. Circadian adaptation to night-shift work by judicious light and darkness exposure. J Biol Rhythms 2002; 17(6):556–567.
45. Burgess HJ, Sharkey KM, Eastman CI. Bright light, dark and melatonin can promote circadian adaptation in night shift workers. Sleep Med Rev 2002; 6(5):407–420.
46. Burgess HJ, Crowley SJ, Gazda CJ, et al. Preflight adjustment to eastward travel: 3 days of advancing sleep with and without morning bright light. J Biol Rhythms 2003; 18(4):318–328.
47. Houpt TA, Boulos Z, Moore-Ede MC. MidnightSun: software for determining light exposure and phase-shifting schedules during global travel. Physiol Behav 1996; 59(3):561–568.
48. Czeisler CA, Johnson MP, Duffy JF, et al. Exposure to bright light and darkness to treat physiologic maladaptation to night work. N Engl J Med 1990; 322(18):1253–1259.
49. Fetveit A, Bjorvatn B. Bright-light treatment reduces actigraphic-measured daytime sleep in nursing home patients with dementia: a pilot study. Am J Geriatr Psychiatry 2005; 13(5):420–423.
50. Middleton B, Stone B, Arendt J. Human circadian phase in 12:12h, 200:<8 lux and 1000:<8 lux light-dark cycles, without scheduled sleep or activity. Neuroscience Letters, 2002, 329, 41–44.
51. Brainard GC, Hanifin JP, Greeson JM, et al. Action spectrum for melatonin regulation in humans: evidence for a novel circadian photoreceptor. J Neurosci 2001; 21(16):6405–6412.
52. Thapan K, Arendt J, Skene DJ. An action spectrum for melatonin suppression: evidence for a novel non-rod, non-cone photoreceptor system in humans. J Physiol 2001; 535(pt 1):261–267.
53. Skene DJ. Optimization of light and melatonin to phase-shift human circadian rhythms. J Neuroendocrinol 2003; 15(4):438–441.
54. Reme C, Reinboth J, Clausen M, et al. Light damage revisited: converging evidence, diverging views? Graefes Arch Clin Exp Ophthalmol 1996; 234(1):2–11.
55. Reme CE, Rol P, Grothmann K, et al. Bright light therapy in focus: lamp emission spectra and ocular safety. Technol Health Care 1996; 4(4):403–413.
56. Kayumov L, Casper RF, Hawa RJ, et al. Blocking low-wavelength light prevents nocturnal melatonin suppression with no adverse effect on performance during simulated shift work. J Clin Endocrinol Metab 2005; 90(5):2755–2761.
57. Stevens RG. Circadian disruption and breast cancer: from melatonin to clock genes. Epidemiology 2005; 16(2):254–258.
58. Jasser SA, Blask DE, Brainard GC. Light during darkness and cancer: relationships in circadian photoreception and tumor biology. Cancer Causes Control 2006; 17(4):515–523.
59. Blask DE, Brainard GC, Dauchy RT, et al. Melatonin-depleted blood from premenopausal women exposed to light at night stimulates growth of human breast cancer xenografts in nude rats. Cancer Res 2005, 65(23):11174–11184.
60. Blask DE, Dauchy RT, Sauer LA, et al. Light during darkness, melatonin suppression and cancer progression. Neuro Endocrinol Lett 2002; 23(suppl 2):52–56.
61. Lissoni P, Chilelli M, Villa S, et al. Five years survival in metastatic non-small cell lung cancer patients treated with chemotherapy alone or chemotherapy and melatonin: a randomized trial. J Pineal Res 2003; 35(1):12–15.
62. Erren TC. Does light cause internal cancers? The problem and challenge of an ubiquitous exposure. Neuro Endocrinol Lett 2002; 23(suppl 2):61–70.
63. Arendt J. Melatonin and human rhythms. Chronobiol Int 2006; 23(1–2):21–37.
64. Deacon S, Arendt J. Adapting to phase shifts, I. An experimental model for jet lag and shift work. Physiol Behav 1996; 59(4–5):665–673.

65. Gibbs M, Hampton S, Morgan L, et al. Predicting circadian response to abrupt phase shift: 6-sulphatoxymelatonin rhythms in rotating shift workers offshore. J Biol Rhythms 2007; 22:368–370.
66. Filipski E, Delaunay F, King VM, et al. Effects of chronic jet lag on tumor progression in mice. Cancer Res 2004; 64(21):7879–7885.
67. Fu L, Lee CC. The circadian clock: pacemaker and tumour suppressor. Nat Rev Cancer 2003; 3(5):350–361.
68. Arendt J. Melatonin: characteristics, concerns, and prospects. J Biol Rhythms 2005; 20(4):291–303.
69. Brzezinski A, Vangel MG, Wurtman RJ, et al. Effects of exogenous melatonin on sleep: a meta-analysis. Sleep Med Rev 2005; 9(1):41–50.
70. Lockley SW, Skene DJ, James K, et al. Melatonin administration can entrain the free-running circadian system of blind subjects. J Endocrinol 2000; 164(1):R1–R6.
71. Hack LM, Lockley SW, Arendt J, et al. The effects of low-dose 0.5-mg melatonin on the free-running circadian rhythms of blind subjects. J Biol Rhythms 2003; 18(5):420–429.
72. Sack RL, Brandes RW, Kendall AR, et al. Entrainment of free-running circadian rhythms by melatonin in blind people. N Engl J Med 2000; 343(15):1070–1077.
73. Herxheimer A, Petrie KJ. Melatonin for the prevention and treatment of jet lag. Cochrane Database Syst Rev 2002; (2):CD001520.
74. Arendt J. Does melatonin improve sleep? Efficacy of melatonin. BMJ 2006; 332(7540):550.
75. Arendt J, Aldhous M, Marks V. Alleviation of jet lag by melatonin: preliminary results of controlled double blind trial. Br Med J (Clin Res Ed) 1986; 292(6529):1170.
76. Revell VL, Burgess HJ, Gazda CJ, et al. Advancing human circadian rhythms with afternoon melatonin and morning intermittent bright light. J Clin Endocrinol Metab 2006; 91(1):54–59.
77. Deacon S Arendt J. Adapting to phase-shifts, II. Effects of melatonin and conflicting light treatment. Physiol Behav 1996; 59:675–682.
78. Hack L.M. Melatonin and Free-Running Circadian Rhythms in the Blind (thesis). Guildford, Surrey: University of Surrey, 2004.
79. Jansen SL, Forbes DA, Duncan V, et al. Melatonin for cognitive impairment. Cochrane Database Syst Rev 2006; (1):CD003802.
80. Riemersma RF. Light and Melatonin: effect on sleep, mood and cognition in demented elderly. Neurobiol Aging 2004; 25(S2):194 (abstr).
81. Haimov I, Lavie P, Laudon M, et al. Melatonin replacement therapy of elderly insomniacs. Sleep 1995; 18(7):598–603.
82. Jan JE, Espezel H, Appleton RE. The treatment of sleep disorders with melatonin. Dev Med Child Neurol 1994; 36(2):97–107.
83. Phillips L, Appleton RE. Systematic review of melatonin treatment in children with neuro-developmental disabilities and sleep impairment. Dev Med Child Neurol 2004; 46(11):771–775.
84. Delagrange P, Boutin JA. Therapeutic potential of melatonin ligands. Chronobiol Int 2006; 23(1–2): 413–418.
85. Wurtman R. Ramelteon: a novel treatment for the treatment of insomnia. Expert Rev Neurother 2006; 6(7):957–964.
86. Arendt J. Safety of melatonin in long-term use. J Biol Rhythms 1997; 12(6):673–681.
87. Herxheimer A. Does melatonin help people sleep? BMJ 2006; 332(7538):373–374.
88. Reiter RJ. Melatonin: clinical relevance. Best Pract Res Clin Endocrinol Metab 2003; 17(2):273–285.
89. Shochat T, Haimov I, Lavie P. Melatonin—the key to the gate of sleep. Ann Med 1998; 30(1):109–114.
90. Mundey K, Benloucif S, Harsanyi K, et al. Phase-dependent treatment of delayed sleep phase syndrome with melatonin. Sleep 2005; 28(10):1271–1278.
91. Rajaratnam SM, Dijk DJ, Middleton B, et al. Melatonin phase-shifts human circadian rhythms with no evidence of changes in the duration of endogenous melatonin secretion or the 24-hour production of reproductive hormones. J Clin Endocrinol Metab 2003; 88(9):4303–4309.
92. Deacon S, English J, Tate J, et al. Atenolol facilitates light-induced phase shifts in humans. Neurosci Lett 1998; 242(1):53–56.
93. Leibenluft E, Feldman-Naim S, Turner EH, et al. Effects of exogenous melatonin administration and withdrawal in five patients with rapid-cycling bipolar disorder. J Clin Psychiatry 1997; 58(9):383–388.
94. Wehr TA, Aeschbach D, Duncan WC, Jr. Evidence for a biological dawn and dusk in the human circadian timing system. J Physiol 2001; 535(pt 3):937–951.
95. Fourtillan JB, Brisson AM, Gobin P, et al. Bioavailability of melatonin in humans after day-time administration of D(7) melatonin. Biopharm Drug Dispos 2000; 21(1):15–22.
96. Suhner A, Schlagenhauf P, Tschopp A, et al. Impact of melatonin on driving performance. J Travel Med 1998; 5(1):7–13.
97. Sasseville A, Paquet N, Sevigny J, et al. Blue blocker glasses impede the capacity of bright light to suppress melatonin production. J Pineal Res 2006; 41(1):73–78.

18 | Description of Hypersomnias

Allison Chan and Emmanuel Mignot

Department of Psychiatry and Behavioral Sciences, Center for Narcolepsy, Stanford University School of Medicine, Stanford, California, U.S.A.

INTRODUCTION

The *International Classification of Sleep Disorders* (ICSD-2) (1) recognizes a vast differential of etiologies of hypersomnolence. Those types of hypersomnolence with a cause of central origin are the focus in this section (Table 1); those due to sleep-related breathing disorders, circadian rhythm sleep disorders, or other causes of disturbed sleep are discussed separately. The main groups of central origin hypersomnias include narcolepsy, recurrent hypersomnia (including Kleine–Levin syndrome and menstrual-related hypersomnia), idiopathic hypersomnia, behaviorally induced insufficient sleep syndrome, hypersomnia due to medical conditions or drugs, nonorganic hypersomnia, and unspecified physiological hypersomnia.

Hypersomnia historically referred to conditions with "increased sleep amounts" (2–4). Over time, however, the term has evolved to embrace all conditions featuring excessive daytime somnolence due to centrally mediated etiologies (5,6). Although other sleep disorders, such as misaligned circadian rhythms or disturbed nocturnal sleep, may be present, they need to be diagnosed and adequately managed before a diagnosis in this category can be confirmed. Similarly, a history of psychiatric and medical disorders, medications, and substance abuse must be ascertained prior to diagnosing hypersomnia of central origin.

NARCOLEPSY

Narcolepsy is characterized as a disorder in which the boundaries of wakefulness and normal sleep, most notably REM sleep, are blurred; features of sleep intrude into the state of wakefulness and vice versa. It has been divided into various categories, including those with cataplexy, those without cataplexy, those due to a medical condition and unspecified forms. Within this section, the different forms will be explored in terms of their defining characteristics. The history and epidemiology will also be discussed.

History and Nomenclature

For many centuries, cases with unexplained excessive daytime sleepiness have been identified and reported. A possible case of narcolepsy was first described in 1672 by Willis. Derived from the Greek words for both "somnolence" and "to seize," the term "narcolepsy" was coined by Gelineau in 1880 to characterize a disorder with episodes of "astasia" (falling) and irresistible sleep attacks. Narcolepsy is characterized as a disorder in which the boundaries of wakefulness and normal sleep, most notably REM sleep, are blurred; features of sleep intrude into the state of wakefulness and vice versa. An association between brief periods of muscle weakness triggered by emotions and excessive somnolence was first reported by Westphal in 1877. Lowenfeld used the term "cataplexy" in 1902 to describe the muscle weakness. The association between hypnagogic hallucinations, cataplexy, sleep paralysis, and excessive daytime somnolence was emphasized by Daniels in 1934. The phrase "narcoleptic tetrad" was first coined in 1957 by Yoss and Daly in reference to these four clinical findings. Sleep-onset rapid eye movement (REM) periods (SOREMPs, nocturnal REM latencies below 20 minutes) were first identified in narcoleptic patients in 1960 by Vogel. Research by Dement and Rechtschaffen further established that disordered REM sleep is key to the pathophysiology of narcolepsy. During the First International Symposium in Narcolepsy, which met in 1975, narcolepsy was recognized as a syndrome defined by excessive daytime somnolence, SOREMPs, cataplexy, and possibly hypnagogic hallucinations and sleep paralysis; however, the etiology remained elusive.

Table 1 *International Classification of Sleep Disorders (ICSD-2)*: Definitions, Prevalence, and Pathophysiology of Narcolepsy and Hypersomnias

Condition	Diagnostic criteria	North American prevalence	Pathophysiology
Narcolepsy with cataplexy	EDS ≥ 3 mo, presence of definite cataplexy (and usually abnormal MSLT results)	0.02–0.067% (well documented)	Hypocretin deficiency; 90% with low CSF Hcrt-1 and HLA-DQB1*0602 positivity
Narcolepsy without cataplexy	EDS ≥ 3 mo, MSLT: mean sleep latency ≤8 min, ≥2 SOREMPs; No or doubtful cataplexy	0.02% if diagnosed. Probably common, several percent if undiagnosed	Unknown, probably heterogeneous; 7–25% with low CSF Hcrt-1, 40% HLA-DQB1*0602 positive
Secondary narcolepsy or Hypersomnia	As above, but due to other known medical conditions (e.g., neurologic, psychiatric)	Unknown	With or without Hcrt deficiency
Periodic hypersomnia (includes Kleine–Levin syndrome and menstrual-related hypersomnia)	Recurrent (>1×/yr) sleepiness (lasting 2–28 days), normal function between occurrences	Rare, probably less than 1/1M	Unknown, probable heterogeneous etiology
Idiopathic hypersomnia—prolonged sleep	EDS ≥ 3 mo, MSLT: short mean sleep latency, <2 SOREMPs; long (≥10 hr) unrefreshing nocturnal sleep	Rare, maybe 0.01–0.02%	Unknown, probable heterogeneous etiology
Idiopathic hypersomnia—normal sleep length	EDS ≥ 3 mo, MSLT: short mean sleep latency, <2 SOREMPs; normal nightly sleep amounts (<10 hr)	Common, unknown prevalence	Unknown, probable heterogeneous etiology
Behaviorally induced insufficient sleep syndrome	EDS ≥ 3 mo, short habitual sleep; typically sleeps longer when off work; sleep extension resolves the sleepiness	Common, unknown prevalence	Physiological consequence of a chronic sleep restriction

EDS, excessive daytime sleepiness; CSF, cerebrospinal fluid; Hcrt: hypocretin; HLA, human leukocyte antigen; MSLT, multiple sleep latency test; SOREMP, sleep-onset rapid eye movement period.

Narcolepsy was first thought to be a genetically determined autoimmune disorder when a link between narcolepsy and the human leukocyte antigen (HLA) DR2 and HLA DQ6 was identified in Japan in 1986 (7). This association was confirmed in 96% of Caucasians diagnosed with narcolepsy, and later shown to be primarily due to DQB1*0602 across multiple ethnic groups (8). Narcoleptics with cataplexy have been found to have DQB1*0602 positivity more often than those without cataplexy; moreover, a positive correlation between DQB1*0602 positivity and severity of cataplexy has been identified (8,9).

In 2000, following on parallel discoveries in animal models (10), most cases of human narcolepsy with cataplexy were found to have low cerebrospinal fluid (CSF) hypocretin-1 (11). Limited postmortem studies found a dramatically decreased number of hypocretin producing cells in the brain of narcoleptic patients (12,13). On the basis of the HLA association, it is hypothesized that narcolepsy-cataplexy may be an autoimmune disorder targeting hypocretin producing cells, a hypothesis still under intense investigation. Importantly, however, only a minority of cases without cataplexy have low CSF hypocretin-1 (14), suggesting either a milder form of hypocretin cell destruction or/and more etiological heterogeneity in cases without cataplexy.

Neurobiology of the Hypocretin/Orexin System
Encoding the precursor of a pair of peptides homologous to secretin, a hypothalamic-specific mRNA was reported by de Lecea et al. in 1998 (15). To denote their resemblance to secretin and their specificity for the hypothalamus, the peptides were named hypocretin-1 and hypocretin-2

(Hcrt-1 and Hcrt-2). Two neuropeptides were identified by Sakurai et al. in 1998 that, when centrally administered to rats, stimulated food intake (16). These peptides bound and activated two related orphan G protein-coupled receptors. From the Greek word "orexis" which means "appetite," the neuropeptides were named orexin A and orexin B. It later became evident that hypocretins and orexins are one and the same. Though hypocretin-2 has a 10-fold lower affinity for Hcrtr 1 versus Hcrtr 2, both hypocretins bind to two G protein-coupled receptors (Hcrtr 1 and Hcrtr 2). Within the hypothalamus are the cell bodies of neurons that produce hypocretin and their dense projections which project widely throughout the brain but predominantly to the locus ceruleus (17).

Four major hypocretin projection pathways have been identified; two project toward the brainstem and the remaining two to the cortex. The two descending pathways impinge on structures that have been recognized to be involved in the occurrence of REM sleep and in sleep/wake regulation. It has been suggested that the hypocretin system's widespread distribution indicates that these neuropeptides participate in various physiologic functions, including endocrine function, sleep-wake cycle, food intake, cardiovascular regulation, and thermoregulation (17). Small and composed of 50 to 100,000 neurons in humans, this neuronal group likely has a regulatory role.

Key Features and Characteristics

Narcolepsy-cataplexy usually manifests during adolescences; in some, the onset is insidious, but in others, it is abrupt. Though a specific trigger may be difficult to isolate, some patients are able to recall specific precipitating events, such as a head trauma, an infection, a bee sting, or an unusual psychological stress. As the name implies, narcolepsy with cataplexy is a syndrome characterized by the presence of both excessive daytime somnolence and cataplexy.

Although sleepiness can be welcome if an individual wants to sleep, it can be pathological when it results in a tendency to fall asleep at inappropriate times. Pathological sleepiness, or excessive daytime somnolence, is often the first symptom to appear in narcolepsy with cataplexy and may be induced by a variety of different factors, including the quality and quantity of one's sleep, drugs, circadian components, environmental stimuli, motivation, and any number of psychiatric, medical, and neurological conditions (18,19).

Physicians must first clarify the words which patients may use to describe their symptoms. Although the term "fatigue" may be used interchangeably in describing one's sleepiness, true fatigue is different in that these patients do not fall asleep if given the opportunity because they lack the physiologic drive to do so. This is in contrast to patients with sleepiness who fall asleep if conditions permit; those who have severe degrees of disease may even be able to sleep under conditions that may not be considered ideal for sleeping (20).

There are many different ways in which sleepiness may be demonstrated. For example, a sleepy person may report that their daytime functioning is suboptimal; they may make mistakes at work or not perform up to their full potential (21,22). In other cases, an individual may have a sense of "decreased subjective alertness" that may be worse after lunch (18). Still others report "sleepability" in terms of their ability to fall asleep in any setting (23).

Some narcoleptics have even demonstrated unintentional periods of sleep during times of desired wakefulness, as during interactive conversation, during intercourse, and while eating. These irresistible periods of sleep are referred to as sleep attacks (18,24). Patients may feel refreshed for a brief period of time after they take a short nap (approximately 10–20 minutes), but then feel sleepy again after a few hours. These individuals have an inability to stay awake or asleep for prolonged periods of time rather than a requirement of increased sleep amounts. The *ICSD-2* requires a daily complaint of sleepiness for a minimum of three months; it must be significant enough to "impair daytime functioning"; three months of daily somnolence is also required for a diagnosis of idiopathic hypersomnia (1).

Essentially pathognomonic for narcolepsy-cataplexy (24–26), cataplexy is characterized by a bilateral loss of muscle tone triggered by strong emotions; it is usually brief in duration, on the order of a few seconds to several minutes (26,27). It often presents within a couple of years from the onset of daytime sleepiness. In mild cases, there may simply be a loss of facial tone, head droop, slurred speech, or jaw drop. Severe attacks are marked by a collapse to the ground. Reflexes cannot be elicited during this event. Cardiac and respiratory muscles are spared; consciousness is maintained. These patients retain complete memory of the event. No sensory deficits are appreciated.

The triggers for cataplexy include laughter, anger, and surprise (26,28). Patients may try to avoid conditions that provoke cataplexy. When the disorder is first beginning to manifest, it is possible, although uncommon, for cataplexy to occur without the typical preceding emotional component. In cases where the diagnosis of cataplexy is in question, as in rare or mild forms or is triggered only by stress, the diagnosis of narcolepsy without cataplexy should be made.

It is important to distinguish genuine cataplexy from normal physiological reactions. Non-narcoleptic patients may report a sense of becoming weak in the knees or collapsing onto the floor when laughing hard. In fact, a sizable portion of the general population has had episodes that appear cataplexy-like in nature, but those events are mild, infrequent, and independent of typical emotional triggers (28). True cataplexy, however, is differentiated in that the muscle weakness is obvious and occurs multiple times in the person's lifetime (26,28).

Questions regarding cataplexy should be framed carefully so as not to lead the patient. It is better to leave questions more open-ended, such as "Does anything unusual happen when you laugh?" rather than "Do you feel weak when you laugh?" An affirmative response should not be considered the end of the matter. Instead, the specific circumstance should be recounted. A detailed account of the first or last episode should also be provided. If the events are not clear or have occurred only once, the diagnosis of cataplexy should not be made.

It is uncommon to witness true cataplectic attacks in the clinic. Severely affected patients may elicit minor facial attacks when they recount emotional episodes. Dr. William Dement recounted his difficulty in eliciting cataplexy in a laboratory setting (29). Telling jokes or funny stories did not work, but when patients were shown episodes of "I Love Lucy," they were observed to collapse on laughing. Subjects were flaccid and without deep tendon reflexes, yet they could move their eyes and breathe normally.

As patients fall asleep or awaken from sleep, they may experience sleep paralysis, which is an inability to move or speak (24,26,30). It usually persists for 10 seconds to several minutes before resolving spontaneously. An external stimulus, like the touch of another person, may also halt the paralysis. Muscles of respiration and eye control are spared, but a sense of fright may be present. This phenomenon is present in approximately 40% to 80% of narcoleptics. Importantly, however, up to 40% to 50% of normal individuals have reported isolated episodes of sleep paralysis, although the symptom is typically mild and rare, and rarely distressful in control subjects (1).

Vivid and realistic hallucinations at sleep onset (hypnagogic) or on awakening (hypnopompic) have been reported in 40% to 80% of narcoleptics (24,26,31). The hallucinations are commonly visual or auditory. Tactile or kinetic hallucinations (as if one were levitating) have also been reported. Normal individuals may also experience these types of hallucinations (30). Often involving a sensation that someone or something is in the room, these hallucinations can be frightening, especially if they occur with sleep paralysis.

Automatic behavior typically manifests in cases of severe sleepiness (24,32). This phenomenon is characterized by an interruption of purposeful activity by a sleep attack or a microsleep episode such that performance is markedly impaired; the individual furthermore demonstrates no recollection of the event. One example is the case where a patient who is sleepy may continue to speak on the phone but in an inarticulate manner. In the case of sleep drunkenness, which is an extreme form of sleep inertia, an individual is profoundly sleepy as he emerges from sleep and manifests confusion. Sleepiness in narcolepsy may be temporarily alleviated by a short nap (32).

Narcoleptic patients with cataplexy are generally not true "hypersomniacs"; indeed, if left alone, patients do not typically sleep a larger amount over a 24-hour period when compared with normal individuals. Rather, patients with narcolepsy are unable to sustain wakefulness for prolonged periods of time. A similar lack of sleep consolidation is also observed at night. About 50% of individuals with narcolepsy with cataplexy have nocturnal sleep that is so disturbed that it is disabling (18,24,25). Narcoleptics experience repeated awakenings and restlessness through the night. Periodic limb movements and nightmares are common (33,34).

Although it is possible to diagnose narcolepsy with cataplexy on clinical findings alone, it is recommended that patients suspected with this disorder undergo a full night polysomnography (PSG) followed by a multiple sleep latency test (MSLT) the next day. The PSG may be significant for a sleep latency of less than 10 min, an increase in the amount of nonrapid eye movement (NREM) stage N1 sleep, and sleep fragmentation. About 25% to 50% of people with this disorder also demonstrate a SOREMP. Two or more SOREMPs and a mean latency to sleep of less than eight minutes are expected on an MSLT as criteria for the diagnosis of narcolepsy. Results of the test should be interpreted cautiously together with the clinical picture. Recommendation for a valid MSLT includes: sufficient sleep prior to daytime testing (total sleep time $\geq$ 6 hour) and the absence of significant sleep-disordered breathing, two criteria that can be difficult to achieve. False positives and negatives are common. A finding of only one SOREMP and a mean latency to sleep of eight minutes or more may be present in about 15% to 25% of patients with cataplexy, particularly in patients who are over 36 years of age. Recent population-based studies have also shown that 1% to 5% of the general population may test positive on the MSLT.

In narcolepsy due to a medical condition, the patient must demonstrate daily excessive daytime somnolence for a minimum of three months and either a definite history of cataplexy or a short mean sleep latency (less than eight minutes) and two SOREMPs on the MSLT. Some of these patients may also manifest sleep paralysis, hypnagogic hallucinations, insomnia, or automatic behavior.

Several medical disorders have been shown to be a direct cause of narcolepsy. Those that have resulted in narcolepsy with cataplexy include neurosarcoidosis, hypothalamic tumors, multiple sclerosis (with plaques in the hypothalamus), autosomal-dominant cerebellar ataxia with deafness, Neimann–Pick type C disease, Norrie's disease, paraneoplastic syndromes with anti-Ma2 antibodies, and perhaps Coffin–Lowry syndrome (35–38). Other medical conditions have resulted in narcolepsy without cataplexy, such as head trauma, multiple system atrophy, Parkinson's disease, myotonic dystrophy, and Prader–Willi syndrome (39–41).

The diagnosis of unspecified narcolepsy is intended for use on a short-term basis. These patients fulfill both clinical and polysomnographic criteria for narcolepsy; however, additional work-up is needed to assess which particular diagnostic category of narcolepsy is most appropriate.

Incidence and Prevalence

Approximately 0.02% to 0.067% of the population in the United States and Western Europe are affected with narcolepsy with cataplexy. In Japan, the prevalence has been reported between 0.16% and 0.18% (42), and in Israel the prevalence of narcolepsy has been reported as 0.0002% (43). Both sexes may be affected equally. The peak onset of symptoms occurs in adolescence with a second peak around the age of 40; about 10% of cases are diagnosed before 10 years old and 5% after 50 years old. Symptoms of narcolepsy are not progressive but usually persist for life.

Although most cases of narcolepsy are sporadic, there have been familial occurrences. In first-degree relatives, the risk of developing narcolepsy with cataplexy is 1% to 2%, which is 10 to 40 times higher than that in the general population. About 4% to 5% of relatives manifest daytime somnolence. Cases of narcolepsy with cataplexy were identified in a number of DQB1*0602 families suggesting that transmittal occurred in an autosomal dominant pattern with high penetrance (44).

In clinical samples, narcolepsy without cataplexy is thought to account for about 10% to 50% of the narcoleptic population. The exact population prevalence of narcolepsy without cataplexy is unknown. A study in the Olmsted County reported a prevalence of 0.016% (45) for diagnosed subjects; whether or not many more mild narcolepsy without cataplexy cases are present in the population is unknown. When systematic MSLT studies are conducted in population samples, approximately 2% of the population meets the diagnostic criteria for narcolepsy without cataplexy (46).

Phylogeny and Animal Models

Various breeds of dogs have been collected at Stanford University to serve as an animal model for narcolepsy-cataplexy. Symptoms have first been noted in dogs at an age equivalent to early adolescence. Similar to that in humans, cataplexy in dogs can be elicited by a strong emotion, as occurs in playing, feeding, or chewing. The dogs maintain alertness during the brief cataplectic event and can even track objects visually if their eyes are open. During the episode, the deep tendon reflexes are lost; they return as the event resolves. Narcoleptic dogs, unlike normal dogs, have been shown to have a sleep latency of less than 5 minutes and short REM latencies when a modified sleep latency test is administered (47).

On the basis of studies on Labrador retrievers and Dobermans, genetic transmission of narcolepsy seems to occur through an identical autosomal recessive mode with complete penetrance. It appears that a mutation in the gene coding for the hypocretin-2 receptor is responsible for canine narcolepsy (48). Preprohypocretin knockout mice were also found to demonstrate behavior consistent with narcolepsy (34). Nevertheless, unsuccessful attempts at breeding affected beagles and poodles suggest that there must be different causes for the canine narcolepsy syndrome other than genetic. Rather, like human narcolepsy, sporadic cases of narcolepsy have low CSF Hypocretin-1 (49).

Social and Economic Factors

Narcoleptics experience multiple consequences from their daytime somnolence. The sleepiness may affect concentration and focus, and thus their performance at school and work may be suboptimal. The risk of accidents is higher in those who are chronically sleepy (50,51) or have a sleep disorder like narcolepsy (52,53). Falling asleep at the wheel is an extremely serious possibility in these individuals; having their driver's license revoked can lead to more than just minor inconveniences. The matter of driving should be discussed and, if deemed appropriate, the patient should be instructed against driving (54,55) and regulatory agencies notified (54). But patients may be reluctant to discuss their symptoms for fear of losing their license. They are also advised against working in an environment where they may injure themselves or others. Yet these more sedentary jobs that may entail sitting, repetitive work, or staring at a computer may be particularly challenging to one struggling with hypersomnia. Employers and teachers should be encouraged to allow these people to schedule 15 to 30 minute long naps. In public, a sleep attack may elicit embarrassment and potentially cause the individual to shun social engagements. Weight gain, loss of confidence, depression, and type 2 diabetes may all occur more frequently in this patient population, particularly in children when disease onset is abrupt (56,57).

RECURRENT HYPERSOMNIA

Kleine–Levin syndrome is a disorder primarily in adolescent boys characterized by periodic hypersomnolence and, more variably compulsive hyperphagia (58). It was first described in 1925 by Kleine (59) and later by Levin in 1936 (60). The duration of each episode is days to weeks. Episodes may occur rarely or multiple times per month and have no clear periodicity. The severity and duration of symptoms may decrease with successive episodes (61,62). Cognitive abnormalities, such as a feeling of derealization, are core to the symptomatology during episodes. Individuals afflicted with this disorder sleep 16 hours or more each day and may eat copious quantities on awakening. While they are awake, they may be hypersexual, withdrawn, dull, confused, and inattentive. Abnormal behavior, such as aggression, irritability, or other odd behavior, may be present, especially if the patient is awakened abruptly. In most cases, the disorder spontaneously remits within 2 to 10 years after onset.

Normal sleep cycling is present on polysomnograms, and MSLTs demonstrate pathologic sleepiness but no evidence of sleep-onset REM. It has been postulated that the disorder may be due to an abnormality of the limbic-hypothalamic pathway. On the basis of an association identified with the HLA DQB1*02, a viral or autoimmune etiology has been suggested.

Menstrual-related hypersomnia occurs within the first few months after menarche. Repeated episodes of hypersomnia tend to persist for approximately one week and spontaneously resolve at the time of menses. Prolonged remission has been observed to occur with use of oral contraceptives, suggesting a hormone imbalance may be responsible for this disorder.

It is important to note that for both of these forms of recurrent hypersomnia, one's sleep and general behavior are normal in between attacks. Psychiatric disorders marked by recurrent episodes of sleepiness, such as bipolar disorder, somatoform disorder, and seasonal affective disorder, must be ruled out. Another consideration is tumors within the third ventricle, like colloid cysts and pedunculated astrocytomas. By intermittently obstructing ventricular flow, these masses may produce vomiting, headaches, paroxysmal impairment of alertness, and sensorial abnormalities.

IDIOPATHIC HYPERSOMNIA WITH AND WITHOUT LONG SLEEP TIME

The hallmark of idiopathic hypersomnia with and without long sleep time is constant, severe excessive daytime somnolence. Those individuals with a long sleep time generally sleep around 12 to 14 hours per night (although a sleep time of greater than 10 hours is sufficient for this group) and may also nap for 3 to 4 hours through the day. Those without a long sleep time sleep may have a major sleep episode that is normal or slightly longer than that seen in normal individuals (but the duration is less than 10 hours); they may inadvertently nap during the day. Sleep fragmentation is not present in either group. They both struggle to awaken in the morning or at the end of their nap (63). Patients report sleep drunkenness, or confusion, on awakening (64). An alarm clock alone is usually insufficient to awaken these people. Peripheral vascular complaints, migraines, and orthostatic hypotension with syncope have been reported to occur in association with this disorder. Sleep paralysis and hypnagogic hallucinations may be present.

Idiopathic hypersomnia is unusual in prepubertal children, and does not show predominance for either gender. Typically, patients with idiopathic hypersomnia with or without long sleep time present with symptoms before the age of 25 years. It appears to have a nonprogressive course; rare spontaneous remission has been noted (3,5). Some cases demonstrating a familial tendency for this disorder have been reported. It is important to differentiate idiopathic hypersomnia with long sleep time from depression with hypersomnia and excessive daytime somnolence.

Both groups of patients demonstrate normal amounts of NREM and REM sleep on PSG, although there may be a greater amount of slow wave sleep (65). Other sleep disorders, such as periodic limb movement disorders and sleep-related breathing disorders, must either be ruled out or appropriately managed before a diagnosis of idiopathic hypersomnia with or without long sleep time may be properly established. An MSLT in either of these patients may demonstrate one or no SOREMPs. Whether or not long sleep time is present, patients with idiopathic hypersomnia have a mean latency to sleep of 6.2 ± 3 minutes. In idiopathic hypersomnia without prolonged daily sleep amounts, an MSLT is mandatory for the diagnosis and must document a mean sleep latency below or equal to eight minutes.

Patients with idiopathic hypersomnia have been studied via spectral analysis of their EEG during sleep. Such research has suggested a decreased sleep pressure, as measured during the first two nocturnal sleep cycles. All subjects studied so far have demonstrated normal levels of hypocretin-1 in the CSF (38,66). Billiard and Dauvilliers have performed neurochemical studies of CSF monoamine metabolites and noted a decrease in noradrenergic metabolites (3). Decreased CSF histamine levels have been identified in a group of idiopathic hypersomnia and narcolepsy patients with normal hypocretin levels (67).

BEHAVIORALLY INDUCED INSUFFICIENT SLEEP SYNDROME

This disorder is present in people who repeatedly acquire suboptimal amounts of sleep to such an extent that their daytime alertness is affected. Although these individuals have no difficulty with sleep onset or sleep maintenance, they continuously subject themselves to sleep deprivation. It is possible for them to manifest hypnagogic hallucinations or sleep paralysis. Secondarily, they may go on to develop poor concentration, fatigue, irritability, malaise, reduced motivation, and restlessness, which are all expected psychological and physiological hallmarks of sleep deprivation. Depression, social withdrawal, and stimulant abuse may occur. Though individuals of any age or gender may develop this problem, adolescents may be slightly more inclined to manifest symptoms as social pressures restrict their sleep; they may report that they sleep for extended periods of time at night on holidays or over the weekend (68,69). It can be challenging to establish a diagnosis of behaviorally induced insufficient sleep syndrome in a patient who physiologically requires particularly large quantities of sleep.

These subjects do not necessarily need to undergo a polysomnogram or MSLT to establish their diagnosis. If they increase their total sleep time and note a subsequent resolution of their symptoms, then the diagnosis is clear. Individuals who have had polysomnographic monitoring demonstrate a high sleep efficiency (usually over 90%), a decreased latency to sleep, and a long sleep time. NREM and REM sleep occur in a normal distribution. Excessive sleepiness and stage N1 and N2 NREM sleep are demonstrated on MSLT.

HYPERSOMNIA DUE TO MEDICAL CONDITION

Some individuals may be hypersomnolent due to an underlying medical or neurological condition. While they do not manifest cataplexy, they may or may not have automatic behavior, sleep paralysis, or hypnagogic hallucinations. MSLT in these people will not demonstrate more than 1 SOREMP or a mean sleep latency less than eight minutes.

Many conditions have been recognized within this category. Hypothyroidism is the most widely known endocrinologic disorder to manifest hypersomnia. Head trauma may also result in this disorder, but it is important to rule out sleep-related breathing disorders, which can also occur as a result of head trauma (28). Hypersomnia can develop after exposure to toxins (e.g., organic solvents, methylchloride, and trichloroethylene) or in certain metabolic conditions (such as chronic renal insufficiency, pancreatic or adrenal insufficiency, or hepatic encephalopathy). As noted previously, genetic conditions, such as fragile X, myotonic dystrophy (30), Prader–Willi, and Niemann Pick type C disease (26,27), may be central mediators of hypersomnolence. It can also be due to infections, like acute disseminated encephalomyelitis (70), diencephalic ischemia (71), sarcoidosis, or central nervous system tumors (24). Some Parkinson's patients have also been noted to manifest daytime sleepiness unrelated to their medications (29).

HYPERSOMNIA DUE TO DRUG OR SUBSTANCE

Excessive daytime somnolence, nocturnal sleep, or daytime napping may occur in individuals who have developed tolerance to or are withdrawing from alcohol (72), prescribed medications (such as antiepileptics (19,73), opioid analgesics (74), gammahydroxybutyric acid, benzodiazepines, or barbiturates (75)), or street drugs (76). Abrupt cessation of stimulants, such as those prescribed for attention deficit disorder or a sleep disorder, can also induce hypersomnia. This problem may occur in alcoholics of any age but tends to be present in abusers of stimulants who are between the ages of 15 and 50 years. If the offending agent is removed and the patient recovers from the aforementioned symptoms, then this diagnosis can be confirmed.

HYPERSOMNIA NOT DUE TO SUBSTANCE OR KNOWN PHYSIOLOGICAL CONDITION

Otherwise referred to as nonorganic hypersomnia, this condition is characterized by unrefreshing, poor quality sleep with excessive daytime somnolence, prolonged napping, or excessive sleep at night. Conversion disorder, atypical depression, bipolar type II disorder, or undifferentiated somatoform disorders are the most commonly associated psychiatric conditions that lead to nonorganic hypersomnia. Schizoaffective disorder, personality disorders, and adjustment disorder are other less well-known psychiatric etiologies. Approximately 5% to 7% of cases of hypersomnia are due to nonorganic hypersomnia. Women between the ages of 20 and 50 years appear to present with this disorder more commonly than men (77).

PHYSIOLOGICAL (ORGANIC) HYPERSOMNIA, UNSPECIFIED

Also known as organic hypersomnia, not otherwise specified, this is a disorder characterized by excessive daytime somnolence present every day for a minimum of three months and an MSLT demonstrating one or no SOREMPs and a mean sleep latency less than eight minutes. A physiological condition is suspected as the etiology, but no other criteria are met.

CONCLUSIONS

Common causes of excessive daytime somnolence in the general population include narcolepsy and idiopathic hypersomnia. These are the fourth most often diagnosed pathologies in sleep disorders clinics, after obstructive sleep apnea, insomnia, and restless legs syndrome. The number of individuals who will be diagnosed with these disorders is likely to increase as the field of sleep medicine expands and appropriate diagnostic measures are performed. The impact of hypersomnolence can be far-reaching. Productivity in school and at work may be compromised. The social stigma some may perceive from this disorder can be debilitating. Serious accidents can occur due to falling asleep on the job or while driving. For all of these reasons, it is imperative for clinicians to perform thorough histories and physical examinations and utilize available studies to elucidate the etiology behind their symptoms and thus provide optimal management strategies.

REFERENCES

1. American Academy of Sleep Medicine. ICSD-2, the international classification of sleep disorders. In: Diagnostic and Coding Manual. 2nd ed. Westchester, IL: American Academy of Sleep Medicine, 2005:79–115.
2. Billiard M. Idiopathic hypersomnia. Neurol Clin 1996; 14:570–582.
3. Billiard M, Dauvilliers Y. Idiopathic hypersomnia. Sleep Med Rev 2001; 5:351–360.
4. Roth B. Narcolepsy and hypersomnia: review and classification of 642 personally observed cases. Schweiz Arch Neurol Neurochir Psychiatr 1976; 119:31–41.
5. Bassetti C, Aldrich MS. Idiopathic hypersomnia. A series of 42 patients. Brain 1997; 120:1423–1435.
6. Dauvilliers Y. Differential diagnosis in hypersomnia. Curr Neurol Neurosci Rep 2006; 6:156–162.
7. Honda Y, Juji T, Matsuki K, et al. HLA-DR2 and Dw 2 in narcolepsy and in other disorders of excessive somnolence without cataplexy. Sleep 1986; 9:133–142.
8. Mignot E, Ling L, Rogers R, et al. Complex HLA-DR and DQ interactions confer risk for narcolepsy–cataplexy in three ethnic groups. Am J Hum Genet 2001; 68:686–699.
9. Mignot E, Hayduk R, Black J, et al. HLA DQB1*0602 is associated with cataplexy in 509 narcoleptic patients. Sleep 1997; 20:1012–1020.
10. Chemelli RM, Willie JT, Sinton CM, et al. Narcolepsy in orexin knockout mice: molecular genetics of sleep regulation. Cell 1999; 98:437–451.
11. Nishino S, Ripley B, Overeem S, et al. Hypocretin (orexin) deficiency in human narcolepsy. Lancet 2000; 355:39–40.
12. Peyron C, Faraco J, Rogers W, et al. A mutation in a case of early onset narcolepsy and a generalized absence of hypocretin peptides in human narcoleptic brains. Nat Med 2000; 6:991–997.
13. Thannickal TC, Moore RY, Nienhuis R, et al. Reduced number of hypocretin neurons in human narcolepsy. Neuron 2000; 27:469–474.
14. Mignot E, Lammers GJ, Ripley B, et al. The role of cerebrospinal fluid hypocretin measurement in the diagnosis of narcolepsy and other hypersomnias. Arch Neurol 2002; 59:1553–1562.
15. de Lecea L, Kilduff TS, Peyron C, et al. The hypocretins: hypothalamus-specific peptides with neuroexcitatory activity. Proc Natl Acad Sci USA 1998; 95:322–327.
16. Sakurai T, Amemiya A, Ishii M, et al. Orexins and orexin receptors: a family of hypothalamic neuropeptides and G protein-coupled receptors that regulate feeding behavior. Cell 1998; 92:573–585.
17. Peyron C, Tighe D, van der Pol A, et al. Neurons containing hypocretin (orexin) project to multiple neuronal systems. J Neurosci 1998; 18:9996–10015.
18. Black J, Brooks SN, Nishino S. Narcolepsy and syndromes of primary excessive daytime somnolence. Semin Neurol 2004; 24:271–282.
19. Guilleminault C, Brooks SN. Excessive daytime sleepiness: a challenge for the practicing neurologist. Brain 2001; 124:1482–1491.
20. Thorpy MJ. Approach to the patient with a sleep complaint. Semin Neurol 2004; 24:225–235.
21. Durmer JS, Dinges DF. Neurocognitive consequences of sleep deprivation. Semin Neurol 2005; 25:117–129.
22. Van Dongen HP, Dinges DF. Sleep, circadian rhythms, and psychomotor vigilance. Clin Sports Med 2005; 24:237–249, vii–viii.
23. Harrsion Y, Horne JA. High sleepability without sleepiness. The ability to fall asleep rapidly without other signs of sleepiness. Neurophysiol Clin 1996; 26:15–20.
24. Overeem S, Mignot E, van Dijk, et al. Narcolepsy: clinical features, new pathophysiologic insights, and future perspectives. J Clin Neurophysiol 2001; 18:78–105.

25. Dauvilliers Y, Billiard M, Montplaisir J. Clinical aspects and pathophysiology of narcolepsy. Clin Neurophysiol 2003; 114:2000–2017.
26. Okun ML, Lin L, Pelin A, et al. Clinical aspects of narcolepsy–cataplexy across ethnic groups. Sleep 2002; 25:27–35.
27. Guilleminault C, Wilson RA, Dement WC. A study on cataplexy. Arch Neurol 1974; 31:255–261.
28. Anic-Labat S, Guilleminault C, Kraemer HC, et al. Validation of a cataplexy questionnaire in 983 sleep-disordered patients. Sleep 1999; 22:77–87.
29. Dement WC. Ambushed by sleep: narcolepsy and other sleep disorders. In: Dement WC, Vaughn C, eds. The Promise of Sleep. New York: Dell Publishing, 1999:194–216.
30. Ohayon MM, Zulley J, Guilleminault C, et al. Prevalence and pathologic associations of sleep paralysis in the general population. Neurology 1999; 52:1194–1200.
31. Ohayon MM, Priest RG, Caulet M, et al. Hypnagogic and hypnopompic hallucinations: pathological phenomena? Br J Psychiatry 1996; 169:459–467.
32. Honda Y. Clinical features of narcolepsy: Japanese experience. In: Honda Y, Juji T, eds. HLA in Narcolepsy. New York: Sringer-Verlag, 1988:24–57.
33. Hong SC, Leen K, Park SA, et al. HLA and hypocretin studies in Korean patients with narcolepsy. Sleep 2002; 25:440–444.
34. Godbout R, Montplaisir J. Nocturnal sleep of narcoleptics: revisited. Sleep 1986; 9:159–161.
35. Arii J, Kanbayashi T, Tanabe Y, et al. A hypersomnolent girl with decreased CSF hypocretin level after removal of a hypothalamic tumor. Neurology 2001; 56:1775–1776.
36. Melberg A, Hetta J, Dahl N, et al. Autosomal dominant cerebellar ataxia deafness and narcolepsy. J Neurol Sci 1995; 134:119–129.
37. Kanbayashi T, Abe M, Fujimoto S, et al. Hypocretin deficiency in Niemann–Pick type C with cataplexy. Neuropediatrics 2003; 34:52–53.
38. Vankova J, Stepanova I, Jech R, et al. Sleep disturbances and hypocretin deficiency in Niemann–Pick disease type C. Sleep 2003; 26:427–430.
39. Guilleminault C, Yuen KM, Gulevich MG, et al. Hypersomnia after head–neck trauma: a medico-legal dilemma. Neurology 2000; 54:653–659.
40. Overeem S, van Hilten JJ, Ripley B, et al. Normal hypocretin-1 levels in Parkinson's disease patients with excessive daytime sleepiness. Neurology 2002; 58:498–499.
41. Martinez-Rodriguez JE, Lin L, Iranzo A, et al. Decreased hypocretin-1 (orexin-A) levels in the cerebrospinal fluid of patients with myotonic dystrophy and excessive daytime sleepiness. Sleep 2003; 26:287–290.
42. Honda Y, Asaka A, Tanimura M, et al. A genetic study of narcolepsy and excessive daytime sleepiness in 308 families with a narcolepsy or hypersomnia proband. In: Guilleminault C, Lugaresi E, eds. Sleep/Wake Disorders: Natural History, Epidemiology, and Long-Term Evolution. New York: Raven Press, 1983:187–199.
43. Aldrich MS. The neurobiology of narcolepsy–cataplexy. Prog Neurobiol 1993; 41:533.
44. Mignot E. Genetic and familial aspects of narcolepsy. Neurology 1998; 50:s16–s22.
45. Silber MH, Krahn LE, Olson EJ. The epidemiology of narcolepsy in Olmsted County, Minnesota: a population-based study. Sleep 2002; 25:197–202.
46. Mignot E, Lin L, Finn L, et al. Correlates of sleep-onset REM periods during the Multiple Sleep Latency Test in community adults. Brain 2006 Apr 5; [Epub ahead of print].
47. Nishino S, Mignot E. Pharmacological aspects of human and canine narcolepsy. Prog Neurobiol 1997; 52:27–78.
48. Lin L, Faraco J, Li R, et al. The sleep disorder canine narcolepsy is caused by a mutation in the hypocretin (orexin) receptor 2 gene. Cell 1999; 98:365–376.
49. Ripley B, Fujiki N, Okura M, et al. Familial and sporadic forms of narcolepsy exist in both humans and canines. Neurobiol Dis 2001; 8:525–534.
50. Gander PH, Marshall NS, Harris RB, et al. Sleep, sleepiness and motor vehicle accidents: a national survey. Aust N Z J Public Health 2005; 29:16–21.
51. Philip P. Sleepiness of occupational drivers. Ind Health 2005; 43:30–33.
52. Broughton WA, Broughton RJ. Psychosocial impact of narcolepsy. Sleep 1994; 17:S45–S49.
53. Findley L, Unverzagt M, Guchu R, et al. Vigilance and automobile accidents in patients with sleep apneas or narcolepsy. Chest 1995; 108:619–624.
54. Black JE, Brooks SN, Nishino S. Conditions of primary excessive daytime sleepiness. Neurol Clin 2005; 23:1025–1044.
55. Douglas NJ. The psychosocial aspects of narcolepsy. Neurology 1998; 50:S27–S30.
56. Kotagal S, Krahn LE, Slocumb N. A putative link between childhood narcolepsy and obesity. Sleep Med 2004; 5:147–150.
57. Daniels L. Narcolepsy. Medicine 1934; 13:1–122.
58. Arnulf I, Zeitzer JM, File J, et al. Kleine–Levin syndrome: a systematic review of 186 cases in the literature. Brain 2005; 128(pt12):2763–2776.

59. Kleine W. Periodische Schlafsucht. Monatsschr Psychiatr Neurol 1925; 57:285–320.
60. Levin M. Periodic somnolence and morbid hunger: a new syndrome. Brain 1936; 58:494–515.
61. Critchley M. Periodic hypersomnia and megaphagia in adolescent males. Brain 1962; 85:627–656.
62. Billiard M. The Kleine Levin syndrome. In: Kryger MH, Roth T, Dement WC, eds. Principles and Practice of Sleep Medicine. Philadelphia: WB Saunders, 1989;377–378.
63. Aldrich MS. The clinical spectrum of narcolepsy and idiopathic hypersomnia. Neurology 1996; 46: 393–401.
64. Roth B, Nevsimalova S, Rechtschaffen A. Hypersomnia with "sleep drunkenness." Arch Gen Psychiatry 1972; 26:456–462.
65. Rechtschaffen A, Dement WC. Narcolepsy and hypersomnia. In Kales A, ed. Sleep: Physiology and Pathology. Philadelphia: JB Lippincott Co., 1969:119–130.
66. Mignot E. Narcolepsy: pharmacology, pathophysiology, and genetics. In: Kryger MH, Roth T, Dement WC, eds. Principles and Practice of Sleep Medicine. 4th ed. Philadelphia, PA: Elsevier Saunders, 2005:761–779.
67. Kanbayashi T, Kodama T, Kondo H, et al. CSF histamine and noradrenaline contents in narcolepsy and other sleep disorders. Sleep 2004; 27:A236.
68. Roehrs T, Zorick F, Sicklesteel J, et al. Excessive daytime sleepiness associated with insufficient sleep. Sleep 1983; 6:319–325.
69. Van Dongen HP, Maislin G, Mullington JM, et al. The cumulative cost of additional wakefulness: dose–response effects of neurobehavioral functions and sleep physiology from chronic sleep restriction and total sleep deprivation. Sleep 2003; 26:117–126.
70. Kubota H, Kanbayashi T, Tanabe Y, et al. A case of acute disseminated encephalomyelitis presenting hypersomnia with decreased hypocretin level in cerebrospinal fluid. J Child Neurol 2002; 17:537–539.
71. Scammell TE, Nishino S, Mignot E, et al. Narcolepsy and low CSF orexin (hypocretin) concentration after a diencephalic stroke. Neurology 2001; 56:1751–1753.
72. Roehrs T, Roth T. Sleep, sleepiness, and alcohol use. Alcohol Res Health 2001; 25:101–109.
73. Blum DE. New drugs for persons with epilepsy. Adv Neurol 1998; 76:57–87.
74. Young-McCaughan S, Miaskowski C. Measurement of opioid-induced sedation. Pain Manage Nurs 2001; 2:132–149.
75. Gault FP. A review of recent literature on barbiturate addiction and withdrawal. Bol Estud Med Biol 1976; 29:5–83.
76. Schweitzer P. Drugs that disturb sleep and wakefulness. In: Kryger MH, Roth T, Dement WC, eds. Principles and Practice of Sleep Medicine. 3rd ed. Philadelphia: WB Saunders; 2000:1176–1196.
77. Vgontzas AN, Bixler EO, Kales A, et al. Differences in nocturnal and daytime sleep between primary and psychiatric hypersomnia: diagnosis and treatment implications. Psychosom Med 2000; 62:220–226.

19 | Pathophysiology, Associations, and Consequences of Hypersomnias

Joan Santamaria

Neurology Service and Multidisciplinary Sleep Disorders Unit, Hospital Clinic of Barcelona, University of Barcelona Medical School, Barcelona, Spain

ETIOLOGY, PATHOPHYSIOLOGY, AND PATHOGENESIS

Sleepiness, like hunger or thirst, is a common experience difficult to define and measure. Sleepiness appears normally during the process of falling asleep as an indicator to the organism that sleep is approaching; it can be prolonged by resisting sleep and disappears after getting enough sleep. These are normal phenomena. Sleepiness, however, becomes abnormal when it is "excessive," that is, when because of its frequency or intensity, it appears under abnormal circumstances and interferes with daytime activities (1). Excessive daytime sleepiness (EDS) may happen despite devoting enough time to sleep. One can realize by reading the above statements that they generate more questions than answers: What does excessive really mean? What is an "abnormal circumstance"? How much sleep is "enough"? What type of daytime activity are we referring to? These questions and the fact that EDS in general develops insidiously explain why patients with EDS take so long to look for medical help, in contrast with other neurological symptoms such as a seizure or a limb palsy.

Terminology

Sleepiness and hypersomnia are terms used in a variety of ways. *Sleepiness* describes at least three different things: the *physiological need state for sleep* (2), also called sleep propensity, which can be objectively measured [for example with a multiple sleep latency test (MSLT)], the *subjective perception of the need for sleep* (3) that can only be assessed by asking the individual, and the *behavioral signs* (yawning, closing of the eyelids, motor slowing, lapses in attention, etc.) that a subject displays when approaching sleep. Not every sleepy patient will show parallel changes in the above three aspects. For example, a subject may fall asleep easily in the MSLT, with behavioral signs of sleepiness but without reporting any sleepiness at all or vice versa. *Hypersomnia* is also used indistinctively to describe *excessive daytime sleepiness, prolonged sleep duration, or both*. Using hypersomnia as synonym of EDS may not be always accurate. Not everybody experiencing sleepiness will fall asleep, particularly if sleepiness is not severe, and on the other hand, people who need ten or more hours of nocturnal sleep (and could be considered as suffering from hypersomnia) may not have EDS at all if they get enough nocturnal sleep. In this chapter we will separate, when possible, each of the different meanings.

Mechanisms of Sleepiness

The neural substrate of sleepiness is not known, despite the large amount of research performed in this area. At least two different approaches have been used to understand how sleep and sleepiness occurs: studies of *sleep regulation* and studies of the *neural circuitry* underlying sleep-wake states.

Studies of Sleep Regulation

The results of these studies indicate that the tendency to fall asleep is not a fixed value; it oscillates continuously due to the interaction of several factors or processes. Some of them act relatively slowly (hours) and others function in a more short-term basis. The two slow-acting ones are the *homeostatic process*, which accumulates sleep propensity during waking and dissipates it with sleep, and the *circadian process*, a clock-like mechanism which tends to limit the appearance of sleep to a time of day where it is more ecologically appropriate (4,5). These two factors constitute the main elements of the *two-process model* of sleep regulation, which postulates that sleep tendency (or its mirror, waking function) at any given moment is the result of the difference between the quantitative state for the homeostatic process and the quantitative state for the circadian process (6). Under a conventional 24-hour schedule sleepiness is highest in the middle of the night with a second peak in the afternoon, whereas alertness is highest in the evening. The model does not tell us, however, how the homeostatic need for sleep is generated and which are the neural substrate and biochemical basis of this regulation. In addition, although the knowledge of the circadian system circuitry, centered in the suprachiasmatic nuclei (SCN) of the hypothalamus (7), is impressive, it is unclear if the SCN function by promoting exclusively an arousal drive that *opposes* the need for sleep (8), by producing both arousing and sleep-promoting signals depending on the time of day (9), or simply by acting as a gate which opens when accumulated sleep exceeds a given threshold and closes whenever accumulated sleep falls below another threshold (10). The neural substrate of the gate and its thresholds is not known. One fundamental problem in understanding how the SCN function in relation to sleep is that there are very little studies recording the activity of their neurons with simultaneous monitoring of the sleep stages. The few studies available suggest that, contrary to previous assumptions, the homeostatic sleep drive and the sleep states influence the discharge pattern of the SCN (11,12).

Researchers studying sleep regulation use protocols that specifically avoid influences from social interaction, work or food schedules, physical activity, etc. in order to unmask the effects of the homeostatic and circadian processes. The focus on these two processes may lead to assume that they are the only factors determining the tendency to fall asleep. There are, however, other *arousing (or sleep-promoting) contextual influences* that, on a more short-term basis, facilitate or hinder the appearance of sleepiness and sleep and may be clinically relevant. For example, it is a common experience that sleep is difficult in the presence of fear, anxiety, or severe pain. Motivation, motor activity, ambient noise, change in temperature, posture, and type of task are other factors present in real life that clearly modify the impact of sleep loss in acute sleep deprivation studies (13) and likely influence the presence of sleepiness in healthy subjects (14) and in patients with sleep disorders. Watching alone a boring TV program favors sleep whereas the presence of other people in the room delays it (15). To complicate it further, one can decide to fight sleepiness by walking instead of remaining seated (a 5-minute walk will prolong sleep latency in the MSLT by a mean of 6 minutes) (16), whereas, if not particularly interested in doing anything, may facilitate sleep by remaining comfortably seated. Contextual factors may vary from one moment to the next and the same situation may not have equal effect on different subjects. The neural circuitry and mechanisms underlying these influences are also unknown, although the hypocretin/orexin system could have a role since it is active during locomotion and its activity promotes arousal (17). Finally, it has been proposed that the individual characteristics of the sleepiness/arousal systems (*sleepiness/arousal "trait"*) of a subject are also responsible for the amount of sleepiness an individual has, both in baseline conditions and in response to sleep deprivation (18–20). In summary, homeostatic, circadian, contextual and individual factors interact, generating the sleep propensity of a subject. The complexity and variety of this interaction in the real world is what makes the measurement of sleepiness so difficult.

A different but complementary view (18,21) proposes that the level of sleepiness is the result of the interaction between two drives: the *drive for sleep* (which includes the homeostatic process, perhaps the circadian process during a portion of the sleep period, sleep-promoting contextual influences and the individual sleepiness/arousal trait) and the *drive for wakefulness* (consisting of the circadian process, other arousal-promoting influences and the individual sleepiness/arousal trait). Excessive sleepiness, therefore, could result from (*i*) a *high sleep drive*, (*ii*) an *arousal level that is too low*, or (*iii*) a *combination of both*. An excessive arousal level, on the other hand, could produce decreased sleep time at night without EDS, as is observed in insomnia patients (22). Whether or not these different possibilities produce different clinical types of sleepiness or insomnia remains to be shown. In this model it is assumed that sleepiness and arousal are not at the opposite ends of a single system but are, instead, two independent systems, one governing arousal—from a high to low level—and another sleep—from a high to low sleep propensity.

Studies of the Neural Circuitry Underlying Sleep-Wake States
The neural mechanisms maintaining sleep and wakefulness are relatively well known. *Wakefulness* is maintained by an intricate network of multiple, parallel, partially redundant

Table 1 Neuronal Systems Promoting Arousal and Sleep

Arousal promoting	Neurotransmitter	Sleep promoting	Neurotransmitter
Basal forebrain	Acetylcholine/glutamate GABA	Basal forebrain/ventrolateral preoptic/median preoptic	GABA/gallamine
Thalamus	Glutamate	Thalamus[a]	GABA
Tuberomammillary	Histamine		
Posterolateral hypothalamus	Hypocretin		
Ventral periaqueductal gray	Dopamine		
Locus coeruleus	Noradrenaline		
Raphe	Serotonin		
Pedunculopontine-laterodorsal	Acetylcholine		
		Nucleus tractus solitarius[a]	?

[a]Low frequency electrical stimulation.
Abbreviation: GABA, γ-aminobutyric acid.
Source: From Ref. 23–25.

systems (23) (Table 1) whose components originate in the cholinergic pontine nuclei, the noradrenergic locus coeruleus, the serotonergic raphe nuclei in *the pons/midbrain junction*, the histaminergic tuberomandibular and hypocretinergic (orexinergic) nuclei in the *posterior hypothalamus*, the cholinergic *basal forebrain*, and the glutamatergic *thalamocortical* systems and probably a dopaminergic ventral periaqueductal gray area in the *midbrain* (24). Cortical areas are activated by widespread projections from these nuclei through different thalamic and extrathalamic pathways and probably cooperate in maintaining arousal (25). Most of these systems are maximally active during wakefulness and are likely responsible for this behavioral state and its electroencephalographic (EEG) correlate. However, the relative weight of each of these systems in producing the arousal level of an individual is not well known since isolated dysfunction of these systems is difficult to identify in humans. In cataplexy, a clinical situation, deactivation of serotoninergic and noradrenergic systems and poor functioning of the hypocretin/orexin systems is not incompatible with alertness, suggesting that the histaminergic system (with perhaps the help of the cholinergic and glutamatergic systems and the dopaminergic one) is able to maintain arousal, at least for the relatively short duration of the cataplectic attack (26). Out of the episodes of cataplexy, narcoleptics may also have periods of normal alertness, suggesting that other arousal systems can produce wakefulness without the help of the hypocretinergic system, although they cannot maintain it for long periods. The SCN also have an important function in maintaining arousal because, after their selective destruction, the other arousal systems are unable to sustain relatively long periods of wakefulness (8,9).

Sleep is associated with activation of the basal forebrain and the hypothalamic ventrolateral preoptic (VLPO) area together with deactivation of arousal systems, but it is not completely clear which goes first. The thalamus, the nucleus tractus solitarius in the lower medulla (23,25) and various cortical areas (premotor, posterior supraorbital, and somesthetic) (27) are also other areas that when stimulated with repetitive low frequency electrical stimuli induce sleep. Although the preoptic area (ventrolateral and median preoptic) has a central role in sleep promotion and some of its neurons show a gradual increase in their firing rates before sleep onset (28), an intriguing fact is that the firing rate of VLPO area neurons during waking does not increase with sleep deprivation; it only increases when the animals actually sleep, suggesting that it is more related to the production of sleep than to the level of sleepiness (29). In sleep-deprived animals, other brain areas, such as the ventral hippocampus, show characteristic sleep discharge patterns in the absence of other signs of sleep (30) and in awake sleep-deprived humans there are decreases in regional brain metabolism, particularly in thalamus and prefrontal and posterior parietal cortices (31), suggesting that sleepiness is probably more a forebrain than a brainstem phenomenon.

The mechanisms governing the transition between sleep and wakefulness are partially disentangled. A "flip-flop" model suggests that the mutual inhibition between arousal and sleep-promoting systems results in stable periods of wakefulness and sleep. For example, activity in the sleep side of the system inhibits the arousal side, which in turn removes the inhibition of the arousal side to the sleep side, stabilizing sleep (29). It is not completely clear, though, how the flip-flop is actually flipped.

Table 2 Sleep Promoting Neurochemical Agents

Adenosine
Interleukin-1β
Prostaglandin D_2
Growth hormone–releasing hormone (GHRH)
Oxidized or reduced glutathione
Nitric oxide

Source: From Ref. 28.

Table 3 Causes of Excessive Sleepiness

1. Insufficient or nonrestorative sleep
    Behaviorally induced insufficient sleep syndrome
    Environmental sleep disorder
    Sleep breathing disorder
        Obstructive sleep apnea
        Primary central sleep apnea
        Cheyne–Stokes breathing pattern
        Sleep-related hypoventilation
2. Hypersomnias of central origin (not due to circadian, sleep-related breathing disorders, or other causes of disturbed nocturnal sleep)
    CNS pathology/dysfunction
        Narcolepsy with cataplexy
        Narcolepsy without cataplexy
        Idiopathic hypersomnia
        Recurrent hypersomnia
        Kleine–Levin syndrome
        Menstrual-related hypersomnia
        Depression
    Hypersomnia due to a medical/neurological disorder
        Hypothyroidism, stroke, neurodegenerative diseases, brain tumor, myotonic dystrophy, head trauma, limbic encephalitis
    Hypersomnia due to drug or substance
        Tolerance to or withdrawal from street drugs or alcohol
        Use or abuse of hypnotic drugs or of sedative compounds
        Cessation of a stimulant prescription
        Smoking cessation
3. Circadian rhythm disorders
    Shift work
    Delayed sleep phase
    Advanced sleep phase
    Irregular sleep-wake patterns
    Jet lag

A fundamental question is—what is the substance(s) or function(s) that accumulates during wakefulness and dissipates during sleep? Several substances (Table 2) (28) and functions, for example, synaptic function (5), which likely accumulate during wakefulness, have been implicated in the generation of sleep propensity. Adenosine has been reported as a key player in inducing sleep via stimulation of the VLPO area. In addition, sleep interruption in rat increases (up to 220%) basal forebrain adenosine levels and correlates with measures of sleepiness (32). The relevance of each of the many implicated substances in explaining the sleepiness of a subject is not yet well understood.

Causes of Excessive Sleepiness

Although the ultimate mechanisms of sleepiness are unknown, EDS has been associated to many causes. They can be categorized into the following types (expanded in Table 3):

1. Insufficient or nonrestorative sleep
    a. Sleep restriction
    b. Sleep fragmentation

2. Hypersomnias of central origin

   a. Central nervous system (CNS) pathology/dysfunction
   b. Hypersomnia due to medical/neurological disorder
   c. Hypersomnia due to drugs
   d. Other (mood disorders)

3. Alterations in the circadian rhythm
4. Sleepiness due to multiple factors

Insufficient or Nonrestorative Sleep

Sleep restriction. Total and partial sleep deprivation in normal subjects produces EDS (6,13). Total sleep deprivation is easy to detect and does not usually represent a diagnostic problem. Partial sleep restriction, however, may be more difficult to recognize either because the patient may underestimate it (33) or because it may coexist with other known causes of sleepiness, such as sleep-disordered breathing (34). EDS appears in normal adults when sleep is curtailed to 3 to 6 hr/night in a dose-response mode (35,36), but deficits in waking performance (measured with the psychomotor vigilance test, PVT) are already recognized when sleep is reduced to less than seven hours as compared to eight or nine hours of sleep (37,38). In addition, sleep deprivation of sufficient severity (<5 hours of sleep/day) in healthy subjects has repeatedly been shown to produce sleepiness and performance deficits that accumulate throughout the duration of the experiment, usually 7 to 14 days (35–38). Whether or not lower levels of sleep restriction (5–7 hours of sleep/day, for up to a week) also produce accumulating waking deficits is not totally clear. One study found that after a decrease the first two to three days, performance remained stable, albeit low, without further reductions (38), whereas in another study waking performance still deteriorated (37). The finding that alertness and performance remain at relatively low levels but in a stable manner could explain why sleep restriction is considered harmless and is so often practiced in modern society (33,38). In the US at least 18% of adults report receiving insufficient sleep and the percentage of men and women who sleep less than 6 hours has increased significantly over the last 20 years (39). Sleep has to compete nowadays with increasing time spent on the Internet and TV viewing as well as growing social, recreational, and work demands.

Studies in healthy adults, not complaining of EDS but showing unusually short sleep latencies on the MSLT (40), showed that sleep extension up to 9 to 10 hr/day produced a clear improvement in daytime sleep propensity in most (but not all) of them, suggesting that they were probably sleep deprived. One study has calculated that the amount of sleep needed to avoid waking deficits is about 8.16 hours (37).

There is significant individual and age-related variability in the responses to sleep disruption or curtailment (41–44). Older subjects do not appear to feel as sleepy as younger ones despite more disrupted sleep and have a lower objective sleep tendency to fall asleep. During chronic partial sleep deprivation some healthy subjects achieved a pathological level of sleepiness, others scored in the borderline range, and others surprisingly had even an alert profile (45).

Behaviorally induced insufficient sleep should be suspected when the patient (*i*) has an unusually high sleep efficiency, (*ii*) reports about two hours more sleep on each weekend day more than each weekday (2), or (*iii*) when the appearance of sleepiness is preceded by a change in the sleep patterns of the patient, particularly a reduction in the usual number of hours of sleep.

Sleep restriction can occur in patients because of medical disorders causing pain, limited mobility, nocturia, dyspnea, etc. and may be a cause of daytime sleepiness. EDS due to sleep restriction may also coexist with other causes of sleepiness, such as sleep disordered breathing, narcolepsy, etc., complicating the diagnosis and treatment of the condition.

It is interesting to know that although, in general, sleep restriction is associated with daytime sleepiness, in some disorders like insomnia or restless leg syndrome there is no such clear relationship between degree of sleep reduction or fragmentation and daytime sleepiness (46,47).

Sleep fragmentation. In healthy subjects, fragmenting sleep experimentally induces daytime sleepiness (48) and prevents the recuperative value of sleep (49). The level of daytime sleepiness in these studies increased directly in relation to the increase in the rate of sleep fragmentation (50), for instance, 1/min interruptions could induce a sleepiness as high as that appearing after total sleep deprivation. Both sleep fragmentation inducing awakenings (with associated total sleep time reduction) and fragmentation inducing only EEG arousals (without reductions in sleep time) increase daytime sleepiness (48,49). In routine practice there is only one condition that can be associated with such a high level of sleep fragmentation and it is obstructive sleep apnea (OSA). (51). In fact, sleep fragmentation has been shown to be more relevant in producing EDS than the oxyhemoglobin desaturations occurring in OSA. In experimentally induced sleep apnea vs. sleep fragmentation without apnea in dogs (52), for prolonged periods, sleep fragmentation alone was responsible for the increase in arousal threshold (sleepiness) and the changes in acute responses to airway occlusion resulting in OSA. However, the relation between sleep fragmentation and EDS in OSA is not simple. Although there is a tendency for higher levels of sleepiness with higher apnea/hypopnea indices (AHIs) (53), this is relatively weak and, for instance, in one large study (54) the mean Epworth Sleepiness Scale (ESS) value in patients with an AHI < 5 was 7.3 whereas it was of only 9.1 in patients with an AHI > 30, but in other studies (55) the ESS was unable to distinguish patients with an AHI > 40 from those with an AHI < 40. Young et al. (56) found that only 22% of the women and 17% of the men with an AHI > 5 reported EDS, based on the answers to three questions [(*i*) feeling excessively sleepy during daytime, (*ii*) waking up unrefreshed, (*iii*) having uncontrollably daytime sleepiness that interferes with daily living]. It appears that at the same level of sleep fragmentation (measured as the sleep apnea index or the arousal index) different patients may have different levels of sleepiness (55,57). The presence of sleep apnea is better considered a risk factor for sleepiness than its only cause (58). Epidemiological studies (59) have found that the AHI is not the best predictor of the complaint of excessive sleepiness in the general population.

Other sleep disorders associated with sleep fragmentation, such as periodic leg movements during sleep, may have a higher arousal index but surprisingly are not indicative of a higher degree of daytime sleepiness (60). Instead, the opposite might be true, indicating perhaps that the sleepiness tendency that a patient has is not a daytime phenomenon only but a 24-hour tendency: patients who are more awake at night are also more awake during daytime.

Hypersomnias of Central Origin
CNS pathology/dysfunction. CNS lesions may produce hypersomnia of sudden or progressive onset, depending upon the type of the lesion. As described above, experimental lesions in the brainstem, hypothalamus and thalamus may produce hypersomnia in animals. In humans, however, some of the lesions either are difficult to find isolated or they do not produce the predicted findings. For example, lesions of the medulla that are compatible with life are unilateral and do not produce hypersomnia. Bilateral lesions of the pontine tegmentum usually produce decreased sleep (61,62) with or without visual or auditory hallucinations rather than hypersomnia. Isolated, bilateral mesencephalic lesions are rarely found and are usually combined with thalamic lesions usually associated with hypersomnia (63). Subthalamic deep brain electrical stimulation has occasionally produced prolonged insomnia, not hypersomnia (64), which improved after repositioning one of the electrodes. Bilateral midline thalamic lesions produce a compulsive presleep behavior without electrophysiological sleep changes during the daytime but with almost normal sleep during nighttime (65,66), emphasizing that the typical behavior that usually accompanies normal sleep may be dissociated from the normal EEG of sleep. In one particular disease, fatal familial insomnia (67), bilateral degeneration of the anterior and dorsomedian thalamus is associated with inability to sleep and generate sleep EEG patterns with severe autonomic disturbances, although a dream-like hallucinatory state, similar to rapid eye movement (REM) sleep behavior disorder and stupor become dominant at the end of the disease. A clinical picture of hypersomnia and cataplexy may occasionally be seen secondary to diencephalic (68) or mesencephalic lesions (69) even with decreased hypocretin cerebrospinal fluid (CSF) levels. Hypothalamic lesions in humans have been associated mostly with hypersomnia (70); in fact, there is not a single reported patient with insomnia due to a hypothalamic lesion, if one excludes the cases with encephalitis lethargica described by von Economo at the beginning of the last century (71).

Narcolepsy, idiopathic hypersomnia, recurrent hypersomnia. Most human cases of narcolepsy with cataplexy are probably due to a loss of hypocretin/orexin neurons in the posterior hypothalamus of unknown cause (72). Levels of hypocretin-1 (Hcrt-1) are decreased (< 110 pcg/mL) in CSF. In narcolepsy without cataplexy CSF levels of Hcrt-1 are usually normal (73) and the possible role of the hypocretinergic transmission is unknown. Since Hcrt-1 CSF levels begin to diminish only when more than 70% of the hypothalamic neurons are destroyed (74) it is possible that less severe degrees of neuron loss could still produce sleepiness and remain undetected in CSF studies. It cannot be excluded that alterations in Hcrt-2, which cannot be measured in CSF, have a role in explaining the EDS in some of these disorders. The cause of idiopathic hypersomnia, which may appear in families, is unknown (75).

Depression. Depressive disorders are associated with reports of severe daytime sleepiness in epidemiological surveys (76). In psychiatric practice, sleepiness is associated with a specific depressive syndrome called *atypical depression*. There are only a few studies assessing sleepiness in depressed patients with objective tests, such as the MSLT (77–79), yielding inconclusive results. Overall, these studies show that most depressed patients with complaints of sleepiness instead display symptoms such as lack of interest, decreased energy, and fatigue that may mimic EDS. One study showed, for example, that among patients initially referred to a sleep center because of EDS and diagnosed with depression 36% had a mildly reduced (less than 10 minutes) mean sleep latency in the MSLT (79). Therefore, it seems that only some depressive patients complaining of EDS had abnormal MSLT values. This is in contrast with the results of a large epidemiological study (16583 adults, 1741 of whom were studied polysomnographically) showing that the presence of a current treatment for depression was the factor most strongly associated with the complaint of EDS (odds ratio: 6.85) (59). This association was four times higher than that for the obstructive apnea/hypopnea index (odds ratio 1.7). Complaints of sleepiness in this study consisted in (*i*) feeling drowsy or sleepy most of the day but managing to stay awake and (*ii*) presence of irresistible sleep attacks during the day.

On the other hand the presence of depression in patients with OSA is frequent. For example 41% of patients with OSA referred to a sleep unit showed depressive symptoms and 39% received antidepressant treatment (80) suggesting a close association between both disorders.

Drugs. EDS may be associated with many drugs. CNS depressant drugs, such as benzodiazepines, barbiturates as well as some antidepressants and antiepileptics are associated with EDS. Drugs acting against histamine-H1 receptors, some β-blockers used as antihypertensives, or dopaminergic drugs may also produce EDS. (2). Diagnosis of drug-related EDS may be easy when sleepiness appears closely related with the administration of the drug, but may be more difficult when it coexists with other common causes of sleepiness, such as sleep restriction, sleep-related breathing disorders, etc.

Circadian Rhythm Disturbances

When individuals choose to be active or are required to work and sleep at times conflicting with the circadian propensity for sleep and alertness, excessive sleepiness and insomnia may appear. Shift workers are especially exposed to this problem. Surveys of the work force engaged in shift or night work have reported more frequent complaints of excessive sleepiness during waking hours than among day workers, and this has been confirmed objectively with EEG recordings (2,81). Apart from shift work, jet lag, advanced sleep phase, and delayed sleep phase syndromes can also be associated with EDS and insomnia, due to the misalignment of the homeostatic drive for sleep with the circadian clock (2).

Sleepiness Caused by Multiple Factors

In clinical practice EDS is often seen associated with a combination of factors, for example, chronically reduced sleep and sleep fragmentation due to OSA. This may explain the situation seen, for example, in some OSA patients with residual sleepiness after continuous positive airway pressure (CPAP) (82). In some neurological disorders, such as Parkinson's disease, EDS may be the result of many factors which may include the use of dopaminergic drugs, the sleep fragmentation produced by the inability to move during the night and the degeneration of sleep-wake-related structures.

Table 4 Genetic Determinants of Sleep Need

- A polymorphism in the PERIOD[3] gene (PER $3^{5/5}$) shortens sleep latency, increases SWS time, slow wave activity, and worsens waking performance after sleep loss in humans (87).
- A functional genetic variation in the gene encoding ADA increases sleep intensity with slower wave activity and less awakenings in humans with the G/A vs. the G/G genotype (88).
- A DAT gene mutation (increasing dopamine transmission) increases locomotor activity, decreases arousal threshold and rest rebound after deprivation, and shortens the rest phase in *Drosophila*. Wake bouts increased and rest time decreased in DAT mutant mice(85,86).
- Two genomics regions in mouse (located in chromosome 13) might contain genes that modify the rate at which SWS need accumulates. Slow wave sleep need (i.e., rate of SWS increases in the absence of SWS) varies greatly between genotypes (89).

Abbreviations: SWS, slow wave sleep; ADA, adenosine deaminase; DAT, dopamine transporter.

PREDISPOSING AND PRECIPITATING FACTORS

EDS is probably more common in modern societies due to the steady rise in work around-the-clock and in automated (boring) work tasks which allow sleepiness to manifest more easily than in jobs with higher amount of physical activity. Epidemiological studies show associations of the complaint of sleepiness with *depression*, AHI, hours of sleep during weekdays, leg cramps or movements during the night (54,59,83) whereas body mass index (BMI), snoring or male sex were associated with EDS in some but not all studies (84).

There is probably a genetic tendency that determines the number of hours that one needs to sleep, the depth of sleep (number of awakenings and threshold for arousals) and the sensitivity to wake deficits produced by sleep deprivation (85–89) (Table 4). These genetic differences in susceptibility to sleep loss could perhaps explain why some patients with an AHI of 30 have sleepiness whereas others with an AHI of 50 do not (90), the different degrees of arousal responses induced by similar apnea episodes (91) or the fact that CPAP does not reduce blood pressure in nonsleepy hypertensive patients (92).

MORBIDITY AND MORTALITY

Adequate alertness is necessary for well-being and performance. Excessive and persisting sleepiness is life-threatening (2) and predisposes an individual to developing serious performance decrements in multiple areas of function, which may have significant consequences in children (39). Sleepiness is associated with substantial morbidity, including adverse effects on job performance (93,94), family relationships (2,95), and quality of life (95,96). Sleepiness is also an important cause of motor vehicle accidents, which occur with greatest frequency in the early morning hours, with a secondary peak in the mid-afternoon, corresponding to the normal biphasic circadian rhythm of sleepiness (93). When evidence of sleepiness was systematically obtained after motor vehicle accidents, it was found to be a causal factor in more than 15% of these accidents (97). Sleepy drivers, despite being able to detect sleepiness, do not seem to react accordingly (98).

The increase in mortality associated with long sleep duration (not EDS) is probable due to multiple mechanisms associated with this behavior rather than to the fact of sleeping more hours itself (99).

ASSOCIATIONS, COMPLICATIONS, AND CONSEQUENCES WITH CONDITIONS/DISORDERS OF ORGAN SYSTEMS

Sleepiness causes a decreased arousal threshold and increased collapsibility in upper airways that may in turn worsen the sleep apnea (52). Medical complications of sleepiness relate mostly with the cause of sleepiness rather than with sleepiness itself. EDS due to OSA may be associated with obesity, hypertension (40), abnormal glucose tolerance, as well as with cardiovascular complications. Sleepiness in older adults is associated with physical functional impairment and decreased exercise frequency, which has implications for continuing physical decline (100).

PSYCHOLOGICAL/PSYCHIATRIC ASSOCIATIONS, COMPLICATIONS, AND CONSEQUENCES

People with hypersomnia may have changes in their mood due to the difficulties in living a normal social or working life. For example, patients with severe narcolepsy with cataplexy or with severe OSA if untreated may have disabling consequences in terms of social life and isolation and may develop loss of confidence and depression (75). The inability to wake up on time in patients with idiopathic hypersomnia with long sleep time may produce important family and work problems, including poor work or school performance. Behaviorally induced insufficient sleep syndrome may cause depression, withdrawal from family life and social activities, with abuse of stimulants. Circadian sleep disorders may produce substance abuse to treat insomnia or sleepiness during conventional waking hours.

CONCLUSIONS

There are multiple causes of excessive sleepiness, which can be categorized into insufficient or nonrestorative sleep (sleep restriction and fragmentation), hypersomnias of central origin, alterations in the circadian rhythm, and sleepiness due to multiple factors. Depression, AHI, hours of sleep during weekdays, and leg cramps or movements during the night are some of the factors that have been associated with the complaint of sleepiness in epidemiological studies. It has been recognized that excessive and persisting sleepiness is life-threatening and has been associated with substantial morbidity, including adverse effects on job performance, family relationships, and quality of life. Sleepiness may worsen sleep apnea and in older adults is associated with physical functional impairment and decreased exercise frequency.

REFERENCES

1. Aldrich MS. Sleep Medicine. New York: Oxford University Press, 1999:113.
2. Roehrs T, Carskadon MA, Dement WC, et al. Daytime sleepiness and alertness. In: Kryger MH, Roth T, Dement WC, eds. Principles and Practice of Sleep Medicine. Philadelphia: Elsevier Saunders, 2005:39–50.
3. Silber MH. The investigation of sleepiness. Sleep Med Clin 2006; 1:1–7.
4. Borbély AA. A two process model of sleep regulation. Hum Neurobiol 1982; 1(3):195–204.
5. Tononi G, Cirelli C. Sleep function and synaptic homeostasis. Sleep Med Rev 2006; 10(1):49–62.
6. Dinges DF, Rogers NL, Baynard MD. Chronic sleep deprivation. In: Kryger MH, Roth T, Dement WC, eds. Principles and Practice of Sleep Medicine. 4th ed. Philadelphia: Elsevier Saunders, 2005:67–50.
7. Gooley JJ, Saper CB. Anatomy of the circadian system. In: Kryger MH, Roth T, Dement WC, eds. Principles and Practice of Sleep Medicine. 4th ed. Philadelphia: Elsevier Saunders, 2005:335–350.
8. Edgar DE, Dement WC, Fuller CA. Effect of SCN lesions on sleep in squirrel monkeys: evidence for opponent processes in sleep-wake regulation. J Neurosci 1993; 13(3):1065–1079.
9. Dijk DJ, Lockley SW. Integration of human sleep-wake regulation and circadian rhythmicity. J Appl Physiol 2002; 92(2):852–862.
10. Daan S, Beersma G, Borbély AA. Timing of human sleep recovery process gated by a circadian pacemaker. Am J Physiol Regul Integr Comp Physiol 1984; 246(2 pt 2):161–183.
11. Deboer T, Vansteensel MJ, Détári L, et al. Sleep states alter activity of suprachiasmatic nucleus neurons. Nat Neurosci 2003; 6(10):1086–1090.
12. Deboer T, Détári L, Meijer JH. Long term effects of sleep deprivation on the mammalian circadian pacemaker. Sleep 2007; 30(3):257–262.
13. Bonnet MH. Acute sleep deprivation. In: Kryger MH, Roth T, Dement WC, eds. Principles and Practice of Sleep Medicine. Philadelphia: Elsevier Saunders, 2005:51–66.
14. De Valck E, Cluydts R, Pirrera S. Effect of cognitive arousal on sleep latency, somatic and cortical arousal following partial sleep deprivation. J Sleep Res 2004; 13(4):295–304.
15. Sharafkhaneh A, Hirshkowitz M. Contextual factors and perceived self-reported sleepiness: a preliminary report. Sleep Med 2003; 4(4):327–331.
16. Bonnet MH, Arand DL. Sleepiness as measured by modified multiple sleep latency test varies as a function of preceding activity. Sleep 1998; 21(5):477–483.
17. Mignot E, Taheri S, Nishino S. Sleeping with the hypothalamus: emerging therapeutic targets for sleep disorders. Nat Neurosci Suppl 2002; 5(suppl):1071–1075.

18. Cluydts R, De Valck E, Verstraeten E, et al. Daytime sleepiness and its evaluation. Sleep Med Rev 2002; 6(2):83–96.

19. Bonnet MH, Arand DL. Performance and cardiovascular measures in normal adults with extreme MSLT scores and subjective sleepiness. Sleep 2005; 28(6):685–693.

20. Tucker AM, Dinges DF, Van Dongen HPA. Trait interindividual differences in the sleep physiology of healthy young adults. J Sleep Res 2007; 16(2):170–180.

21. Johns M. Rethinking the assessment of sleepiness. Sleep Med Rev 1998; 2(1):3–15.

22. Stepanski E, Zorick F, Roehrs T, et al. Daytime alertness in patients with chronic insomnia compared with asymptomatic control subjects. Sleep 1988; 11(1):54–60.

23. Jones BE. From waking to sleeping: neuronal and chemical substrates. Trends Pharmacol Sci 2005; 26 (11):578–586.

24. Lu J, Jhou TC, Saper CB. Identification of wake-active dopaminergic neurons in the ventral periaqueductal gray matter. J Neurosci 2006; 26(1):193–202.

25. Siegel J. The Neural Control of Sleep and Waking. New York: Springer, 2002.

26. John J, Wu MF, Boehmer LN, et al. Cataplexy-active neurons in the hypothalamus: implications for the role of histamine in sleep and waking behavior. Neuron 2004; 42(4):619–634.

27. Peñaloza-Rojas JH, Elterman M, Olmos N. Sleep induced by cortical stimulation. Exp Neurol 1964; 10:140–147.

28. McGinty D, Szymusiak R. Sleep-promoting mechanisms in mammals. In: Kryger MH, Roth T, Dement WC, eds. Principles and Practice of Sleep Medicine. Philadelphia: Elsevier Saunders, 2005:169–184.

29. Saper CB, Chou TC, Scammell TE. The sleep switch: hypothalamic control of sleep and wakefulness. Trends Neurosci 2001; 24(12):726–731.

30. Friedman L, Bergmann BM, Rechtschaffen A. Effects of sleep deprivation on sleepiness, sleep intensity, and subsequent sleep in the rat. Sleep 1997; 1(4):360–391.

31. Thomas M, Sing H, Belenky G, et al. Neural basis of alertness and cognitive performance impairments during sleepiness. I. effects of 24 h of sleep deprivation on waking human regional brain activity. J Sleep Res 2000; 9(4):335–352.

32. McKenna JT, Tartar JL, Ward CP, et al. Sleep fragmentation elevates behavioral, electrographic and neurochemical measures of sleepiness. Neuroscience 2007; 146(4):1462–1473.

33. Banks S, Dinges DF. Behavioral and physiologic consequences of sleep restriction. J Clin Sleep Med 2007; 3(5):519–528.

34. Pack AI, Maislin G, Staley B, et al. Impaired performance in commercial drivers. Role of sleep apnea and short sleep duration. Am J Resp Crit Care Med 2006; 174(4):446–454.

35. Carskadon MA, Dement WC. Cumulative of sleep restriction on daytime sleepiness. Psychophysiology 1981; 18(2):107–113.

36. Dinges DF, Pack F, Williams K, et al. Cumulative sleepiness, mood disturbance, and psychomotor vigilance performance decrements during a week of sleep restricted to 4-5 hours per night. Sleep 1997; 20(4):267–277.

37. Van Dongen HPA, Maislin G, Mullington JM, et al. The cumulative cost of additional wakefulness: dose-response effects on neurobehavioral functions and sleep physiology from chronic sleep restriction and total sleep deprivation. Sleep 2003; 26(3):117–126.

38. Belenky G, Wesensten NJ, Thorne DR, et al. Patterns of performance degradation and restoration during sleep restriction and subsequent recovery: a sleep dose-response study. J Sleep Res 2003; 12 (1):1–12.

39. Colten HR, Altevogt BM, eds. Committee on Sleep Medicine and Research. Sleep Disorders and Sleep Deprivation: An Unmet Public Health Problem. Washington, D.C.: National Academies Press, 2006.

40. Rohers T, Shore E, Papineau K, et al. A two-week sleep extension in sleepy normals. Sleep 1996; 19 (7):576–582.

41. Leproult R, Colecchia EF, Berardi AM, et al. Individual differences in subjective and objective alertness during sleep deprivation are stable and unrelated. Am J Physiol Regul Comp Physiol 2003; 284(2):280–290.

42. Dijk DJ, Duffy JF, Riel E, et al. Ageing and the circadian and homeostatic regulation of human sleep during forced desynchrony of rest, melatonin and temperature rhythms. J Physiol 1999; 516(pt 2):611–627.

43. Buysse DH, Monk TH, Carrier J, et al. Circadian patterns of sleep, sleepiness and performance in older and younger adults. Sleep 2005; 28(11):1365–1376.

44. Adam M, Rétey JV, Khatami R, et al. Age-related changes in the time course of vigilant attention during 40 hours without sleep in men. Sleep 2006; 29(1):55–57.

45. Van Dongen HV, Baynard MD, Maislin G, et al. Systematic interindividual differences in neurobehavioral impairment from sleep loss: evidence of trait-linked differential vulnerability. Sleep 2004; 27(3):423–433.

46. Lichstein KL, Wilson NW, Noe SL, et al. Daytime sleepiness in insomnia: behavioral, biological and subjective indices. Sleep 1994; 17(8):693–702.
47. Bonnet MH, Arand DL. The consequences of a week of insomnia II: patients with insomnia. Sleep 1998; 21(4):359–368.
48. Stepanski E. The effect of sleep fragmentation on daytime function. Sleep 2002; 25(3):268–276.
49. Levine B, Roehrs T, Stepanski E, et al. Fragmenting sleep diminishes its recuperative value. Sleep 1987; 10(6):590–599.
50. Bonnet MH, Arand DL. Clinical effects of sleep fragmentation versus sleep deprivation. Sleep Med Rev 2003; 7(4):297–310.
51. Stepanski E, Lamphere J, Badia P, et al. Sleep fragmentation and daytime sleepiness. Sleep 1984; 7(1): 18–26.
52. Brooks D, Horner RL, Kimoff RJ, et al. Effect of sleep apnea versus sleep fragmentation on responses to airway occlusion. Am J Respir Crit Care Med 1997; 155(5):1609–1617.
53. Chervin RD, Aldrich MS. Characteristics of apneas and hypopneas during sleep and relation to excessive daytime sleepiness. Sleep 1998; 21(8):799–806.
54. Gottlieb DJ, Whitney CW, Bonekat WH, et al. Relation of sleepiness to respiratory disturbance index. Am J Rev Respir Crit Care Med 1999; 159(2):502–507.
55. Sauter C, Asenbaum S, Popovic R, et al. Excessive daytime sleepiness in patients suffering from different levels of obstructive sleep apnea syndrome. J Sleep Res 2000; 9(3):293–301.
56. Young T, Palta M, Dempsey J, et al. The occurrence of sleep-disordered breathing among middle-aged adults. N Eng J Med 1993; 328(17):1230–1235.
57. Poceta JS, Timms RM, Jeong D, et al. Maintenance of wakefulness test in obstructive sleep apnea syndrome. Chest 1992; 101(4):893–897.
58. Pack AI. Advances in sleep-disordered breathing. Am J Respir Crit Care Med 2006; 173(1):7–15.
59. Bixler EO, Vgontzas AN, Lin HM, et al. Excessive daytime sleepiness in a general population sample: the role of sleep apnea, age, obesity, diabetes, and depression. J Clin Endocrinol Metab 2005; 90(8):4510–4515.
60. Chervin RD. Periodic leg movements and sleepiness in patients evaluated for sleep-disorderd breathing. Am J Respir Crit Care Med 2001; 164(8 pt 1):1454–1458.
61. Autret A, Laffont F, de Toffol B, et al. A syndrome of REM and Non-REM sleep reduction and lateral gaze paresis after medial tegmental pontine stroke. Arch Neurol 1988; 45(11):1236–1242.
62. Forcadas MI, Zarranz JJ. Insomnio y alucinaciones tras lesions vasculares del tegmento protuberancial en el hombre. Neurologia 1994; 9(6):211–223.
63. Bogousslavsky J, Regli F, Uske A. Thalamic infarcts: clinical syndromes, etiology, and prognosis. Neurology 1988; 38(6):837–848.
64. Monaca C, Ozsancak C, Defebvre L, et al,. Transient insomnia induced by high-frequency deep brain stimulation in Parkinson disease. Neurology 2004; 62(7):1232–1233.
65. Guilleminault C, Quera-Salva MA, Goldberg MP. Pseudo-hypersomnia and pre-sleep behavior with bilateral paramedian thalamic lesions. Brain 1993; 116(pt 6):1549–1563.
66. Bassetti C, Mathis J, Gugger M, et al. Hypersomnia following paramedian thalamic stroke: a report of 12 patients. Ann Neurol 1996; 39(4):471–480.
67. Lugaresi E, Medori R, Montagna P, et al. Fatal familial insomnia and dysautonomia with slecetive degeneration of thalamic nuclei. N Eng J Med 1986; 315(16):997–1003.
68. Aldrich MS, Naylor MW. Narcolepsy associated with lesions of the diencephalons. Neurology 1989; 39(11):1505–1508.
69. Scammell TE, Nishino S, Mignot E, et al. Narcolepsy and low CSF orexin (hypocretin) concentration after a diencephalic stroke. Neurology 2001; 56(12):1751–1753.
70. Beal MF, Kleinman GM, Ojemann RG, et al. Gangliocytoma of third ventricle: hyperphagia, somnolence, and dementia. Neurology 1981; 31(10):1224–1228.
71. von Economo C. Sleep as a problem of localization. J Nerv Ment Dis 1930; 71:249–259.
72. Dauvilliers Y, Arnulf I, Mignot E. Narcolepsy with cataplexy. Lancet 2007; 369(9560):499–511.
73. Mignot E, Lammers GJ, Ripley B, et al. The role of cerebrospinal fluid hypocretin measurement in the diagnosis of narcolepsy and other hypersomnias. Arch Neurol 2002; 59(10):1553–1562.
74. Gerashchenko D, Murillo-Rodriguez E, Lin L, et al. Relationship between CSF hypocretin levels and hypocretin neuronal loss. Exp Neurol 2003; 184(2):1010–1016.
75. American Academy of Sleep Medicine. International Classification of Sleep Disorders: Diagnostic and Coding Manual. 2nd ed. Westchester, Illinois: American Academy of Sleep Medicine, 2005.
76. Ohayon MM, Caulet M, Philip P, et al. How sleep and mental disorders are related to complaints of daytime sleepiness. Arch Intern Med 1997; 157(22):2645–2652.
77. Nofzinger EA, Thase ME, Reynolds CF III, et al. Hypersomnia in bipolar depression: a comparison with narcolepsy using the multiple sleep latency test. Am J Psychiatry 1991; 148(9):1177–1181.
78. Reynolds CF III, Coble PA, Kupfer DJ, et al. Application of the multiple sleep latency test in disorders of excessive sleepiness. Electroencephalogr Clin Neurophysiol 1982; 53(4):443–452.

79. Billiard M, Dolenc L, Aldaz C, et al. Hypersomnia associated with mood disorders: a new perspective. J Psychosomatic Res; 38(suppl 1):41–47.
80. Schwartz DJ, Kohler WC, Karatinos G. Symptoms of depression in individuals with obstructive sleep apnea may be amenable to treatment with continuous positive airway pressure. Chest 2005; 128(3):1304–1309.
81. Torsvall L, Akersdet T, Gillander K, et al. Sleep on the night shift: 24hr EEG monitoring of spontaneous sleep/wake behavior. Psychophysiology 1989; 26(3):352–358.
82. Santamaria J, Iranzo A, Montserrat JM, et al. Persistent sleepiness in CPAP treated obstructive sleep apnea patients: evaluation and treatment. Sleep Med Rev 2007; 11(3):195–207.
83. Breslau N, Roth T, Rosenthal L, et al. Daytime sleepiness: an epidemiological study of young adults. Am J Public Health 1997; 87(10):1649–1653.
84. Pallesen S, Nordhus IH, Omvik S, et al. Prevalence and risk factors of subjective sleepiness in the general adult population. Sleep 2007; 30(5):619–624.
85. Kume K, Kume S, Park SK, et al. Dopamine is a regulator of arousal in the fruit fly. J Neurosci 2005; 25(32):7377–7383.
86. Wisor JP, Nishino S, Sora I, et al. Dopaminergic role in stimulant induced wakefulness. J Neurosci 2001; 21(5):1787–1794.
87. Viola AU, Archer SN, James LM et al. PER3 polymorphism predicts sleep structure and waking performance. Curr Biol 2007; 17(7):613–618.
88. Rétey JV, Adam M, Honegger E, et al. A functional genetic variation of adenosine deaminase affects the duration and intensity of deep sleep in humans. Proc Nat Acad Sci 2005; 102(43):1576–1681.
89. Franken P, Chollet D, Tafti M. The homeostatic regulation of sleep need is under genetic control. J Neurosci 2001; 21(8):2610–2621.
90. Barbe F, Mayoralas LR, Duran J, et al. Treatment with continuous positive airway pressure is not effective in patients with sleep apnea but no daytime symptoms. A randomized controlled trial. Ann Int Med 2001; 134(11):1015–1023.
91. Rees K, Spence DP, Earis JE. Arousal responses from apneic events during non-rapid-eye-movement sleep. Am J Respir Crit Care Med 1995; 152(3):1016–1021.
92. Robinson GV, Smith DM, Langford BA et al. Continuous positive airway pressure does not reduce blood pressure in nonsleepy hypertensive OSA patients. Eur Resp J 2006; 27(6):1229–1235.
93. Mitler, MM, Carskadon MA, Czeisler CA, et al. Catastrophes, sleep, and public policy: consensus report. Sleep 1988; 11(1):100–109.
94. Akerstedt T. Sleepiness as a consequence of shift work. Sleep 1988; 11(1):17–34.
95. Roth T, Roehrs TA. Etiologies and sequelae of excessive daytime sleepiness. Clin Ther 1996; 18(4): 562–576.
96. Briones BN, Adams M, Strauss C, et al. Relationship between sleepiness and general health status. Sleep 1996; 19(7):583–588.
97. Horne, JA, Reyner LA. Sleep related vehicle accidents. BMJ 1995; 310(6979):565–567.
98. Nabi H, Guéguen A, Chiron M, et al. Awareness of driving while sleepy and road traffic accidents: prospective study in GAZEL cohort. BMJ 2006; 333(7558):75; [Epub 2006 June 2003].
99. Grandner Ma, Drummond SPA. Who are the long sleepers? Towards an understanding of the mortality relationship. Sleep Med Rev 2007; 11(5):341–360.
100. Chasens ER, Sereika SM, Weaver T, et al. Daytime sleepiness, exercise, and physical function in older adults. J Sleep Res 2007; 16(1):60–65.

20 | Types of Hypersomnias

Seiji Nishino

Department of Psychiatry and Behavioral Sciences, Sleep and Circadian Neurobiology Laboratory & Center for Narcolepsy, Stanford University School of Medicine, Stanford, California, U.S.A.

INTRODUCTION

Somnolence is a complex state, impacted by multiple determinants such as quantity and quality of prior sleep, circadian time, drugs, attention, motivation, environmental stimuli, and various medical, neurological, and psychiatric conditions. Clearly, somnolence is welcomed when sleep is desired, but at other times often becomes an unwanted symptom. Pathological or inappropriate somnolence is clinically termed hypersomnia or excessive daytime sleepiness (EDS). Subjects with hypersomnia are unable to stay alert and awake during the major waking episodes of the day, resulting in unintended lapses into sleep.

Sleepiness may vary in severity and is more likely to occur in boring, monotonous situations that require no active participation. In some cases, sleepiness is associated with large increases in the total daily amount of sleep without any genuine feeling of restoration. In other cases, sleepiness can be alleviated temporarily by naps but recurs shortly thereafter. In most cases, excessive sleepiness is a chronic symptom. It must occur for at least three months prior to diagnosis.

In the second revision of the *International Classification of Sleep Disorders* (ICSD-2) (1), hypersomnia of central origin was defined as a category of hypersomnia not due to a circadian rhythm sleep disorder, a sleep-related breathing disorder (SRBD), or other causes of disturbed nocturnal sleep. Other sleep disorders may be present, but they must first be properly treated prior to establishing diagnoses in this category. Under this category, 12 diseases/conditions (including two unspecified categories) are listed (Table 1).

In this chapter, demographic, clinical features as well as known pathophysiology of these hypersomnias will be presented.

GENERAL CONSIDERATIONS IN THE EVALUATION OF SLEEPINESS

The severity of daytime sleepiness can be quantified subjectively using severity scales such as the Epworth sleepiness scale (2), and objectively using the multiple sleep latency test (MSLT) (3) and the maintenance of wakefulness test (MWT) (4). These measures are, however, poorly correlated with each other and must be used with appropriate clinical judgment (5,6).

The MSLT measures the physiological tendency to fall asleep (i.e., sleep latency) and to document sleep-onset rapid eye movement periods (SOREMPs) in quiet situations. MSLT evaluations are now required in the *ICSD-2* for the diagnosis of narcolepsy and idiopathic hypersomnia (and highly recommended in the diagnosis of narcolepsy with cataplexy) (1). It should be noted that the MSLT has not been validated as a diagnostic test in children less than eight years of age.

In the context of diagnosing hypersomnia and narcolepsy, the MSLT must be conducted during the day following a documented adequate night of sleep and after two weeks of regular sleep. In the *ICSD-2*, a mean MSLT sleep latency below eight minutes is used to document sleepiness for diagnostic purposes (1). This value has been shown to be the best cutoff in the context of diagnosing narcolepsy (7). Importantly, however, a significant portion of the general population may have a mean sleep latency equal to or less than eight minutes, especially if the nocturnal sleep is not normalized prior to the MSLT (8). The results of the MSLT should thus be carefully interpreted in the presence of a significant complaint of daytime sleepiness.

In contrast, the presence of multiple SOREMPs during the MSLT is a more specific finding than a mean sleep latency less than or equal to eight minutes, although a very small portion of adult normal sleepers (less than 2%) also experience multiple SOREMPs during the MSLT (8). Multiple SOREMPs during the MSLT have also been reported more frequently in other sleep disorders such as sleep apnea (8). The MWT measures the ability to maintain

Table 1 Classification (Second Revision of the *International Classification of Sleep Disorders*) of Hypersomnias of Central Origin

1. Narcolepsy with cataplexy[a]
2. Narcolepsy without cataplexy[a]
3. Narcolepsy due to medical condition
4. Narcolepsy, unspecified
   (This diagnosis is used on a temporary basis when the patient meets clinical and MSLT criteria for narcolepsy, but further evaluation is required to determine the specific diagnostic category for narcolepsy.)
5. Recurrent hypersomnia
   Kleine–Levin syndrome
   Menstrual-related hypersomnia
6. Idiopathic hypersomnia with long sleep time[a]
7. Idiopathic hypersomnia without long sleep time[a]
8. Behaviorally induced insufficient sleep syndrome
9. Hypersomnia due to medical condition
10. Hypersomnia due to drug or substance
11. Hypersomnia not due to a substance or known physiological condition (nonorganic hypersomnia)
12. Physiological (organic) hypersomnia, unspecified (organic hypersomnia)
    (Disorders that satisfy clinical and MSLT criteria for hypersomnolence and are believed to be due to physiological conditions but do not meet criteria for other hypersomnolence conditions are classified here.)

[a]Clinical characteristics of some frequent hypersomnias are summarized in Table 2.
Source: From Ref. 1.

wakefulness in quiet situations (4). It is mostly used to objectively document an ability to stay awake and fight sleeping, for example, following stimulant treatment of hypersomnia. Subjective scales like the Epworth directly measure the impact of the symptom on daily life (2). It is particularly useful in diagnosing idiopathic hypersomnia with prolonged sleep time because the MSLT may not be easy to conduct and may be difficult to interpret. In all cases where a diagnosis of hypersomnia is to be made, a review of psychiatric history, drug and medication use, and an assessment of other sleep and medical disorders should be performed.

NARCOLEPSY WITH CATAPLEXY

Narcolepsy with cataplexy is characterized by EDS and cataplexy (9). Frequently occurring ancillary symptoms include sleep paralysis, hypnagogic hallucinations, and disturbed nocturnal sleep (9). Many of the symptoms of narcolepsy are due to an unusual proclivity to transition rapidly from wakefulness into rapid eye movement (REM) sleep and to experience dissociated REM sleep events (9). Thanks to significant progress in studies using animal models of narcolepsy (10,11), major portions of the pathophysiology of human narcolepsy have been revealed: a large majority of narcolepsy-cataplexy is associated with hypocretin ligand (hypothalamic neuropeptide) deficiency (12,13), possibly because of the postnatal loss of hypocretin-containing neurons (14,15). Since narcolepsy-cataplexy is strongly associated with a specific human leukocyte antigen (HLA) (i.e., HLA-DQB1*0602), an immune-mediated etiology for hypocretin deficiency has also been suggested (but not proved) (9).

Demographics

Narcolepsy with cataplexy affects 0.02% to 0.18% of the United States and Western European population (9). A lower prevalence has been reported in Israel, whereas narcolepsy may be slightly more frequent in Japan (0.16% to 0.18%). Both genders seem affected, with a slight preponderance of males. Narcolepsy is observed at any age but very rarely before five years of age.

There is also a low prevalence of familial cases: the risk of a first-degree relative developing narcolepsy with cataplexy is approximately 1% to 2% (16). When compared with the population prevalence, however, this indicates a 10- to 40-fold increase in risk. This increased risk cannot be explained solely by HLA gene effects, suggesting the existence of other genetic factors (16). Multiplex families with more than two patients with narcolepsy-cataplexy are exceptional. Most of the multiplex families (60% to 100%) are also HLA-DQB1*0602 positive (16). Interestingly, one report has found familial cases to be more often HLA-DQB1*0602 negative and with normal cerebrospinal fluid (CSF) hypocretin-1, suggesting a different etiology (Table 2) (13).

Table 2 Clinical Characteristics of Narcolepsy (With and Without Cataplexy) and Idiopathic Hypersomnia

Type of hypersomnia	Daytime sleepiness Duration	Awaken refreshed	Other symptoms	MSLT Sleep latency	SOREMPs	HLA-DQB1[a]*0602 positivity	Low CSF hypocretin levels (<110 pg/mL)
Narcolepsy with cataplexy	Short (<30 min)	(+)	Cataplexy REM sleep-related symptoms	<8 min[a]	≥2	>90%	85–90% >90% in HLA positive
Narcolepsy without cataplexy	Short (<30 min)	(+)	Cataplexy (−) REM sleep-related symptoms	<8 min[a]	≥2	40–50%	10–20% (almost all are HLA positive)
Idiopathic hypersomnia with long sleep time	Long (>30 min)	(−)	Cataplexy (−) REM sleep-related symptoms (−) Prolonged nighttime sleep (>10 hr) Autonomic nervous system dysfunction	<8 min[a]	≤1	No consistent results	Normal
Idiopathic hypersomnia without long sleep time	Varied	(−)	Cataplexy (−) REM sleep-related symptoms (−) No prolonged nighttime sleep (<10 hr) Autonomic nervous system dysfunction	<8 min[a]	≤1	No consistent results	Normal

[a]Less than 8 minutes (instead of 5 minutes) is considered for the second revision of *ICSD*.

Key Symptoms and Signs

EDS is usually the most disabling symptom and the first to occur (9). It is characterized by repeated episodes of naps or lapses into sleep across daytime. Patients with narcolepsy typically sleep for a short duration and awaken refreshed, but within two or three hours begin to feel sleepy again. The pattern repeats itself throughout the day. Sleepiness is more likely to occur in boring, monotonous situations that require no active participation, such as watching television. Sudden and often irreversible sleep attacks may also occur in unusual situations such as eating, walking, or driving. Sleep attacks usually occur within a background of overall sleepiness.

Sleepiness in narcolepsy varies in severity and is not easily distinguishable from the sleepiness caused by insufficient sleep or other sleep disorders (9). In cases where sleepiness is severe, a symptom called "automatic behavior" is occasionally observed: The patient continues an activity in a semiautomatic fashion without memory or consciousness. A patient may, for example, continue to write sentences in a letter or work on the computer, but the output will be nonsensical.

Cataplexy, a unique characteristic of narcolepsy, is characterized by sudden loss of bilateral muscle tone provoked by strong emotions that are usually positive, such as laughter, pride, elation, or surprise (9). Negative emotions such as anger may also occasionally be a trigger. Cataplexy can be localized, or it can include all skeletal muscle groups. The lower or upper limbs, neck, mouth, or eyelids may be regionally affected. Most commonly affected areas include the knees, face, and neck. Blurred vision may occur and may reflect oculomotor involvement. Respiratory muscles are never affected, but a feeling of choking may result from the occurrence of cataplexy in an awkward position. The duration of cataplexy is usually short, ranging from a few seconds to several minutes at most, and recovery is immediate and complete. Cataplexy may vary in pattern, frequency, and severity. The loss of muscle tone ranges from a mild sensation of weakness with head drop, facial sagging, jaw weakness, slurred speech, and buckling of the knees, to complete postural collapse with a fall to the ground. Twitches and jerks may occur, particularly in the face, as the patient is trying to fight the episode. In severe episodes, it usually takes several seconds before a complete state of muscle weakness is reached, preventing serious injuries in the majority of instances. When mild, the weakness may not be very noticeable, for example, a simple drooping of the eye or of the corner of the mouth. Cataplexy may sometimes be followed by sleep. The frequency of cataplexy shows wide interpersonal variation. Some patients exhibit only rare attacks a few times annually, while others may suffer countless attacks in a single day. In very rare cases, strong emotional triggers may provoke multiple episodes of cataplexy in succession, a phenomenon known as status cataplecticus. Episodes of status cataplecticus can last for many minutes, and sometimes up to an hour. The use of adrenergic/serotoninergic antidepressant medications (including tricyclic antidepressants) almost always ameliorates cataplexy with a short latency (9). Episodes of status cataplecticus are most often observed when these medications are withdrawn, resulting in a rebound cataplexy.

Sleep paralysis, hypnagogic hallucinations, and nocturnal sleep disruption commonly occur in patients with narcolepsy (9). These symptoms, however, also occasionally occur in normal people and in patients with other sleep disorders.

Hypnagogic hallucinations are vivid perceptual experiences typically occurring at sleep onset, often with realistic awareness of the presence of someone or something, and include visual, tactile, kinetic, and auditory phenomena. The accompanying emotional effect is often fear or dread. Hallucinatory experiences, such as being caught in a fire, being about to be attacked by a stranger, or flying through the air, are commonly reported. Recurrent hypnagogic hallucinations are experienced by 40% to 80% of patients with narcolepsy. Some normal sleepers may experience hypnagogic or hypnopompic (occurring upon waking) hallucinations a few times in their life; to be a significant symptom, these must occur regularly. Sleep paralysis is a transient, generalized inability to move or to speak during the transition between sleep and wakefulness. The patient usually regains muscular control within several minutes. Sleep paralysis is a frightening experience, particularly when initially experienced, and is often accompanied by a sensation of inability to breathe. Episodes often occur with hypnagogic hallucinations, and thus the frightful emotional experience is intensified.

Sleep paralysis is experienced by 40% to 80% of narcoleptic patients. Occasional episodes of sleep paralysis may be experienced by normal people. To be considered a significant symptom, sleep paralysis should occur regularly. Narcoleptic patients may report memory lapses (especially during automatic behavior without awareness of sleepiness), and may show inappropriate activity and poor adjustment to abrupt environmental demands. Other symptoms may include ptosis, blurred vision, and diplopia (either as a result of sleepiness or cataplexy). Nocturnal sleep disruption occurs in approximately 50% of narcoleptics and can even be the presenting symptom. Most typically, sleep maintenance rather than sleep-onset insomnia is seen. It is often a very disabling symptom that may exacerbate all other symptoms. Narcolepsy is often associated with increased body mass, and more rarely, obesity, especially when untreated (17).

Onset, Ontogeny, and Clinical Course

Onset almost always occurs after five years of age and most typically between the ages of 15 and 25 (9). Sleepiness is usually the first symptom to appear. Cataplexy most often occurs within a year of onset, but in rare instances may precede the onset of sleepiness or commence up to 40 years later. Hypnagogic hallucinations, sleep paralysis, and disturbed nocturnal sleep often manifest later in the course of the disease.

Current evidence suggests that most cases of narcolepsy with cataplexy are associated with the loss of approximately 50,000 to 100,000 hypothalamic neurons containing the neuropeptide hypocretin/orexin (14,15). The lack of hypocretin can be best assessed by measuring CSF hypocretin-1 (orexin-A) (12,13). Using this test, approximately 90% of patients with narcolepsy with cataplexy, almost all with HLA-DQB1*0602, have dramatically decreased CSF levels (13). Because narcolepsy with cataplexy is HLA associated, it is believed, but not proven, that the cause of most cases is an autoimmune destruction of hypocretin cells that generally occurs during adolescence.

When left untreated, severe narcolepsy can be socially disabling and isolating; patients may gain weight, fail at school, lose jobs, and avoid social interactions 25 (9). Patients lose confidence, and depression often occurs. Type II diabetes mellitus may be more frequent in patients with this disorder (18).

Risk Factors

Genetic and nongenetic predisposing factors are suspected. At the genetic level, narcolepsy with cataplexy is very tightly associated with the HLA subtypes DR2/DRB1*1501 and DQB1*0602 (19). These two subtypes are always found together in Caucasians and Asians, but in African Americans, DQB1*0602 is more specifically associated with narcolepsy. Almost all patients with cataplexy are positive for DQB1*0602 when compared with 12% to 38% of the general population, and HLA positivity is tightly associated with hypocretin ligand deficiency. The cause of the hypocretin cell destruction is unknown, but involvement of an immune-mediated mechanism is suggested. In twin studies, only 5 of 17 monozygotic twin pairs (29%) with narcolepsy were reported as concordant, indicating the importance of environmental factors (16).

Many precipitating factors have been suggested in case reports but have not been proven to be involved. Among the most commonly reported triggers are head trauma, an abrupt change in sleep-wake patterns, sustained sleep deprivation, and an unspecified viral illness.

Ten percent of narcolepsy with cataplexy patients have normal CSF hypocretin-1 (12,13), which suggests either that CSF levels do not perfectly reflect brain hypocretin neurotransmission or that narcolepsy with cataplexy can be caused by factors other than hypocretin deficiency.

NARCOLEPSY WITHOUT CATAPLEXY

In the *ICSD-2*, narcolepsy without cataplexy is described separately from narcolepsy with cataplexy (meets narcolepsy diagnostic criteria, but with the absence of cataplexy) (1). This change is mostly due to recent progress in nosological understanding. The majority of narcolepsy without cataplexy is not associated with hypocretin ligand deficiency (13,20).

Demographics

The population prevalence is unknown. Narcolepsy without cataplexy cases represents 10% to 50% of the narcoleptic population. A study of diagnosed narcoleptic patients in Olmsted County, Minnesota has indicated that 0.02% of the population were diagnosed with narcolepsy without cataplexy (21). Population-based studies have shown that approximately 1% to 3% of adults may have multiple SOREMPs during random MSLTs. Recurrent sleep paralysis or hypnagogic hallucinations similarly affect approximately 4% of the normal population (22). As multiple SOREMPs and abnormal REM sleep events are also observed in association with other sleep disorders, for example, sleep apnea or behaviorally induced insufficient sleep syndrome (8), it is difficult to assess the true prevalence of narcolepsy without cataplexy (diagnosed and undiagnosed) with currently available data. Both the sexes can be affected at any age.

Relatives of patients with narcolepsy with cataplexy may be more likely to experience partial narcolepsy symptoms compatible with the diagnosis of narcolepsy without cataplexy.

Key Symptoms and Signs

EDS in narcolepsy without cataplexy is most typically associated with naps that are refreshing in nature, while nocturnal sleep is normal or moderately disturbed without excessive amounts of sleep. Sleep paralysis, hypnagogic hallucinations, and/or automatic behavior may be present. In a meta-analysis, the mean MSLT sleep latency in narcolepsy was 3.1 ± 2.9 minutes. An essential feature of the diagnosis is the presence of a mean sleep latency less than or equal to eight minutes and greater than or equal to two SOREMPs on an MSLT.

Symptoms often associated with narcolepsy without cataplexy are memory lapses (especially during automatic behavior without awareness of sleepiness), inappropriate activity, and poor adjustment to abrupt environmental demands. Other symptoms include ptosis, blurred vision, and diplopia. Unambiguous cataplexy is not present, but cataplexy-like episodes may be reported. These include atypical sensations of muscle weakness triggered by unusual emotions such as stress, sex, or intense activity/exercise; long episodes of tiredness that do not fit the classical description of cataplexy; and episodes that have occurred only a few times over the course of a lifetime. Nocturnal sleep disruption with frequent awakenings may occur. When severe insomnia is observed, diagnosis may be difficult as the symptoms or abnormal MSLT results could be secondary to sleep deprivation.

Onset, Ontogeny, and Clinical Course

Onset of narcolepsy without cataplexy typically occurs during adolescence. When the patient is young, however, it is always possible that cataplexy will develop later in the course of the disease, necessitating a change in diagnosis to narcolepsy with cataplexy.

The cause of most cases is unknown. In a minority of cases of narcolepsy without cataplexy, the disease is associated with the loss of hypocretin-containing neurons (14), as described for narcolepsy with cataplexy. The lack of hypocretin can be best assessed by measuring CSF hypocretin-1, and using this test, 10% to 15% of patients without cataplexy, almost all with HLA-DQB1*0602, have decreased CSF levels (13). Hypocretin deficiency is most often suspected if the patient is young and still developing the symptoms, or if the subject has significant sleep paralysis/hypnagogic hallucination and an MSLT with very short sleep latency and three or four SOREMPs. In most other cases, however, CSF hypocretin-1 is normal, suggesting another cause for the disorder. Surprisingly, some investigators have reported increased HLA-DQB1*0602 positivity as in narcolepsy with cataplexy, raising the possibility that some cases share a common HLA-associated pathophysiology (19,23). In the only postmortem study of one case with narcolepsy without cataplexy, the number of hypocretin cells was decreased but not as much as in narcolepsy with cataplexy cases (14). Possibly, a partial lesion of hypocretin-containing cells that does not result in a complete loss of CSF hypocretin could be involved.

Whether or not narcolepsy without cataplexy represents a true continuum with narcolepsy with cataplexy, sharing a common pathophysiology is unknown. Most likely, the condition as described is etiologically heterogeneous and its frequency in case series is highly dependent on the diagnostic criteria used by each clinician.

When left untreated, narcolepsy is socially disabling and isolating. Patients have a tendency to fail at school and are often dismissed from their job. Driving may be avoided for fear of car accidents. The inability to sleep at night may further contribute to a loss of control these patients have over their schedule. Depression is common.

Risk Factors

Genetic and nongenetic predisposing factors are suspected but not known. At the genetic level, there is some controversy regarding a possible association with HLA subtypes DR2 and DQB1*0602, as in narcolepsy with cataplexy. In a case series of narcolepsy without cataplexy, approximately 40% of these subjects are HLA-DQB1*0602 positive versus 12% to 25% in most control populations (19). Problematically, however, subjects are frequently HLA-typed to assist in the diagnosis of narcolepsy and it is possible that the increase in HLA frequency is a result of selection bias. CSF hypocretin studies have shown that a small percentage of these cases are hypocretin deficient, these being almost always DQB1*0602 positive (13). There is thus a definite overlap with narcolepsy with cataplexy, but the extent (a few percent to 20%) is unknown. Environmental precipitating factors are suspected from case reports but have never been proven to be involved in the triggering of narcolepsy. Among the most commonly reported triggers have been head trauma or an unspecified viral illness.

NARCOLEPSY DUE TO MEDICAL CONDITION

Several cases of narcolepsy in association with brain tumors have been reported. Narcolepsy has also been reported in patients with multiple sclerosis, encephalitis, cerebral ischemia, cranial trauma, brain tumor, and cerebral degeneration (24–27). Hypothalamic sarcoidosis has caused narcolepsy in at least two cases, although neither had cataplexy (24,28). Symptomatic narcolepsies are also present in children affected with Niemann–Pick type C disease (29). A recent report described patients with paraneoplastic anti-Ma antibodies who have hypothalamic inflammation, sleepiness, and cataplexy (30,31). Melberg and colleagues have described a Swedish family with autosomal dominant cerebellar ataxia, deafness, and narcolepsy (25). Affected members gradually develop chronic sleepiness and cataplexy in young adulthood.

In the *ICSD-2*, narcolepsy with or without cataplexy associated with these conditions is classified under "narcolepsy due to medical condition," and a significant underlying medical or neurological disorder must account for EDS and/or cataplexy (1).

Demographics

The cause of narcolepsy in these cases is assumed to be due to a coexisting medical or neurological disorder. Therefore, various diseases may cause narcolepsy and demographic features may also be varied.

In a recent meta-analysis (32), 116 symptomatic cases of secondary narcolepsy reported in literature were collated. All cases meet *ICSD* criteria for narcolepsy due to medical condition (32). As several authors previously reported, inherited disorders ($n = 38$), tumors ($n = 33$), and head trauma ($n = 19$) were the three most frequent causes of symptomatic narcolepsy. Of 116 cases, 10 were associated with multiple sclerosis and one case with acute disseminated encephalomyelitis. Relatively rare cases were reported with vascular disorders ($n = 6$), encephalitis ($n = 4$), neurodegeneration ($n = 1$), and heterodegenerative disorder (three cases in a family).

EDS without cataplexy or other REM sleep abnormalities is also often associated with these neurological conditions and defined as symptomatic cases of EDS (*ICSD-2*: hypersomnia due to medical condition).

Key Symptoms and Signs

Daytime sleepiness in these cases may be of variable severity. Sleep paralysis, hypnagogic hallucination, insomnia, or automatic behavior may or may not be present. Key features of common symptomatic cases of narcolepsy are listed.

Narcolepsy without cataplexy, as documented with the MSLT, has been reported in some cases of Parkinson's disease. MSLT results in Parkinson's disease may be due to insufficient treatment at night that results in insufficient sleep and resulting daytime sleepiness (insomnia due to medical condition). Treatment of Parkinson's disease with dopaminergic agonists can also induce daytime sleepiness (hypersomnia due to drug or substance). In other cases, however, narcolepsy without cataplexy is likely of central origin and should be classified in this section.

The issue of posttraumatic hypersomnia is often fraught with medicolegal difficulties. Cases of hypersomnia or even narcolepsy with cataplexy have been documented, and head trauma has also been reported to increase sleep apnea. As a result, control of other potential sleep disorders is necessary prior to this diagnosis, and use of MSLT documentation of sleepiness and SOREMPs is important.

Genetic disorders such as Niemann–Pick type C, Norrie disease, and Coffin–Lowry syndrome have been reported to be associated with primary daytime somnolence and, in some cases, cataplexy (32). Genetic disorders associated with narcolepsy and abnormal breathing during sleep include myotonic dystrophy and Prader–Willi syndrome and may be associated with both sleep apnea and hypersomnia (32). Sleep-onset REM periods are often present during the MSLT. Narcolepsy due to medical condition should only be diagnosed if the excessive somnolence and SOREMPs are still present during the MSLT after adequate therapeutic control of sleep apnea. Low CSF hypocretin-1 has been reported in some cases (33).

Vascular, infectious, inflammatory, neoplastic, and neurodegenerative lesions of the brain may produce documented daytime sleepiness with SOREMPs and, more rarely, cataplexy (32). Similarly, narcolepsy due to medical condition should only be diagnosed if the excessive somnolence and SOREMPs are independent of sleep apnea or any other sleep disorder.

Onset, Ontogeny, and Clinical Course

Onset and clinical courses are also significantly varied depending on the causative disease. Although it is sometimes difficult to rule out comorbidity of idiopathic narcolepsy in some cases, a review of the literature reveals numerous unquestionable cases of symptomatic narcolepsy (32). These include cases with HLA negativity and/or late onset cases, and cases in which the occurrence of the narcoleptic symptoms paralleled the rise and fall of the causative disease. Interestingly, a review of these cases with symptomatic narcolepsy (especially those with brain tumors) clearly indicates that the hypothalamus is most often involved (32): analysis of 33 symptomatic cases of narcolepsy associated with brain tumor illustrated a clear picture that the pituitary, suprasellar or the optic chasm are most often (70%) involved, while the brainstem lesions are much less frequently causative, found in only 10% of these cases.

CSF hypocretin-1 measurements were also carried out in a limited number of symptomatic cases of narcolepsy. Reduced CSF hypocretin-1 levels were seen in most symptomatic narcolepsy cases with various etiologies (32). EDS/cataplexy in these cases is sometimes reversible, with an improvement of the causative neurological disorder and an improvement of the hypocretin status.

Risk Factors

The risk factors for this condition are not well understood. As stated above, hypothalamic involvement (hypocretin deficiency in some cases) is suggested, but no systematic study about the association with HLA types and its predisposition has been done (32).

RECURRENT HYPERSOMNIA

Demographics

Recurrent hypersomnia is rare. Roughly 200 cases have been reported in the literature to date (34–37). The male-to-female ratio is about 4:1 in Kleine–Levin syndrome, with a more balanced male-to-female ratio in cases where recurrent sleepiness is the only symptom. Familial cases of Kleine–Levin syndrome are rare, and previously reported cases include atypical conditions (34). Occasionally, the presence of mood disorders in family members of patients is reported.

Another form of recurrent hypersomnia is menstrual-related periodic hypersomnia, in which EDS occurs during the several days prior to menstruation (38,39). The prevalence of this syndrome has not been well characterized.

Key Symptoms and Signs

Recurrent hypersomnia (Kleine–Levin is the best-characterized recurrent hypersomnia) is characterized by recurrent episodes of hypersomnia often associated with other symptoms that typically occur weeks or months apart (34–37). Episodes usually last a few days to several weeks and appear one to ten times a year. Episodes are often preceded by prodromes such as fatigue or headache lasting a few hours. Patients may sleep as long as 16 to 18 hours per day, waking or getting up only to eat and void. Urinary incontinence does not occur. Body weight gain of a few kilograms is often observed during the episode. Cognitive abnormalities such as feelings of unreality, confusion, and hallucinations may occur. Behavioral abnormalities such as binge eating, hypersexuality, irritability, and aggressiveness may be present. Patients may respond verbally, but often unclearly or aggressively, when aroused by strong stimuli during the episode. The simultaneous occurrence of all these symptoms is the exception rather than the rule, and in some cases, isolated recurrent hypersomnia may be the only symptom. Amnesia, transient dysphoria, or elation with insomnia may signal the termination of an episode. To be characterized as recurrent hypersomnia, sleep and general behavior must be normal between episodes.

Physical examination is sometimes remarkable for the presence of a reddish face with severe perspiration. Social and occupational impairment during attacks is often severe but can be variable depending on the frequency, severity, and duration of episodes.

- A diagnosis of Klein–Levin syndrome should be reserved for cases in which recurrent episodes are clearly associated with behavioral abnormalities. These may include binge eating; hypersexuality; abnormal behavior such as irritability, aggression, and odd behavior; and cognitive abnormalities such as feeling of unreality, confusion, and hallucinations.
- Recurrent episodes of sleepiness that occur in association with the menstrual cycle may be indicative of the menstrual-associated sleep disorder. The disease occurs within the first months after menarche. Episodes generally last one week, with rapid resolution at the time of menses. Hormonal imbalance is likely since oral contraceptives usually lead to prolonged remission.

Onset, Ontogeny, and Clinical Course

Early adolescence is the usual age of onset. A somewhat older age of onset has been reported in females. The course of recurrent hypersomnia is characterized by recurrent episodes of severe sleepiness, lasting up to several weeks, but with normal functioning between episodes (34–37). Long-term follow-up studies of patients with Kleine–Levin syndrome are lacking. Case report reviews suggest a typically benign course, with episodes lessening in duration, severity, and frequency over one to several years. However, long-term follow-up after the last episode is frequently lacking, making it difficult to conclude that the disorder has completely resolved. In rare cases, episodes have been shown to recur over a period of 10 to 20 years. Complications are mainly social and occupational. In rare cases, subjects have been reported to choke while eating voraciously during the episode and to suffer cardiopulmonary arrest.

Postmortem examination of the central nervous system has been performed in only four cases with inconsistent findings (34). One subject showed significant perivascular lymphocytic infiltrations in the hypothalamus, amygdala, and grey matter of the temporal lobes. A mild, localized encephalitis was suggested. The second and third cases showed similar lesions in other locations—the thalamus in one case, the diencephalon and the midbrain in the other. In the fourth case, a smaller locus coeruleus and decreased pigmentation in the substantia nigra were reported. The symptoms typically observed in Kleine–Levin syndrome may be of hypothalamic origin. However, hypothalamic and pituitary functions have generally been normal. A possible exception is the recent finding of moderately decreased CSF hypocretin-1 during the episodes (40). MRI evaluation is unremarkable. An autoimmune basis for the disorder is suggested clinically (onset occurs during adolescence, often in conjunction with an infection) and by the recently reported association with HLA-DQB1*0201 (41). The pathophysiology of these disorders is completely unknown. Hypothalamic dysfunction has long been suggested but is not established. All examinations of hypothalamic function performed to date have been normal.

Likewise, the etiology of menstrual-related periodic hypersomnia is not known, but presumably, the symptoms are related to hormonal changes. Some cases of menstrual-related hypersomnia have responded to the blocking of ovulation with estrogen and progesterone (birth control pills) (42).

Risk Factors

The frequency of HLA-DQB1*0201 was recently found to be increased in patients with Kleine–Levin syndrome (41). A flu-like illness or an infection of the upper airway is occasionally found immediately prior to the onset of the first episode. Other less frequently reported triggering events include acute drunkenness, seasickness, head trauma, sunstroke, or general anesthesia.

IDIOPATHIC HYPERSOMNIA WITH LONG SLEEP TIME

Idiopathic hypersomnia is an incompletely defined disorder characterized by EDS (43,44). Traditionally, this diagnosis has been used as a nosological haven for individuals with excessive somnolence but lacking the classic features of narcolepsy or another disorder known to cause EDS (such as sleep apnea). Without doubt, many patients have been diagnosed with idiopathic hypersomnia, when, in fact, they suffered from other disorders, such as narcolepsy without cataplexy, delayed sleep phase syndrome, or upper airway resistance syndrome (45). Roth (46) described monosymptomatic (EDS) and polysymptomatic (EDS, prolonged nocturnal sleep time, marked difficulty with awakening) forms of idiopathic hypersomnia. Others have suggested that the category of idiopathic hypersomnia is heterogeneous, including individuals with EDS but with or without one or more of the other features of Roth's polysymptomatic form (44). Idiopathic hypersomnia is believed to be less common than narcolepsy, but estimation of prevalence is obviously elusive because strict diagnostic criteria are lacking and no specific biological marker has been identified.

In the *ICSD-2* (1), two types of idiopathic hypersomnia are classified depending on the length of the sleep time.

Demographics

The disorder seems to be less frequently diagnosed now than it had been, with recent studies suggesting a ratio of 1 patient with idiopathic hypersomnia for every 10 with narcolepsy in a series from sleep disorders centers. There is no indication of gender predominance. Pediatric cases are rare. Idiopathic hypersomnia may be familial. An autosomal dominant mode of inheritance has been suggested.

Key Symptoms and Signs

Idiopathic hypersomnia with long sleep time is characterized by constant and severe excessive sleepiness with prolonged but non-refreshing naps of up to three or four hours, a prolonged major sleep episode, and great difficulty waking up either in the morning or at the end of a nap (44). The major sleep episode is prolonged to at least 10 hours (typically 12 to 14 hours), with few or no awakenings. Post-awakening confusion (sleep drunkenness) is often reported. For many researchers, idiopathic hypersomnia should only be diagnosed in the presence of long sleep time and is a unique disease entity. More recently, the term idiopathic hypersomnia has been used to include subjects with hypersomnolence without increased sleep. In the current diagnostic classification, these two variants have been separated.

Subjects typically do not awaken to alarm clocks and frequently use special devices or procedures to wake up. Significant sleep paralysis or hypnagogic hallucinations are typically not present. Associated symptoms suggesting a dysfunction of the autonomic nervous system, including headaches, orthostatic hypotension with syncope, and Raynaud's phenomenon are not uncommon. Idiopathic hypersomnia has an unpredictable response to stimulants. Lack of efficacy, tolerance, and side effects such as headache, tachycardia, and irritability are common.

Onset, Ontogeny, and Clinical Course

The onset of idiopathic hypersomnia usually occurs before 25 years of age. Once established, the disorder is stable in severity and long lasting, although spontaneous improvement can occur. Complications are most commonly seen in social and professional functions.

Neurochemical studies measuring monoamine metabolites and hypocretin-1 in the CSF have been so far inconclusive. Preliminary results have shown normal CSF hypocretin-1 concentrations in patients with idiopathic hypersomnia.

The etiology of the disorder is not known, but viral illnesses, including Guillain–Barre syndrome, hepatitis, mononucleosis, and atypical viral pneumonia may herald the onset of sleepiness in a subset of patients. EDS may occur as part of the acute illness, but it persists after the other symptoms subside. Rarely, familial cases are known to occur, with increased frequency of HLA-Cw2 and HLA-DR11 (47). Some of these patients have associated symptoms suggesting autonomic nervous system dysfunction, including orthostatic hypotension, syncope, vascular headaches, and peripheral vascular complaints. Most patients with idiopathic hypersomnia have neither a family history nor an obvious associated viral illness. Little is known about the pathophysiology of idiopathic hypersomnia. No animal model is available for study. Neurochemical studies using CSF have suggested that patients with idiopathic hypersomnia may have altered noradrenergic and histaminergic system function, but no alterations of the hypocretin system were observed in most patients (48–51).

Risk Factors

A familial, probably genetic predisposition to both hypersomnia and psychiatric disorders has been reported. In contrast to narcolepsy, the disorder is not known to be HLA associated and no consistent precipitating factor has been identified.

IDIOPATHIC HYPERSOMNIA WITHOUT LONG SLEEP TIME

Previously, idiopathic hypersomnia was diagnosed only in the presence of long sleep time. More recently, however, the term idiopathic hypersomnia includes subjects with hypersomnolence without increased sleep (43,44). Currently, these two disorders are separated.

Demographics

Not known (see sect. "Idiopathic Hypersomnia with Long Sleep Time").

Key Symptoms and Signs

The major clinical feature of idiopathic hypersomnia without long sleep time is a complaint of constant and severe EDS (43,44). Daytime sleepiness results in unintended naps that are generally of non-refreshing nature. Cataplexy is absent. The major sleep episode (e.g., nighttime) is either normal or slightly prolonged (less than 10 hours), usually with few or no awakenings. Mean sleep latency in idiopathic hypersomnia has been shown to be 6.2 ± 3.0 minutes. For a diagnosis of idiopathic hypersomnia without long sleep time, an MSLT documents a mean sleep latency less than or equal to eight minutes and one or no SOREMPs in the face of generally normal nocturnal sleep (at least six hours of nocturnal sleep prior to the MSLT). Patients sometimes have great difficulty waking up in the morning and from naps. Post-awakening confusion (sleep drunkenness) is sometimes reported.

Sleep drunkenness is common. Associated symptoms suggesting a dysfunction of the autonomic nervous system may be present, including headaches, which may be migrainous in quality; fainting episodes (syncope); orthostatic hypotension; and peripheral vascular complaints (Raynaud's type phenomena with cold hands and feet). Idiopathic hypersomnia has an unpredictable response to stimulants such as amphetamines, methylphenidate, or modafinil. Stimulant side effects such as headache, tachycardia, and irritability are commonly reported.

Onset, Ontogeny, and Clinical Course

The onset of idiopathic hypersomnia typically occurs before age 25. Once established, the disorder is stable in severity and long lasting, although spontaneous improvement has been reported in a few subjects. Complications are mostly social and professional. These include poor work/school performance, reduced earnings, and loss of employment. The cause of idiopathic hypersomnia is unknown (see also sect. "Idiopathic Hypersomnia with Long Sleep Time").

Risk Factors

Not known (see also sect: "Idiopathic Hypersomnia with Long Sleep Time").

BEHAVIORALLY INDUCED INSUFFICIENT SLEEP SYNDROME

The most common cause of daytime sleepiness is insufficient sleep, which may reflect poor sleep "hygiene" (behaviors impacting sleep) or self-imposed or socially dictated sleep deprivation (52–54).

Demographics

It affects people of all ages and both sexes. It may be more frequent in adolescence, when sleep need is high but social pressure and delayed sleep phase often lead to chronically restricted sleep.

Key Symptoms and Signs

Behaviorally induced insufficient sleep syndrome occurs when an individual persistently fails to obtain the amount of sleep required to maintain normal levels of alertness and wakefulness (53,54). The individual engages in voluntary, albeit unintentional, chronic sleep deprivation. Examination reveals unimpaired or above-average ability to initiate and maintain sleep, with little or no psychopathology. Physical examination reveals no medical explanation for the patient's sleepiness. A detailed history of the current sleep pattern reveals a substantial disparity between the need for sleep and the amount actually obtained. Its significance is unappreciated by the patient. A markedly extended sleep time on weekend nights as compared with weekday nights is also suggestive of this disorder. A therapeutic trial of a longer major sleep episode can reverse the symptoms. Additional symptoms such as sleep paralysis and hypnagogic hallucination may occur.

Depending on chronicity and extent of sleep loss, individuals with this condition may develop irritability, concentration and attention deficits, reduced vigilance, distractibility, reduced motivation, anergia, dysphoria, fatigue, restlessness, incoordination, and malaise. Secondary symptoms may become the main focus of the patient, serving to obscure the primary cause of the difficulties. Psychologically and somatically normal individuals who chronically obtain less sleep than they physiologically require typically experience sleepiness during waking hours. Situational factors may, on occasion, make it impossible to obtain adequate sleep. Individuals should not be classified here unless they are unaware of the role sleep debt plays in their clinical complaint.

Onset, Ontogeny, and Clinical Course

This condition results in increased daytime sleepiness, concentration problems, lowered energy level, and malaise. If unchecked, behaviorally induced insufficient sleep syndrome may cause depression and other psychological difficulties, with poor work performance and withdrawal from family and social activities occurring. Abuse of stimulants may also occur. Traffic accidents or injury at work may take place.

Symptoms are due to normal physiological and psychological responses to sleep deprivation. Sleep restriction studies in normal volunteers have shown that even mild sleep restriction (e.g., six hours of nocturnal sleep per night) results in a corresponding decrease in performance and increased sleepiness. Conversely, in some long sleepers, extending sleep to nine hours often results in improved performance. The diagnosis of insufficient sleep may thus be especially difficult to make in subjects who have an unusual need for large amounts of sleep.

Risk Factors

Social, cultural, and psychological factors may dispose the individual to search for causes other than the obvious one.

HYPERSOMNIA DUE TO MEDICAL CONDITION

EDS is often associated with disorders of the central or peripheral nervous systems and is a clinical feature of many toxic or metabolic encephalopathic processes. These disorders often present with other symptoms and signs, but EDS may dominate the picture, particularly in chronic cases. Structural brain lesions, including strokes, tumors, cysts, abscesses, hematomas, vascular malformations, hydrocephalus, and multiple sclerosis plaques are known to produce EDS (32). Somnolence may result either from direct involvement of discrete brain regions (especially the brainstem, reticular formation, or midline diencephalic structures) or because of effects on sleep continuity (e.g., nocturnal seizure activity or secondary SRBDs).

EDS is a frequent sequela of encephalitis or head trauma. Victims of "encephalitis lethargica," described by Von Economo in the early twentieth century, were found to have lesions in the midbrain, subthalamus, and hypothalamus. Additionally, posttraumatic narcolepsy with cataplexy is well documented (55). Epileptic patients may suffer from EDS as a consequence of medication effects or, less obviously, because of nocturnal seizure activity (56). EDS may be associated with numerous infectious agents affecting the central nervous system, including bacteria, viruses, fungi, and parasites. Perhaps the best known is trypanosomiasis, which is called "sleeping sickness" because of the prominent hypersomnia. Sleepiness may occur with acute infectious illness, even without direct invasion of the nervous system, and may be mediated by cytokines, including interferon, interleukins, and tumor necrosis factor (57). EDS may also persist chronically after certain viral infections (58).

Sleep disruption and EDS are common in neurodegenerative disorders, including Parkinson's disease, Alzheimer's disease, and other dementias, as well as multiple system atrophy (59–61). Patients with neuromuscular disorders or peripheral neuropathies may also develop EDS because of associated SRBD (central or obstructive apnea), pain, or periodic limb movements of sleep (PLMS) (62). Patients with myotonic dystrophy often suffer from EDS even in the absence of sleep-disordered breathing (63).

Demographics

As for the cases with narcolepsy due to medical condition, a number of hypersomnia cases (without cataplexy and REM sleep abnormality) associated with various neurological conditions have appeared in the literature (32).

The causative diseases include focal/generalized central nervous system (CNS) invasion, as in cerebral tumors, brain infections, vascular diseases, head trauma, and neurodegenerative disorders (Alzheimer's disease, Parkinson's disease), and CNS diseases mediated with neuroimmune mechanisms such as inflammatory and demyelinating diseases.

This category likely consists of heterogeneous conditions and includes less well-defined cases of hypersomnia. Demographic features may also vary depending on the causative diseases.

The prevalence of the disease is not known, but a recent review counted only 71 cases in the literature (32). However, the prevalence of these symptomatic EDS cases appeared to be much higher, considering the progress in therapeutic medicine for emergency and CNS diseases and the fact that applying standardized polygraphic assessments (all-night polygraphic recordings followed by MSLT) was sometimes difficult under many of these neurological conditions.

Key Symptoms and Signs

Daytime sleepiness may be of variable severity and may resemble either that of narcolepsy (i.e., refreshing effects of naps) or of idiopathic hypersomnia with long sleep time (i.e., long sleep episode and unrefreshing sleep). If an MSLT is performed, the results obtained must not qualify for narcolepsy without cataplexy. Similarly, cataplexy must not be present. Sleep paralysis, hypnagogic hallucination, or automatic behavior may or may not be present. In the case of disorders associated both with sleep apnea and with central hypersomnia, a diagnosis of hypersomnia due to medical condition should be made only if hypersomnia persists after adequate treatment of the sleep-disordered breathing. Hypersomnia secondary to psychiatric disorders, drugs of abuse, or the effects of prescribed medications are classified elsewhere. Hypersomnia due to medical condition is diagnosed only if the medical condition is judged to be directly causing the hypersomnia.

Onset, Ontogeny, and Clinical Course/Risk Factors

The pathophysiology of the disease appears to be heterogeneous and is largely understudied. Multiple complex interactions may also be present. As an example, preexisting obstructive sleep apnea may predispose to a cerebral infarct that may exacerbate the sleep apnea, causing further sleepiness and impaired recovery from the stroke. Further studies are needed to determine how sleep disorders interact with other diseases.

CSF hypocretin-1 measurements were also carried out in a limited number of symptomatic cases of EDS. Reduced CSF hypocretin-1 levels were seen in most symptomatic EDS cases with various etiologies (32). EDS in these cases is sometimes reversible, with an improvement of the causative neurological disorder and the hypocretin status. It is also noted that in some symptomatic cases with EDS (with Parkinson's disease and thalamic infarction), hypocretin status was in the normal range.

Since CSF hypocretin-1 measures are still experimental, cases with sleep abnormalities are habitually selected for CSF hypocretin-1 measures. Therefore, it is still not known whether all or a large majority of cases with low CSF hypocretin-1 levels with CNS interventions exhibit EDS.

A recent study suggests that histamine neurotransmission may be impaired in patients with symptomatic ESD as is also seen in narcolepsy and idiopathic hypersomnia cases.

HYPERSOMNIA DUE TO DRUG OR SUBSTANCE

Demographics

Excessive nocturnal sleep, daytime sleepiness, or excessive napping can occur secondary to substance use or prescribed medication (64). Hypersomnia due to substance (substance abuse) may also be associated with tolerance to or withdrawal from various prescribed or street drugs and alcohol (65–67).

Onset is usually 15 to 50 years of age for stimulant abuse and is more variable for alcohol abuse.

If hypersomnia is believed to be secondary to the medical prescription of a drug, a separate classification applies (medication). Hypersomnia or daytime sleepiness may be the result of the abrupt cessation of a previously prescribed stimulant. Stimulants in this context are typically prescribed for attention deficit hyperactivity disorder or for a sleep disorder. Withdrawal is often observed in the context of a reevaluation. Hypersomnia is often associated with the prescription of sedative compounds, such as high doses of sedative antiepileptic medications, which result in daytime sleepiness (64). Similar side effects occur frequently with opioid analgesic agents. Tolerance to the sedative effects often occurs with time.

Key Symptoms and Signs

Excessive nocturnal sleep, daytime sleepiness, or excessive napping is believed to be secondary to substance use or medical prescription. If narcolepsy or hypersomnia existed prior to stimulant abuse, the category should not be used. Problems at work and/or unemployment are frequently associated with EDS secondary to substance use.

Hypersomnia is observed in the context of a prescribed medication: it is often associated with the prescription of sedative drugs or withdrawal from prescribed stimulants. Sleepiness may or may not be documented objectively. Drugs involved may be sedative hypnotics, antiallergic agents (e.g., antihistamines), analgesics (e.g., opioids), antiepileptic agents, antihypertensive agents (e.g., α-2 clonidine-like compounds), stimulants, anti-Parkinsonian compounds (e.g., dopaminergic agonists), antidepressants (e.g., trazodone, doxepin), other psychotropic agents (e.g., neuroleptics, anxiolytics), cardiovascular compounds, anti-inflammatory drugs, anti-infectious agents (e.g., some antiviral drugs), and anticancer agents (68–71).

Onset, Ontogeny, and Clinical Course/Risk Factors

Sedative compounds have been suggested to increase sleep apnea. Sleepiness in association with the administration of a sedative compound may be due, in part, to the exacerbation of sleep apnea or another sleep disorder.

HYPERSOMNIA NOT DUE TO SUBSTANCE OR KNOWN PHYSIOLOGICAL CONDITION (NONORGANIC HYPERSOMNIA)

Demographics

Hypersomnia not due to substance or known physiological condition (but due to psychiatric conditions) explains 5% to 7% of hypersomnia cases. Causative psychiatric conditions include mood disorders, conversion or undifferentiated somatoform disorder, and, less frequently, other mental disorders such as schizoaffective disorder, adjustment disorder, or personality disorders (64,72–75). Females are more susceptible than men, and 20 to 50 years is the typical age range. Familial patterns are known, except for certain psychiatric disorders (e.g., bipolar disorder type 2).

Key Symptoms and Signs

Excessive nocturnal sleep, daytime sleepiness, or excessive napping is reported; sleep is perceived as non-restorative and generally of poor quality. Patients are often intensely focused on their hypersomnia, and psychiatric symptoms typically become apparent only after prolonged interviews or psychometric testing. Poor work attendance, spending full days in bed once or twice a week, or abruptly leaving work because of a perceived need to sleep is characteristic of this type of hypersomnia.

Hypersomnia associated with a major depressive episode: Hypersomnia in the context of depression is a frequent feature of atypical depression and bipolar type II disorder (recurrent major depressive episodes with hypomanic episodes). MSLT results are normal, but long hours spent in bed are reported. In hypersomnia as a conversion disorder or as an undifferentiated somatoform disorder, pseudo-hypersomnia or pseudo-narcolepsy is characteristic, sometimes even with reports of pseudocataplexy. In hypersomnia associated with seasonal affective disorder (SAD), daytime fatigue, loss of concentration, hypersomnia, increased appetite for carbohydrates, and weight gain are reported.

Onset, Ontogeny, and Clinical Course/Risk Factors

Mean age of onset is usually in the third decade in both sexes. Hypersomnia may or may not resolve spontaneously or with treatment. Treating successfully the accompanying psychiatric disorder does not always lead to a resolution of the associated hypersomnia. Complications are mostly social and occupational.

Nocturnal sleep may be fragmented, contributing to daytime sleepiness and unrefreshing sleep. In hypersomnia associated with other psychiatric disorders, the complaint is typically associated with lack of interest and social withdrawal. Energy level is decreased, and there is a tendency to stay long hours in bed without sleeping deeply, rather than a true increase in sleep propensity.

PHYSIOLOGICAL (ORGANIC) HYPERSOMNIA, UNSPECIFIED

These conditions meet the clinical and MSLT criteria for hypersomnia, are suspected of having a physiological etiology, and do not meet criteria for the other types of hypersomnia.

CONCLUSIONS

Excessive daytime somnolence is a prevalent problem in medical practice and in society in general. It exacts a great cost in terms of quality of life, personal and public safety, and productivity. EDS can be caused by various conditions/pathophysiology, including circadian rhythm disorders, SRBDs, or other causes of disturbed nocturnal sleep. Several different types of hypersomnia of central origin, such as narcolepsy (with and without cataplexy), recurrent hypersomnia, idiopathic hypersomnia (with and without long sleep time), behaviorally induced insufficient sleep syndrome, narcolepsy/hypersomnia due to medical condition, hypersomnia due to drug and substance, and nonorganic hypersomnia have been described and classified. Various methods have been developed to assess EDS (although each of them has limitations), and one of the objective polytrophic measures for sleep tendency and REM sleep abnormalities (i.e., MSLT) has been included in the diagnostic criteria for EDS of central origin. The causes of EDS are myriad, and a careful evaluation is needed to determine the classification in any individual case. Although much progress has been made in discovering the pathophysiology of narcolepsy in humans (i.e., hypocretin ligand deficiency), much more remains to be understood and far less is known about other primary conditions of EDS. However, there is no doubt that detailed evaluations and descriptions of these cases will help to uncover their pathophysiology and to establish better treatments.

REFERENCES

1. American Academy of Sleep Medicine, . International Classification of Sleep Disorders: Diagnostic and Coding Manual. 2nd ed. Illinois: American Academy of Sleep Medicine, 2005.
2. Johns M. A new method for measuring daytime sleepiness. The Epworth sleepiness scale. Sleep 1991; 14:540–545.
3. Carskadon MA, Dement WC, Mitler MM, et al. Guidelines for the multiple sleep latency test (MSLT): a standard measure of sleepiness. Sleep 1986; 9:519–524.
4. Mitler MM, Walsleben J, Sangal RB, et al. Sleep latency on the maintenance of wakefulness test (MWT) for 530 patients with narcolepsy while free of psychoactive drugs. Electroencephalogr Clin Neurophysiol 1998; 107(1):33–38.
5. Johns MW. Sleepiness in different situations measured by the Epworth sleepiness scale. Sleep 1994; 17 (8):703–710.
6. Chervin RD, Aldrich MS, Pickett R, et al. Comparison of the results of the Epworth sleepiness scale and the multiple sleep latency test. J Psychosom Res 1997; 42(2):145–155.
7. Moscovitch A, Partinen M, Guilleminault C. The positive diagnosis of narcolepsy and narcolepsy's borderland. Neurology 1993; 43:55–60.
8. Aldrich MS, Chervin RD, Malow BA. Value of the multiple sleep latency test (MSLT) for the diagnosis of narcolepsy. Sleep 1997; 20(8):620–629.
9. Nishino S, Mignot E. Pharmacological aspects of human and canine narcolepsy. Prog Neurobiol 1997; 52:27–78.
10. Lin L, Faraco J, Li R, et al. The sleep disorder canine narcolepsy is caused by a mutation in the hypocretin (orexin) receptor 2 gene. Cell 1999; 98(3):365–376.
11. Chemelli RM, Willie JT, Sinton CM, et al. Narcolepsy in orexin knockout mice: molecular genetics of sleep regulation. Cell 1999; 98:437–451.
12. Nishino S, Ripley B, Overeem S, et al. Hypocretin (orexin) deficiency in human narcolepsy. Lancet 2000; 355(9197):39–40.
13. Mignot E, Lammers GJ, Ripley B, et al. The role of cerebrospinal fluid hypocretin measurement in the diagnosis of narcolepsy and other hypersomnias. Arch Neurol 2002; 59(10):1553–1562.
14. Thannickal TC, Moore RY, Nienhuis R, et al. Reduced number of hypocretin neurons in human narcolepsy. Neuron 2000; 27(3):469–474.
15. Peyron C, Faraco J, Rogers W, et al. A mutation in a case of early onset narcolepsy and a generalized absence of hypocretin peptides in human narcoleptic brains. Nat Med 2000; 6(9):991–997.
16. Mignot E. Genetic and familial aspects of narcolepsy. Neurology 1998; 50(suppl 1):S16–S22.
17. Schuld A, Hebebrand J, Geller F, et al. Increased body-mass index in patients with narcolepsy. Lancet 2000; 355(9211):1274–1275.
18. Honda Y, Doi Y, Ninomiya R, et al. Increased frequency of non-insulin-dependent diabetes mellitus among narcoleptic patients. Sleep 1986; 9(1):254–259.
19. Mignot E, Hayduk R, Black J, et al. HLA DQB1*0602 is associated with cataplexy in 509 narcoleptic patients. Sleep 1997; 20(11):1012–1020.
20. Kanbayashi T, Inoue Y, Chiba S, et al. CSF hypocretin-1 (orexin-A) concentrations in narcolepsy with and without cataplexy and idiopathic hypersomnia. J Sleep Res 2002; 11(1):91–93.
21. Silber MH, Krahn LE, Olson EJ, et al. The epidemiology of narcolepsy in Olmsted County, Minnesota: a population-based study. Sleep 2002; 25(2)197–202.
22. Fukuda K, Miyasita A, Inugami M, et al. High prevalence of isolated sleep paralysis: kanashibari phenomenon in Japan. Sleep 1987; 10(3):279–286.
23. Honda Y, Juji T, Matsuki K, et al. HLA-DR2 and Dw2 in narcolepsy and in other disorders of excessive somnolence without cataplexy. Sleep 1986; 9:133–142.
24. Aldrich MS, Naylor MW. Narcolepsy associated with lesions of the diencephalon. Neurology 1989; 39: 1505–1508.
25. Melberg A, Ripley B, Lin L, et al. Hypocretin deficiency in familial symptomatic narcolepsy. Ann Neurol 2001; 49(1):136–137.
26. Arii J, Kanbayashi T, Tanabe Y, et al. A hypersomnolent girl with decreased CSF hypocretin level after removal of a hypothalamic tumor. Neurology 2001; 56(12):1775–1776.
27. Scammell TE, Nishino S, Mignot E, et al. Narcolepsy and low CSF orexin (hypocretin) concentration after a diencephalic stroke. Neurology 2001; 56(12):1751–1753.
28. Malik S, Boeve BF, Krahn LE, et al. Narcolepsy associated with other central nervous system disorders. Neurology 2001; 57(3):539–541.
29. Challamel MJ, Mazzola ME, Nevsimalova S, et al. Narcolepsy in children. Sleep 1994; 17:S17–S20.
30. Overeem S, Dalmau J, Bataller L, et al. Hypocretin-1 CSF levels in anti-Ma2 associated encephalitis. Neurology 2004; 62(1):138–140.
31. Rosenfeld MR, Eichen JG, Wade DF, et al. Molecular and clinical diversity in paraneoplastic immunity to Ma proteins. Ann Neurol 2001; 50(3):339–348.

32. Nishino S, Kanbayashi T. Symptomatic narcolepsy, cataplexy and hypersomnia, and their implications in the hypothalamic hypocretin/orexin system. Sleep Med Rev 2005; 9(4):269–310.

33. Nevsimalova S, Vankova J, Stepanova I, et al. Hypocretin deficiency in Prader-Willi syndrome. Eur J Neurol 2005; 12(1):70–72.

34. Arnulf I, Zeitzer JM, File J, et al. Kleine-Levin syndrome: a systematic review of 186 cases in the literature. Brain 2005; 128(pt 12):2763–2776.

35. Critchley M. Periodic hypersomnia and megaphagia in adolescent males. Brain 1962; 85:627–656.

36. Takahashi Y. [Clinical studies of periodic somnolence: analysis of 28 personal cases]. Seishin Shinkeigaku Zasshi 1965; 67(9):853–889.

37. Mayer G, Leonhard E, Krieg J, et al. Endocrinological and polysomnographic findings in Kleine-Levin syndrome: no evidence for hypothalamic and circadian dysfunction. Sleep 1998; 21(3):278–284.

38. Billiard M, Guilleminault C, Dement WC. A menstruation-linked periodic hypersomnia. Kleine-Levin syndrome or new clinical entity? Neurology 1975; 25(5):436–443.

39. Sachs C, Persson HE, Hagenfeldt K. Menstruation-related periodic hypersomnia: a case study with successful treatment. Neurology 1982; 32(12):1376–1379.

40. Dauvilliers Y, Baumann CR, Carlander B, et al. CSF hypocretin-1 levels in narcolepsy, Kleine-Levin syndrome, and other hypersomnias and neurological conditions. J Neurol Neurosurg Psychiatry 2003; 74(12):1667–1673.

41. Dauvilliers Y, Mayer G, Lecendreux M, et al. Kleine-Levin syndrome: an autoimmune hypothesis based on clinical and genetic analyses. Neurology 2002; 59(11):1739–1745.

42. Bamford CR. Menstrual-associated sleep disorder: an unusual hypersomniac variant associated with both menstruation and amenorrhea with a possible link to prolactin and metoclopramide. Sleep 1993; 16(5):484–486.

43. Billiard M, Dauvilliers Y. Idiopathic Hypersomnia. Sleep Med Rev 2001; 5(5):349–358.

44. Aldrich M. The clinical spectrum of narcolepsy and idiopathic hypersomnia. Neurology 1996; 46:393–401.

45. Guilleminault C, Stoohs R, Clerk A, et al. A cause of excessive daytime sleepiness. The upper airway resistance syndrome. Chest 1993; 104(3):781–787.

46. Roth B. Narcolepsy and hypersomnia. Arch Neurol Psychiatr 1976; 119:31–41.

47. Montplaisir J, Poirier G. HLA in disorders of excessive daytime sleepiness without cataplexy in Canada. In: Honda Y, Juji T, eds. HLA in Narcolepsy. New York: Springer-Verlag, 1988:186–190.

48. Montplaisir J, de Champlain J, Young SN, et al. Narcolepsy and idiopathic hypersomnia: biogenic amines and related compounds in CSF. Neurology 1982; 32(11):1299–12302.

49. Faull KF, Thiemann S, King RJ, et al. Monoamine interactions in narcolepsy and hypersomnia: a preliminary report. Sleep 1986; 9(1):246–249.

50. Faull KF, Guilleminault C, Berger PA, et al. Cerebrospinal fluid monoamine metabolites in narcolepsy and hypersomnia. Ann Neurol 1983; 13(3):258–263.

51. Kanbayashi T, Kodama T, Hondo H, et al. CSF histamine and noradrenaline contents in narcolepsy and other sleep disorders. Sleep 2004; 27(suppl):A236 (abstr).

52. Carskadon MA, Dement WC. Effects of total sleep loss on sleep tendency. Percept Mot Skills 1979; 48(2):495–506.

53. Roehrs T, Zorick F, Sicklesteel J, et al. Excessive daytime sleepiness associated with insufficient sleep. Sleep 1983; 6(4):319–325.

54. Van Dongen HP, Maislin G, Mullington JM, et al. The cumulative cost of additional wakefulness: dose-response effects on neurobehavioral functions and sleep physiology from chronic sleep restriction and total sleep deprivation. Sleep 2003; 26(2):117–126.

55. Francisco GE, Ivanhoe CB. Successful treatment of post-traumatic narcolepsy with methylphenidate. Am J Phys Med Rehabil 1996; 75(1):63–65.

56. Manni R, Tantara A. Evaluation of sleepiness in epilepsy. Clin Neurophysiol 2000; 111(suppl 2):S111–S114.

57. Toth LA, Opp MR. Sleep and infection. In: Lee-Chiong TL, Sateia MJ, Carskadon MA, eds. Sleep Medicine. Philadelphia: Hanley and Belfus, 77–83.

58. Guilleminault C, Mondini S. Mononucleosis and chronic daytime sleepiness. A long-term follow-up study. Arch Intern Med 1986; 146(7):1333–1335.

59. Askenasy JJ. Sleep in Parkinson's disease. Acta Neurol Scand 1993; 87(3):167–170.

60. Chokroverty S. Sleep and degenerative neurologic disorders. Neurol Clin 1996; 14(4):807–826.

61. Trenkwalder C. Sleep dysfunction in Parkinson's disease. Clin Neurosci 1998; 5(2):107–114.

62. George CFP. Neuromuscular disorders. In: Kryger MH, Roth T, Dement WC, eds. Principles and Practice of Sleep Medicine. 3rd ed. Philadelphia: W. B. Saunders, 2000:1087–1092.

63. Gibbs JW 3rd, Ciafaloni E, Radtke RA. Excessive daytime somnolence and increased rapid eye movement pressure in myotonic dystrophy. Sleep 2002; 25(6):662–665.

64. Guilleminault C, Brooks SN. Excessive daytime sleepiness: a challenge for the practising neurologist. Brain 2001; 124(pt 8):1482–1491.

65. Gault FP. A review of recent literature on barbiturate addiction and withdrawal. Bol Estud Med Biol 1976; 29(2–3):75–83.

66. Roehrs T, Roth T. Sleep, sleepiness, and alcohol use. Alcohol Res Health 2001; 25(2):101–109.

67. Thompson PM, Gillin JC, Golshan S, et al. Polygraphic sleep measures differentiate alcoholics and stimulant abusers during short-term abstinence. Biol Psychiatry 1995; 38(12):831–836.

68. Blum DE. New drugs for persons with epilepsy. Adv Neurol 1998; 76:57–87.

69. Oppenheimer JJ, Casale TB. Next generation antihistamines: therapeutic rationale, accomplishments and advances. Expert Opin Investig Drugs 2002; 11(6):807–817.

70. Roehrs T, Bonahoom A, Pedrosi B, et al. Nighttime versus daytime hypnotic self-administration. Psychopharmacology (Berl) 2002; 161(2):137–142.

71. Young-McCaughan S, Miaskowski C. Definition of and mechanism for opioid-induced sedation. Pain Manag Nurs 2001; 2(3):84–97.

72. Billiard M, Dolenc L, Aldaz C, et al. Hypersomnia associated with mood disorders: a new perspective. J Psychosom Res 1994; 38(suppl 1):41–47.

73. Nofzinger EA, Thase ME, Reynolds CF 3rd, et al. Hypersomnia in bipolar depression: a comparison with narcolepsy using the multiple sleep latency test. Am J Psychiatry 1991; 148(9):1177–1181.

74. Nishino S, Taheri S, Black J, et al. The neurobiology of sleep in relation to mental illness. In: Charney DS, Nestler EJ, eds. Neurobiology of Mental Illness. New York: Oxford University Press, 2004:1160–1179.

75. Rosenthal NE, Sack DA, Gillin JC, et al. Seasonal affective disorder. A description of the syndrome and preliminary findings with light therapy. Arch Gen Psychiatry 1984; 41(1):72–80.

21 | Diagnostic Tools for Hypersomnias

Jose Mendez
Sleep Disorders Center and Division of Child Neurology, Mayo Clinic, Rochester, Minnesota, U.S.A.

Suresh Kotagal
Division of Child Neurology, Mayo Clinic, Rochester, Minnesota, U.S.A.

Sleepiness is an awake condition that is associated with an increased tendency to fall asleep. For many years, the measurement of sleepiness has remained a challenge for sleep clinicians and researchers alike. This topic is so significant that it has even warranted consideration as the possible "holy grail of sleep medicine." (1). There are many challenges in the clinical assessment of sleepiness. To start with, sleepiness is frequently confused with fatigue, which refers to a lack of physical energy and a sense of exhaustion following physical activity. Second, we have the issue of subjective underestimation of sleepiness by those who are excessively sleepy. Third, can data from neurophysiological and neuropsychological studies obtained from sleep deprivation experiments in healthy subjects be extrapolated to sleepiness due to actual sleep disorders? Further, the correlation between subjective (questionnaires) and objective measures of sleepiness [multiple sleep latency test (MSLT)/maintenance of wakefulness test (MWT)] is suboptimal. Finally, physiological measurements obtained in the quiet environment of the sleep laboratory may not be representative of sleepiness encountered in day-to-day, real-life situations like driving or desk work. These shortcomings notwithstanding, a substantial body of information has been gathered on the measurement of sleepiness, a synopsis of which is presented hereunder.

The clinical evaluation and management of daytime sleepiness starts with a comprehensive sleep history and medical examination, followed when indicated by appropriate laboratory diagnostic procedures. Gender and age influence sleepiness—in a survey of 1562 women and 1351 men of a mean age of 46.6 years ± 7.9 years enrolled in the Wisconsin Sleep Cohort Study, worse perceived sleepiness was significantly related to female gender, younger age, higher sleep debt, and worse scores on the Stanford sleepiness scale (SSS) (2).

HISTORY AND PHYSICAL EXAMINATION

Daytime History

Physiological daytime napping is common before the age of five years, so it is difficult to identify a pathologically sleepy preschool-age child. In a school-age child, however, habitually falling asleep in the classroom, while being driven in an automobile, at the dinner table, while watching television, or while reading should arouse suspicion of significant daytime sleepiness. Since sleepiness impacts the prefrontal cortex, mood swings and inattentiveness, which are consequences of frontal lobe dysfunction, may coexist. Sleepy teens may show declining grades, chronic absence from school, and vulnerability to accidents/near miss accidents. There may also be a gradual increase in the consumption of caffeinated beverages or nicotine. Adults with significant sleepiness may show involuntary napping in socially inappropriate situations like talking or eating. Their performance at work may also suffer. Periods of hypersomnia lasting 10 to 14 days in teenagers in association with hyperphagia or hypersexual behavior may suggest the Kleine–Levin syndrome (3). Inadequate sleep hygiene, substance abuse, and drug-seeking behavior may also mimic a primary disorder of vigilance like narcolepsy/idiopathic hypersomnia. A medication history for prescription and over-the-counter agents is therefore critical. Low self-esteem, sadness, and social withdrawal may suggest underlying depression. Cataplexy may be relatively subtle in childhood, and thus easily overlooked. Leading questions may need to be asked about cataplexy, hypnagogic hallucinations, and sleep paralysis. It is also important to inquire what impact daytime sleepiness has had on the quality of life.

Nighttime History

The history should assess bedtime, sleep onset time, sensorimotor disturbance suggestive of restless legs syndrome, bedtime rituals, habitual snoring, mouth breathing, nocturnal awakenings and associated behavior, heartburn, periods of observed apnea, parasomnias or seizures, bed wetting, and how alert the person feels upon awakening in the morning.

Physical Examination

The height, weight, body mass index, occipitofrontal head circumference, and blood pressure should be recorded. Obstructive sleep apnea (OSA) may be associated with poor weight gain during infancy and with obesity in older children. The patient should be assessed for craniofacial abnormalities like micrognathia, dental malocclusion, enlarged tongue size, and midface hypoplasia. A deviated nasal septum, swollen inferior turbinates, tonsillar hypertrophy, and mouth breathing may also be seen in children with OSA. Consultation with an otolaryngologist may be required to exclude adenoidal hypertrophy. Brainstem anomalies like the Chiari type II malformation can be associated with hoarseness of the voice, decreased gag reflex, and abnormal tendon reflexes. Neuromuscular disorders like myotonic dystrophy are associated with chronic obstructive hypoventilation due to a combination of oropharyngeal muscle weakness leading to airway collapse, combined with diminished respiratory muscle excursion. Home videos, when available, also provide valuable clues to cataplexy, nocturnal seizures, and parasomnias.

SUBJECTIVE ASSESSMENT TOOLS

Questionnaire surveys of sleepiness are useful in epidemiological research and also serve as screening instruments in clinical practice. Because sleep is a multidimensional phenomenon, subjective, unidimensional measures like the Epworth sleepiness scale (ESS) and the SSS correlate only weakly with objective measures of sleepiness like the MSLT.

Epworth Sleepiness Scale

The ESS is the most widely self-administered questionnaire in sleep clinical practice (4). It has been validated in a variety of clinical scenarios and proven to be reliable (5–8). Eight questions estimate the patient's chance of dozing off on a zero to three scale during common activities such as while sitting and reading, watching television, sitting inactive in a public place, as a passenger in a car, lying down in the afternoon, sitting talking to somebody, after lunch, and while driving after stopping for a few minutes at a traffic light (Table 1). The maximum score is 24, and values up to 10 are physiologic and that above 12 correlate with pathological daytime sleepiness. In the original description by Johns, the questionnaire was administered to 188 adults, including 30 healthy controls and 150 patients with sleep disorders consisting of primary snoring, OSA, narcolepsy, idiopathic hypersomnia, insomnia, and periodic limb movement disorder (4). The ages of the subjects ranged from 18 to 78, with men outnumbering women in the snoring, OSA, and periodic limb movement disorder groups. The controls showed a mean ESS score of 5.9 ± 2.2, with no significant gender difference. All patients with narcolepsy and idiopathic hypersomnia had higher ESS scores (>10) than controls. Scores >16 were felt to reflect severe sleepiness. One drawback of the ESS is that patients frequently underestimate the severity of their own

Table 1   The Stanford Sleepiness Scale

---

1 Feeling active and vital; wide awake
2 Functioning at a high level, but not at peak; able to concentrate
3 Relaxed; awake; not at full alertness; responsive
4 A little foggy; not at peak level; let down
5 Foggy; beginning to lose interest in remaining awake; slowed down
6 Sleepy; preferring to lie down; fighting sleep; woozy
7 Almost in reverie; sleep onset soon; lost struggle to remain awake

---

This is a quick way to assess how alert you are feeling. If it is during the day when you go about your business, ideally you would want a rating of one. Take into account that most people have two peak times of alertness daily, at about 9 am and 9 pm. Alertness wanes to its lowest point at around 3 pm; after that it begins to build again. Rate your alertness at different times. A rating of seven is an indication that you have a serious sleep debt and you need more sleep.

Table 2 The Epworth Sleepiness Scale

Situation	Chance of dozing			
	Never	Slight	Moderate	High
	0	1	2	3
Sitting and reading				
Watching TV				
Sitting inactive in a public place, e.g., a theater or a meeting				
As a passenger in a car for an hour without a break				
Lying down to rest in the afternoon when circumstances permit				
Sitting and talking to someone				
Sitting quietly after lunch without alcohol				
In a car, while stopped for a few minutes in traffic				

How likely are you to doze off and fall asleep in the following situations, in contrast to just feeling tired? This refers to your usual way of life in recent times. Even if you have not done some of the things recently, try to work out how they would have affected you. Use the following scale to choose the most appropriate number for each situation:
0 = would never doze
1 = slight chance of dozing
2 = moderate chance of dozing
3 = high chance of dozing

sleepiness. Others have difficulty distinguishing sleepiness from fatigue. Though used occasionally in teenagers, the ESS has not been validated in this age group.

Stanford Sleepiness Scale

In this self-rating scale, patients are asked to choose from one to seven statements that best describe their level of sleepiness at a specific time of the day (9). It reliably measures the effects of partial sleep deprivation, though not performance after sleep deprivation (Table 2). As with the ESS, there can be subjective underestimation of sleepiness. There are no reference values, and the scale has not been validated against other physiological measures. The SSS does not capture the true, multidimensional nature of sleepiness (10). It does show a high correlation with visual analog scales of mood (11). Broughton (12) found that while the SSS scores reliably reflected performance decrements following acute partial sleep deprivation, they did not accurately reflect the effects of cumulative sleep loss or the overwhelming sleepiness seen in narcolepsy-cataplexy.

Karolinska Sleepiness Scale

Developed in 1990 by Akerstedt and Gillberg (13), this scale has been frequently applied in the occupational health field. It uses a nine-point scale that ranges from one being very alert to nine being very sleepy and trying hard to stay awake. Patients are asked to rate their sleepiness in the five minutes immediately prior to taking the test. A score of seven or more denotes pathological sleepiness.

Pittsburgh Sleep Quality Index

This is a 19-item, self-rated questionnaire that has special utility in older adults across all health care settings. Seven "component" scores are generated in subjective sleep quality, sleep latency, sleep duration, habitual sleep efficiency, sleep disturbances, use of sleeping medications, and daytime dysfunction. A global score of greater than five has a diagnostic sensitivity of 89.6% and specificity of 86.5% from the standpoint of distinguishing good sleepers from poor sleepers (14). The test can be used for baseline and longitudinal follow-up of a cohort. The Pittsburgh sleep quality index (PSQI) has good internal consistency and a reliability coefficient of 0.83 (Cronbach).

Children's Sleep Habits Questionnaire

This is a validated 45-item, parent questionnaire in which daytime sleepiness is included as one of eight domains (15). The questionnaire was validated in a sample of 469 children of 4 to 10 years of age. Items are rated on a three-point scale: usually, sometimes, and rarely. The higher the score, the more disturbed the sleep.

OBJECTIVE ASSESSMENT

Actigraphy

The actigraph measures linear acceleration and translates physical motion into a numeric representation, which is sampled frequently, e.g., every 0.1 second, and is aggregated at a constant interval or epoch, to be then displayed graphically. The actigraph is generally attached to the left (nondominant) wrist. Muscle activity is frequent during wakefulness and infrequent during sleep. To draw valid conclusions, data should be recorded for one to three weeks at a time and matched with simultaneously maintained logs of sleep-wake function. Visual inspection of the raw actigraphy data is recommended. On the basis of the presence or absence of muscle activity, one can determine whether an individual is awake or asleep at a given time. When combined with the sleep logs, the total time in bed, total sleep time, sleep efficiency, sleep onset time, and awakening time can be reliably estimated (16). There is good correlation with polysomnogram-based scoring of sleep and wakefulness; a trained actigraph scorer can distinguish sleep from wakefulness with 91% to 93% accuracy in adults (ages 20–30 years) and 91.4% to 96.5% accuracy in adolescents [ages 10–16 years (17)]. The level of agreement may diminish as sleep becomes more fragmented because of intrinsic sleep disorders. Wrist actigraphy is a useful adjunct in the assessment of insomnia, circadian rhythm sleep disorders, daytime sleepiness, and restless legs syndrome/periodic limb movement disorder as it provides longitudinal, qualitative, and semiquantitative information about sleep-wake function in the home environment. It also has utility in measuring the outcome in intervention trials of sleep disorders of children and adults. One limitation is not being able to distinguish wakefulness from sleep if the patient is lying quietly awake in bed without movement; another limitation is that actigraphy is also unable to distinguish sleep stages.

Overnight Oximetry

Overnight oximetry analysis is a screening tool for sleep-disordered breathing (18), a frequent cause of daytime sleepiness. Oximetry data must be visually inspected and interpreted by clinicians knowledgeable in distinguishing artifact from the "saw-toothed" (cyclical) oscillations in the oxyhemoglobin saturation that are caused by apneas/hypopneas. Gries and Brooks, in a normative study of 350 healthy subjects (19), noted a mean overnight oxygen saturation (sat 50) of 96.5%, with values decreasing slightly with age. The sat 50 ranged from 96.8% in the 1- to 10-year age group to 95.1 in subjects over age 60. It was not influenced by age, gender, or ethnicity. The mean value of the lowest overnight oxygen saturation in healthy subjects is 90.4%. There is no difference in saturation values obtained from applying the sensors over the ear or the finger tip, but recorded values may be lower from that over the toes. The sensitivity and specificity of oximetry in the diagnosis of OSA are dependent on its severity—in a study of 41 subjects with suspected OSA, Cooper et al. found that for those with apnea-hypopnea index (AHI) > 25, the sensitivity was 100% and specificity was 95% (20). When the AHI was >15, the sensitivity and specificity fell to 75% and 86%, respectively, and when the AHI was >5, the sensitivity and specificity dropped to 60% and 80%, respectively. A normal overnight oximetry essentially excludes moderate/severe obstructive sleep apnea-hypopnea syndrome (OSAHS) but does not exclude mild OSA or upper airway resistance syndrome (UARS), nor does it rule out etiologies of sleepiness that are unrelated to sleep-disordered breathing. In a study of 250 Irish patients, Deegan and McNicholas (21) were able to establish a diagnosis of OSA on the basis of patient history and oximetry in a third of the patients, thus highlighting the value of overnight oximetry, a diagnostic tool in sleepiness related to sleep-disordered breathing. In a study of 995 third-grade students from Germany, Urschitz et al. (22) found that an oxygen saturation nadir below 90% (from presumed OSA) was associated with a significantly higher likelihood of impairment of scores in mathematics (odds ratio 2.28).

Nocturnal Polysomnography

The definitive test for a sleep-related breathing disturbance is attended nocturnal polysomnography (PSG). Clinical assessment by a sleep specialist prior to the PSG is recommended to optimally tailor the study to the clinical question.

PSG is routinely indicated in diagnosing OSA, hypoventilation syndromes, central sleep apnea, and suspected Cheyne–Stokes breathing (23). Patients with systolic or diastolic heart failure or those with coronary artery disease with symptoms of sleep-disordered breathing also need nocturnal PSG. There are also a number of other disorders with sleep-related breathing disturbances in which PSG provides additional clinical perspective and assistance in management, but it is not essential for diagnosis of such disorders. These include chronic obstructive pulmonary disease, asthma, cystic fibrosis, myopathies like myotonic dystrophy, as well as amyotrophic lateral sclerosis and poliomyelitis.

PSG is also indicated for determining optimal continuous positive airway pressure (CPAP) settings in patients with confirmed OSA—generally when the baseline PSG shows a respiratory disturbance index (RDI) > 15 per hour, or RDI of >5 with presence of excessive daytime sleepiness. Follow-up PSG may be indicated during long-term follow-up if there is a greater than 10% weight gain or weight loss and CPAP seems to be losing effectiveness (23). Traditionally, a full-night diagnostic polysomnogram has been performed for the evaluation of sleep-related breathing disorders, followed, if necessary, by a full-night titration of CPAP or bi-level positive airway pressure breathing (BPAP). Because PSG is expensive and inconvenient, alternatives continue to be sought. One validated modification is split-night PSG, which combines an initial diagnostic segment with a latter-half CPAP titration during the same night—the first half serves as baseline or the diagnostic segment, while the second half is for titrating CPAP to an optimum level (24). The initial diagnostic segment needs to be at least 120 minutes long and should include rapid eye movement (REM) sleep in the supine position. The CPAP titration segment should be at least 180 minutes in duration, with documentation of elimination/near elimination of sleep-disordered breathing by adjustments in positive airway pressure levels.

In the investigation of disorders leading to daytime sleepiness such as narcolepsy, idiopathic hypersomnia, and periodic hypersomnia (Kleine–Levin syndrome), the nocturnal polysomnogram is helpful in excluding disorders such as OSA that may lead to daytime sleepiness. Patients with narcolepsy may exhibit a sleep onset REM period (SOREMP), which is defined as REM sleep within 15 minutes of sleep onset. Others may show a short nocturnal REM latency of <70 minutes. During the symptomatic phase, patients with periodic hypersomnia may show decreased sleep efficiency, decreased slow-wave sleep, and a shortened initial REM latency.

PSG is also helpful in the investigation of nocturnal spells. This includes nocturnal seizures as well as REM and non-REM (NREM) sleep parasomnias. The hypermotor clinical semiology of the nocturnal frontal lobe may mimic parasomnias such as sleep terrors. An expanded, 16-channel electroencephalographic montage with synchronized digital video monitoring should be utilized when evaluating a patient with nocturnal spells. During the record review process, the electroencephalogram (EEG) tracing should be observed at a slow speed of 10 mm/sec to detect epileptiform transients like spikes and sharp waves that may otherwise appear compressed and difficult to visualize at the traditional paper speed of 30 mm/sec.

The EEG, eye movements, chin and leg electromyogram (EMG), electrocardiogram (ECG), oxygen saturation, snoring intensity, nasal pressure/nasal airflow, and thoracic and abdominal respiratory effort are monitored simultaneously. Esophageal pressure monitoring, though a reliable tool in suspected UARS, is somewhat invasive and, for the most part, has been supplanted by nasal pressure transducers. End-tidal CO_2 measurements are useful in children with suspected hypoventilation related to obesity, neuromuscular disorders, Down syndrome, and Prader–Willi syndrome. Approximately 10% of patients with an AHI < 5 during the first night will have an AHI $\geq$ 5 during a second polysomnogram. Therefore, if clinical suspicion is high, a second polysomnogram may be indicated if the first study is negative. For most patients, however, a single night's recording provides sufficient information.

While standard polysomnographic measurements like an elevated AHI and obstructive apnea index predict daytime sleepiness, the study of respiratory cycle–related electro-encephalographic changes may be an additional measure of sleep fragmentation (25).

Multiple Sleep Latency Test

When used in conjunction with sleep history, examination, and nocturnal PSG, the MSLT is the "gold standard" for the assessment of daytime sleepiness in adults and children (26). The strengths of the test lie in its intuitive design (sleepy individuals are more likely to fall asleep than those who are not sleepy), its reliability, and the availability of normative data across various ages. It has also been validated in conditions such as sleep loss, sleep disruption, and hypnotic and alcohol use (27). One major indication for the MSLT is suspected narcolepsy or idiopathic hypersomnia. For the MSLT to be valid, the procedure must have a polysomnogram performed the night before, which helps to exclude disorders such as OSA and periodic limb movement disorder, which may also be associated with daytime sleepiness. The lower age limit till which one can apply the MSLT seems to be around six years—physiological daytime napping can occur up to the age of five years. The adult normal values were established from a sample of 13 subjects (mean age 35.5 years $\pm$ 10.3 years, 9/13 female). As far as possible, the total sleep time on the PSG must approximate that observed at home. Wrist actigraphy obtained over one to two weeks prior to the MSLT helps ensure that the patient has received adequate sleep at night on a regular basis. All medications that impact sleep such as benzodiazepines, psychostimulants, antidepressants, and barbiturates must be stopped at least two weeks prior to the MSLT. Drugs with very long half-lives such as fluoxetine need to be discontinued for three to four weeks owing to their enduring tendency for suppressing REM sleep. Since sleep latency in children and adolescents is very closely linked to the Tanner stage of sexual development, physical examination to evaluate the stage of sexual maturation is important.

The MSLT is commenced 1.5 to 3 hours after the final morning awakening. At least six hours of sleep must have been recorded on the nocturnal polysomnogram if the MSLT is being conducted to rule out narcolepsy. The patient is dressed in street clothes. The test consists of the provision of five nap opportunities at two hourly intervals, e.g., 0900 hours, 1100 hours, 1300 hours, 1500 hours, and 1700 hours. Central and occipital EEG (C3-O1, C4-O2), eye movements (right outer canthus to left outer canthus), and chin EMG need to be recorded. One of the eye movement sensors is placed slightly above the outer canthus, and the other slightly below the outer canthus. This arrangement facilitates capture of both horizontal and vertical eye movements. The time constant for the electrooculogram (EOG) should be long enough to allow for the recording of slow rolling eye movements that typically herald the onset of NREM sleep. Baseline biocalibration signals are recorded prior to commencing each trial. At the designated hour, lights are turned off, the patient is advised to relax, close the eyes, and try to fall asleep while the electrophysiological parameters are being monitored. If no sleep occurs, the nap opportunity is terminated 20 minutes following "lights out," and the patient is designated as having a sleep latency of 20 minutes (the maximum). If the patient falls asleep, the test is continued for 15 minutes after sleep onset. Sleep is scored in 30-second epochs. The time interval between "lights out" and electroencephalographic sleep onset is designated the sleep latency. A mean of the sleep latency (MSL) is derived from averaging the sleep latency of the five nap opportunities. Reference values for the MSL at various ages are listed in Table 3. If clinically indicated, a urine drug screen may be obtained in between the MSLT nap opportunities to exclude the possibility of drug-induced sleepiness.

Besides serving as an objective measure of sleep propensity, the MSLT also helps in determining whether the transition from wakefulness is into NREM or REM sleep. A SOREMP is defined as the occurrence of REM sleep within 15 minutes of sleep onset. About 80% of patients with narcolepsy show two or more SOREMPs during the MSLT. False positives may occur in patients with severe OSA who have suppression of nocturnal REM sleep with a consequent daytime REM sleep rebound. False negatives may occur in the early stages of evolution of narcolepsy in childhood when the patient may manifest daytime sleepiness but

Table 3 Age-Specific Normal Values for the Multiple Sleep Latency Test

Age/Tanner	Mean sleep latency (time in minutes)	Standard Deviation (minutes)
Stage of sexual development		
Tanner stage 1	18.8	1.8
Tanner stage 2	18.3	2.1
Tanner stage 3	16.5	2.8
Tanner stage 4	15.5	3.3
Tanner stage 5	16.2	1.5
Older adolescents	15.8	3.5
Adults	13.3	4.3

Data for children and adolescents adapted from the first night of three successive nocturnal polysomnographic recordings.
Source: Adapted from Ref. 28.

not the requisite two or more SOREMPs (29). The diagnostic sensitivity of the MSLT for the diagnosis of narcolepsy has been estimated around 61%, while the diagnostic specificity when two or more SOREMPs are present is around 94%. If the presence of two or more SOREMPs is combined with a MSL <5 minutes, then the diagnostic specificity rises to 97%. Similar data are unavailable in the pediatric population.

The MSLT has high test-retest reliability when conducted in normal healthy adult subjects who have been studied over a 4- to 14-month period (0.97), and also shows good inter-scorer reliability. One drawback is that the MSL in preadolescent children may actually be over 20 minutes, and the artificial truncation of the nap opportunity at 20 minutes may limit adequate assessment of the sleep propensity in this age group. Another limitation of the MSLT is its "floor" effect—e.g., in pathologically sleepy subjects with MSL <5 minutes, it cannot help determine whether an individual with a MSL of 2 minutes is somehow different from an individual with MSL of 1 minute. The normal values for the MSLT were derived from the study of healthy, sleep-deprived subjects, thus, its application to subjects with sleep disorders also poses limitations—we do not know whether sleepiness resulting from sleep deprivation and that due to sleep disorders are qualitatively identical. The MSLT can control for environmental variables such as light, ambient temperature, and noise, but it cannot control for internal psychological factors like motivation and anxiety that might also impact sleep latency.

Maintenance of Wakefulness Test

This test is a mirror image opposite of the MSLT (26). It is a test of daytime alertness and measures the ability to stay awake during the daytime in a darkened, quiet environment. Electrodes are applied for monitoring the EEG, eye movements, and chin EMG in a manner identical to the MSLT. The patient is provided four opportunities to stay awake in a darkened, quiet room at two hourly intervals, starting at 1.5 to 3 hours after the final morning awakening. The patient sits in street clothes and is advised to "sit still and remain awake for as long as possible." Sleep is scored in 30-second epochs. Each trial ends after 40 minutes if no sleep occurs or after three epochs of unequivocal sleep. The latter is defined as three consecutive epochs of stage 1 sleep or one epoch of any other sleep stage. As in the MSLT, patients undergoing the MWT show their shortest MSL around 1300 hours. The physiological MSL on the MWT is 30.4 ± 11.2 minutes. The upper limit of the 95% confidence interval is 40 minutes. Using 20-minute MWT trials, Mitler et al. (29) found that subjects with narcolepsy were able to stay awake only for an average of 6 minutes as compared with 19 minutes in normal control subjects. The MWT is useful in monitoring response to therapy in daytime sleepiness when the patient is being treated with psychostimulants (narcolepsy), CPAP (OSA), and in instances where one needs to ensure adequate daytime alertness for occupational reasons (airline pilots, truck drivers, etc.). The drawback is that normative data are limited. It is unclear whether the MWT correlates reliably with alertness in the real-life day-to-day setting.

Portable Monitoring Devices

Various systems are now available that seek to improve convenience and comfort by recording only a limited number of cardiorespiratory parameters, with some of these devices designed for home use without a technologist in attendance. The proper role for these portable monitors remains a matter of significant debate. A comprehensive review of the data conducted jointly by the American Academy of Sleep Medicine, American College of Chest Physicians, and American Thoracic Society led to the conclusion that there was insufficient evidence to support the use of limited, portable monitoring devices in an *unattended* (performed in the home; no technologist present) manner for ruling in or ruling out OSAHS (30). On the other hand, *attended* (performed in the sleep laboratory; technologist present) use may be a whole-night, diagnostic option, provided the data are manually reviewed by qualified personnel, applied to patients without significant comorbid conditions, and not used for titration of CPAP. The Center for Medicare presently mandates that for CPAP reimbursement purposes, the diagnosis of OSA must be established by a facility-based polysomnogram, not in the home or mobile facility. In instances where there is a high pretest probability of finding OSA, a limited channel, attended cardiorespiratory study that monitors airflow/nasal pressure, respiratory effort, ECG, and oxygen saturation may suffice. Current recommendations do not support the use of unattended sleep recording for diagnosing OSA.

OTHER SCREENING OR ADJUNCTIVE TOOLS

Sleep specialists remain challenged in developing ambulatory diagnostic tools that are sensitive, valid, and reliable measures of impairment in performance due to sleepiness (Table 4). Practice effect from repeated measurements, impact of time of the day on performance, internal motivation of the subject, and length and nature of the task (novel, or dull and boring) also impact performance on these tasks. The psychomotor vigilance test (PVT) developed by Dinges and Powell (31,32) and standard deviation on lane position during the Systems Technology, Inc. (sti-sim) driving simulator test seem to have the greatest effect size (33,34) and clinical applicability.

The PVT was developed in 1985 as a measure of sustained attention. It has subsequently been found to be sensitive to the effects of sleepiness in the clinical arena. The PVT is presented on a computer screen as a series of random images of white dots that appear sequentially on a black screen. They are seen only for a short period of time, e.g., 50 milliseconds. The subject is asked to press a button as fast as possible whenever the object appears on the screen. The interstimulus interval is random. The mean reaction time is a measure of motor speed and is calculated from the number of correct responses. The entire test takes about 20 minutes. Performance accuracy is surmised from the number of lapses. On functional magnetic resonance imaging, fast reaction times on the PVT correlate with activation of the frontoparietal cortex (right middle frontal gyrus, right inferior parietal lobe, and left inferior parietal lobe) (32). Handheld computer versions of some PVT tests are also available now. Of the various test instruments available, PVT is the most sensitive to sleep restriction, the most reliable, and the least subject to practice effect upon repeat testing.

Spectral analysis of the EEG alpha, theta, and delta power density combined with the recording of slow rolling eye movements (heralding the onset of stage 1 NREM sleep) also correlates with sleepiness as measured on visual vigilance test. Torsvall and Akerstedt have found that just prior to dozing off, healthy subjects show an increase in the slow eye movements and EEG power in the delta and theta range (35).

Table 4 Outcome Measures and Their Sensitivity to Sleep Restriction

Outcome measure	Sensitivity index	Significant
Sleep latency	0.961	Yes
PVT—speed	0.954	Yes
Sti-sim lane deviation	0.591	Yes
10-choice reaction time—speed	0.510	Yes
Sti-sim lane position	0.502	Yes
Wilkinson 4-choice reaction time—speed	0.496	Yes
Stanford sleepiness scale	0.482	Yes
Serial addition, subtraction—speed	0.467	Yes
10-choice reaction time—percent correct	0.425	Yes
Saccadic velocity, FIT	0.328	No
Syn work	0.314	No
Sti-sim—number of accidents	0.280	No
Stroop color naming—speed	0.271	No
Stroop color naming—percent correct	0.252	No
Serial addition, subtraction—percent correct	0.246	No
Time estimation	0.235	No
Wilkinson 4-choice reaction time—percent correct	0.231	No
Latency to pupil constriction—FIT	0.229	No
Running memory—percent correct	0.210	No
Code substitution—speed	0.177	No
Running memory—speed	0.166	No
Logical reasoning—percent correct	0.164	No
Initial pupil diameter—FIT	0.139	No
Amplitude of pupil constriction—FIT	0.101	No
Logical reasoning—speed	0.074	No

Sensitivity index is the ratio of effect size to the confidence interval range.
A "yes" in the "significant" column indicates that the effect size for the corresponding measure was significantly greater than zero ($p < 0.05$).
Abbreviations: FIT, fitness impairment tester; PVT, psychomotor vigilance test.
Source: Adapted from Ref. 33.

NEW DIAGNOSTIC TOOLS

Pulse Transit Time

Nasal pressure transducers are semiquantitative and capable of detecting a greater number of respiratory events than nasal thermistors. The diagnostic yield of even the nasal pressure transducers is however limited in children owing to the tendency of children with sleep-disordered breathing to sleep with the mouth held partially open. Additionally, some arousals are mediated at subcortical rather than cortical levels, manifesting only as K-complexes or transient acceleration of the heart rate. These subcortical arousals correlate with abrupt reductions in the pulse transit time (PTT), which is defined as the time taken by the arterial pressure wave to travel from the aortic valve to the periphery. It is recorded as the time delay between the R wave of the ECG and the arrival of the corresponding pulse at the finger (Fig. 1). The value is approximately 200 to 300 milliseconds. Arousals, whether cortical or subcortical, are associated with increased blood pressure and heart rate and thus a transient reduction in the PTT. For both adults and children, the assessment of PTT increases the diagnostic yield of PSG (36,37).

Cyclic Alternating Patterns

Cyclic alternating pattern (CAP) is a periodic EEG pattern seen during NREM sleep that is characterized by sequences of transient electrocortical events that are distinct from the background EEG activity and recur at up to one-minute intervals (Fig. 2) (38,39). CAPs correlate with sleep instability, sleep disturbance, or both. They may be seen during stages 1, 2, 3, or 4 of NREM sleep. Each CAP sequence is composed of two phases—A and B. Each phase is of two

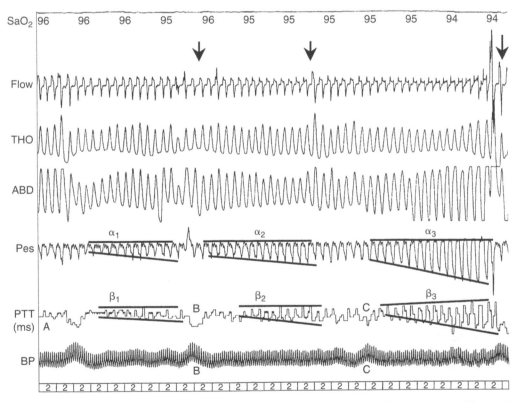

Figure 1 Example of how pulse transit time can enhance the recognition of microarousals. The respiratory events correspond to obstructive hypopneas ended by cortical microarousals (*arrows*). This figure demonstrates SaO$_2$, thoracic (THO) and abdominal (ABD) inductance plethysmography, Pes, PTT, and BP using a Finapres. Notice the progressive increase in negative Pes from obstructive apnea terminates with an abrupt increase in BP, a arousal (*arrow*), and a corresponding, transient decrease in PTT (*arrowhead*). *Abbreviations*: Pes, esophageal pressure; PTT, pulse transit time; BP, blood pressure; EMG, electromyogram; ECG, electrocardiogram. *Source*: Adapted from: Ref. 37.

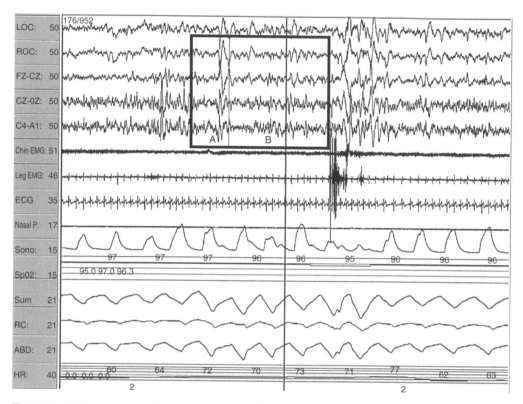

Figure 2 CAP shown on a bipolar montage. The high-voltage repetitive elements constitute phase A of CAP, whereas the intervening lower-amplitude periods constitute phase B. The combination of one phase A and one phase B is termed a CAP cycle. *Abbreviations*: ABD, abdominal inductance plethysmogram; C4-A1, right central–left mastoid electroencephalogram; CAP, cyclic alternating pattern; Cz-Oz, midline central–occipital electroencephalogram; Fz-Cz, midline frontal–midline central electroencephalogram; HR, heart rate; LOC, left outer canthus; Nasal P, nasal pressure; RC, chest inductance plethysmogram; ROC, right outer canthus; Sono, snore channel.

seconds or more in duration. The A phase is composed of high-amplitude transients that may include K-complexes, high-amplitude delta, polyphasic bursts of delta and theta, vertex sharp transients, or K-alpha complexes. The key is that the A phase stands out from the background. The B phase is the intervening, lower-amplitude background that separates two A phases, and may be 2 to 60 seconds long. CAP sequences are a series of CAPs put together. The significance of CAPs is that A phases are associated with cortical, autonomic, and motor activation and thus represent arousal or prearousal phenomena. Correlation of CAPs with daytime sleepiness has not yet been established, but is a fertile area for research. In patients with OSA, the presence of excessive CAPs may serve as a marker of unstable flow and help guide CPAP titration (40).

Yet another method appears to be quantifying cycle-related electroencephalographic changes (25). A comparison of the practical utility, sensitivity, and specificity of PTT, CAP, and respiratory cycle–related EEG changes in the adults and children has not yet been done.

Hypocretin Assay

Hypocretin is a peptide secreted by the dorsolateral hypothalamus. The hypocretin-secreting neurons have widespread projections to the ventral forebrain and the brainstem, and enhance alertness as well as locomotor activity, together with suppression of appetite. Autopsy of patients with narcolepsy has shown marked reduction in hypocretin neurons in the region of the dorsolateral hypothalamus (41). The downregulation of hypocretin secretion is thus a key finding in patients with narcolepsy. Nishino et al. have shown that patients with narcolepsy show reduced cerebrospinal fluid (CSF) levels of hypocretin-1, i.e., below 100 pg/mL, with healthy controls showing mean levels of 280.3 ± 33 pg/mL and controls with other neurological disorders showing mean levels of 260.5 ± 37 pg/mL (42). The reduction in CSF hypocretin-1 is seen specifically in subjects with narcolepsy-cataplexy, and not in narcolepsy without cataplexy or in idiopathic hypersomnia. The assay is most useful in patients with suspected narcolepsy-cataplexy who are already being treated with psychopharmacological agents such as methylphenidate or fluoxetine that cannot be safely discontinued for diagnostic PSG and MSLT. In narcolepsy-cataplexy patients who are positive for the HLA DQB1*0602 haplotype, the diagnostic sensitivity of low CSF hypocretin is 94% (42).

ADDENDUM

The Pediatric Daytime Sleepiness Scale is a useful, eight-item questionnaire that has been validated in 11- to 15-year-olds (43). Each item is scored on a 0–4 point scale. The mean score is 15.3, +/− 6.2. The Cleveland Adolescent Sleepiness Questionnaire is another useful tool that has been validated in 11- to 17-year-old subjects (44). It is a 16-item scale, with responses to each item being rated on a 1–5 scale.

CONCLUSIONS

A comprehensive sleep history and physical examination are the first step in the clinical evaluation and management of a patient with daytime sleepiness. Subjective assessment tools such as the ESS, SSS, Karolinska sleepiness scale, PSQI, and the children's sleep habits questionnaire serve as instruments to guide the clinician in evaluating the patient's sleep and/or level of daytime sleepiness. Actigraphy, overnight oximetry, nocturnal PSG, MSLT, MWT, and portable monitoring devices provide the clinician with objective measures to identify sleep-wake patterns or sleep disorders and/or document levels of daytime sleepiness. Other tools such as the PVT, pulse transit time, CAP, and hypocretin assays further assist the clinician in his or her diagnosis and management of sleep disorders.

REFERENCES

1. Bliwise DL. Is the measurement of sleepiness the holy grail of sleep medicine? Am J Res Crit Care Med 2001; 163:1517–1519.
2. Kim H, Young T. Subjective daytime sleepiness: dimensions and correlates in the general population. Sleep 2005; 28(5):625–634.
3. Galosh N, Kesler A, Vainstein G, et al. Clinical and polysomnographic characteristics of 34 patients with Kleine Levin syndrome. J Sleep Res 2001; 10:337–341.
4. Johns MW. A new method for measuring daytime sleepiness: the Epworth sleepiness scale. Sleep 1991; 14:540–545.
5. Johns M, Hocking B. Daytime sleepiness and sleep habits of Australian workers. Sleep 1997; 20:844–849.
6. Johns MW. Reliability and factor analysis of the Epworth sleepiness scale. Sleep 1992; 15:376–381.
7. Johns MW. Daytime sleepiness, snoring, and obstructive sleep apnea. The Epworth sleepiness scale. Chest 1993; 103:30–36.
8. Johns MW. Sleepiness in different situations measured by the Epworth Sleepiness Scale. Sleep 1994; 17:703–710.
9. Hoddes EDW, Zarcone V. The development and use of the Stanford Sleepiness Scale. Psychophysiology 1972; 9:150.
10. Maclean AW, Fekken CG, Saskin P, et al. Psychometric evaluation of the Stanford Sleepiness Scale. J Sleep Res 1992; 1:35–39.
11. Surridge-David M, Maclean AW, Coulter M, et al. Mood changes following an acute delay of sleep. Psychiatry Res 22:149–158.
12. Broughton R. Performance and evoked potential measures of various states of daytime sleepiness. Sleep 1982; 5:S135–S146.
13. Akerstedt T, Gillberg M. Subjective and objective sleepiness in the active individual. Int J Neurosci 1990; 52:29–37.
14. Buysse DJ, Reynolds CF III, Monk TH, et al. The Pittsburgh Sleep Quality Index: a new instrument for psychiatric practice and research. Psychiatry Res 1989; 28(2):193–213.
15. Owens JA, Spirito A, McGuinn M. The Children's Sleep Habits Questionnaire(CSHQ): psychometric properties of a survey instrument for school-aged children. Sleep 2000; 23(8):1.

16. Littner M, Kushida CA, Anderson WM, et al. Practice parameters for the role of actigraphy in the study of sleep and circadian rhythms: an update for 2002. Sleep 2003; 26(3):337–341.

17. Sadeh A, Sharkey KM, Carskadon MA. Activity based sleep-wake identification. An empirical test and methodological issues. Sleep 1994; 17:201–207.

18. Netzer N, Eliasson AH, Netzer C, et al. Overnight pulse oximetry for sleep disordered breathing in adults. Chest 2001; 120:625–633.

19. Gries RE, Brooks LJ. Normal oxyhemoglobin saturation during sleep. Chest 1996; 110:1489–1492.

20. Cooper BG, Veale D, Griffiths CJ, et al. Values of nocturnal oxygen saturation as a screening test for sleep apnea. Thorax 1991; 46(8):586–588.

21. Deegan PC, McNicholas WT. Predictive value of clinical features for the diagnosis of obstructive sleep apnea. Eur Respir J 1996; 9:117–224.

22. Urschitz MS, Wolff J, Sokollik C, et al. Nocturnal arterial oxygen saturation and academic performance in a community sample of children. Pediatrics 2005; 115:e204–e209.

23. Kushida CA, Littner MR, Morgenthaler T, et al. Practice parameters for the indications for polysomnography and related procedures: an update for 2005. Sleep 2005; 28(4):499–521.

24. Kushida CA, Littner MR, Hirschkowitz M, et al. Practice parameters for the use of continuous and bi-level positive airway pressure devices to treat adult patients with sleep related breathing disturbances. Sleep 2006; 29(3):375–380.

25. Chervin RD, Weatherly RA, Ruzicka DL, et al. Subjective sleepiness polysomnographic correlates in children scheduled for adenotonsillectomy vs. other surgical care. Sleep 2006; 29:495–503.

26. Littner MR, Kushida C, Wise M, et al. Practice parameters for the clinical use of the multiple sleep latency test and the maintenance of wakefulness test. Sleep 2005; 1 28(1):113–121.

27. Kotagal S, Goulding P. The laboratory assessment of daytime sleepiness. J Clin Neurophysiol 1996; 13(3):208–218.

28. Carskadon MA. The second decade. In: Guilleminault C, ed. Sleeping and Waking Disorders. Indications and Techniques. Menlo Park: Addison Wrsley, 1982:99–125.

29. Mitler MM, Gujavarty KS, Browman CP. Maintenance of wakefulness test: a polysomnographic technique for evaluation and treatment efficacy in patients with excessive somnolence. Electro-encephalogr Clin Neurophysiol 1982; 53(6):658–661.

30. Chesson AL, Barry RB, Pack A. American Academy of Sleep Medicine, American Thoracic Society, American College of Chest Physicians. Practice parameters for the use of portable monitoring devices in the investigation of suspected obstructive sleep apnea in adults. Sleep 2003; 26(7):907–913.

31. Dinges DF, Powell JW. Microcomputer analyses of performance on a portable, simple visual RT task during sustained operations. Beh Res Meth Instr Com 1985; 17:652–655.

32. Drummond SPA, Bischoff-Grethe A, Dinges DF, et al. The neural basis of the psychomotor vigilance task. Sleep 2005; 28:1059–1068.

33. Balkin TJ, Bliese PD, Belenky G, et al. Comparative utility of instruments for monitoring sleepiness-related performance decrements in the operational environment. J Sleep Res 2004; 13:219–227.

34. Balkin T, Thorne D, Sing H, et al. Effects of sleep schedules on commercial driver performance. Report No. DOT-MC-00-133. Washington, D.C.: U.S. Department of Transportation, Federal Motor Carrier Safety Administration, 2000.

35. Torsvall L, Akerstedt T. Extreme sleepiness: quantification of EOG and spectral EEG parameters. Int J Neurosci 1988; 38(3–4):435–419.

36. Pitson DJ, Stradling JR. Autonomic markers of arousal during sleep in patients undergoing investigation for obstructive sleep apnea, their relationship to EEG arousal, respiratory events and subjective sleepiness. J Sleep Res 1998; 7:53–59.

37. Pepin J-L, Delavie N, Pin I, et al. Pulse transit time improves detection of sleep respiratory events and microarousals in children. Chest 2005; 127:722–730.

38. Parrino L, Halasz P, Tassinari CA, et al. CAP, epilepsy and motor events during sleep: the unifying role of arousal. Sleep Med Rev 2006; 10:267–285.

39. Terzano MG, Parrino L, Sherieri L, et al. Atlas, rules, and recording techniques for the scoring of cyclic alternating pattern (CAP) in human sleep. Sleep Med 2001; 2(6):537–553.

40. Thomas RJ. Cyclic alternating pattern and positive airway pressure titration. Sleep Med 2002; 3: 315–322.

41. Thannickal TC, Moore RY, Nienhuis R, et al. Reduced number of hypocretin neurons in human narcolepsy. Neuron 2000; 27:469–474.

42. Nishino N, Ripley B, Overeem S, et al. Low cerebrospinal fluid hypocretin (orexin) and altered energy homeostasis in human narcolepsy. Ann Neurol 2001; 50:381–388.

43. Drake C, Nickel C, Burduvali E, et al. The pediatric daytime sleepiness scale (PDSS): sleep habits and school outcomes in middle school children. Sleep 2003; 26(4):455–458.

44. Spilsbury JC, Drotar D, Rosen CL, et al. The Cleveland Adolescent Sleepiness Questionnaire: a new measure to assess excessive daytime sleepiness in adolescents. J Clin Sleep Med 2007; 3(6):603–612.

22 | Diagnostic Algorithm for Hypersomnias

Yves Dauvilliers

Service de Neurologie, Hôpital Gui-de-Chauliac and INSERM U888, Montpellier, France

INTRODUCTION

Sleep disorders are common in the general population, and a complaint of excessive daytime sleepiness (EDS) is one of the primary symptoms of these disorders. Sleepiness, defined as the propensity to enter in sleep, is a normal behavioral and physiological state after a prolonged wakefulness period. In contrast, EDS is pathological and defined as the propensity to fall asleep at inappropriate times. EDS is a common symptom in the general population but still often insufficiently recognized. In our modern society, consequences of EDS may be important causing an alteration in the quality of life, an impairment in work performance, and also increasing the risk of accidents at work or while driving (1–4).

Chronic hypersomnia is defined by a constant complaint of EDS, which occurs everyday for at least three months. Hypersomnia syndromes affect 5% to 15% of individuals, with a higher prevalence for men in relation to sleep apnoea syndromes (5,6). Although poor nocturnal sleep could be suspected as an etiology of hypersomnia, EDS is frequently the cardinal symptom of many sleep disorders as reported in the revised International Classification of Sleep Disorders (ICSD-2) (6). Considerable progress has been made in the identification of different types of hypersomnia in the last few years; however, a tendency to overdiagnose sleep-related breathing disorders in patients with EDS still persist. Physicians dispose of several methods to affirm the existence of daytime somnolence and to diagnose in between the different causes of hypersomnia, but most of them are insufficiently recognized (7–10). The steps of the evaluation of patients with hypersomnia disorders are reviewed in this chapter, and symptoms and other features that may point to a particular diagnosis are emphasized.

CLINICAL VIGNETTE

A 13-year-old boy came to a sleep disorders center for evaluation of EDS. He presented with severe daytime somnolence impairing school performance and sports activities starting at age 11, with a progressive gradation of EDS. At age 13, he reported continuous drowsiness and daytime sleepiness without any sleep attacks. Naps were long (more than one hour), unrefreshing, and never associated with dreams. The Epworth sleepiness scale (ESS) (11) score was 23 out of a possible 24 points. Nocturnal sleep was considered normal, starting at 9:30 p.m. and ending at 7 a.m. without any experience of awakening. Morning awakening was often laborious with frequent difficulties in reacting adequately to external stimuli. However, during weekends and holidays, his night sleep was uninterrupted and prolonged till 11 a.m. with normal alertness at awakening. No abnormal change in body mass index and no particular circumstances at onset of symptoms were noted.

After intensive interview, he recalled positive experiences of rare episodes of sudden head and arms dropping while eating, or weakness of legs while walking, but never after laughter or surprise. No somesthetic, auditory, or visual hypnagogic or hypnopompic hallucinations were reported; sleep paralysis was also absent. Physical examination was unremarkable.

Clinical interview of both parents confirmed their son's severe EDS with a normal nighttime sleep but the parents could not agree about the presence of episodes of loss of muscle tone. In addition, the mother reported experiences of frequent episodes of EDS since she was 20 years old with an ESS score to date at 12 out of 24 points. She never experienced hallucinations, sleep paralysis, or cataplexy.

To objectively assess EDS and to provide clues to its etiology, a polysomnogram (PSG) followed by a multiple sleep latency test (MSLT) (12) was performed. Results revealed a relatively normal sleep at night with sleep and rapid eye movement (REM) sleep latencies at 12 and 68 minutes, respectively. Sleep efficiency was 92.4%, with 28.2% of slow wave sleep and 24.4% of REM sleep. There were 32 awakenings of more than one minute and the microarousal index was 7.8/hr. The periodic limb movement (PLM) index when awake was 8.9/hr and 10.8/hr during sleep and including only 0.7/hr of PLM associated with microarousals. The apnea-hypopnea index was 2.1/hr and mean SaO_2 was 97.7%, without any episode of desaturation below 90%. The MSLT revealed a short mean sleep latency at 3.4 minutes and three sleep-onset REM periods (SOREMPs). HLA typing was DRB1*1501, DQB1*0602.

In summary, the clinical phenotype of EDS was atypical for the diagnosis of narcolepsy mainly in the absence of short and refreshing naps, hypnagogic hallucinations, and sleep paralysis. The presence of episodes of loss of muscle tone was considered as doubtful or atypical cataplexy-like episodes due to its rarity and its absence of emotional triggering factors. Finally, the PSG followed by MSLT objectively demonstrated the presence of EDS with a mean sleep latency less than eight minutes and more than two SOREMPs that led to the final diagnosis of narcolepsy without cataplexy.

The diagnosis of narcolepsy in children is challenging because the symptoms of narcolepsy may be difficult to distinguish from those of idiopathic hypersomnia (IH) (7,8). The number and duration of daytime naps and the refreshing characteristics of sleep episodes are fairly nonspecific features that are not always easily distinguishable from narcolepsy as compared with other etiologies of chronic hypersomnia. EDS may also be characterized by behavioral problems such as hyperactivity and inattentiveness. It is also important to note that the ESS is not validated for children given that it assesses circumstances that may not yet be experienced by children. Regarding the presence of REM sleep abnormalities, the narcoleptic tetrad is not frequently found in children and cataplexy is not always easy to pinpoint. Those symptoms may also occur later in the course of the disease. Finally, the indication for the measurement of cerebrospinal fluid (CSF) hypocretin-1 level is still debated in clinical practice. In this specific case, the lumbar puncture was refused by both the patient and parents.

KEY STEPS IN THE DIAGNOSIS OF THE DISORDERS

In presence of a complaint of EDS, a clinical interview combined with questionnaires and tests is necessary to distinguish fatigue, somnolence, and vigilance impairment, to diagnose hypersomnia syndromes and to differentiate between their different etiologies.

First Step
Phenotype of EDS
The first step is to precisely determine the phenotype of the chief complaint by clinical interview with details on sleep quantity and sleep quality, including the duration and quality of the nocturnal sleep period, the number and duration of daytime naps, and the refreshing characteristics of those sleep episodes (Fig. 1). During the clinical interview, the presence of multiple pauses, slowed responses, repetitive ptosis, pupillary constriction, loss of neck extensor tone, and yawning argue for the complaint of EDS. Patients with EDS typically complain of drowsiness that interferes with daytime activities, unavoidable napping, or both, with a large variability between patients. Daytime sleepiness may occur daily, only on several consecutive days, or in an intermittent mode. When EDS occurs, it may be permanent, only during inactivity or with recurrence typically at two-hour intervals. Sleep episodes could be irresistible, of short duration, and associated with dreaming (13). The method of awakening should also be determined, whether it is spontaneous, with an alarm, or by a family member (7,8,14).

The age at onset of EDS, the existence of circumstances at its onset, and the factors that led to exacerbation or improvement also need to be reviewed (7,10,13). In cases of long-standing sleep problems, it is necessary to ask why the patient is seeking help at the present time.

Differentiating EDS and "fatigue" or "tiredness" is frequently needed for the consultation (15). EDS as previously mentioned is characterized by an urge to sleep with an

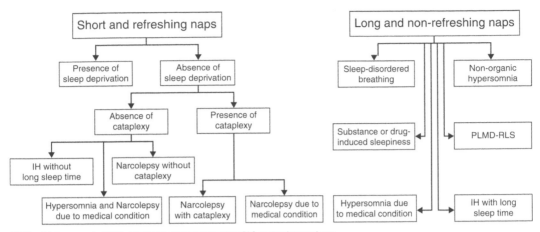

Figure 1 Clinical algorithm for chronic hypersomnia.

IH, idiopathic hypersomnia; PLMD, periodic limb movement disorders; RLS, restless legs syndrome

aggravation by rest and with possible improvement by sleep. Fatigue is also a prevalent complex phenomenon characterized by impairment in concentration and memory, lack of motivation, and an impression of low-energy; all conditions partially improved by rest. In contrast to EDS, fatigue fails to lead to rapid onset of sleep in daytime naps. As acute fatigue frequently occurs in healthy subjects under particular conditions, only chronic fatigue is considered a pathological symptom. Unfortunately, many patients and practitioners use the term "fatigue" in place of "sleepiness" to describe these two different symptoms that may also coexist.

The phenotype of EDS is of importance in term of etiologies of chronic hypersomnias. For example, except in children, the refreshing value of short naps is of significant diagnostic value for narcolepsy (10,16). In contrast, in IH with long sleep time, awakening after nighttime or daytime sleep is extremely difficult (17). Accordingly, age at onset in both narcolepsy and IH is mostly young as compared with obstructive sleep apnea and PLM disorder.

Severity of EDS
EDS can occur in various degrees. In mild sleepiness, a subject might fall asleep while reading a paper. However, sleepiness may also be characterized by episodes of irresistible sleep, sleep attacks or unconscious lapses occurring while talking, eating, or driving. Severe sleepiness may lead the patient to a significant risk for accidents and may have a major impact on performance and cognitive functions and the person's quality of life (1–4). Narcolepsy is classically reported as one of the most severe conditions of EDS.

The severity of the condition may help in differentiating the etiology of hypersomnia. Several sleep questionnaires should be used to quantify the severity of the complaint and to assess different aspects of sleepiness. All questionnaires require a correct perception by the subject of his or her own sleepiness and they do not rely on any objective parameter of sleepiness.

The ESS is the most widely used, with a score greater than 10 supporting a complaint of hypersomnia (11). This scale measure the average sleep propensity on eight soporific situations over a recent period of time. Other sleepiness scales such as the Stanford sleepiness scale (18), the Karolinska sleepiness scale (19), and visual analog scales may be used to measure the sleepiness state at a particular time. However, these latter scales are more useful for research purposes.

Associated Symptoms and Treatments
Once the main complaint is delineated, details concerning other sleep disturbances are necessary to evaluate other types of problems that are not mutually exclusive:

The presence of insomnia, abnormal movements, or behaviors during sleep or during nocturnal awakenings need to be reviewed systematically (7,8,10).

A comprehensive sleep history includes questions about the presence or absence of cataplexy, hypnagogic or hypnopompic hallucinations, sleep paralysis, and automatic behavior. Other symptoms such as snoring, nocturia, headache, discomfort of the extremities during periods of inactivity and/or repetitive nocturnal agitation need to be investigated.

A thorough characterization of the daily schedule, including the usual bedtime and estimated time to sleep onset, the number and timing of awakenings, the time of final awakening, and morning and daytime symptoms, are also required. Information regarding sleep habits and the environment may also disclose other important contributing factors. It is important to obtain detailed sleep-wake schedules with a comparison of the patient's weekday and weekend schedules. A sleep diary may be helpful to estimate the regularity of the sleep-wake schedule.

A specific interview on past medical history, family history, and social history should always be conducted.

As in other fields of medicine, other medical conditions need to be screened, and a general physical examination is essential to consider the correct diagnosis. Patients with neurological, cardiological, rheumatological, and other organ system-related disorders may note sleepiness and fatigue as a result of the disease process and/or treatment.

A psychiatric assessment is also frequently needed in cases of hypersomnia. In that context, the degree of sleep disturbances varies with the severity of the underlying illness.

Finally, current and past medication use and other substances also need to be considered.

Bed Partner Interview

The evaluation of a history from the patient's bed partner is often useful since many sleep problems are not evident to the patient or their existence is denied by the patient. Indeed, some patients may over-report their degree of sleepiness and note EDS even during periods of normal alertness, while other individuals may under-report periods of EDS. In particular cases, it could be of interest to compare sleepiness scale scores (such as the ESS) completed by the patient and the bed partner. The bed partner can also comment on the intensity of snoring, duration and frequency of apneas, and the presence of nocturnal behaviors or events.

Second Step

In cases of a clinical suspicion of hypersomnia, the condition needs to be confirmed or excluded through objective measurements. In other cases of an uncertain clinical diagnosis, differential diagnoses are proposed and polysomnographic studies are performed to arrive at a definitive diagnosis whenever it is possible.

Polysomnography Followed by a MSLT

A PSG during the night following by a MSLT is highly recommended to objectively quantify the level of daytime sleepiness. The MSLT is the most frequent objective test of sleepiness used in clinical practice. The MSLT consists of five nap opportunities, scheduled at two-hour intervals, starting 1.5 to 3 hours after awakening (12). Subjects need to discontinue psychotropic medications at least two weeks (depending on the half-life) before the date of the test. Subjects are asked to lie in a quiet, darkened and comfortable bedroom during the test and are instructed not to resist sleep. Each test is terminated after a 15-minute sleep period or after 20 minutes if the patient does not fall asleep. According to standardized guidelines, the MSLT is the best scientifically validated objective test to detect EDS in several clinical conditions but also in normal subjects under sleep restriction or sleep extension. In addition, the MSLT had a high test-retest reliability in normal subjects and also in pathological conditions (1,20).

Sleep latencies are measured with a mean sleep latency below eight minutes confirming the EDS (6) (Fig. 2). Latencies below five minutes indicate severe sleepiness (1). The MSLT is considered normal if sleep occurs after a mean sleep latency of 10 minutes. Between these two values, the interpretation should take into account the clinical status of the patient. Several normal subjects without any symptoms of EDS experienced low MSLT latencies while others

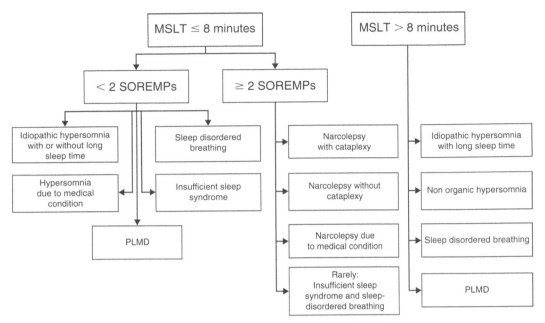

MSLT, multiple sleep latency test; SOREMPs, sleep-onset REM periods; PLMD, periodic limb movement disorder

Figure 2 Multiple sleep latency test (MSLT) algorithm for chronic hypersomnia.

with a clear complaint of EDS did not fall asleep during the MSLT. The subjective perception of sleep propensity differs from the ability to switch from wakefulness to sleep. In addition, there is a poor correlation between ESS and MSLT results (20), indicating that ESS and MSLT measure different components of sleepiness. In contrast to the MSLT performed in only one given situation that includes several alerting factors (e.g., effects of stress, temperature, light, noise), the ESS measures the mean subjective sleep propensity over a prolonged period.

A SOREMP defined as the occurrence of REM sleep within 15 minutes after sleep onset has also been evaluated, with a higher risk of being narcoleptic in the presence of at least two SOREMPs on the MSLT; these findings, however, are not highly specific or sensitive (1). Data also suggest that a 20-minute cutoff would be better especially with aging (21). Some clinicians use the 20-minute cutoff to define SOREMPs during daytime sleep but this procedure is not in accordance with guidelines. Finally, a study revealed that both men and women with SOREMPs are also frequent in the general population (22).

Polysomnography Followed by a MWT
An alternative of MSLT is the maintenance of wakefulness test (MWT) (1,23). This test objectively assesses the patient's ability to maintain wakefulness rather than the drive to fall asleep. The patient is seated comfortably in bed, with low lighting placed behind with instructions to try to stay awake. During two or four daytime 20- or 40-minute sessions depending on the protocol used, the patient is asked to stay awake as long as possible (1,23). The test ends either after 15 seconds of any stage of sleep, indicating the insufficient ability to fight against sleep. MWT results show evidence of a "ceiling effect" in subjects with normal levels of wakefulness; however, this effect is less pronounced in the 40-minute protocol. Therefore, specific recommendations include a four-trial 40-minutes MWT protocol with a mean sleep latency at 30.4 ± 11.2 min found in normal controls. Cutoffs from 12 to 19 minutes (limit of the 95% confidence interval) are considered as abnormal (1,23,24). Scores between 10 and 40 minutes are of uncertain significance. The MWT test is rarely used as a real test of sleepiness but rather to measure the effectiveness of treatment especially for research or legal purposes (in cases of driver's license suspension). The MWT provides a more sensitive indicator of variation of sleepiness and alertness than the MSLT. Both MSLT and MWT do measure degrees of sleepiness but due to a weak correlation between the results of these tests, they certainly measure different abilities (23,24). Indeed, the MSLT seems to measure physiological sleepiness in relation to the sleep drive while MWT measures alertness in relation to the wake drive.

24-hour Continuous Polysomnography
In rare circumstances, a 24-hour continuous PSG recording would be necessary to assess the degree of sleepiness. This is especially the case in IH with long sleep time. In the latter condition, the MSLT latency is longer than in narcolepsy, sometime in the normal range and may be somewhat questionable. First, it may be difficult to wake up the patient in preparation for the test or to keep the patient awake between naps; second, and of more concern, awaking the patient in the morning in view of the first MSLT session precludes documenting the abnormally prolonged night sleep, which is of major diagnostic value (8,17). In this sense it is more relevant to perform a 24-hour continuous PSG on an ad lib sleep-wake protocol to document a major sleep episode at night (more than 10 hours) and a daytime sleep episode (at least one nap of more than one hour) but this procedure still needs standardization and validation (8,17).

Third Step
In particular cases, a third step of investigation is necessary to define the etiology of hypersomnia. Although frequently used in research, all tests detailed below are not widely used in the clinical assessment of patients with hypersomnia.

Measurement of Hypocretin-1 in Cerebrospinal Fluid
As the diagnosis is generally clear in cases of narcolepsy with cataplexy, the measurement of CSF hypocretin-1 is currently reserved for specialized indications and after usual diagnostic procedures.

The indications for measurement of CSF hypocretin-1 may include the following situations (25):

The MSLT results are equivocal (e.g., a long mean sleep latency or one SOREMP on the MSLT).

Individuals are affected with severe or complex psychiatric, neurological, or medical disorders that may compromise the validity of the clinical interview (especially for cataplexy).

Individuals are already taking psychotropic medications (e.g., anticataplectics or stimulants) and are unwilling to stop these medications.

Young children (e.g., <6–8 years old) who are unable to follow MSLT instructions, but there are some limitations due to ethical issues.

Individuals (e.g., without insurance coverage) who cannot afford polysomnographic testing.

CSF hypocretin-1 levels lower than 110 pg/mL or one-third of mean normal control values are alternatively proposed as highly specific (99%) and sensitive (87–89%) for cases with clear-cut cataplexy and highly specific (99%) but not sensitive (16%) for cases with mild, atypical, or absent cataplexy, and for cases with familial or human leukocyte antigen (HLA)-negative narcolepsy (26,27).

HLA Typing
The presence of the HLA DQB1*0602 genotype in patients is only a supportive criterion for the diagnosis of narcolepsy and is no longer in the inclusion criteria for narcolepsy in the revised classification of sleep disorders (6). The diagnosis of narcolepsy is reinforced by the presence of HLA DRB1*1501-DQB1*0602 alleles, found in 80% to 95% of Caucasian narcoleptics and in only 20% of the general population (28).

Other Tests
Performance tests including the psychomotor vigilance test (PVT) and driving simulation tasks could be used to assess alertness, and to measure the neurocognitive impairment that results from EDS (29,30).

Psychomotor tasks that measure simple or complex reaction time may also be used, in which variation in scores reflect different degrees of sleepiness (31). However, these tests do not measure the sleep propensity per se, and are mostly used in research.

Cognitive evoked potential recordings may be performed in particular cases to evaluate sleep inertia upon awakening (32). Long latency cortical event-related evoked potentials were found in several conditions of hypersomnia but with a large degree of intersubject variability. However, the measurement of these evoked potentials are useful in assessing the sleep inertia in forced awakenings paradigms (33).

Brain computed tomography (CT) scan and/or magnetic resonance imaging (MRI) could be performed in cases of clinical suspicion of a hypersomnia associated with a neurological condition (7,8).

IMPORTANT DIAGNOSTIC FEATURES AND CRITERIA TO DIFFERENTIATE DISORDER TYPES

Narcolepsy with Cataplexy

Clinical Features

Daytime sleepiness. In a majority of patients with narcolepsy, EDS is the first symptom to appear, occurring mainly in childhood or in young adulthood (34). It is also the most severe symptom and the most frequent cause for consultation (16,35).

The sleep episodes characteristic of EDS are (25):

Often irresistible, despite the patient making desperate efforts to fight against sleepiness;

Usually of short duration, depending on environmental factors;

Frequently associated with dreaming;

Typically capable of restoring normal vigilance for one to several hours. The refreshing value of short naps is of significant diagnostic value, except in children who are frequently tired upon awakening (13,14).

Severe sleepiness can also lead to unconscious microsleep episodes or lapses, and to a semiautomatic continuation of behavior, such as inappropriate words in a conversation, continuing to automatically write out-of-topic or unreadable words, or driving to an inappropriate location (16,25).

Cataplexy. A history of sudden muscle weakness with buckling of the knees, laxity of the neck or jaw muscles, or complete loss of muscle tone favor the presence of cataplexy (16,35,36). However, the latter condition is triggered by emotional factors, most often by positive emotions such as laughter, repartee, good surprise and rarely by anger, but almost never by stress, fear, or physical effort (16,35). Patients remain fully conscious during the episode. Deep tendon reflexes are transiently abolished during cataplexy, while the H-reflex is absent (37).

The clinician should inquire specifically about incomplete forms of cataplexy (limited to facial muscles or to the upper or lower limbs, with dysarthria, facial flickering, jaw tremor, head dropping, dropping objects, or unlocking of the knees) since the patient does not necessarily see them as pathological (16,35,36).

The duration of cataplexy varies from a second to one or two minutes. Its frequency varies from less than one episode per year to several episodes per day. Cataplexy worsens with poor sleep and fatigue. Patients may also rarely experience "status cataplecticus" with continual cataplectic episodes, lasting several hours and confining the subject to bed (38). It can occur spontaneously but more often upon withdrawal from anticataplectic antidepressant drugs.

In most patients, cataplexy occurs within the same year as EDS, but the general course of narcolepsy varies from one subject to another. Cataplexy is specific to narcolepsy and is the best diagnostic marker for the disease.

Other symptoms of dissociated REM sleep. Episodes of partial or total paralysis at the onset or termination of sleep (sleep paralysis) and dreamlike auditory, visual, or tactile hallucinations occurring at sleep onset (hypnagogic) or upon awakening (hypnopompic) may also suggest narcolepsy. Sleep paralysis is characterized by an inability to move the limbs or the head either at sleep onset or upon awakening. Hallucinations are sometimes so scary that the subject becomes fearful of going to bed and resorts to reassuring behaviors. Sleep paralysis can be associated with hypnagogic hallucinations.

Sleep-related hallucinations and sleep paralysis are not specific for narcolepsy, present in 20% of the general population (39), but are more severe and are more frequently reported in around 50% of patients with narcolepsy (16).

Other clinical features. Several other features may be observed in narcolepsy but are of less diagnostic value.

A higher body mass index with a rapid weight gain at narcolepsy onset may be observed, especially in children (40).

A poor sleep at night and parasomnias including sleep talking and REM sleep behavior disorder are frequently observed in narcoleptic patients (41).

Depression is reported in up to 35% of cases (42,43).

Familial component: Up to 10% of narcolepsy cases are familial with several relatives affected with narcolepsy plus cataplexy. In addition, in 10% to 30% of families first or second degree relatives are affected with an attenuated phenotype characterized by isolated recurrent daytime naps and/or lapses into sleep (44,46).

Laboratory Features

Polysomnography plus MSLT. The diagnosis of narcolepsy with cataplexy is essentially clinical, but requires whenever possible a nocturnal PSG recording followed by a MSLT. The aim of the nighttime PSG is to eliminate other causes of daytime sleepiness and to assess for the presence of sufficient sleep (at least six hours) before the MSLT. In addition, the nighttime PSG may show a shortened REM sleep latency (less than 15 minutes) in 40% of cases, a fragmentation in REM sleep with imperfect loss of muscle tone, an increased percentage of non-REM (NREM) stage 1 sleep and a relative augmentation in slow wave sleep at the end of the night. PLMs are also frequent in narcoleptic patients, especially with advancing age (16).

The MSLT should document a mean sleep onset latency equal or less than eight minutes and two or more SOREMPs (6). This latter criterion may, however, be absent in elderly patients with clear-cut cataplexy (21).

CSF hypocretin-1 measurement. CSF hypocretin-1 levels lower than 110 pg/mL or one-third of mean normal control values are alternatively proposed as a highly specific (and definite) and sensitive criteria in sporadic cases with clear-cut cataplexy and positive HLA DQB1*0602.

HLA typing. The presence of the HLA DRB1*1501-DQB1*0602 alleles, found in 80% to 95% of Caucasian narcoleptics and only 20% of the general population, is only a supportive criterion (28). Those alleles are neither necessary, nor sufficient for the development of the disease, especially in the cases of familial narcolepsy. As in other HLA-associated disorders, associations are complex and the HLA DQB1*0301 allele was also found to increase susceptibility to narcolepsy whereas DQB1*0601 allele appears protective; these effects are nevertheless far weaker than those of DQB1*0602 (28).

Diagnostic criteria for narcolepsy with cataplexy
  A. Complaint of EDS occurring almost daily for at least three months (6).
  B. Definite history of cataplexy, defined as sudden and transient (less than two minutes) episodes of loss of muscle tone, generally bilateral, triggered by emotions (most reliably laughing and joking) with preserved consciousness.
  C. Diagnosis should, whenever possible, be confirmed by nocturnal polysomnography (with a minimum of six hours slept) followed by a day-time multiple sleep latency tests: Mean daytime sleep latency is less or equal to eight minutes and two or more sleep onset in REM periods. Alternatively, hypocretin-1 levels in the CSF are less or equal to 110 pg/mL, or one third of mean control values.
  D. The hypersomnia is not better explained by another sleep disorder, medical or neurological disorder, mental disorder, medication use, or substance use disorder.

Narcolepsy without Cataplexy

Clinical Features

Narcolepsy without cataplexy has been described as a phenotypic variant of narcolepsy with cataplexy and is individualized as a diagnostic entity in the new ICSD-2 (6). Apart from cataplexy, the clinical diagnostic criteria are similar to that of narcolepsy with cataplexy, with frequent associated REM abnormalities such as hypnagogic hallucinations and sleep paralysis (7,8).

The prevalence of narcolepsy without cataplexy when compared with narcolepsy with cataplexy is still a subject to debate, initially considered as a ratio from 2–3 to 10, respectively (6,16); more recent data argue for a largely higher frequency in the general population (22).

Laboratory Features
PSG plus MSLT are required to ascertain the diagnosis of narcolepsy without cataplexy, reporting the presence of a mean sleep onset latency equal or less than eight minutes and two or more SOREMPs (6).

The association with HLA DQB1*0602 is weaker and the decrease in CSF hypocretin-1 level is less frequently encountered.

Diagnostic criteria for narcolepsy without cataplexy
A. Complaint of EDS occurring almost daily for at least three months (6).
B. Typical cataplexy is not present, although doubtful or atypical cataplexy-like episodes may be reported.
C. Diagnosis must be confirmed by nocturnal polysomnography (with a minimum of six hours slept) followed by a day-time multiple sleep latency tests: Mean daytime sleep latency is less or equal to eight minutes and two or more sleep onset in REM periods.
D. The hypersomnia is not better explained by another sleep disorder, medical or neurological disorder, mental disorder, medication use, or substance use disorder.

Narcolepsy due to Medical Condition
Narcolepsy can rarely occur as part of other medical conditions and in these cases are referred to as symptomatic or secondary narcolepsies (6). The medical condition produces narcolepsy in the presence or absence of cataplexy and without any effect of treatment. The MSLT is needed in most of the cases and allows the clinician to differentiate objective EDS from fatigue.

Clinical Features
The cause of narcolepsy due to medical condition is a coexisting medical or neurological disorder. The problem is to recognize the underlying condition that definitely causes narcolepsy. Rare cases of secondary cataplexy have been reported in patients with brain lesions located in the posterior hypothalamus, the mesencephalon, and the pons (47,48). Brain lesions may be caused by tumor, multiple sclerosis, encephalitis, cerebral ischemia, head trauma, and neurodegeneration (47,48). In addition, symptomatic narcolepsy without cataplexy can be observed in muscular dystrophy and rarely in Parkinson's disease and multiple system atrophy (49,50). Finally, young children suffering from the Niemann–Pick disease type C may present with symptomatic narcolepsy.

In addition to EDS with variable degrees of severity, the presence of cataplexy needs to be checked. The diagnosis could be essentially clinical in the presence of clear-cut cataplexy.

Laboratory Features
In cases with an absence of cataplexy, the diagnosis of narcolepsy must be confirmed by a PSG followed by a MSLT reporting the presence of a mean daytime sleep latency of less than or equal to eight minutes and two or more SOREMPs. Finally, the determination of hypocretin-1 levels in the CSF represents a sufficient alternative criterion for the diagnosis (6).

Diagnostic criteria for narcolepsy due to medical condition
A. Complaint of EDS occurring almost daily for at least three months (6).
B. One of the following is observed:
  i. Definite history of cataplexy, defined as sudden and transient (less than two minutes) episodes of loss of muscle tone, generally bilateral, triggered by emotions (most reliably laughing and joking) with preserved consciousness.
  ii. If cataplexy is not present or is very atypical, nocturnal polysomnography (with a minimum of six hours slept) followed by a day-time multiple sleep latency tests

must demonstrate a mean daytime sleep latency of less or equal to eight minutes with two or more sleep onset in REM periods.

    iii. Hypocretin-1 levels in the CSF are less or equal to 110 pg/mL, or one third of mean control values, provided the patient is not comatose.

C.   A significant underlying medical or neurological disorder accounts for the daytime sleepiness.

D.   The hypersomnia is not better explained by another sleep disorder, mental disorder, medication use, or substance use disorder.

Idiopathic Hypersomnia with Long Sleep Time

IH is a rare condition of EDS, approximately ten times less frequent than narcolepsy with cataplexy (6,17). IH remains a relatively poorly defined condition due to the absence of specific symptoms such as cataplexy or sleep apnea. This hypersomnia still needs clarification and new methods of investigation to make the accurate diagnosis (7,8). The age of onset varies from childhood to young adulthood (17,51,52). There is no gender predominance. Family cases are frequent, in the range from 25% to 60% without any clear mode of inheritance proposed. The psychosocial and professional consequences appear similar to those found in narcolepsy (53).

Clinical Features

Nighttime and daytime sleepiness. IH with long sleep time is characterized by three major symptoms (7,8,17,51,52):

A constant daily excessive sleepiness and unwanted naps, longer (more than one hour) and less irresistible than in narcolepsy, and nonrefreshing irrespective of their duration.

Nighttime sleep is uninterrupted and prolonged with more than 10 hours of sleep. Extended total sleep time, whenever possible, mainly during holidays and weekends, is frequently above 12 hours.

Awakening after nighttime or daytime sleep is laborious with frequent difficulties to react adequately to external stimuli upon awakening for up to three hours. This state is referred to as "sleep drunkenness" or "sleep inertia," and sleep never restores normal alertness (8,17). Episodes of automatic behavior can occur during this "drowsy state" especially in the morning, with frequent amnesia following these episodes (4).

Other symptoms. Although cataplexy needs to be absent, sleep paralysis, and hypnagogic or hypnopompic hallucinations are rare but may be present as in other sleep disorders or in the general population.

Neurological and psychological evaluations are necessary and need to be normal to exclude differential diagnoses of other hypersomnias (8,17). However, mood changes are frequently reported in these patients, but they never reach the point of major depression.

Headache (mainly migraine or tension-type) and manifestations of neurovegetative impairment with cold hands and feet, orthostatic hypotension or syncope have been reported in patients with IH with long sleep time (51). However, all those nonspecific symptoms have little if any diagnostic value.

Laboratory Features

Diagnosis is mostly clinical. However, PSG plus MSLT are required to assess the objective EDS, to ascertain the diagnosis, and to rule out some other causes of hypersomnia especially narcolepsy, PLM disorder, and sleep apnea syndrome (8,17). PSG demonstrates normal sleep except for its prolonged duration. Sleep efficiency is above 90%. NREM sleep and REM sleep are in normal proportions and the microarousal index is less than 10/hr.

Sleep apnea or PLM (index >10/hr) disorder should theoretically be absent, but may be acceptable in rare cases of an early onset of IH and the late occurrence of these other disorders. In cases in which there are numerous microarousals (>10/hr) during the night, the upper airway resistance syndrome should be suspected, which requires a new sleep recording with esophageal pressure monitoring to evaluate transpleural pressure.

Theoretically, the MSLT demonstrates a mean sleep latency of less than eight minutes with less than two SOREMPs as reported in the ICSD-2 (6). However, MSLT latency might be longer than in narcolepsy. As previously mentioned, it is more relevant to perform a 24-hour continuous PSG on an ad lib sleep-wake protocol to document a major sleep episode at night (more than 10 hours) and daytime sleep episodes (at least one nap of more than one hour) but this procedure still awaits standardization and validation (8,17).

Cognitive evoked potentials recording could be performed to evaluate sleep inertia upon awakening (8,17,32,33). Brain CT scan and/or MRI could be of interest and need to be normal to exclude the possibility of hypersomnia associated with a neurological disorder (8,17). In contrast to narcolepsy, HLA typing and/or CSF hypocretin-1 levels are of no help in the positive diagnosis of IH.

Diagnostic criteria for idiopathic hypersomnia with long sleep time
A. Complaint of EDS occurring almost daily for at least three months (6).
B. Prolonged nocturnal sleep time (more than 10 hours) documented by interview, actigraphy or sleep logs. Waking up in the morning or at the end of naps is almost always laborious.
C. Nocturnal polysomnography has excluded other causes of daytime sleepiness.
D. Nocturnal polysomnography demonstrates a short sleep latency and a major sleep period that is prolonged to more than 10 hours in duration.
E. If a multiple sleep latency test is performed following polysomnography, a mean sleep latency of less than eight minutes, and fewer than two sleep onset in REM periods are found.
F. The hypersomnia is not better explained by another sleep disorder, medical or neurological disorder (especially head trauma), mental disorder, medication use, or substance use disorder.

Idiopathic Hypersomnia without Long Sleep Time
The age of onset, familial component, and psychosocial and professional consequences are similar to those found in IH with long sleep time (8,17,53). The prevalence of this condition is unknown.

Clinical Features
IH without long sleep time remains a poorly clinically defined condition due to the absence of specific symptoms such as cataplexy or sleep apnea. IH without long sleep time is characterized by isolated EDS. Daytime sleep episodes may be more irresistible and more refreshing than in IH with long sleep time, establishing a bridge with narcolepsy without cataplexy (8,17,51,52).

Nocturnal sleep is normal, sometimes prolonged (more than six hours but less than 10 hours) but mostly refreshing. "Sleep inertia" or "sleep drunkenness" are rarely reported. Cataplexy is always absent. Sleep paralysis and hypnagogic or hypnopompic hallucinations are rare, but may be present as in other sleep disorders or in the general population. Mood changes are also frequently reported as they are in IH with long sleep time.

Laboratory Features
PSG plus MSLT are necessary to assess objective EDS and to ascertain the diagnosis. Nighttime PSG results are the same as those observed for IH with long sleep time. An MSLT is required for the diagnosis and demonstrates a mean sleep latency of less than eight minutes with less than two SOREMPs. MSLT results remain closer to narcolepsy in terms of mean sleep latency, in contrast to IH with long sleep time (8,17).

A 24-hour continuous PSG recording on an ad lib sleep-wake protocol and cognitive evoked potential recordings are not relevant for this condition (8,17). As in IH with long sleep time, HLA typing and/or CSF hypocretin-1 levels are of no help in the positive diagnosis of IH without long sleep time. Finally, neurological and psychological evaluations, brain CT scan, and/or MRI could be of interest in terms of ruling out differential diagnoses.

Diagnostic criteria for idiopathic hypersomnia without long sleep time

A. Complaint of EDS occurring almost daily for at least three months (6).
B. Normal nocturnal sleep (greater than 6 but less than 10 hours) documented by interview, actigraphy, or sleep logs.
C. Nocturnal polysomnography has excluded other causes of daytime sleepiness
D. Nocturnal polysomnography demonstrates a major sleep period that is normal in duration (greater than 6 but less than 10 hours)
E. A multiple sleep latency test following polysomnography demonstrates a mean sleep latency of less than eight minutes and fewer than two sleep onset in REM periods.
F. The hypersomnia is not better explained by another sleep disorder, medical or neurological disorder, mental disorder, medication use, or substance use disorder.

Recurrent Hypersomnia

Clinical Features

Recurrent hypersomnia is an exceptional condition, affecting primarily teenagers and characterized by recurrent episodes of excessive sleep (at least 16 hours per day) lasting from a few days to several weeks (6). Episodes are typically separated by weeks or months, during which time normal sleep patterns are observed. Recurrent hypersomnia results in major disturbances in social and family life. Its prognosis is unclear but the evolution throughout life is favorable in most cases, with a progressive disappearance of symptoms after 5 to 10 years duration.

The best-characterized recurrent hypersomnia is Kleine–Levin syndrome (KLS), a rare disorder defined by constant hypersomnia and cognitive (feelings of unreality and confusion) and behavioral disturbances with overeating (in up to 80% of cases) and less frequently hypersexuality during symptomatic episodes (54–56). KLS cases are more frequent in men (60–80%) with a mean age at onset of 15 years. Frequent triggering factors such as infections, head trauma, or alcohol have been reported. A review suggests that KLS appears to be more severe in women (55).

Recurrent hypersomnia can also occur in relation to menstruation; in this case it is referred to as "menstrual-related hypersomnia" (57). This condition generally occurs within the first months after menarche. The duration of the episodes is generally one week with a rapid ending at the time of menses. Oral contraceptives are frequently effective for treatment and may also help in the positive diagnosis assessment.

Laboratory Features

Diagnosis is mainly clinical. To confirm hypersomnia and to exclude epilepsy and organic pathology, electroencephalographic and polysomnographic recordings, as well as cerebral imaging are necessary.

The presence of the HLA DQB1*0201 genotype in patients is only a poor supportive criterion, reported in an isolated study (27). In addition, a decrease in CSF hypocretin-1 levels in KLS during symptomatic episodes when compared with the asymptomatic period has been reported, implicating a possible transient alteration in functional hypocretin neurotransmission (56).

Diagnostic criteria for recurrent hypersomnia (including Kleine–Levin syndrome and menstrual-related hypersomnia.)

A. Recurrent episodes of EDS of two days to four weeks duration (6).
B. Episodes recur at least once a year
C. The patient has normal alertness, cognitive functioning, and behavior between attacks.
D. The hypersomnia is not better explained by another sleep disorder, medical or neurological disorder, mental disorder, medication use, or substance use disorder.

Behaviorally Induced Insufficient Sleep Syndrome

As sleep deprivation is very common in our modern society, patients with a complaint of EDS should always be asked about their sleep-wake schedules with a comparison of weekday and weekend schedules. Insufficient sleep is the most frequent cause of EDS. In addition, patients who are chronically insufficient in their sleep amounts become used to their impairment and are less likely to assess their potential sleepiness (6,58).

Clinical Features
This syndrome is a disorder that occurs in an individual who fails to obtain sufficient nocturnal sleep required to support normally alert wakefulness for at least three months (6). The individual is in fact chronically sleep deprived on his own will, but without being aware of it. The subject is generally an active or overactive 40-year-old man, with responsibilities and a high cultural level. As the sleep debt develops, the individual starts suffering from EDS in the afternoon, in the evening or after meals (29,58). Patients report that they sleep five to six hours nightly on weekdays, and 9 hours during the weekends. They have difficulty rising in the morning and sometimes experience sleep drunkenness-like episodes (29,58). Work and cognitive performance may be impaired. The patient may also complain about increasing levels of subjective fatigue, mood deterioration, muscular pain, gastrointestinal unrest, and visual disturbances. Children may exhibit hyperactivity rather than sleepiness. Symptoms disappear on weekends and during the holidays. Sleep diaries and actigraphy may be helpful to precisely determine sleep-wake schedules with naps and to verify longer nighttime sleep on weekends.

The diagnosis is mainly established during the clinical interview. In cases of suspected associated pathology, such as respiratory disturbances during sleep, a polysomnographic recording may be indicated. In insufficient sleep syndrome, polysomnography shows a good sleep efficiency (>90%) and short sleep latency, indicative of a sleep rebound.

Diagnostic criteria for behaviorally induced insufficient sleep syndrome
    A. Complaint of excessive sleepiness, or in prepubertal children a complaint of behavioral abnormalities suggesting sleepiness, occurring almost daily for at least three months (6).
    B. Habitual sleep episode, established using history, actigraphy, or sleep logs is usually shorter than expected from age-adjusted normative data.
    C. When the habitual sleep schedule is not maintained (weekends or vacation time), patients will sleep considerably longer than usual.
    D. If diagnostic polysomnography is performed (not required for diagnosis), sleep latency is less than 10 minutes and sleep efficiency greater than 90%. During the MSLT, a short mean sleep latency of less than eight minutes (with or without multiple SOREMPs) may be observed.
    E. The hypersomnia is not better explained by another sleep disorder, medical or neurological disorder, mental disorder, medication use, or substance use disorder.

Hypersomnia Due to Medical Condition
A medical condition may produce hypersomnia in absence of associated cataplexy and without any effect of treatment (6). EDS is mostly associated with other symptoms of the underlying condition. Nighttime sleep is frequently fragmented by periods of wakefulness. The MSLT is needed in most of the cases and allows one to differentiate objective EDS from fatigue. If performed, the MSLT must demonstrate a mean sleep latency of less than eight minutes and fewer than two SOREMPs (6).

Hypersomnia Associated with Neurological Disorders
Several neurological disorders may cause EDS with large variabilities in terms of severity and phenotype. Brain tumors, encephalitis, or stroke-provoking lesions or dysfunction in the thalamus, hypothalamus, or brainstem can cause hypersomnia that may mimic clinical symptoms of IH with long sleep time but with frequent alteration in sleep continuity (7,8,47,59). Neurodegenerative conditions such as Alzheimer's disease, Parkinson's disease, or multiple system atrophy are also frequently associated with hypersomnia (50). Although intrinsic hypersomnia exists in those neurological disorders, other etiologies of hypersomnia such as sleep apnoea syndromes, drugs, and PLMs need first to be excluded.

Several genetic disorders (Norrie disease, Niemann–Pick type C, Prader–Willi syndrome, myotonic dystrophy) may be associated with central hypersomnia but also with sleep-related breathing disorders that lead to EDS (7,8,49).

Post-traumatic hypersomnia is another etiology of neurological hypersomnia (6). Abnormal sleepiness may be observed within 6 to 18 months following head trauma. Clinical symptoms may be similar to IH with long sleep time, but with poor sleep efficiency and frequent association with headaches, memory loss, and lack of concentration (60). Post-traumatic complaints of EDS have been associated with variable degrees of impaired daytime functioning. Patients who had been in a coma for 24 hours, had a head fracture, or had undergone immediate neurosurgical procedures may have higher scores of subjective and objective EDS (60,61).

Hypersomnia Associated with Infectious Disorders

Patients with infectious mononucleosis, Guillain Barré syndrome, pneumonia, hepatitis, or Whipple's disease may develop a hypersomnia syndrome that may mimic clinical symptoms of IH with long sleep time several months after the acute infection (62,63).

Human African trypanosomiasis (HAT) which is due to the transmission of trypanosomes by tsetse flies is a frequent cause of severe hypersomnia in Western Africa (*Trypanosoma brucei gambiense*) and Eastern Africa (*Trypanosoma brucei rhodesiense*) (64,65). After an extensive immune reaction during the initial stage, severe sleep and wakefulness impairment follows and the disorder at this point is referred to as "sleeping sickness." The possibility of HAT needs to be assessed in travelers and individuals migrating from Africa with EDS who may export the disease to the Western world. Given the increase in global tourism, it is important for clinicians to keep in mind that hypersomnia can easily be screened and evaluated during a routine clinical interview.

Hypersomnia Associated with Metabolic or Endocrine Disorders

Hypersomnia in diabetes, hepatic encephalopathy, hypothyroidism, and acromegaly are rarely reported. Sleep-related breathing and PLM disorders, frequently associated with these conditions, may also explain the relative frequency of such hypersomnias (6–8,10).

Diagnostic criteria for hypersomnia due to medical condition

A. Complaint of EDS occurring almost daily for at least three months (6).
B. A significant underlying medical or neurological disorder accounts for the daytime sleepiness.
C. If an MSLT is performed following nocturnal polysomnography (with a minimum of six hours slept), the mean sleep latency is less than eight minutes with no more than one SOREMP.
D. The hypersomnia is not better explained by another sleep disorder, mental disorder, medication use, or substance use disorder.

Hypersomnia Due to Drug or Substance

Patients affected with medical disorders may report sleepiness, but also fatigue as a result of treatment for their disorders (6). Hypersomnias secondary to sedative-hypnotic drugs or stimulant withdrawal exist and are easily recognized during a clinical interview. Numerous medications are potentially responsible for EDS, at least hypnotic, anxiolytic, antidepressant, neuroleptic, antihistaminic, antiepileptic (except for lamotrigine), and anti-Parkinsonism drugs. However, the relationship between the current use of drugs and the complaint of EDS is not always easy to ascertain. Dosing of drugs, drug-drug interactions, liver or renal impairments, and individual susceptibility may explain the large variability in the EDS phenotype. Several substances including alcohol yield sedative effects, which also depend on the dosage and individual susceptibility (66).

Diagnosis is mainly clinical; blood or urine drug screens may be necessary in particular cases.

Diagnostic Criteria For Hypersomnia Due to Drug or Substance (Abuse)

A. Complaint of daytime sleepiness or excessive sleep (6).
B. Complaint is believed to be secondary to current use, recent discontinuation, or prior prolonged use of drugs.
C. Hypersomnia is not better explained by another sleep disorder, medical or neurological disorder, mental disorder, or medication use.

Diagnostic Criteria For Hypersomnia Due to Drug or Substance (Medications)
   A.   Complaint of daytime sleepiness or excessive sleep (6).
   B.   Complaint is associated with current use, recent discontinuation, or prior prolonged use of a prescribed medication.
   C.   Hypersomnia is not better explained by another sleep disorder, medical or neurological disorder, mental disorder, or substance use disorder.

Hypersomnia not Due to a Substance or Known Physiological Condition

This entity also named "nonorganic hypersomnia" condition refers to several causes of hypersomnia including depressive disorder, seasonal affective disorder (SAD), abnormal personality traits, and conversion episodes (6). Most of the patients affected with psychiatric disorders suffered from insomnia; however, some (mainly with atypical depression) may also present with a complaint of EDS.

Clinical Features
The complaint of EDS may be rather similar to that of patients with IH with long sleep time, except that it may vary from day to day and is often associated with poor and fragmented sleep at night (7,8,17,67). In that sense, insomnia and EDS are frequently associated, especially in cases of depression. Chronic insomnia may be a precursor, symptom, residual symptom, or adverse effect of depression or its treatment. However, EDS may also be a precursor, symptom, or adverse effect of depression.

Hypersomnia associated with seasonal affective disorder (SAD) is considered a clinical subtype of nonorganic hypersomnia. SAD is characterized by the fall and winter recurrence of depressive episodes, with remission of symptoms in spring and summer (68). Patients with winter depression report hypersomnia, fatigue, loss of energy, carbohydrate craving, change in appetite and weight gain. Light therapy for 30 days in the morning, effective in this condition, may also help in the positive diagnosis assessment.

Laboratory Features
Polysomnographic studies in hypersomnia with mood disorders are rare and show a long time in bed without sleep that lead to a low sleep efficiency (67–70). The MSLT does not demonstrate a shortened mean sleep latency when compared with normal controls (67–70). In addition, REM sleep is totally absent during daytime naps in depressed patients. Finally, 24-hour continuous polysomnography reveals a lower total sleep time and decreased slow wave sleep in these patients (67). Therefore, the complaint of sleepiness appears to be related to the lack of interest, social withdrawal, and decreased energy, which are inherent in the depressed condition, rather than related to an increase in sleep propensity or REM sleep propensity. A diagnosis of fatigue appears more likely in this condition, although no objective criteria of fatigue are currently available.

Diagnostic criteria for hypersomnia not due to substances or known physiological condition (non-organic hypersomnia)
   A.   Complaint of EDS or excessive sleep (6).
   B.   Complaint is temporally associated with a psychiatric diagnosis.
   C.   Polysomnographic monitoring demonstrates both of the following:
         i. Reduced sleep efficiency and increased frequency and duration of awakenings
         ii. Variable, often normal, mean sleep latencies on the MSLT
   D.   The hypersomnia is not better explained by another sleep disorder, medical or neurological disorder, medication use, or substance use disorder.

Hypersomnias of Noncentral Origins
Sleep-Related Breathing Disorders
Sleep-related breathing disorders are the most frequent etiology of EDS, which may vary from falling asleep in relaxing situations to a major symptom that can be responsible for automobile- or work-related accidents (6,71). Questioning patients who complain of sleepiness about other

associated symptoms such as loud snoring, obesity, headaches, hypertension, fatigue in the morning, nocturia, reduced libido, and witnessed episodes of apnea provide essential clinical information for the diagnosis of sleep-related breathing disorders.

Sleep-Related Movement Disorders
Sleep-related movement disorders include two main conditions, restless legs syndrome (RLS) and periodic limb movement disorder (PLMD) (6,72,73). Patients or bed partners may complain of movements before or during sleep. Nocturnal sleep disturbances and/or complaints of EDS are frequently reported in these conditions. A clinical interview should address symptoms such as nocturnal agitation and discomfort of the extremities during periods of inactivity that are relieved with movement. However, the relationship between PLMD and EDS is still subject to debate.

Circadian Rhythm Sleep Disorders
Circadian rhythm sleep disruption may lead to insomnia but also to EDS or both (6,74). In particular cases of shift workers, both insufficient sleep and circadian disruptions lead to a frequent complaint of EDS. A thorough characterization of the daily schedule is always required in the determination of the etiology of chronic hypersomnia. A sleep diary may be helpful to precisely assess the regularity of sleep-wake schedule.

DIFFERENTIAL DIAGNOSIS FOR EACH DISORDER TYPE

Narcolepsy with Cataplexy
In the presence of frequent and clear-cut cataplexy, the clinical diagnosis of narcolepsy with cataplexy is easy. However, when cataplexy is predominant, narcolepsy could be misdiagnosed as a psychiatric condition, an epileptic variant, syncope, a drop attack, or an attack of a histrionic nature. Pseudonarcolepsy and pseudocataplexy are equivalent to a conversion disorder. Cases of malingering can also be seen when seeking disability benefits, leave from work, or to obtain a prescription of stimulants (6,16).

Other forms of hypersomnia may confound the diagnosis of narcolepsy with cataplexy: narcolepsy without cataplexy (especially when cataplexy is rare and not clear-cut), sleep-disordered breathing, IH, recurrent hypersomnia, PLMD, hypersomnia associated with depression and chronic sleep deprivation.

Hypersomnias in other medical conditions: Narcolepsy can occur in genetic, medical, or neurological conditions and are referred to as symptomatic or secondary narcolepsies.

Narcolepsy without Cataplexy
IH without long sleep time: In clinical terms, it is almost impossible to differentiate patients affected with IH without long sleep time and those with narcolepsy without cataplexy. However, associated REM abnormalities such as hypnagogic hallucinations and sleep paralysis are less frequent and severe in IH patients. The final diagnosis is easy to determine with the MSLT procedure, which demonstrates the presence of two or more SOREMPs in cases of narcolepsy without cataplexy only. A continuum between narcolepsy without cataplexy and IH without long sleep time is however possible.

IH with long sleep time: Patients affected with IH with long sleep time frequently report long (typically one to two hours) and nonrefreshing naps that contrast with the short and refreshing naps of narcoleptic patients. However in children, the phenotype of EDS in narcolepsy is not always clear-cut.

Other forms of hypersomnia may confound the diagnosis of narcolepsy without cataplexy: narcolepsy with cataplexy (in cases of atypical cataplexy), sleep-disordered breathing, recurrent hypersomnia, PLMD, hypersomnia associated with depression, and chronic sleep deprivation.

Idiopathic Hypersomnia with Long Sleep Time

IH with long sleep time remains a relatively poorly defined and rare condition, with many differential diagnoses. The final diagnosis rests on the exclusion of other causes of hypersomnias.

- IH without long sleep time: The absence of prolonged nocturnal sleep time and sleep inertia makes the difference.
- Behaviorally induced insufficient sleep syndrome in long sleepers: A long sleeper sleeps more than the typical amount of sleep in his normative age group. In the condition of behaviorally induced insufficient sleep, the individual has difficulty arising in the morning and begins suffering from EDS in the afternoon or after meals. A detailed history of the patient's current sleep-wake schedule is needed for the diagnosis. Patients report that they sleep two to three hours less on weekday nights when compared with weekend nights. Symptoms disappear on weekends and during the holidays. Subjects with IH with long sleep time do not report any improvement of EDS after prolonged sleeping for days.
- Nonorganic hypersomnia: This condition is a main clinical differential diagnosis of IH with long sleep time. It is often difficult to rule out hypersomnia associated with depression while some patients may have mood changes that do not qualify for the diagnosis of affective disorders (Diagnostic and Statistical Manual of Mental Disorders, DSM-IV). Questions assessing mood are always necessary to identify patients with sleep disorders associated with mood disorders. The sleep-wake schedule may also provide clues to the diagnosis, since there is frequent variability in this schedule with psychiatric conditions. Finally, polysomnography reveals lower total sleep time and percentage of slow wave sleep in nonorganic hypersomnia when compared with the IH condition.
- Sleep-disordered breathing including the upper airway resistance syndrome: Before ascertaining the diagnosis of IH, sleep-disordered breathing syndromes need to be excluded. Sleep apnea-hypopnea syndrome is easily diagnosed by routine polysomnography. On the other hand, the upper airway resistance syndrome needs more complex investigation (75). Patients affected are nonobese men or women, with complaints of EDS, snoring (especially in men) and frequent fatigue upon awakening. Clinical examination often reveals a triangular face, a small chin, an arched palate, a class II malocclusion and a retroposition of the mandible.
- PLMD: This disorder associates a sleep complaint (insomnia and/or hypersomnia) and/or daytime fatigue, with polysomnographic demonstration of periodic, highly stereotyped limb movements during sleep (PLMS), exceeding more than 15 per hour in adults. PLMD must be interpreted in the context of a patient's related complaint, with an important overlap between symptomatic and asymptomatic patients according to the index of PLMS.
- Narcolepsy Without Cataplexy: (see above)
- Hypersomnia due to medical condition: Several medical conditions may produce hypersomnia and mimic IH. Genetic, neurological, infectious, and metabolic disorders need to be reviewed during a detailed medical history before establishing the definitive diagnosis of hypersomnia.
- Hypersomnia due to drug or substance: Hypersomnia secondary to the abuse of sedative-hypnotic drugs or to the abrupt cessation of stimulant drugs are easily recognized during a clinical interview.
- Chronic fatigue syndrome: This syndrome is characterized by persistent or relapsing fatigue that does not resolve with sleep or rest (76). However, patients have frequent difficulties in clearly distinguishing excessive sleepiness from fatigue. In addition to fatigue, patients report myalgia, anxiety, fever, headaches, and cognitive alterations. Chronic fatigue syndrome is not a cause of chronic hypersomnia but is part of the differential diagnosis.

Idiopathic Hypersomnia Without Long Sleep Time

This condition results in the same diagnostic differential as for IH with long sleep time.

Recurrent Hypersomnia

Organic central nervous system disorder: The recurrence of episodes of EDS may be caused by brain tumors (mainly within the third ventricle), head trauma, or encephalitis, and is referred to as "secondary recurrent hypersomnia" (6). A neurological examination is therefore required in all cases of recurrent hypersomnia.

Recurrent episodes of hypersomnia may be found in the context of psychiatric disorders such as bipolar disorder or somatoform disorder (6). Hypersomnia associated with depression is rarely characterized as a recurrent hypersomnia.

Other forms of hypersomnia rarely confound the diagnosis of recurrent hypersomnia: narcolepsy, sleep-disordered breathing, IH, PLMD, and chronic sleep deprivation.

Behaviorally Induced Insufficient Sleep Syndrome

Other forms of hypersomnia may confound the diagnosis of behaviorally induced insufficient sleep syndrome: narcolepsy, sleep-disordered breathing, IH, PLMD, recurrent hypersomnia, and hypersomnia associated with depression.

Circadian rhythm sleep disorders: These disorders should be considered in patients with complaints of nocturnal insomnia and daytime sleepiness (6,74). Patients with delayed sleep phase syndrome frequently complain of difficulty waking up, morning sleepiness, and difficulty falling asleep at night. Symptoms are worse on days when the patient must awaken by a set time to be at school or work. Patients with advanced sleep phase syndrome may complain of evening sleepiness and early morning awakening. It is important to obtain detailed sleep-wake schedules with a comparison of the patient's weekday and weekend schedules to differentiate those conditions.

Hypersomnia Due to Medical Condition

Other forms of hypersomnia may confound the diagnosis of hypersomnia due to medical condition: narcolepsy, sleep-disordered breathing, IH, recurrent hypersomnia, PLMD, hypersomnia associated with depression, and chronic sleep deprivation.

However, the main problem in this diagnostic category is to recognize the underlying medical condition that is responsible for the hypersomnia.

Hypersomnia Due to Drug or Substance

All causes of hypersomnia need to be ruled out before establishing the diagnosis of hypersomnia due to drug or substance. Blood or urine drug screens may be necessary in particular cases.

Hypersomnia Not Due to a Substance or Known Physiological Condition

Other forms of hypersomnia may confound the diagnosis of hypersomnia not due to a substance or known physiological condition: narcolepsy, sleep-disordered breathing, PLMD, IH, recurrent hypersomnia, and chronic sleep deprivation.

As the MSLT does not demonstrate a shortened mean sleep latency in this condition when compared with normal controls, the chronic fatigue syndrome must also be proposed as an important differential diagnosis (6–8,10,76).

CONCLUSIONS

EDS is a frequent complaint in modern societies. As drowsiness and naps may be limited to sedentary situations in which falling asleep is socially acceptable, EDS can also contribute to impaired performance, accidents at work or while driving, and disturbances of mood and social adjustment.

Clinicians should always question their patients with a complaint of EDS for potentially insufficient sleep, insomnia, medical or psychiatric conditions, and drug use. Physicians have several methods at their disposal to distinguish sleepiness from fatigue, to affirm the existence of daytime somnolence, and to appropriately diagnose the different causes of hypersomnia. There is no doubt that progress has been made in the identification of the different phenotypes of chronic hypersomnia. However, a tendency to overdiagnose sleep-disordered breathing in patients with EDS still persists. As several of the other causes of chronic hypersomnia are rare, insufficiently recognized, or poorly defined, there is a definite need to further develop sleep laboratory investigations to assess the correct diagnosis of hypersomnia and to propose the most effective treatment. Lastly, studies at the genetic, biological, and pharmacological levels are also needed to further our understanding of the pathophysiology of chronic hypersomnia and to develop specific treatments in the future.

REFERENCES

1. Arand D, Bonnet M, Hurwitz T, et al. The clinical use of the MSLT and MWT. Sleep 2005; 28(1):123–144.
2. Hays JC, Blazer DG, Foley DJ. Risk of napping: excessive daytime sleepiness and mortality in an older community population. J Am Geriatr Soc 1996; 44(6):693–698.
3. Daniels E, King MA, Smith IE, et al. Health-related quality of life in narcolepsy. J Sleep Res 2001; 10(1):75–81.
4. Kales A, Soldatos CR, Bixler EO, et al. Narcolepsy–cataplexy. II. Psychosocial consequences and associated psychopathology. Arch Neurol 1982; 39(3):169–171.
5. Guilleminault C, Tilkian A, Dement WC. The sleep apnea syndromes. Ann Rev Med 1976; 27:465–484.
6. American Academy of Sleep Medicine. International Classification of Sleep Disorders, 2nd Edition: Diagnostic and Coding Manual. Westchester, Illinois: American Academy of Sleep Medicine, 2005.
7. Dauvilliers Y. Differential diagnosis in hypersomnia. Curr Opin Neurol Neurosci 2006; 6:156–162.
8. Dauvilliers Y, Billiard M. Chronic hypersomnia. In: Guilleminault C, ed. Excessive Sleepiness: Sleep Medicine Clinics. Philadelphia: W.B. Saunders 2006; 1(1):79–88.
9. Silber M. The investigation of sleepiness. In: Guilleminault C, ed. Excessive Sleepiness: Sleep Medicine Clinics. Philadelphia: W.B. Saunders 2006; 1(1):1–7.
10. Guilleminault C, Brooks SN. Excessive daytime sleepiness: a challenge for the practising neurologist. Brain 2001; 124(pt 8):1482–1491.
11. Johns MW. A new method for measuring daytime sleepiness: the Epworth sleepiness scale. Sleep 1991; 14:540–545.
12. Carskadon MA, Mitler MM, Roth T. Guidelines for the Multiple Sleep Latency Test (MSLT): a standard measure of sleepiness. Sleep 1986; 9:519–524.
13. Hood B, Bruck D. A comparison of sleep deprivation and narcolepsy in terms of complex cognitive performance and subjective sleepiness. Sleep Med 2002; 3(3):259–266.
14. Roehrs T, Zorick F, Wittig R, et al Alerting effects of naps in patients with narcolepsy. Sleep 1986; 9(1 pt 2):194–199.
15. Shen J, Barbera J, Shapiro CM. Distinguishing sleepiness and fatigue: focus on definition and measurement. Sleep Med Rev 2006; 10(1):63–76.
16. Dauvilliers Y, Billiard M, Montplaisir J. Clinical aspects and pathophysiology of narcolepsy. Clin Neurophysiol 2003; 114(11):2000–2017.
17. Billiard M, Dauvilliers Y. Idiopathic hypersomnia. Sleep Med Rev 2001; 5(5):349–358.
18. Hoddes E, Zarcone V, Smythe H, et al. Quantification of sleepiness: a new approach. Psychophysiology 1973; 10(4):431–436.
19. Akerstedt T, Gillberg M. Subjective and objective sleepiness in the active individual. Int J Neurosci 1990; 52(1–2):29–37.
20. Benbadis SR, Mascha E, Perry MC, et al. Association between the Epworth sleepiness scale and the multiple sleep latency test in a clinical population. Ann Intern Med 1999; 130(4 pt 1):289–292.
21. Dauvilliers Y, Gosselin A, Paquet J, et al. Effect of age on MSLT results in patients with narcolepsy-cataplexy. Neurology 2004; 62(1):46–50.
22. Mignot E, Lin L, Finn L, et al. Correlates of sleep-onset REM periods during the Multiple Sleep Latency Test in community adults. Brain 2006; 129(pt 6):1609–1623.
23. Doghramji K, Mitler MM, Sangal RB, et al. A normative study of the maintenance of wakefulness test (MWT). Electroencephalogr Clin Neurophysiol 1997; 103(5):554–562.
24. Sangal RB, Thomas L, Mitler MM. Maintenance of wakefulness test and multiple sleep latency test. Measurement of different abilities in patients with sleep disorders. Chest 1992; 101(4):898–902.
25. Dauvilliers Y, Arnulf I, Mignot E. Narcolepsy with cataplexy. Lancet 2007; 369(9560):499–511.
26. Mignot E, Lammers GJ, Ripley B, et al. The role of cerebrospinal fluid hypocretin measurement in the diagnosis of narcolepsy and other hypersomnias. Arch Neurol 2002; 59(10):1553–1562.
27. Dauvilliers Y, Baumann CR, Carlander B, et al. CSF hypocretin-1 levels in narcolepsy, Kleine–Levin syndrome, and other hypersomnias and neurological conditions. J Neurol Neurosurg Psychiatry 2003; 74(12):1667–1673.

28. Mignot E, Lin L, Rogers W, et al. Complex HLA-DR and -DQ interactions confer risk of narcolepsy-cataplexy in three ethnic groups. Am J Hum Genet 2001; 68(3):686–699.

29. Van Dongen HP, Maislin G, Mullington JM, et al. The cumulative cost of additional wakefulness: dose-response effects on neurobehavioral functions and sleep physiology from chronic sleep restriction and total sleep deprivation. Sleep 2003; 26(2):117–126.

30. Findley LJ, Suratt PM, Dinges DF. Time-on-task decrements in "steer clear" performance of patients with sleep apnea and narcolepsy. Sleep 1999; 22(6):804–809.

31. Dinges DF, Kribbs NB. Performing while sleepy: effects of experimentally induced sleepiness. In: Monk TM, ed. Sleep, Sleepiness and Performance. Chichester, England: John Wiley and Sons, 1991: 97–128.

32. Sangal RB, Sangal JM. Measurement of P300 and sleep characteristics in patients with hypersomnia: do P300 latencies, P300 amplitudes, and multiple sleep latency and maintenance of wakefulness tests measure different factors? Clin Electroencephalogr 1997; 28(3):179–184.

33. Bastuji H, Garcia-Larrea L. Evoked potentials as a tool for the investigation of human sleep. Sleep Med Rev 1999; 3(1):23–45.

34. Dauvilliers Y, Montplaisir J, Molinari N, et al. Age at onset of narcolepsy in two large populations of patients in France and Quebec. Neurology 2001; 57(11):2029–2033.

35. Overeem S, Mignot E, van Dijk JG, et al. Narcolepsy: clinical features, new pathophysiologic insights, and future perspectives. J Clin Neurophysiol 2001; 18(2):78–105.

36. Anic-Labat S, Guilleminault C, Kraemer HC, et al. Validation of a cataplexy questionnaire in 983 sleep-disorders patients. Sleep 1999; 22(1):77–87.

37. Guilleminault C. Cataplexy. In: Guilleminault C, Dement W, Passouant P, eds. Narcolepsy. New York: Spectrum, 1976:125–143.

38. Poryazova R, Siccoli M, Werth E, et al. Unusually prolonged rebound cataplexy after withdrawal of fluoxetine. Neurology 2005; 65(6):967–968.

39. Ohayon MM. Prevalence of hallucinations and their pathological associations in the general population. Psychiatry Res 2000; 97(2–3):153–164.

40. Kotagal S, Krahn LE, Slocumb N. A putative link between childhood narcolepsy and obesity. Sleep Med 2004; 5(2):147–150.

41. Nightingale S, Orgill JC, Ebrahim IO, et al. The association between narcolepsy and REM behavior disorder (RBD). Sleep Med 2005; 6(3):253–258.

42. Roth B, Nevsimalova S. Depresssion in narcolepsy and hypersommia. Schweiz Arch Neurol Neurochir Psychiatry 1975; 116(2):291–300.

43. Vandeputte M, de Weerd A. Sleep disorders and depressive feelings: a global survey with the Beck depression scale. Sleep Med 2003; 4(4):343–345.

44. Mignot E. Genetic and familial aspects of narcolepsy. Neurology 1998; 50(2 suppl 1):S16–S22.

45. Billiard M, Pasquie-Magnetto V, Heckman M, et al. Family studies in narcolepsy. Sleep 1994; 17(8 suppl):S54–S59.

46. Dauvilliers Y, Blouin JL, Neidhart E, et al. A narcolepsy susceptibility locus maps to a 5 Mb region of chromosome 21q. Ann Neurol 2004; 56(3):382–388.

47. Autret A, Lucas B, Mondon K, et al. Sleep and brain lesions: a critical review of the literature and additional new cases. Neurophysiol Clin 2001; 31:356–375.

48. Nishino S, Kanbayashi T. Symptomatic narcolepsy, cataplexy and hypersomnia, and their implications in the hypothalamic hypocretin/orexin system. Sleep Med Rev 2005; 9(4):269–310.

49. Gibbs JW, Ciafaloni E, Radtke RA. Excessive daytime somnolence and increased rapid eye movement pressure in myotonic dystrophy. Sleep 2002; 25(6):662–665.

50. Arnulf I, Konofal E, Merino-Andreu M, et al. Parkinson's disease and sleepiness: an integral part of PD. Neurology 2002; 58:1019–1024.

51. Aldrich MS. The clinical spectrum of narcolepsy and idiopathic hypersomnia. Neurology 1996; 46:393–401.

52. Bassetti C, Aldrich MS. Idiopathic hypersomnia. A series of 42 patients. Brain 1997; 120:1423–1435.

53. Broughton R, Nevsimalova S, Roth B. The socioeconomic effects (including work, education, recreation and accidents) of idiopathic hypersomnia. Sleep Res 1978; 7:217.

54. Critchley M. Periodic hypersomnia and megaphagia in adolescent males. Brain 1962; 85:627–656.

55. Arnulf I, Zeitzer JM, File J, et al. Kleine–Levin syndrome: a systematic review of 186 cases in the literature. Brain 2005; 128(pt 12):2763–2776.

56. Dauvilliers Y, Mayer G, Lecendreux M, et al. Kleine–Levin syndrome: an autoimmune hypothesis based on clinical and genetic analyses. Neurology 2002; 59:1739–1745.

57. Billiard M, Guilleminault C, Dement WC. A menstruation-linked periodic hypersomnia. Kleine–Levin syndrome or new clinical entity? Neurology 1975; 25:436–443.

58. Carskadon MA, Dement WC. Cumulative effects of sleep restriction on daytime sleepiness. Psychophysiology 1981; 18:107–113.

59. Guilleminault C, Quera-Salva MA, Goldberg MP. Pseudo-hypersomnia and pre-sleep behaviour with bilateral paramedian thalamic lesions. Brain 1993; 116:1549–1563.
60. Guilleminault C, Yuen KM, Gulevich MG, et al. Hypersomnia after head-neck trauma: a methodological dilemma. Neurology 2000; 54:653–659.
61. Masel BE, Scheibel RS, Kimbark T, et al. Excessive daytime sleepiness in adults with brain injuries. Arch Phys Med Rehabil 2001; 82(11):1526–1532.
62. Voderholzer U, Riemann D, Gann H, et al. Transient total sleep loss in cerebral Whipple's disease: a longitudinal study. J Sleep Res 2002; 11:321–329.
63. Guilleminault C, Mondini S. Mononucleosis and chronic daytime sleepiness. A long-term follow-up study. Arch Intern Med 1986; 146(7):1333–1335.
64. Buguet A, Bisser S, Josenando T, et al. Sleep structure: a new diagnostic tool for stage determination in sleeping sickness. Acta Trop 2005; 93:107–117.
65. Buguet A, Bourdon L, Bouteille B, et al. The duality of sleeping sickness: focusing on sleep. Sleep Med Rev 2001; 5:139–153.
66. Roehrs T, Roth T. Sleep, sleepiness, sleep disorders and alcohol use and abuse. Sleep Med Rev 2001; 5:287–297.
67. Billiard M, Dolenc L, Aldaz C, et al. Hypersomnia associated with mood disorders: a new perspective. J Psychosom Res 1994; 38:41–47.
68. Rosenthal NE, Sack DA, Gillin JC, et al. Seasonal affective disorder. A description of the syndrome and preliminary findings with light therapy. Arch Gen Psychiatry 1984; 41:72–80.
69. Nofzinger EA, Thase ME, Reynolds CF, et al. Hypersomnia in bipolar depression: a comparison with narcolepsy using the multiple sleep latency test. Am J Psychiatry 1991; 148:1177–1181.
70. Vgontzas AN, Bixler EO, Kales A, et al. Differences in nocturnal and daytime sleep between primary and psychiatric hypersomnia: diagnostic and treatment implications. Psychosom Med 2000; 62(2):220–226.
71. Young T, Palta M, Dempsey J, Skatrud J, et al.. The occurrence of sleep-disordered breathing among middle-aged adults. N Engl J Med 1993; 328:1230–1235.
72. Hening WA. Subjective and objective criteria in the diagnosis of the restless legs syndrome. Sleep Med 2004; 5:285–292.
73. Nicolas A, Lesperance P, Montplaisir J. Is excessive daytime sleepiness with periodic leg movements during sleep a specific diagnostic category? Eur Neurol 1998; 40:22–26.
74. Wagner DR. Disorders of the circadian sleep-wake cycle. Neurol Clin 1996; 14(3):651–670.
75. Guilleminault C, Stoohs R, Clerk A, et al.. A cause of excessive daytime sleepiness. The upper airway resistance syndrome. Chest 1993; 104:781–787.
76. Prins JB, van der Meer JW, Bleijenberg G. Chronic fatigue syndrome. Lancet 2006; 367(9507):346–355.

23 | Treatment of Hypersomnias

Mark E. Dyken

Department of Neurology, University of Iowa College of Medicine, Iowa City; Department of Neurology Sleep Disorders Center, University of Iowa Hospitals and Clinics, Iowa City, Iowa, U.S.A.

Thoru Yamada

Department of Neurology, University of Iowa College of Medicine, Iowa City; Division of Clinical Electrophysiology, University of Iowa Hospitals and Clinics, Iowa City, Iowa, U.S.A.

Mohsin Ali

Department of Neurology, SUNY Upstate Medical University, Syracuse, New York, U.S.A.

INTRODUCTION

This chapter focuses on treatment of the hypersomnias of central origin as defined in the second edition of the *International Classification of Sleep Disorders* (ICSD-2; Fig. 1) (1). Rational therapy begins with an understanding of the normal anatomy, physiology, and neurochemistry of central wake/sleep mechanisms.

BASIC WAKE SYSTEMS

The ascending reticular activating system, defined in part through Bremer's "isole" preparations and the early studies of Moruzzi and Magoun, promotes wakefulness through monoaminergic and cholinergic neurotransmitter systems (2–4). Monoaminergic elements include the hypothalamic histaminergic tuberomammillary nucleus (TMN) and the brainstem noradrenergic locus coeruleus (LC) (5,6). The cholinergic system functions through the pedunculopontine/lateral dorsal tegmental nuclear complex (PPN/LDTN) and is composed of "rapid eye movement (REM) sleep-off" and "REM sleep-on" cells that are respectively most active during wakefulness and REM sleep (7).

The PPN/LDTN has two waking pathways, leading to diffuse cortical projections (Fig. 2) (8). A ventral hypothalamic system excites the TMN and the orexin/hypocretin neurons in the perifornical lateral nucleus of the hypothalamus, which relay to cholinergic basal forebrain cells, while a dorsal thalamic route stimulates nonspecific midline and intralaminar nuclei, inhibiting the reticular nucleus of the thalamus.

BASIC SLEEP ONSET SYSTEMS

A hypothalamic "sleep switch" was first suggested by von Economo's encephalitis lethargica investigations (9–11). Sleep onset can be envisioned as resulting from excitation of nuclei in the preoptic area of the hypothalamus (the ventrolateral and median preoptic nuclei) (11–13). These nuclei use inhibitory neurotransmitters [γ-aminobutyric acid (GABA) and galanin] in reciprocal inhibitory relays with the aforementioned waking centers, and in direct thalamic projections (Fig. 3) (12–15).

A gradual inhibition of REM sleep-off cells, which involve the PPN/LDTN, leads to disinhibition of GABAergic reticular thalamic nuclei that generate non–rapid eye movement (NREM) sleep through intrathalamic connections to limbic forebrain structures that include the orbitofrontal cortex (Fig. 3) (16). Sleep is also facilitated by the solitary tract nucleus, utilizing unknown neurotransmitters, through direct connections with the hypothalamus, amygdala, and other forebrain structures (17).

In addition, serotonergic neurons in the midline (raphe) of the medulla, pons, and mesencephalon of the brainstem help modulate sleep (14). Although lesions of the caudal midbrain and pontine raphe lead to insomnia, as they are necessary for the initiation of sleep,

HYPERSOMNIAS OF CENTRAL ORIGIN

**Not due to a Circadian Rhythm Sleep Disorder
Sleep Related Breathing Disorder, or
Other Cause of Disturbed Nocturnal Sleep**

1. Narcolepsy with Cataplexy

2. Narcolepsy without Cataplexy

3. Narcolepsy Due to Medical condition

4. Narcolepsy Unspecified

5. Recurrent Hypersomnia
   Kleine-Levin Syndrome
   Menstrual-Related Hypersomnia

6. Idiopathic Hypersomnia with Long Sleep Time

7. Idiopathic Hypersomnia without Long Sleep Time

8. Behaviorally Induced Insufficient Sleep Syndrome

9. Hypersomnia Due to Medical Condition

10. Hypersomnia Due to Drug or Substance

11. Hypersomnia Not Due to Substance or Known Physiological Condition
    (Nonorganic Hypersomnia, NOS)

12. Physiological (Organic) Hypersomnia, Unspecified (Organic Hypersomnia, NOS)

Figure 1 Hypersomnias of central origin. *Abbreviation*: NOS, not otherwise specified. *Source*: From Ref. 1.

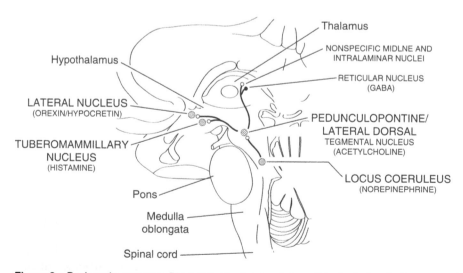

Figure 2 Basic wake systems. Diagrammatic representation of the brainstem in the parasagittal plane showing the proposed mechanism and structures involved in the generation of wakefulness. Cholinergic cells in the pedunculopontine/laterodorsal tegmental nuclear complex have two waking pathways, leading to diffuse cortical projections. A ventral hypothalamic system excites the tuberomammillary and the orexin/hypocretin neurons in the perifornical lateral nucleus of the hypothalamus, which relay to cholinergic basal forebrain cells, while a dorsal thalamic route stimulates nonspecific midline and intralaminar nuclei (while inhibiting the reticular nucleus of the thalamus). Open circle, facilitatory; closed circle, inhibitory. *Source*: Modified from Ref. 8, Figure 1.

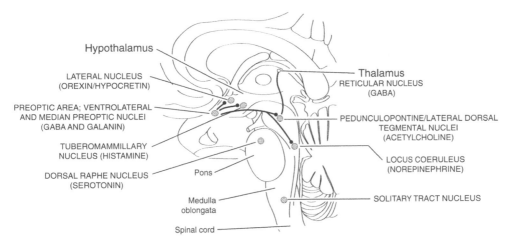

Figure 3 Basic sleep onset systems. Diagrammatic representation of the brainstem in the parasagittal plane showing the proposed mechanism and structures involved in sleep onset. Excited nuclei in the preoptic area of the hypothalamus (the ventrolateral and median preoptic nuclei) use inhibitory neurotransmitters (GABA and galanin) in reciprocal inhibitory relays with waking centers, and in direct thalamic projections. Gradual inhibition of REM sleep-off cells, which function through the PPN/LDTN, leads to disinhibition of GABAergic reticular thalamic nuclei that generate NREM sleep through intrathalamic connections to limbic forebrain structures that include the orbitofrontal cortex. Sleep is also facilitated by the solitary tract nucleus, utilizing unknown neurotransmitters, through direct connections with the hypothalamus, amygdala, and other forebrain structures. Serotonergic neurons in the midline (raphe) of the medulla, pons, and mesencephalon of the brainstem help modulate sleep. Open circle, facilitatory; closed circle, inhibitory. *Abbreviations*: GABA, γ-aminobutyric acid; PPN/LDTN, pedunculopontine/lateral dorsal tegmental nucleus; NREM, non–rapid eye movement. *Source*: Modified from Ref. 8, Figure 1.

these serotonergic cells actually decrease their firing rate during the onset of slow wave sleep, and cease firing during REM sleep (18,19).

PHARMACOLOGIC THERAPY

Narcolepsy

The Standards of Practice Committee of the American Academy of Sleep Medicine (AASM) provides a periodically updated list of medicines recognized for the treatments of hypersomnolence associated with narcolepsy. The list has included modafinil, amphetamines, and amphetamine-like drugs (methylphenidate), whereas sodium oxybate, non-sedating tricyclic antidepressants (TCAs, protriptyline), selective serotonin reuptake inhibitors (SSRIs, fluoxetine), and monoamine oxidase inhibitors (MAOIs, selegiline) have been suggested for the auxiliary symptoms of cataplexy, sleep paralysis, and hypnagogic/hypnopompic hallucinations (Table 1) (21).

Hypersomnolence

In 1931, Doyle and Daniels first recommended the use of ephedrine for the treatment of hypersomnolence associated with narcolepsy (22). Ephedrine is a direct-acting sympathomimetic, isolated from the *Ephedra vulgaris* plant, with α_1-adrenergic agonist properties.

Amphetamine and amphetamine-like drugs. In 1935, Prinzmetal and Bloomberg suggested treating narcolepsy with the indirect-acting sympathomimetic amphetamine (phenylisopropylamine) as it was safer and cheaper than ephedrine and had efficacy on both sleepiness and cataplexy (23). Amphetamine, synthesized in 1897 and recognized as a stimulant by Alles in 1929, has a chemical structure similar to the endogenous catecholamines, dopamine (DA) and norepinephrine (NE) (Fig. 4) (24). Amphetamine is highly lipid soluble, well absorbed (with peak serum levels reached within 2 hours), and undergoes hepatic catabolism with renal excretion.

Table 1 Medications Commonly Used in the Treatment of Narcolepsy

Medications commonly used in the treatment of narcolepsy	Usual adult daily doses (maximums)	Medication class	Major side effects
Amphetamine	30 mg (100 mg)	Stimulant, amphetamine	Insomnia, restlessness, tachycardia, psychotic episodes, dizziness, diarrhea, constipation, hypertension, impotence
Amphetamine (sustained release)	30 mg (100 mg)	a	a
Methamphetamine	40 mg (80 mg)	a	a
Methylphenidate	30 mg (100 mg)	Stimulant, otherwise not defined	Nervousness, insomnia, anorexia, nausea, dizziness, hypertension, hypersensitivity reactions, tachycardia, headache, neuroleptic malignant syndrome
Modafinil	200 mg (400 mg)	Stimulant, otherwise not defined	Headache, nausea, eosinophilia, diarrhea, dry mouth, anorexia
GHB (sodium oxybate, Xyrem)	9 g in two divided doses	A naturally occurring metabolite; anticataplectic and anti-other REM-related symptoms	Sedation, headache, nausea, dizziness, headache, confusion, vomiting, enuresis
Protriptyline (non-sedating TCA; other TCAs are usually sedating; characteristics except dose are otherwise similar among TCAs such as imipramine)	10 mg (60 mg)	TCA; anticataplectic and anti-other REM-related symptoms	Orthostatic hypotension, hypertension, seizures, headache, anticholinergic symptoms, impotence, impaired liver function, myocardial infarction, stroke
Fluoxetine	20 mg (80 mg)	SSRI; anticataplectic and anti-other REM-related symptoms	Asthenia, nausea, diarrhea, anorexia, insomnia, tremor, anxiety, somnolence
Selegiline	20 mg (40 mg)	MAO inhibitor; stimulant and anti-cataplectic and anti-other REM-related symptoms	Nausea, dizziness, confusion, tremor, orthostatic hypotension, diet-induced hypertension

[a]same as with amphetamines.
Abbreviations: GHB, γ-hydroxybutyrate; REM, rapid eye movement sleep; TCA, tricyclic antidepressant; SSRI, selective serotonin reuptake inhibitor; MAO, monoamine oxidase.
Source: Modified from Ref. 20.

Amphetamine and amphetamine-like drugs promote wakefulness through dopaminergic, mesolimbocortical projections from the mesencephalic ventral tegmental area of Tsai and the medial substantia nigra (25,26). Dopaminergic projections from the midbrain to the basolateral and corticomedial amygdalar nuclei establish extensive cortical connections through the lamina terminalis and/or amygdalofugal pathways (27). Stimulation of the basolateral nucleus results in an arousal response that is independent from that elicited by the reticular formation. As DA reuptake is important in the elimination of DA from the cortex and limbic forebrain, it is likely that the wakefulness effects of amphetamines and amphetamine-like drugs operate through DA terminals in these areas (28).

Amphetamine and amphetamine-like drugs inhibit uptake and enhance release of DA and NE through nerve terminal transporter (T) molecules (DAT/NET) (29). Normally, these transporters move the neurotransmitters from outside to inside the cell; amphetamines reverse

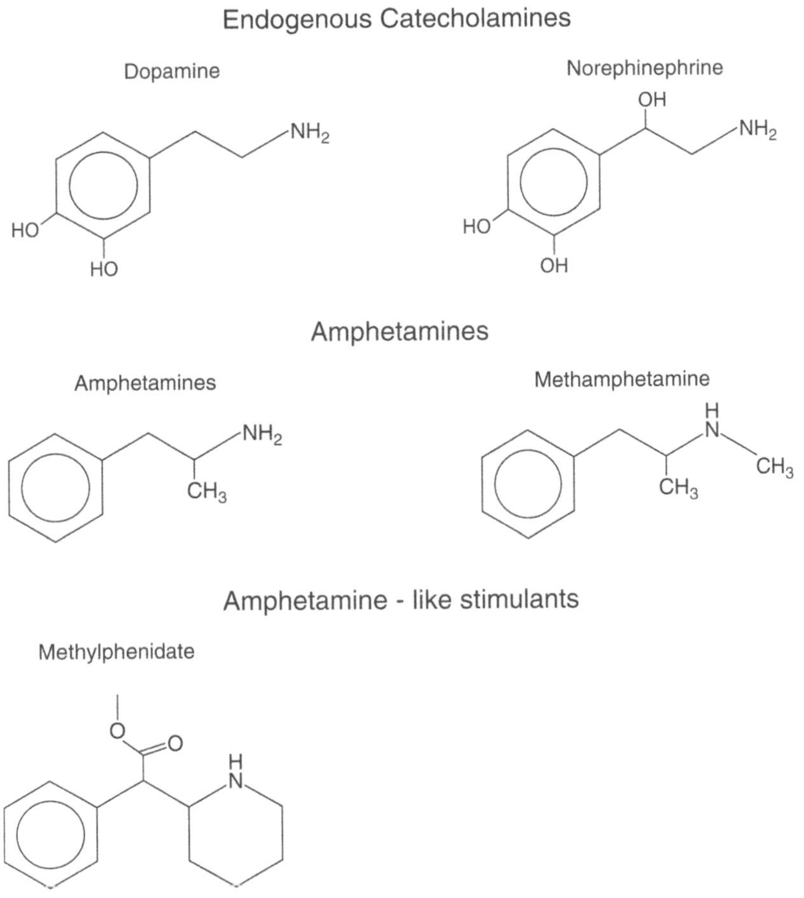

Endogenous Catecholamines

Dopamine

Norephinephrine

Amphetamines

Amphetamines

Methamphetamine

Amphetamine - like stimulants

Methylphenidate

Figure 4 Comparison of chemical structures of endogenous catecholamines with amphetamines and amphetamine-like stimulants. *Source*: Modified from Ref. 38, Figure 38.1.

this process (30). In addition, sequestration of DA into neuronal synaptic vesicles depends on vesicular monoamine transporter 2 (VMAT2). Amphetamines inhibit vesicular uptake of DA by mechanisms that include directly binding to VMAT2 (31). The primary dopaminergic effect of amphetamines appears to be on wakefulness as DAT ligands promote electroencephalography (EEG) arousal patterns, whereas NET ligands reduce REM sleep (25).

Amphetamines *Dextroamphetamine and methamphetamine.* The effects of amphetamine and amphetamine derivatives are often isomer specific. D-Amphetamine (dextroamphetamine) is four times more potent than L-amphetamine in inducing EEG arousal (32). In the synthesis of methamphetamine, an additional methyl group placed on the amine of amphetamine may improve central nervous system (CNS) penetration and increase wakefulness (Fig. 4) (33).

Amphetamines, classified as Schedule II substances under the Controlled Substances Act of 1970, have the potential for abuse and adverse cardiovascular, cerebrovascular, and psychiatric effects (34). Mesencephalic dopaminergic cells project widely to the frontal, temporal, parietal, and occipital cortices and may lead to side effects by stimulating non–wake-promoting areas in striatum and nucleus accumbens (35). Additional adverse effects might be realized through alterations in VMAT2 storage of other monoamine neurotransmitters, such as histamine and serotonin (31).

At high doses, amphetamines can cause free radical–mediated neurotoxicity. In dopaminergic neurons, damage from peroxynitrite can be reduced by antioxidants or L-carnitine (36). Nevertheless, even at these higher doses, amphetamine success rate in adequately treating hypersomnolence in narcolepsy only ranges from 65% to 85% (34,37).

In addition, coadministration of amphetamine and MAOIs should be avoided as MAOIs impair hepatic removal of amphetamine and potentiate its negative effects (38). Although chlorpromazine prolongs amphetamine half-life and chlordiazepoxide and diazepam increase amphetamine tissue levels, the central effects of these psychotropic medications may ameliorate the otherwise untoward behavioral correlates of amphetamine (39).

Amphetamine-like drugs   *Methylphenidate.* The amphetamine-like compound methylphenidate, a piperazine derivative of amphetamine, retains the amphetamine benzene core and ethylamine side chain (Fig. 4). In 1959, Yoss and Daly recommended it as a milder stimulant for the treatment of narcolepsy (40). Methylphenidate is almost completely absorbed after oral administration, has a half-life of approximately three hours, and is 90% excreted in the urine. It is available as a racemic mixture, but the single-isomer form (D-methylphenidate, or dexmethylphenidate) is most effective for treating hypersomnolence (32).

Methylphenidate has abuse potential and is classified as a Schedule II substance. Side effects are similar to amphetamines and include appetite suppression and weight loss, and also dose-related cardiac dysrhythmias, elevated blood pressure, and hyperthermia (41). Nevertheless, of the amphetamine-like drugs, it may have the best profile for reducing hypersomnolence, with relatively minimal tolerance, psychosis, hepatic, and cardiovascular problems. At recommended doses, its use in children does not appear to impair behavior, academic performance, or growth (42).

Pemoline. Pemoline, another amphetamine-like drug, although less effective than amphetamines, had low abuse potential, and could be taken as a single daily dose (43). Nevertheless, because of liver toxicity and rare reports of death, it is no longer routinely used (44).

Modafinil. Modafinil (2-diphenylmethylsulfinyl acetamide), a nonamphetamine, nonsympathomimetic, racemic mix of two active isomers, was specifically designed for treating hypersomnolence in narcolepsy. It is rapidly absorbed, has a half-life of 11 to 14 hours, and is primarily metabolized in the liver (45). Modafinil has replaced amphetamine-like stimulants as a first-line therapy in narcolepsy because of proven subjective and objective efficacy, relatively few cardiovascular side effects, and its low abuse potential (classified as a Schedule IV substance) (46,47).

Modafinil sites of action include the hypothalamus (anterior and lateral nuclei, and the TMN) and cingulate cortex, but its mechanism of action is not clear (47). Although α_1-adrenergic antagonists inhibit its wakefulness effects, modafinil does not bind to α_1-adrenergic receptors in vivo or have the otherwise expected anticataplectic and/or hypertensive effects (48).

Modafinil has low, but highly specific DAT binding, and does not promote wakefulness in DAT knockout mice. Nevertheless, high doses of modafinil do not produce behaviors stereotypic of dopaminergic drugs. In addition, DA inhibitors do not prevent the motor activity typically seen after large doses of modafinil (25,49,50). Although modafinil potentiates noradrenergic inhibition of sleep active neurons in the hypothalamic ventrolateral preoptic nucleus, it does not have the anticataplectic effects expected of an adrenergic agent (51,52).

Finally, serotonin antagonists can reduce GABA release and sleepiness (53). Modafinil increases striatal serotonin metabolism, resulting in reduced cortical GABA, which could theoretically disinhibit wake-promoting orexin/hypocretin neurons.

A double blind study showed 200 to 400 mg of modafinil per day significantly reduced sleepiness in narcolepsy, and was well tolerated, with headaches and nausea being the most frequent side effects (54). In animal studies, doses of modafinil greater than 800 mg/day cause less irritability, agitation, rebound hypersomnolence, and adverse blood pressure effects than amphetamines (55,56). In humans, modafinil has few negative effects on cortisol, melatonin, or growth hormone levels, and although drug tolerance and dependency are limited, there are cocaine-like reinforcing effects in animals (57,58).

REM-Related Symptoms
Narcolepsy is associated with pathologic REM sleep mechanisms, clinically evidenced as cataplexy, sleep paralysis, and hypnagogic/hypnopompic hallucinations. As such, rational treatment of these auxiliary symptoms begins with a basic understanding of the anatomy, physiology, and neurochemistry association with REM sleep, where there is a deficiency of wake-promoting neuropeptides in the lateral nucleus of the hypothalamus (59,60). These lateral nuclear peptides have been alternately named orexins/hypocretins because of

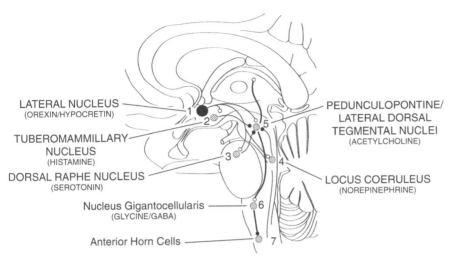

LATERAL NUCLEUS
(OREXIN/HYPOCRETIN)

TUBEROMAMMILLARY
NUCLEUS
(HISTAMINE)

DORSAL RAPHE NUCLEUS
(SEROTONIN)

Nucleus Gigantocellularis
(GLYCINE/GABA)

Anterior Horn Cells

PEDUNCULOPONTINE/
LATERAL DORSAL
TEGMENTAL NUCLEI
(ACETYLCHOLINE)

LOCUS COERULEUS
(NOREPINEPHRINE)

Figure 5 Diagrammatic representation of the brain and brainstem in the parasagittal plane showing the basic proposed mechanism and structures involved in generation of REM-sleep phenomena in narcolepsy with cataplexy. The paucity of hypocretin (orexin) cells in the lesioned lateral nucleus of the hypothalamus (1) results in a loss of what otherwise would have been wake-promoting effects on the tuberomammillary nucleus (2), the dorsal pontine raphe nucleus (3), the locus coeruleus (4), and the PPN/LDTN (5). This leaves cholinergic REM sleep-on related cells in the PPN/LDTN (5) uninhibited, allowing some of them to polysynaptically stimulate the nucleus gigantocellularis (6) (one of the medial groups of reticular nuclei in the medulla oblongata), which then causes a glycine and GABA-mediated hyperpolarization of anterior horn cells (7) in the spinal cord, resulting in atonia. Open circle, facilitatory; closed circle, inhibitory. *Abbreviation*: PPN/LDTN, pedunculopontine/lateral dorsal tegmental nucleus. *Source*: Modified from Ref. 8, Figure 1.

simultaneous discovery by different groups. The paucity of orexin/hypocretin effect results in a loss of wake promotion on the TMN, dorsal raphe (DR), LC, and PPN/LDTN (Fig. 5) (59–61).

During REM-related symptoms, there is evidence that inactivation of the DR and LC leads to disinhibition of cholinoceptive REM sleep-on cells, which function through the PPN/LDTN (61–63). REM sleep-on cells project rostrally (in the pontine reticular formation) to several thalamic nuclei with cortical relays (64). Caudally directed pathways from the PPN/LDTN to medial medullary reticular nuclei activate the nucleus gigantocellularis, which produces REM-related atonia through glycine and GABA-mediated inhibition of α–motor neurons (26,65,66).

During REM sleep, medial pontine reticular formation generates pontine-geniculo-occipital (PGO) spikes and the PPN/LDTN complex acts as their "output" to the forebrain (67). PGO spikes allowed McCarley and Hobson to propose the activation-synthesis hypothesis that correlates REM physiology to dream (68,69). PGO spikes are associated with REM, and vestibular, motor, and middle-ear-muscle phasic activity. The entire brain is made aware of this activity through a "corollary discharge system", which, according to the "isomorphism postulate," is subsequently realized as dream and the hallucinatory phenomena that may occur with cataplexy and sleep paralysis (68–70).

Amphetamine and amphetamine-like drugs. At high doses the adrenergic effects of the amphetamine and amphetamine-like drugs can reduce REM sleep–related phenomena such as cataplexy (52). This is rationalized by the fact that NET ligands can reduce REM sleep, while inhibition of noradrenergic LC cells lead to REM sleep (25). Nevertheless, the frequent side effects associated with higher doses of the amphetamines and amphetamine-like drugs often limit the usefulness of these phenomena (29).

Tricyclic antidepressants. TCAs have been the most common treatment for cataplexy. A cholinergic hypersensitivity in the pons, medial medulla, and/or basal forebrain may predispose narcoleptics to such REM-related phenomena (71). The anticataplectic effects of TCAs appear to result from their reduction of adrenergic reuptake, which leads to inhibition of the caudally directed cholinergic mesencephalic mechanisms responsible for atonia (52).

In addition, the inhibitory effects of TCAs on the cytochrome P-450 system can reduce metabolism of amphetamine/methylphenidate, allowing successful therapy using relatively low drug doses when these medicines are used in combination (72,73). Nevertheless, this could also potentiate the hypertensive, and the undesirable, behavioral effects of amphetamines. The anticholinergic effects of TCA (sedation and impotence) can also limit their utility (73).

γ-Hydroxybutyrate (sodium oxybate, Xyrem). Frequent unavoidable naps may reduce overall sleep pressure at night, leading to the frequent symptom of insomnia (74). As such, consolidating nocturnal sleep might lead to improvements in both sleepiness and cataplexy (75). This is one mechanism hypothesized for γ-hydroxybutyrate (GHB). GHB, prescribed as sodium oxybate (Xyrem), is a GABA precursor, which has been approved for treating both sleepiness and cataplexy (75,76). Nevertheless, at higher doses, there are reports of urinary incontinence in 14%, and nausea and dizziness in 33%. Historically, it has been abused as a recreational drug, is well known for an association with date rape, and has the potential for causing respiratory depression, coma, and death (77). Although GHB, as a Xyrem preparation, is classified as a Schedule III substance, its illicit use subjects an individual to the penalties for a Schedule I substance (the most restrictive schedule of the Controlled Substances Act).

Selective serotonin reuptake inhibitors (fluoxetine). Serotonin, through a complex mechanism, facilitates the onset of slow wave sleep. Some therapeutic benefits in narcolepsy with cataplexy may result from a serotonin-induced increase in total nocturnal sleep time (18,19,78). SSRIs, such as fluoxetine, can also have adrenergic effects that inhibit REM mechanisms (79,80). Nevertheless, SSRIs at higher doses often lead to side effects that limit their utility.

Monoamine oxidase inhibitors (selegiline). The AASM's Standards of Practice Committee considers selegiline as a potentially effective treatment for both sleepiness and cataplexy (21). It is a potent, irreversible MAO-B inhibitor, whose mechanism of action is probably dopaminergic, as it is metabolized to amphetamine and methamphetamine (81,82). Doses up to 30 mg provide comparable effects to D-amphetamine in reducing hypersomnolence. Although it has low abuse potential, it is not frequently used, because of expense, and side effects such as diet-induced hypertension.

Mazindol. Mazindol, an imidazoline derivative, has high affinity for DAT and NET, and the ability to block DA and NE reuptake (83). Consequently, dopaminergic and adrenergic mechanisms appear to explain mazindol's effectiveness in treating both sleepiness and cataplexy using 2 to 6 mg/day (84,85). Although it has a low abuse potential, side effects at higher doses can cause nausea, vomiting, nervousness, tremor, constipation, urinary retention, and angioneurotic edema.

Bupropion. Bupropion is an antidepressant that inhibits DA and NE reuptake and has limited serotoninergic effects (86). It has been reported to be useful in treating sleepiness in narcoleptics with atypical depression.

Recurrent Hypersomnias

The recurrent hypersomnias described in the *ICSD-2* are the Kleine-Levin syndrome (KLS) and menstrual-related hypersomnia (MRH) (1).

Kleine-Levin Syndrome

The KLS was first described by Antimoff in 1898, detailed by Willi Kleine in 1925, clearly summarized by Max Levin in 1929, and formally named the Kleine-Levin syndrome by Critchley and Hoffmann in 1942 (87). Originally described, and perhaps more common, in males, KLS is characterized by periods of hypersomnia, hyperphagia, and encephalopathy, can last several weeks, and may recur up to 10 times a year. Spells tend to improve over four years, and rarely continue after 10 to 20 years (1).

The neurologic examination (other than cognitive concomitants) and brain magnetic resonance imaging (MRI) are generally normal, but single photon emission computed tomography (SPECT) scans have shown reduced thalamic blood flow (1,88). Case reports of

KLS associated with head trauma, encephalitis, stroke, and reduced cerebrospinal fluid (CSF) orexin/hypocretin levels support autopsy evidence of hypothalamic injury (although endocrinologic studies suggesting reduced hypothalamic dopaminergic tone have been inconsistent) (89–94).

Unsatisfactory therapeutic interventions have been attempted using TCAs, SSRIs, neuroleptics, and electroconvulsive therapy. Stimulants may improve sleepiness and lithium (especially in posttraumatic KLS) may reduce the frequency, severity, and length of relapses (89,95). In one study, effective treatment of hypersomnolence was reported in five of eight patients who received lithium, and in three of eight who received carbamazepine, whereas modafinil was deemed "partially effective" in 10 patients, with a "good response" in four (96).

Menstrual-Related Hypersomnia

MRH may be a variant of KLS, with recurrent hypersomnolent episodes occurring within the first months after menarche (1,97). Episodes usually last one week and rapidly resolve after menses. MRH may relate to hormone imbalance, as oral contraceptives usually lead to prolonged remission. A suspected elevation in 5-hydroxyindolacetic acid turnover has led some investigators to consider progesterone as a treatment option (97). In a subject with low CSF 5-hydroxyindolacetic and homovanillic acid, sleepiness resolved after ovulation was inhibited, using a combination of 50 µg ethinylestradiol and 2.5 mg lynestrenol (98).

Idiopathic Hypersomnia

Bedrich Roth provided the initial criteria that distinguished idiopathic hypersomnia (IH) from narcolepsy, and sleepiness because of drug, metabolic, endocrinologic, and brain injury (99). The *ICSD*-2 describes two variants of IH; one with long sleep time, and another without long sleep time (1). Patients with long sleep time have prolonged, uninterrupted, and non-refreshing 10 to 20 hour nocturnal sleep periods, whereas in IH without long sleep time the major sleep period is greater than 6 hours and less than 10 hours.

It is a lifelong problem, with genetic concomitants, and begins relatively early in life (100). IH is due to a dysfunction of NREM sleep mechanisms, characterized by unwanted episodes of NREM onset sleep, difficulties in waking, and sleep drunkenness (100–102).

Hypothalamic dysfunction is suspected given the frequent autonomic concomitants of migraine headaches, orthostasis, syncope, and Raynaud's syndrome (103). Although CSF studies have shown normal orexin/hypocretin levels, deficiencies of histamine have been reported (104).

Traditionally, IH has been treated with similar doses of amphetamine and methylphenidate used for narcolepsy. To address morning sleep drunkenness, small doses of stimulants have been given in the evening, although successful timing of administration is problematic (103). In one study, 50% of patients given 2 mg of slow-release melatonin at bedtime reported improvements (104). The response to stimulants is variable, and relatively ineffective, often leading to the use of high doses and frequent headache, tachycardia, irritable mood, and drug tolerance.

There have been reports that modafinil can reduce subjective and objective sleepiness, with few side effects and low abuse potential (46). Some experts consider modafinil the treatment of choice and recommend an initial dose of 100 mg, gradually titrating (as needed) to a maximum of 400 mg/day (46,105).

Hypersomnia due to a Medical Condition

Medical and neurologic conditions that cause hypersomnia, through direct effects on wake/sleep mechanisms, include neurodegenerative diseases, head trauma, encephalitis, genetic disorders, stroke, and brain tumors (1,106). When cataplexy is a symptom, the diagnosis of narcolepsy because of medical condition is given.

Neurodegenerative Disorders

Subtypes of neurodegenerative disorders, typified by Parkinson's disease, includes Alzheimer's disease, and frontotemporal and Lewy body dementia (106–108). In Parkinson's disease, degeneration of dopaminergic cells in the substantia nigra and cholinergic neurons in the basal forebrain may lead to hypersomnolence.

Petit et al. warn that drug regimens for hypersomnolence in dementia must be highly individualized, and suggest an initial 2.5 mg dose of methylphenidate, with 2.5 to 5 mg increments, as needed, every three to five days, using b.i.d. (am and noon) dosing schedules (typically 5 mg q. am to 30 mg b.i.d.) (109). Modafinil can also be considered, using an initial morning dose of 100 mg, with 100 mg increments every five to seven days, in b.i.d. dosing regimens, ranging from 100 mg q. am to 400 mg/day (as 400 mg q. am, or 200 mg b.i.d.).

Posttraumatic Hypersomnia
Posttraumatic hypersomnia has been reported in mild head injury without loss of consciousness, and during recovery from posttraumatic coma [where early polysomnographic (PSG) return of normal sleep-wake cycling and sleep spindles is a good prognostic sign] (110–112). Amphetamines have been reported to improve hypersomnolence in some patients recovering from posttraumatic coma (110,112).

Genetic Disorders
Genetic disorders associated with hypersomnolence include Niemann-Pick type C disease, Norrie's disease, Prader–Willi syndrome, myotonic dystrophy, Moebius syndrome, and fragile X syndrome (1,113,114). In Niemann-Pick disease type C, sleepiness may result from hypothalamic accumulation of unesterified cholesterol and sphingolipids, and subsequent orexin/hypocretin deficiency (113). In myotonic dystrophy, loss of serotonin in the dorsal raphe nucleus and dysfunction of the hypothalamic (orexin/hypocretin) system are potential sources of sleepiness (114,115).

Stroke
Bassetti indicates that treating stroke-related hypersomnolence is difficult, but improvements have been reported in bilateral mesodiencephalic paramedian infarction using 200 mg of modafinil (116,117). In addition, the gains reported in early poststroke rehabilitation using methylphenidate (5–30 mg/day), and levodopa (100 mg/day), may in part be related to improved alertness (118,119). In hypersomnolent poststroke patients with affective concomitants, bromocriptine (20–40 mg/day) may improve sleepiness, apathy, and problematic presleep behavior (120).

Endocrine Disorders
Hypothyroidism typifies hypersomnia secondary to endocrine disorder. Hypothyroidism can cause a significant reduction in slow wave sleep that is reversible with treatment of hypothyroidism itself (121).

Hypersomnia Not due to Substance or Known Physiologic Condition
These are psychiatric conditions related to mood, personality, adjustment, and schizoaffective disorders (1). Clinical and pathologic subtypes include hypersomnia associated with a major depressive episode (atypical depression and bipolar type II disorder) and conversion disorder (or as an undifferentiated somatoform disorder). Treatment of these disorders is often based on aggressively addressing the primary psychiatric diagnosis and utilizing behavioral therapies.

NONPHARMACOLOGIC THEORY

Behavioral Therapy
Good sleep hygiene is a mandatory part of treating hypersomnolence. It is a positive set of habitual sleep-related behaviors that involve exercise, appropriate diet (in regard to meal size, frequency, and composition), regular sleep-wake schedules, and a proper sleep environment (with optimal dark-light contrast and temperature and noise level control). Good sleep hygiene utilizes behavioral interventions that include cognitive, sleep restriction, stimulus control, and relaxation therapies (122). Specific strategies vary with diagnosis, symptom severity, health-related factors, and individual patient goals.

Formal individualized counseling can minimize the overall impact of sleepiness, while maximizing an individual's strengths. Great benefits in home, academic, and occupational settings can be derived by learning a priority system to develop an organized, highly structured daily routine with well-defined and reasonably attainable goals, while avoiding monotonous and potentially hazardous tasks that include evening, night, shifting, and 24-hour work schedules.

Behaviorally Induced Insufficient Sleep Syndrome
The behaviorally induced insufficient sleep syndrome is due to voluntary, but unintentional, chronic sleep deprivation (1). Patients are preoccupied with presumed etiologies (other than insufficient sleep) and symptoms of irritability, malaise, and poor concentration. The treatment goal of longer nocturnal sleep is achieved using cognitive therapy to change faulty beliefs and attitudes about sleep and to prevent excessive monitoring of symptoms.

Treatment options also include restriction of time in bed to actual sleeping time. Initially, mild sleep deprivation leads to more efficient/consolidated nocturnal sleep. Patients who nap frequently can have difficulty initiating sleep restriction therapy (123). A single 10- to 20-minute nap, taken 12 hours after waking, can reduce hypersomnolence, with minimal negative effects on nocturnal sleep in some individuals (124).

Narcolepsy
In narcolepsy, naps completed immediately prior to planned activities can have a synergistic effect with medications (125). Short, 20-minute naps can provide up to 2 hours of refractory wakefulness. It can be difficult to awaken from longer naps that extend into NREM N3 (formerly stages 3 and 4) sleep, as the effects of sleep inertia, evidenced as reduced alertness, confusional arousals, and sleep drunkenness, can last for several hours (126).

Insomnia, intrinsic to disorders such as narcolepsy, can predispose to negative conditioning (learning to associate the bed with expectations of poor sleep). Stimulus control therapy can be used to associate the bedroom with good sleep expectations, by teaching avoidance of negative thoughts/activities in bed, going to bed only when sleepy, and getting out of bed when unable to sleep for any prolonged period of time.

Disorders such as narcolepsy and IH have been associated with endogenous depression and secondary mood disorders (because of factors such as social isolation) (127,128). Behavioral approaches may be helpful when combined with pharmacologic treatments and psychotherapeutic techniques to address depression (103). Relaxation therapy can help manage the stress that can reduce deep sleep, while improving mood and concentration (124). Stress management may also reduce the anxiety that can act as a trigger for cataplexy.

Hypersomnias due to Drug or Substance
Hypersomnias due to drug or substance include abuse and cessation of stimulants and sedative-hypnotic drugs (1). Although treatment is centered on withdrawal from offending agents, aggressively addressing psychosocial issues is critical for long-term success.

Bright Light Therapy
Seasonal Affective Disorder
Hypersomnia associated with seasonal affective disorder (SAD) is characterized by increased appetite, weight gain, and depression. SAD is related to elevated melatonin levels secondary to seasonal reduction in sunlight exposure to retinohypothalamic pathways (1). A single, 30- to 40-minute session of bright light therapy [BLT, sitting 1 foot from a box utilizing white, fluorescent light, with ultraviolet (UV) wavelengths filtered out, at an illuminance of 10,000 lux], upon awakening, has shown a remission rate in up to 75% of patients studied (129,130). Therapeutic melatonin suppression is afforded with a raised, and downward-tilting light source (illuminating the lower retina), which also allows for comfortable reading and desk work (131).

For patients who are initially unable to awaken at a desired time, treatment can start at their habitual waking time, and gradually be moved to their desired waking time as therapy takes effect (132). Studies using BLT in nonseasonal depression suggest that a therapeutic response should be appreciated within the first week of treatment (133).

Oculoretinal damage has not been reported in patients who are not on medications and have normal oculoretinal examinations (134). Nevertheless, UV, short-wavelength visible light up to 500 nm, and infrared illumination can damage the cornea, lens, and retina. Adverse retinal effects can also be exacerbated by concomitant use of some antidepressants, antipsychotics, antiarrhythmics, and antibiotics. An ophthalmologic examination should precede BLT, as evidence of retinal disease may be a contraindication for therapy (135). In addition, studies using BLT in nonseasonal depression suggest hypomania as another potential side effect (133).

EQUIPMENT

Sleep Diary and the Epworth Sleepiness Scale

Successful therapy can be qualified and quantified by comparing introspective measures of sleepiness, using tools such as a sleep diary and the Epworth Sleepiness Scale (ESS), before and after treatment (Figs. 6 and 7) (136,137). The ESS is a short and simple self-report scale of

	Mon. a.m.	Tues. a.m.	Wed. a.m.	Thurs. a.m.	Fri. a.m.	Sat. a.m.	Sun. a.m.
1. What time did you go to bed last night?							
2. How many minutes did it take you to fall asleep?							
3. How many times did you wake up?							
4. How many total minutes did the awakenings keep you awake?							
5. What time did you wake up?							
6. What time did you get out of bed?							
Please use Wakefulness key below to answer the following questions:	Mon. p.m.	Tues. p.m.	Wed. p.m.	Thurs. p.m.	Fri. p.m.	Sat. p.m.	Sun. p.m.
1. How awake were you in the morning?							
2. How awake were you in the afternoon?							
3. How awake were you in the evening?							
4. Did you nap today? When and for how long?							

Level of Wakefulness key:

1 - Very sleepy
2 – Fairly sleepy
3 – Mix of sleepy and alert feelings
4 – Fairly alert
5 – Very alert

Figure 6   Example of a typical week-at-a-glance sleep diary. *Source*: From Ref. 136.

THE EPWORTH SLEEPINESS SCALE

Name: _____

Today's date: _____ Your age (years): _____

Your sex (male = M; female = F): _____

How likely are you to doze off or fall asleep in the following situations, in contrast to feeling just tired? This refers to your usual way of life in recent times. Even if you have not done some of these things recently try to work out how they would have affected you. Use the following scale to choose the *most appropriate number* for each situation:

0 = would *never* doze
1 = *slight* chance of dozing
2 = *moderate* change of dozing
3 = *high* chance of dozing

Situation	Chance of dozing
Sitting and reading	_____
Watching TV	_____
Sitting, inactive in a public place (e.g. a theater or a meeting)	_____
As a passenger in a car for an hour without a break	_____
Lying down to rest in the afternoon when circumstances permit	_____
Sitting and talking to someone	_____
Sitting quietly after a lunch without alcohol	_____
In a car, while stopped for a few minutes in the traffic	_____

Thank you for your cooperation

Figure 7 The Epworth Sleepiness Scale. *Source*: From Ref. 137.

---

sleepiness that correlates with the multiple sleep latency test (MSLT) and is useful in determining treatment efficacy (137–139).

The Maintenance of Wakefulness Test

The maintenance of wakefulness test (MWT) is an MSLT variant that is performed while the patient attempts to maintain wakefulness. The MWT provides an objective measure of treatment efficacy that may more accurately translate to a work situation when compared with the MSLT (140). The AASM Standards of Practice Committee recommends the MWT begin two hours after awakening from overnight sleep (141). It consists of four, 40-minute naps; each nap separated from the next by a 2-hour interval. A mean sleep latency less than eight minutes is abnormal, whereas values between 8 and 40 minutes are of uncertain value.

The use of an MWT has been approved in some occupations where sleepiness is hazardous, to justify a change in employment, and to support disability (142–144). No sleep is the strongest evidence for a patient's ability to maintain wakefulness; nevertheless, Mitler et al. warn that a "normal" MWT does not necessarily guarantee safety in regard to hypersomnolence (145).

Brain Imaging and Electroencephalography

In some hypersomnias, because of a medical condition, imaging of the brain and routine EEG may be of prognosticating value. In posttraumatic coma with hypersomnolence, radiographic evidence of hydrocephalus predicts poor treatment response (112). In Alzheimer's disease, clinical progression, secondary to degeneration of cholinergic neurons in the basal forebrain, often correlates with EEG loss of sleep spindles, slow waves, and REM sleep patterns (146).

ADJUNCTIVE AND ALTERNATIVE THERAPY

Caffeine

Caffeine was chemically defined in 1819, and has been utilized in the form of coffee to treat general sleepiness since the 1600s (147). It is used daily by up to 85% of Americans to address morning sleep inertia (148,149). Caffeine is a xanthine derivative that inhibits sleep by blocking adenosine A_1 receptors (150). Adenosine, a degradation product of adenosine triphosphate, inhibits cholinergic neurons in the brainstem, thalamus, and basal forebrain and induces slow wave sleep (151). Caffeine's site of action is believed to be the basal forebrain, as adenosine levels are elevated here after prolonged sleep deprivation.

Caffeine has a half-life from 3 to 5 hours, with peak blood levels reached 30 to 60 minutes after oral intake (152). It delays sleep onset and reduces delta sleep, total sleep time, and sleep efficiency. Six cups of strong coffee has similar wakefulness effects as 5 mg of dextroamphetamine, and in young, healthy sleep-deprived people, 600 mg of caffeine has similar effects to 400 mg of modafinil in improving performance (153,154).

For doses greater than 4 mg/kg, caffeine can lead to nausea, diarrhea, cramps, nervousness, and insomnia (152,155). Moderate to heavy coffee use has been associated with bladder cancer, irritable bowel syndrome, exacerbation of fibrocystic breast disease, and possible cardiovascular risks. Fatalities using greater than 10 g in enema formulations have occurred. Sudden withdrawal, after regimens as low as 235 mg/day, can lead to headache, reduced mood, and sleepiness (156). Rapid development of tolerance makes caffeine ineffective for chronic treatment of many disorders of hypersomnolence, including narcolepsy and IH (152).

FUTURE RESEARCH

Potential Therapies
Orexin/Hypocretin
Hypersomnia associated with hypothalamic dysfunction and orexin/hypocretin levels less than 110 pg/mL (or 30% of controls) has been reported in narcolepsy, and many medical and neurologic conditions, including infections, sarcoidosis, paraneoplastic syndromes, head trauma, brain tumors, multiple sclerosis, and dementia (1,92,113,114,157–159). In narcoleptic animals, central and systemic administration of orexin/hypocretin can normalize sleep-wake patterns and prevent cataplectic-like events (160,161).

Fetal Transplantation
Symptoms produced in animals by lesioning the preoptic area of the hypothalamus can also be reversed by transplantation of healthy fetal tissue (162). In addition, lateral hypothalamic, orexin/hypocretin containing cells from newborn rats have shown long-term viability when injected into the pontine reticular formation of adult animals (163).

Immunization
The high association of specific human leukocyte class II antigens in narcolepsy with cataplexy (subtype allele DQB1*0602) and KLS (reports of significantly greater DQB1*0201 homozygosity compared to controls) suggests that a genetic predisposition to autoimmune disease may be an etiologic factor in a variety of hypersomnolence disorders (164–166). Abnormal genetic coding in orexin/hypocretin systems may predispose to virally mediated alterations, leaving the lateral hypothalamus prone to autoimmune injury.

Histaminergics and Thyrotropin-Releasing Hormone
A deficiency of histamine in narcolepsy may lead to a relative denervation hypersensitivity of inhibitory H_3 autoreceptors (166). Although central injection of histamine and H_1 agonists promote wakefulness, side effects are prohibitive. Nevertheless, an H_3 antagonist, thioperamide, has been found to produce significant wakefulness in narcoleptic mice (167).

Finally, canine studies suggest thyrotropin-releasing hormone and its analogues have the potential to significantly increase wakefulness and decrease cataplexy in narcolepsy (168,169).

CONCLUSIONS

Rational treatment regimens for the hypersomnias of central origin are based on understanding the normal anatomy, physiology, and neurochemistry of central wake/sleep mechanisms. Dysfunction localized to the hypothalamus, brainstem, thalamus, and cortex has led to pharmacologic interventions based on deficits in endogenous monoaminergic, cholinergic, and orexin/hypocretin systems. In addition, a synergistic treatment efficacy is afforded through the judicious incorporation of a variety of behavioral therapeutic techniques. Strong consideration must also be given to problems that might arise secondary to medication side effects, and other concomitant medical, neurologic, psychologic, and primary sleep disorders.

In the future, for patients poorly responsive to routine therapeutic interventions, specific fetal neuronal transplantations may prove beneficial. Finally, recent research has allowed the hypothesis that some disorders of hypersomnolence may result from a genetic predisposition to autoimmune disease (164–166). It is possible that aberrant genetic coding of elements in the orexin/hypocretin system allows a susceptibility to inducible, possibly virally mediated changes, leaving cells in the hypothalamus susceptible to autoimmune attack. In the future, genetic screening of high-risk individuals might also justify treatment regimens, which include prophylactic immunosuppression.

REFERENCES

1. American Academy of Sleep Medicine, . International Classification of Sleep Disorders: Diagnostic and Coding Manual. 2nd ed. Westchester: American Academy of Sleep Medicine, 2005:79–115.
2. Bremer F. Cerveau "isole" et physiologie du sommeil. C R Soc Biol (Paris) 1929; 102:1235.
3. Moruzzi G, Magoun HW. Brain stem reticular formation and activation of the EEG. Electro-encephalogr Clin Neurophysiol 1949; 1:455.
4. Jovet M. The role of monoamines and acetylcholine-containing neurons in the regulation of the sleep-waking cycle. Ergebn Physiol 1972; 64:165.
5. Sherin JE, Elmquist JK, Torrealba F, et al. Innervation of histaminergic tuberomammillary neurons by GABAergic and galaninergic neurons in the ventrolateral preoptic nucleus of the rat. J Neurosci 1998; 18:4705–4721.
6. Aston-Jones G, Chiang C, Alexinsky T. Discharge of noradrenergic locus coeruleus neurons in behaving rats and monkeys suggests a role in vigilance. Prog Brain Res 1991; 88:501–520.
7. Woolf NJ, Butcher LL. Cholinergic systems in the rat brain: III. Projections from the pontomesencephalic tegmentum to the thalamus, tectum, basal ganglia, and basal forebrain. Brain Res Bull 1986; 16:603–637.
8. Dyken ME, Yamada T. Narcolepsy and disorders of excessive somnolence. In: Ballard RD, Lee-Chiong TL Jr, eds. Primary Care: Clinics in Office Practice. Philadelphia: Elsevier Saunders, 2005: 389–413.
9. Saper CB, Chou TC, Scammel TE. The sleep switch: hypothalamic control of sleep and wakefulness. Trends Neurosci 2001; 24:726–731.
10. Von Economo C. Encephalitis Lethargica: Its Sequelae and Treatment. London: Oxford University Press, 1931.
11. Sherin JE, Shiromani PJ, McCarley RW, et al. Activation of ventrolateral preoptic neurons during sleep. Science 1996; 271:216–219.
12. Steininger T, Gong H, McGinty D, et al. Subregional organization of preoptic area/anterior hypothalamic projections to arousal-related monoaminergic cell groups. J Comp Neurol 2001; 429:638–653.
13. Gritti I, Mariotti M, Mancia M. Gabaergic and cholinergic basal forebrain and preoptic-anterior hypothalamic projections to the mediodorsal nucleus of the thalamus of the cat. Neuroscience 1998; 85:149–178.
14. Nitz D, Siegel JM. GABA release in the dorsal raphe nucleus. Role in the control of REM sleep. Am J Physiol 1997; 273:R451–R455.
15. Nitz D, Siegel JM. GABA release in the locus coeruleus as a function of sleep/wake state. Neuroscience 1997; 78:795–801.
16. Steriade M, Domich L, Oakson G, et al. The deafferented reticular thalamic nucleus generates spindle rhythmicity. J Neurophysiol 1987; 57:260–273.
17. Ricardo JA, Koh ET. Anatomical evidence of direct projections from the nucleus of the solitary tract to the hypothalamus, amygdala, and other forebrain structures in the rat. Brain Res 1978; 153:1.
18. Markand ON, Dyken ML. Sleep abnormalities in patients with brain stem lesions. Neurology 1976; 26:769.
19. McGinty D, Harper R. Dorsal raphe neurons: depression of firing during sleep in cats. Brain Res 1976; 101:569–575.
20. Littner M, Johnson SF, McCall MV, et al. Standards of Practice Committee. Practice parameters for the treatment of narcolepsy: an update for 2000. Sleep 2001; 24(4):451–466.

21. Morgenthaler TI, Kapur VK, Brown T, et al. Practice parameters for the treatment of narcolepsy and other hypersomnias of central origin. Sleep 2007; 30:1705–1711.
22. Doyle JB, Daniels LE. Symptomatic treatment for narcolepsy. JAMA 1931; 96:1370–1372.
23. Prinzmetal M, Bloomberg W. The use of benzedrine for the treatment of narcolepsy. JAMA 1935; 105:2051–2054.
24. Alles GA. The comparative physiological actions of d 1-beta-phenylisopropylamines: pressor effects and toxicity. J Pharmacol Exp Ther 1933; 47:339–354.
25. Nishino S, Mao J, Sampathkumaran R, et al. Increased dopaminergic transmission mediates the wake-promoting effects of CNS stimulants. Sleep Res Online 1998; 1:49–61.
26. Afifi AK, Bergman RA. Reticular formation, wakefulness, and sleep. In: Afifi AK, Bergman RA, eds. Functional Neuroanatomy: Text and Atlas. 2nd ed. New York: McGraw-Hill Medical, 2005: 398–406.
27. Kaelber WW, Afifi AK. Nigro-amygdaloid fiber connections in the cat. Am J Anat 1977; 148: 129–135.
28. Nissbrandt N, Engberg G, Pileblad E. The effects of GBR 12909, a dopamine re-uptake inhibitor, on monoaminergic neurotransmission in rat striatum, limbic forebrain, cortical hemispheres, and substantia nigra. Naunyn Schmiedebergs Arch Pharmacol 1991; 344:16–28.
29. Kuczenski R, Segal DS. Neurochemistry of amphetamine. In: Cho AD, Segel DS, eds. Psychopharmacology, Toxicology, and Abuse. San Diego: Academic Press, 1994:81–113.
30. Sulzer D, Chen TK, Lau YY, et al. Amphetamine redistributes dopamine from synaptic vesicles to the cytosol and promotes reverse transport. J Neurosci 1995; 15:4102–4108.
31. Gonzalez AM, Walther D, Pazos A, et al. Synaptic vesicular monoamine transporter expression: distribution and pharmacologic profile. Brain Res Mol Brain Res 1994; 22:219–226.
32. Kanbayashi T, Nishino S, Honda K, et al. Differential effects of D- and L-amphetamine isomers on dopminergic transmission: implication for the control of alertness in canine narcolepsy. Sleep Res 1997; 26:383.
33. Fujimori M, Himwich HE. Electroencephalographic analyses of amphetamine and its methoxy derivatives with reference to their sites of EEG alerting in the rabbit brain. Int J Neuropharmacol 1969; 8:601–613.
34. Mitler MM, Erman M, Hajdukovic R. The treatment of excessive somnolence with stimulant drugs. Sleep 1993; 16:203–206.
35. Seiden L, Sabol KE, Ricaurte GA. Amphetamine: effects on catecholamine systems and behavior. Annu Rev Pharmacol Toxicol 1993; 32:639–667.
36. Virmani A, Gaetani F, Imam S, et al. The protective role of L-carnitine against neurotoxicity evoked by drug of abuse, methamphetamine, could be related to mitochondrial dysfunction. Ann N Y Acad Sci 2002; 965:225–232.
37. Mitler MM, Hajdukovic RM. Relative efficacy of drugs for the treatment of sleepiness in narcolepsy. Sleep 1991; 14:218–220.
38. Nishino S, Mignot E. Wake-promoting medications: basic mechanisms and pharmacology. In: Kryger MH, Roth T, Dement WC, eds. Principles and Practice of Sleep Medicine. 4th ed. Philadelphia: Elsevier Saunders, 2005:468–483.
39. Parkes JD. Central nervous system stimulant drugs. In: Thorpy M, ed. Handbook of Sleep Disorders. New York: Marcel Dekker, 1990:755–778.
40. Yoss RE, Daly DD. Treatment of narcolepsy with Ritalin. Neurology 1959; 9:171–173.
41. Honda Y, Hishakawa Y, Takahashi Y. Long-term treatment of narcolepsy with methylphenidate (Ritalin). Curr Ther Res Clin Exp 1979; 25:288–298.
42. Klein RG, Mannuzza S. Hyperactive boys almost grown up. III. Methylphenidate effects on ultimate height. Arch Gen Psychiatry 1988; 45:1131–1134.
43. Honda Y, Hishikawa Y. Effectivenes of pemoline in narcolepsy. Sleep Res 1970; 8:192.
44. Nehra A, Mullick F, Ishak KG, et al. Pemoline-associated hepatic injury. Gastroenterology 1990; 99:1517–1519.
45. Robertson P, DeCory HH, Madan A, et al. In vitro inhibition and induction of human hepatic cytochrome P450 enzymes by modafinil. Drug Metab Dispos 2000; 28:664–671.
46. Bastuji H, Jovet M. Successful treatment of idiopathic hypersomnia and narcolepsy with modafinil. Prog Neuropsychopharmacol Biol Psychiatry 1988; 12:695–700.
47. Saper CB, Scammell TE. Modafinil: a drug in search of a mechanism. Sleep 2004; 27:11–12.
48. Duteil J, Rambert FA, Pessonnier J, et al. Central α 1-adrenergic stimulation in relation to the behaviour stimulating effect of modafinil: studies with experimental animals. Eur J Pharmacol 1990; 180:49–58.
49. Mignot E, Nishino S, Guilleminault C, et al. Modafinil binds to the dopamine uptake carrier site with low affinity. Sleep 1994; 17:436–437.

50. Simon P, Hemet C, Ramassamy C, et al. Non-amphetaminic mechanisms of stimulant locomotor effect of modafinil in mice. Eur Neuropsychopharmacol 1995; 5:509–514.
51. Gallopin T, Luppi PH, Rambert FA, et al. Effect of the wake-promoting agent modafinil on sleep-promoting neurons from the ventrolateral preoptic nucleus: an in vitro pharmacologic study. Sleep 2004; 27:19–25.
52. Mignot E, Renaud A, Nishinao S, et al. Canine cataplexy is preferentially controlled by adrenergic mechanisms: evidence using monoamine selective uptake inhibitors and release enhancers. Psychopharmacology 1993; 113:76–82.
53. Tanganelli S, Fuxe K, Ferraro L, et al. Inhibitory effects of the psychoactive drug modafinil on gamma-aminobutyric acid outflow from the cerebral cortex of the awake freely moving guinea pig. Arch Pharmacol 1992; 345:461–465.
54. U.S. Modafinil in Narcolepsy Multicenter Study Group, . Randomized trial of modafinil for the treatment of pathological somnolence in narcolepsy. Ann Neurol 1998; 43:88–97.
55. Edgard DM, Seidel WF. Modafinil induces wakefulness without intensifying motor activity or subsequent rebound hypersomnolence in the rat. J Pharmacol Exp Ther 1997; 283:757–769.
56. Hermant JF, Rambert FA, Deuteil J. Lack of cardiovascular effects after administration of modafinil in conscious monkeys. Fundam Clin Pharmacol 1991; 5:825.
57. Brun J, Chamba G, Khalfallah Y, et al. Effect of modafinil on plasma melatonin, cortisol and growth hormone rhythms, rectal temperature and performance in healthy subjects during a 36 h sleep deprivation. J Sleep Res 1998; 7:105–114.
58. Gold LH, Balster RH. Evaluation of the cocaine-like discriminative stimulus effects and reinforcing effects of modafinil. Psychopharmacology 1996; 126:286–292.
59. Nishino S, Ripley B, Overeem S, et al. Hypocretin (orexin) deficiency in human narcolepsy. Lancet 2000; 355:39–40.
60. Sakurai T, Amemiya A, Ishii M, et al. Orexins and orexin receptors: a family of hypothalamic neuropeptides and G protein-coupled receptors that regulate feeding behavior. Cell 1998; 92:573–583.
61. Peyron C, Tighe DK, van den Pol AN, et al. Neurons containing hypocretin (orexin) project to multiple neuronal systems. J Neurosci 1998; 18:9996–10015.
62. Aston-Jones G, Chiang C, Alexinsky T. Discharge of noradrenergic locus coeruleus neurons in behaving rats and monkeys suggests a role in vigilance. Prog Brain Res 1991; 88:501–520.
63. McGinty DJ, Harper R. Dorsal raphe neurons: depression of firing during sleep in cats. Brain Res 1976; 101:569–575.
64. Sakai K, Koyama Y. Are there cholinergic and non-cholinergic paradoxical sleep-on neurons in pons? Neuroreport 1996; 7:2449–2453.
65. Sakai K, Sastre JP, Salvert D, et al. Tegmentoreticular projections with special reference to the muscular atonia during paradoxical sleep in cat: an HRP study. Brain Res 1979; 176:233–254.
66. Kodama T, Lai YY, Siegel JM. Enhancement of acetylcholine release during REM sleep in the caudomedial medulla as measured by in vivo microdialysis. Brain Res 1992; 580:348–350.
67. Vertes RP. Brain stem generation of hippocampal EEG. Prog Neurobiol 1982; 19:159–186.
68. Hobson JA, McCarley RW, Pivik RT, et al. Selective firing by cat pontine brain stem neurons in desynchronized sleep. J Neurophysiol 1974; 37:497–511.
69. Hobson JA, McCarley RW. The brain as a dream state generator: an activation-synthesis hypothesis of the dream process. Am J Psychiatry 1977; 134:1335–1348.
70. Hong CC, Potkin SG, Antrobus JS, et al. REM sleep eye movement counts correlate with visual dream imagery in dreaming: a pilot study. Psychophysiology 1997; 34:377–381.
71. Kilduff TS, Bowersox SS, Kaitin KI, et al. Muscarinic cholinergic receptors and the canine model of narcolepsy. Sleep 1986; 9:102–106.
72. Burrell JM, Black M, Wharton RN, et al. Inhibition of imipramine metabolism by methylphenidate. Fed Proc 1969; 28:418.
73. Carlton PL. Potentiation of the behavioral effects of amphetamines by imipramine. Psychopharmacologia 1961; 2:364–376.
74. Harsh J, Pezka J, Hartwig G, et al. Night-time sleep and daytime sleepiness in narcolepsy. J Sleep Res 2000; 9:309–316.
75. Mamelak M, Black J, Montplaisir J, et al. A pilot study on the effects of sodium oxybate on sleep architecture and daytime alertness in narcolepsy. Sleep 2004; 27:1327–1334.
76. Cook H. A randomized, double blind, placebo-controlled multicenter trial comparing the effects of three doses of orally administered sodium oxybate with placebo for the treatment of narcolepsy. Sleep 2002; 25:42–49.
77. Spillane J, Camejo M. GHB overdoses and deaths in south Florida. In: Community Epidemiology Work Group. Epidemiologic Trends in Drug Abuse. Vol. 2. Rockville: National Institute on Drug Abuse, 1998:432–436. (NIH publication no. 99-4527.)

78. Autret A, Minz M, Beillevaire T, et al. Clinical and polygraphic effects of d.1 5 HTP on narcolepsy-cataplexy. Biomedicine 1977; 27:200–203.

79. Montplaisir J, Godbout R. Serotoninergic reuptake mechanisms in the control of cataplexy. Sleep 1986; 9:280–284.

80. Frey J, Darbonne C. Fluoxetine suppresses human cataplexy: a pilot study. Neurology 1994; 44: 707–709.

81. Hublin C, Partinen M, Heinonen EH, et al. Selegiline in the treatment of narcolepsy. Neurology 1994; 44:2095–2101.

82. Reynolds GP, Elsworth JD, Blau K, et al. Deprenyl is metabolized to methamphetamine and amphetamine in man. Br J Clin Pharmacol 1978; 6:542–544.

83. Wallace AG. AN 448 Sandoz (mazindol) in the treatment of obesity. Med J Aust 1976; 1:343.

84. Vespignani H, Barroche G, Escaillas JP, et al. Importance of mazindol in the treatment of narcolepsy. Sleep 1984; 7:274–275.

85. Iijima S, Sugita Y, Teshima Y, et al. Therapeutic effects of mazindol on narcolepsy. Sleep 1986; 9: 265–268.

86. Rye DB, Dihenia B, Bliwise DL. Reveral of atypical depression, sleepiness, and REM-sleep propensity in narcolepsy with buproprion. Depress Anxiety 1998; 7:92–95.

87. Afifi AK, Bergman RA. Reticular formation, wakefulness, and sleep: clinical correlates. In: Afifi AK, Bergman RA, eds. Functional Neuroanatomy: Text and Atlas. 2nd ed. New York: McGraw-Hill Medical, 2005:407–410.

88. Huang YS, Guilleminault C, Kao PF, et al. SPECT findings in the Kleine-Levin syndrome. Sleep 2005; 28:955–960.

89. Gill RG, Young JPR, Thomas DJ. Kleine-Levin syndrome. Report of two cases with onset of symptoms precipitated by head trauma. Br J Psychiatry 1988; 152:410–412.

90. Fenzi F, Simonati A, Crosato F, et al. Clinical features of Kleine-Levin syndrome with localized encephalitis. Neuropediatrics 1993; 24(5):292–295.

91. Drake ME. Kleine-Levine syndrome after multiple cerebral infarctions. Psychosomatics 1987; 28: 329–333.

92. Dauvilliers Y, Baumann CR, Carlander B, et al. CSF hypocretin-1 levels in narcolepsy, Kleine-Levin syndrome, and other hypersomnias and neurological conditions. J Neurol Neurosurg Psychiatry 2003; 74:1667–1673.

93. Chesson AL Jr, Levine SN, Kong LS, et al. Neuroendocrine evaluation in Kleine-Levin syndrome: evidence of reduced dopaminergic tone during periods of hypersomnolence. Sleep 1991; 14(3): 226–232.

94. Mayer G, Leonhard E, Krieg J, et al. Endocrinological and polysomnographic findings in Kleine-Levin syndrome: no evidence for hypothalamic and circadian dysfunction. Sleep 1998; 21:278–284.

95. Poppe M, Friebel D, Reuner U, et al. The Kleine-Levin syndrome: effects of treatment with lithium. Neuropediatrics 2003; 34,113–119.

96. Dauvilliers Y, Mayer G, Lecendreux M, et al. Kleine-Levin syndrome; An autoimmune hypothesis based on clinical and genetic analyses. Neurology 2002; 59:1739–1745.

97. Billiard M, Guilleminault C, Dement, WC. A menstruation-linked periodic hypersomnia. Kleine-Levin syndrome or new clinical entity? Neurology 1975; 25:436–443.

98. Sachs C, Persson HE, Hagenfeldt K. Menstrual-related periodic hypersomnia: a case study with successful treatment. Neurology 1982; 32:1376–1379.

99. Roth B. On the dissociation of sleep inhibition. Neurol Psychiat Ceskoslov 1954; 17:18–26 (in Czech).

100. Poirier G, Montplaisir J, Decary F, et al. HLA antigens in narcolepsy and idiopathic central nervous system hypersomnolence. Sleep 1986; 9:153–158.

101. Roth B, Bruhova s, Lehovsky M. REM sleep and NREM sleep in narcolepsy and hypersomnia. Electroencephalogr Clin Neurophysiol 1969; 26:176–182.

102. Roth B, Nevsimalova S, Rechtschaffen A. Hypersomnia with "sleep drunkenness." Arch Gen Psychiatry 1972; 26:456–462.

103. Bassetti C, Aldrich MS. Idiopathic hypersomnia. A series of 42 patients. Brain 1997; 120:1423–1435.

104. Billiard M, Dauvillier Y. Idiopathic hypersomnia. Sleep Med Rev 2001; 5:351–360.

105. Bassetti C, Pelayo R, Guilleminault C. Idiopathic Hypersomnia. In: Kryger MH, Roth T, Dement WC, eds. Principles and Practice of Sleep Medicine. 4th ed. Philadelphia: Elsevier Saunders, 2005:791–800.

106. Arnulf I, Konofal E, Merino-Andreu M, et al. Parkinson's disease and sleepiness: an integral part of PD. Neurology 2002; 58:1019–1024.

107. Harper DG, Stopa EG, McKee AC, et al. Differential circadian rhythm disturbances in men with Alzheimer disease and frontotemporal degeneration. Arch Gen Psychiatry 2001; 58:353–360.

108. Grace JB, Walker MP, McKeith IG. JA comparison of sleep profiles in patients with dementia with Lewy bodies and Alzheimer's disease. Int J Geriatr Psychiatry 2000; 15:1028–1033.

109. Petit D, Montplaisir J, Boeve BF. Alzheimer's disease and other dementias. In: Kryger MH, Roth T, Dement WC, eds. Principles and Practice of Sleep Medicine. 4th ed. Philadelphia: Elsevier Saunders, 2005:853–862.
110. Culebras A. Other neurological disorders. In: Kryger MH, Roth T, Dement WC, eds. Principles and Practice of Sleep Medicine. 4th ed. Philadelphia: Elsevier Saunders, 2005:879–888.
111. Ron S, Algom D, Hary D, et al. Time-related changes in the distribution of sleep stages in brain-injured patients. Electroencephalogr Clin Neurophysiol 1980; 48:432–441.
112. Guilleminault C. Post-traumatic hypersomnia. Course 3AS.007. 52nd Annual Meeting of the American Academy of Neurology, San Diego, California, 2000.
113. Vankova J, Stepanova I, Jech R, et al. Sleep disturbances and hypocretin deficiency in Niemann-Pick disease type C. Sleep 2003; 26:427–430.
114. Martinez-Rodriguez JE, Lin L, Iranzo A, et al. Decreased hypocretin-1 (Orexin-A) levels in the cerebrospinal fluid of patients with myotonic dystrophy and excessive daytime sleepiness. Sleep 2003; 26:287–290.
115. Ono S, Takahashi K, Jinnai K, et al. Loss of serotonin-containing neurons in the raphe of patients with myotonic dystrophy: a quantitative immunohistochemical study and relation to hypersomnia. Neurology 1998; 50:535–538.
116. Bassetti CL. Sleep and stroke. In: Kryger MH, Roth T, Dement WC, eds. Principles and Practice of Sleep Medicine. 4th ed. Philadelphia: Elsevier Saunders, 2005:811–830.
117. Bastuji H, Nighoghossian N, Salord F, et al. Mesodiencephalic infarct with hypersomnia: sleep recording in two cases. J Sleep Res 1994; 3(suppl 1):16.
118. Grade C, Redford B, Chrostowski J, et al. Methylphenidate in early poststroke recovery. A double-blind, placebo-controlled study. Arch Phys Med Rehab 1998; 79:1047–1050.
119. Scheidtmann K, Fries W, Muller F, et al. Effect of levodopa in combination with physiotherapy on functional recovery after stroke: a prospective, randomized, double-blind study. Lancet 2001; 358:787–790.
120. Catsman-Berrevoets CE, Harskamp F. Compulsive pre-sleep behavior and apathy due to bilateral thalamic stroke. Neurology 1988; 38:647–649.
121. Ruiz-Primo E, Jurado JL, Solis H, et al. Polysomnographic effects of thyroid hormones in primary myxedema. Electroencephalogr Clin Neurophysiol 1982; 53:559–564.
122. Morin CM. Psychological and behavioral treatments for primary insomnia. In: Kryger MH, Roth T, Dement WC, eds. Principles and Practice of Sleep Medicine. 4th ed. Philadelphia: Elsevier Saunders, 2005:726–737.
123. Bonnet MH, Balkin TJ, Dinges DF, et al. The use of stimulants to modify performance during sleep loss: a review by the Sleep Deprivation and Stimulant Task Force of the American Academy of Sleep Medicine. Sleep 2005; 28:1163–1187.
124. Jacobs GD. Establishing sleep-promoting habits. In: Brown T, ed. Say Good Night to Insomnia. New York: Henry Holt, 1998:97.
125. Rogers AE, Aldrich MS, Lin X. A comparison of three different sleep schedules for reducing daytime sleepiness in narcolepsy. Sleep 2001; 24:385–391.
126. Achermann P, Werth E, Dijk DJ, et al. Time course of sleep inertia after nighttime and daytime sleep episodes. Arch Ital Biol 1995; 134:109–119.
127. Honda Y, Asaka A, Tanimura M, et al. A genetic study of narcolepsy and excessive daytime sleepiness in 308 families with a narcolepsy or hypersomia proband. In: Guilleminault C, Lugaresi E, eds. Sleep/Wake Disorders: Natural History, Epidemiology, and Long-Term Evolution. New York: Raven Press, 1983:187–198.
128. Guilleminault C, Pelayo R. Idiopathic central nervous system hypersomnia. In: Kryger MH, Roth T, Dement WC, eds. Principles and Practice of Sleep Medicine. 3rd ed. Philadelphia: WB Saunders, 2000:687–692.
129. Terman JS, Terman M, Schlager DS, et al. Efficacy of brief intense light exposure for treatment of winter depression. Arch Gen Psychiatry 1998; 55:875–882.
130. Lam RW, Levitt AJ, eds. Canadian Consensus Guidelines for the Treatment of Seasonal Affective Disorder. Vancouver, British Columbia: Clinical and Academic Publishing, 1999.
131. Glickman G, Hanifin JP, Rollag MD, et al. Inferior retinal light exposure is more effective than superior retinal exposure in suppressing melatonin in humans. J Biol Rhythms 2003; 18:71–79.
132. Terman M, Terman JS. Light therapy. In: Kryger MH, Roth T, Dement WC, eds. Principles and Practice of Sleep Medicine. 4th ed. Philadelphia: Elsevier Saunders, 2005:1424–1442.
133. Tuunainen A, Kripke DF, Endo T. Light therapy for non-seasonal depression. Cochrane Database Syst Rev. 2004;(2):CD004050 (review).
134. Gallin PF, Terman M, Reme CE, et al. Ophthalmologic examination of patients with seasonal affective disorder, before and after bright light therapy. Am J Ophthalmol 1995; 119:202–210.
135. Gallin PF, Terman M, Reme DE, et al. The Columbia Eye Examination for Users of Light Treatment. New York: New York State Psychiatric Institute, 1993.

136. Dyken ME, Yamada T. Approach to the patient with sleep disorders. In: Biller J, ed. Practical Neurology. 2nd ed. Philadelphia: Lippincott Williams & Wilkens, 2002:100.

137. Johns MW. A new method for measuring daytime sleepiness: the Epworth Sleepiness Scale. Sleep 1991; 14(6):540–545.

138. Johns MW. Reliability and factor analysis of the Epworth Sleepiness Scale. Sleep 1992; 15:376–381.

139. Chervin RD, Aldrich MS, Pickett R, et al. Comparison of the results of the Epworth Sleepiness Scale and the Multiple Sleep Latency Test. J Psychosom Res 1997; 42:145–155.

140. Johns MW. Sensitivity and specificity of the multiple sleep latency test (MSLT), the Maintenance of Wakefulness Test and the Epworth Sleepiness Scale: failure of the MSLT as a gold standard. J Sleep Res 2000; 9:5–11.

141. A review by the MSLT and MWT Task Force of the Standards of Practice Committee of the American Academy of Sleep Medicine. The clinical use of the MSLT and MWT. Sleep 2005; 28:127–143.

142. Pakola SJ, Dinges DF, Pack AI. Review of regulations and guidelines for commercial and noncommercial drivers with sleep apnea and narcolepsy. Sleep 1995; 18:787–796.

143. Anfield RN. Americans with disabilities Act of 1990. A primer of Title I provisions for occupational health care professionals. J Occup Med 1992; 34:503–509.

144. Federal Aviation Administration (FAA), . Sleep Apnea Evaluation Specifications. Federal Aviation Administration specification letter dated October 6, 1992. Washington, DC: US Department of Transportation; 1992.

145. Mitler MM, Carskadon MA, Hirshkowitz M. In: Kryger MH, Roth T, Dement WC, eds. Principles and Practice of Sleep Medicine. 4th ed. Philadelphia: Elsevier Saunders, 2005:1417–1423.

146. Frolich L. The cholinergic pathology in Alzheimer's disease: discrepancies between clinical experience and pathophysiological findings. J Neural Transm 2002; 109:1003.

147. Angrist B, Sudilovsky A. Central nervous system stimulants: historical aspects and clinical effects. In: Iversen LL, Iversen SD, Snyder SH, eds. Handbook of Psychopharmacology. Vol. 11. New York: Plenum Press, 1976:99–165.

148. National Sleep Foundation, . 2001 "Sleep in America" Poll. Washington, DC: National Sleep Foundation, 2001.

149. Van Dongen HP, Price NJ, Mjllington JM, et al. Caffeine eliminates psychomotor vigilance deficits from sleep inertia. Sleep 2001; 24:813–819.

150. Porkka-Heiskanen T, Strecker RE, Thakkar M, et al. Adenosine: a mediator of the sleep-inducing effects of prolonged wakefulness. Science 1997; 276:1265–1268.

151. Strecker RE, Morairty S, Thakkar MM, et al. Adenosinergic modulation of basal forebrain and preoptic/anterior hypothalamic neuronal activity in the control of behavioral state. Behav Brain Res 2000; 115:183–204.

152. Mitler MM, O'Malley MB. Wake-promoting medications: efficacy and adverse effects. In: Kryger MH, Roth T, Dement WC, eds. Principles and Practice of Sleep Medicine. 4th ed. Philadelphia: Elsevier Saunders, 2005:484–498.

153. Parkes JD, Dahlitz M. Amphetamine prescription. Sleep 1993; 16:201–202.

154. Wesenten NJ Belenky G, Kautz MA, et al. Maintaining alertness and performance during sleep deprivation: modafinil versus caffeine. Psychopharmacology (Berl) 2002; 159:238–247.

155. Nawrot P, Jordan S, Eastwood J, et al. Effects of caffeine on human health. Food Addit Contam 2003; 20:1–30.

156. Silverman K, Evans SM, Strain EC, et al. Withdrawal syndrome after the double-blind cessation of caffeine consumption. N Engl J Med 1992; 327:1109–1114.

157. Mignot E, Lammers GJ, Ripley B, et al. The role of cerebrospinal fluid hypocretin measurement in the diagnosis of narcolepsy and other hypersomnia. Arch Neurol 2002; 59:1553–1562.

158. Kubota H, Kanbayashi T, Tanabe Y, et al. A case of acute disseminated encephalomyelitis presenting hypersomnia with decreased hypocretin level in cerebrospinal fluid. J Child Neurol 2002; 17: 537–539.

159. Autret A, Lucas B, Mondon K, et al. Sleep and brain lesions: a critical review of the literature and additional new cases. Neurophysiol Clin 2001; 31:356–375.

160. Mieda M, Willie JT, Hara J, et al. Orexin peptides prevent cataplexy and improve wakefulness in an orexin neuron-ablated model of narcolepsy in mice. Proc Natl Acad Sci U S A 2004; 101:4649–4654.

161. Fujiki N, Ripley B, Yoshida Y, et al. Effects of IV and ICV hypocretin-1 (orexin A) in hypocretin receptor-2 gene mutated narcoleptic dogs and IV hypocretin-1 replacement therapy in a hypocretin-ligand-deficient narcoleptic dog. Sleep 2003; 6:953–959.

162. John J, Kumar V, Gopinath G. Recovery of sleep after fetal preoptic transplantation in the medial preoptic area-lesioned rat. Sleep 1998; 21:601–606.

163. Munillo-Rodrigez E, Arias-Carrion O, Xu M, et al. Time course of survival of hypocretin neuronal transplants into the pons of adult rats. Sleep 2004; 27(suppl):A239 (abstr).

164. Scammell TE. The neurobiology, diagnosis, and treatment of narcolepsy. Ann Neurol 2003; 53: 157–166.

165. Nishino S, Ripley B, Overeem S, et al. Hypocretin (orexin) deficiency in human narcolepsy. Lancet 2000; 355:39–40.
166. Nishino S, Sakurai S, Nevisimalova S, et al. CSF histamine content is decreased in hypocretin-deficient human narcolepsy. Sleep 2002; 25(suppl):A476.
167. Shiba T, Fujiki N, Wisor JP, et al. Wake promoting effects of thioperamide, a histamine H_3 antagonist in orexin/ataxin-3 narcoleptic mice. Sleep 2004; 27(suppl):A241.
168. Nishino S, Arrigoni J, Kanbayashi T, et al. TRH and its analogs significantly reduce canine cataplexy. Sleep Res 1995; 24A:352.
169. Riehl J, Honda K, Kwan M, et al. Chronic oral administration of CG-3703, a thyrotropin releasing hormone analog, increases wake and decreases cataplexy in canine narcolepsy. Neuropsychopharmacology 2000; 23:34–45.

24 | Special Considerations for Treatment of Hypersomnias

Yutaka Honda
Neuropsychiatric Research Institute, Shinjuku-ku, Tokyo, Japan

Makoto Honda
Sleep Disorder Research Project, Tokyo Institute of Psychiatry, Setagaya-ku, Tokyo, Japan

SIDE EFFECTS OF TREATMENT

Adverse Effects of Treatment Drugs in Short-Term Use

Short-Term Use of Psychostimulants

Psychostimulants, such as methylphenidate and dextroamphetamine, are effective in controlling the somnolence of narcolepsy (1–3). However, they often show side effects due to stimulation of the sympathetic nervous system. Constitutional factors may contribute to the development and severity of side effects. These include dry mouth, headache, palpitations, sweating, tremor, anorexia, gastritis, nausea, insomnia, irritation, and hyperactivity (3,4). The half-life of methylphenidate is approximately three to four hours, and administration twice a day, in the morning and at lunchtime, is recommended. Pemoline has a longer half-life of about 12 hours and can be used in one dose in the morning. It has less sympathetic nervous system stimulation and longer effectiveness as compared with methylphenidate (5–8). However, because of its association with idiosyncratic hepatic failure leading to transplantation or death, it is no longer available in the United States. Half-lives of amphetamine and methamphetamine are reported to be 8 to 20 hours (7,9,10). Development of paradoxical somnolence may occasionally appear, usually 15 minutes after ingestion of psychostimulants (11–13). Such somnolence usually lasts for less than half an hour, and then an awakening effect appears and lasts for several hours depending on the half-life of the drug. Ingestion of one tablet of psychostimulant one hour before the scheduled time of awakening in the morning may help reduce this effect. After a short sleep, the patients can awake feeling refreshed at a scheduled time in the morning. In rare cases, the paradoxical sleepiness effect of psychostimulants is severe and lasts for an entire day (6). In such cases, administration of psychostimulants is useless. Modafinil has little effect on the sympathetic nervous system and lacks most of the short-term side effects (14–17). Its half-life is about 12 hours. Amphetamine and methamphetamine show little short-term side effects. They have a longer half-life of more than 20 hours (7,9,18). Selegiline, also known as l-deprenyl, is a selective monoamine oxidase (MAO)-B inhibitor. This drug has been used for daytime sleepiness, but it also has more frequent hepatic side effects (19,20).

Short-Term Use of Tricyclic Antidepressants

Imipramine was first recognized as a potent tricyclic anticataplectic drug (21). Other tricyclic drugs, including desmethylimipramine, protriptyline, and amitriptyline, were clinically tested for their potency against cataplexy (22,23). Later, clomipramine was found to be the most potent anticataplectic drug (24,25). Short-term side effects include dry mouth, constipation, aggravation of glaucoma, nausea, and impotence (26). Cataplexy and dreadful hypnagogic hallucinations are often very distressing to the patients, and continuation of tricyclic drugs is preferred in spite of minor side effects.

Some selective serotonin reuptake inhibitor (SSRI) agents, such as fluvoxamine (27) and fluoxetine (28), have limited anticataplectic effects. Sodium oxybate, or γ-hydroxybutyrate (GHB), was recently rerecognized as a treatment for both daytime somnolence and cataplexy of narcolepsy. Adverse effects include nausea, dizziness, headache, and, less frequently, sleepwalking, enuresis, vomiting, fatigue, nightmares, abdominal pain, diarrhea, and anorexia (29–33).

Adverse Effects of Other Treatment Drugs

The prevalence of periodic limb movements in sleep (PLMS) is higher in narcoleptic patients than in the general population. Dopaminergic drugs, such as levodopa, and dopamine agonists (e.g., ropinirole, pramipexole) are effective in treating PLMS. However, they often result in nausea, orthostatic hypotension, insomnia, and daytime fatigue. There is no documented effect of these drugs in treating excessive daytime sleepiness and may instead be associated with daytime somnolence (34).

Adverse Effects of Treatment Drugs in Long-Term Use

Long-Term Adverse Effects of Psychostimulants

Psychostimulants have been used for many years for the treatment of narcolepsy. Adequate control of somnolence in the daytime is usually possible. However, this control is not always possible because of side effects and nonadherence. The awakening effects of psychostimulants should not be extended beyond evening meals to minimize remaining brain concentrations of the drugs at night to ensure a sound night's sleep. The most serious long-term side effect is the development of mental symptoms of psychosis, which are not very rare (12,35–40). Special attention for psychiatric symptoms is required for the patients under psychostimulant medication. Individual interviewing of patients should be done at least every two to three months to detect any pathological change of mental state as early as possible.

Initial stages of a psychotic state are the ideas of observation and reference. Activation of hypnagogic hallucinations is another early change. If these initial signs are left unnoticed, development of auditory and/or tactile hallucinations with delusions in the daytime may ensue. In some patients, aggravation of preexisting schizophrenic psychosis may develop.

On the other hand, intensified hypnagogic hallucinations may progress into the daytime hours and show a hallucinatory paranoid state, usually of a nature of fantasy-like ideations. They may appear without stimulant medications (41). Such a delusional state of a fantasy-like nature can be considered as a naturally occurring unique psychosis (narcoleptic psychosis). The development of psychosis appears most frequently within the first one year of the start of psychostimulants (36) (Fig. 1). Predisposing factors should be considered. When psychotic state occurs, psychiatric treatment should be initiated immediately. If this treatment is

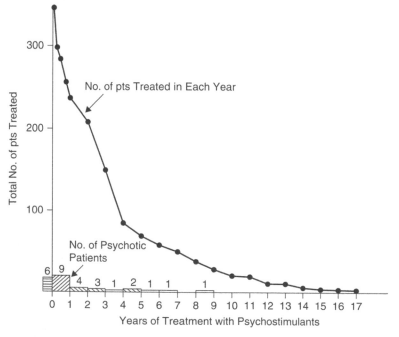

Figure 1   The shaded area shown at the bottom of the graph indicates the frequency of psychotic states. The highest peak of nine psychotic patients was observed within the initial one year of treatment. Note that six patients were psychotic before the initiation of treatment. *Source*: From Ref. 36.

neglected or too late, daytime hallucinatory paranoid states may become aggravated and more intensive psychiatric treatments are usually required.

We conducted a study on the 30- to 40-year follow-up of 329 narcoleptics and 100 patients with idiopathic hypersomnia without long sleep time, who visited our clinic during 1955 to 1995 (42). Among the responses, 73% answered that they had been taking psychostimulants (methylphenidate and/or pemoline) regularly. Major tolerable somatic adverse effects were dryness of mouth (36%), paradoxical sleepiness effect (13%), palpitations (12%), gastritis (8%), and sweating (5%). Frequencies of patients with psychotic symptoms among all narcoleptic patients were 1.5% for the transient ideas of reference, 0.7% for the development of hypnagogic hallucinations into a daytime hallucinatory paranoid state, and 1.0% for daytime auditory hallucinations and delusions. Once established, treatment of the hallucinatory paranoid state is often difficult. On rare occasions, schizophrenia mimics narcolepsy (43). Generally speaking, the severity of sleepiness in narcolepsy gradually decreases in the long course of time with the disease. Daily dose of psychostimulants for patients with long-term treatment for about 20 years can be reduced to find a new optimal dose. Some narcoleptic patients who had been successfully treated with psychostimulants may complain of worsening of daytime sleepiness after middle age. In many of such cases, complications with sleep-related breathing disorders, PLMS, and restless legs syndrome (RLS) may have developed. Reevaluation of patients by nocturnal polysomnography (PSG) is needed in cases with worsening of daytime sleepiness.

Tolerance to psychostimulants is rare. There are little or no evidence of abuse or addiction to these drugs in narcoleptic patients. On the other hand, abuse of methylphenidate is a newly recognized problem among the younger generations. Some nonnarcoleptic youngsters with personality disorders seek excessive amount of psychostimulants for pleasure and satisfaction. Such abusers are usually multiple-drug abusers, and they may try to cheat physicians by complaining of narcoleptic symptoms to obtain methylphenidate. They crush the methylphenidate into powder, purify it by evaporating it with alcohol, and then inhale the crystallized methylphenidate through the nose (sniffing or snorting). No such abusive use of psychostimulants has been reported among narcoleptic patients.

Hepatic toxicity of pemoline has been reported in England where excess amount of pemoline was administered to children with attention-deficit hyperactivity disorder. However, the use and need of pemoline to treat narcolepsy is rare in European countries and in the United States because of the reasons discussed above. Use of pemoline to treat narcolepsy is officially permitted only in Japan. In my clinical experience in Japan with several hundred narcoleptic patients for more than 30 years, no hepatic problems leading to the discontinuation of pemoline has ever been experienced. Some rare patients who had disturbed liver function showed improvement of their liver function during the treatment with pemoline.

Long-Term Adverse Effects of Tricyclic Antidepressants

Long-term side effects of tricyclics include the development of tolerance in some patients. Sudden discontinuation of tricyclics often provokes rebound or aggravation of cataplexy and even status cataplecticus. Addition of a serotonin norepinephrine reuptake inhibitor (SNRI), such as milnacipran, or a further increase of clomipramine may be of some help in such cases for a while. In severe cases, a high dose (200 mg) of clomipramine can be no more effective. In such case, a careful discontinuation of the tricyclic for one month under hospital care is helpful. Usually, the effectiveness of the tricyclic against cataplexy recovers. Afterwards, a much smaller dose of clomipramine (25–50 mg) becomes effective again to treat the cataplexy. On the other hand, in the long course of time for some 20 years or more, cataplexy, hypnagogic hallucinations, and sleep paralysis may subside and disappear in half of the narcoleptic patients. The amount of tricyclics can be reduced, and finally, no more may be needed. On the other hand, daytime sleepiness and disturbed nocturnal sleep persist much longer, but the severity usually becomes less. Idiopathic hypersomnia patients without long sleep time show higher effectiveness of psychostimulants against daytime somnolence as compared with narcolepsy, and daytime sleepiness may disappear more frequently and earlier.

Tricyclics are known to aggravate PLMS and RLS. Although physicians interested in sleep apnea and PLMS often prefer discontinuation of tricyclics, aggravation of cataplexy and hypnagogic hallucinations may result, and the daily activities of the patients are more likely to be disturbed. Decreasing the dose or discontinuation of tricyclics should be done with extreme care in narcoleptic patients with PLMS and RLS.

AGE AND GENDER EFFECTS OF TREATMENT

There are no major age effects of treatment, with the exception of some recent reports regarding the possibility of sudden death in children and adolescents with cardiac disease who were taking dextroamphetamine. With respect to gender, family studies revealed no sex differences in the frequency of birth of patients with narcolepsy (44). In outpatient sleep clinics, however, male dominance is typically found. This may be due to the sex differences of social functioning. Social regulations are stricter for working male narcoleptic patients. Teratology studies performed in animals do not provide any harmful changes to the fetus. The use of tricyclics during the pregnancy of depressive patients did not increase teratology. However, narcoleptic pregnant women may prefer to discontinue or minimize the use of psychostimulants and tricyclics during pregnancy, especially in the early stages of pregnancy. Scheduled pregnancy is recommended. Cataplexy with sudden loss of facial as well as bodily muscle tone may produce awkwardness and despair more frequently in female narcoleptic patients, limiting social interactions and posing a significant safety risk, particularly if a woman has a cataplectic attack in an unfamiliar environment.

DRIVING RISK AND MEDICOLEGAL ASPECTS

A driver's license is typically suspended or revoked when the diagnosis of narcolepsy and/or sleep-related breathing disorders is established in some countries. However, the regulations vary from country to country, and are less severe in other countries.

In the United States, the regulations differ by state, with California having the strictest regulations. When a physician identifies a narcoleptic patient, narcolepsy is classified as a disorder characterized by lapses of consciousness, and a confidential morbidity report is submitted to the state department of health services. The department of motor vehicles is notified, and a doctor's certification is indispensable to attest to the patient's ability to safely operate a motor vehicle before his or her driving privileges can be restored.

The regulations on sleepy drivers vary among European countries. In the United Kingdom, an initial version of the regulatory document restricted the application of the regulation to "sleepiness leading to a sudden and disabling event at wheel." But this was later changed to "excessive awake time sleepiness." A sleep-related breathing disorder is not specifically mentioned, but "sleep disorders" appear in the section on respiratory disorders.

In Sweden, a medical certificate is mandatory to apply for a driver's license, and it is usually completed by the general practitioner. This must be renewed after the age of 65 years for license holders, which therefore indicates that the physician decides whether a patient is fit to drive.

In Belgium, a questionnaire must be completed on the initial application for a license. If, at a later date, a sleep-related breathing disorder is diagnosed, the driver must send his or her license to the licensing authority, but the license may be reissued when he or she is able to provide a medical certificate stating that the disorder has been adequately treated.

In Switzerland, federal law authorizes (but does not enforce) a physician to report any individual judged to be medically unable to drive to the vehicle-licensing authority.

Other European countries that have specific regulations to suspend the driver's license of a sleepy driver are France, Spain, and Sweden. In Japan, the use of the diagnostic terms, e.g., "narcolepsy" and "sleep apnea syndrome" were deleted from the initial draft of the traffic regulations. Only the severity of daytime sleepiness as defined by Epworth sleepiness scale or subjective report whether they fell asleep more than three times per week under adequate nocturnal sleep schedules is used as the criterion to consider suspension of a driver's license. At the time of renewing driver's license, all drivers must complete an inquiry form to report whether or not they experience intolerable daytime sleepiness more than three times a week. If more than three episodes of sleepiness is reported, a doctor's certification for the patient as a safe driver is required before renewal of a driver's license. Narcoleptic patients under regular treatment are less likely to fit to these criteria, and they rarely cause traffic accidents.

On the other hand, no regulations on sleepy driving were enforced in Portugal, Austria, Denmark, Finland, Germany, Norway, Switzerland, Greece, and Ireland at the time of survey in 2002 (45). In these countries, the general rules concerning fitness to drive apply. There are no uniformly accepted regulations within Europe concerning driver's license for sleep-related breathing disorders and narcolepsy.

A regular comment from physicians is that patients with sleep-related breathing disorders are more dangerous before they have been diagnosed compared with after they have commenced treatment. Therefore, the law by itself may be insufficient to reduce the risk related to disorders causing sleepiness. The sleep disorders mentioned in the law represent only a minority of the causes of sleepiness while driving. Therefore, it is unfair to penalize patients who, in addition, may be better informed and thus more cautious than the occasionally sleepy "normal" drivers.

The present California regulations raise serious concerns regarding confidentiality between doctor and patients. California's mandatory reporting requirement may defeat the very purpose it is designed to achieve, if it causes persons with narcolepsy or other sleep disorders to avoid seeking diagnosis and treatment. The sleepy, undiagnosed patient may hesitate to visit a sleep clinic to avoid suspension or revocation of his or her driver's license, and if the license is revoked, the patient may become hostile toward the physician who diagnosed the disorder and this may impede successful disease management.

The confidential trust between patients and physicians is always important. Strict adherence to a regular medication regimen needs to be encouraged by the physician. Finally, from a practical point of view, it appears that education and training of the professionals involved in traffic safety plays a critical role. Specific regulations concerning the diagnosis of sleep disorders would be meaningless if the police and other law enforcement officials are not aware of the details.

If they undergo proper management of their disorder, narcoleptic patients are no longer dangerous to themselves or society. Adherence of patients to their prescribed medication regimen is most important. Regulations developed for a specific diagnosis are usually not practical. Instead, it is the severity of sleepiness while driving that is important. Also, the patient's adherence to regular medical follow-up visits and the regular use of adequate dosages of medications are important. The severity criteria for narcolepsy and other sleep disorders also need to be documented.

OTHER CONSIDERATIONS FOR TREATMENT: PSYCHOSOCIAL PROBLEMS OF HYPERSOMNIA PATIENTS

Special attention on the mental state of patients is always needed in the treatment of narcolepsy and hypersomnia. The major problem that disturbs the life of patients with these disorders is the daily recurrence of intolerable daytime sleepiness. The patients fail to remain awake at work, at home, during examinations, and while participating in recreational activities. Patients cannot maintain alertness even at very important occasions. A pitiful example of this behavior was described by one of my male narcoleptic patients, who mentioned that his girlfriend disappeared while he unintentionally slept at the movies. Because of daily, frustrating failures, narcoleptic patients often lose friendships and are often forced to change jobs. The patients often feel frustrated and depressed and become pessimistic about their future. But in the long run, the patients become much more accustomed to their sleepiness, and it becomes an accepted part of their daily life. However, a small proportion of narcoleptic patients may deny their sleepiness, even while the electroencephalogram (EEG) is showing sleep patterns. This is called the "denial of sleepiness" in narcolepsy and may indicate long-standing excessive sleepiness in the past that they consider their baseline state. While completing a sleepiness questionnaire such as the Epworth sleepiness scale, narcoleptic patients sometimes deny sleepiness and their answers are unreliable. After initiation of treatment, these patients often become aware of what is a normal level of alertness and start complaining about their sleepiness. They often develop a unique personality change called "narcoleptoid personality" (1), characterized by decreased psychic tension, denial of sleepiness, and low self-esteem. The patients remain passive, do not want to become assertive, appear good natured, and do not resist contrary opinions of others during conversations.

Narcoleptic patients are often regarded as idle and unreliable. They are often chased out of their jobs, sent to local posts, or dismissed. These personality characteristics remain even after the treatment of their sleepiness and cataplexy with administration of psychostimulants and tricyclics, respectively.

Psychosocial support and personal counseling, including information on the activities of patients' self-help groups, are recommended for patients with narcolepsy or other hypersomnias. Depression is often observed in untreated narcoleptic patients, and it may not be the side effect of the treatment.

Prejudice among general public and the lack of knowledge among patients themselves regarding narcolepsy are common. When informed by television, magazines, and mass media, patients are afraid and reluctant to be diagnosed as having narcolepsy. The diagnosis of narcolepsy often carries with it a caricature of an idle, sleepy fellow with a psychiatric illness, especially in rural areas. Propagation of knowledge about narcolepsy and other hypersomnias as treatable diseases among the general population and government officials is desperately needed.

Information on the activities of patients' self-help organizations, e.g., Japan Narcolepsy Association (44) and American Narcolepsy Network, is also important.

Regular follow-up of patients, at least every two to three months, is essential to evaluate the patients' mental status, to assess adverse effects of treatment, and to screen for other concomitant sleep conditions, such as sleep-related breathing disorders.

Other than medications, scheduled naps and a regular sleep-wake schedule are strongly recommended. Sufficient nocturnal sleep may prevent the development of psychotic side effects of the psychostimulants.

CONCLUSIONS

The psychostimulants (e.g., modafinil, methylphenidate, dextroamphetamine) are generally well tolerated and effective in treating the daytime sleepiness associated with narcolepsy and other hypersomnias. Psychosis is the most serious long-term side effect observed with psychostimulant use. Tricyclic antidepressants (e.g., imipramine, clomipramine) and some SSRI agents are effective in controlling cataplexy. Tolerance to the tricyclic antidepressants may develop in some patients; they may aggravate PLMS and RLS, and rebound effects may be provoked with sudden discontinuation of this class of medications. The newer drug sodium oxybate appears effective in treating both daytime somnolence and cataplexy of narcolepsy. Narcoleptic pregnant women may prefer to limit or stop use of psychostimulant and tricyclic medications during pregnancy, even though conclusive evidence of untoward effects of these medications to the developing fetus is lacking. Driving privileges are typically suspended or revoked with diagnoses of narcolepsy or other hypersomnias, though regulations vary from country to country and even by state in the United States. However, the severity of sleepiness while driving is more important than any specific sleep-related diagnosis. Careful follow-up and adherence to treatment regimens are critical for any patient with narcolepsy or other hypersomnia.

REFERENCES

1. Honda Y. Clinical features of narcolepsy: Japanese experiences. In: Honda Y, Juji T, eds. HLA in Narcolepsy. Heidelberg: Springer-Verlag, 1988:24–57.
2. Mitler MM, Aldrich M, Kooh G, et al. Narcolepsy and its treatment with stimulants. ASDA standards of practice. Sleep 1994; 17:352–371.
3. Mitler MM, Shafor R, Hajdukovik R, et al. Treatment of narcolepsy: objective studies on methylphenidate, pemoline and protriptyline. Sleep 1986; 9:260–264.
4. Auger RR, Goodman SH, Silber MH, et al. Risks of high-dose stimulants in the treatment of disorders of excessive somnolence: a case-control study. Sleep 2005; 28:667–672.

5. Sasaki T, Aoyama T, Kotaki H, et al. Non-linear disposition of d-methylphenidate in hypersomniac patients and healthy volunteers. Abstract of 17th Congress of Collegium Internationale Neuro-Psychopharmacologium. Kyoto, Japan, 1990:129.

6. Sasaki T, Kotaki H, Aoyama T, et al. Plasma concentration of methylphenidate and clinical symptoms. Ann Rep Pharmacopsychiatry Res 1995; 21:115–122. (in JPN)

7. Kotaki H. Pharmacokinetics of psychostimulants. In: Inoue S, Okuma T, Hishikawa Y, eds. Handbook of Somnology. Tokyo: Asakura Shoten, 1994:366–374. (in JPN)

8. Nishihara K, Kohda Y, Saitoh Y, et al. Determination of pemoline in plasma, plasma water, mixed saliva, and urine by high performance liquid chromatography. Ther Drug Monit 1994; 6:232–237.

9. Mitler MM, Hajdukovic R, Erman M. Treatment of narcolepsy with methamphetamine. Sleep 1993; 16:306–317.

10. Dauvilliers Y, Billiard M, Montplaisir J. Clinical aspects and pathophysiology of narcolepsy. Clin Neurophysiol 2003; 114:2000–2017.

11. Tecce JJ, Cole JO. Amphetamine effects in man: paradoxical drowsiness and lowered electrical brain activity (CNV). Science 1974; 185(149):451–453.

12. Honda Y, Hishikawa Y, Takahashi Y. Long-term treatment of narcolepsy with methylphenidate (Ritalin®). Curr Ther Res 1979; 25(2):288–298.

13. Honda Y, Hishikawa Y. A long-term treatment of narcolepsy and excessive daytime sleepiness with pemoline (Betanamin®). Curr Ther Res 1980; 27(3):429–441.

14. Billiard M, Besset A, Montplaisir J, et al. Modafinil: a double-blind multicenter study. Sleep 1994; 17(8):S107–S112.

15. U.S. Modafinil in Narcolepsy Multicenter Study Group. Randomized trial of modafinil for the treatment of pathological somnolence in narcolepsy. Ann Neurol 1998; 43:88–97.

16. U.S. Modafinil in Narcolepsy Multicenter Study Group. Randomized trial of modafinil as a treatment for the excessive daytime somnolence of narcolepsy. Neurology 2000; 54:1166–1175.

17. Schwartz JR, Feldman NT, Bogan RK, et al. Dosing regimen of modafinil for improving daytime wakefulness in patients with narcolepsy. Clin Neuropharmacol 2003; 26:252–257.

18. Shindler J, Schachter M, Brincat S, et al. Amphetamine, mazindol and fencamfamin in narcolepsy. BMJ 1985; 290:1167–1170.

19. Hublin C, Partinen M, Heinonen E, et al. Selegiline in the treatment of narcolepsy. Neurology 1994; 44:2095–2101.

20. Mayer G, Meier-Ewert K. Selegiline hydrochloride treatment in narcolepsy. A double-blind, placebo-controlled study. Clin Neuropharmacol 1995; 18:306–319.

21. Akimoto H, Honda Y, Takahashi Y. Pharmacotherapy in narcolepsy. Dis Nerv Syst 1960; 21:1–3.

22. Takahashi Y, Honda Y. Pharmacotherapy in narcolepsy II: effects of thymoleptics and some other psychotropic drugs. Seishin Igaku 1964; 6(10):775–784.

23. Honda Y. Treatment of narcolepsy. Saishin Igaku 1965; 20(9):2464–2472.

24. Honda Y. Treatment of narcolepsy. In: Hirai T, Hara T, Hozaki H, eds. Treatment of Psychiatric Disorders. Tokyo: Kanehara Publishing, 1972:327–333. (in JPN)

25. Guilleminault C, Raynal D, Takahashi S, et al. Evaluation of short-term and long-term treatment of the narcolepsy syndrome with clomipramine hydrochloride. Acta Neurol Scand 1976; 54:71–87.

26. Takahashi Y, Honda Y. Side effects of psychostimulants and thymoleptics in their long-term administration to the narcoleptics – laboratory findings with special reference to electrocardiographic changes. Ann Rep Pharmacopsychiatry Res 1970; 2:145.

27. Schachter M, Parkes JD. Fluvoxamine and clomipramine in the treatment of cataplexy. J Neurol Neurosurg Psychiatry 1980; 43:171–174.

28. Langdon N, Bandak S, Shindler J, et al. Fluoxetine in the treatment of cataplexy. Sleep 1986; 9:371–372.

29. Broughton R, Mamela K. The treatment of narcolepsy-cataplexy with nocturnal gamma-hydroxybutyrate. Can J Neurol Sci 1977; 6:1–6.

30. Mamelak K, Scharf M, Woods M. Treatment of narcolepsy with gamma-hydroxybutyrate. A review of clinical and sleep laboratory findings. Sleep 1986; 9:285–289.

31. U.S. Xyrem® Multicenter Study Group. A randomized, double-blind, placebo-controlled multicenter trial comparing the effects of three doses of orally administered sodium oxybate with placebo for the treatment of narcolepsy. Sleep 2002; 25:42–49.

32. U.S. Xyrem® Multicenter Study Group. A 12-month, open-label multicenter extension trial of orally administered sodium oxybate for the treatment of narcolepsy. Sleep 2003; 26:31–35.

33. U.S. Xyrem® Multicenter Study Group. Sodium oxybate demonstrates long-term efficacy for the treatment of cataplexy in patients with narcolepsy. Sleep Med 2004; 5:119–123.

34. Montplaisir J, Allen RP, Walters AS, et al. Restless legs syndrome and periodic limb movements during sleep. In: Kryger H, Roth T, Dement WC, eds. Principles and Practice of Sleep Medicine. 4th ed. Philadelphia: Elsevier Saunders, 2005:839–852.

35. Eisenberg M, Woods L. Narcolepsy with psychosis: report of two cases. Mayo Clin Proc 1962; 37:561–566.

36. Honda Y, Takahashi Y. The psychosis–like states in narcolepsy during long-term treatment with psychostimulants. Ann Rep Pharmacopsychiatry Res 1971; 3:164–169.
37. Honda Y, Takahashi Y. Experience of long-term treatment of narcolepsy with psychostimulants: effectiveness and problems. Ann Rep Pharmacopsychiatry Res Found 1997; 28:54–59.
38. Honda Y. Application of DSM-III diagnostic criteria to narcoleptic patients with hallucinatory-paranoid states. J Clin Psychiatry 1982; 11:239–246.
39. Young D, Scoville W. Paranoid psychosis in narcolepsy and the possible danger of benzedrine treatment. Med Clin North Am 1938; 22:637–646.
40. Nishiyama A, Honda Y, Suzuki J, et al. Hallucinosis developed in the course of treatment of narcolepsy. Clin Psychiatry (Seishin Igaku) 1966; 6:485–491. (in JPN)
41. Utena H. On the hallucinations of narcolepsy. Psychiatr Neurol Japonica 1939; 43:373–395.
42. Honda Y, Asaka A, Tanimura M, et al. A genetic study of narcolepsy and excessive sleepiness in 308 families with a narcolepsy or hypersomnia proband. In: Guilleminault C, Lugaresi E, eds. Sleep/Wake Disorders, Natural History, Epidemiology and Long-Term Evolution. New York: Raven Press, 1983:187–199.
43. Hicks JA, Shapiro CM. Pseudo-narcolepsy, case report. J Psychiatry Neurosci 1999; 24(4):348–350.
44. Honda Y. Activities of the Japan Narcolepsy Association (A NPO self-help group of the Japanese narcoleptic patients). Jpn J Clin Psychiatry (Rinsho Seishin Igaku) 1983; 12:1525–1530. (in JPN)
45. McNicholas WT, Levy PW, De Backer N, et al. Public health and medicolegal implications of sleep apnea. Eur Respir J 2002; 20:1594–1609.

25 | Description of Sleep-Related Breathing Disorders

Linda Snyder and Stuart F. Quan

Arizona Respiratory Center, University of Arizona, Tucson, Arizona, U.S.A.

HISTORY

Sleep-related breathing disorders (SRBDs) are an important public health problem associated with significant morbidity. Disorders of breathing during sleep exist along a spectrum of respiratory disturbances including conditions resulting in complete or partial upper airway obstruction, those that alter breathing patterns and those that lead to hypoventilation or hypoxemia. Initial descriptions of abnormal breathing during sleep can be traced to ancient historians. However, medical knowledge concerning SRBD dates back to the early 19th century, when the clinical observation of a pattern of breathing called Cheyne–Stokes was described (1,2). Subsequently, clinical descriptions of patients with obesity and excessive sleepiness were noted. In 1956, Burwell and colleagues applied the term "Pickwickian syndrome" to describe individuals with obesity, hypersomnolence, and chronic hypoventilation, because of the similar description of a character in the Dickens' story, *The Posthumous Papers of the Pickwick Club* (3). Subsequent investigations of patients with the Pickwickian syndrome by Gastaut and coworkers in 1966 discovered that cessation of respiration during sleep in these patients was due to intermittent upper airway obstruction (4). This work is credited as the initial recognition of obstructive sleep apnea (OSA) as a distinct clinical syndrome. In subsequent years, the connection between nocturnal obstructive respiratory events and daytime sleepiness became generally accepted with Guilleminault and coworkers in 1976 describing the OSA syndrome as a disorder with daytime sleepiness and obstructive apneas on polysomnography (PSG) (5). This was followed shortly thereafter by reports indicating that partial airway obstruction or hypopneas during sleep could produce clinical symptoms identical to those previously attributed only to apnea (6,7). Consequently, OSA syndrome became known as obstructive sleep apnea hypopnea (OSAH) syndrome. More recently, Guilleminault and colleagues described a group of patients who had daytime sleepiness, but no apneas or hypopneas on PSG (8). More detailed physiologic investigation using esophageal manometry demonstrated episodes of increasingly negative intrathoracic pressure without reductions in tidal volume. These findings were evidence of periodic increased upper airways resistance. This led to the appellation of "upper airways resistance syndrome" (UARS) to describe these patients and the use of "respiratory effort–related arousals (RERAs)" as the corresponding nomenclature for these episodes of increased upper airways resistance.

Although current therapeutic approaches will be discussed in subsequent chapters, the history of OSA and OSAH treatment is punctuated by three landmarks. In the early 1970s, the first therapeutic intervention for this condition was described in two case reports noting successful treatment of OSA using tracheostomy to bypass the upper airway obstruction (9,10). In 1981, the concept of therapeutic enlargement of the upper airway by removal of some of the soft palate and lateral pharyngeal wall tissues was introduced by Fujita in his description of uvulopalatopharyngoplasty (11). In the same year, the seminal work of Sullivan and colleagues was published, describing the reversal of OSA by nasal continuous positive airway pressure (CPAP), a technique that pneumatically splints the upper airway, thus maintaining patency (12).

On the basis of this rich historical background, the last two decades have noted a substantial increase in our knowledge concerning SRBD, particularly OSA/OSAH. An important epidemiologic study published by Young and colleagues in 1993 revealed an unexpectedly high prevalence of OSAH in adults, providing strong evidence of its potentially large public health impact (vide infra) (13). More recent studies have emphasized its importance in children as well (14). From a historical perspective, neurocognitive and quality of life issues were the initial concerns that elevated the visibility of OSA/OSAH among clinicians. These linkages now are better described along with putative mechanisms. The 1970s were marked by increasing reports of the association between OSA/OSAH and hypertension. Now there are numerous recent studies that provide strong evidence of the role of OSA/ OSAH as an independent risk factor for hypertension and cardiovascular disease (15–19). Furthermore, recent data implicate OSA/OSAH as possible contributing risk factors for diabetes mellitus and gastroesophageal reflux (20,21). All of these issues will be discussed in more detail in subsequent chapters. Finally, the increasing recognition of OSA/OSAH has led to the description of other conditions that affect breathing during sleep. This has resulted in the use of the term "sleep-related breathing disorders" as the general category for all of the conditions outlined in the following section.

NOMENCLATURE

The first diagnostic classification of sleep and arousal disorders was published in the journal Sleep in 1979. This was followed by the publication of the *International Classification of Sleep Disorders* (*ICSD*) in 1990. In 2002, the American Academy of Sleep Medicine noted significant advances in the field of sleep medicine, which led to an international effort to substantially revise the *ICSD*. In 2005, the *International Classification of Sleep Disorders-2* (*ICSD-2*) was published (22). In *ICSD-2*, the broad category of SRBDs encompasses the following five groups: (*i*) central sleep apnea syndromes (CSA), (*ii*) OSA syndromes, (*iii*) sleep-related hypoventilation/hypoxemic syndromes, (*iv*) sleep-related hypoventilation/hypoxemia due to medical conditions, and (*v*) other sleep-related breathing disorders.

Central Sleep Apnea Syndromes
CSA syndromes are divided into six subcategories: the idiopathic form, or primary CSA, and five other with defined underlying causes. These latter five disorders are CSA secondary to Cheyne–Stokes breathing pattern or periodic breathing, CSA due to high-altitude periodic breathing, CSA due to a medical condition exclusive of Cheyne–Stokes respiration, CSA due to a drug or substance, and primary sleep apnea of infancy.

Obstructive Sleep Apnea Syndromes
The OSA syndromes are divided into adult and pediatric forms. Consistent with *ICSD-2*, references to the OSA syndromes in this chapter will include patients having apneas, hypopneas, and upper airway resistance syndrome.

Sleep-Related Hypoventilation/Hypoxemic Syndromes
This group includes two subcategories, the idiopathic sleep-related nonobstructive alveolar hypoventilation syndrome and the congenital central alveolar hypoventilation syndrome. Alternate names for the idiopathic disorder are central alveolar hypoventilation or primary alveolar hypoventilation.

Sleep-Related Hypoventilation/Hypoxemia due to Medical Conditions
In this group are three subcategories of medical conditions that lead to sleep-related hypoventilation or hypoxemia: pulmonary parenchymal or vascular pathology, lower airways obstruction, and neuromuscular and chest wall disorders. The obesity-hypoventilation syndrome (OHS) is included in this category.

Other Sleep-Related Breathing Disorder
This category is used for forms of SRBD that cannot be classified elsewhere or do not clearly fit into one of the above categories but are felt to be disorders of respiratory sleep disturbance.

    The remainder of this chapter will focus on the key features and characteristics, incidence and prevalence, animal models, and social and economic consequences of three of the most important and more common SRBDs: OSA syndromes, CSA secondary to Cheyne–Stokes breathing pattern, and the OHS.

KEY FEATURES AND CHARACTERISTICS

Obstructive Sleep Apnea Syndromes

In OSA syndrome, there are frequent repetitive episodes of complete (apnea) or partial (hypopnea) upper airway obstruction during sleep, but not always leading to reduction in oxygen saturation. In adults, these episodes last a minimum of 10 seconds, during which there is effort to breathe and can occur at any stage of sleep. Generally, OSA is felt to be present when there are five or more episodes per hour of sleep (22). Most affected individuals have a mixture of both apneic and hypopneic events during their sleep. Frequently, bed partners note loud, disruptive snoring, breathing pauses, or episodes of choking or gasping in the night. Excessive daytime sleepiness and chronic fatigue are very commonly present symptoms, although in some patients the primary symptom is insomnia (23). Individuals often complain of feeling unrested with a headache upon awakening in the morning. OSA is often present concurrently with a number of other medical conditions including hypertension, athero-sclerotic cardiovascular disease, stroke, diabetes mellitus, depression, and gastroesophageal reflux (23).

OSA is increasingly recognized in children (14). However, because of the child's increased respiratory rate, the minimum event duration is the length of two breath cycles. Although there is as yet no consensus on the minimum event frequency, a number of studies consider that one or more apnea or hypopnea events per hour of sleep is diagnostic of OSA in a child (22). Moreover, hypopneas are the predominant event type rather than the mixture of frank apnea and hypopneas observed in adults. Like adults, children with OSA may present with loud snoring and excessive daytime sleepiness. Frequently, however, they paradoxically exhibit hyperactive behavior. Poor school performance also is frequently observed (24). Hypertension and cor pulmonale have been noted in children with OSA as well.

The major predisposing factor for OSA is obesity (13). Men are more often afflicted than women in a ratio of approximately 2:1 (25). Also OSA is more common in certain craniofacial phenotypes such as micrognathia and brachycephaly, which are associated with upper airway narrowing (26). Other medical conditions such as hypothyroidism, acromegaly, and myotonic dystrophy increase the risk for OSA as well. Finally, OSA exhibits familial aggregation suggesting that there is a genetic predisposition (26). It is unclear however, whether this reflects the heritability of obesity, craniofacial bone structure, ventilatory control, or another unknown factor.

In children, the primary risk factor is tonsillar hypertrophy (27). However, similar to adults, obesity and craniofacial phenotypes are risk factors. OSA also frequently occurs in some congenital conditions such as Pierre Robin and Down syndromes (26).

Central Sleep Apnea Associated with Cheyne–Stokes Breathing Pattern

Cheyne–Stokes breathing during sleep occurs if there are at least three consecutive cycles of a cyclical crescendo and decrescendo change in breathing amplitude, and there are five or more central sleep apneas or hypopneas per hour of sleep or the cyclic crescendo and decrescendo change in breathing amplitude has a duration of at least 10 consecutive minutes (22). CSA with Cheyne–Stokes breathing generally occurs in the setting of impairment in left ventricular function or cerebrovascular disease (28–30). Although CSA with Cheyne–Stokes breathing occurs more commonly in those with severe left ventricular dysfunction, it can be observed in those with milder heart disease as well (31). In addition to symptoms of the underlying disorder, individuals may complain of nonrestorative sleep, morning headaches, paroxysmal nocturnal dyspnea, snoring, and daytime sleepiness or fatigue.

Obesity-Hypoventilation Syndrome

This condition is usually defined as a combination of obesity (body mass index > 30 kg/m^2) and awake hypercapnia ($PaCO_2 > 45$ mmHg) in the absence of other known causes of hypoventilation (22). The clinical presentation may be similar to that of OSA syndrome as patients may present with excessive daytime sleepiness, fatigue, or morning headaches. Patients with OHS also have daytime hypercapnia and hypoxemia, which leads to the development of pulmonary hypertension and cor pulmonale (32).

INCIDENCE AND PREVALENCE

Obstructive Sleep Apnea Syndromes

There is little available data documenting the incidence of OSA in adults. However, the Cleveland Family Study evaluated 286 eligible patients to determine the five-year incidence of SRBD and the influence of risk factors (33). The five-year incidence was 10% for OSA defined as >15 apneas or hypopneas per hour (apnea-hypopnea index, AHI) and 16% for OSA with an AHI > 5. In this study, the incidence of OSA was greater in men and in those who were obese, but these effects diminished and eventually became inconsequential with increasing age. The incidence of OSA in children is unknown. An important contribution to understanding the prevalence of OSA among middle-aged adults was published in 1993 by Young and colleagues (13). In this study, the estimated prevalence of OSA, defined as an AHI on polysomnography of five or higher, was 9% for women and 24% for men. In addition, this study estimated that 2% of women and 4% of men met the minimal diagnostic criteria for the OSA syndrome (an AHI of 5 or higher and daytime hypersomnolence). In addition to the Wisconsin Cohort Study, there have been two additional large cohort studies in predominantly white men and women from Pennsylvania and Spain that utilized in-laboratory polysomnography and similar methodology and design (34–36). On the basis of the average of prevalence estimates from these three studies, approximately 1 of every 5 adults has at least mild OSA and 1 of every 15 has at least moderate OSA (25). Recent investigations in nonwhite populations also have shown a similarly high prevalence of OSA. Ip and colleagues studied 784 Hong Kong men and estimated the prevalence of OSA syndrome (defined as an AHI > 5) to be 4.1% (37). Another study of middle-aged Korean men and women noted that the prevalence of polysomnographic OSA (AHI > 5) was 27% in men and 16% in women; for the OSA syndrome (AHI > 5 with excessive daytime sleepiness), its prevalence was 4.5% in men and 3.2% in women (38). Recently, a study of healthy urban Indian males 35 to 65 years of age reported the prevalence of polysomnographic OSA was 19.5%, and that of OSA syndrome was 7.5% (39). Prevalence data for OSA in African-Americans are limited and conflicting. Redline et al. reported that young African-American subjects (<25 years old) were almost twice as likely to have OSA than Caucasians (40). Studies by Ancoli-Israel and coworkers found that it is twice as likely for African-Americans over age 65 years to have severe OSA than Caucasians over 65 years (41). However, in the multicenter Sleep Heart Health Study, the prevalence of OSA was not higher in African-Americans compared with Caucasians (42).

It has long been recognized that OSA is more common in men than women. Initial estimates from clinic-derived populations suggested that the gender disparity may be as high as 10:1. However, more recent data from general population cohorts suggest that the prevalence of OSA in men is two to three times that in women (25). The prevalence is much lower in premenopausal women and is less in postmenopausal women taking hormone replacement therapy (35). Furthermore, the gender difference in OSA prevalence appears to narrow with age (35).

In population studies, the frequency of OSA increases progressively with age. Some population-based studies note that OSA prevalence is higher in adults over age 65 years (43). However, there are other studies that do not find this, but suggest a plateau in OSA prevalence at some point after age 65 years (34,42).

The prevalence of childhood OSA is estimated to be approximately 2% (25). The peak prevalence occurs at age two to eight years and it appears that it occurs with equal frequency among boys and girls.

Central Sleep Apnea Associated with Cheyne–Stokes Breathing Pattern

CSA secondary to Cheyne–Stokes breathing pattern is the most common form of CSA that is clinically observed. The prevalence in the general population is low, but it is increased in patients with congestive heart failure and stroke (44). This SRBD has a strikingly higher prevalence in patients with heart failure as compared with those with normal left ventricular function (28,45). Two studies involving 81 and 450 patients with heart failure reported prevalence rates of 40% and 33%, respectively (31,46). In a study of 45 acutely ill patients with left ventricular ejection fractions of less than 45% admitted to a heart failure unit, 62% had CSA secondary to Cheyne–Stokes breathing pattern (47). Its prevalence in stroke is approximately

10% (29). Cheyne–Stokes breathing pattern is generally seen in patients who are male and over age 60 years of age.

Obesity-Hypoventilation Syndrome

The prevalence of the OHS is unknown. A recent study of severely obese hospitalized patients found that 31% had daytime hypercapnia unexplained by other disorders (48). Nearly half the patients in this study with a body mass index 50 kg/m^2 or greater had chronic daytime hypoventilation suggesting it is common in obese individuals but frequently unrecognized.

PHYLOGENY AND ANIMAL MODELS

Given the significant clinical relevance of OSA, there is great interest in understanding the pathophysiologic mechanisms underlying the consequences of OSA. There is no one ideal animal model for the study of SRBDs. The animal studies currently under investigation include two canine models, two rodent models (rat and mouse), an obese pig model, and a feasibility study in monkeys (49–57). The two canine models are the English bulldog as the model of spontaneously occurring upper airway obstruction and the tracheostomized dog as the model of induced upper airway occlusion. The pathogenesis of OSA in the English bulldog is similar to that observed in humans (49). The English bulldog has significant body obesity and an anatomically narrowed pharyngeal airway and exhibits obstructive breathing particularly during REM sleep, making it a natural animal model of OSA in humans. This model is useful for investigations into the pathogenesis and progression of OSA and allows studies regarding effects of drugs on upper airway dilator activity. The induction of OSA in dogs by intermittent airway occlusion during nocturnal sleep was reported in 1994 (57). This experimental model of repeated airway occlusion during sleep is a powerful tool for investigating the sequelae of OSA. In 1997, an important study using this model demonstrated that OSA causes systemic hypertension (52).

One of the major manifestations of OSA is repeated hypoxia during sleep. Acute hypoxia leads to increases in sympathetic outflow, which is followed by acute hypertension. The experimental work of Fletcher and colleagues using a rodent model of chronic-intermittent hypoxia has allowed examination of the chronic cardiovascular response to intermittent hypoxia (56). In addition, there is a murine model of OSA produced by induction of hypoxia at sleep onset and removal of hypoxia in response to arousal (54). This pattern is thus similar to the sequence of repetitive hypoxic events occurring with in patients with SRBD. These rodent models of chronic-intermittent hypoxia have expanded our knowledge about the mechanisms that contribute to the development of the hypertensive response in humans with OSA who have repeated episodes of nocturnal hypoxemia.

Other models of OSA currently being investigated are the obese Vietnamese potbellied pig and obese miniature pigs (51). There is no primate model of sleep-disordered breathing; however, one study reports the ability to create a spontaneously reversible OSA syndrome in the monkey (50).

SOCIAL AND ECONOMIC FACTORS

Obstructive Sleep Apnea Syndromes

SRBDs are common and many cases remain undiagnosed and untreated. The economic burden of untreated OSA syndrome is substantial (58–60). Patients with OSA syndrome have an increased risk of motor vehicle crashes, increased rate of work-related injuries and reduced work productivity, all of which lead to significant human and financial costs. Moreover, patients with OSA syndrome and OHS have more physician visits and hospitalizations and higher health care costs than matched controls during the 5 to 10 years preceding the diagnosis of a SRBD (61–63). It has also been noted that in children with OSA syndrome, use of health care services are higher than matched controls in the year prior to diagnosis (64). Sassani and colleagues specifically evaluated costs associated with OSA syndrome-related motor vehicle collisions (65). On the basis of their analysis, estimates of annual OSA syndrome-related collision costs, collisions, and fatalities are $15.9 billion, 810,000 collisions, and 1400 fatalities, respectively. All of these studies highlight the substantial cost implications, in terms of human life and health care expenditures of untreated sleep-disordered breathing. Three studies from Canada show a reduction in health care expenditures with treatment in OSA syndrome and OHS (62,66,67). In addition, CPAP therapy reduces motor vehicle collisions and number of missed days of work (68,69). Sassani and coworkers estimated that CPAP treatment in patients with OSA syndrome could reduce collision costs annually by $11.1 billion and save nearly 1000 lives (65). A recent study by Ayas and colleagues concluded that CPAP therapy for patients with moderate-to-severe OSA syndrome is an efficient use of health care resources (70).

One of the major clinical consequences of SRBDs is daytime sleepiness, which impairs social functioning and work performance and leads to a large socioeconomic burden on the community. Several studies have shown that patients with sleep-disordered breathing have impairment in many aspects of health-related quality of life including physical and emotional health and social functioning, and this impairment is comparable to that observed in other chronic diseases like diabetes mellitus, arthritis or hypertension (71,72). There are a number of studies that demonstrate that CPAP is an effective short-term and long-term therapy for improving the health status, quality of life and neuropsychologic deficits of patients with OSA syndrome (73,74). A meta-analysis of seven randomized controlled trials where CPAP was compared with either placebo or conservative management in the treatment of mild-to-moderate OSA syndrome indicated that CPAP significantly reduced subjective daytime sleepiness and improved objective daytime wakefulness but did not affect objective daytime sleepiness (75).

In 2006, the Cochrane Database of Systematic Reviews published an analysis of 36 trials comparing CPAP with controls or an oral appliance in adults with OSA (76). The overall results demonstrate that in patients with moderate-to-severe OSA, CPAP therapy can lead to a reduction in symptoms of sleepiness and several improvements in quality of life, cognitive function, and depression measures. CPAP is recommended as an option for improving quality of life in patients with OSA (77).

Central Sleep Apnea Associated with Cheyne–Stokes Breathing Pattern

Congestive heart failure is a major health issue with huge medical, social, and economic consequences. CSA associated with Cheyne–Stokes breathing pattern is seen in 30% to 80% of patients with advanced congestive heart failure (31,46,47). There are reports that show central sleep apnea is an independent risk factor for death or cardiac transplantation in these patients (44). The main reason for treating central sleep apnea in patients with congestive heart failure is the potential to improve cardiac function, reduce morbidity and mortality, and improve quality of life. These improvements could have important social and economic consequences. The recent multicenter Canadian Positive Airway Pressure (CANPAP) trial was conducted to determine whether CPAP would improve CSA, morbidity, mortality, and cardiovascular function in heart failure patients with CSA receiving optimal medical therapy for heart failure (78). Although CPAP in this study did not affect survival, transplant free survival, or quality of life, it did attenuate CSA and improve cardiovascular function. Larger randomized trials are needed in patients with heart failure and CSA to determine whether there is a beneficial effect of CPAP on survival in these patients.

Obesity-Hypoventilation Syndrome

Much less is known about the health care utilization and cost for patients with OHS. In a study from Canada, patients with OHS during the five years prior to diagnosis had more physician visits and were more likely to be hospitalized than patients with simple obesity (62). Two years after the diagnosis was made and treatment started, patients had a significant reduction in health care utilization and hospitalizations.

CONCLUSIONS

In the past four decades since the initial description of OSA syndrome by Gastaut and colleagues, there has been a rapid expansion of our knowledge concerning the spectrum, prevalence rates, pathophysiology, treatment and health impact of all SRBDs. SRBDs are common, occurring in both genders, in all ages and across all ethnic and racial groups. They are underdiagnosed and undertreated, and represent a significant public health problem with important social and economic ramifications on society.

REFERENCES

1. Cheyne J. A case of apoplexy in which the fleshy part of the heart was converted into fat. Dublin Hosp Rep 1818; 2:216–223.
2. Stokes W. The Diseases of the Heart and Aorta. Dublin: Hodges and Smith, 1854.
3. Burwell CS, Robin ED, Whaley RD, et al. Extreme obesity associated with alveolar hypoventilation: a Pickwickian syndrome. Am J Med 1956; 21:811–818.
4. Gastaut H, Tassinari CA, Duron B. Polygraphic study of the episodic diurnal and nocturnal (hypnic and respiratory) manifestations of the Pickwick syndrome. Brain Res 1966; 1:167–186.
5. Guilleminault C, Tilkian A, Dement WC. The sleep apnea syndromes. Annu Rev Med 1976; 27:465–484.
6. Block AJ, Boysen PG, Wynne JW, et al. Sleep apnea, hypopnea and oxygen desaturation in normal subjects. A strong male predominance. N Engl J Med 1979; 300:513–517.
7. Gould GA, Whyte KF, Rhind GB, et al. The sleep hypopnea syndrome. Am Rev Respir Dis 1988; 137: 895–898.
8. Guilleminault C, Stoohs R, Clerk A, et al. A cause of excessive daytime sleepiness. The upper airway resistance syndrome. Chest 1993; 104:781–787.
9. Kryger M, Quesney LF, Holder D, et al. The sleep deprivation syndrome of the obese patient. A problem of periodic nocturnal upper airway obstruction. Am J Med 1974; 56:530–539.
10. Lugaresi E, Coccagna G, Mantovani M, et al. Effect of tracheotomy in hypersomnia with periodic respiration. Electroencephalogr Clin Neurophysiol 1971; 30:373–374.
11. Fujita S, Conway W, Zorick F, et al. Surgical correction of anatomic abnormalities in obstructive sleep apnea syndrome: uvulopalatopharyngoplasty. Otolaryngol Head Neck Surg 1981; 89:923–934.
12. Sullivan CE, Issa FG, Berthon-Jones M, et al. Reversal of obstructive sleep apnoea by continuous positive airway pressure applied through the nares. Lancet 1981; 1:862–865.
13. Young T, Palta M, Dempsey J, et al. The occurrence of sleep-disordered breathing among middle-aged adults. N Engl J Med 1993; 328:1230–1235.
14. Guilleminault C, Lee JH, Chan A. Pediatric obstructive sleep apnea syndrome. Arch Pediatr Adolesc Med 2005; 159:775–785.
15. Yaggi HK, Concato J, Kernan WN, et al. Obstructive sleep apnea as a risk factor for stroke and death. N Engl J Med 2005; 353:2034–2041.
16. Nieto FJ, Young TB, Lind BK, et al. Association of sleep-disordered breathing, sleep apnea, and hypertension in a large community-based study. Sleep Heart Health Study. JAMA 2000; 283:1829–1836.
17. Bixler EO, Vgontzas AN, Lin HM, et al. Association of hypertension and sleep-disordered breathing. Arch Intern Med 2000; 160:2289–2295.
18. Peppard PE, Young T, Palta M, et al. Prospective study of the association between sleep-disordered breathing and hypertension. N Engl J Med 2000; 342:1378–1384.
19. Budhiraja R, Quan SF. Sleep-disordered breathing and cardiovascular health. Curr Opin Pulm Med 2005; 11:501–506.
20. Zanation AM, Senior BA. The relationship between extraesophageal reflux (EER) and obstructive sleep apnea (OSA). Sleep Med Rev 2005; 9:453–458.
21. Punjabi NM, Shahar E, Redline S, et al. Sleep-disordered breathing, glucose intolerance, and insulin resistance: the Sleep Heart Health Study. Am J Epidemiol 2004; 160:521–530.
22. Medicine AAoS, . The Interntional Classicfication of Sleep Disorders: Diagnostic and Coding Manual. Westchester, IL: American Academy of Sleep Medicine, 2005.
23. Flemons WW. Clinical practice. Obstructive sleep apnea. N Engl J Med 2002; 347:498–504.
24. Gozal D. Sleep-disordered breathing and school performance in children. Pediatrics 1998; 102:616–620.
25. Young T, Peppard PE, Gottlieb DJ. Epidemiology of obstructive sleep apnea: a population health perspective. Am J Respir Crit Care Med 2002; 165:1217–1239.
26. Pack AI. Advances in sleep-disordered breathing. Am J Respir Crit Care Med 2006; 173:7–15.
27. Marcus CL. Sleep-disordered breathing in children. Am J Respir Crit Care Med 2001; 164:16–30.
28. Bradley TD, Floras JS. Sleep apnea and heart failure: Part II: central sleep apnea. Circulation 2003; 107:1822–1826.
29. Mohsenin V. Sleep-related breathing disorders and risk of stroke. Stroke 2001; 32:1271–1278.
30. Javaheri S. Central sleep apnea in congestive heart failure: prevalence, mechanisms, impact, and therapeutic options. Semin Respir Crit Care Med 2005; 26:44–55.
31. Javaheri S, Parker TJ, Liming JD, et al. Sleep apnea in 81 ambulatory male patients with stable heart failure. Types and their prevalences, consequences, and presentations. Circulation 1998; 97:2154–2159.
32. Olson AL, Zwillich C. The obesity hypoventilation syndrome. Am J Med 2005; 118:948–956.

33. Tishler PV, Larkin EK, Schluchter MD, et al. Incidence of sleep-disordered breathing in an urban adult population: the relative importance of risk factors in the development of sleep-disordered breathing. JAMA 2003; 289:2230–2237.
34. Duran J, Esnaola S, Rubio R, et al. Obstructive sleep apnea-hypopnea and related clinical features in a population-based sample of subjects aged 30 to 70 yr. Am J Respir Crit Care Med 2001; 163:685–689.
35. Bixler EO, Vgontzas AN, Lin HM, et al. Prevalence of sleep-disordered breathing in women: effects of gender. Am J Respir Crit Care Med 2001; 163:608–613.
36. Bixler EO, Vgontzas AN, Ten Have T, et al. Effects of age on sleep apnea in men: I. Prevalence and severity. Am J Respir Crit Care Med 1998; 157:144–148.
37. Ip MS, Lam B, Lauder IJ, et al. A community study of sleep-disordered breathing in middle-aged Chinese men in Hong Kong. Chest 2001; 119:62–69.
38. Kim J, In K, You S, et al. Prevalence of sleep-disordered breathing in middle-aged Korean men and women. Am J Respir Crit Care Med 2004; 170:1108–1113.
39. Udwadia ZF, Doshi AV, Lonkar SG, et al. Prevalence of sleep-disordered breathing and sleep apnea in middle-aged urban Indian men. Am J Respir Crit Care Med 2004; 169:168–173.
40. Redline S, Tishler PV, Hans MG, et al. Racial differences in sleep-disordered breathing in African-Americans and Caucasians. Am J Respir Crit Care Med 1997; 155:186–192.
41. Ancoli-Israel S, Klauber MR, Stepnowsky C, et al. Sleep-disordered breathing in African-American elderly. Am J Respir Crit Care Med 1995; 152:1946–1949.
42. Young T, Shahar E, Nieto FJ, et al. Predictors of sleep-disordered breathing in community-dwelling adults: the Sleep Heart Health Study. Arch Intern Med 2002; 162:893–900.
43. Ancoli-Israel S, Kripke DF, Klauber MR, et al. Sleep-disordered breathing in community-dwelling elderly. Sleep 1991; 14:486–495.
44. Pepin JL, Chouri-Pontarollo N, Tamisier R, et al. Cheyne-Stokes respiration with central sleep apnoea in chronic heart failure: proposals for a diagnostic and therapeutic strategy. Sleep Med Rev 2006; 10:33–47.
45. Arzt M, Bradley TD. Treatment of sleep apnea in heart failure. Am J Respir Crit Care Med 2006; 173: 1300–1308.
46. Sin DD, Fitzgerald F, Parker JD, et al. Risk factors for central and obstructive sleep apnea in 450 men and women with congestive heart failure. Am J Respir Crit Care Med 1999; 160:1101–1106.
47. Tremel F, Pepin JL, Veale D, et al. High prevalence and persistence of sleep apnoea in patients referred for acute left ventricular failure and medically treated over 2 months. Eur Heart J 1999; 20: 1201–1209.
48. Nowbar S, Burkart KM, Gonzales R, et al. Obesity-associated hypoventilation in hospitalized patients: prevalence, effects, and outcome. Am J Med 2004; 116:1–7.
49. Hendricks JC, Kline LR, Kovalski RJ, et al. The English bulldog: a natural model of sleep-disordered breathing. J Appl Physiol 1987; 63:1344–1350.
50. Philip P, Gross CE, Taillard J, et al. An animal model of a spontaneously reversible obstructive sleep apnea syndrome in the monkey. Neurobiol Dis 2005; 20:428–431.
51. Tuck SA, Dort JC, Olson ME, et al. Monitoring respiratory function and sleep in the obese Vietnamese pot-bellied pig. J Appl Physiol 1999; 87:444–451.
52. Brooks D, Horner RL, Kozar LF, et al. Obstructive sleep apnea as a cause of systemic hypertension. Evidence from a canine model. J Clin Invest 1997; 99:106–109.
53. Fenik P, Ogawa H, Veasey SC. Hypoglossal nerve response to 5-HT3 drugs injected into the XII nucleus and vena cava in the rat. Sleep 2001; 24:871–878.
54. Tagaito Y, Polotsky VY, Campen MJ, et al. A model of sleep-disordered breathing in the C57BL/6J mouse. J Appl Physiol 2001; 91:2758–2766.
55. Sica AL, Greenberg HE, Ruggiero DA, et al. Chronic-intermittent hypoxia: a model of sympathetic activation in the rat. Respir Physiol 2000; 121:173–184.
56. Fletcher EC. Invited review: physiological consequences of intermittent hypoxia: systemic blood pressure. J Appl Physiol 2001; 90:1600–1605.
57. Kimoff RJ, Makino H, Horner RL, et al. Canine model of obstructive sleep apnea: model description and preliminary application. J Appl Physiol 1994; 76:1810–1817.
58. Kapur V, Blough DK, Sandblom RE, et al. The medical cost of undiagnosed sleep apnea. Sleep 1999; 22:749–755.
59. Hillman DR, Murphy AS, Pezzullo L. The economic cost of sleep disorders. Sleep 2006; 29:299–305.
60. Wittmann V, Rodenstein DO. Health care costs and the sleep apnea syndrome. Sleep Med Rev 2004; 8:269–279.
61. Ronald J, Delaive K, Roos L, et al. Health care utilization in the 10 years prior to diagnosis in obstructive sleep apnea syndrome patients. Sleep 1999; 22:225–229.
62. Berg G, Delaive K, Manfreda J, et al. The use of health-care resources in obesity-hypoventilation syndrome. Chest 2001; 120:377–383.
63. Smith R, Ronald J, Delaive K, et al. What are obstructive sleep apnea patients being treated for prior to this diagnosis? Chest 2002; 121:164–172.

64. Reuveni H, Simon T, Tal A, et al. Health care services utilization in children with obstructive sleep apnea syndrome. Pediatrics 2002; 110:68–72.
65. Sassani A, Findley LJ, Kryger M, et al. Reducing motor-vehicle collisions, costs, and fatalities by treating obstructive sleep apnea syndrome. Sleep 2004; 27:453–458.
66. Albarrak M, Banno K, Sabbagh AA, et al. Utilization of healthcare resources in obstructive sleep apnea syndrome: a 5-year follow-up study in men using CPAP. Sleep 2005; 28:1306–1311.
67. Bahammam A, Delaive K, Ronald J, et al. Health care utilization in males with obstructive sleep apnea syndrome two years after diagnosis and treatment. Sleep 1999; 22:740–747.
68. George CF. Reduction in motor vehicle collisions following treatment of sleep apnoea with nasal CPAP. Thorax 2001; 56:508–512.
69. Ellen RLB, Palayew SM, Molnar F, et al. Systematic review of motor vehicle crash risk in persons with sleep apnea. J Clin Sleep Med 2006; 2:193–200.
70. Ayas NT, FitzGerald JM, Fleetham JA, et al. Cost-effectiveness of continuous positive airway pressure therapy for moderate to severe obstructive sleep apnea/hypopnea. Arch Intern Med 2006; 166:977–984.
71. D'Ambrosio C, Bowman T, Mohsenin V. Quality of life in patients with obstructive sleep apnea: effect of nasal continuous positive airway pressure—a prospective study. Chest 1999; 115:123–129.
72. Finn L, Young T, Palta M, et al. Sleep-disordered breathing and self-reported general health status in the Wisconsin Sleep Cohort Study. Sleep 1998; 21:701–706.
73. Sin DD, Mayers I, Man GC, et al. Can continuous positive airway pressure therapy improve the general health status of patients with obstructive sleep apnea?: a clinical effectiveness study. Chest 2002; 122:1679–1685.
74. Lloberes P, Marti S, Sampol G, et al. Predictive factors of quality-of-life improvement and continuous positive airway pressure use in patients with sleep apnea-hypopnea syndrome: study at 1 year. Chest 2004; 126:1241–1247.
75. Marshall NS, Barnes M, Travier N, et al. Continuous positive airway pressure reduces daytime sleepiness in mild to moderate obstructive sleep apnoea: a meta-analysis. Thorax 2006; 61:430–434.
76. Giles TL, Lasserson TJ, Smith BJ, et al. Continuous positive airways pressure for obstructive sleep apnoea in adults. Cochrane Database Syst Rev 2006; CD001106.
77. Kushida CA, Littner MR, Hirshkowitz M, et al. Practice parameters for the use of continuous and bilevel positive airway pressure devices to treat adult patients with sleep-related breathing disorders. Sleep 2006; 29:375–380.
78. Bradley TD, Logan AG, Kimoff RJ, et al. Continuous positive airway pressure for central sleep apnea and heart failure. N Engl J Med 2005; 353:2025–2033.

26 | Pathophysiology, Associations, and Consequences of Sleep-Related Breathing Disorders

Gina H. Chen and Christian Guilleminault

Sleep Disorders Center, Stanford University School of Medicine, Stanford, California, U.S.A.

INTRODUCTION

Sleep provides a permissive state for uncovering breathing difficulties. Sleep apnea was first described independently by Gastaut, Tassinari, and Duron in France and by Jung and Kuhlo in Germany in 1965 (1). In 1972, Guilleminault evaluated a 10-year-old boy with excessive daytime sleepiness (EDS) and unexplained hypertension whose polysomnography showed an apnea index of 55 and esophageal pressure (Pes) of 80 to 120 cm H2O (1). The patient was treated with tracheostomy and his symptoms and hypertension subsequently improved. Since then, major strides have been achieved to understand the natural history, pathophysiology, and consequences of sleep-related breathing disorders (SRBD). The nosology of SRBD as defined by the *International Classification of Sleep Disorders*, second edition (ICSD-2) spans an array of disorders that result in variable degrees of upper airway obstruction. Additionally, all other breathing abnormalities occurring in sleep, including central apnea and hypoventilation, are included in SRBD (2).

Primary central sleep apnea is characterized by recurrent cessation of respiration during sleep without associated ventilatory effort. A high ventilatory response to hypercapnea appears to be a predisposing factor, with low normal arterial $PaCO_2$ during wakefulness (typically less than 40 mmHg). Arterial $PaCO_2$ levels below the $PaCO_2$ apnea threshold will lead to a cessation in respiratory efforts and resultant central apnea. Individuals with higher ventilatory response to $PaCO_2$ tend to have lower arterial $PaCO_2$ to start with, and consequently, a smaller increase in ventilation is required to reach the apnea threshold. In these individuals, there is more instability of respiratory control system during transition from wakefulness to sleep, and the polysomnogram will demonstrate more than five episodes of cessation of ventilatory effort and ventilation for 10 seconds or longer during the onset of non–rapid eye movement (NREM) sleep. In contrast, Cheyne-Stokes breathing is characterized by apnea and/or hypopnea alternating with prolonged hyperpneas in a crescendo-decrescendo pattern. Typically, Cheyne-Stokes pattern is observed during NREM sleep. Individuals who chronically hyperventilate during wakefulness and sleep are predisposed to this breathing pattern. Their $PaCO_2$ is closer to their apneic threshold than individuals without Cheyne-Stokes breathing. The central apnea arises out of arousals where there is an augmentation of ventilatory effort, driving the $PaCO_2$ to below the apneic threshold leading to apnea. Cheyne-Stokes breathing pattern typically has a ventilatory-apneic cycle time of greater than 45 seconds, in contrast to primary central sleep apnea, which is typically less than 45 seconds. The most important predisposing factors are congestive heart failure (CHF), strokes, and possibly, renal failure. In CHF, Cheyne-Stokes breathing is associated with poor prognosis.

Sleep-related nonobstructive alveolar hypoventilation is also termed "central alveolar hypoventilation," "primary alveolar hypoventilation," or "idiopathic central alveolar hypoventilation." Individuals can present with diurnal as well as nocturnal hypoventilation with normal lung mechanics. There is a blunted chemoresponsiveness with consequent decreased alveolar ventilation and tidal volume resulting in hypercapnea and hypoxemia. Hypoventilation is most pronounced during rapid eye movement (REM) sleep.

The *ICSD-2* includes many respiratory disorders during sleep under the classification of SRBD. However, in the clinical setting, many clinicians use SRBD to describe breathing abnormalities found in sleep. More specifically, SRBD is often equated with obstructive sleep apnea (OSA), as it is the most common sleep breathing disorder. Given the high prevalence of OSA and upper airway resistance syndrome (UARS), the remainder of this chapter will focus on these two disease entities.

According to the *ICSD-2*, OSA is characterized by repetitive episodes of complete or partial upper airway closure during sleep (2). Complete airway obstruction for 10 seconds or more is termed "apnea." In general, there are three different types of apnea—central, obstructive, and mixed. Mixed apnea begins with central apnea but terminates in an obstructive apnea, and partial airway obstruction is termed a "hypopnea." The severity of OSA is based on apnea-hypopnea index (AHI), which is the number of apneas and hypopneas that occur in an hour. It has been empirically determined that AHI of five or greater is abnormal in adults, and furthermore, mild OSA has an AHI of 5 to less than 15, moderate OSA is 15 to 30 and severe is more than 30. UARS is classified under OSA in the most recent edition of ICSD. The original description of UARS included patients whose AHI was less than 5 but had EDS, which improved after treatment for upper airway obstruction (3). In this patient population, respiratory effort–related arousals (RERAs) can be measured by measuring esophageal pressures, which reflect intrathoracic pressures, that is, inspiratory effort. RERAs are arousals associated with episodes of high inspiratory efforts, which do not meet the criteria for either apnea or hypopnea. Usually, there is a crescendo pattern of progressively increasing inspiratory effort followed by an arousal, termed a "Pes crescendo." In children, polysomnographic findings of OSA are defined by the *ICSD-2* as one or more scoreable respiratory events per hour, and a scoreable event is an apnea or hypopnea of at least two respiratory cycles long.

ETIOLOGY, PATHOPHYSIOLOGY, AND PATHOGENESIS

Normal Physiology

During wakefulness, pharyngeal muscles including genioglossus, levator palatine, and palatoglossus muscles show phasic inspiratory activity (4). These muscle activities, coupled with tonic activation of the tensor palatine muscle, counteract the negative intraluminal pressure generated with each inspiratory effort via the diaphragm. The airway patency is maintained by neuromuscular activation of the aforementioned muscles. More importantly, the pharyngeal muscle is able to rapidly react, initiating contraction prior to diaphragmatic activation. Consequently, they contract the negative inspiratory pressure generated by the diaphragm, preventing upper airway collapse (5). Furthermore, there is reflex pharyngeal dilatory muscle activity in genioglossus, tensor palatine, levator palatine, and palatoglossus in response to brief pulses of negative intraluminal pressure (6–8). Both tonic activation and phasic activation of the pharyngeal muscles are decreased in sleep, producing a reduction in the airway lumen (9). In addition, sleep produces a decrease in the magnitude and an increase in the latency of the pharyngeal reflex to brief impulses of negative pressure (10). Consequently, the delay in the dilator muscles reflex means that at onset of inspiration, as the diaphragm contracts generating a negative inspiratory pressure, there is no compensation to the resistive load generated (11).

Additionally, the resting lung volumes and ventilatory response to hypoxia and hypercapnia are blunted in sleep (12–14). This results in a 2 to 8 mmHg rise in carbon dioxide during sleep in normal subjects. As described by Dempsey et al., there is instability in breathing during sleep onset, which is dependent on the change in ventilatory response to the change in $PaCO_2$ and the magnitude of the $PaCO_2$ change from wake to sleep (15). With sleep onset, there is an abrupt, brief increase in airway resistance, as well as an increase in $PaCO_2$ (16). Normally, there is stabilization of breathing shortly after sleep onset, if sleep stabilizes and there are no arousals. Upper airway resistance initially increases with sleep onset but decreases after the initial abrupt increase (17). This is secondary to a fall in diaphragmatic and intercostals muscle activities and an initial fall in genioglossus and tensor palatini muscle activities, as well as a subsequent recruitment of genioglossus muscle after two to three breaths (18–20). The tensor palatini activity, however, continues to fall as long as sleep is maintained (21,22). During sleep onset, the decrease in genioglossus and tensor palatini is more pronounced in the older than in the younger male subjects. Greater decrements in activity during sleep onset and decrease in recruitment during sleep contribute to the pathogenesis of OSA and UARS (23).

Obstructive Sleep Apnea and Upper Airway Resistance Syndrome

Although in the ICSD upper airway resistance syndrome is grouped with OSA, there is clear difference in the degree of pathophysiology. In patients with OSA, there are several factors which, when coupled with the physiologic changes in normal sleep, predispose them to airway obstruction. OSA patients are more likely to have an anatomically smaller airway during sleep. This may be coupled with increased pharyngeal fat pads further narrowing the airway, rendering it vulnerable to increased intraluminal pressure (24). Additionally, this patient population may have increased activation of pharyngeal dilator muscles during wakefulness, and therefore, there is a relatively larger reduction in muscle activation during sleep (25). Lastly, there is a significant reduction in the degree and speed of the pharyngeal reflex activation in response to brief impulses of negative intraluminal pressure, further incapacitating OSA patients to counteract upper airway collapse. Maximal negative intraluminal pressure occurs during midinspiration. However, on endoscopic examinations of OSA patients, the minimal cross-sectional area of the airway occurs at end expiration. Consequently, if there is a delay in the reflex activation of the dilator muscles, there is increased likelihood of airway obstruction.

It has been proposed that chronic snoring and continuous trauma to the pharyngeal muscles may lead to permanent lesions and neuropathy causing the decrease, and potentially lack of, reflex response and activation of the muscles (26). Biopsies from OSA patients demonstrated atrophy and an abnormal distribution of fiber types. Frieberg et al. showed progressive lesions consistent with a polyneuropathy in the palatopharyngeal muscles of OSA patients, and the degree of abnormalities correlated with the severity of OSA (27). His group further found increased density in sensory nerve terminals of the soft palate (28). Larrson et al. found pathologically increased thresholds for temperature sensitivity on the tonsillar pillars in patients with OSA (29). Guilleminault et al. demonstrated decreased sensitivity to pressure in the larynx and velopharynx in patients with airway obstruction (30). Patients with OSA also have more type IIA and less type IIB and type I muscle fibers than normal controls, where type IIA are fast fiber with intermediate fatigue resistance (31,32). Heavy resistance training, such as breathing in against an obstruction every night, will preferentially produce type II hypertrophy to resist fatigue (33). Carrera et al. studied obese and nonobese OSA patients with matched controls (34). They found that the obese patients' muscle endurance was indistinguishable from that of control; however, the nonobese patients, at diagnosis, had increased fatigability. In the treated continuous positive airway pressure (CPAP) patients, they did not see an increase in fatigability. In a prior study, they demonstrated the reversibility of the structural and functional changes in OSA patients treated with CPAP, suggesting perhaps that some of the changes seen in OSA are a consequence of untreated disease rather than a primary cause of OSA (35).

For patients with intact sensory input from upper airway sensors and appropriate motor nerve conduction, they may present with UARS or chronic snoring. Guilleminault et al. have shown similar two-point discrimination in the palate of patients with UARS and control. Consequently, there is a better perception of airway size change, and in turn, a faster reflex response is triggered, when compared to OSA patients. This faster response may lead to a subcortical activation, manifested as cyclic alternating patterns on the electroencephalography (EEG) (36,37). With a stronger and broader activation, an alpha EEG arousal may ensue (38).

Nasal obstruction appears to contribute to abnormal airflow, contributing to sleep fragmentation. In normal subjects, there was greater ventilation with nasal breathing than oral, suggesting nasal breathing may have stimulatory effect on either respiration or pharyngeal muscle tone (39,40). In a number of studies, normal subjects with increased nasal resistance displayed an increase in arousals and/or awakenings and less slow wave sleep on their polysomnograms (41–43). There is no clear correlation between increased nasal resistance and increased AHI (44), although there appears to be a higher incidence of increased nasal resistance in patients with either snoring or OSA (45,46). Overall, it appears that minor breathing impairments, such as increased nasal resistance, can lead to UARS (47).

PREDISPOSING AND PRECIPITATING FACTORS

There are a number of risk factors associated with increased upper airway obstruction. In addition to age, male gender has been consistently associated with a two- to threefold increased risks of sleep apnea (48,49). Hormonal differences are theorized to be the reason for the gender difference. A woman's risk changes with pregnancy and menopause. Both have increased rates of OSA. In the Wisconsin Sleep Cohort study, postmenopausal women have three times the risks of having moderate to severe OSA as compared with premenopausal women, independent of body mass index (BMI) or age (50). In the Sleep Heart Health Study, 2994 postmenopausal women aged 50 years or older showed that those who used hormone replacement therapy (HRT) were half as likely to have OSA as compared with those without HRT (51).

Obesity is a common risk factor. The degree of BMI and neck circumference and waist-to-hip ratio has been correlated to the prevalence and the severity of OSA (52). In a longitudinal study, it was found that a 10% increase in weight was associated with a sixfold increase in the risk for developing OSA (53). A 3% change in AHI is expected for each 1% increase in BMI, and similar change in the opposite direction is noted with decrease in BMI. However, not all patients with OSA are obese. Craniofacial and upper airway anatomy can play a significant role, especially in the Asian population and in the pediatric population (54). Dimorphism of the mandibular or maxillary bony structure or abnormality of soft tissue plays a major role in the development of OSA (55,56). Lam et al. looked at 239 consecutive patients (164 Asian and 75 Caucasian) and found that Mallapati score, thyromental angle, neck circumference as well as age and BMI were the best predictors of OSA (57). In children, syndromes associated with craniofacial abnormalities, such as Peirri-Robin, Apert, Down syndrome, are associated with OSA. Some studies have shown increased incidence of OSA in certain ethnic groups. For example, Pacific Islanders and Mexican-Americans as well as African Americans appear to have increased risk for developing OSA (58–60). Whether this is related to craniofacial features, or familial tendency for OSA, as was reported in some Caucasian families, remains unclear (61,62).

Lastly, there is a strong correlation between chronic rhinitis or nasal obstruction and OSA. Young et al. noted that patients with nasal congestion are 1.8 times more likely to have moderate to severe OSA (63). Similarly, Kramer et al. compared 10 patients with EDS and nonallergic rhinitis with 16 age and BMI matched patients and found that these patients have higher AHI and lower mean oxygen saturation compared to the controls (64). For children, there is a complex interaction between nasal breathing and maxillomandibular growth. Increased nasal resistance and oral breathing will impair maxillomandibular growth and lead to smaller jaw and airways (65–67). Additionally, enlarged adenoids and tonsils during childhood will often lead to mouth breathing, which can cause abnormal growth of the lower face and jaw resulting in "adenoidal facies," predisposing the child to development of OSA (68).

MORBIDITY AND MORTALITY

Snoring and EDS are common complaints by patients or their bed partners. Snoring can start anytime in one's life, but most commonly it starts at puberty. It becomes worse and positionally dependent as one gets older and as one gains weight. There can be complaints of dry mouth, teeth grinding, and sleeping separately from bed partners. EDS can be attributed to sleep fragmentation with frequent arousals caused by airflow limitations. As a consequence, there is decreased slow wave and REM sleep. Often times with frequent arousals, the patient is not aware of wakening, but has a sense of nonrestorative sleep in the morning. A subpopulation of patients will present with sleep maintenance insomnia where they complain of waking up multiple times during the night without a clear cause. This usually occurs after an apneic episode that ends in an arousal where the patient wakes up and is conscious of the awakening (69). If the arousals occur during stage N3 sleep, sleepwalking and night terrors may result. During REM sleep, nightmares with themes of repetitive drowning or choking may occur. Morning headaches, which resolve within an hour of awakening, may indicate nocturnal hypercarbia and increased intracranial pressure. Nocturia has been reported by male OSA patients and is felt to be related to elevated plasma levels of atrial natriuretic peptide and catecholamine (70,71). Symptoms of gastroesophageal reflex may worsen during sleep secondary to larger negative intrathoracic pressure during inspiration. The increased negative intrathoracic pressure can increase intra-abdominal pressure resulting in acid reflux.

Although sleep bruxism is classified as a parasomnia by *ICSD-2*, its presence should prompt a search for SRBD. Jaw muscle relaxation during sleep contributes to tongue retrusion and decrease airway patency. In the apneic patient the coactivation of jaw-opening and jaw-clenching muscles prevents pharyngeal collapse (72,73). Experimentally induced micro-arousals can evoke bruxism (74–76).

Symptoms of OSA overlap with those of UARS, although there are some very important differences (77). Sleep onset insomnia and sleep maintenance insomnia tend to be more common in patients with UARS secondary to behavioral conditioning of frequent arousal (78). Instead of sleepiness, this patient group complains of fatigue, in addition to headaches and irritable bowel syndrome, and is often misdiagnosed with chronic fatigue syndrome or fibromyalgia or adult attention deficit syndrome (79,80). Autonomic dysfunction such as cold hands and feet, lightheadedness, and orthostatic hypotension are reported, and are also seen in patients with UARS. It appears lower blood pressure is commonly associated with UARS whereas hypertension is commonly seen in OSA patients (81–83). Cognitive function such as short-term memory can also be affected. Epworth Sleepiness Scale gives a measurement of the patient's propensity to fall asleep in certain circumstances (84). However, the degree of daytime sleepiness does not necessarily correlate with severity of sleep apnea (85,86).

ASSOCIATIONS, COMPLICATIONS, AND CONSEQUENCES

Cognitive Function

Cognitive impairment in patients with OSA has been demonstrated in a number of studies. There are cognitive deficits concerning memory, attention, executive function, and motor abilities (87–89). The cause of cognitive dysfunction in OSA is not quite clear. Some hypothesize it is related to hypoxemia (90,91) while others point to EDS (92,93). More recent studies have suggested impairment of executive functions, motor and visuoconstructive abilities may be related to severity of hypoxemia, whereas the attention and memory deficit may be due to EDS secondary to sleep fragmentation (94,95). These impairments improve after treatment with CPAP. The degree of recovery is not absolute and the patients studied have been varied (96,97). Lastly, there have been studies, which suggest increased prevalence of Alzheimer's disease with sleep apnea, while others have shown prevalence of sleep apnea being more common in multi-infarct dementia (98,99).

Stroke

The prevalence of OSA among stroke patients is greater than 60%, in contrast to the 4% in the middle-aged adult population (100–102). Whether OSA serves as a risk factor in itself, independent of hypertension, cardiac arrhythmias, hyperlipidemia, and diabetes is not clear. Cross-sectional studies have demonstrated an increase in the risk of stroke in SRBD patients comparable in magnitude to the effects of other cardiovascular risks (103,104). Marler et al. showed that the presence of SRBD in a patient who had a prior stroke is at increased risk of having a second event upon wakening from sleep (105). It appears that during the early morning hours, this patient population had more significant desaturations occurring with apneic episodes than during REM sleep. More recently, Yaggi et al. conducted an observational cohort study to examine the role of obstructive sleep apnea in the development of first time stroke event in patients referred to the sleep clinic for suspected SRBD (106). They excluded patients with prior history of stroke, myocardial infarction, tracheostomy, and patients referred for evaluation other than suspected SRBD. Although 58% of the diagnosed patients received CPAP therapy, 31% achieved weight reduction of 10% or more, and 15% underwent upper airway surgery, they still found an increased incidence of stroke in this patient group, independent of other cardiovascular and cerebrovascular risk factors. This suggests there may be other factors than just hypoxemia and hypertension contributing to strokes in patients with OSA. Interestingly, the hazard ratio for stroke or death seems to increase with increasing AHI. In this particular study, there was not enough power to see if CPAP treatment would significantly alter the risk. Other studies have demonstrated CPAP therapy can reverse hypercoagulability (107,108) and hemodynamic changes (109,110).

Cardiac Consequences

Hypertension

The prevalence of hypertension is higher than expected in patients with OSA (111,112). The association has been known since 1970s; however, it was not until recently that several studies showed OSA to be an independent risk factor for hypertension (83,113). The Wisconsin Sleep Cohort Study examined the development of hypertension as a function of OSA and found the unadjusted odds ratio for developing hypertension was 4.5 in patients with AHI greater than 15. When adjusted for age, sex, smoking, body habitus, and alcohol consumption, the odds ratio was 2.9. The mechanism of OSA causing hypertension is unclear. There is evidence of increased sympathetic tone during sleep as well as during daytime (114,115), and the hemodynamic profile during sleep is primarily dictated by the duration and severity of apnea (116,117). Repeat apnea and hypoxia, and hypercapnia and swings in intrathoracic pressure lead to activation of sympathetic system which leads to increased heart rate, cardiac output, peripheral vascular resistance, and increased tubular sodium reabsorption. This increase in sympathetic activity persists into daytime, when patients are breathing normally (118). Baroreflex and chemoreflex dysfunctions (119,120), vasoconstrictor effects of nocturnal endothelin release (121) and endothelial dysfunction (122) are felt to contribute to the persistence of hypertension. Although CPAP treatment results in marked reduction in nocturnal sympathetic activity and modulates blood pressure surges during sleep (123), the effect on daytime blood pressure is less clear. Most studies showed small to moderate decreases (109,124).

Coronary Artery Disease

OSA frequently occurs in patients with coronary artery diseases and is generally associated with nocturnal angina and nocturnal ST-T segment depression (125). OSA is an independent risk factor for ischemic heart disease (126). The ST-T segment depression correlates with oxyhemoglobin desaturation and severity of OSA (127,128). It is postulated that the ischemic changes are likely related to increased myocardial oxygen requirements during the postapneic period with blood pressure and heart rate surges (129). In the study by Milleron et al., there was a reduction in the risk of cardiovascular death and acute coronary syndrome in patients treated with CPAP compared to a matched number of patients who declined treatment (130).

Congestive Heart Failure

OSA has been associated with congestive heart failure (CHF). Possible mechanism linking OSA and CHF is hypertension and its effects on the left ventricular function (138). The increase in sympathetic tone, the surges in the blood pressure and the wall stress, together with the metabolic derangements and the hypoxic effect of OSA come together to further stress an already diseased heart. CPAP have shown to improve ejection fraction (131). In the Sleep Heart Health Study, OSA was noted to be an independent risk factor for CHF, where patients with AHI greater than 11 have an odds ratio of 2.38 of having CHF. OSA has been correlated with both systolic and diastolic dysfunction. In the normotensive patients with OSA, left ventricular hypertrophy was more common than right heart failure (132,133). Cheyne-Stokes respirations (CSR) occur in patients with CHF, as mentioned earlier in this chapter. This patient group has increased carbon dioxide (PCO_2) chemosensitivity and hyperventilates during wakefulness resulting in a lower PCO_2 apneic threshold (134,135).

PSYCHOLOGIC OR PSYCHIATRIC ASSOCIATIONS, COMPLICATIONS, AND CONSEQUENCES

Obstructive Sleep Apnea

Excessive Daytime Sleepiness

Excessive daytime sleepiness (EDS) or fatigue is the most common complaint in OSA. Sleepiness can range from mild, such as feeling drowsy during an afternoon meeting to falling asleep at the wheel. The National Sleep Foundation 2000 Omnibus Sleep in America Poll found 43% of adults report sleepiness that interferes with their daily activities a few days per month.

Twenty percent of adults report experiencing this degree of sleepiness at least a few days a week (136). Powell et al. demonstrated a decrease in performance secondary to sleepiness can be worse than that associated with alcohol intoxication (137). It is important to inquire about sleepiness in relationship to operation of machinery, as accidents tend to occur with sleepiness and slower reaction time. Hakkanen et al. studied a cohort of professional truck drivers, 40% of long-haul drivers reported difficulties staying alert during at least 20% of their drives, and 20% admitted to dozing off at least twice while driving (138). There have been a multitude of studies linking OSA with EDS and motor vehicle accidents (139,140). In the United States, more than 50,000 motor vehicle accidents are attributed to driving while sleepy (141). It is important to obtain detailed history as patients may not always describe sleepiness nor admit to it. Associated problems include neurocognitive function decline, slower reaction time, and more difficulty executing tasks. Performance may not always be the best indicator as motivation can often transiently override sleepiness.

Various methods to assess sleepiness have been developed. The Stanford Sleepiness Scale and the Karolinska Sleepiness Scale assess the momentary degree of alertness or sleepiness (142,143). They are useful in tracking symptoms during a given time. The Epworth Sleepiness Scale offers a more appropriate method for assessing global sleepiness (84). It consists of eight questions and each is scored with a degree of severity. A multiple sleep latency test (MSLT) has been used to attempt to quantify degree of sleepiness. It is usually performed after a normal polysomnogram (144). A sleep onset latency of greater than 10 minutes is normal; less than 8 minutes suggests pathological sleepiness. Between 8 and 10 minutes is a "gray" area. The maintenance of wakefulness is another similar test, but the subject is asked to stay awake (145). This test is frequently used in legal battles.

Other Symptoms

Some patients complain of difficulty concentrating, short-term memory recall deficit, or clumsiness in tasks requiring dexterity (146). Intellectual impairments can be detected on neuropsychological testing (147). Mood swings, aggressiveness, irritability, anxiety, and depression can also be part of the presentation. Studies comparing community-recruited subjects with low levels of sleep disordered breathing to patients with OSA showed that impairment effects are proportional to the severity of OSA (148).

Sexual dysfunction is often reported in one third of the patient population with OSA, and will improve with treatment, unless there are other underlying pathological factors. Dry mouth in the morning is another complaint, with 74% of patients reporting a dry mouth and 36% reporting drooling. This is secondary to congested nasal passage with resultant mouth breathing frequently seen in patients with OSA.

Upper Airway Resistance Syndrome

Many of the symptoms in UARS overlap with those in OSA. However, there are some important differences. Chronic insomnia tends to be more common in patients with UARS (149). Many patients complain of sleep onset as well as sleep maintenance insomnia. This is thought to be a result of conditioning, as a consequence of frequent sleep disruption. Fatigue is a more likely complaint than sleepiness. Gold et al. emphasized that patients with UARS tend to have more complaints of functional somatic problems such as headaches, sleep-onset insomnia, and irritable bowel syndrome (79). Unfortunately, many times the patients are misdiagnosed with chronic fatigue syndrome or fibromyalgia, attention deficit or psychiatric disorder (80). Autonomic dysfunction is seen more often in patients with UARS than in those with OSA. Patients complain of cold hands and feet, and a quarter of them will complain of lightheadedness. Hypotension can be associated with UARS and can account for the lightheadedness (81).

CONCLUSIONS

SRBD is a group of very broadly defined disorders that relates to abnormalities of respiration during sleep. The most prevalent SRBD are OSA and UARS. The diagnosis of these disorders requires recognition of the vast constellation of signs and symptoms with which a patient may present. Even when the presenting symptom is insomnia, one cannot immediately rule out

SRBD. There are health and economic consequences to unrecognized and untreated SRBD secondary to the multiple organs potentially affected by these disorders. OSA and UARS should specifically be considered a systemic disease. Involvement of the cerebral and cardiovascular as well as neurocognitive and endocrine systems appears to be just a few of the potential far-reaching effects of OSA and UARS. Much has been elucidated regarding the pathophysiology of SRBD; however, much remains to be discovered. CPAP treatment clearly has beneficial outcomes, but the specific situations are yet to be defined.

REFERENCES

1. Krieger M, Roth T, Dement W, eds. Principles and Practice of Sleep Medicine. Philadelphia, PA: Elsevier, 2005:7–9.
2. American Academy of Sleep Medicine. The International Classification of Sleep Disorders. 2nd ed. Westbrook, IL: The American Academy of Sleep Medicine, 2005.
3. Guilleminault C, Stoohs R, Clerk A, et al. A cause of excessive daytime sleepiness: the upper airway resistance syndrome. Chest 1993; 104:781–787.
4. Horner R. Motor control of the pharyngeal musculature and implications for the pathogenesis of obstructive sleep apnea. Sleep 1996; 19:827–853.
5. Dick T, Van Launtern E. Fiber subtype distribution of pharyngeal dilator muscles and diaphragm in the cat. J Appl Physiol 1990; 68:2237–2240.
6. Horner R, Innes J, Morrell M, et al. The effect of sleep on reflex genioglossus muscle activation by stimuli of negative airway pressure in humans. J Physiol 1994; 476:141–145.
7. Wheatley J, Mezzanotte W, Tangel D, et al. Influence of sleep on genioglossus muscle activation by negative pressure in normal men. Am Rev Respir Dis 1993; 148:597–605.
8. Horner R, Innes J, Murphy K, et al. Evidence for reflex upper airway dilator muscle activation by sudden negative airway pressure in man. J Physiol 1991; 436:15–29.
9. Morrell M, Arabi Y, Zahn B, et al. Progressive retropalatal narrowing preceding obstructive apnea. Am J Respir Crit Care Med 1998; 158:1974–1981.
10. Wheatley J, Tangel D, Mezzanotte W, et al. Influence of sleep on response to negative airway pressure of tensor palatini muscle and retropalatal airway. J Appl Physiol 1993; 75:2117–2124.
11. Morrell M, Browne H, Adams L, et al. The respiratory response to inspiratory resistive loading during rapid eye movement sleep in humans. J Physiol 2000; 526:195–202.
12. Hudgel D, Martin R, Johnson B, et al. Mechanics of the respiratory system and breathing pattern during sleep in normal humans. J Appl Physiol 1984; 56(1):133–137.
13. Douglas N, White D, Weil J, et al. Hypoxic ventilatory response decreases during sleep in normal men. Am Rev Respir Dis 1982; 125(3):286–289.
14. Dempsey J, Smith C, Przybylowski T, et al. The ventilatory responsiveness to CO_2 below eupnoea as a determinant of ventilatory stability in sleep. J Physiol 2004; 560:1–11.
15. Dempsey J, Skatrud J, Smith C. Powerful stabilizing effect of CO_2 during CPAP treatment. Sleep 2005; 28:12–13.
16. Colrain I, Trinder J, Fraser G, et al. Ventilation during sleep onset. J Appl Physiol 1987; 63:2067–2074.
17. Kay A, Trinder J, Kim Y. Changes in airway resistance during sleep onset. J Appl Physiol 1994; 76:1600–1607.
18. Edstrom L, Larsson H, Larsson L. Neurogenic efforts on the plaltopharyngeal muscle in patients with obstructive sleep apnea: a muscle biopsy study. J Neurol Neurosurg Psychiatry 1992; 55:916–920.
19. Woodson B, Wooten M. A multisensor solid-state pressure manometer to identify the level of collapse in obstructive sleep apnea. Otolaryngol Head Neck Surg 1992; 107(5):651–656.
20. Worsnop C, Kay A, Kim Y, et al. Effect of age on sleep onset-related changes in respiratory pump and upper airway muscle function. J Appl Physiol 2000; 88:1831–1839.
21. Nguyen A, Jobin V, Payne R, et al. Laryngeal and velopharyngeal sensory impairment in obstructive sleep apnea. Sleep 2005; 28(5):585–593.
22. Boyd J, Petrof B, Hamid Q, et al. Upper airway muscle inflammation and denervation changes in obstructive sleep apnea. Am J Respir Crit Care Med 2004; 170:541–546.
23. Tangle D, Mezzanotte W, White D. Influence of sleep on tensor palatini EMG and upper airway resistance in normal men. J Appl Physiol 1991; 70:2574–2581.
24. Horner R, Mohiaddin R, Lowell D, et al. Sites and sizes of fat deposits around the pharynx in obese patients with obstructive sleep apnea and weight matched controls. Eur Respir J 1989; 2:613–622.
25. Mezzanotte W, Tangel D, White D. Waking geioglossal electromyogram in sleep apnea patients versus normal controls (a neuromuscular compensatory mechanism). J Clin Invest 1992; 89:1572–1579.
26. Kimoff R, Sforza E, Champagne V, et al. Upper airway sensation in snoring and obstructive sleep apnea. Am J Respir Crit Care Med 2001; 164:250–255.

27. Frieberg D, Answed T, Borg K. Histological indications of a progressive snorer disease in upper airway muscle. Am Respir Crit Care Med 1998; 157:586–593.
28. Frieberg D, Gazelius B, Hokfelt T, et al. Abnormal afferent nerve endings in the soft palatal mucosa of sleep apnoics and habitual snorers. Regul Pept 1997; 71:29–36.
29. Larrson H, Carlsson-Norlander B, Lindblad L, et al. Temperature thresholds in the oropharynx of patients with obstructive sleep apnea syndrome. Am Rev Respir Dis 1992; 146:1246–1249.
30. Guilleminault C, Li K, Chen N, et al. Two-point palatal discrimination in patients with upper-airway resistance syndrome, obstructive sleep apnea sydrome, and normal control subjects. Chest 2002; 122:866–870.
31. Series F, Simoneau S, St Pierre S, et al. Characteristics of the genioglossus and musculus uvulae in sleep apnea hypopnea syndrome and in snorers. Am J Respir Crit Care Med 1996; 153:1870–1874.
32. Smirne S, Iannaccone S, Ferini-Strambi L, et al. Muscle fiber type and habitual snoring. Lancet 1991; 337:597–599.
33. Fry A. The role of resistance exercise intensity on muscle fiber adaptations. Sports Med 2004; 34: 663–679.
34. Carrera M, Barbe F, Sauleda J, et al. Effects of obesity upon genioglossus structure and function in obstructive sleep apnea. Eur Respir J 2004; 23:425–429.
35. Carrera M, Barbe F, Sauleda J, et al. Patients with obstructive sleep apnea exhibit genioglossus dysfunction that is normalized after treatment with continuous positive airway pressure. Am J Respir Crit Care Med 1999; 159:1960–1966.
36. Terzano M, Parrino L, Chervin R, et al. Atlas, rules and recording techniques for the scoring of the cyclic alternating pattern (CAP) in human sleep. Sleep Med 2001; 2:537–554.
37. Altas Task Force of the American Sleep Disorders Association. EEG arousals: scoring rules and examples: a preliminary report from the Sleep Disorders Atlas Task Force of the American Sleep Disorders Association. Sleep 1992; 15:173–184.
38. Bao G, Guilleminault C. Upper airway resistance syndrome—one decade later. Curr Opin Pulm Med 2004; 10:461–467.
39. McNicholas W, Coffey M, Boyle T. Effects of nasal airflow on breathing during sleep in normal humans. Am Rev Respir Dis 1993; 147:620–623.
40. Basner R, Simon P, Schwartzstein R, et al. Breathing route influences upper airway muscle activity in awake normal adults. J Appl Physiol 1989; 66:1766–1771.
41. Zwillich C, Pickett C, Westbrook P. Sleep and breathing disturbance secondary to nasal obstruction. Otolaryngol Head Neck Surg 1981; 89:804–810.
42. Taasan V, Wynne J, Cassissi N, et al. The effect of nasal packing on sleep disordered breathing and nocturnal oxygen desaturation. Laryngoscope 1981; 91:1163–1172.
43. Lavis P, Fischel J, Zomer J, et al. The effects of partial and complete mechanical occlusion of the nasal passages on sleep structure and breathing in sleep. Acta Otolaryngol 1983; 95:161–166.
44. DeVito A. The importance of nasal resistance in obstructive sleep apnea syndrome: a study with positional rhinomanometry. Sleep Breath 2001; 5:3–11.
45. Ohki M, Ushi N, Kanazawa H, et al. Relationship between oral breathing and nasal obstruction in patients with obstructive apnea. Acta Otolaryngol 1996; 523:228–230.
46. Lofaso F, Coste A, D'Ortho M, et al. Nasal obstruction as a risk factor sleep apnoea syndrome. Eur Respir J 2000; 16:639–643.
47. Chen W, Kushida C. Nasal obstruction in sleep-disordered breathing. Otolaryngol Clin North Am 2003; 36:437–460.
48. Bixler E, Bgontzas A, Lin H, et al. Prevalence of sleep-disordered breathing in women: effects of gender [see comment]. Am J Respir Crit Care Med 2001; 163:608–613.
49. Olson L, King M, Hensley M, et al. A community study of snoring and sleep-disordered breathing. Prevalence. Am J Respir Crit Care Med 1995; 152(2):711–716.
50. Young T, Finn L, Austin D, et al. Menopausal status and sleep-disordered breathing in the Wisconsin Sleep Cohort study. Am J Respir Crit Car Med 2003; 167:1181–1185.
51. Shahar E, Redline S, Young T, et al. Hormone replacement therapy and sleep-disordered breathing. Am J Respir Crit Care Med 2003; 167:1186–1192.
52. Newman A, Nieto F, Guidry U, et al. Relation of sleep-disordered breathing to cardiovascular disease risk factors: the Sleep Heart Health Study. Am J Epidemiol 2001; 154(1):50–59.
53. Peppard P, Young T, Palta M, et al. Longitudinal study of moderate weight change and sleep-disordered breathing. JAMA 2000; 284:3015–3021.
54. Li K, Kushida C, Powell N, et al. Obstructive sleep apnea syndrome: a comparison between Far-East Asian and white men. Larungoscope 2000; 100:1689–1693.
55. Dempsey J, Skatrud J, Jacques A, et al. Anatomic determinants of sleep-disordered breathing across the spectrum of clinical and nonclinical male subjects. Chest 2002; 122:840–851.
56. Schwab R, Gupta K, Gefter W, et al. Upper airway and soft tissue anatomy in normal subjects and patients with sleep-disordered breathing. Am J Respir Crit Care Med 1995; 152:1673–1589.

57. Lam B, Ip M, Tench E, et al. Craniofacial profile in Asian and white subjects with obstructive sleep apnea. Thorax 2005; 60(6):504–510.
58. Grunstein R, Lawrence S, Spies J, et al. Snoring in paradise—the Western Samoa Sleep Survey. Eur Respir J 1989; 2(suppl 5):4015.
59. Schmid-Mowara W, Coultas D, Wiggins C, et al. Snoring in Hispanic-American population: risk factors and association with hypertension and other morbidity. Arch Intern Med 1990; 150:597.
60. Redline S, Hans M, Parcharktam N, et al. Differences in the age distribution and risk factors for sleep-disordered breathing in blacks and whites. Am J Respir Crit Care Med 1994; 149:577.
61. Guilleminault C, Partinen M, Hollman N, et al. Familial aggregates in obstructive sleep apnea syndrome. Chest 1995; 107:1545.
62. Redline S, Tishler P, Tosteson T, et al. The familial aggregation of obstructive sleep apnea. Am J Respir Crit Care Med 1995; 151:682–687.
63. Young T, Finn L, Kim H. Nasal obstruction as a risk factor for sleep-disordered breathing. The University of Wisconsin Sleep and Respiratory Research Group. J Allergy Clin Immunnol 1997; 99(2): S757–S762.
64. Kramer M, De la Chaux R, Fintelmann R, et al. NARES: a risk factor for obstructive sleep apnea? Am J Otolaryngol 2004; 25(3):173–177.
65. O'Ryan F, Gallagher D, LaBanc J, et al. The relation between nasorespiratory function and dentofacial morphology: a review. Am J Orthod 1982; 82:403–410.
66. Cheng M, Enlow D, Papsidero M, et al. Developmental effects of impaired breathing in the face of the growing child. Angle Orthod 1988; 58:309–320.
67. Woodside D, Linder-Aronson S, Lundstrom A, et al. Mandibular and maxillary growth after changed mode of breathing. Am J Orthod Dentofacial Orthop 1991; 100:1–18.
68. Riley R, Powell N, Li K, et al. Surgery and obstructive sleep apnea: long-term clinical outcomes. Otolaryngol Head Neck Surg 2000; 122:415–421.
69. Guilleminault C, Stoohs R, Quera-Salva M. Sleep-related obstructive and nonobstructive apneas and neurological disorders. Neurology 1992; 42:53–60.
70. Guilleminault C. Obstructive sleep apnea syndrome: a review. Psychiatr Clin North Am 1987; 4:607.
71. Baruzzi A, Riva R, Cirignotta F, et al. Atrial natriuretic peptide and catecholamines in obstructive sleep apnea syndrome. Sleep 1991; 1:83.
72. Fuller D, Mateika J, Fregosi R. Co-activation of tongue protrudor and retractor muscles during chemoreceptor stimulation in the rat. J Physiol 1998; 507:265–276.
73. Fuller D, Williams J, Janssen P, et al. Effects of co-activation of tongue protrudor and retractor muscles on tongue movement and pharyngeal airflow mechanics in the rat. J Physiol 1999; 519:601–613.
74. Sjoholm T, Lowe A, Miyamoto K, et al. Sleep bruxism in patients with sleep-disordered breathing. Arch Oral Biol 2000; 45:889–896.
75. Macaluso GM, Guerra P, Di Giovanni G, et al. Sleep bruxism is a disorder related to periodic arousals during sleep. J Dent Res 1998; 77:565–573.
76. Ohayon M, Li K, Guilleminault C. Risk factors for sleep bruxism in the general population. Chest 2001; 119:53–61.
77. Guilleminault C, Bassiri A. Clinical features and evaluation of obstructive sleep apnea-hypopnea syndrome and the upper airway resistance syndrome. In: Kriger M, Roth T, Dement W, eds. Principles and Practice of Sleep Medicine. 4th ed. Philadelphia: WB Saunders, 2004.
78. Guilleminault C, Palombini L, Poyares D, et al. Chronic insomnia, postmenopausal women, and SDB, part 2: comparison of non drug treatment trails in normal breathing and UARS postmenopausal women complaining of insomnia. J Psychosom Res 2002; 53:617–623.
79. Gold A, Dipalo F, Gold M, et al. The symptoms and signs of upper airway resistance syndrome: a link to the functional somatic syndromes. Chest 2003; 123:87–95.
80. Lewin D, Pinto M. Sleep disorders and ADHD: shared and common phenotypes. Sleep 2004; 27:188–189.
81. Guilleminault C, Faul J, Stoohs R. Sleep-disordered breathing and hypotension. Am J Respir Crit Care Med 2001; 164:1242–1247.
82. Guilleminault C, Khramtsov A, Stoohs R, et al. Abnormal blood pressure in prepubertal children with sleep-disordered breathing. Pediatr Res 2004; 55:76–84.
83. Peppard P, Young T, Palta M, et al. Prospective study of the association between sleep-disordered breathing and hypertension. N Engl J Med 2000; 342:1378–1384.
84. Johns M. A new method for measuring daytime sleepiness: the Epworth Sleepiness Scale. Sleep 1991; 14:540–545.
85. Chervin R, Aldrich M, Pickett R, et al. Comparison of the results of the Epworth Sleepiness Scale and the multiple sleep latency test. J Psychosom Rev 1997; 42:145–155.
86. Olson L, Cole M, Ambrogetti A. Correlations among Epworth sleepiness scores, multiple sleep latency tests and psychological symptoms. J Sleep Res 1998; 7:248–253.
87. Berard M, Montplaisir F, Richer I, et al. Obsructive sleep apnea syndrome: pathogenesis of neuropsychological deficits. J Clin Exp Neuropsychol 1991; 13:950–964.

88. Naegele B, Thouvard V, Pepin J, et al. Deficits of cognitive executive function in patients with sleep apnea syndrome. Sleep 1995; 18:43–52.

89. Findley L, Suratt P, Dinges D, et al. Time-on task decrements in steer clear performance of patients with sleep apnea and narcolepsy. Sleep 1999; 22:804–809.

90. Findley L, Barth J, Posers D, et al. Cognitive impairment in patients with obstructive sleep apnea and associated hypoxemia. Chest 1986; 90:686–690.

91. Berry D, Webb W, Block A, et al. Nocturnal hypoxemia and neuropsychological variables. J Clin Exp Neuropsychol 1986; 8:229–238.

92. Telakiivi T, Kajaste S, Partinen M, et al. Cognitive function middle-aged snorers and controls: role of excessive daytime somnolence and sleep related hypoxic events. Sleep 1988; 11:545–462.

93. Valencia-Flores M, Bliwise D, Guilleminault C, et al. Cognitive function in patient with sleep apnea after acute nocturnal nasal continuous positive airway pressure treatment: sleepiness and hypoxemia effect. J Clin Exp Neuropsychol 1996; 18:197–210.

94. Berard M, Montplaisir J, Richer F, et al. Nocturnal hypoxemia as a determinant of vigilance impairment in sleep apnea syndrome. Chest 1991; 100:367–370.

95. Doran S, Van Dongen H, Dinges D. Sustained attention performance sleep deprivation: evidence of state instability. Arch Ital Biol 2001; 139:253–267.

96. Ferini-Strambi L, Baietto C, Di Gioia M, et al. Cognitive dysfunction in patients with obstructive sleep apnea: partial reversibility after continuous positive airway pressure. Brain Res Bull 2003; 61: 87–92.

97. Kotterba S, Rasche K, Widdig W, et al. Neuropsychological investigations and event-related potentials in obstructive sleep apnea syndrome before and during CPAP therapy. J Neurol Sci 1998; 159: 45–50.

98. Hoch C, Reynolds C III, Kupfer D, et al. Sleep disordered breathing in normal and pathological aging. J Clin Psyciatry 1986; 47:499–503.

99. Erkinjuntti T, Partinen M, Sulkava R, et al. Sleep apnea in multi-infarct dementia and Alzheimer's disease. Sleep 1987; 19:419–425.

100. Mohsenin V, Valor R. Sleep apnea in patients with hemispheric stroke. Arch Phys Med Rehabil 1995; 76:71–76.

101. Dyken M, Somers V, Yamada T, et al. Investigating the relationship between stroke and obstructive sleep apnea. Stroke 1996; 27:401–407.

102. Bassetti C, Aldrich M. Sleep apnea in acute cerebrovascular diseases: final report on 128 patients. Sleep 1999; 22:217–223.

103. Spriggs D, French J, Murdy J, et al. Snoring increases the risk of stroke and adversely affects prognosis. QJM 1992; 82:555–562.

104. Smirne S, Palazzi S, Zucconi M, et al. Habitual snoring as a risk factor for acute vascular disease. Eur Respir J 1993; 6:1357–1361.

105. Marler J, Price T, Clark G, et al. Morning increase in onset of ischemic stroke. Stroke 1989; 20:473–476.

106. Yaggi H, Concato J, Kernan W, et al. Obstructive sleep apnea as a risk factor for stroke and death. N Engl J Med 2005; 353:2034–2041.

107. Bokinsky G, Miller M, Ault K, et al. Spontaneous platelet activation and aggregation during obstructive sleep apnea and its response to therapy with nasal continuous positive airway pressure: a preliminary investigation. Chest 1999; 108:625–630.

108. Chin K, Ohi M, Kita H, et al. Effects of NCPAP therapy on fibrinogen levels in obstructive sleep apnea syndrome. Am J Respir Crit Care Med 1996; 153:1972–1976.

109. Becker H, Jerrentrup A, Ploch T, et al. Effects of nasal continuous positive airway pressure treatment on blood pressure in patients with obstructive sleep apnea. Circulation 2003; 107:68–73.

110. Diomedi M, Placidi F, Cupini L, et al. Cerebral hemodynamic changes in sleep apnea syndrome and effect of continuous positive airway pressure treatment. Neurology 1998; 51:1051–1056.

111. Kales A, Bixler E, Cadieux R, et al. Sleep apnoea in a hypertensive population. Lancet 1984; 2: 1005–1008.

112. Fletcher E, DeBehnke R, Lovoi M, et al. Undiagnosed sleep apnea in patients with essential hypertension. Ann Intern Med 1985; 103:190–195.

113. Lavie P, Herer P, Hoffstein V. Obstructive sleep apnea syndrome as a risk factor for hypertension: population study. BMJ 2000; 320:479–482.

114. Somers V, Dyken M, Mark A, et al. Sympathetic nerve activity during sleep in normal humans. N Engl J Med 1993; 328:303–307.

115. Carlson J, Hedner J, Elam M, et al. Augmented resting sympathetic activity in awake patients with obstructive sleep apnea. Chest 1993; 103:1763–1768.

116. Somers V, Dyken M, Clary M, et al. Sympathetic neural mechanisms in obstructive sleep apnea. J Clin Invest 1995; 96:1897–1904.

117. Portalupppi F, Provini F, Cortelli P, et al. Undiagnosed sleep-disordered breathing among male nondippers with essential hypertension. J Hypertens 1997; 15:1227–1233.

118. Narkiewicz K, Montano N, Cogliati C, et al. Altered cardiovascular variability in obstructive sleep apnea. Circulation 1998; 98:1071–1077.
119. Narkiewicz K, De Borne P, Pesek C, et al. Selective potentiation of peripheral chemoreflex sensitivity in obstructive sleep apnea. Circulation 1999; 99:1183–1189.
120. Carlson J, Hedner J, Sellgren J, et al. Depressed baroreflex sensitivity in patients with obstructive sleep apnea. Am J Respir Crit Care Med 1996; 154:1490–1496.
121. Phillips G, Narkiewicz K, Pesek C, et al. Effects of obstructive sleep apnea on endothelin-1 and blood pressure. J Hypertens 1999; 17:61–66.
122. Kato M, Roberts-Thomson P, Phillips G, et al. Impairment of endothelium-dependent vasodilation resistance vessels in patients with obstructive sleep apnea. Circulation 2000; 102:2607–2610.
123. Ali N, Davies R, Fleetham J, et al. The acute effects of continuous positive airway pressure and oxygen saturation on blood pressure during obstructive sleep apnea. Chest 1992; 102:1526–1532.
124. Dimsdale J, Loredo J, Profant J. Effect of continuous positive airway pressure on blood pressure: a placebo trial. Hypertension 2000; 35:144–147.
125. Leung R, Bradley T. Sleep apnea and cardiovascular disease. Am J Respir Crit Care Med 2001; 161:2147–2165.
126. Partinen M, Guilleminault C. Daytime sleepiness and vascular morbidity at seven-year follow up in obstructive sleep apnea patients. Chest 1990; 97:27–32.
127. Hanly P, Sasson Z, Zuberi N, et al. ST-T segment depression during sleep in obstructive sleep apnea. Am J Cardiol 1993; 71:1341–1345.
128. Peled N, Abinader E, Pillar G, et al. Nocturnal ischemic events in patients with obstructive sleep apnea syndrome and ischemic heart disease; effects of continuous positive air pressure treatment. J Am Coll Cardiol 1999; 34:1744–1749.
129. Parish J, Somers V. Obstructive sleep apnea and cardiovascular disease. Mayo Clin Proc 2004; 79:1036–1046.
130. Milleron O, Pilliere R, Foucher A, et al. Benefits of obstructive sleep apnea treatment in coronary artery disease: long-term prognosis. A long-term follow-up study. Eur Heart J 2004; 25:728–734.
131. Kaneko Y, Floras J, Usui K, et al. Cardiovascular effects of continuous positive airway pressure in patients with heart failure and obstructive sleep apnea. N Engl J Med 2003; 348:1233–1241.
132. Hedner J, Ejnell H, Caidahl K. Left ventricular hypertrophy independent of hypertension in patients with obstructive sleep apnea. J Hypertens 1990; 8:941–946.
133. Fung J, Li T, Choy D, et al. Severe obstructive sleep apnea is associated with left ventricular diastolic dysfunction. Chest 2002; 121:422–429.
134. Ponikowski P, Chua T, Piepoli M, et al. Chemoreceptor dependence of very low frequency rhythms in advanced chronic heart failure. Am J Physiol 1997; 272(1):H438–H447.
135. Naughton M, Benard D, Tam A, et al. Role of hyperventilation in the pathogenesis of central sleep apnea in patients with congestive heart failure. Am Rev Respir Dis 1993; 148:330–338.
136. Guilleminault C, Brooks S. Excessive daytime sleepiness, a challenge for the practicing neurologist. Brain 2001; 124:1482–1491.
137. Powell N, Riley R, Schechtman K, et al. A comparative model: reaction time performance in sleep-disordered breathing versus alcohol-impaired controls. Laryngoscope 1999; 109:1648–1654.
138. Hakkanen J, Summala H. Sleepiness at work among commercial truck drivers. Sleep 2000; 23:49–57.
139. George C, Nickerson P, Hanly P, et al. Sleep apnoea patients have more automobile accidents. Lancet 1987; 2:447.
140. Findley L, Unverzadt M, Surratt P. Automobile accidents in patients with obstructive sleep apnea. Am Rev Respir Dis 1988; 138:337–340.
141. Mahowald M. Eyes wide shut. The dangers of sleepy driving. Minn Med 2000; 83:25–30.
142. Hoddes E, Dement W, Zarcone V. The development and use of the Stanford Sleepiness Scale. Psychophysiology 1972; 9:150.
143. Akerstedt T. Wide awake at odd hour. Stockholm: Swedish Council for Work Life Research, 1996.
144. Carskadon M, Dement W, Mitler M, et al. Guidelines for the multiple sleep latency test (MSLT): a standard measure of sleepiness. Sleep 1986; 9:519–562.
145. Doghramji K, Mitler M, Sangal R, et al. A normative study of the maintenance of wakefulness test. Electroencephalogr Clin Neurophysiol 1997; 103:554–562.
146. Grunstein R, Stenlof J, Hedner J, et al. Impact of self-reported breathing disturbances on psychosocial performance in the Swedish obese subjects (SOS) study. Sleep 1995; 18:635–643.
147. Greenberg G, Watson R, Deptula D. Neuropsychological dysfunction in sleep apnea. Sleep 1987; 10:254.
148. Engleman H, Douglas N. Sleep 4: sleepiness, cognitive function, and quality of life in obstructive sleep apnoea/hypopnoea syndrome. Thorax 2004; 59:618–622.
149. Guilleminault C, Palombini L, Ddalva P, et al. Chronic insomnia, premenopausal women and sleep disordered breathing, part 2: comparison of nondrug treatment trials in normal breathing and UARS postmenopausal women complaining of chronic insomnia. J Psychosom Res 2002; 53:617–623.

27 | Types of Sleep-Related Breathing Disorders

Murali Maheswaran
Center for Sleep Disorders, Skagit Valley Medical Center, Mount Vernon, Washington, U.S.A.

CENTRAL SLEEP APNEA SYNDROMES

Central sleep apnea (CSA) syndromes consist of a heterogeneous group of disorders in which respiratory effort is diminished or absent because of withdrawal of central respiratory drive (1,2). These disorders can be classified into a hypercapnic and a non-hypercapnic group on the basis of awake $PaCO_2$. In the hypercapnic group, they have an already blunted respiratory drive that is further reduced during sleep, resulting in central sleep apnea usually from syndromes such as central alveolar hypoventilation or neuromuscular weakness. In the non-hypercapnic group, central sleep apnea is induced when arterial $PaCO_2$ levels are below the $PaCO_2$ apnea threshold, leading to cessation in ventilatory effort, which can occur in such disorders as congestive heart failure (CHF), neurological diseases, and high-altitude periodic breathing (1). But it may also be seen in the absence of any underlying medical illness, which is called idiopathic central sleep apnea or primary central sleep apnea (1,3).

PRIMARY CENTRAL SLEEP APNEA

Demographics
The population prevalence is unknown, but the consensus is that the disorder is very rare and occurs more commonly in middle-aged to elderly individuals. Some studies have shown a higher incidence in men than in women, but this has not been consistent. The patients are typically thinner than those with obstructive sleep apnea, but they can still be relatively overweight (1,4).

Key Symptoms and Signs
Patients may complain of excessive daytime sleepiness, frequent arousals and awakening during sleep, awakening with shortness of breath or insomnia complaints. Witnessed apneas can be detected with or without snoring.

Onset, Ontogeny, and Clinical Course
The onset is unknown, but it seems to be more common in middle-aged to elderly individuals. The cause is also unknown, but in a study by Xie et al., recurrent primary central sleep apnea during non–rapid eye movement (NREM) N2 (formerly stage 2) sleep was triggered by relative degree of hyperventilation and hypocapnia (1).

Primary central sleep apnea can lead to excessive daytime sleepiness and insomnia, but there has not been any evidence to suggest that apneas lead to cardiovascular consequences such as hypertension or cor pulmonale. Oxygen desaturations are less severe than in Cheyne–Stokes breathing because the duration of cycle time (typically 20–40 seconds) is shorter and the chemoresponsiveness of the respiratory system is higher (4).

Risk Factors
Risk factors are not known, but it has been more prevalent in middle-aged to elderly individuals and in men.

CENTRAL SLEEP APNEA DUE TO CHEYNE–STOKES BREATHING PATTERN

Demographics
Central sleep apnea associated with Cheyne–Stokes breathing is markedly more prevalent in men older than 60 years(3). There is also high correlation of CSA in patients with CHF and strokes. Patients with CHF and a left ventricular ejection fraction (LVEF) <40% have a 30% to

50% likelihood of having CSA (5). CSA in patients with strokes has been estimated to be between 6% and 28% (6–8). Even in patients with strokes, there is a higher incidence with LVEF $\leq$40% and nocturnal hypocapnia (6). In a study conducted by Sin et al., there was almost a fourfold greater adjusted risk in men than in women (9).

Key Symptoms and Signs
Presenting features include excessive daytime sleepiness, insomnia, awakening short of breath, and frequent arousals, but more commonly it is detected at bedside in those who are being treated for CHF or stroke.

Onset, Ontogeny, and Clinical Course
The onset is not clear, although it probably occurs after onset of medical disorders such as CHF or stroke. Cheyne–Stokes breathing is commonly associated with poor prognosis in patients with CHF especially in the presence of a high apnea-hypopnea index (AHI) $\geq$ 30 in clinically stable patients with moderate to severe CHF (10). Predictors of mortality in patients with systolic heart failure are CSA, right ventricular dysfunction, and low diastolic blood pressure (11).

Risk Factors
Risk factors include male sex, increasing age, lower mean $PaCO_2$ during wakefulness, and atrial fibrillation (9,12). In a study by Sin et al., men had an almost fourfold greater adjusted risk for CSA than women. $PaCO_2 \leq$ 38 mmHg was associated with 4.3-fold increase compared with normocapnic or hypercapnic patients. In addition, patients >60 years of age had 2.4 times the risk of having CSA than those younger (9).

CENTRAL SLEEP APNEA DUE TO HIGH-ALTITUDE PERIODIC BREATHING

Demographics
High-altitude periodic breathing occurs during NREM sleep probably because of inadequate hypoxic ventilatory drive secondary to higher chemoresponsiveness of the carotid body (13). It can occur in all ages and all sexes, but it may be more common in men because of higher chemoresponsiveness (14,15). Normal subjects, after ascent to high altitudes >2500 m, often develop acute mountain sickness (AMS) characterized by insomnia, nausea, vomiting, headaches, dizziness, and loss of appetite. Subjects more likely to develop AMS tend to have pronounced nocturnal hypoxemia (14). Approximately 40% to 50% subjects ascending rapidly from low altitude to 4200 m develop AMS (13). There is a high prevalence of periodic breathing in those developing AMS. Almost all subjects ascending higher than 7600 m will have periodic breathing (3). There has been no data suggesting differing prevalence within ethnic groups, but there is a form of chronic mountain sickness seen primarily in Tibetans and South American Indians of the Andes (16).

Key Symptoms and Signs
These include insomnia, frequent nighttime awakenings, feeling unrefreshed in the morning, excessive daytime sleepiness, shortness of breath upon awakening, increased wake after sleep onset, and decreased sleep efficiency (17).

Onset, Ontogeny, and Clinical Course
High-altitude periodic breathing is described as three or four breaths of increasing and decreasing amplitude separated by periods of apnea associated with varying oxygen saturations (18). It generally occurs during stage 1 and 2 sleep and is worse with rapidity of ascent and at higher elevations. Periodic breathing is usually worse during the first night. Diagnostic criteria require recent ascent to altitude of at least 4000 m (3).

Risk Factors
A predisposing factor is increased ventilatory chemoresponsiveness, primarily a high hypoxic ventilatory response that leads to hyperventilation resulting in hypocapnic alkalosis that inhibits ventilation during sleep (3).

CENTRAL SLEEP APNEA DUE TO MEDICAL CONDITION NOT CHEYNE–STOKES

Demographics
Demographics are not known. The majority of these individuals have brain stem lesions of vascular, neoplastic, degenerative, demyelination, or traumatic origin as well as cardiac or renal etiologies (3). Leung et al. found that there was a marked increase in prevalence of atrial fibrillation in idiopathic central sleep apnea in the absence of CHF. Twenty-seven percent of the patients with idiopathic central sleep apnea had atrial fibrillation compared with 1.7% and 3.3% with sleep apnea and no apnea, respectively (19).

Key Symptoms and Signs
These are similar to those with primary central sleep apnea such as excessive daytime sleepiness, frequent arousals and awakenings during sleep, and insomnia, but the patients have additional symptoms and signs reflective of their underlying etiology.

Onset, Ontogeny, and Clinical Course
Onset occurs after resulting lesions to the brain stem. Central sleep apnea worsens with progressive brain stem dysfunction.

Risk Factors
Risk factors include neurological disorders involving the brain stem and cardiac disorders such as atrial fibrillation.

CENTRAL SLEEP APNEA DUE TO DRUG OR SUBSTANCE

Demographics
There does not seem to be a sex bias, and familial pattern is unknown. The prevalence is likely increasing because of concurrent increasing use of long-acting opioid along with a higher prevalence of undiagnosed sleep-disordered breathing (SDB) (20). In a study by Wang et al., they found that 30% of stable methadone maintenance treatment patients had central sleep apnea (21).

Key Symptoms and Signs
These are similar to patients with primary central sleep apnea. Stable methadone maintenance patients have significantly lower sleep efficiency, less slow-wave sleep (SWS), and rapid eye movement (REM) sleep. Teichtahl et al. also found these patients to have increased sleep latency, higher arousal index, and less total sleep time, although it did not reach statistical significance (22).

Onset, Ontogeny, and Clinical Course
Onset usually occurs after taking a long-acting opioid regularly for at least two months. The most common opioid causing central sleep apnea is methadone, but it can also occur in other opioids such as time release morphine or hydrocodone (3). Methadone has been shown to decrease hypoxic and hypercapnic respiratory drive and cause hypoventilation. There is partial tolerance to respiratory depression caused by methadone over a period of five to eight months (22). Long-term opioids most commonly cause central sleep apnea, but other breathing patterns include ataxic breathing, biot respiration, obstructive hypoventilation and hypopneas, usually prolonged secondary to delayed arousal responses, and periodic breathing (20). There is a three- to fourfold increase in mortality in methadone maintenance patients compared with normals, and half of the deaths usually occur in the first two to three weeks of methadone use because of high dose and blood levels (21). But Wang et al. found that only 12% of cases of CSA in methadone maintenance treatment were associated with elevated methadone blood concentrations, thus, the pathogenesis of CSA in these patients is likely multifactorial and may be related to abnormalities in the central brain stem respiratory pathway as well as central and peripheral control mechanisms (21).

Risk Factors
Heroin, cocaine, and amphetamine use can cause brain damage, thus affecting central respiratory centers and increasing likelihood of CSA in patients taking long-acting opioids (21).

PRIMARY SLEEP APNEA OF INFANCY

Demographics
The prevalence of primary sleep apnea in infancy is inversely related to gestational age. In the second edition of the *International Classification of Sleep Disorders* (ICSD-2), it is documented that 92% of preterm infants are symptom free by 37 weeks of gestational age and 98% by 40 weeks of gestational age, and 25% of infants weighing <2500 g and 84% weighing <1000 g experience symptomatic apnea during the neonatal period (3). The Collaborative Home Infant Monitoring Evaluation Study Group consisted of 1079 infants (classified as healthy-term infants) and six groups of those at risk for sudden infant death syndrome (SIDS) who had 718,358 hours of continuous monitoring during the first six months after birth. Of healthy asymptomatic full-term infants, 2.3% had at least one apnea event ≥30 seconds and a heart rate <60 bpm for at least 10 seconds, while these events occurred in 33% of symptomatic preterm infants and 20% of asymptomatic preterm infants. When including apneas of at least 20 seconds and bradycardia as defined by heart rate <60 bpm for at least 5 seconds or <80 bpm for at least 15 seconds in infants <44 weeks post conception age and a heart rate <50 bpm for at least 5 seconds or <60 bpm for at least 15 seconds in infants at least 44 weeks post conception age, then up to 43% of healthy asymptomatic full-term infants had these abnormalities (23).

Key Symptoms and Signs
These include witnessed apneas (central, obstructive, or mixed), color change, choking or gagging, hypotonia, bradycardia, or the need for intervention such as stimulation or resuscitation (3,24).

Onset, Ontogeny, and Clinical Course
In preterm infants, primary sleep apnea of infancy is more likely to occur between days 2 and 7. Apneas and bradycardia decrease by 37 to 43 weeks post conception age, but it may persist for several weeks thereafter (3,25). Usually long-term outcomes for uncomplicated apnea in premature or term infants are excellent. Such practices as supine sleep position, safe sleeping environments, and elimination of exposure to tobacco smoke have decreased the risk of SIDS (25).

Risk Factors
Apnea in infancy can be exacerbated or precipitated by other medical conditions such as hypoxemia due to lung abnormalities, anemia, acid reflux, metabolic disturbances, drugs, or anesthesia (3). Infants born to substance-abusing mothers have been shown to increase the risk of SIDS by 5- to 10-fold, reduce hypercapnic and hypoxic ventilatory responsiveness, and increase prevalence of periodic breathing (22). Home cardiorespiratory monitoring is not recommended to prevent SIDS, but it can be warranted for premature infants who have experienced altered life-threatening events, tracheostomies, or anatomic abnormalities that make them vulnerable to airway compromise or neurological or metabolic disorders affecting respiratory centers of infants with symptomatic chronic lung disease (25).

OBSTRUCTIVE SLEEP APNEA SYNDROMES

SDB associated with upper airway obstruction describes a spectrum of breathing abnormalities including snoring, upper airway resistance syndrome, and obstructive sleep apnea/hypopnea syndrome. Despite airway obstruction, breathing effort continues but ventilation is impaired. Adult and pediatric patients may clinically present differently. The pediatric population can present with inattentiveness, hyperactivity, and behavioral issues.

OBSTRUCTIVE SLEEP APNEA, ADULT

Demographics
Age
The prevalence of SDB has been wide ranging in literature published depending on populations studied and criteria used. Estimates are anywhere from 3% to 28% as defined by an AHI $\geq$ 5 and as high as 62% as defined by a respiratory disturbance index (RDI) $\geq$ 10 in community-dwelling elderly (26–36). Although OSA increases from childhood, a study by Bixler et al. has shown that the largest increase of obstructive sleep apnea is in middle age (45–64 years), which then levels off and even decreases in the elderly (31). In addition, the most common age group susceptible to increased mortality and morbidity seems to be middle-aged men, especially those who have concomitant medical problems such as hypertension and vascular disease (31,37).

Ethnicity
SDB was twice as prevalent in African-Americans <25 years of age than in Caucasians. Although African-Americans had a higher RDI at younger ages, they tended to have a similar RDI as compared to Caucasians between the 50 to 60 years age group and an even lower RDI compared with Caucasians older than 60 (38).

Various studies have also been conducted in other ethnic groups such as Asians and Hispanics. On the basis of a population survey, it has been estimated that 16.3% of U.S. Hispanics and racial minorities have OSA as compared with 4.9% non-Hispanic whites aged 40 to 64 years (27). On the basis of a community study of middle-aged Chinese men, approximately 8.8% had an AHI $\geq$ 5% and 4.1% had OSA with an AHI $\geq$ 5 (39). Although this is similar to some studies conducted in middle-aged Caucasians, the severity of SDB in Far East Asians seems to be less correlated with obesity than in Caucasians (40,41).

Craniofacial anatomy in Asians seems to play a great role in those who develop OSA. Although Far East Asian men with OSA have an elongated soft palate, inferiorly positioned hyoid, and decreased cranial base flexure similar to Caucasians, they differ in that they have significantly decreased cranial base dimensions (shorter anterior cranial base and more acute cranial base flexure), which in turn may cause a reduction in pharyngeal airway (42–44). African-Americans, on the other hand, have significantly greater tongue area than Caucasians that in turn reduces the airway because of base of the tongue obstruction (38).

Gender
A community sample showed that SDB was 2:1 (males: females) on the basis of a RDI $\geq$ 15 (45). Another study showed that male prevalence was 24% as compared with 9% on the basis of an AHI $\geq$ 5 (28). Postmenopausal women and those over 55 years of age had a greater likelihood to develop SDB and were 2.6 times more likely than premenopausal women to have SDB defined by an AHI $\geq$ 5 and 3.5 times more likely with SDB defined with AHI $\geq$ 15 (46). Those premenopausal women with SDB tended to be obese (45,46). Interestingly, women were two to three times less likely to report OSA symptoms such as snoring, gasping, witnessed apneas, and snorting (45). The prevalence of SDB (AHI $\geq$15) in hormone replacement therapy users was approximately half of that in nonusers, and this association seemed to be most significant among 50- to 60-year-old women (33).

Key Symptoms and Signs
These include excessive daytime sleepiness, snoring, witnessed apneas, gasping, choking, snorting, frequent awakenings, unrefreshed sleep, daytime fatigue, impaired memory and concentration, dry mouth and drooling, increased sweating, panic attacks, sexual dysfunction, morning headaches, and sleep bruxism. Other associated features include obesity, especially neck circumference, systemic hypertension, sleep fragmentation, insomnia, pulmonary hypertension, gastroesophageal reflux disease, sleep-related cardiac arrhythmias, nocturnal angina, and impaired quality of life (47–49).

Onset, Ontogeny, and Clinical Course
OSA can occur in any age but is more prevalent during middle age (45–64 years). OSA tends to worsen in time but seems to level off in the elderly (31). There can be grave consequences for

not treating OSA. OSA is associated with conditions such as hypertension and cardiovascular and cerebrovascular diseases that are leading causes of mortality in adults. Also, OSA can cause daytime sleepiness and impaired cognition, thus contributing to motor vehicle accidents, job-related accidents, and potentially decreasing work efficiency at the job, thereby playing a role of great public health and economic importance (26).

Risk Factors
These include obesity associated particularly with central body fat distribution and large neck circumference. OSA can occur in nonobese individuals with craniofacial abnormalities such as mandibular and maxillary hypoplasia and increased pharyngeal soft or lymphoid tissue such as tonsillar hypertrophy. Other risk factors include nasal obstruction, endocrine abnormalities such as hypothyroidism and acromegaly, menopause, alcohol use before sleep, and family history (47,50). Smoking is a possible risk factor. In a study by Wetter et al., they found current smokers to be three times more likely to have OSA than nonsmokers and former smokers (51).

OBSTRUCTIVE SLEEP APNEA, PEDIATRIC

Demographics
In the pediatric population, the prevalence is estimated to be approximately 2% in otherwise normal young children (3,52). The prevalence of OSA in children between the ages of 2 and <18 years ranges from 0.7% to 3% and habitual snoring in children ranges from 3.2% to 12.1% according to a literature review conducted by Schecter (53). This number seems to be even higher in children with first-degree relatives with OSA. Approximately 40% of these children snored, and 12.2% of the pediatric first-degree relatives had symptoms highly suggestive of OSA (52).

Ethnicity
There seems to be a higher prevalence in the pediatric population among African-Americans than Caucasians. According to Redline et al., African-American children <18 years of age are 3.5 times more likely to have SDB than Caucasians. The strongest risk factors in this pediatric population (<18 years) tested were obesity, African-Americans, and those with both upper and lower respiratory problems (54). The prevalence of other pediatric ethnic groups is unknown.

Key Symptoms and Signs
Clinical features include nocturnal symptoms such as snoring, apnea, labored breathing, paradoxical breathing, restlessness, sleeping in unusual positions such as neck hyperextension or seated, and enuresis. Daytime symptoms include excessive daytime sleepiness, morning headaches, fatigue, mouth breathing, nasal obstruction, hyponasal speech, similar symptoms associated with attention-deficit hyperactivity disorder (ADHD), aggression, social withdrawal, and poor school performance (55).

Onset, Ontogeny, and Clinical Course
The peak incidence of OSA occurs between two to five years of age, although the disease may not be diagnosed until years later (26). If OSA is left untreated, then cognitive, behavioral, cardiovascular, and growth complications can occur. Cognitive and behavioral complications are common and may include developmental delay, ADHD, learning problems, and aggression (3). OSA should be in the differential diagnosis for children with growth impairment or failure to thrive that is unexplained by other medical conditions. Cardiovascular complications include pulmonary hypertension, cor pulmonale, and systemic hypertension (56).

Risk Factors
These include adenotonsillar hypertrophy, obesity, neuromuscular disorders associated with muscular hypotonia and hypertonia, family history, craniofacial abnormalities, and genetic abnormalities causing midface hypoplasia, micrognathia, and small nasopharynx such as

Down syndrome and Pierre Robin sequence. Other less common risk factors include larygomalacia, pharyngeal flap surgery, sickle cell disease, and structural malformations of the brain stem such as chiari malformations (26,57). African-American race and children with respiratory problems are also risk factors. In a study by Redline et al., they found that children with SDB significantly reported coughing, occasional or persistent wheezing, sinus problems, and physician-diagnosed asthma (54).

SLEEP-RELATED HYPOVENTILATION/HYPOXEMIC SYNDROMES

Hypoventilation refers to reduction of alveolar ventilation accompanied by hypoxemia and hypocapnia. Sleep-related nonobstructive alveolar hypoventilation can occur from birth, in an idiopathic form in patients with normal lung mechanical properties or more commonly associated with other medical disorders that alter the mechanical properties of the lung, chest wall, and respiratory muscles.

SLEEP-RELATED NONOBSTRUCTIVE ALVEOLAR HYPOVENTILATION, IDIOPATHIC

Demographics
Demographics are not known. The idiopathic form of alveolar hypoventilation is very rare but appears to be more common in men. It is characterized by decreased alveolar ventilation and blunted chemoresponsiveness resulting in hypercapnia, hypoxemia, and frequent arousals not associated with medical or neurological disorders, medication use, substance use, or other sleep disorders (3,58). Additional diagnostic criteria recommended by the Respiratory Failure Research Committee of the Japanese Ministry of Health and Welfare are chronic hypercapnia ($PaCO_2 \geq 45$ torr), exacerbation of hypoxemia during sleep, improvement of hypercapnia after voluntary hyperventilation, and body mass index < 30 kg/m^2 (58).

Key Symptoms and Signs
Patients often report excessive daytime sleepiness, frequent arousals, awakenings during sleep, insomnia, and headaches upon awakening (3).

Onset, Ontogeny, and Clinical Course
The onset often appears in adolescence or early adulthood. The course is usually slowly progressive and can lead to pulmonary and cardiac consequences such as cor pulmonale, peripheral edema, cardiac arrhythmias (brady-tachycardia), pulmonary hypertension, heart failure, and polycythemia. Hypoventilation is worse during REM sleep. Idiopathic non-obstructive hypoventilation is believed to result from failure of chemical respiratory control system, possibly because of lesions of medullary chemoreceptors that are too small to be seen in magnetic resonance imaging (3,58).

Risk Factors
Male sex may be a risk factor, and central nervous system depressant use such as alcohol, anxiolytics, and hypnotics may worsen hypoventilation (3).

CONGENITAL CENTRAL ALVEOLAR HYPOVENTILATION SYNDROME

Demographics
Congenital central alveolar hypoventilation syndrome (CCAHS) is an extremely rare disorder characterized by a failure of the autonomic control of breathing (3). These infants have severe hypoventilation during sleep, which is most marked during SWS (59). There has been an association with CCAHS and Hirschsprung's disease in approximately 16% of patients, neural crest tumors such as ganglioneuroblastomas, neuroblastomas, and ganglioneuromas, and a large majority of patients (>90%) with CCAHS have been identified with a PHOX2B mutation (3,59,60).

In a French registry survey, it was determined that the incidence of CCAHS in France was approximately 1 per 200,000 live births and the median age at diagnosis was 3.5 months prior to 1995 and has improved to <2 weeks over the last five years (59). The French registry included 70 patients, while an international survey published in 2003 consisted of 196 patients (59,61). CCAHS is believed to occur equally among both sexes and ethnic groups, but in the French registry, there was a male: female sex ratio of 0.7 (3,59). The two-year mortality was significantly greater in men in the French population (59).

Key Symptoms and Signs
Patients generally have adequate ventilation while awake unless disorder is severe, but during sleep they exhibit shallow breathing, cyanosis, and apneas. Breath-holding spells, poor basal body temperature regulation, sporadic profuse sweating episodes with cool extremities, and feeding difficulties with esophageal dysmotility have been described anecdotally (62).

Onset, Ontogeny, and Clinical Course
Congenital central alveolar hypoventilation usually presents at birth, but diagnosis may not be made until weeks to months later. A few rare cases present later at two to four years of age, which are associated with hypothalamic and endocrine abnormalities, but it is unclear if this subgroup represents an entirely different syndrome. If adequately managed, then prolonged survival and overall good quality of life have been described (62). If this disorder is not detected early or not adequately managed, then complications such as cor pulmonale, heart failure, pulmonary hypertension, and cardiac arrhythmias can result in death. It is recommended that infants with congenital central alveolar hypoventilation should be evaluated very frequently to assess for growth, speech, and mental and motor development and have detailed cardiac and pulmonary evaluations with echocardiogram, Holter monitor, periodical pulmonary function tests, and overnight respiratory physiology laboratory studies to monitor adequacy of ventilation (62). Cognitive function can be normal if effectively managed.

Risk Factors
Risk factors are unknown, but there are associated abnormalities such as Hirschsprung's disease, neural tumors, dysphagia due to abnormal esophageal motility, and ocular problems such as strabismus (63).

SLEEP-RELATED HYPOVENTILATION/HYPOXEMIA DUE TO PULMONARY PARENCHYMAL OR VASCULAR PATHOLOGY

Demographics
Demographic associations between sleep hypoventilation/hypoxemia and pulmonary parenchymal or vascular disease are unknown and not yet established (3).

Key Symptoms and Signs
Diseases shown to cause sleep-related hypoventilation/hypoxemia due to pulmonary parenchymal or vascular pathology include interstitial lung disease, primary and secondary hypertension, sickle cell anemia, and other hemoglobinopathies (3). Hypoxemia in these cases occurs in the absence of upper airway obstruction. Patients with interstitial lung disease can have very disrupted and fragmented sleep resulting in decrease of REM or SWS. Hypoxemia, cough, and several respiratory reflexes can produce arousals, and excessive daytime sleepiness and insomnia can occur (64).

Onset, Ontogeny, and Clinical Course/Risk Factors
Patients with interstitial lung disease have a rapid shallow breathing pattern while awake, which is thought to be a reflex response to stiff lungs mediated by vagal afferents. Breathing frequency during NREM sleep has been shown to be higher than normal (64,65). Marked hypoxemia can occur during REM sleep and contribute to development of pulmonary hypertension, polycythemia, and cardiac arrhythmias. Rafanan et al. found that 77% of the 13 patients they studied with primary pulmonary hypertension had marked nocturnal hypoxemia and spent greater than 25% of total sleep time with $SpO_2 < 90\%$ (66). Higher rates

of painful sickle cell crisis in children have been associated with hypoventilation/hypoxemia. A study by Hargrave et al. found significant associations between a decrease in pain rate and higher mean SaO$_2$, higher minimum SaO$_2$, and decreased percentage of sleep study with SaO$_2$ < 90% (67). Nocturnal oxygen desaturation in children and adolescents with sickle cell disease have been described, and it is believed to occur in part to abnormalities in oxyhemoglobin affinity (68).

SLEEP-RELATED HYPOVENTILATION/HYPOXEMIA DUE TO LOWER AIRWAY OBSTRUCTION

Demographics
Chronic obstructive pulmonary disease (COPD) has been estimated to affect 14 to 16 million individuals and is the fourth leading cause of morbidity and mortality in the United States (3,69).

Key Symptoms and Signs
COPD has been associated with nocturnal hypoxemia, poor sleep quality, frequent arousals and disrupted sleep, and decreased total sleep time. Sleep disturbance can be related to nocturnal cough, wheezing, and shortness of breath. Excessive daytime sleepiness and insomnia can be common. Klink et al. found that insomnia occurred in 39% and excessive daytime sleepiness in 12% of those who had either complaints of coughing or wheezing, and the prevalence increased to 53% and 23%, respectively, if both symptoms were present (70).

Onset, Ontogeny, and Clinical Course/Risk Factors
Some studies have shown that nocturnal hypoxemia in COPD patients with daytime PaO$_2$ > 60 mmHg is associated with shorter survival than in patients without COPD. This transient hypoxemia has been well documented in patients with COPD during REM sleep, and these patients may benefit by low-flow nocturnal oxygen acutely by lowering pulmonary artery pressure and decreasing or eliminating transient hypoxemia during REM sleep (71,72). Transient hypoxemia during REM sleep probably results from a combination of alveolar hypoventilation and gas exchange abnormalities due to REM sleep muscle atonia and changes in respiratory control. In a study by Fletcher et al., 27% of COPD patients with PaO$_2$ ≥ 60 mmHg had nocturnal REM-associated hypoxia (73). The consequences of sleep-related hypoventilation/hypoxia in patients with lower airway obstruction are pulmonary hypertension, cor pulmonale, cardiac arrhythmias, polycythemia, and neurocognitive dysfunction (3). Patients with moderate and severe COPD have been shown to have neuropsychological deficits mostly affecting cognitive functions such as reasoning and perceptual motor integration, although memory may be spared. In severe cases, delirium can occur because of severe hypoxemia or hypercapnia (74).

Risk factors for COPD include cigarette smoking, environmental exposure to occupational dusts, chemicals, and pollutants. There is a greater risk to have sleep-related hypoventilation/hypoxemia in patients with greater worsening of pulmonary functions resulting in hypercapnia with PaCO$_2$ > 45mmHg and those with lower awake PaO$_2$ (3).

SLEEP-RELATED HYPOVENTILATION/HYPOXEMIA DUE TO NEUROMUSCULAR AND CHEST WALL DISORDERS

Demographics
Neuromuscular and chest wall disorders include muscular dystrophies, inflammatory and metabolic myopathies, neuromuscular junction disorders such as myasthenia gravis and Lambert–Eaton syndrome, diaphragmatic paralysis or paresis, postpolio syndrome, amytrophic lateral sclerosis, polyneuropathies such as Guillain–Barre syndrome and Charcot–Marie–Tooth disease, spinal cord injury, obesity, and congenital or idiopathic kyphoscoliosis. The demographics of sleep-related hypoventilation/hypoxemia reflect that of these underlying neuromuscular or chest wall disorders.

Key Symptoms and Signs

Signs and symptoms include excessive daytime sleepiness, fatigue, frequent arousals, snoring, apneas, morning headaches, exertional dyspnea, and orthopnea (75). Insomnia can occur in patients with muscle pain and cramps or painful polyneuropathies. In neuromuscular disorders, sleep disturbances are secondary to involvement of respiratory muscles, phrenic and intercostal nerves, or neuromuscular junctions of the respiratory and oropharyngeal muscles.

Onset, Ontogeny, and Clinical Course/Risk Factors

The onset of sleep hypoventilation/hypoxemia depends on the onset and progression of the underlying neuromuscular or chest wall disorders. The more severe the respiratory muscle weakness (intercostals, diaphragm, and accessory muscles), the greater the hypoxemia, particularly in REM sleep. Predictive properties of nocturnal hypoxemia include vital capacity percentage predicted and percentage fall in vital capacity when changing from erect to supine position and reduced awake oxyhemoglobin saturation (76). Hypoxemia during REM sleep is related to diaphragmatic weakness along with a combination of upper airway narrowing and ventilation/perfusion abnormalities, especially those with atelectasis, which is common in those with progressed neuromuscular or chest wall disorders (76). Sleep-related hypoventilation/hypoxemia can contribute to pulmonary hypertension, cor pulmonale, heart failure, and cardiac arrhythmias. Risk factors include obesity and family history.

SLEEP APNEA/SLEEP-RELATED BREATHING DISORDER, UNSPECIFIED

This diagnosis is reserved for forms of sleep-related breathing disorders (SRBDs) that do not meet exact criteria of the SRBDs mentioned previously. This diagnosis can be used until further workup may better delineate these SRBDs to meet the criteria of the other SRBD types.

CONCLUSIONS

Types of SRBDs include primary central sleep apnea; central sleep apnea due to Cheyne–Stokes breathing pattern, high-altitude periodic breathing, medical conditions, or drug or substance; primary sleep apnea of infancy; obstructive sleep apnea of adults and children; sleep-related nonobstructive alveolar hypoventilation of idiopathic type; CCAHS; sleep-related hypoventilation/hypoxemia due to pulmonary parenchymal or vascular pathology, lower airways obstruction, or neuromuscular and chest wall disorders; and sleep apnea/SRBD of unspecified type. The central sleep apnea syndromes are characterized by decrease of central respiratory drive resulting in reduction or cessation or respiratory effort, and can be divided into hypercapnic and non-hypercapnic types on the basis of awake $PaCO_2$. Obstructive sleep apnea syndromes are disorders that involve partial or complete blockage of the upper airway. Sleep-related hypoventilation/hypoxemic syndromes involve a reduction of alveolar ventilation accompanied by hypoxemia and hypocapnia. Lastly, any SRBD that does not meet any of the criteria of the aforementioned types of disorders is classified as sleep apnea/SRBD of unspecified type.

REFERENCES

1. Xie A, Wong B, Phillipson E, et al. Interaction of hyperventilation and arousal in the pathogenesis of idiopathic central sleep apnea. Am J Respir Crit Care Med 1994; 150:489–495.
2. Bradley TD, McNicholas WT, Rutherford R, et al. Clinical and physiologic heterogeneity of the central sleep apnea syndrome. Am Rev Respir Dis 1986; 134:217–221.
3. American Academy of Sleep Medicine. International Classification of Sleep Disorders: Diagnostic and Coding Manual. 2nd ed. Illinois: American Academy of Sleep Medicine, 2005.
4. Eckert DJ, Jordan AS, Merchia P, et al. Central sleep apnea pathophysiology and treatment. Chest 2007; 131:595–607.
5. Javaheri S, Parker TJ, Wexler L, et al. Occult sleep-disordered breathing in stable congestive heart failure. Ann Intern Med 1995; 122:487–492.

6. Nopmaneejumruslers C, Kanedo Y, Hajek V, et al. Cheyne-stokes respiration in stroke: relationship to hypocapnia and occult cardiac dysfunction. Am J Respir Crit Care Med 2005; 171:1048–1052.

7. Nachtmann A, Siebler M, Rose G, et al. Cheyne-stokes respiration in ischemic stroke. Neurology 1995; 45: 820–821.

8. Wessendorf TE, Teschler H, Wang YM, et al. Sleep-disordered breathing among patients with first-ever stroke. J Neurol 2000; 247:41–47.

9. Sin DS, Fitzgerald F, Parker JD, et al. Risk factors for central and obstructive sleep apnea in 450 men and women with congestive heart failure. Am J Respir Crit Care Med 1999; 160:1101–1106.

10. Lanfranchi PA, Braghiroli A, Bosimini E, et al. Prognostic value of nocturnal Cheyne-Stokes respiration in chronic heart failure. Circulation 1999; 99:1435–1440.

11. Javaheri S, Shukla R, Zeigler H, et al. Central sleep apnea, right ventricular dysfunction, and low diastolic blood pressure are predictors of mortality in systolic heart failure. J Am Coll Cardiol 2007; 49:2028–2034.

12. Javaheri S, Parker TJ, Liming JD, et al. Sleep apnea in 81 ambulatory male patients with stable heart failure. Circulation 1998; 97:2154–2159.

13. Rosen JM. High altitude disease in adults. 2006.

14. Erba P, Anastasi S, Senn O, et al. Acute mountain sickness is related to nocturnal hypoxemia but not to hypoventilation. Eur Respir J 2004; 24:303–308.

15. Schneider M, Bernasch D, Weymann J, et al. Acute mountain sickness: influence of susceptibility, preexposure and ascent rate. Med Sci Sports Exerc 2002; 34:1886–1891.

16. Monge CC, Whittembury J. Chronic mountain sickness. Johns Hopkins Med J 1976; 139(suppl):87.

17. Anholm J, Powles A, Downey R, et al. Operation Everest II: arterial oxygen saturation and sleep at extreme simulated altitude. Am Rev Respir Dis 1992; 145:817–826.

18. Burgess K, Johnson P, Edwards N. Central and obstructive sleep apnea during ascent to high altitude. Respirology 2004; 9:222–229.

19. Leung R, Huber M, Rogge T, et al. Association between atrial fibrillation and central sleep apnea. Sleep 2005; 28(12):1543–1546.

20. Farney R, Walker J, Cloward T, et al. Sleep disordered breathing associated with long-term opioid therapy. Chest 2003; 123:632–639.

21. Wang D, Teichtahl H, Drummer O, et al. Central sleep apnea in stable methadone maintenance treatment patients. Chest 2005; 128:1348–1356.

22. Teichtahl H, Prodromidis A, Miller B, et al. Sleep-disordered breathing in stable methadone programme patients: a pilot study. Addiction 2001; 96:395–403.

23. Ramanathan R, Corwin M, Hunt C, et al. Cardiorespiratory events recorded on home monitors: comparison of healthy infants with those at increased risk for SIDS. JAMA 2001; 285:2199–2207.

24. National institutes of health consensus development conference on infantile apnea and home monitoring, Sept 29 to Oct 1, 1986. Pediatrics 1987; 79:292–299.

25. American Academy of Pediatrics. Apnea, sudden infant death syndrome, and home monitoring. Pediatrics 2003; 111:914–917.

26. Young T, Peppard P, Gottlieb D. Epidemiology of obstructive sleep apnea. Am J Respir Crit Care Med 2002; 165:1217–1239.

27. Kripke DF, Ancoli-Isreal S, Klauber MR, et al. Prevalence of sleep-disordered breathing in ages 40–64 years: a population based survey. Sleep 1997; 20:65–76.

28. Young T, Palta M, Dempsey J, et al. The occurrence of sleep-disordered breathing among middle-aged adults. N Engl J Med 1993; 328:1230–1235.

29. Young TB, Evans L, Finn L, et al. Estimation of the clinically diagnosed proportion of sleep apnea syndrome in middle-aged men and women. Sleep 1997; 20:705–706.

30. Ancoli-Isreal S, Kripke DF, Klauber MR, et al. Sleep-disordered breathing in community-dwelling elderly. Sleep 1991; 14:486–495.

31. Bixler EO, Vgontzas AN, Ten Have T, et al. Effects of age on sleep apnea in men. Am J Respir Crit Care Med 1998; 157:144–148.

32. Bixler EO, Vgontzas AN, Lin HM, et al. Prevalence of sleep-disordered breathing in women: effects of gender. Am J Respir Crit Care Med 2001; 163:608–613.

33. Shahar E, Redline S, Young T, et al. Hormone replacement therapy and sleep-disordered breathing. Am J Respir Crit Care Med 2003; 167:1186–1192.

34. Bearpark H, Elliot L, Grunstein R, et al. Occurrence and correlates of sleep-disordered breathing in the Australian town of Busselton: a preliminary analysis. Sleep 1993; 16:S3–S5.

35. Gislason T, Almqvist M, Eriksson G, et al. Prevalence of sleep apnea syndrome among Swedish men: an epidemiological study. J Clin Epidemiol 1988; 41:571–576.

36. Duran J, Esnaola S, Rubio R, et al. Obstructive sleep apnea-hypopnea and related clinical features in a population-based sample of subjects aged 30 to 70 yr. Am J Respir Crit Care Med 2001; 163:685–689.

37. Strohl KP, Redline S. Recognition of obstructive sleep apnea. Am J Respir Crit Care Med 1996; 154: 279–289.

38. Redline S, Tishler PV, Hans MG, et al. Racial differences in sleep-disordered breathing in African-Americans and Caucasians. Am J Respir Crit Care Med 1997; 155:186–192.

39. Ip MSM, Lam B, Lauder IJ, et al. A community study of sleep-disordered breathing in middle-aged Chinese men in Hong Kong. Chest 2001; 119:62–69.

40. Li KK, Powell NB, Kushida C, et al. A comparison of Asian and white patients with obstructive sleep apnea. Laryngoscope 1999; 109:1937–1940.

41. Ong K, Clerk A. Comparison of the severity of sleep-disordered breathing in Asian and Caucasian patients seen at a sleep disorders center. Respir Med 1998; 92:843–848.

42. Li KK, Kushida C, Powell NB, et al. Obstructive sleep apnea syndrome: a comparison between far-east Asian and white men. Laryngoscope 2000; 110:1689–1693.

43. Steinberg B, Fraser B. The cranial base in obstructive sleep apnea. J Oral Maxillofac Surg 1995; 53: 1150–1154.

44. Enlow DH, Kuroda T, Lewis AB. The morphological and morphogenetic basis for craniofacial form and pattern. Angle Orthod 1971; 41:161–188.

45. Redline S, Kump K, Tishler PV, et al. Gender differences in sleep disordered breathing in a community-based sample. Am J Respir Crit Care Med 1994; 149:722–726.

46. Young T, Finn L, Austin D, et al. Menopausal status and sleep-disordered breathing in the Wisconsin sleep cohort study. Am J Respir Crit Care Med 2003; 167:1181–1185.

47. Sleep-related breathing disorders in adults: recommendations for syndrome definition and measurement techniques in clinical research: the report of an American Academy of Sleep Medicine Task Force. Sleep 1999; 22:667–689.

48. Malhotra A, White D. Obstructive sleep apnea. Lancet 2002; 360:237–245.

49. Abad V, Guilleminault C. Neurological perspective on obstructive and nonobstructive sleep apnea. Semin Neurol 2004; 24:261–269.

50. Young T, Skatrud J, Peppard P. Risk factors for obstructive sleep apnea in adults. JAMA 2004; 291: 2013–2016.

51. Wetter D, Young T, Bidwell T, et al. Smoking as a risk factor for sleep-disordered breathing. Arch Intern Med 1994; 154:2219–2224.

52. Orchinsky A, Rao M, Lotwin I, et al. The familial aggregation of pediatric obstructive sleep apnea syndrome. Arch Otolaryngol Head Neck Surg 2002; 128:815–818.

53. Schecter MS. Technical report: diagnosis and management of childhood obstructive sleep apnea syndrome. Pediatrics 2002; 109(4):e69.

54. Redline S, Tishler P, Schluchter M, et al. Risk factors for sleep-disordered breathing in children. Am J Respir Crit Care Med 1999; 159:1527–1532.

55. Bandla P, Brooks L, Trimarchi T, et al. Obstructive sleep apnea syndrome in children. Anesthesiol Clin North America 2005; 23:535–549.

56. Sterni L, Tunkel D. Obstructiv sleep apnea in children: an update. Pediatr Clin North Am 2003; 50: 427–443.

57. American Thoracic Society. Standards and indications for cardiopulmonary sleep studies in children. Am J Respir Crit Care Med 1996; 153:866–878.

58. Hara J, Fujimura M, Myou S, et al. Primary alveolar hypoventilation syndrome complicated with antiphospholipid syndrome. Intern Med 2005; 44:987–989.

59. Trang H, Dehan M, Beaufils F, et al. The French congenital central hypoventilation syndrome registry. Chest 2005; 127:72–79.

60. Amiel J, Laudier B, Attie-Bitach T, et al. Polyalanine expansion and frameshift mutations of the paired-liked homeobox gene PHOX2B in congenital central hypoventilation syndrome. Nat Genet 2003; 33:459–461.

61. Vanderlaan M, Holbrook CR, Wang M, et al. Epidemiologic survey of 196 patients with congenital central hypoventilation syndrome. Pediatr Pulmonol 2004; 37:217–229.

62. American thoracic society consensus statement. Idiopathic congenital central hypoventilation syndrome: diagnosis and management. Am J Respir Crit Care Med 1999; 160:368–373.

63. O'Brien L, Holbrook C, Vanderlaan M, et al. Autonomic function in children with congenital central hypoventilation syndrome and their families. Chest 2005; 128:2478–2484.

64. Padilla R, West P, Lertzman M, et al. Breathing during sleep in patients with interstitial lung disease. Am Rev Respir Dis 1985; 132:224–229.

65. Bye P, Issa F, Berthon-Jones M, et al. Studies of oxygenation during sleep in patients with interstitial lung disease. Am Rev Respir Dis 1984; 129:27–32.

66. Rafanan A, Golish J, Dinner D, et al. Nocturnal hypoxemia is common in primary pulmonary hypertension. Chest 2001; 120:894–899.

67. Hargrave D, Wade A, Evans J, et al. Nocturnal oxygen saturation and painful sickle cell crisis in children. Blood 2003; 101:846–848.

68. Needleman J, Franco M, Varlotta L, et al. Mechanism of nocturnal oxyhemoglobin desaturation in children and adolescents with sickle cell disease. Pediatr Pulmonol 1999; 28:418–422.

69. Sanders M, Newman A, Haggerty C, et al. Sleep and sleep-disordered breathing in adults with predominately mild obstructive airway disease. Am J Respir Crit Care Med 2003; 167:7–14.
70. Klink M, Dodge R, Quan S. The relation of sleep complaints to respiratory symptoms in a general population. Chest 1994; 105:151–154.
71. Fletcher E, Donner C, Midgren B, et al. Survival in COPD patients with a daytime PaO_2 greater than 60 mm hg with and without nocturnal oxyhemoglobin desaturation. Chest 1992; 101:649–655.
72. Fletcher E, Levin D. Cardiopulmonary hemodynamics during sleep in subjects with chronic obstructive pulmonary disease: the effect of short and long term oxygen. Chest 1984; 85:6–14.
73. Fletcher E, Miller J, Divine G, et al. Nocturnal oxyhemoglobin desaturation in COPD patients with arterial oxygen tensions above 60 mm hg. Chest 1987; 92:604–608.
74. Grant I, Heaton R, McSweeney A, et al. Brain dysfunction in COPD. Chest 1980; 77:308–309.
75. Labanowski M, Schmidt-Nowara W, Guilleminault C. Sleep and neuromuscular disease: frequency of sleep-disordered breathing in a neuromuscular disease clinic population. Neurology 1996; 47: 1173–1180.
76. Bye P, Ellis E, Issa F, et al. Respiratory failure and sleep in neuromuscular disease. Thorax 1990; 45: 241–247.

28 | Diagnostic Tools for Sleep-Related Breathing Disorders

James A. Rowley and M. Safwan Badr

Division of Pulmonary, Critical Care & Sleep Medicine, Wayne State University School of Medicine, Detroit, Michigan, U.S.A.

HISTORY AND PHYSICAL EXAMINATION

A complete sleep history should be obtained on all patients suspected of having a sleep-related breathing disorder (SRBD). The sleep history should include questions regarding the patient's sleep habits (such as time to bed, time out of bed) and symptoms of other common sleep disorders, especially insomnia, restless leg syndrome and narcolepsy, which can frequently coexist with a SRBD. A full medical history should be obtained as a diagnosis of congestive heart failure or neurologic disease may indicate the presence of Cheyne–Stokes respiration as the underlying cause of the SRBD. Likewise, a complete list of medications should be ascertained as many medications may affect sleep and/or respiration. The list includes sedatives, hypnotics, narcotics, and stimulants. A family history of SRBD should be sought as obstructive sleep apnea [OSA, formerly referred to as the obstructive sleep apnea-hypopnea syndrome (OSAHS)] appears to display a familial aggregation (1,2). Finally, a complete history of alcohol and/or tobacco use, which worsens OSA, should also be obtained (3).

Symptoms suggestive of a SRBD are generally divided into two groups: nocturnal and daytime. Snoring is the most common nocturnal complaint and is generally described as loud, irregular, habitual, and disturbing to a bed or room partner (who sometimes moves out of the bedroom to avoid the noise). If there is no regular bed or room partner, the patient should be asked if there has been any other recent occasion in which he or she has shared a room or if there are other people in the house that have heard the patient snore from other rooms. A bed or room partner will also often notice pauses in the snoring or breathing (witnessed apneas) that may end with a snorting sound. Other nocturnal symptoms include gasping, gagging, or choking sensations, restless sleep, and frequent unexplained awakenings. It should be noted that while the presence of a nocturnal symptom such as snoring is associated with an increased likelihood of having an SRBD, in general, symptoms, whether alone or in combination, are only mildly predictive of the presence of a SRBD in a sleep clinic population, given that the nocturnal symptoms are prevalent in patients presenting to a sleep clinic (4–8).

The most common daytime symptom is excessive sleepiness. Several studies suggest that the degree of sleepiness, whether measured using the Epworth Sleepiness Scale (9) or the multiple sleep latency test (MSLT) (10), directly correlates with the degree of sleep-disordered breathing (11,12). However, sleepiness is not a universal finding in patients with SRBD, even patients with moderate-to-severe disease (13). Patients also frequently complain of fatigue, tiredness, and lack of energy. Interestingly, in one investigation, when asked to choose their most significant symptom, more patients chose lack of energy (40%) compared to sleepiness (22%) (14). Therefore, these symptoms should be sought in all patients presenting with suspected SRBD, especially if they deny daytime sleepiness. Other daytime symptoms include morning headache, morning dry or sore throat, and problems with memory, vigilance, attention, and/or concentration.

The physical examination of the patient with a suspected SRBD generally starts with measures of body habitus. The body mass index and neck circumference both are predictive of the presence and severity of OSA (15–17) and are the most commonly used measures of body habitus. However, it should be noted that most other measures of body habitus, including measures such as waist-hip ratio and skin-fold thicknesses, are also predictive of OSA (15).

The physical examination of the patient with a suspected SRBD is concentrated on the upper airway examination. A common finding in children and thin adults with suspected OSA is tonsillar enlargement. Other upper airway findings that have been associated with OSA

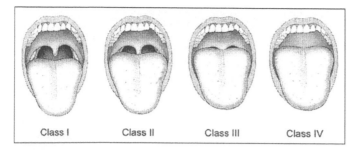

Figure 1 The Mallampati classification scale. During the assessment, the patients are instructed to open their mouth as wide as possible, while protruding the tongue as far as possible. Class I: tonsillar pillars, soft palate, and entire uvula visible; Class II: only soft palate and portion of uvula visible; Class III: only soft palate visible; Class IV: only hard palate visible. *Source*: From Ref. 22.

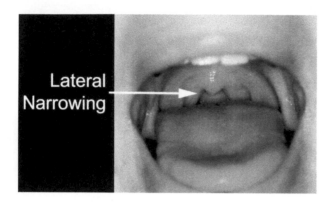

Figure 2 A view of the pharynx demonstrating lateral narrowing. Lateral narrowing is defined by the presence of bands of tissue impinging into the posterior pharyngeal space. *Source*: From Ref. 18.

include an overjet (horizontal relationship of upper and lower central incisors), retrognathia, tongue and/or uvula enlargement, a low-lying palate, a high-arched palate, and a high Mallampati score (18–21).

Two physical examination findings have been found to be independent predictors of the presence of OSA: the Mallampati score (Fig. 1) and lateral narrowing (Fig. 2). The Mallampati score is a simple airway-classification scheme developed to identify patients at risk for difficult intubation. In one study, each 1-point increase in the Mallampati score was associated with a two-fold increase in the odds of having OSA and a 5-point increase in the apnea-hypopnea index (AHI) (22). Lateral narrowing is the finding of airway narrowing by the lateral pharyngeal walls. In a study of 420 subjects with suspected OSA, it was found that narrowing of the airway by the lateral pharyngeal walls and tonsillar enlargement are independent predictors for the presence of OSA after controlling the body mass index and neck circumference, but only in men (18). The reason for the gender difference in the occurrence of lateral narrowing is unclear.

Two groups of investigators have published predictive models for OSA on the basis of physical examination findings. The first included morphometric measures comprising palatal height, overjet, and the maxillary and mandibular intermolar distances in addition to body mass index (19). However, the body mass index accounted for the majority of the predictive ability of the model. In a more recent investigation, researchers combined pharyngeal grade (as measured by the Mallampati classification), the degree of overbite, and the cricomental space into a decision rule (21). Of interest, the authors found that a cricomental space of greater than 1.5 cm excluded OSA with a 100% negative predictive value. It should be noted that neither of these models have been independently tested in a sleep clinic population; therefore, their overall usefulness for a sleep clinician has not been determined.

SUBJECTIVE ASSESSMENT TOOLS

One approach to the problem of distinguishing patients with a high likelihood of OSA from those with a low likelihood of OSA has been the development of clinical prediction models that calculate the probability that a patient referred to a sleep laboratory has OSA. The majority of these models combine self-reported OSA symptoms with demographic and anthropometric variables to discriminate between patients with and without OSA (4,6,8,17,23–30). In addition, two other studies (see above section, History and Physical Examination) utilized only anthropometric/physical examination findings to predict the likelihood of OSA (19,21). Several general comments can be made about the prediction models. The most important is that these models are of limited utility because while the models have sensitivities that are generally >80%, the specificities are generally <60%. Therefore, the likelihood ratios are in a range (0.2–5.0) that does not significantly increase or decrease the posttest probability of the presence of OSA. This would be particularly true for a sleep laboratory with a high pretest probability of disease (8).

A major limitation of these models is that the majority of the models were created in sleep clinic populations; therefore, they were specifically created to determine which patients who already had symptoms suggestive of OSA were most likely to have OSA. Therefore, the models may have limited utility and validity in broader populations of patients, such as a primary care practice. Only two models were created using data from non-sleep clinic populations, one from an epidemiologic cohort (6) and one from a primary care population (28). Other limitations of the studies included: single-center studies in the majority; data from limited numbers of women and minorities included in the model; and it was unclear if consecutive patients were enrolled and/or exclusion criteria were applied to exclude some patients.

The limitations of these models were shown in an investigation in which four of the models were prospectively tested in a consecutive group of 370 patients referred to a sleep center (8). In this study, no patients were excluded, a large number of women were enrolled (48%), and the pretest probability was high (67%). In general, the models had lower likelihood ratios than in the original studies (positive likelihood ratios 1.1–1.7), poor positive predictive values, and performed worse in women as compared to men. Therefore, the clinical prediction models tested are not sufficiently accurate to discriminate between patients with and without OSA. Lower likelihood ratios have also been found in other studies in which a prediction model was used in a population other than the original reported population (25,30).

However, the same investigation found that the models may be more helpful in identifying high-risk patients (AHI > 20; positive likelihood ratios 2.6–5.6), though at the risk of losing sensitivity. Therefore, the prediction models could be used to identify patients at the highest risk of OSA. This approach may be helpful in identifying OSA in a high-risk group such as commercial truck drivers (31), to identify a group of patients for an alternative ambulatory management algorithm (32), or for identifying patients most likely to need continuous positive airway pressure (CPAP) and therefore excellent candidates for split-night polysomnography (see below, Objective Assessment Tools). This approach has been studied by one group that combined a questionnaire prediction model with overnight oximetry, resulting in improved sensitivity and specificity (31,33).

The major barrier limiting the use of prediction models is that they lack the sensitivity to serve as a screening test and the specificity to obviate, or minimize, the need for further testing. In fact, the current medical insurance reimbursement system in the United States requires measurement of sleep time and the number of events per hour of sleep as a prerequisite for payment by insurance and for CPAP therapy to be authorized. Nevertheless, prediction models may become increasingly useful as the cost of sleep services occupies a larger portion of health care costs. It is plausible that a patient with "high probability" for sleep apnea can be directed to a disease management model that is based on a "decision to treat" rather than the diagnostic label. However, the development of a disease management model requires robust clinical trials.

OBJECTIVE ASSESSMENT TOOLS

Overnight polysomnography is the most widely used test for the diagnosis of SRBDs in the United States. Practice parameters developed by the American Academy of Sleep Medicine for the use of polysomnography have been updated and the reader is referred to these parameters for a detailed review (34). This section will review the elements of polysomnography and the different types of sleep studies that are performed for the diagnosis and management of SRBD.

Table 1 Parameters Recorded During Polysomnography

Use		Channels
Sleep stage scoring and arousal detection	Standard	Central, frontal, and occipital EEG Right and left EOG Chin EMG
Respiratory event detection	Standard	Flow: nasal pressure transducer Effort: esophageal manometry, inductance plethysmography Pulse oximetry
	Pediatric Studies	End-tidal CO_2
Leg movement detection	Standard	Right and left anterior tibialis EMG
Arrhythmia detection	Standard	ECG, chest lead

Abbreviations: EEG, electroencephalogram; EOG, electrooculogram; EMG, electromyogram; ECG, electrocardiogram; CO_2, carbon dioxide

During polysomnography, multiple physiologic parameters are continuously monitored and recorded (Table 1). The recording of at least three electroencephalograms (EEGs) (one central, one occipital, and one frontal lead), a chin electromyogram, and bilateral electrooculograms is required to score sleep and wake states (35). An electrocardiogram (ECG) (generally a chest lead) is used to monitor the cardiac rate and rhythm. Bilateral anterior tibialis muscle electromyograms are recorded to assess leg movements. Respiratory parameters generally include flow channel (both oronasal thermal sensors and nasal pressure transducers), thoracic and abdominal effort channels (ideally inductance plethysmography), snoring channel, and continuous pulse oximetry (35). For sleep studies in children, it is also recommended that end-tidal carbon dioxide monitoring should also be performed as many children present with obstructive hypoventilation rather than obstructive apneas and hypopneas (36).

Airflow through the upper airway can be measured by a variety of methods (37). Most of the available methods are adequate for detecting apneas (the absence of flow) but have varying ability to detect hypopneas (reduction in flow). The pneumotachometer, which measures airflow by measuring the pressure drop across a linear resistance, is considered the gold standard for measuring and quantifying airflow through the upper airway. Tidal volume can be computed by integration of the flow signal. However, the use of the pneumotachometer requires collection of all exhaled air via a closed breathing circuit; thus, it is primarily used in the research setting.

Nasal pressure transducers detect nasal airflow by the same physical principles of closed-circuit pneumotachometers, namely detecting pressure drop across a linear resistance albeit in an open circuit design. Therefore, nasal pressure transducers can detect changes in nasal flow, quantitatively. However, oral breathing can degrade the quality of the signal. Furthermore, there is a nonlinear relationship between pressure changes measured at the nares and actual airflow such that nasal pressure underestimates airflow at low flow rates and overestimates airflow at high flow rates (38,39). Accuracy can be increased by taking the square root transformation of the nasal pressure signal (38) though this is not routinely performed in clinical practice. Nasal pressure transducers are more sensitive than thermal sensors in detecting hypopneas (40) (Fig. 3), resulting in an increased AHI for polysomnograms with airflow recorded using nasal pressure transducers versus thermal sensors (41,42). In addition, nasal pressure transducers have the added advantage of being able to detect inspiratory flow limitation (43). Inspiratory flow limitation, when associated with an arousal, characterizes a respiratory effort–related arousal (RERA), which is considered a hallmark of the upper airway resistance syndrome (37,41,43,44). Recent guidelines recommend that nasal pressure transducers are the optimal sensor to detecting hypopneas (35).

Airflow can also be measured indirectly by differentiating the tidal volume signal obtained via respiratory inductance plethysmography (RIP). RIP is based on the detection of changes in the volume of the chest and abdomen over the breathing cycle, with the sum of the measurements providing an estimate of tidal volume if calibration is maintained (45). RIP is a reasonable methodology for detecting hypopneas when there is at least a 50% reduction in the

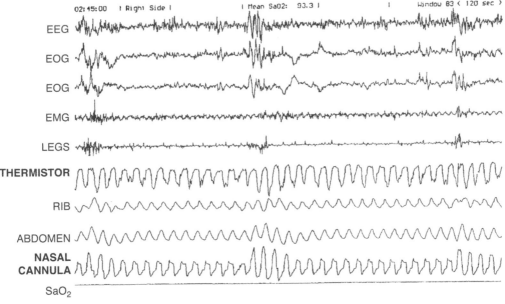

Figure 3 A 120-second epoch from a sleep study in one subject. On the nasal cannula channel, there is evidence of two episodes of decreased flow with inspiratory flow limitation that results in two corresponding separate arousals, consistent with hypopneas. Note that there is no clear decrease in the flow as measured by the thermistor. *Abbreviations*: EEG, electroencephalogram; EOG, electrooculogram; EMG, chin electromyogram; LEGS, bilateral leg electromyogram; THERMISTOR, temperature-sensitive measure of airflow; RIB, chest wall movement; ABDOMEN, abdominal wall movement; NASAL CANNULA, flow-sensitive measure of nasal airflow; SaO2, oxygen saturation. *Source*: From Ref. 40.

sum signal and it has also been used to detect inspiratory flow limitation during sleep (37,46,47). A major problem with these devices is that accurate calibration is not maintained over the course of the sleep study, especially in obese patients and if body position is changed, thereby decreasing the usefulness of the sum signal in the detection of respiratory events.

Thermal sensors (either thermistors or thermocouples), which measure changes in the temperature of air moving in and out of the nose and mouth, provide a qualitative assessment of airflow that is not well correlated with actual amplitude; thus, while these devices can detect the absence of flow, they are not considered reliable for the detection of relative decreases in amplitude required to detect hypopneas (48). Thermal sensors have recently been recommended as the sensor to detect apneas (35).

Respiratory effort has traditionally been monitored by measuring rib cage and abdominal movement using piezo sensors or strain gauges. These devices provide qualitative information on changes in rib cage and abdominal movement and cannot be used to reliably distinguish between central and obstructive events, particularly hypopneas (37,49). In contrast, measurement of pleural pressure using an esophageal pressure monitor (esophageal manometry), is considered the gold standard for measuring respiratory effort. The use of esophageal pressure monitoring has two major clinical applications. First, it can be used to verify central apnea and hypopnea episodes with a high degree of certainty (49). Second, esophageal pressure monitoring is necessary to detect RERAs and the upper airway resistance syndrome (37,50). The recently updated guidelines on polysomnography recommend either esophageal manometry or inductance plethysmography for the detection of respiratory effort (35).

As the identification of a hypopnea generally requires a desaturation of 3% to 4%, the accuracy of the oximeter is important. However, different oximeters have different sampling frequencies [ranging from 0.08 to 10 Hz (51)] and algorithms used to record oxygen saturation. Memory storage and methods of automated analysis of the oxygen saturation also vary between devices. Two studies demonstrate that the AHI will vary in the same subject when different oximeters are used (52,53), indicating that the oximeter acquisition parameters could be an important determinant of its ability to increase or reduce the probability of OSA in any given subject. Other studies indicate that there is night-to-night variability in oximetry results (54) and that the body mass index influences the likelihood ratios of oximetry alone for diagnosing OSA (55). Therefore, the limitations of these devices need to be understood by sleep physicians and technologists.

Many laboratories continue to determine the effective CPAP or bilevel positive airway pressure (BPAP) setting by performing full-night titration studies, during which the pressure is incrementally increased until the sleep-disordered breathing (apneas and hypopneas) is eliminated. The reader is referred to practice parameters on this subject (56,57). The goal of a positive pressure titration is to determine a CPAP or BPAP setting that eliminates the sleep-disordered breathing in all stages of sleep and in all body positions. Most laboratories increase the pressure to eliminate not only apneas and hypopneas (with a goal AHI < 5 events/hour) but also snoring and snoring-related arousals. In addition to the standard parameters already mentioned, many laboratories also record the flow obtained from the positive pressure unit. As an adjunct to positive pressure titration, equations that predict the optimal CPAP setting have been described (58,59). One of these equations was found to increase the likelihood of CPAP titration success (as defined as the number of studies with a final positive pressure level associated with an AHI < 5 events/hour) but it did not accurately predict the prescribed CPAP setting (60).

As many sleep laboratories have long waiting periods for an overnight sleep study, split-night polysomnography is frequently performed (61) for patients who are diagnosed with OSA. In split-night polysomnography, at least the first two hours of study are performed as a diagnostic study; if the AHI during the first portion of the study is 40 events/hour or greater (or ≥ 20 events/hour based on clinical judgment), a positive pressure titration is performed for the remainder of the night. This approach has been found to be accurate for diagnosing SRBD and determining the optimal positive pressure setting in the majority of patients without a difference in adherence in CPAP use (61–63).

OTHER SCREENING OR ADJUNCTIVE TOOLS

Because of the high prevalence of SRBD, the high cost, and technical requirements of in-laboratory polysomnography and the limited availability of sleep centers in some but not all countries (64), alternative approaches to the diagnosis of SRBD have been widely investigated in the last several years. The most common of these approaches is the use of portable monitoring. The term portable monitoring encompasses a variety of monitors that can record from as few as one physiologic parameter (channel) to as many as those in standard in-laboratory polysomnography. To provide consistency, the American Academy of Sleep Medicine defined four types of monitors: type 1 is defined as in-laboratory standard polysomnography; type 2, comprehensive portable polysomnography (similar number of channels as type 1 monitors including EEG; there is limited evidence for these devices and they will not be discussed further); type 3, generally four channels, including flow, effort, ECG, and oximetry; type 4, limited monitoring with generally 1–2 channels, and often oximetry alone (65). Portable monitors also vary in other ways. For instance, depending on the monitor, flow can be measured by nasal pressure transducers, thermistor, or RIP. Some monitors include automated scoring routines without the ability for editing results while others allow editing of the scoring. Finally, the criteria used for automatically scoring hypopneas may vary between devices (51).

There are several limitations to the available evidence for the use of portable monitors (51). First, while there are several portable monitors available for use, there are a limited number of high-quality studies on any given monitor. Second, the patient population in most studies was primarily white men without significant comorbidities; thus, the utility of these devices in women, other ethnic groups, and in patients with comorbidities is unclear. In addition, there is no evidence that they can be used in patients with suspected central sleep-disordered breathing as most studies excluded patients suspected of having this type of SRBD. Furthermore, many studies did not clearly enroll consecutive patients, limiting the generalizability of the results. Finally, the majority of portable monitors have been studied simultaneously with in-laboratory polysomnography in an attended setting. Few have actually assessed actual home use of the monitors. This consideration is important as the utility of a portable monitor in part depends on both the ease of use by the patient (the device can be put on and started without significant training) and the failure rate of recording (as lost signals cannot be fixed during the study as there is no attended monitoring by a technologist).

Ideally, a monitor that has a high sensitivity and high specificity in detecting OSA compared with the gold standard of in-laboratory polysomnography would be optimal. Likelihood ratios, or the likelihood that a given test result would be expected in a patient with the disorder compared to the likelihood that that same result would be expected in a patient without the disorder, have been increasingly used to assess the performance of these monitors. Likelihood ratios have advantages over sensitivity and specificity measures because they are less likely to change with disease prevalence, they can be calculated for several levels of the symptom/sign or test, and they can be used to calculate posttest probability for a target disorder. Depending on the pretest odds of the probability of the patient having OSA, the posttest probability of patients having OSA as assessed by type 3 monitors can be low or high (66–73). As described above, these monitors generally record at least four channels, including airflow, thoracic effort, oximetry, and ECG. As there is no EEG to measure sleep time, the devices calculate a respiratory disturbance index (RDI) using study time as the denominator. In general, several studies show positive likelihood ratios that ranged from 5.1 to 23.8 with negative likelihood ratios that ranged from 0.03 to 0.15. Three studies used different RDI cutoffs to reduce or increase the likelihood of OSA; while this methodology varies the posttest probability of patients having OSA, it results in some patients (22–37%) without a positive or negative result. Type 3 monitors have the potential to either reduce or increase the probability of OSA in a given patient when used in the attended setting but the utility in an unattended setting has not been established.

The use of oximetry as the primary signal for detecting OSA has been extensively studied (25,33,74–80) primarily because of its simplicity. The studies used a variety of oximetry criteria to detect OSA, including desaturation indices at different ΔSaO_2 cutoffs (2–4%), time spent with a saturation <90%, and a delta index that describes the variability of the oxyhemoglobin saturation over the course of the night, making comparisons between devices difficult. Five high-level evidence studies reported both high (>5.0) and low likelihood (<0.02) ratios (25,33,75,76,79), indicating that the oximetry device used both increased and reduced the probability that a patient had an abnormal AHI. However, to achieve these results, these studies used multiple cutoffs with the result that up to 49% of the patients were not classified. In general, the evidence suggests that oximetry devices can be used to either reduce or increase the probability of OSA in the attended setting. However, because of the limitations of oximetry devices outlined in the prior section and the fact that there is limited data for use of oximetry in the unattended environment, guidelines state that oximetry alone is not an acceptable diagnostic modality for diagnosing or excluding OSA (81,82).

Based upon the available evidence, guidelines have been recently updated regarding the use of portable monitors in the diagnosis of OSA (82). For patients with a high pretest probability of moderate to severe OSA, Type 3 monitors may be used as an alternative to polysomnography in the unattended setting. Physicians should recognize the following limitations: the studies need to be scored and reviewed manually, the patient should not have any significant comorbidity (particularly significant pulmonary disease or congestive heart failure), and that a negative study should be followed by a full Type 1 sleep study. Based upon the available evidence, the guidelines state that both Type 2 and Type 4 monitors should not be used in either the attended or unattended settings. Based upon recent evidence, the Center for Medicare and Medicaid Services recently decided to reimburse unattended portable monitoring as an alternative to full, attended polysomnography.

In conclusion, portable monitoring, particularly with type 3 devices, has the potential to change the process by which most patients are diagnosed with OSA. Instead of being referred for a full type 1 study, patients, particularly those with a high pretest probability of disease, could have a home study; if OSA is confirmed, the patient could be referred directly for a CPAP titration study. A negative study in a patient with a high pretest probability would be followed by a full type 1 study to confirm the absence of OSA. To identify high-risk patient, the prediction models discussed in section "Subjective Assessment Tools," could be used. This combined approach has been studied by one group that combined the questionnaire prediction model with overnight oximetry, resulting in improved sensitivity and specificity (31,33). However, further studies in which specific algorithms are tested and portable monitoring is performed in the home are needed. In addition, outcome studies need to be performed to show that a home-based approach results in similar efficacy of treatment. One such study has been published and showed no difference in outcome (80). Finally, studies examining whether an algorithm that includes home monitoring is cost-effective also need to be performed, especially given that an older study found full in-laboratory testing was more cost-effective than home testing (83).

NEW DIAGNOSTIC TOOLS

Termination of apnea or hypopnea is often associated with transient arousal from sleep. Repetitive arousals lead to sleep fragmentation and daytime sleepiness. Visual inspection of the cortical EEG is time-consuming and fraught with subjective variability. Therefore, development of objective, even if indirect, markers of arousal would be greatly beneficial. Changes in heart rate or blood pressure may serve as reliable surrogates of arousal, even if cortical changes are minimal or absent (84).

One technique for detecting acute changes in blood pressure is pulse transit time (PTT), an indirect method of measuring beat-to-beat blood pressure change (84–87). Pulse-transit time reflects the interval from the ECG R-wave until the pulse pressure wave reaches the finger. The normal interval is about 250 milliseconds, and is determined primarily by the stiffness/tension in the arterial walls and hence blood pressure. Accordingly, an increase in blood pressure leads to increased arterial wall stiffness, a faster pulse wave, and a shorter PTT. The essential components required to measure beat-to-beat are three thoracic electrodes and a modified oximeter finger probe. Several studies have shown that PTT is a sensitive marker of the arousal process in normal subjects. PTT has not yet been incorporated in commercial polysomnographic recordings; however, it is of potential benefit and can be applied in an objective, reproducible, and automated fashion.

Transient arousals from sleep are associated with increased bursts of sympathetic nerve activity in adults that lead to increased heart rate, blood pressure, and peripheral vasoconstriction. Peripheral arterial tonometry (PAT) is a new technique that uses a plethysmographic technique to measure the peripheral vasoconstriction. PAT uses a finger-mounted pneumo-optical sensor that measures the digital arterial pulse wave volume. Attenuation of the PAT signal indicates digital vasoconstriction and can be used as a marker for arousals associated with respiratory events (88,89). The PAT signal has been combined with pulse oximetry and wrist actigraphy in a wrist-worn portable monitor that is being studied as a home-based methodology for the diagnosis of OSA. In laboratory-based investigations comparing the PAT device with standard polysomnography performed simultaneously, there is excellent correlation between the PAT index and the AHI with high sensitivities and specificities (90,91). The PAT device has also been studied in the home and was found to have a high positive likelihood ratio for diagnosing moderate OSA (92).

CONCLUSIONS

A complete sleep history and physical examination that includes comprehensive assessment of the visible areas of the oropharynx should be conducted on all patients with suspected SRBDs. Clinical prediction models are the main subjective assessment tools for SRBD that have been studied; however, the studies are limited and none of the tools have been widely accepted. In terms of objective assessment tools, overnight polysomnography is the most widely used test for the diagnosis of SRBD in the United States, while portable monitoring is rapidly emerging as a technology that has the potential of changing the current diagnostic algorithm for SRBD. Lastly, the measurement of PTT and PAT are new techniques that show promise in the evaluation of patients with SRBD.

REFERENCES

1. Redline S, Tishler PV, Tosteson TD, et al. The familial aggregation of obstructive sleep apnea. Am J Respir Crit Care Med 1995; 151:682–687.
2. Palmer LJ, Redline S. Genomic approaches to understanding obstructive sleep apnea. Respir Physiol Neurobiol 2003; 135(2–3):187–205.

3. Scrima L, Broudy M, Nay KN, et al. Increased severity of obstructive sleep apnea after bedtime alcohol ingestion: diagnostic potential and proposed mechanism of action. Sleep 1982; 5(4):318–328.
4. Crocker BD, Olson LG, Saunders NA, et al. Estimation of the probability of disturbed breathing during sleep before a sleep study. Am Rev Respir Dis 1990; 142:14–18.
5. Deegan PC, McNicholas WT. Predictive value of clinical features for the obstructive sleep apnoea syndrome. Eur Respir J 1996; 9(1):117–124.
6. Kump K, Whalen C, Tishler PV, et al. Assessment of the validity and utility of a sleep-symptom questionnaire. Am J Respir Crit Care Med 1994; 150:735–741.
7. Olson LG, King MT, Hensley MJ, et al. A community study of snoring and sleep-disordered breathing. Symptoms. Am J Respir Crit Care Med 1995; 152(2):707–710.
8. Rowley JA, Aboussouan LS, Badr MS. The use of clinical prediction formulas in the evaluation of obstructive sleep apnea. Sleep 2000; 23:929–938.
9. Johns MW. A new method for measuring daytime sleepiness: the Epworth sleepiness scale. Sleep 1991; 14(6):540–545.
10. Carskadon MA, Dement WC. The multiple sleep latency test: what does it measure? Sleep 1982; 5 (suppl 2):S67–S72.
11. Punjabi NM, O'hearn DJ, Neubauer DN, et al. Modeling hypersomnolence in sleep-disordered breathing. A novel approach using survival analysis. Am J Respir Crit Care Med 1999; 159(6): 1703–1709.
12. Gottlieb DJ, Whitney CW, Bonekat WH, et al. Relation of sleepiness to respiratory disturbance index: the Sleep Heart Health Study. Am J Respir Crit Care Med 1999; 159(2):502–507.
13. Kapur VK, Baldwin CM, Resnick HE, et al. Sleepiness in patients with moderate to severe sleep-disordered breathing. Sleep 2005; 28(4):472–477.
14. Chervin RD. Sleepiness, fatigue, tiredness, and lack of energy in obstructive sleep apnea. Chest 2000; 118(2):372–379.
15. Young T, Palta M, Dempsey J, et al. The occurrence of sleep-disordered breathing among middle-aged adults. N Engl J Med 1993; 328:1230–1235.
16. Young T, Palta M, Badr MS. Sleep-disordered breathing (letter). N Engl J Med 1993; 329:1429–1430.
17. Flemons WW, Whitelaw WA, Brant R, et al. Likelihood ratios for a sleep apnea clinical prediction rule. Am J Respir Crit Care Med 1994; 150:1279–1285.
18. Schellenberg JB, Maislin G, Schwab RJ. Physical findings and the risk for obstructive sleep apnea. Am J Respir Crit Care Med 2000; 162:740–748.
19. Kushida CA, Efron B, Guilleminault C. A predictive morphometric model for the obstructive sleep apnea syndrome. Ann Intern Med 1997; 127:581–587.
20. Guilleminault C, Stoohs R, Kim YD, et al. Upper airway sleep-disordered breathing in women. Ann Intern Med 1995; 122(7):493–501.
21. Tsai WH, Remmers JE, Brant R, et al. A decision rule for diagnostic testing in obstructive sleep apnea. Am J Respir Crit Care Med 2003; 167(10):1427–1432.
22. Nuckton TJ, Glidden DV, Browner WS, et al. Physical examination: Mallampati score as an independent predictor of obstructive sleep apnea. Sleep 2006; 29:903–908.
23. Williams AJ, Yu G, Santiago S, et al. Screening for sleep apnea using pulse oximetry and a clinical score. Chest 1991; 100:631–635.
24. Viner S, Szalai JP, Hoffstein V. Are history and physical examination a good screening test for sleep apnea? Ann Intern Med 1991; 115:356–359.
25. Gyulay S, Olson LG, Hensley MJ, et al. A comparison of clinical assessment and home oximetry in the diagnosis of obstructive sleep apnea. Am Rev Respir Dis 1993; 147:50–53.
26. Maislin G, Pack AI, Kribbs NB, et al. A survey screen for prediction of apnea. Sleep 1995; 18:158–166.
27. Pradhan PS, Gliklich RE, Winkelman J. Screening for obstructive sleep apnea in patients presenting for snoring surgery. Laryngoscope 1996; 106(11):1393–1397.
28. Netzer NC, Stoohs RA, Netzer CM, et al. Using the Berlin Questionnaire to identify patients at risk for the sleep apnea syndrome. Ann Intern Med 1999; 131(7):485–491.
29. Rodsutti J, Hensley M, Thakkinstian A, et al. A clinical decision rule to prioritize polysomnography in patients with suspected sleep apnea. Sleep 2004; 27(4):694–699.
30. Hussain SF, Fleetham JA. Overnight home oximetry: can it identify patients with obstructive sleep apnea-hypopnea who have minimal daytime sleepiness? Respir Med 2003; 97(5):537–540.
31. Gurubhagavatula I, Maislin G, Nkwuo JE, et al. Occupational screening for obstructive sleep apnea in commercial drivers. Am J Respir Crit Care Med 2004; 170(4):371–376.
32. Mulgrew AT, Fox N, Ayas NT, et al. Diagnosis and initial management of obstructive sleep apnea without polysomnography: a randomized validation study. Ann Intern Med 2007; 146(3):157–166.
33. Gurubhagavatula I, Maislin G, Pack AI. An algorithm to stratify sleep apnea risk in a sleep disorders clinic population. Am J Respir Crit Care Med 2001; 164(10 pt 1):1904–1909.
34. Kushida CA, Littner MR, Morgenthaler T, et al. Practice parameters for the indications for polysomnography and related procedures: an update for 2005. Sleep 2005; 28(4):499–521.

35. Iber C, Ancoli-Israel S, Chesson AL Jr., et al. The AASM Manual for the Scoring of Sleep and Associated Events. Westchester, IL: American Academy of Sleep Medicine, 2007.
36. Katz ES, Marcus CL. Diagnosis of obstructive sleep apnea syndrome in infants and children. In: Sheldon SH, Ferber R, Kryger MH, eds. Principles and Practice of Pediatric Sleep Medicine. Philadelphia, PA: Elsevier Saunders, 2005:197–210.
37. American Academy of Sleep Medicine Task Force. Sleep-related breathing disorders in adults: recommendations for syndrome definition and measurement techniques in clinical research. The Report of an American Academy of Sleep Medicine Task Force. Sleep 1999; 22(5):667–689.
38. Farre R, Rigau J, Montserrat JM, et al. Relevance of linearizing nasal prongs for assessing hypopneas and flow limitation during sleep. Am J Respir Crit Care Med 2001; 163(2):494–497.
39. Montserrat JM, Farre R, Ballester E, et al. Evaluation of nasal prongs for estimating nasal flow. Am J Respir Crit Care Med 1997; 155(1):211–215.
40. Norman RG, Ahmed MM, Walsleben JA, et al. Detection of respiratory events during NPSG: nasal cannula/pressure sensor versus thermistor. Sleep 1997; 20(12):1175–1184.
41. Ayappa I, Norman RG, Krieger AC, et al. Non-invasive detection of respiratory effort-related arousals (RERAs) by a nasal cannula/pressure transducer system. Sleep 2000; 23(6):763–771.
42. Ballester E, Badia JR, Hernandez L, et al. Nasal prongs in the detection of sleep-related disordered breathing in the sleep apnoea/hypopnoea syndrome. Eur Respir J 1998; 11(4):880–883.
43. Hosselet JJ, Norman RG, Ayappa I, et al. Detection of flow limitation with a nasal cannula/pressure transducer system. Am J Respir Crit Care Med 1998; 157(5 pt 1):1461–1467.
44. Hosselet J, Ayappa I, Norman RG, et al. Classification of sleep-disordered breathing. Am J Respir Crit Care Med 2001; 163(2):398–405.
45. Carry PY, Baconnier P, Eberhard A, et al. Evaluation of respiratory inductive plethysmography: accuracy for analysis of respiratory waveforms. Chest 1997; 111(4):910–915.
46. Loube DI, Andrada T, Howard RS. Accuracy of respiratory inductive plethysmography for the diagnosis of upper airway resistance syndrome. Chest 1999; 115(5):1333–1337.
47. Kaplan V, Zhang JN, Russi EW, et al. Detection of inspiratory flow limitation during sleep by computer assisted respiratory inductive plethysmography. Eur Respir J 2000; 15(3):570–578.
48. Farre R, Montserrat JM, Rotger M, et al. Accuracy of thermistors and thermocouples as flow-measuring devices for detecting hypopnoeas. Eur Respir J 1998; 11(1):179–182.
49. Boudewyns A, Willemen M, Wagemans M, et al. Assessment of respiratory effort by means of strain gauges and esophageal pressure swings: a comparative study. Sleep 1997; 20(2):168–170.
50. Guilleminault C, Stoohs R, Clerk A, et al. A cause of excessive daytime sleepiness. The upper airway resistance syndrome. Chest 1993; 104(3):781–787.
51. Flemons WW, Littner MR, Rowley JA, et al. Home diagnosis of sleep apnea: a systematic review of the literature. An evidence review cosponsored by the American Academy of Sleep Medicine, the American College of Chest Physicians, and the American Thoracic Society. Chest 2003; 124(4): 1543–1579.
52. Zafar S, Ayappa I, Norman RG, et al. Choice of oximeter affects apnea-hypopnea index. Chest 2005; 127(1):80–88.
53. Davila DG, Richards KC, Marshall BL, et al. Oximeter's acquisition parameter influences the profile of respiratory disturbances. Sleep 2003; 26(1):91–95.
54. Fietze I, Dingli K, Diefenbach K, et al. Night-to-night variation of the oxygen desaturation index in sleep apnoea syndrome. Eur Respir J 2004; 24(6):987–993.
55. Nakano H, Ikeda T, Hayashi M, et al. Effect of body mass index on overnight oximetry for the diagnosis of sleep apnea. Respir Med 2004; 98(5):421–427.
56. Kushida CA, Littner MR, Hirshkowitz M, et al. Practice parameters for the use of continuous and bilevel positive airway pressure devices to treat adult patients with sleep-related breathing disorders. Sleep 2006; 29(3):375–380.
57. Kushida CA, Chediak A, Berry RB, et al. Clinical guidelines for the manual titration of positive airway pressure in patients with obstructive sleep apnea. J Clin Sleep Med 2008; 4:157–171.
58. Series F, Marc I. Efficacy of automatic continuous positive airway pressure therapy that uses an estimated required pressure in the treatment of the obstructive sleep apnea syndrome. Ann Intern Med 1997; 127(8 pt 1):588–595.
59. Hoffstein V, Mateika S. Predicting nasal continuous positive airway pressure. Am J Respir Crit Care Med 1994; 150(2):486–488.
60. Rowley JA, Tarbichi AG, Badr MS. The use of a predicted CPAP equation improves CPAP titration success. Sleep Breath 2005; 9(1):26–32.
61. Sanders MH, Kern NB, Costantino JP, et al. Adequacy of prescribing positive airway pressure therapy by mask for sleep apnea on the basis of a partial-night trial. Am Rev Respir Dis 1993; 147:1169–1174.
62. Sanders MH, Black J, Costantino JP, et al. Diagnosis of sleep-disordered breathing by half-night polysomnography. Am Rev Respir Dis 1991; 144(6):1256–1261.

63. Strollo PJ Jr., Sanders MH, Costantino JP, et al. Split-night studies for the diagnosis and treatment of sleep-disordered breathing. Sleep 1996; 19(10 suppl):S255–S259.
64. Flemons WW, Douglas NJ, Kuna ST, et al. Access to diagnosis and treatment of patients with suspected sleep apnea. Am J Respir Crit Care Med 2004; 169(6):668–672.
65. Ferber R, Millman R, Coppola M, et al. Portable recording in the assessment of obstructive sleep apnea. ASDA standards of practice. Sleep 1994; 17(4):378–392.
66. White DP, Gibb TJ, Wall JM, et al. Assessment of accuracy and analysis time of a novel device to monitor sleep and breathing in the home. Sleep 1995; 18(2):115–126.
67. Verse T, Pirsig W, Junge-Hulsing B, et al. Validation of the POLY-MESAM seven-channel ambulatory recording unit. Chest 2000; 117(6):1613–1618.
68. Ficker JH, Wiest GH, Wilpert J, et al. Evaluation of a portable recording device (Somnocheck) for use in patients with suspected obstructive sleep apnoea. Respiration 2001; 68(3):307–312.
69. Ballester E, Solans M, Vila X, et al. Evaluation of a portable respiratory recording device for detecting apnoeas and hypopnoeas in subjects from a general population. Eur Respir J 2000; 16(1):123–127.
70. Man GC, Kang BV. Validation of a portable sleep apnea monitoring device. Chest 1995; 108(2):388–393.
71. Emsellem HA, Corson WA, Rappaport BA, et al. Verification of sleep apnea using a portable sleep apnea screening device. South Med J 1990; 83(7):748–752.
72. Zucconi M, Ferini-Strambi L, Castronovo V, et al. An unattended device for sleep-related breathing disorders: validation study in suspected obstructive sleep apnoea syndrome. Eur Respir J 1996; 9(6):1251–1256.
73. Redline S, Tosteson T, Boucher MA, et al. Measurement of sleep-related breathing disturbances in epidemiologic studies. Assessment of the validity and reproducibility of a portable monitoring device. Chest 1991; 100(5):1281–1286.
74. Series F, Marc I, Cormier Y, et al. Utility of nocturnal home oximetry for case finding in patients with suspected sleep apnea hypopnea syndrome. Ann Intern Med 1993; 119:449–453.
75. Stoohs R, Guilleminault C. MESAM 4: an ambulatory device for the detection of patients at risk for obstructive sleep apnea syndrome (OSAS). Chest 1992; 101(5):1221–1227.
76. Vazquez JC, Tsai WH, Flemons WW, et al. Automated analysis of digital oximetry in the diagnosis of obstructive sleep apnoea. Thorax 2000; 55(4):302–307.
77. Yamashiro Y, Kryger MH. Nocturnal oximetry: is it a screening tool for sleep disorders? Sleep 1995; 18(3):167–171.
78. Golpe R, Jimenez A, Carpizo R, et al. Utility of home oximetry as a screening test for patients with moderate to severe symptoms of obstructive sleep apnea. Sleep 1999; 22(7):932–937.
79. Esnaola S, Duran J, Infante-Rivard C, et al. Diagnostic accuracy of a portable recording device (MESAM IV) in suspected obstructive sleep apnoea. Eur Respir J 1996; 9(12):2597–2605.
80. Whitelaw WA, Brant RF, Flemons WW. Clinical usefulness of home oximetry compared with polysomnography for assessment of sleep apnea. Am J Respir Crit Care Med 2005; 171(2):188–193.
81. Chesson AL Jr., Berry RB, Pack A. Practice parameters for the use of portable monitoring devices in the investigation of suspected obstructive sleep apnea in adults. Sleep 2003; 26(7):907–913.
82. Collop NA, Anderson WA, Boehlecke B, et al. Clinical guidelines for the use of unattended portable monitors in the diagnosis of obstructive sleep apnea in adult patients. J Clin Sleep Med 2007; 3:737–747.
83. Chervin RD, Murman DL, Malow BA, et al. Cost-utility of three approaches to the diagnosis of sleep apnea: polysomnography, home testing, and empirical therapy. Ann Intern Med 1999; 130(6):496–505.
84. Pitson DJ, Stradling JR. Autonomic markers of arousal during sleep in patients undergoing investigation for obstructive sleep apnoea, their relationship to EEG arousals, respiratory events and subjective sleepiness. J Sleep Res 1998; 7(1):53–59.
85. Pitson DJ, Sandell A, van den HR, et al. Use of pulse transit time as a measure of inspiratory effort in patients with obstructive sleep apnoea. Eur Respir J 1995; 8(10):1669–1674.
86. Pitson DJ, Stradling JR. Value of beat-to-beat blood pressure changes, detected by pulse transit time, in the management of the obstructive sleep apnoea/hypopnoea syndrome. Eur Respir J 1998; 12(3):685–692.
87. Pepin JL, Delavie N, Pin I, et al. Pulse transit time improves detection of sleep respiratory events and microarousals in children. Chest 2005; 127(3):722–730.
88. Grote L, Zou D, Kraiczi H, et al. Finger plethysmography—a method for monitoring finger blood flow during sleep disordered breathing. Respir Physiol Neurobiol 2003; 136(2–3):141–152.
89. O'Donnell CP, Allan L, Atkinson P, et al. The effect of upper airway obstruction and arousal on peripheral arterial tonometry in obstructive sleep apnea. Am J Respir Crit Care Med 2002; 166(7):965–971.
90. Ayas NT, Pittman S, MacDonald M, et al. Assessment of a wrist-worn device in the detection of obstructive sleep apnea. Sleep Med 2003; 4(5):435–442.
91. Bar A, Pillar G, Dvir I, et al. Evaluation of a portable device based on peripheral arterial tone for unattended home sleep studies. Chest 2003; 123(3):695–703.
92. Pittman SD, Ayas NT, MacDonald MM, et al. Using a wrist-worn device based on peripheral arterial tonometry to diagnose obstructive sleep apnea: in-laboratory and ambulatory validation. Sleep 2004; 27(5):923–933.

29 | Diagnostic Algorithm for Sleep-Related Breathing Disorders

Gang Bao
Alvarado Sleep Disorders Center and Alvarado Hospital, San Diego, California, U.S.A.

INTRODUCTION

Sleep-related breathing disorders (SRBDs) describe all disorders due to breathing problems in sleep. The *International Classification of Sleep Disorders*, 2nd edition (*ICSD-2*) categorizes the disorders according to their causes, breathing patterns, or age groups (adult or pediatric) (1). In clinical practice, obstructive sleep apnea (OSA) is far more commonly diagnosed than other types of SRBDs. Even so, it is assumed that OSA is still underdiagnosed. It is possible that some types of the SRBDs or other sleep disorders are less familiar to health care providers or even to sleep specialists, therefore, are mislabeled and treated as OSA. There are a few new SRBD entities proposed to the sleep medicine community, but not included in *ICSD-2*, such as complex sleep apnea (CompSA), that may possibly be considered in the future version of the ICSD. This chapter intends to provide readers with a logical and step-by-step tool for daily clinical practice on the basis of *ICSD-2*; therefore, newly proposed disease entities such as CompSA will not be discussed here.

SRBD is a spectrum of breathing disorders recognized gradually over the history of sleep medicine. First, OSA was described (2), and gradually, other disorders were identified clinically and reported in the literature. The sleep medicine community has accepted the term SRBD as a group of disorders caused by breathing abnormalities during sleep but with different pathophysiologic mechanisms. In the general medical practice, OSA is by far the most common SRBD, it presents in 4% adult men and 2% women who are both with clinical symptoms and with an apnea-hypopnea index of 5 or higher on the polysomnogram (3). If using the apnea-hypopnea index of 5 per hour or higher alone, it could affect as much as 24% of adult men and 19% of the women. Although there are limited data regarding the prevalence of OSA in the pediatric population, the study from the Cleveland cohort indicates that at least 5% of children suffer from OSA, and another 15% have primary snoring (4). The prevalence for other SRBDs is even less defined due to the lack of studies, partly due to their low prevalence compared to OSA.

CLINICAL VIGNETTE

A 43-year-old Caucasian man with a long history of loud snoring was referred by his primary care physician for evaluation. He has been otherwise healthy but complained of feeling tired and groggy in the mornings after getting up despite seven to eight hours of sound sleep every night. He usually went to bed at 10 p.m., falling asleep within 10 minutes and waking up a few times at night with a dry mouth and sometimes choking and gasping for air. He fell back to sleep immediately after using the bathroom at night. His awakening time was 6 a.m. and he worked between 7 a.m. and 4 p.m. as a construction worker. After work he felt extremely tired especially the last year or so, unable to help with household tasks such as yard work, and also quit going to the gym, which he used to enjoy; he subsequently gained 30 pounds of weight. He often fell asleep in the couch watching television in the evenings and ended up napping 1 hour or longer. On the weekends, he usually slept 10 to 12 hours at night, still feeling groggy afterward. He denied any driving problems but admitted feeling sleepy or even dozing off occasionally when driving long distances. His wife confirmed that he snored loudly especially when sleeping on his back and after consumption of alcohol. He often ceased breathing for 10 to 20 seconds before making a noisy snoring sound. His Epworth Sleepiness Scale (ESS) score was 14 out of a possible 24 points.

He has been married for 20 years and has two teenage girls aged 18 and 15 years. The younger girl also snores at night. He does not smoke but drinks two beers at dinnertime three to four times a week. He remembered his father snored and suffered from high blood pressure and diabetes mellitus. He took Afrin for nasal congestions when needed and went to his doctor for physicals once a year. He had a tonsillectomy when he was 5 years old.

On physical examination, the patient showed a well-developed and nourished white gentleman in no acute distress. He was 5 ft 11 in. tall and weighted 230 lbs. His body mass index (BMI) was 32.1 kg/m². His blood pressure was 140/88 mmHg, pulse 78 per minute. He had a long facial structure and some retrognathia. His nose was narrowed and had significant turbinate enlargement bilaterally with a slightly deviated septum to the left. Oral examination showed a high-arched hard palate, and the airway was Mallampati class 4. His tonsils were absent, the uvula was elongated and enlarged, the soft palate was low, and the pharynx area was crowded. He had very crowded teeth in the front and signs of teeth grinding. He showed a 5-mm overjet of the upper teeth against the lower teeth. The size of the tongue was large and could not sit flat within the lower jaw. The temporomandibular joint (TMJ) had bilateral click sounds when chewing. His neck was short and thick; the circumference was 44 cm. His chest, abdomen, and peripheral examinations were unremarkable.

The patient went through a diagnostic polysomnography of over 440 minutes, showing sleep onset latency at 5 minutes, and rapid eye movement (REM) sleep onset latency at 210 minutes, with 56% non–rapid eye movement (NREM) sleep stage 1, 28% stage 2, 9% stage 3, and 7% REM sleep. The respiratory disturbance index (RDI) was 56, and the lowest oxygen saturation was 82%. His sleep efficiency was 67%. His periodic limb movement index was 0.

On the basis of clinical data, the patient was diagnosed as having severe OSA and treated with a continuous positive airway pressure (CPAP) device after titration; weight loss was also recommended to the patient.

KEY STEPS IN THE DIAGNOSIS OF THE DISORDER

Clinical Complaints and Symptoms
Snoring
In adult populations, snoring is reported in 50% of men and 25% of women (5). Snoring indicates turbulence of the airflow in the upper airway. Although there is a term called primary snoring, the majority of the snorers have airway narrowing during sleep; therefore, snoring should not be considered as a nuisance (6). Snoring usually is worse after consumption of alcohol and in the supine position. In children, snoring is never normal; therefore, further evaluation for SRBDs should be initiated (7).

Excessive Daytime Sleepiness
Many patients with SRBDs present with excessive daytime sleepiness (EDS). The best-known and clinically widely used tool is the ESS (8), which has been validated clinically (9,10). It contains eight questions related to daily activities; a score below 9 is considered normal, 10 or above indicates EDS. However, some patients consider themselves rather tired or fatigued than sleepy; therefore they rate their ESS score low even though they may have a severe SRBD. On the other hand, a typical insomnia patient will give an extremely low score of 0 to 2 to express his or her difficulty initiating sleep at any time. The severity of EDS can vary from falling asleep all the time, dozing off in front of the television or while reading, driving difficulties with especially long distances, feeling tired in the evening; or taking additional naps during the daytime.

Witnessed Apnea
Often reported by bed partners or family members, witnessed apnea is highly suggestive of the presence of OSA (11–13). Some bed partners are scared and therefore initiate the clinical evaluation.

Insomnia
Sleep maintenance insomnia is especially associated with SRBD. While patients with SRBD can present with sleep onset insomnia, the sleep maintenance insomnia is more indicative of SRBD

(14,15). Waking up many times with choking or gasping for air, a dry mouth, or frequent nighttime urination (16) further suggests possible airway problems during sleep.

Mouth Breathing and Dry Mouth
Due to upper airway obstruction, OSA patients can complain of breathing through the mouth and a dry mouth, especially after waking up at night. Often they will have symptoms of nasal allergies and congestion (17–19), even during the day.

Weight Gain
Weight gain is common in OSA patients due to an inability to exercise when sleepy and tired, also due to metabolic changes associated with OSA. Weight gain can also contribute to the development or worsening of OSA (20).

Neuropsychological Symptoms
Mood swings, depression, lack of interest, memory deterioration, and morning headaches all suggest consequences of poor quality of sleep related to SRBDs (21–23).

Medication
For people addicted to pain medications, especially in a large amount and chronically, central apnea due to drugs and substance should be considered (24,25).

Other histories suggestive of SRBD include a family history of OSA or snoring (26), and hypertension (27–34). For patients with heart failure (35–37), chronic renal disease (38,39), or stroke (40–42), central sleep apneas are common as either a Cheyne-Stokes or a non-Cheyne-Stokes breathing (non-CSB) pattern.

Physical Examination
- High blood pressure
- Obesity and BMI > 25
- Nasal congestion
- Craniofacial abnormality: midface hypoplasia, retrognathia, or micrognathia (43,44)
- High Mallampati classification (45,46)
- Pharyngeal tissue enlargement: tonsillomegaly, large uvula, low soft palate, and lateral narrowing (47)
- Jaw and denture abnormalities: high-arched hard palate, overjet, overbite, open bite, crowded teeth
- Large neck circumference (48), anterior cervical-spine fusion, enlarged thyroid tissues
- Abnormal chest wall and breathing weakness, diaphragmatic weakness
- Neurological abnormalities: quadriplegia or paraplegia, kyphoscoliosis

For children with SRBDs, the clinical presentations may be different from those of adults. A different approach may be necessary (49,50).

Diagnostic Polysomnography
Overnight polysomnography is considered the standard for the diagnosis of an SRBD (51). The in-laboratory attended polysomnography (type 1 monitoring) has been challenged recently by several organizations as the use of portable monitoring studies showed comparable sensitivity and specificity but at lower cost. Type 2 monitors include a minimum of seven channels, including electroencephalography (EEG), electro-oculography (EOG), chin electromyography (EMG), electrocardiography (ECG) or heart rate, airflow, respiratory effort, and oxygen saturation; type 3 monitors include a minimum of four channels: airflow, respiratory movement, heart rate or EKG, and oxygen saturation; type 4 monitors have one or two parameters such as oxygen saturation with/without airflow. Some health maintenance organizations (HMO) and U.S. Department of Veterans Affairs (VA) systems have implemented portable monitoring systems for the diagnosis of SRBDs, in an effort to cut the cost and shorten the waiting time for the sleep study.

Split-night polysomnography is used to complete the diagnostic and CPAP titration process in one night. Split-night polysomnography starts with at least two hours of recording of sleep without CPAP, and if there are a significant number of apneas and hypopneas and/or oxygen desaturation, CPAP will be applied throughout the rest of the night. In some cases, if patients do not show significant apneas and hypopneas during the first two hours or the CPAP titration is suboptimal, a full night of CPAP titration is then necessary.

IMPORTANT DIAGNOSTIC FEATURES AND CRITERIA TO DISTINGUISH DISORDER TYPES

Primary Central Sleep Apnea
Central sleep apnea could present similar to OSA with frequent awakenings, EDS, witnessed apneas, or even snoring, especially in CompSA, when the obstructive component is present.
Diagnostic Criteria (1)
Complaints of EDS, insomnia, short of breath waking up; with polysomnographic findings of five or more central apneas per hour; and absence of another sleep disorder, medical or neurological disorders, or medication/substance use.

Cheyne-Stokes Breathing Pattern
CSB is often seen in congestive heart failure, stroke, and renal failure. Polysomnographic features include recurrent central apnea and hypopnea alternating with crescendo-decrescendo hyperpneas, generally considered as a CO_2-drive-dependent respiration in central respiratory control.
Diagnostic Criteria (1)
Characteristic crescendo-decrescendo patterns of central apneas/hypopneas on polysomnography with frequent arousals and disturbances from sleep; suffering heart failure, stroke, or renal failure; and absence of another sleep disorder, medical or neurological disorders, medication or substance use.

High-Altitude Periodic Breathing
This disorder occurs in high altitude above 7600 m and sometimes at lower than 5000 m. High-altitude periodic breathing is associated with frequent awakenings, poor quality of sleep, and a sense of suffocation, and it often improves when the altitude is lowered.
Diagnostic Criteria (1)
At higher than 4000 m above the sea level with central apneas five or more per hour on polysomnography, usually during NREM sleep.

Central Sleep Apnea due to Medical Condition not Cheyne-Stokes
This disorder is characterized as a non-CSB pattern with central apnea and hypopnea in neurologic, cardiac, and renal diseases. It is only distinguishable by polysomnography.

Central Sleep Apnea due to Drug or Substance
Diagnostic Criteria (1)
At least two months of regular opioid use with central apneas five or more per hour or periodic breathing defined by 10 or more per hour crescendo-decrescendo pattern of hyperpneas with central apneas/hypopneas and arousals or disturbed sleep.

Primary Sleep Apnea of Infancy (Formerly Primary Sleep Apnea of Newborn)
Diagnostic Criteria (1)
Apnea of prematurity. The patient is younger than 37 weeks conceptional age, with presence of central apneas of 20 seconds or longer; if less than 20 seconds, must be accompanied by clinical symptoms, such as bradycardia, hypoxemia, or others requiring nursing intervention. The conditions are not attributable to other sleep disorders or medical, neurological disorders.

Apnea of infancy. In a patient older than 37 weeks conceptional age with central apneas 20 seconds or longer, or less than 20 seconds but having bradycardia, cyanosis, pallor, or marked hypotonia.

Obstructive Sleep Apnea Syndromes, Adult
Diagnostic Criteria (1)
Symptoms reported by the patient or bed partner including daytime sleepiness, fatigue; nighttime insomnia, loud snoring, breath holding, gasping, or choking; with polysomno- graphic findings of five or more respiratory events per hour, including apnea, hypopnea, or respiratory effort–related arousals (RERAs). The conditions are not due to other sleep disorder, medical or neurological disorders.

Obstructive Sleep Apnea Syndromes, Pediatric
Diagnostic Criteria (1)
Reported abnormal breathing during sleep, such as snoring, difficulty breathing, with clinical signs (paradoxical inward rib-cage motion, movement arousals, diaphoresis, neck hyper- extension) and physical or mental disturbances (enuresis, morning headaches, EDS, delayed growth), as well as polysomnographic findings of one or more apnea/hypopnea episodes per hour (over two respiratory cycles, not 10 seconds as in adult). Other diagnostic features include desaturation with respiratory events, hypercapnia, negative esophageal pressure swings.

Sleep-Related Hypoventilation/Hypoxemic Syndromes
Sleep-Related Nonobstructive Alveolar Hypoventilation, Idiopathic
Diagnostic Criteria (1)
Periodic breathing abnormalities longer than 10 seconds during sleep with desaturation and arousals not due to other conditions such as lung diseases, neuromuscular or skeletal problems, and absence of another sleep disorder, medical neurological, medication or substance use.

Congenital Central Alveolar Hypoventilation Syndrome
Diagnostic Criteria (1)
Onset since birth with shallow breathing, cyanosis, and apneas during sleep; absent or diminished response to hypoxia and hypercapnia, worse during sleep than during wakeful- ness shown on polysomnography; without presence of another sleep disorder, medical or neurological disorders, or substance use.

Sleep-Related Hypoventilation/Hypoxemia due to Medical Condition
Sleep-Related Hypoventilation/Hypoxemia due to Pulmonary Parenchymal or Vascular Pathology
Diagnostic Criteria (1)
Lung parenchymal (such as interstitial pulmonary fibrosis) or pulmonary vascular diseases (such as pulmonary HTN) as a cause of hypoxemia and polysomnographic findings of (*i*) SpO_2 < 90% for more than five minutes or 30% of total sleep time, or abnormally high/increased $PaCO_2$ during sleep compared to wakefulness and (*ii*) no other sleep disorder, medical or neurological disorders can be attributable to the conditions.

Sleep-Related Hypoventilation/Hypoxemia due to Lower Airways Obstruction
Diagnostic Criteria (1)
Hypoxemia with abnormal forced expiratory volume/forced vital capacity ratio (FEV1/FVC ratio) of less than 70% on the pulmonary function test, together with polysomnographic findings of SpO_2 < 90% for more than five minutes or 30% of total sleep time, or abnormally high/increased $PaCO_2$ during sleep compared to wakefulness.

Sleep-Related Hypoventilation/Hypoxemia due to Neuromuscular and Chest Wall Disorders
Diagnostic Criteria (1)
Neuromuscular or chest wall abnormalities causing hypoxemia and polysomnographic findings of SpO_2 < 90% for more than five minutes or 30% of total sleep time, or abnormally high/increased $PaCO_2$ during sleep compared to wakefulness.

Other Sleep-Related Breathing Disorders

Sleep Apnea/Sleep-Related Breathing Disorder, Unspecified

For conditions do not fit any of the above categories of diagnosis but clearly due to breathing problems in sleep.

DIFFERENTIAL DIAGNOSIS FOR EACH DISORDER TYPE

Primary Central Sleep Apnea

Polysomnography and an arterial blood gas often are needed to differentiate OSA, CSB pattern, sleep-related hypoventilation/hypoxic syndrome, and other SRBDs. Polysomnography shows respiratory effort when apneas/hypopneas occur in OSA; and a crescendo-decrescendo respiration pattern and history of heart failure, stroke, or renal failure make a diagnosis of CSB clear. In sleep-related hypoventilation/hypoxic syndrome, an arterial blood gas demonstrates hypercapnia during wakefulness, and polysomnography reveals significant desaturations during sleep that are worse during REM sleep.

Cheyne-Stokes Breathing Pattern

A crescendo-decrescendo respiration pattern on polysomnography and history of heart failure, stroke, or renal failure are the key differential features for CSB pattern. Often the crescendo-decrescendo respiration is longer than 45 seconds.

High-Altitude Periodic Breathing

This disorder characteristically occurs after ascending to at least 4000 m above sea level and polysomnography shows central apneas shorter than 34 seconds.

Central Sleep Apnea due to Medical Condition not Cheyne-Stokes

Similar medical conditions but without a CSB pattern, should be differentiated from primary CSA, as the treatment of the medical conditions may improve the patients' sleep.

Central Sleep Apnea due to Drug or Substance

This condition is often missed from the patient's history taking. Polysomnography shows central apneas not different from other types of CSA.

Primary Sleep Apnea of Infancy (Formerly Primary Sleep Apnea of Newborn)

This type of SRBD should be readily differentiable from other disorders on the basis of the unique age group, the time of onset, and polysomnographic findings.

Adult Obstructive Sleep Apnea

For majority of adult OSA cases, the diagnostic process is straightforward. However, for cases either atypical or equivocal, emphasis should lay on identifying subsets of OSA, especially in non-obese patients or those with upper airway resistance syndrome (UARS), and avoiding misdiagnosis of other diseases labeled as OSA, which is a tendency in our daily practice when OSA occupies the majority of our sleep medicine practice. Even the most experienced sleep specialists can have difficulty differentiating leg movements caused by arousals from respiratory events, resulting in mislabeling periodic limb movement in sleep (PLMS) as OSA. A thorough sleep history is important to recognize restless legs syndrome (RLS) and PLMS, before jumping into OSA as the diagnosis.

For people with EDS, insufficient sleep (due to short sleep time, delayed sleep phase, or shift work), narcolepsy (with and without cataplexy), and idiopathic hypersomnia need to be ruled out. In most cases, a patient history about routine bedtime schedule and total sleep time over 24 hours can help identify insufficient sleep problems. A history about the patient's day- and nighttime symptoms, such as cataplexy, sleep paralysis, and hypnagogic hallucinations, together with human leukocyte antigen (HLA) typing for DQB1*0602, and polysomnographic evidence of disturbances in sleep; a multiple sleep latency test (MSLT) with a sleep onset less than eight minutes and two or more sleep-onset REM periods (SOREMPs); and low cerebrospinal fluid (CSF) levels of hypocretin-1 ($\leq$110 pg/mL) are features for the diagnosis of narcolepsy. OSA, PLMS, and REM sleep behavior disorder (RBD) are also more prevalent in narcolepsy patients; therefore, the presence of those disorders do not exclude the diagnosis for narcolepsy.

Idiopathic hypersomnia is a diagnosis of exclusion, meaning the diagnosis can only be made when all other sleep disorders are ruled out, and the patient demonstrates EDS.

Pediatric Obstructive Sleep Apnea

For the pediatric population, the diagnosis of OSA still lacks standardization. The *ICSD-2* improved the diagnostic criteria by listing some symptoms and clinical signs to look for in the diagnosis of pediatric OSA. One point that needs to be kept in mind is that the presentations of pediatric OSA are different than those for adult OSA. The differential diagnosis includes attention deficit/hyperactive disorder (ADD, ADHD). It is speculated that 25% of ADD/ADHD children could suffer from pediatric OSA. Narcolepsy usually presents with EDS in teen age; a history of typical cataplexy can help the clinical diagnosis. Sometimes cataplexy will not occur until several months to one year later; a polysomnogram with a following MSLT can establish the diagnosis. Childhood RLS and periodic limb movement disorder are usually not difficult to differentiate from OSA, and a thorough clinical history regarding the sleep habits and pattern can help make the diagnosis. For children presenting with hypersomnolence, OSA needs to be ruled out before a diagnosis of idiopathic hypersomnia can be made as the diagnosis of exclusion. If the child has history of brain injury or central nervous system (CNS) infections, posttraumatic hypersomnia may be the diagnosis after OSA is ruled out by a sleep study including MSLT.

CONCLUSIONS

SRBDs are the most common sleep disorders in sleep medicine practice. To recognize each type of the disorders and to differentiate them from each other have a direct impact on patient care and treatment success. A tendency to label everyone with OSA is misleading and should be avoided by taking a thorough clinical history and a physical examination other than being solely dependent on a sleep study. Continued education to improve our understanding about SRBD is important to keep up with the rapidly growing and changing field of sleep medicine.

REFERENCES

1. American Academy of Sleep Medicine. International Classification of Sleep Disorders, 2nd ed. Diagnostic and Coding Manual, Westchester, Illinois: American Academy of Sleep Medicine, 2005.
2. Gastaut H, Tassinari, Duran B. Polygraphic study of the episodic diurnal and nocturnal (hypnic and respiratory) manifestations of the Pickwick syndrome. Brain Res 1966; 1(2):167–186.
3. Young T, Palta M, Dempsey J, et al. The occurrence of sleep-disordered breathing among middle-aged adults. N Engl J Med 1993; 328(17):1230–1235.
4. Rosen CL, Storfer-Isser A, Taylor HG, et al. Increased behavioral morbidity in school-aged children with sleep-disordered breathing. Pediatrics 2004; 114(6):1640–1648.
5. Netzer NC, Hoegel JJ, Loube D, et al. Prevalence of symptoms and risk of sleep apnea in primary care. Chest 2003; 124(4):1406–1414.
6. Guilleminault C, Lee JH. Does benign "primary snoring" ever exist in children? Chest 2004; 126(5): 1396–1398.
7. American Academy of Pediatrics, . Clinical practice guideline: diagnosis and management of childhood obstructive sleep apnea syndrome. Pediatrics 2002; 109(4):704–712.
8. Johns MW. A new method for measuring daytime sleepiness: the Epworth sleepiness scale. Sleep 1991; 14(6):540–545.
9. Johns MW. Reliability and factor analysis of the Epworth Sleepiness Scale. Sleep 1992; 15(4):376–381.
10. Sharafkhaneh A, Hirshkowitz M. Contextual factors and perceived self-reported sleepiness: a preliminary report. Sleep Med 2003; 4(4):327–331.

11. Flemons WW, Whitelaw WA, Brant R, et al. Likelihood ratios for a sleep apnea clinical prediction rule. Am J Respir Crit Care Med 1994; (5);150:1279–1285.
12. Maislin G, Pack AI, Kribbs NB, et al. A Survey screen for prediction of apnea. Sleep 1995; 18(3):158–166.
13. Young T, Shahar E, Nieto FJ, et al. Predictors of sleep-disordered breathing in community-dwelling adults: the Sleep Heart Health Study. Arch Intern Med 2002; 162(8):893–900.
14. Krell SB, Kapur VK. Insomnia complaints in patients evaluated for obstructive sleep apnea. Sleep Breath 2005; 9(3):104–110.
15. Krakow B, Melendrez D, Ferreira E, et al. Prevalence of insomnia symptoms in patients with sleep-disordered breathing. Chest 2001; 120(6):1923–1929.
16. Hajduk IA, Strollo PJ Jr., Jasani RR, et al. Prevalence and predictors of nocturia in obstructive sleep apnea-hypopnea syndrome—a retrospective study. Sleep 2003; 26(1):61–64.
17. Lofaso F, Coste A, d'Ortho MP, et al. Nasal obstruction as a risk factor for sleep apnoea syndrome. Eur Respir J 2000; 16(4):639–643.
18. Rombaux P, Liistro G, Hamoir M, et al. Nasal obstruction and its impact on sleep-related breathing disorders. Rhinology 2005; 43(4):242–250.
19. Canova CR, Downs SH, Knoblauch A, et al. Increased prevalence of perennial allergic rhinitis in patients with obstructive sleep apnea. Respiration 2004; 71(2):138–143.
20. Peppard PE, Young T, Palta M, et al. Longitudinal study of moderate weight change and sleep-disordered breathing. JAMA 2000; 284(23):3015–3021.
21. Guilleminault C, Eldridge FL, Tilkian L, et al. Sleep apnea syndrome due to upper airway obstruction: a review of 25 cases. Arch Intern Med 1977; 137(3)296–300.
22. Mosko S, Zetin M, Glen S, et al. Self-reported depressive symptomatology, mood ratings, and treatment outcome in sleep disorders patients. J Clin Psychol 1989; 45(1):51–60.
23. Ohayan MM. The effects of breathing-related sleep disorders on mood disturbances in the general population. J Clin Psychiatry 2003; 64(10):1195–200; quiz, 1274–1276.
24. Farney RJ, Walker JM, Cloward TV, et al. Sleep-disordered breathing associated with long-term opioid therapy. Chest 2003; 123(2):632–639.
25. Wang D, Teichtahl H, Drummer O, et al. Central sleep apnea in stable methadone maintenance treatment patients. Chest 2005; 128(3):1348–1356.
26. Redline S, Tishler PV, Tosteson TD, et al. The familial aggregation of obstructive sleep apnea. Am J Respir Crit Care Med 1995; 151(3):682–687.
27. Fletcher EC, DeBehnke RD, Lovoi MS, et al. Undiagnosed sleep apnea in patients with essential hypertension. Ann Intern Med 1985; (2):190–195.
28. Hla KM, Young TB, Bidwell T, et al. Sleep apnea and hypertension. A population-based study. Ann Intern Med 1994; 120(5):382–388.
29. Worsnop CJ, Naughton MT, Barter CE, et al. The prevalence of obstructive sleep apnea in hypertensives. Am J Respir Crit Care Med 1998; 157(1):111–115.
30. Lavie P, Herer P, Hoffstein V. Obstructive sleep apnoea syndrome as a risk factor for hypertension: population study. BMJ 2000; 320(7233):479–482.
31. Grote L, Ploch T, Heitmann J, et al. Sleep-related breathing disorder is an independent risk factor for systemic hypertension. Am J Respir Crit Care Med 1999; 160(6):1875–1882.
32. Bixler EO, Vgontzas AN, Lin HM, et al. Association of hypertension and sleep-disordered breathing. Arch Intern Med 2000; 160(15):2289–2295.
33. Peppard PE, Young T, Palta M, et al. Prospective study of the association between sleep-disordered breathing and hypertension. N Engl J Med 2000; 342(19):1378–1384.
34. Nieto FJ, Young TB, Lind BK, et al. Association of sleep-disordered breathing, sleep apnea, and hypertension in a large community-based study. Sleep Heart Health Study. JAMA 2000; 283(14):1829–1836. Erratum in: JAMA 2002; 288(16):1985.
35. Javaheri S, Parker TJ, Liming SD, et al. Sleep apnea in 81 ambulatory male patients with stable heart failure. Types and their prevalences, consequences, and presentations. Circulation 1998; 97(21): 2154–2159.
36. Sin DD, Fitzgerald F, Paker JD, et al. Risk factors for central and obstructive sleep apnea in 450 men and women with congestive heart failure. Am J Respir Crit Care Med 1999; 160(4):1101–1106.
37. Bradley TD, Floras JS. Sleep apnea and heart failure. Part II: central sleep apnea. Circulation 2003; 107 (13):1822–1826.
38. Hanly PJ, Pierratos A. Improvement of sleep apnea in patients with chronic renal failure who undergo nocturnal hemodialysis. N Engl J Med 2001; 344(2):102–107.
39. Venmans BJW, van Kralingen KW, Chandi DD, et al. Sleep complaints and sleep disordered breathing in hemodialysis patients. Neth J Med 1999; 54(5):207–212.
40. Dyken ME, Somers VK, Yamada T, et al. Investigating the relationship between stroke and obstructive sleep apnea. Stroke 1996; 27(3):401–407.
41. Turkington PM, Bamford J, Wanklyn P, et al. Prevalence and predictors of upper airway obstruction in the first 24 hours after acute stroke. Stroke 2002; 33(8):2037–2042.

42. Yaggi HK, Concato J, Kenan WN, et al. Obstructive sleep apnea as a risk factor for stroke and death. N Engl J Med 2005; 353(19):2034–2041.
43. Zonato AI, Martinho FL, Bittencourt LR, et al. Head and neck physical examination: comparison between nonapneic and obstructive sleep apnea patients. Laryngoscope 2005; 115(6):1030–1034.
44. Tsai WH, Remmers JE, Brant R, et al. A decision rule for diagnostic testing in obstructive sleep apnea. Am J Respir Crit Care Med 2003; 167(10):1427–1432.
45. Nuckton TJ, Glidden DV, Brwoner WS, et al. Physical examination: Mallampati score as an independent predictor of obstructive sleep apnea. Sleep 2006; 29(7):903–908.
46. Liistro G, Rombaux P, Belge C, et al. High Mallampati score and nasal obstruction are associated risk factors for obstructive sleep apnoea. Eur Respir J 2003; 21(2):248–252.
47. Schellenberg JB, Maislin G, Schwab RJ. Physical findings and the risk for obstructive sleep apnea. The importance of oropharyngeal structures. Am J Respir Crit Care Med 2000; 162(2):740–748.
48. Kushida CA, Efron B, Guilleminault C. A predictive morphometric model for the obstructive sleep apnea syndrome. Ann Intern Med 1997; 127(8):581–587.
49. Guilleminault C, Huang YS, Glamann C, et al. Adenotonsillectomy and obstructive sleep apnea in children: a prospective survey. Otolaryngol Head Neck Surg 2007; 136(2):169–175.
50. Halbower AC, Ishman SL, McGinley BM. Childhood obstructive sleep-disordered breathing: a clinical update and discussion of technological innovations and challenges. Chest 2007; 132(6):2030–2041.
51. Chessen AL Jr., Berry RB, Pack A. American Academy of Sleep Medicine: Practice parameters for the use of portable monitoring devices in the investigation of suspected obstructive sleep apnea in adults. Sleep 2003; 26(7):907–913.

30 | Positive Airway Pressure Treatment of Sleep-Related Breathing Disorders

Brian Boehlecke

Division of Pulmonary and Critical Care Medicine, University of North Carolina at Chapel Hill, Chapel Hill, North Carolina, U.S.A.

INTRODUCTION

The defining feature of obstructive sleep apnea (OSA) is episodic total or partial upper airway obstruction during sleep. These episodes are usually associated with oxyhemoglobin desaturations of varying severity and brief electroencephalographically defined arousals (microarousals) (1,2). OSA is a risk factor for symptoms of poor quality sleep, e.g., excessive daytime sleepiness and impaired mood, as well as for impaired performance on various neurobehavioral tests, e.g., vigilance tests and simulated driving (3–5). There is also evidence associating OSA with hypertension, insulin resistance, and cardiovascular disease including myocardial infarction and stroke (6–8). Individuals with OSA also appear at increased risk for motor vehicle crashes (9). These consequences are all thought to be related to the sleep disruption and/or the hypoxemia associated with the episodes of upper airway obstruction. Therefore, treatment has focused on methods to reduce or abolish the episodes of upper airway obstruction. When the condition was first recognized, tracheostomy was the only effective means to alleviate this obstruction. However, in 1981 the novel idea of splinting the upper airway open with continuous positive airway pressure (CPAP) was introduced (10). This remains the mainstay of treatment today. When accepted and used regularly by a patient with OSA, CPAP is almost always highly effective in abolishing or dramatically reducing the frequency of upper airway obstructive events and the symptom of excessive daytime sleepiness (11,12). It is less clearly established that this treatment as now applied reliably ameliorates all the other symptoms and morbidity described above (13,14). This may be in part due to a lack of close correspondence between the frequency of sleep-disordered breathing (SDB) events as defined by current criteria (15) and the severity of the physiologic abnormalities underlying the symptoms and morbidity associated with OSA. Reviews have provided detailed discussions of the evidence on effectiveness and some questions that remain unanswered (16,17). This chapter will describe the basis for the use of positive airway pressure (PAP) therapy for OSA and some of the factors that appear to influence the outcomes obtained.

RATIONALE AND MECHANISM OF ACTION

Upper airway luminal cross-sectional area is determined by the net balance of forces tending to narrow the airway (e.g., extraluminal tissue positive pressure and intraluminal negative pressure during inspiration) and those tending to maintain or expand the airway size (e.g., intrinsic airway wall stiffness and contraction of various airway dilator muscles) (18). Patients with OSA appear to maintain airway patency while awake by maintaining increased activity of upper airway dilator muscles compared with that in healthy persons, but this activity decreases during sleep predisposing the airway to narrow or collapse. Anatomic narrowing from enlarged tonsils or tongue, peripharyngeal fat deposition, or facial bony structural characteristics may predispose the airway to collapse at a net pressure, which would maintain patency in the absence of such structural narrowing. By maintaining intraluminal airway pressure above atmospheric pressure at all times during the respiratory cycle, CPAP provides a "pneumatic splint" which opposes the forces tending to narrow the airway. Radiographic and magnetic resonance imaging have demonstrated that intraluminal positive pressure increases upper airway cross-sectional area especially laterally (19,20). This does not appear to be due to stimulation of dilator muscle activity that actually diminishes when positive pressure is applied (21). CPAP also tends to increase lung volume including that at the end of expiration (functional residual capacity), which in turn appears to increase airway size (22). This may in part be due to physical stretching of the upper airway resulting in dilation and/or stiffening of the walls. Since airway collapse in patients with OSA has been shown to occur at the end of expiration (23), maintaining a balance of forces that promotes airway patency is necessary throughout the respiratory cycle. Therefore, when bilevel positive airway pressure (BPAP) is used to lower the average pressure as a means to improve patient comfort and acceptance, the pressure during expiration must be maintained high enough to prevent airway closure prior to the start of inspiration.

APPLIED PHYSICS AND MODES OF POSITIVE AIRWAY PRESSURE DEVICES

Positive pressure is maintained in the upper airway throughout the respiratory cycle by including the upper airway as part of a chamber (CPAP mask-upper airway) that allows egress to ambient air only through a restricted "controlled leak." The CPAP mask usually fits over the nose and seals the face such that air may exit to the room only through a restricted expiratory port. Through a separate large diameter hose the CPAP "blower" supplies airflow into the mask that is at all times greater than the flow out of the chamber including that exiting to the lower airways during inspiration. Therefore during inspiration some of the flow from the blower exits the chamber as the inspiratory airflow into the lower airways while the remainder exits the mask through the expiratory port. During expiration, airflow from the lungs/lower airways and the CPAP "blower" combine to exit the mask through the expiratory port. Maintaining an outward flow from the mask through the restricted expiratory port at all times maintains a positive pressure (i.e., greater than ambient) inside the mask and upper airway throughout the respiratory cycle. During inspiration the CPAP blower must increase its airflow output to compensate for the airflow leaving the mask-upper airway chamber and entering the lower airways and lungs. During expiration the blower can decrease its output since air is also entering the mask-upper airway chamber from the lungs/lower airways. Most currently available CPAP devices can provide a signal that tracks the blower airflow output and thus is proportional to the inspiratory and expiratory airflow generated by the patient's breathing. This V_{est} signal can be displayed and recorded to provide an indirect measure of respiratory airflow while the patient is wearing the CPAP mask. This signal can be used by a sleep technologist to detect total cessation of flow (apnea), reduction in flow (hypopnea), or flattening of the flow profile suggestive of increased upper airway resistance during a therapeutic CPAP titration trial. The signal can also be used in an algorithm that controls adjustments of pressure maintained by an autoadjusting PAP device. Some patients perceive the increased airway pressure during expiration as an unpleasant sensation of difficulty exhaling, which is worse the higher the pressure that is maintained by the CPAP device. This has lead to various methods to try to decrease the pressure during expiration to improve patient tolerance. Bilevel pressure devices provide for separate settings for the pressure maintained during inspiration and during expiration. The device can initiate a change in mask pressure from the prescribed inspiratory level to a lower prescribed expiratory level when the patient's inspiratory flow ceases. Other devices provide partial reductions in mask pressure during a portion of expiration (expiratory pressure relief or C-FLEX®) with the amount of pressure reduction proportional to the rate of the patient's expiratory flow. Mask pressure returns to the single prescribed pressure near the end of expiration.

The continuous airflow from the CPAP blower washes out CO_2 exhaled by the patient into the mask so rebreathing of CO_2 generally does not occur. However, this flow also dilutes any supplemental oxygen supplied into the mask so that the fractional concentration of oxygen inhaled by the patient will be lower for a given supplemental oxygen flow rate when the patient is using a CPAP device than it is for that same oxygen flow rate while the patient is breathing without CPAP (assuming similar overall ventilation). Therefore, to maintain adequate oxyhemoglobin saturation during CPAP use in patients with intrinsic lung disorders requiring supplemental oxygen while awake, oxygen flow rates higher than those used during the daytime may be needed.

Mask upper airway chamber pressure can only be maintained near the desired prescribed pressure if there is limited egress of air from the chamber (i.e., a limited "leak"). Pressure may still be maintained despite some leak from an inadequately sealed mask by an increased airflow from the CPAP blower and currently available CPAP devices include the capacity to sense and compensate for mask leaks. However, if the patient opens his/her mouth while wearing a nasal mask, a very large leak is produced and pressure cannot be maintained. Also, the high airflow produced by the CPAP blower's attempt to compensate for the leak is uncomfortable to the patient and may create a sense of suffocation due to the Venturi effect of flow in the upper airway and out the mouth. Mouth opening during the night while asleep may cause microarousals or frank awakenings and also lead to drying of the nasal and oral mucosa due to the large volume of air passing through. This is especially true if the CPAP blower supplied air is inadequately humidified.

SLEEP LABORATORY TITRATION OF CPAP FOR OSA

Ideally the "optimal" CPAP pressure would abolish all sleep disordered breathing (SDB) events and clinically significant oxyhemoglobin desaturations. However the pressure needed to achieve the complete elimination of all SDB events may not be acceptable to the patient. Also problems with the interface used to deliver the CPAP such as discomfort, persistent irritating air leaks, or a sense of claustrophobia may cause the patient to reject the therapy or use it only intermittently thereby reducing or eliminating the benefit. Therefore the goal of CPAP titration is to try to identify the optimal conditions for the application of CPAP, i.e., a pressure that is effective in reducing the frequency of SDB events to a clinically acceptable level with attention to other factors including the type of interface and other attendant factors such as addition of humidification and/or supplemental oxygen needed to achieve maximal benefits for the patient.

A patient's initial experience with CPAP has been shown to be a major determinant of acceptance or rejection of the treatment and the adherence to long-term use (24). Identifying the best interface and adjusting it appropriately to minimize discomfort and leaks during titration is critical. No one type of interface has proven to be ideal for all patients. If an adequate seal cannot be achieved with the standard nasal masks available, nasal pillows or one of the oxygen cannula-like nasal interfaces should be tried. A crossover study found that a nasal interface is associated with fewer adverse effects and better sleep quality during the first 3 weeks of therapy (25). However, individual preference is still a key factor in choice of interface. For patients who cannot maintain mouth closure, a full-face mask is effective in maintaining CPAP pressure whereas other means such as chin straps and mouth guards are less so. However, acceptance of a full-face mask is lower possibly due to the added bulk and increased potential for causing claustrophobia (26). A device to deliver CPAP orally has been found to be efficacious, but acceptance was limited by upper airway drying or "rain out" of moisture in the tubing if heated humidification was used (27).

The factors that predict long-term clinical improvement on CPAP are not fully understood. Apnea-hypopnea index (AHI) severity and microarousals were not correlated with subjective improvement on CPAP as measured by the Stanford Sleepiness Scale and the Medical Outcomes Study Short Form-36 (SF-36) quality-of-life score or an objective measure of sleepiness (maintenance of wakefulness test (MWT)) (28). Therefore, elimination of all SDB events may not be necessary to produce a clinically acceptable benefit. However, improvement in these measures did correlate with the number of 4% desaturations and minimum SpO_2 on the diagnostic study suggesting that severity of hypoxemic events is an important factor in determining the clinical impact of SDB. Other studies have indicated that patient acceptance may not be determined by the absolute reduction in SDB event-associated arousals, but by the overall improvement in sleep quality on CPAP. This in turn may be strongly influenced by factors affecting tolerance of the CPAP itself and improvement in physiologic variables not reflected in the AHI alone. Whittle and coworkers (29) found that the increase in N3 sleep (formerly slow wave sleep (SWS)) but not the number of respiratory events or arousals correlated with the subsequent use and subjective sleepiness on CPAP. However, a controlled trial did not show an increase in SWS on CPAP compared with placebo level CPAP after 2 weeks of treatment (30). Therefore, the effect of CPAP on sleep quality as manifest by the amount of SWS may not be an important factor. Drake and coworkers (31) found that an increase in sleep efficiency (SE) during CPAP titration compared with the diagnostic night was the only significant predictor of objectively measured adherence with CPAP after controlling for indices of severity of SDB and sleep quality during the diagnostic night. Patients whose SE increased used their machines an average of two hours more per night than those without an increase in SE. Thus, factors that affect sleep quality while using CPAP in addition to the frequency of SDB events are likely to be important in determining its overall effectiveness.

Drying of the upper airway is a significant side effect of CPAP and can lead to intermittent use or discontinuation. It is reported by up to 70% of users (32). Heated humidification has been shown to reduce subjective complaints of dryness and to improve the refreshing quality of sleep on CPAP (33). It has thus been advocated for use during all CPAP titrations (34). However, patients reported no significant improvement in subjective quality of sleep with heated humidification and did not clearly indicate a preference for it (35). Use of heated humidification is clearly indicated for patients with prior complaints of nasal dryness and those who experience unacceptable drying with standard humidifiers, but depending on cost considerations, may not be necessary for all patients.

Despite the lack of perfect correlation between reduction of currently used objective measures of the severity of SDB (the AHI and the frequency/severity of desaturations) on effective CPAP pressure and subjective improvement, reduction of the AHI to less than 15 and abolishment of desaturations below 88% is a desirable goal for titration. It is likely that achieving this level of therapeutic response will produce significant improvement in daytime sleepiness and reduce the risk of cardiovascular disease in patients with moderate-to-severe OSA. Early studies showed that effective CPAP pressure was related to the AHI and the patient's body mass index (BMI) and neck circumference. These findings suggested that effective CPAP pressure would be determined by the severity of OSA as mediated through factors related to obesity. However, others have found no relation between baseline AHI and effective CPAP pressure but have noted an association with oral or craniofacial structural characteristics (36). Interestingly, the mean SpO_2 was found to be the best predictor of CPAP pressure needed in these studies.

If sleep quality on CPAP is likely a major factor in both patient acceptance, adherence to treatment, and clinical improvement in symptoms, titration to eliminate arousals that are not associated with respiratory events scorable as apneas or hypopneas by current American Academy of Sleep Medicine (AASM) criteria (15) may be useful. When nasal pressure cannulae are used to identify respiratory events a spectrum of electroencephalographic (EEG) changes are noted to be associated with the termination of respiratory events (37). Lack of understanding of the clinical consequences of these various EEG findings may partly explain the poor correlation of the reduction in the AHI as a measure of success in CPAP titration and the clinical improvement or adherence with treatment. Of note was that titration to eliminate flow limitation indicated by flattening of the CPAP airflow profile resulted in increased subsequent home use (7.3 hours vs. 6.0 hours per night) compared with titration to an endpoint of elimination of only overt apneas and hypopneas (38).

Patient acceptance and adherence to CPAP treatment is also strongly influenced by psychosocial factors including patient understanding of the condition, their perception of the health consequences, and cognitive constructs such as locus of control and self-efficacy (32). Including psychosocial variables in the model produces the best multivariate prediction of adherence. A systematic educational program for patients appears to increase utilization (39). It is important to set reasonable expectations for the beneficial effects as well as possible adverse effects of CPAP, to pay careful attention to mask fitting and acclimatization before starting the trial, and to be sensitive and attentive to individual patient circumstances during the titration. As stated by Engleman, "...the emphasis is shifted from the numeric value to the patient's perceptions of these values" as the most important factor for a successful titration outcome (32). Increased frequency of contact with health care providers also improves adherence (40) but a study found access to computerized answers to frequently asked questions and guidelines for managing problems resulted in equivalent use and functional status at 30 days to that resulting from greater access to the care provider (41).

Optimal pressure for reduction in SDB events will also vary with attendant circumstances such as patient sleeping position, use of respiratory depressant medications, herbals or alcohol, and presence and severity of nasal obstruction. Even with seemingly unchanged clinical conditions a difference of −2 to +3 cm water between pressures thought to be "optimal" by the monitoring technician was noted on two successive night titrations (42). Thus, too much attention to achieving an ideal pressure from the perspective of reduction in AHI while overlooking other factors influencing patient comfort and acceptance may be counter productive.

The use of autoadjusting CPAP machines makes continuously adjusted pressures during in-laboratory titrations and unattended home titrations possible. Both of these situations offer theoretical and potential practical advantages over the traditional titration by a sleep laboratory technologist. A study (43) compared three methods of initiating and maintaining CPAP treatment for patients with moderate to severe OSA: (1) autotitration pressure throughout, (2) autotitration pressure for one week followed by a fixed pressure (95th percentile) thereafter and, (3) fixed pressure determined by an algorithm based on neck size and frequency of 4% oxyhemoglobin desaturations. All three groups showed similar large improvements in subjective daytime sleepiness reported on the Epworth Sleepiness Scale (ESS) and increased ability to stay awake on the MWT after 6 months of treatment. The authors concluded that the method of determining CPAP pressure makes no significant difference to clinical outcome. Interestingly although not statistically significant, the patients on autotitration for the entire period averaged 5.49 hours use per night, those on a fixed pressure after one week averaged 4.9 hours, and those on an algorithm derived pressure averaged only four hours nightly use. This suggests that autotitration may be slightly better tolerated than fixed pressure. However it also indicates that nightly use longer than four hours was not associated with a detectable additional beneficial effect on subjective or objective sleepiness.

A study compared OSA patients' subjective evaluations of three different autoadjusting positive pressure devices used in random order for four-week periods (44). All patients had been on a fixed CPAP pressure for at least three years. Only approximately half of the patients preferred an autoadjusting device over fixed CPAP. Of note, there was a significant difference in subjective comfort and usage rate between the three devices with one of them being used on only 59% of trial nights for an average of five hours while the other two were used 96% to 100% of nights for an average of 6.8–7.1 hours. Despite these differences in use there were no differences between the quality of life (QOL) scores on the SF-36 questionnaire or sleepiness scores on the ESS reported by patients while using the three devices nor were the scores different from those while on fixed CPAP. Acceptance and use of an autoadjusting CPAP device initiated at home in patients suspected of having OSA has been suggested as a diagnostic test for OSA (45). Only one patient out of 36 who agreed to continue using the device after a two-week trial and who had used it for at least two hours per night during the trial did not have OSA later confirmed by polysomnography (PSG) (false positive rate of 5%). However, patients were excluded from the trial if they had any diagnosis, which might explain "some of the symptoms" they reported. Also, there was a false negative rate of 23% (9 of 40). Interestingly, in blinded efficacy trails of CPAP in patients with OSA using "sham CPAP" control arms, patient acceptance, and usage of the sham CPAP set at subtherapeutic pressure levels was equivalent to that for the effective level of CPAP (13,30). Thus, patient acceptance and usage are not established as valid criteria to determine the presence or absence of clinically significant OSA. Providing a therapeutic CPAP device to patients without directly establishing the presence of clinically significant SDB is not justified at the present time (46).

Unattended autoadjusting device titration without EEG monitoring cannot distinguish respiratory events occurring while the patient is awake (e.g., apneas following swallowing) nor can the current equipment distinguish central from obstructive respiratory events. While central apneas (CAs) can be associated with arousals and thus produce similar sleep-related symptoms to those resulting from obstructive events, increases in CPAP pressure in response to CAs may in some instances increase their frequency or severity and can worsen the arousals. If the titration is unattended, whether arousals are associated with SDB events is not determined so this aspect of the clinical impact of the SDB cannot be factored into the clinical decision on the need for CPAP or the optimal pressure. Some risks of adverse effects of autotitration including arrhythmias have been reported (47). Practice parameters for use of autotitrating devices have been issued by the AASM (48). Autotitration is not recommended for patients with congestive heart failure (CHF), significant lung disease such as chronic obstructive pulmonary disease (COPD), daytime hypoxemia, and respiratory failure from any cause, or prominent nocturnal desaturations other than from OSA (e.g., obesity hypoventilation syndrome). A review of the literature by this author found that the agreement between the AHI measured by the diagnostic mode of the autotitrating machines versus that from standard scoring of the PSG was often not good. The limits of agreement in optimum pressure (a measure roughly equivalent to a determination of the 95% confidence limits for the difference between the two measures) was as high as -20.7 to $+24.6$ cm water in one study and usually ranged from -10 to -15 for the lower limit to $+10$ to $+18$ for the upper limit in the others. A direct comparison of two autotitrating machines (49) found that the limits of agreement for therapeutic pressure were -3 to $+9$ cm water. There was no correlation of the magnitude of the difference with patient demographic characteristics, indices of severity of OSA or lung function, so there was no basis for selection of a subset of patients for whom agreement would have been better.

One study reported good results with patient self-titration at home using a starting pressure from a prediction formula (50). The limits of agreement for optimal pressure between the self-titration and laboratory titration were -3 to $+4$ cm water. There was no significant difference during the five-week trial periods between use of the self-titration optimal pressure and the one determined in the laboratory on measures of QOL or reported sleepiness. However, all patients had had the laboratory titration before starting home CPAP. Also all patients had 30 minutes of education from the technologist and a call from a research assistant during each arm of the study. At least four hours of use was achieved in the two arms in 86 and 87% of patients indicating an unusually high rate of adherence likely resulting from these interventions. Thus, the efficacy of this method in less supportive situations is not established. Others have developed algorithms to estimate the CPAP pressure needed based on the AHI and neck circumference (51,52). The difference between a reference pressure based on an average over 28 nights on an autotitrating device and one derived from the algorithm was similar to that between the reference pressure and one determined by a single-night titration (53). There was no difference on ESS scores or nightly hours of use after 11 months between patients initiated on CPAP after an in-laboratory titration and those treated using an algorithm derived pressure, but the assignment of patients was not random. A study using a portable monitoring device in the home found 17% of 101 patients with OSA had an AHI > 10/hr while using CPAP at the pressure prescribed from a laboratory titration trial three months previously (54). Those who were obese and had a high AHI at diagnosis were more likely to have the persistently elevated AHI on CPAP. Interestingly a greater percentage of those with a persistently elevated AHI compared with those without this finding had had a mask "problem" noted by the technologist during the laboratory study (47% vs. 14%, $p < 0.004$). Also there was no difference in reported mood, QOL, or ESS scores between those with and without persistently elevated AHI suggesting an equivalent clinical response in both groups. Thus, achieving an "optimal" CPAP pressure during a titration may not be critical for determining a pressure that will produce an acceptable therapeutic response. Adequate attention to mask fit and comfort during a CPAP titration is important to obtaining an adequate therapeutic pressure.

In-laboratory titration currently provides the best environment for a good initial experience with CPAP as well as for establishing the "optimal" CPAP pressure. The technologist can detect and fix interface leaks, change interfaces, and add heated humidification to maximize patient comfort and acceptance. They can switch to bilevel pressure machines if needed for patent tolerance. Also they can detect oxyhemoglobin desaturations and arousals occurring without associated "scorable" disordered breathing events and adjust the PAP and/or add supplemental oxygen as needed to eliminate arousals and maintain acceptable levels of saturation. Finally and perhaps most importantly the technologist can correct patient misapprehensions about the CPAP titration and provide reassurance and encouragement during this initial experience with the device. This support may prove to be a critical factor in determining patients' initial acceptance or rejection of PAP and their willingness to persevere and adhere to therapy during the initial home acclimatization period.

SPLIT-NIGHT TITRATIONS

Because of limited sleep laboratory availability and the cost of a second full night for PAP titration, many facilities attempt to establish the diagnosis and severity of OSA in the first portion of the night and then perform a PAP titration during the latter portion, i.e., a split-night

(SN) study. Guidelines for use of this method have been published by the AASM (55). The Academy recognizes that the SN study is usually adequate but indicates that full-night attended PSG is still considered the preferred approach (34). Studies have compared the CPAP pressures established as adequate for treatment after a SN study with those after a full-night titration and the clinical outcomes of patients treated with the pressures so obtained (56). Pressures determined from SN studies are usually similar to those from full-night studies but may be lower for patients with mild to moderate OSA who may not manifest the maximal severity of their condition during the first portion of the night. Clinical outcomes assessed at approximately two years after initiation of treatment showed no difference between those prescribed CPAP from a SN titration and those prescribed from a full-night titration (57). Also in the study of the adequacy of prescribed CPAP pressure at 3 months (54), a persistent AHI > 10 was no more common in those who had had their CPAP pressure determined from a SN study than in those whose pressure was determined from a full-night study.

AASM Criteria for utilizing a CPAP titration after a partial night diagnostic study include the following: (*i*) An AHI > 40/hr or 20–40/hr if clinically warranted due to severe oxyhemoglobin desaturations or repetitive long obstructions. (*ii*) A minimum of two hours of diagnostic PSG (note current Medicare guidelines require 2 hours of recorded sleep but CMS has proposed to eliminate this requirement). (*iii*) CPAP titration carried out for more than three hours. (*iv*) CPAP is documented to eliminate or nearly eliminate respiratory events during both rapid eye movement (REM) and non-REM (NREM) sleep including when the patient is supine. If these criteria are not met, the AASM recommends that a full-night titration be done.

ACCEPTANCE AND ADHERENCE TO PAP TREATMENT

Although PAP is efficacious for reducing the frequency of SDB events to within or near the normal range in most patients with OSA, the limiting factor for effectiveness is patients' acceptance and adherence to its use. Reported acceptance rates vary widely with maximal values approximately 75% to 80% (58,59). Continued use for at least four hours per night for at least five nights per week has been found to be present in less than 50% (60). Objective measures of use from CPAP device recordings of time with power on or time at prescribed mask pressure show that many patients significantly over-report usage. Somewhat surprisingly severity of OSA as measured by AHI is not the major determinant of use. Those with more severe OSA by AHI do have a tendency toward higher acceptance and usage with the severity of the symptom of daytime sleepiness being an important factor (61). The patient's perception of the risk to his/her well-being posed by the OSA and the patient's own decision (rather than a family member's or partner's) to seek treatment are also important. Use in the first week of treatment is predictive of longer-term use (24) so it is important to attend promptly to any unwanted side effects that may reduce initial tolerability. High pressure may cause discomfort for some patients but evidence is lacking that use of bilevel pressure or autotitrating devices significantly increase adherence (34). A small study suggested that a type of expiratory pressure relief (C-FLEX®) may increase adherence over three months compared with standard CPAP (62) but more evidence is needed to substantiate this. Although the evidence is mixed, adherence does not appear to be diminished by pressure determination from a SN versus a full-night titration (63).

SIDE EFFECTS

There are numerous side effects that may compromise patient adherence to treatment, but fortunately most are relatively minor and if detected promptly can be managed effectively thereby preventing the patient from discontinuing CPAP. Common problems associated with the interface are mask leak and discomfort from pressure points. These can usually be remedied by checking that the mask is of the correct size and has been fitted properly including proper headgear adjustment. If this does not remedy the problem, changing to another style mask or an intranasal interface (nasal pillows or other type) may be necessary. Claustrophobia may also be managed by switching to an intranasal interface. Rhinitis and/or rhinorrhea are common especially in those with preexisting allergic rhinitis. Intranasal steroids or antihistamine sprays are helpful and intranasal ipratropium bromide spray may reduce rhinorrhea if that is the predominant feature. Heated humidification is often helpful in reducing nasal drying, which may be the cause of the rhinitis. Although higher pressures may sometimes cause rhinitis, the author's experience has not shown reduction in pressure to be effective treatment in most instances even when possible without adversely affecting control of the SDB. Mouth leak is another common problem and this may respond to a chin strap or to a reduction in pressure. This problem seems especially difficult in patients with prior upper airway surgery, e.g., uvulopalatopharyngoplasty, perhaps due to compromise of the ability of the soft palate to seal against the tongue and reduce transmission of the nasal pressure to the mouth. When intractable mouth leak is present use of a full face mask covering the mouth obviates the problem. Oral interfaces have been developed but adherence does not seem to be improved over more conventional interfaces (64).

BENEFITS OF TREATMENT/INDICATIONS FOR TREATMENT

Numerous studies have shown that PAP treatment improves subjective sleepiness in patients with severe OSA (11,12,16). Evidence for an effect on objective measures of sleepiness (multiple sleep latency test [MSLT] and/or MWT) that differs from that on placebo or conservative treatment is less robust. Self-reported QOL using the SF-36 and/or the Functional Outcomes of Sleep Questionnaire also improves on PAP treatment in patients with severe OSA. However, other aspects of neurobehavioral performance and psychologic status such as cognitive processing, executive functioning and mood do not consistently show changes different from those observed on placebo or conservative therapy (65). Individual suscepti- bility to impairment of performance associated with sleep loss/disruption appears to vary significantly perhaps explaining why some individuals may manifest impairment with only slight residual sleep disturbance while on therapy (66). Also changes in the central nervous system that develop over many years as a consequence of OSA may be reversible only slowly if at all and thus may not show improvement in studies of relatively short duration. On the other hand, a large beneficial effect of CPAP on performance on a driving simulator may be evident after only a few days of treatment (67). There is also good evidence that actual driving performance of persons with OSA improves such that the risk of motor vehicle crashes decreases on therapy compared with that prior to therapy (68).

An important potential benefit of PAP therapy is a reduction of the long-term risk of cardiovascular morbidity and mortality, which appears to be associated with OSA (69). PAP therapy may contribute to the reduction in several risk factors for cardiovascular disease. Several studies show reestablishment of the normal pattern of nocturnal "dipping" of blood pressure and/or improvement in daytime blood pressure after initiation of PAP pressure (70–72). Treatment effects appear most likely in those with severe OSA and uncontrolled hypertension and are less likely in persons with mild to moderate OSA, especially those who do not report excessive sleepiness (73,74). PAP therapy has also been shown to improve many of the physiologic and biochemical abnormalities associated with long-term risk of cardiovascular morbidity and mortality including increased sympathetic nervous system activation, endothelial dysfunction, increased levels of C-reactive protein, and glucose intolerance (75). Substantial direct evidence that PAP treatment of OSA reduces fatal and/or nonfatal cardiac events was lacking until recently. Marin et al. (76) followed men (264 healthy, 377 snorers without OSA [AHI < 5], 403 with untreated mild-moderate OSA [AHI 5–30] without severe daytime sleepiness), 235 with untreated severe OSA (AHI > 30 or 5–30 with severe daytime sleepiness), and 372 with severe OSA treated with CPAP for a mean of 10.1 years. Fatal and nonfatal cardiac event rates per 100 person years were both significantly higher in those with untreated severe OSA than those in the healthy men (1.05 vs. 0.3, $p < 0.0001$ and 2.13 vs. 0.45, $p < 0.0001$, respectively). However, rates for those with severe OSA treated with CPAP were not different from those of the healthy men (0.35 and 0.64, respectively). Rates for 52 men with severe OSA started on CPAP but using it < four hours per night at three months and so switched to alternate therapies including various surgical procedures ($n = 33$) or no specific treatment ($n = 11$) had rates of fatal and nonfatal events not different from those without treatment (0.9 and 1.9, respectively). Interestingly, the rates for the snorers and the untreated mild-moderate OSA groups were not significantly different from those of the healthy men. Although not from a randomly assigned blinded treatment study, these results provide substantial direct evidence that risk of cardiovascular events is increased in those with severe OSA and decreased in that group if they are able to adhere to CPAP therapy for at least four hours per night.

Because the underlying pathophysiologic mechanisms may differ among the various clinical impairments associated with OSA use of a single index such as the AHI to assess severity and/or adequacy of CPAP therapy may not be valid. Vascular conditions associated with OSA such as hypertension may be more closely related to bursts of sympathetic activation and arousals associated with disordered breathing events while metabolic abnormalities such as insulin resistance may be more closely related to hypoxic stress from periodic oxyhemoglobin desaturations (77). Some neurobehavioral impairments may also be related to hypoxemia whereas sleepiness appears more related to sleep disruption and even one night without CPAP increases self-perceived sleepiness in patients with OSA (78). One night of recovery sleep on CPAP improved subjective and objective sleepiness after seven days off CPAP. Supplemental oxygen therapy can ameliorate desaturations in patients with OSA but does not improve sleep architecture whereas CPAP does, including decreased sleep stage shifts and increased REM sleep (30).

The findings cited above support the prescription of PAP to all patients with severe OSA, i.e., an AHI > 30 with a vigorous effort by the health care provider to facilitate tolerance and adherence, especially for those with excessive daytime sleepiness, and/or additional cardiovascular risk factors. It is also usually indicated for those with moderate OSA (AHI 15–30) with symptoms of excessive daytime somnolence. Clinical judgment must be used for those without reported excessive daytime sleepiness but other conditions or risk factors, which may be exacerbated by untreated OSA. This judgment many partially depend on the patient's perception of risk and motivation for adherence to treatment. A patient should not be denied a trial of CPAP if clinically indicated solely based concerns by the physician about the patient's likely adherence to treatment. On the other hand, for patients with this level of severity of OSA, vigorous pursuit of alternate modes of therapy for OSA and optimization of other therapies for potentially related conditions (e.g., antihypertensives) may be the most beneficial therapeutic strategy if the patient is unwilling or unable to adhere to an effective pressure level and usage rate of PAP therapy.

A cost-effectiveness analysis (79) based on the impact of CPAP treatment of moderate to severe OSA on motor vehicle crashes indicated that treatment is cost effective with an incremental cost-effectiveness ratio (ICER), the incremental cost per unit increment in quality-adjusted life-years, of only $314 from a societal perspective, which considers indirect costs (e.g., lost productivity and insurance administrative costs) as well as direct medical costs. Even when only direct medical costs are considered, the ICER is $3354, which compares very favorably with other preventive therapies in common use and publicly funded. Persons with only mild OSA (AHI 5–15) without excessive sleepiness may often be treated most effectively with alterative therapies, but until results of controlled long-term outcome studies are available, evidence for this approach is lacking. Current AASM Practice Parameters (34) recommends CPAP as an option for these patients.

CONCLUSIONS

PAP is an efficacious treatment for moderate to severe OSA, which quickly improves the symptoms associated with sleep disruption and reduces the risk of motor vehicle crashes in patients who adhere to therapy. A reduction in long-term risk of cardiovascular morbidity associated with OSA may also occur, especially in those with additional risk factors. Acceptance and adherence limit its overall effectiveness but patient education programs and prompt attention by the health care provider to medically minor but annoying side effects can improve patient tolerance. Despite the minor nature of most side effects this therapy should only be applied to those for whom a diagnosis has been established by a sleep study using validated methodology. Benefits to those with milder disease are less certain and may vary partly due to imprecision of the currently used measures of severity and to individual differences in susceptibility to sleep disruption. Therefore clinical judgment of a health care provider experienced in treating patients with SDB should still be the determining factor in applying this treatment.

REFERENCES

1. Olson EJ, Moore WR, Morganthaler TI, et al. Obstructive sleep apnea-hypopnea syndrome. Mayo Clin Proc 2003; 78(12):1545–1552.
2. White DP. Sleep apnea. Proc Am Thorac Soc 2006; 3:124–128.
3. Chugh DK, Dinges DF. Mechanisms of sleepiness in obstructive sleep apnea. In: Pack AI, ed. Sleep Apnea: Pathogenesis, Diagnosis and Treatment, Lung Biology in Health and Disease. New York: Marcel Dekker, 2002:265–285.
4. Mazza S, Pepin JL, Naegele B, et al. Most obstructive sleep apnoea patients exhibit vigilance and attention deficits on an extended battery of test. Eur Respir J 2005; 25:75–80.
5. Turkington P, Sircar M, Allgar V, et al. Relationship between obstructive sleep apnoea, driving simulator performance, and risk of road traffic accidents. Thorax 2001; 56:800–805.
6. Robinson GV, Stradling JR, Davies RJO. Sleep 6: obstructive sleep apnoea/hypopnoea syndrome and hypertension. Thorax 2004; 59:1089–1094.
7. Ip MSM, Lam B, Ng MMT, et al. Obstructive sleep apnea is independently associated with insulin resistance. Am J Respir Crit Care Med 2002; 165(5):670–676.
8. Lavie P. Pro: sleep apnea causes cardiovascular disease. Am J Respir Crit Care Med 2004; 169(2):148–149.
9. George CFP. Sleep 5: driving and automobile crashes in patients with obstructive sleep apnoea/hypopnoea syndrome. Thorax 2004; 59:804–807.
10. Sullivan CE, Issa FG, Berthon-Jones M, et al. Reversal of obstructive sleep apnoea by continuous positive airway pressure applied through the nares. Lancet 1981; 1:862–865.
11. Patel SR, White DP, Malhotra A, et al. Continuous positive airway pressure therapy for treating sleepiness in a diverse population with obstructive sleep apnea. Results of a meta-analysis. Arch Intern Med 2003; 163:565–571.
12. Marshall NS, Barnes M, Travier N, et al. Continuous positive airway pressure reduces daytime sleepiness in mild to moderate obstructive sleep apnoea: a meta-analysis. Thorax 2006; 61:430–434.
13. Marshall NS, Neill AM, Campbell AJ, et al. Randomised controlled crossover trial of humidified continuous positive airway pressure in mild obstructive sleep apnoea. Thorax 2005; 60:427–432.
14. Monasterio C, Vidal S, Duran J, et al. Effectiveness of continuous positive airway pressure in mild sleep apnea-hypopnea syndrome. Am J Respir Crit Care Med 2001; 164:939–943.
15. American Academy of Sleep Medicine. Sleep-related breathing disorders in adults: recommendations for syndrome definition and measurement techniques in clinical research. The Report of an American Academy of Sleep Medicine Task Force. Sleep 1999; 22:667–689.
16. Gay P, Weaver T, Loube D, et al. Evaluation of positive airway pressure treatment for sleep related breathing disorders in adults. Sleep 2006; 29(3):381–401.
17. Giles TL, Lasserson TJ, Smith BJ, et al. Continuous positive airways pressure for obstructive sleep apnoea in adults. The Cochrane Database of Systematic Reviews 2006, Issue 1, Art. No.: CD001106. pub2. DOI:10.1002/14651858. CD001106.pub2.
18. White DP. Sleep apnea. Proc Am Thorac Soc 2006; 3:124–128.
19. Abbey NC, Block AJ, Green D, et al. Measurement of pharyngeal volume by digitized magnetic resonance imaging. Effect of nasal continuous positive airway pressure. Am Rev Respir Dis 1989; 140:717–723.
20. Schwab RJ, Pack AI, Gupta KB, et al. Upper airway and soft tissue structural changes influences by CPAP in normal subjects. Am J Respir Crit Care Med 1996; 154:1106–1116.
21. Alex CG, Aronson RM, Onal E, et al. Effects of continuous positive airway pressure on upper airway and respiratory muscle activity. J Appl Physiol 1987; 62:2026–2030.
22. Hoffstein V, Zamel N, Phillipson EA. Lung volume dependence of cross-sectional area in patients with obstructive sleep apnea. Am Rev Respir Dis 1984; 130:175–178.
23. Schwab RJ, Gefter WB, Hoffman EA, et al. Dynamic upper airway imaging during awake respiration in normal subjects and patients with sleep disordered breathing. Am Rev Respir Dis 1993; 148:1385–1400.
24. Weaver TE, Kribbs NB, Pack AI, et al. Night-to-night variability in CPAP use over the first three months of treatment. Sleep 1997; 20:278–283.
25. Massie CA, Hart RW. Clinical outcomes related to interface type in patients with obstructive sleep apnea/hypopneas syndrome who are using continuous positive airway pressure. Chest 2003; 123(4):1112–1118.
26. Mortimer IL, Whittle AT, Douglas AJ. Comparison of nose and face mask CPAP therapy for sleep apnea. Thorax 1998; 53:290–292.
27. Beecroft J, Zanon S, Lukie D, et al. Oral continuous positive airway pressure for sleep apnea. Effectiveness, patient preference, and adherence. Chest 2003; 124:2200–2208.
28. Kingshott RN, Vennell M, Hoy C, et al. Predictors of improvement in daytime function outcome with CPAP therapy. Am J Respir Crit Care Med 2000; 161:866–871.
29. Whittle AT, Douglas NJ. Does the physiological success of CPAP titration predict clinical success? J Sleep Res 2000; 9(2):201–206.

30. Loredo JS, Ancoli-Israel S, Kim EJ, et al. Effect of continuous positive airway pressure versus supplemental oxygen on sleep quality in obstructive sleep apnea: a placebo-CPAP-controlled study. Sleep 2006; 29(4):564–571.
31. Drake CL, Day R, Hudgel D, et al. Sleep during titration predicts continuous positive airway pressure compliance. Sleep 2003; 26(3):308–311.
32. Engleman HM, Wild MR. Improving CPAP use by patients with the sleep apnoea/hypopneas syndrome (SAHS). Sleep Med Rev 2003; 7(1):81–99.
33. Massie CA, Hart RW, Peralez K, et al. Effects of humidification on nasal symptoms and compliance in sleep apnea patients using continuous positive airway pressure. Chest 1999; 116:403–408.
34. Kushida CA, Littner MR, Hirshkowitz M, et al. Practice parameters for the use of continuous and bilevel positive airway pressure devices to treat adult patients with sleep-related breathing disorders. Sleep 2006; 29(3):375–380.
35. Wiest GH, Harsch IA, Fuchs FS, et al. Initiation of CPAP therapy for OSA: does prophylactic humidification during CPAP pressure titration improved initial patient acceptance and comfort? Respiration 2002; 69(5):406–412.
36. Akashiba T, Kosaka N, Yamamoto H, et al. Optimal continuous positive airway pressure in patients with obstructive sleep apnoea: role of craniofacial structure. Respir Med 2001; 95:393–397.
37. Thomas RJ. Arousals in sleep-disordered breathing: patterns and implications. Sleep 2003; 26(8): 1042–1047.
38. Meurice JC, Paquereau J, Denjean A, et al. Influence of correction of flow limitation on continuous positive airway pressure efficiency in sleep apnoea/hypopnoea syndrome. Eur Respir J 1998; 11(5): 1121–1127.
39. Hoy CJ, Vennelle M, Kingshott RN, et al. Can intensive support improve continuous positive airway pressure use in patients with the sleep apnea/hypopnea syndrome? Am J Respir Crit Care Med. 1999; 159(4 pt 1):1096–1100.
40. Palmer S, Selvaraj S, Dunn C, et al. Annual review of patients with sleep apnea/hypopnea syndrome—a pragmatic randomised trial of nurse home visit versus consultant clinic review. Sleep Med 2004; 5(1):61–65.
41. Taylor Y, Eliasson A, Andrada T, et al. The role of telemedicine in CPAP compliance for patients with obstructive sleep apnea syndrome. Sleep Breath 2006; Epub March 28, 2006; DOI: 10.1007/sll325-006-0059-9. Accessed 8/23/06.
42. Wiest GH, Fuchs FS, Harsch IA, et al. Reproducibility of a standardized titration procedure for the initiation of continuous positive airway pressure therapy in patients with obstructive sleep apnoea. Respiration 2001; 68(2):145–150.
43. West SD, Jones DR, Stradling JR. Comparison of three ways to determine and deliver pressure during nasal CPAP therapy for obstructive sleep apnoea. Thorax 2006; 61:226–231.
44. Nolan GM, Ryan S, O'Connor TM, et al. Comparison of three auto-adjusting positive pressure devices in patients with sleep apnoea. Eur Respir J 2006; 28:159–164.
45. Senn O, Brack T, Russi EW, et al. A continuous positive airway pressure trial as a novel approach to the diagnosis of the obstructive sleep apnea syndrome. Chest 2006; 129:67–75.
46. Collop NA. Blue light special on CPAP, aisle 11. Chest 2006; 129:6–7.
47. Juhasz J, Schillen J, Ubrigkeit A, et al. Unattended continuous positive airway pressure titration. Clinical relevance and cardiorespiratory hazards of the method. Am J Respir Crit Care Med 1996; 154:359–365.
48. Littner M, Hirshkowitz M, Davila D, et al. Practice parameters for the use of auto-titrating continuous positive airway pressure devices for titrating pressures and treating adult patients with obstructive sleep apnea syndrome. Sleep 2002; 25(2):143–147.
49. Kessler R, Weitzenblum E, Chaouat A, et al. Evaluation of unattended automated titration to determine therapeutic continuous positive airway pressure in patients with obstructive sleep apnea. Chest 2003; 123:704–710.
50. Fitzpatrick MF, Alloway CE, Wakeford TM, et al. Can patients with obstructive sleep apnea titrate their own continuous positive airway pressure? Am J Respir Crit Care Med 203; 167(5):716–722.
51. Hoffstein V, Mateika S. Predicting nasal continuous positive airway pressure. Am J Respir Crit Care Med 1994; 150:486–488.
52. Stradling JR, Hardinge M, Smith DM. A novel, simplified approach to starting nasal CPAP therapy in OSA. Respir Med 2004, 98(2):155–158.
53. Stradling JR, Hardinge M, Paxton J, et al. Relative accuracy of algorithm-based prescription of nasal CPAP in OSA. Respir Med 2004; 98(2):152–154.
54. Baltzan MA, Kassissia I, Elkholi O, et al. Prevalence of persistent sleep apnea in patients treated with continuous positive airway pressure. Sleep 2006; 29(4):557–563.
55. American Sleep Disorders Standard of Practice Committee, Chesson A. Practice parameters for the indications for polysomnography and related procedures. Sleep 1997; 20:406–422.

56. Sanders MH, Kern NB, Costantino JP, et al. Adequacy of prescribing positive airway pressure therapy by mask for sleep apnea on the basis of a partial-night trial. Am Rev Respir Dis 1993; 147:1169–1174.
57. McArdle N, Grove A, Devereux G, et al. Split-night versus full-night studies for sleep apnoea/hypopnoea syndrome. Eur Respir J 2000; 15:670–675.
58. Rauscher H, Popp W, Wonke T, et al. Acceptance of CPAP therapy for sleep apnea. Chest 1991; 100: 1019–1023.
59. Meurice JC, Dore P, Paquereou J, et al. Predictive factors of long-term compliance with nasal continuous positive airway pressure treatment in sleep apnea syndrome. Chest 1994; 105:429–433.
60. Kribbs NB, Pack AI, Kline LR, et al. Objective measurement of patterns of nasal CPAP use by patients with obstructive sleep apnea. Am Rev Respir Dis 1993; 147:887–895.
61. McArdle N, Devereux G, Heidomejad H, et al. Long-term use of CPAP therapy for sleep apnea/hypopnea syndrome. Am J Respir Crit Care Med 1999; 159:1108–1114.
62. Aloia MS, Stanchina M, Arnedt JT, et al. Treatment adherence and outcomes in flexible vs. standard continuous positive airway pressure therapy. Chest 2005; 127:2085–2093.
63. Jokic R, Klimaszewski A, Sridhar G, et al. Continuous positive airway pressure requirement during the first month of treatment in patients with severe obstructive sleep apnea. Chest 1998; 114:1061–1069.
64. Anderson FE, Kingshott RN, Taylor DR, et al. A randomized crossover efficacy trial of oral CPAP (Oracle) compared with nasal CPAP in the management of obstructive sleep apnea. Sleep 2003; 26:721–726.
65. Henke KG, Grady JJ, Kuna ST. Effect of nasal continuous positive airway pressure on neuro-psychological function in sleep apnea-hypopnea syndrome. Am J Respir Crit Care Med 2001; 163(4): 911–917.
66. Van Dongen H, Baynard MD, Maislin G, et al. Systematic interindividual differences in neurobehavioral impairment from sleep loss: evidence of trait-like differential vulnerability. Sleep 2004; 27(3):423–433.
67. Turkington P, Sircar M, Saralaya D, et al. Time course of changes in driving simulator performance with and without treatment in patients with sleep apnoea hypopnoea syndrome. Thorax 2004; 59:56–59.
68. George C. Reduction in motor vehicle collisions following treatment of sleep apnoea with nasal CPAP. Thorax 2001; 56:508–512.
69. Ayas NT, Mancini GBJ, Fleetham J. Does CPAP delay the development of cardiovascular disease in patients with obstructive sleep apnoea hypopnoea? Thorax 2006; 61:459–460.
70. Pepperell JCT, Ramdassingh-Dow S, Crosthwaite N, et al. Ambulatory blood pressure after therapeutic and subtherapeutic nasal continuous positive airway pressure for obstructive sleep apnea: a randomized parallel trial. Lancet 2002; 359:204–210.
71. Campos-Rodriguez F, Grilo-Reina A, Perez-Ronchel J, et al. Effect of continuous positive airway pressure on ambulatory BP in patients with sleep apnea and hypertension. A placebo-controlled trial. Chest 2006; 129:1459–1467.
72. Norman D, Loredo JS, Nelesen RA, et al. Effects of continuous positive airway pressure versus supplemental oxygen on 24-hour ambulatory blood pressure. Hypertension 2006; 47:840–845.
73. Becker HF, Jerrentrup A, Ploch T, et al. Effect of nasal continuous positive airway pressure treatment on blood pressure in obstructive sleep apnea. Circulation 2003; 107:68–73.
74. Robinson GV, Smith DM, Langford BA, et al. Continuous positive airway pressure does not reduce blood pressure in nonsleepy hypertensive OSA patients. Eur Respir J 2006; 27:1229–1235.
75. Pack AI. Advances in sleep-disordered breathing. Am J Respir Crit Care Med 2006; 173:7–15.
76. Marin JM, Carrizo SJ, Vincente E, et al. Long-term cardiovascular outcomes in men with obstructive sleep apnoea-hypopnoea with or without treatment with continuous positive airway pressure: an observational study. Lancet 2005; 365:1046–1053.
77. Sulit L, Storfer-Isser A, Kirchner HL, et al. Differences in polysomnography predictors for hypertension and impaired glucose tolerance. Sleep 2006; 29(6):777–783.
78. Yang Q, Phillips CL, Melehan KL, et al. Effects of short-term CPAP withdrawal on neurobehavioral performance in patients with obstructive sleep apnea. Sleep 2006; 29(4):545–552.
79. Ayas NT, FitzGerald M, Fleetham JA, et al. Cost-effectiveness of continuous positive airway pressure therapy for moderate to severe obstructive sleep apnea/hypopnea. Arch Intern Med 2006; 166: 977–984.

31 | Noninvasive Ventilation Treatment of Sleep-Related Breathing Disorders

Ramon Farré

Unit of Biophysics & Bioengineering, School of Medicine, University of Barcelona—IDIBAPS, Barcelona, and CIBER de Enfermedades Respiratorias (CIBERES), Bunyola, Spain

Joan Escarrabill

UFIS Respiratòria (Chest Division) Hospital Universitari de Bellvitge, L'Hospitalet, Spain

Josep M. Montserrat

Sleep Lab, Hospital Clinic, IDIBAPS, Barcelona, and CIBER de Enfermedades Respiratorias (CIBERES), Bunyola, Spain

INTRODUCTION

The most effective treatment to avoid the sleep disturbances characterizing patients with obstructive sleep apnea (OSA) is the application of a constant positive pressure at the airway opening (CPAP) by means of a nasal mask. Although OSA is the most prevalent sleep related breathing disorder (SRBD), a non-negligible proportion of SRBD patients suffer from ventilation disturbances requiring nocturnal ventilatory support different from CPAP. On the one hand, in some patients, OSA is accompanied by alterations that compromise adequate ventilation. For instance, OSA patients with concurrent morbid obesity or chronic obstructive pulmonary disease (COPD) may require not only a CPAP to splint the collapsible upper airway but also a mechanical ventilatory support to overcome the increased mechanical load to breathing associated with these concurrent disorders. On the other hand, patients with non-OSA sleep breathing disturbances such as Cheyne–Stokes breathing may also require noninvasive ventilatory support to compensate for an insufficient inspiratory drive during sleep.

RESPIRATORY MECHANICS DURING SPONTANEOUS BREATHING

From a mechanical viewpoint, spontaneous inspiration is a maneuver where a pump (breathing muscles) applies the level of energy (pressure) that a fluid (air) requires to flow through a resistance (airways) and to inflate an elastic compartment (lung and chest). Figure 1 shows a simplified model of the mechanics of the respiratory system. P_{mus} is the driving pressure exerted by the inspiratory muscles to generate an inspiratory flow V'. The respiratory system resistance (R) is mainly due to airway resistance, with a small tissue resistance component. The respiratory elastance (E), which is the reciprocal of respiratory compliance, is determined by the elastic properties of the lung and chest wall tissues. P_{ao} is the pressure at the airway opening, which is zero (atmospheric reference level) in spontaneous breathing.

The pressure P_R required to generate an airflow V' through the respiratory resistance R is $P_R = R \cdot V'$. The pressure P_E necessary to produce an inspiration of volume V in a respiratory elastance E is $P_E = E \cdot V$. Figure 2 (top) shows an example of the inspiratory flow recorded in a spontaneous breathing subject and the volume computed by integrating flow. Figure 2 (center) depicts the values of P_R corresponding to the inspiratory V' for two typical values of respiratory resistance: a normal subject (5 cmH$_2$O·s/L) and an obstructive patient (15 cmH$_2$O·s/L) (1,2). P_R exhibits the same time course as flow, attaining a maximum value of ≈ 7 cmH$_2$O in the case of $R = 15$ cmH$_2$O·s/L. Figure 2 (bottom) shows the P_E corresponding to the inspiratory volume V for two typical values of respiratory elastance in a normal subject and in a restrictive patient (20 cmH$_2$O/L and 40 cmH$_2$O/L, respectively). P_E exhibits an increasing value along inspiration, reflecting the time course of volume. The end-inspiratory value of P_E is ≈ 25 cmH$_2$O in the case of $E = 40$ cmH$_2$O/L.

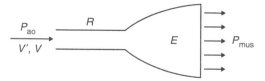

Figure 1 Simplified model of the respiratory mechanics during inspiration. V' and V are inspiratory flow and volume, respectively. P_{mus} is the driving pressure exerted by the inspiratory muscles. P_{ao} is the pressure at the airway opening. R and E are total respiratory system resistance and elastance, respectively.

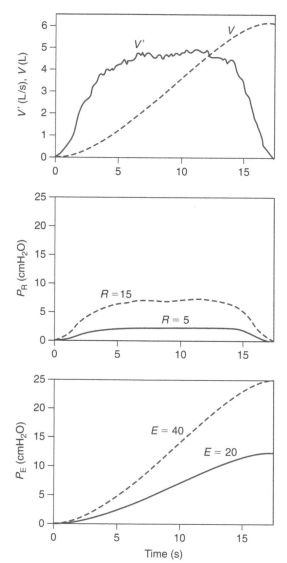

Figure 2 (*Top*): Inspiratory flow (V') and corresponding volume (V) recorded in a spontaneously breathing subject. (*Center*): Resistive pressure (P_R) required to generate the flow V' (top) in case of a respiratory resistance of 5 cmH$_2$O·s/L (normal) and of 15 cmH$_2$O·s/L (obstruction). (*Bottom*): Elastic pressure (P_E) required to generate the volume V (top) in case of a respiratory elastance of 20 cmH$_2$O/L (normal) and of 40 cmH$_2$O/L (restriction).

The equation of movement for the simple respiratory model in Figure 1 indicates that the muscle pressure required for the inspiration is

$$P_{mus} = P_R + P_E = R \cdot V' + E \cdot V \tag{1}$$

For given values of R and E, the magnitude of achieved ventilation (V' and V) depends on P_{mus}. As indicated by the equation of motion, to keep the level of ventilation, the P_{mus} applied by the inspiratory pump should increase in case of obstruction (R increased) and/or in case of restriction (E increased). This is illustrated in Figure 3, showing the values of the inspiratory muscle pressure required to obtain the ventilation in Figure 2 (top) for different combinations of R and E. The peak of P_{mus}, which is ≈ 12 cmH$_2$O for normal $R = 5$ cmH$_2$O·s/L and E = 20 cmH$_2$O/L, increases up to ≈ 28 cmH$_2$O in the simulated patient with obstruction ($R = 15$ cmH$_2$O·s/L) and restriction (E = 40 cmH$_2$O/L).

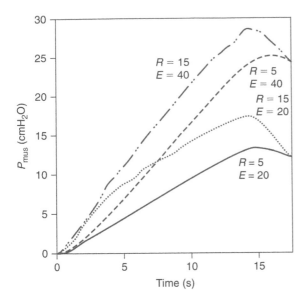

Figure 3 Inspiratory muscles pressure (P_{mus}) required to generate the flow and volume inspiration in Figure 2 (*top*) in case of different values of respiratory resistance (R; in cmH$_2$O·s/L) and elastance (E; in cmH$_2$O/L).

Ventilatory failure ensues when the muscle pump is unable to maintain the required ventilation. This situation could be due to pump failure because of reduced neural drive (e.g., Cheyne–Stokes breathing) or because the inspiratory muscles are unable to generate enough force (e.g., neuromuscular diseases). Ventilatory failure could also appear when a normal breathing pump cannot produce the augmented pressure demands owing to an increase in the mechanical load because of a rise in R and/or E (e.g., obesity, COPD, thoracic cage abnormalities). A combination of pump weakness and increased respiratory load also may result in ventilatory failure.

VENTILATORY SUPPORT

Noninvasive mechanical ventilation (NIMV) is a ventilatory support procedure aimed at helping the patient to maintain an adequate level of alveolar ventilation. NIMV consists in using an artificial air pump to cooperate with the patient's inspiratory muscles. NIMV can be applied by artificially imposing a negative pressure around the chest wall (negative pressure ventilation). This procedure, which requires an iron lung, cuirass or a poncho, considerably reduces patient comfort and in most cases the patient needs a caregiver to adapt the device. Therefore, negative pressure devices are not useful for long-term application during sleep. Alternatively, NIMV can be applied by connecting a positive pressure generator at the airway opening, for instance by means of a nasal mask. Given its easier application and greater comfort, particularly during sleep, positive NIMV is the most widespread method of providing nocturnal ventilatory support in SRBD.

In addition to giving artificial support to unload inspiration, NIMV can also be employed to simultaneously provide an expiratory pressure. Nocturnal application of a positive expiratory pressure can be useful in increasing lung volume in patients with reduced functional residual capacity (e.g., obese patients in supine) or in reducing work of breathing by avoiding expiratory flow limitation (e.g., in supine COPD patients (3)). Moreover, combination of inspiratory and expiratory pressure is a way of simultaneously applying CPAP and ventilatory support, which could be of interest in patients suffering from both OSA and chronic respiratory failure or obesity requiring NIMV.

In contrast to the situation of spontaneous breathing, where only one ventilation pump is operating (eq. 1), during NIMV there are two generators acting simultaneously: the inspiratory muscles and the ventilator. If P_{ao} is the airway opening pressure applied by a ventilator, the equation of movement is in this case:

$$P_{ao} + P_{mus} = R \cdot V' + E \cdot V \qquad (2)$$

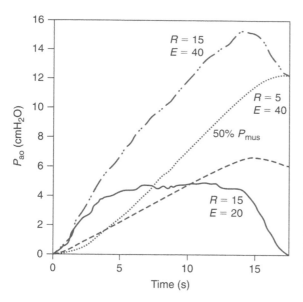

Figure 4 Pressure support required at the airway opening (P_{ao}) to generate the flow and volume inspiration in Figure 2 (*top*) in case of increased values of respiratory resistance (R; in $cmH_2O \cdot s/L$) and/or elastance (E; in cmH_2O/L), and in case that muscle pressure is reduced by 50% owing to muscle weakness. In all cases it is assumed that muscle pressure is the one corresponding to normal R (5 $cmH_2O \cdot s/L$) and E (20 cmH_2O/L).

indicating that inspiratory flow (V') and volume (V) depend on the addition of P_{ao} and P_{mus}. Figure 4 shows the values of pressure support ($P_{ao} = R \cdot V' + E \cdot V - P_{mus}$) required in case of increased R and/or E (Fig. 3) while maintaining the muscle effort corresponding to the baseline R (5 $cmH_2O \cdot s/L$) and E (20 cmH_2O). Figure 4 also shows the P_{ao} required when, owing to muscle weakness or reduced neural drive, the patient's P_{mus} is reduced by 50%. As indicated by Figure 4, both the magnitude and waveform of the pressure support (P_{ao}) required depend on the cause originating the need for ventilatory support.

NIMV allows the patient to increase ventilation while maintaining inspiratory effort or, alternatively, to maintain ventilation by reducing the activity of his/her inspiratory muscles. The actual effect of ventilatory support would depend on the type and magnitude of the pressure applied at the airway opening. Given that conventional ventilators are usually set to operate in volume- or pressure-preset modes, the patient has a reduced control of ventilation (V' and V). Moreover, the effectiveness of NIMV would also depend on the synchrony between the mechanical ventilator and patient muscles. A lack of synchrony may result in patient discomfort, consequent low adherence, and loss of clinical effectiveness.

VOLUME-PRESET AND PRESSURE-PRESET NIMV

One of the conventional ventilator types used in NIMV is designed to insufflate a given preset volume of air into the lung during each inspiration (volume-preset mode). These ventilators are usually based on a piston pump with an adjustable volume stroke and with a predefined pattern of speed inflation. By presetting V' and V in a patient with given R and E, the right hand side ($R \cdot V' + E \cdot V$) of the equation of movement (eq. 2) is fixed and, consequently, the left hand side of the equation ($P_{ao} + P_{mus}$) is also determined. Accordingly, the P_{ao} applied by the ventilator is the one necessary to complement the P_{mus} so that the sum attains the fixed value: the higher the patient effort, the lower the ventilator action. When the patient reduces the activity of the inspiratory muscles, the ventilator increases the applied P_{ao}. This mode of assisted ventilation has the advantage that patient ventilation (V', V) is ensured.

Another type of ventilation used in NIMV is based on a pressure-preset mode. In this case the ventilator, usually based on a servo-controlled blower, is designed to apply a given pattern of inspiratory and expiratory pressures. P_{ao} being fixed for a patient with given R and E, equation (2) shows that the magnitude of ventilation (V', V) depends on patient effort (P_{mus}). This mode of assisted ventilation has the advantage of providing a preset value of inspiratory P_{ao} to unload the respiratory muscles. Accordingly, the amount of pressure support provided by the ventilator is independent of patient effort.

LIMITATIONS OF VOLUME- AND PRESSURE-PRESET NIMV

Volume- and pressure-preset are the most widely used modes of NIMV because of their simplicity and proven effectiveness. However, one potential limitation of these conventional NIMV modes is that the patient has reduced control of ventilation. In the case of volume-preset ventilation, the patient completely loses his/her control over the flow and volume pattern, which requires patient adaptation to avoid fighting against the ventilator. In pressure-preset ventilation, the patient maintains a degree of control over the ventilation waveform. Indeed, when the pressure support (P_{ao}) is lower than the pressure required (Fig. 4), the patient can simply reduce his/her effort. Nevertheless, if P_{ao} exceeds the pressure required the patient would experience an inspiration (V' and V) greater than expected. This situation is clearly found at the beginning of inspiration, where the required pressure support tends to be lower (Fig. 4). Accordingly, a suitable design of the inspiratory ramp of P_{ao} could improve patient comfort.

A decisive factor in the successful application of ventilatory support is the correct detection of the beginning and the end of inspiration to synchronize the ventilator with the breathing cycle of the patient. A false positive detection of the beginning of patient inspiration would result in a ventilator inspiration when the patient is not ready for it (for instance during expiration), causing the patient to fight against the ventilator. In the case of false negative detection the patient would be unsupported during the inspiration. Incorrect detection of the end of inspiration would result in the cessation of ventilator support in the final phase of the inspiration or in prolonged ventilator insufflation when the patient is already in the expiratory phase (another situation of patient-ventilator fight). A certain reduction in ventilator synchrony, although uncomfortable, could be tolerated by the awake patient. However, the need for a suitable ventilator-patient synchrony is particularly important when NIMV is applied during sleep since a minor lack of synchrony could result in disruption of sleep architecture.

OTHER MODES OF NIMV

Designing ventilation modes that are more complex than volume- and pressure-preset has been possible by incorporating transducers and microprocessors into the ventilators. Indeed, a microprocessor-controlled ventilator is able to acquire the V' and P_{ao} signals and to process them in real time so that the pressure support is applied at the airway opening according to a predefined pattern.

A conceptually important advance in this regard was the definition of proportional assist ventilation (4). This is a ventilatory support mode that avoids the problems arising from machine synchronization, and that applies an airway pressure that is fully controlled by the patient. Instead of presetting a given inspiratory pressure or volume waveform, proportional assist ventilators apply a P_{ao} that is designed to be proportional to P_{mus}. To this end, the applied pressure is proportional to the inspiratory flow and to the inspiratory volume ($P_{ao} = k_1 \cdot V' + k_2 \cdot V$). k_1 and k_2 represent the amounts of respiratory resistance and elastance, respectively, which the ventilator is unloading from the patient's inspiratory muscle. The main advantage of proportional assist ventilation is that the ventilator works as an extension of the patient's respiratory muscles, which could improve comfort and adherence. Indeed, the flow and volume patterns are always under patient control. There is no lack of synchrony between the ventilator and the patient and the ventilator work is adapted to the ventilatory requirements of the patient. The performance of proportional assist ventilation is illustrated by Figure 5, showing the nasal pressure and flow and the esophageal pressure recorded in a patient on proportional assist ventilation. As expected, the nasal pressure applied by the ventilator followed the same pattern as the breathing effort (assessed by esophageal pressure). The greater the patient effort, the greater the nasal pressure support applied. Consequently, the ventilator acted under the full control of the patient. However, this ventilation mode runs the risk of under-assistance in case of patients with reduced inspiratory activity, which is particularly likely during sleep, or with auto positive end expiratory pressure (which is expected in COPD and in obese patients). Moreover, the proportional ventilation actually applied may be affected by technical problems such as air leaks and incorrect empirical setting of k_1 and k_2 (5). Although proportional assist ventilation has been successfully tested in research studies, its effectiveness in routine application for NIMV during sleep has not been confirmed to date.

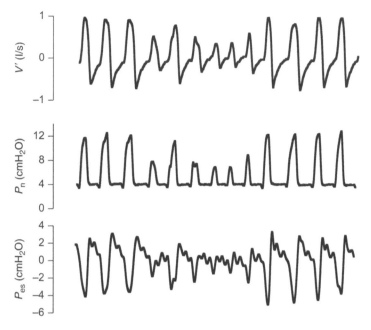

Figure 5 Nasal pressure (P_n), flow (V') and esophageal pressure (P_{es}) in a patient subjected to proportional assist ventilation through a nasal mask.

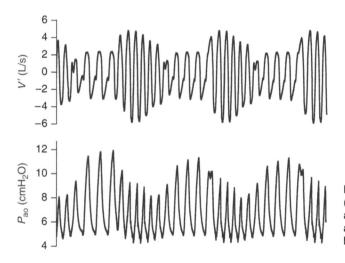

Figure 6 Flow (V') and nasal pressure (P_{ao}) recorded in a bench study when an adaptive pressure ventilator was applied to a patient model simulating Cheyne–Stokes breathing.

Adaptive pressure support was recently proposed as a novel procedure to help nocturnal ventilation in patients with unstable central drive such as those exhibiting Cheyne–Stokes breathing (6). The rationale for this kind of NIMV is to incorporate the advantages of volume- and pressure-preset ventilators simultaneously. Indeed, the ventilator operates in a pressure-preset mode (which in theory cannot guarantee a fixed ventilation) in such a way that the magnitude of pressure support in the different cycles is automatically adjusted to ensure a preset ventilation (6). Figure 6 illustrates the operation of an adaptive ventilator when connected to a respiratory system model simulating a patient with Cheyne–Stokes breathing. The flow signal exhibits the characteristic crescendo-decrescendo pattern. As expected, the nasal pressure support applied by the ventilator was automatically adapted to provide greater support during the cycles with reduced patient breathing activity. The pressure applied by this kind of ventilator greatly contrasts with that applied by a conventional pressure-preset ventilator (equal nasal support in each cycle regardless of the patient breathing amplitude).

TECHNICAL OPTIMIZATION OF ROUTINE NIMV

One improvement implemented in the conventional volume- and pressure-preset ventilation is that the ventilator automatically: (*i*) estimates the unintended air leak caused by an imperfect sealing between the mask and patient skin, and (*ii*) compensates the amount of flow delivered to the patient (7). Another possibility of improving conventional NIMV is that the ventilator allows the modification of the rising time and waveform of the inspiratory pressure to optimize patient comfort (8). Microprocessor-controlled ventilators can also improve the detection of the start and end of patient effort for a better synchronization of the machine and inspiratory muscle action (9).

In addition to improving the technical characteristics of ventilators, optimizing nocturnal NIMV at home also requires quality control of the equipment. Studies have shown that the quality assessment of home ventilators is not well defined (10,11) and that the actual ventilation provided by ventilators at home could be markedly different from the prescribed settings (12). Such a difference could arise from the fact that: (*i*) the machine does not perform in accordance with the settings in the control panel (13,14), or (*ii*) because the patient/caregiver voluntarily or involuntarily modifies the ventilator settings (12,15). Given that NIMV at home is a treatment provided by a machine that is not under the direct and constant supervision of expert staff for a long period of time, quality control of NIMV at home will provide the patient with a ventilatory support closer to the one prescribed to him/her and will reassure both the patient and the physician concerning the adequacy of the patient's treatment.

NIMV IN PATIENTS WITH SRBD

NIMV is scarcely employed in patients with OSA because CPAP is extremely effective in normalizing the upper airway and the sleep of these patients. However, some OSA patients requiring a high nasal pressure may not tolerate CPAP despite the fact that this technique is able to avoid his/her nocturnal upper airway obstructions. Such intolerance could be due to the fact that application of a high level of CPAP markedly increases lung volume, thereby reducing the efficiency of inspiratory muscles and increasing patient discomfort. OSA patients who do not tolerate CPAP are candidates to be treated with positive NIMV in the pressure support mode. Indeed, in these patients the inspiratory pressure applied by the ventilator is not designed to unload the breathing muscles but to split the collapsible upper airway in a way similar to CPAP. Application of an expiratory pressure lower than inspiratory pressure facilitates expiration to a lung volume close to functional residual capacity and decreases discomfort. A nasal pressure lower in expiration than inspiration allows the upper airway to be open since the tendency to airway collapse is reduced during expiration (16).

Based on the fact that the pressure required to keep the upper airway open is lower during expiration than inspiration (17), some variants of pressure support ventilation specially adapted for OSA treatment have been designed. One of these variants consists in the application of a flow-dependent positive nasal pressure (16). According to the Starling model describing the collapsible upper airway (17), the pressure applied by the ventilator consists in the addition of two terms: (*i*) a constant value set to account for the critical (closure) pressure of the upper airway, and (*ii*) a pressure component proportional to flow to account for the resistive pressure drop in the upper airway segment (16). Other variants of bilevel pressure support adapted to OSA patients are based on releasing expiratory pressure (18). As NIMV could be better tolerated than CPAP, it allows the therapeutic rescue of patients who do not tolerate CPAP or in whom CPAP is not sufficiently effective. However, there are no data available to support the hypothesis that bilevel pressure is better than CPAP for treating the general OSA population (19,20).

A significant proportion of OSA presents with obesity. OSA patients with severe obesity could require a nasal pressure treatment not only to avoid upper airway collapse (CPAP) but also as a support to offset the ventilatory effects induced by obesity. Indeed, an excessive accumulation of fat impedes ventilation because of a reduction in functional residual capacity and an increase in respiratory resistance and elastance (Fig. 4). The effects of obesity on ventilation are particularly relevant in supine posture, resulting in nocturnal hypoventilation, particularly during rapid eye movement (REM) sleep (21,22). Accordingly, patients with obesity hypoventilation syndrome with daytime hypercapnia may benefit from nocturnal NIMV (23,24). If the obesity hypoventilation syndrome coexists with OSA, NIMV should be titrated so that: (*i*) expiratory pressure normalizes functional residual capacity, (*ii*) the obstruction of the upper airway disappears, and (*iii*) sufficient inspiratory support is provided to a respiratory system with increased load (Fig. 4).

Patients with unstable inspiratory drive during sleep also require NIMV to normalize ventilation (Fig. 4). This is the case, for instance, in congestive heart failure patients with Cheyne–Stokes respiration (25) that is characterized by recurrent increments and reductions in ventilation. As a result of their periodic breathing pattern during sleep, these patients experience oxygen desaturations, arousals, and altered sleep architecture with symptoms very similar to those found in OSA (daytime somnolence, fatigue and insomnia). Some studies have reported that CPAP was effective in these patients (26,27). However, given the unstable nature of Cheyne–Stokes breathing, a conventional NIMV (providing the same level of support in every cycle) is not the most suitable treatment. Rather, a NIMV variant such as adaptive ventilation (Fig. 6) capable of providing a level of support tailored to the needs of each individual breathing cycle could be of more interest (28,29).

NOCTURNAL NIMV IN OTHER PATHOLOGIES

Nocturnal NIMV is routinely applied in a large number of patients with no specific sleep pathologies. These patients suffer from a variety of respiratory disorders that in most cases require ventilatory support during sleep. Most of these patients are able to maintain spontaneous breathing during daytime. Nevertheless, they require nocturnal ventilatory support owing to the mechanical disadvantage of the supine posture, the disappearance of the voluntary compensatory breathing mechanisms during sleep, or to the physiological sleep-induced reduction in central drive and muscular tone. The pathologies of non-OSA patients receiving mainly nocturnal NIMV at home can be classified into two main categories: (*i*) thoracic cage abnormalities including early-onset kyphoscoliosis, tuberculosis sequelae, obesity hypoventilation syndrome, and sequelae of lung resection; and (*ii*) neuromuscular diseases such as muscular dystrophy, motor neuron disease (mainly amyotrophic lateral sclerosis), postpolio kyphoscoliosis, central hypoventilation, spinal cord damage and phrenic nerve paralysis. Daytime hypercapnia, repetitive hospital admissions, or daytime symptoms (e.g., cephalgia and fatigue) are the main indicators of NIMV in these patients. It is important to take into consideration that these patients usually need a close support during the first days of NIMV. Sleep studies are necessary to monitor the improvement in physiological parameters. However, clinical improvement under NIMV has been reported in some of these patients despite sleep disruption observed by polysomnography (30).

As estimated by an extended study carried out in 2001–2002 covering 16 European countries, the estimated prevalence of home NIMV in non-OSA patients was 6.6 per 100,000 people (10). Given the increasing tendency toward the application of home NIMV, it is expected that the number of non-OSA patients on nocturnal NIMV is considerably higher than the estimated figure of >21,500 in 2002. However, more studies are required to precisely determine the adequate indication criteria of NIMV, particularly taking into account the current tendency to prescribe long-term NIMV to COPD patients.

CONCLUSIONS

Patients with SRBD may be afflicted with ventilatory disturbances requiring nocturnal ventilatory support apart from positive airway pressure. Ventilatory failure can occur due to pump failure (i.e., reduced neural drive or inability of the inspiratory muscles to generate enough force) or when a normal breathing pump cannot produce the augmented pressure demands owing to an increase in the mechanical load because of a rise in resistance or elastance. NIMV is a ventilatory support procedure designed to help the patient maintain an adequate level of alveolar ventilation, and volume-preset and pressure-preset represent two NIMV modes. There are additional new advances in ventilation modes, including proportional assist ventilation and adaptive pressure support, as well as technical improvement in conventional volume- and pressure-preset ventilation. Lastly, NIMV has utility in some patients with SRBD and other pathologies, such as thoracic cage abnormalities and neuromuscular disease.

REFERENCES

1. Farre R, Gavela E, Rotger M, et al. Noninvasive assessment of respiratory resistance in severe chronic respiratory patients with nasal CPAP. Eur Respir J 2000; 15:314–319.
2. Navajas D, Alcaraz J, Peslin R, et al. Evaluation of a method for assessing respiratory mechanics during noninvasive ventilation. Eur Respir J 2000; 16:704–709.
3. Dellaca RL, Rotger M, Aliverti A, et al. Noninvasive detection of expiratory flow limitation in COPD patients during nasal CPAP. Eur Respir J 2006; 27:983–991.
4. Younes M. Proportional assist ventilation, a new approach to ventilatory support. Theory Am Rev Respir Dis 1992; 145:114–120.
5. Farre R, Mancini M, Rotger M, et al. Oscillatory resistance measured during noninvasive proportional assist ventilation. Am J Respir Crit Care Med 2001; 164:790–794.
6. Teschler H, Dohring J, Wang YM, et al. Adaptive pressure support servo-ventilation: a novel treatment for Cheyne–Stokes respiration in heart failure. Am J Respir Crit Care Med 2001; 164:614–619.
7. Mehta S, McCool FD, Hill NS. Leak compensation in positive pressure ventilators: a lung model study. Eur Respir J 2001; 17:259–267.
8. Prinianakis G, Delmastro M, Carlucci A, et al. Effect of varying the pressurisation rate during noninvasive pressure support ventilation. Eur Respir J 2004; 23:314–320.
9. Richard JC, Carlucci A, Breton L, et al. Bench testing of pressure support ventilation with three different generations of ventilators. Intensive Care Med 2002; 28:1049–1057.
10. Lloyd-Owen SJ, Donaldson GC, Ambrosino N, et al. Patterns of home mechanical ventilation use in Europe: results from the Eurovent survey. Eur Respir J 2005; 25:1025–1031.
11. Farre R, Lloyd-Owen SJ, Ambrosino N, et al. Quality control of equipment in home mechanical ventilation: a European survey. Eur Respir J 2005; 26:86–94.
12. Farre R, Navajas D, Prats E, et al. Performance of mechanical ventilators at the patient's home: a multicentre quality control study. Thorax 2006; 61:400–404.
13. Lofaso F, Fodil R, Lorino H, et al. Inaccuracy of tidal volume delivered by home mechanical ventilators. Eur Respir J 2000; 15:338–341.
14. Battisti A, Tassaux D, Janssens JP, et al. Performance characteristics of 10 home mechanical ventilators in pressure-support mode: a comparative bench study. Chest 2005; 127:1784–1792.
15. Farre R, Giro E, Casolive V, et al. Quality control of mechanical ventilation at the patient's home. Intensive Care Med 2003; 29:484–486.
16. Farré R, Peslin R, Montserrat JM, et al. Flow-dependent positive airway pressure to maintain airway patency in sleep apnea-hypopnea syndrome. Am J Respir Crit Care Med 1998; 157:1855–1863.
17. Gold AR, Schwartz AR. The pharyngeal critical pressure: the whys and hows of using nasal continuous positive airway pressure diagnostically. Chest 1996; 110:1077–1088.
18. Nilius G, Happel A, Domanski U, et al. Pressure-relief continuous positive airway pressure vs constant continuous positive airway pressure: a comparison of efficacy and compliance. Chest 2006; 130:1018–1024.
19. Kushida CA, Littner MR, Hirshkowitz M, et al. Practice parameters for the use of continuous and bilevel positive airway pressure devices to treat adult patients with sleep-related breathing disorders. Sleep 2006; 29(3):375–380.
20. Gay P, Weaver T, Loube D, et al. Evaluation of positive airway pressure treatment for sleep related breathing disorders in adults. Sleep 2006; 29(3):381–401.
21. Jubber AS. Respiratory complications of obesity. Int J Clin Pract 2004; 58(6):573–580.
22. Olson AL, Zwillich C. The obesity hypoventilation syndrome. Am J Med 2005; 118(9):948–956.
23. Masa JF, Celli BR, Riesco JA, et al. The obesity hypoventilation syndrome can be treated with noninvasive mechanical ventilation. Chest 2001; 119(4):1102–1107.
24. Storre JH, Seuthe B, Fiechter R, et al. Average volume-assured pressure support in obesity hypoventilation: a randomized crossover trial. Chest 2006; 130:815–821.
25. Javaheri S, Parker TJ, Wexler L, et al. Occult sleep-disordered breathing in stable congestive heart failure. Ann Intern Med 1995; 122:487–492.
26. Davies RJO, Harrington KJ, Ormerod OJM, et al. Nasal continuous positive airway pressure in chronic heart failure with sleep disordered breathing. Am Rev Respir Dis 1993; 147:630–634.
27. Naughton MT, Benard DC, Liu PP, et al. Effect of nasal CPAP on sympathetic activity in patients with heart failure and central sleep apnea. Am J Respir Crit Care Med 1995; 152:473–479.

28. Pepperell JC, Maskell NA, Jones DR, et al. A randomized controlled trial of adaptive ventilation for Cheyne–Stokes breathing in heart failure. Am J Respir Crit Care Med 2003; 168:1109–1114.
29. Pepin JL, Chouri-Pontarollo N, Tamisier R, et al. Cheyne–Stokes respiration with central sleep apnoea in chronic heart failure: proposals for a diagnostic and therapeutic strategy. Sleep Med Rev 2006; 10:33–47.
30. Bach JR, Robert D, Leger P, et al. Sleep fragmentation in kyphoscoliotic individuals with alveolar hypoventilation treated by NIPPV. Chest 1995; 107:1552–1558.

32 | Surgical Treatment of Sleep-Related Breathing Disorders

Donald M. Sesso

Department of Otolaryngology/Head and Neck Surgery, Stanford University Medical Center, Stanford, California, U.S.A.

Nelson B. Powell and Robert W. Riley

Department of Otolaryngology/Head and Neck Surgery, Stanford University Medical Center and Department of Behavioral Sciences, Division of Sleep Medicine, Stanford University School of Medicine, Stanford, California, U.S.A.

INTRODUCTION

Snoring, upper airway resistance syndrome (UARS), obstructive sleep apnea (OSA), and obstructive sleep apnea-hypopnea syndrome (OSAHS) are collectively referred to as sleep-related breathing disorders (SRBD). These terms describe a partial or complete obstruction of the upper airway during sleep. Patency of the pharyngeal airway is maintained by two opposing forces: negative intraluminal pressure and the activity of the upper airway musculature. Anatomical or central neural abnormalities can disrupt this delicate balance and result in compromise of the upper airway. This reduction of airway caliber may cause sleep fragmentation and subsequent behavioral derangements, such as excessive daytime sleepiness (EDS) (1–3). The goal of medical and surgical therapy is to alleviate this obstruction and increase airway patency.

The first therapeutic modality employed to treat SRBD was surgery. Kuhlo described placement of a tracheotomy tube in an attempt to bypass upper airway obstruction in Pickwickian patients (4). Although effective, tracheotomy does not address the specific sites of pharyngeal collapse and is not readily accepted by most patients. These sites include the nasal cavity/nasopharynx, oropharynx, and hypopharynx. Often, multilevel obstruction is present. Consequently, the surgical armamentarium has evolved to create techniques that correct the specific anatomical sites of obstruction. To eliminate SRBD, it is necessary to alleviate all levels of obstruction in an organized and safe protocol. The surgeon must counsel the patient regarding all surgical techniques, risks, complications, and alternative medical therapies prior to intervention.

Medical management is often considered the primary treatment of SRBD; however, there are exceptions. Treatment may consist of weight loss, avoidance of alcohol and sedating medications, and manipulation of body position during sleep (5–9). Currently, continuous positive airway pressure (CPAP) or bilevel positive airway pressure (BPAP) devices are the preferred methods of treatment and the standard to which other modalities are compared. The efficacy of CPAP has clearly been demonstrated, but a subset of patients struggle to comply with or accept CPAP therapy (10–13). Patients who are unwilling or unable to comply with medical treatment may be candidates for surgery.

RATIONALE FOR SURGICAL TREATMENT

The rationale for surgical treatment of SRBD is to alleviate the pathophysiologic and neurobehavioral derangements associated with upper airway obstruction. The goal is to achieve outcomes that are equivalent to those of medical management. Ideally, this would include an improved quality of life with a reduction in cardiopulmonary and neurologic morbidity (14–17).

Table 1 Surgical Indications

Apnea-hypopnea index (AHI) $\geq 20^a$ events/hr of sleep
Oxygen desaturation nadir <90%
Esophageal pressure (P_{es}) more negative than −10 cmH$_2$O
Cardiovascular derangements (arrhythmia, hypertension)
Neurobehavioral symptoms [excessive daytime sleepiness (EDS)]
Failure of medical management
Anatomical sites of obstruction (nose, palate, tongue base)

^{a}Surgery may be indicated with an AHI < 20 if accompanied by excessive daytime fatigue.
Source: From Ref. 18.

Table 2 Relative Contraindications to Surgery

Severe pulmonary disease
Unstable cardiovascular disease
Morbid obesity
Alcohol or drug abuse
Psychiatric instability
Unrealistic expectations

Source: From Ref. 18.

SURGICAL INDICATIONS

Surgical indications are listed in Table 1. Those patients whose apnea-hypopnea index (AHI) is less than 20 may still be candidates for surgery. Surgery is considered appropriate if these patients have associated EDS, which results in altered daytime performance or comorbidities as recognized by the Center for Medicare and Medicaid Services (including stroke and ischemic heart disease). For those patients whose EDS is not explained by the severity of their sleep apnea or resolved with CPAP therapy, consideration may be given to obtaining a multiple sleep latency test (MSLT) or the maintenance of wakefulness test (MWT) to determine other etiologies of sleepiness (18,19). In these patients, surgery is unlikely to be beneficial. Other factors exist, which could predict poor surgical outcomes, and are considered relative contraindications to surgery. These factors are listed in Table 2. All patients require a comprehensive evaluation to determine if they meet the criteria for surgery. Polysomnography and a history and physical examination are essential to make this determination.

MEDICAL AND SURGICAL EVALUATION

Proper screening and selection of patients for surgery is vital to achieve successful outcomes and to minimize postoperative complications. The preoperative evaluation requires a comprehensive medical history, head and neck examination, polysomnography, fiberoptic nasopharyngolaryngoscopy, and lateral cephalometric analysis. A thorough review of this data can determine the extent of SRBD severity, uncover comorbidities, and assist in risk management. Furthermore, this systematic approach will identify probable anatomic sites of obstruction. Armed with this information, a safe, site-specific surgical protocol can be presented to the patient.

PHYSICAL EXAMINATION

A complete physical exam with vital signs, weight and neck circumference should be performed on every patient. Specific attention is focused in the regions of the head and neck that have been well described as potential sites of upper airway obstruction, such as the nose, palate, and base of tongue (20–25). Nasal obstruction can occur as a result of alar collapse, turbinate hypertrophy, and septal deviation or sinonasal masses. These can be identified on anterior rhinoscopy. The oral cavity should be examined for periodontal disease, dental occlusion and any lesions, including torus mandibulae or torus palatinus. Examination of the oropharyngeal and hypopharyngeal regions includes a description of the palate, lateral pharyngeal walls, tonsils, and tongue base. A variety of grading systems, such as the Mallampati system, have been developed to establish a standard of describing the degree of obstruction caused by these structures (26,27). However, it was Fujita, who first proposed a classification system to define the levels of upper airway obstruction in OSA patients (28,29). Examination of the larynx is required in all patients ideally by nasopharyngolaryngoscopy.

POLYSOMNOGRAM

A polysomnogram (PSG) is an integral part of the preoperative evaluation. The surgeon must carefully review the PSG, with particular attention focused on the AHI and oxygen desaturation nadir. This data will guide appropriate surgical treatment, as well as preoperative and postoperative management. As with any intervention, a postoperative PSG is needed to assess a patient's response to surgery. Failure to obtain this study may result in an inadequately treated patient.

FIBEROPTIC NASOPHARYNGOLARYNGOSCOPY

Fiberoptic examination provides a detailed view of the entire upper airway. In particular, the larynx can be more closely observed for such abnormalities as an omega-shaped epiglottis, vocal fold paralysis, or obstructing lesions. The airway is examined at rest as well as during provocative maneuvers. One such technique, Müller's maneuver, has been evaluated by Sher et al. to identify potential sites of obstruction and to predict surgical success (30). This test involves inspiration against a closed oral and nasal airway, while keeping the glottis open. Photodocumentation of findings may prove useful for surgical planning and patient education (Fig. 1).

Besides identifying obstruction, fiberoptic examination assists in the preoperative planning by determining the difficulty of intubation. This information can be invaluable to both the surgeon and anesthesiologist, as they determine the best method to intubate a patient.

CEPHALOMETRIC ANALYSIS

The lateral cephalogram is the most cost-effective radiographic study of the bony facial skeleton and soft tissues of the upper airway. Using these landmarks, Riley et al. were first to describe anthropomorphic measurements that can be performed to ascertain skeletal facial

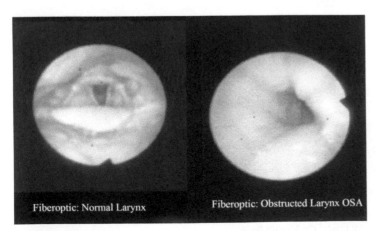

Fiberoptic: Normal Larynx   Fiberoptic: Obstructed Larynx OSA

Figure 1 Fiberoptic laryngoscopy. View of the normal larynx. Note that the entire vocal folds can be visualized (*left*). Müller's maneuver results in collapse of the velopharyngeal and hypopharyngeal airway. The vocal folds are completely obscured by redundant soft tissue in a patient with OSA (*right*).

abnormalities (31). Magnetic resonance imaging (MRI) and computed tomography (CT) scanning have proven to be effective radiographic studies; however, these tools are often reserved for investigational studies due to expense and time (32–34). Although not as detailed as CT scan or MRI, the cephalogram allows measurement of the length of the soft palate, posterior airway space (PAS), skeletal proportions, and hyoid position. Studies have shown the cephalogram to be valid in assessing obstruction, and in fact, it compares favorably to three-dimensional volumetric computed tomographic scans of the upper airway (35). The cephalogram, as with other imaging modalities, may underestimate the degree of obstruction, since they are not obtained while the patient is sleeping.

SURGICAL TREATMENT PHILOSOPHY

The goal of surgical treatment is to alleviate upper airway obstruction and its associated neurobehavioral symptoms and morbidities. No longer is a 50% reduction in the AHI deemed acceptable (Table 3). Rather, the objective is to treat to cure (normalization of respiratory events and elimination of hypoxemia). This can only be accomplished if a thorough and systematic evaluation is performed on every patient.

Since multilevel obstruction may exist, it may be necessary to treat more than one site. Failure to recognize or treat all anatomical levels will lead to persistent obstruction. Thus, the surgeon must be committed to treating the entire upper airway.

Once a surgical plan has been formulated, this must be communicated to the patient and our medical colleagues. Successful treatment of a SRBD patient typically requires a multidisciplinary team. This team will assist in the preoperative and postoperative course to minimize risk and potential complications. Prior to any intervention, the surgeon must discuss all treatment options and the associated risks and complications with the patient. Only after the patient fully understands the process and has consented to surgery can the treatment plan proceed.

A surgeon has numerous procedures available within their armamentarium to treat SRBD. Selecting the appropriate surgery for a patient can be challenging. However, we have created a two-phase surgical protocol (Powell–Riley surgical protocol) as a logically directed plan to treat the specific areas of upper airway obstruction (36,37). This protocol (Table 4) as well as other surgical techniques (Table 5) will be discussed in this chapter.

Table 3 Powell–Riley Definition of Surgical Responders

Apnea-hypopnea index (AHI) < 20 events/hr of sleep[a]
Oxygen desaturation nadir ≥ 90%
Excessive daytime sleepiness (EDS) alleviated
Response equivalent to CPAP on full-night titration

[a]A reduction of the AHI by 50% or more is considered a cure if the preoperative AHI is less than 20.
Source: From Ref. 18.

Table 4 Powell–Riley Protocol Surgical Procedures

Phase I
 Nasal surgery (septoplasty, turbinate reduction, nasal valve grafting)
 Tonsillectomy
 Uvulopalatopharyngoplasty (UPPP) or uvulopalatal flap (UPF)
 Mandibular osteotomy with genioglossus advancement
 Hyoid myotomy and suspension
 Temperature-controlled radiofrequency (TCRF)[a]—turbinates, palate, tongue base
Phase II
 Maxillomandibular advancement osteotomy (MMO)
 Temperature-controlled radiofrequency (TCRF)[a]—tongue base

[a]TCRF is typically used as an adjunctive treatment. Select patients may choose TCRF as primary treatment.

Table 5 Alternative Upper Airway Surgical Techniques

Pharyngeal obstruction
Temperature-controlled radiofrequency (TCRF)
Pillar® palatal implant system
Laser-assisted uvulopalatoplasty (LAUP)
Injection snoreplasty
Hypopharyngeal obstruction
Genial bone advancement trephine system (GBAT™)
Repose™ genioglossus advancement hyoid myotomy (GAHM)
Temperature-controlled radiofrequency (TCRF)
Midline glossectomy and lingualplasty
Airway bypass surgery
Tracheotomy

POWELL–RILEY TWO-PHASE SURGICAL PROTOCOL

This protocol consists of two distinct phases. The procedures included in each phase are listed in Table 4. Developed to prevent unnecessary surgery, this method is a conservative surgical approach to the SRBD patient. Phase II surgery has documented success rates exceeding 90%; however, a substantial number of patients may not need such extensive surgery (38,39). In fact, patients have a realistic chance to be cured by phase I surgery alone. However, it is difficult to predict surgical outcomes for an individual patient. Conservative surgery (phase I) is therefore recommended initially with the plan to perform postoperative PSG to assess response to surgery. Those patients who are incompletely treated would then be considered for phase II surgery. As with any treatment protocol, exceptions may occur. There are certain cases in which phase II surgery may be the appropriate first step, as in nonobese patients with marked mandibular deficiency and normal palates (40).

Phase I surgery is directed towards the three potential sites of upper airway obstruction (nose, palate, and tongue base). Neither dental occlusion nor the facial skeleton is altered. Clinical response is determined by PSG. The PSG is obtained four to six months following surgery to allow for adequate healing. Patients who have persistent SRBD are offered phase II surgery.

Phase II surgery refers to maxillomandibular advancement osteotomy (MMO) or bimaxillary advancement. MMO helps clear hypopharyngeal obstruction, which would be the only region incompletely treated by phase I. This is the only procedure that physically creates more room for the tongue to be advanced anteriorly, thus enlarging the PAS.

SURGICAL PROTOCOL OUTCOMES

Previously, reducing the AHI by 50% was considered a cure for SRBD. However, most researchers and clinicians no longer consider this parameter valid. Rather, surgical intervention aims to attain the results obtained by CPAP therapy. Consequently, a more comprehensive criterion was established to determine surgical success or cure (Table 3).

Clinical response to phase I surgery ranges from 42% to 75% (38,41–45). Our published data have shown that approximately 60% of all patients are cured with phase I surgery (38). Factors that portend less successful outcomes are a mean respiratory disturbance index (RDI) greater than 60, oxygen desaturation below 70%, mandibular deficiency (sella nasion point B $<75°$), and morbid obesity (body mass index [BMI] $> 33 \text{ kg/m}^2$). However, it is imprudent to discount phase I surgery in these patients, since a reasonable percentage may not need more aggressive surgery (37).

Incomplete treatment by phase I surgery is primarily due to persistent hypopharyngeal obstruction. Phase II surgery (MMO) would then be offered to those patients who have been incompletely treated by phase I surgery. MMO is a more aggressive surgery, which requires more intensive operative and postoperative care. Patients must be prepared for a recovery period of 4 to 6 weeks. Despite a longer convalescence period, documented success rates of MMO exceed 90% (38,46–49).

SURGICAL PREPARATION—RISK MANAGEMENT

Ensuring that a patient is medically stable for the operative procedure can reduce the risk of postoperative complications. This would include obtaining the appropriate laboratory, cardiopulmonary, and radiographic tests. In patients with existing comorbid medical conditions (diabetes, hypothyroidism, cardiovascular disease, and pulmonary disease), consultation with the appropriate medical specialist should be sought.

Preoperative CPAP can alleviate the issues associated with sleep deprivation and may reduce the risk of postobstructive pulmonary edema. Consequently, all patients who are tolerant of CPAP are encouraged to use this modality for at least two weeks prior to surgery (50). In 1988, Powell et al. recommended the use of preoperative CPAP for all patients who have an RDI greater than 40 and an oxygen desaturation of 80% or less. According to this protocol, the surgeon must consider insertion of a temporary tracheotomy for those patients with severe OSA (RDI greater than 60 and/or SaO_2 less than 70%) who are intolerant of CPAP therapy (51). Tracheotomy is rarely needed at our center and must be determined on a case-by-case basis.

SURGICAL PROCEDURES—PHASE I

Nasal Reconstruction

A patent nasal airway is essential to normal respiration and sleep. Obstruction can increase airway resistance and result in mouth breathing. Opening of the mouth rotates the mandible posteriorly, which in turn allows the tongue to prolapse into the PAS and narrow the hypopharyngeal airway. Nasal obstruction can occur due to septal deviations, incompetent nasal valves, or enlarged turbinates. A multitude of techniques (septoplasty, alar grafting, and turbinate reduction) exist to treat nasal obstruction. These techniques and their results have been well established in the head and neck literature. The choice of procedure depends on surgeon preference and experience.

Nasal reconstruction can improve quality of life and may improve OSA in select patients (52,53). In addition, improvement of the nasal airway may improve a patient's tolerance of nasal CPAP (54). Rarely, however, will alleviating nasal obstruction cure OSA.

While most treatments of the nasal cavity are well established, treatment of the turbinates is an evolving technique. Our preferred method is submucosal turbinoplasty with a radiofrequency probe. Submucosal turbinoplasty can be performed with radiofrequency or a microdebrider. Radiofrequency is rarely associated with complications such as bleeding or crusting. However, the ultimate goal of reducing submucosal erectile tissue, while preserving the ciliated, surface mucosa is the same (55,56).

Uvulopalatopharyngoplasty/Uvulopalatal Flap

Uvulopalatopharyngoplasty (UPPP) was introduced by Ikematsu for the treatment of habitual snoring (57). Subsequently, this technique was adapted to treat SRBD and snoring by Fujita et al. in 1981 (29). Since this time, many variations have been developed to treat the obstructing tissues of the soft palate, lateral pharyngeal walls, and tonsils.

UPPP is an excellent technique to alleviate isolated retropalatal (Table 6) obstruction (Fujita type I). Performed under general anesthesia, a portion of the palate, uvula, lateral pharyngeal walls, and tonsils may be removed (Fig. 2). Unfortunately, due to the intensity of postoperative pain and variable cure rates there is often a stigma associated with UPPP.

A metaanalysis of the cure rate of UPPP was performed by Sher et al. in 1996. UPPP was found to have a success rate of 39% for curing OSA (46). Unrecognized hypopharyngeal

Table 6 Fujita Classification of Obstructive Regions

Type I palate (normal base of tongue)
Type II palate and base of tongue
Type III base of tongue (normal palate)

Source: From Ref. 28.

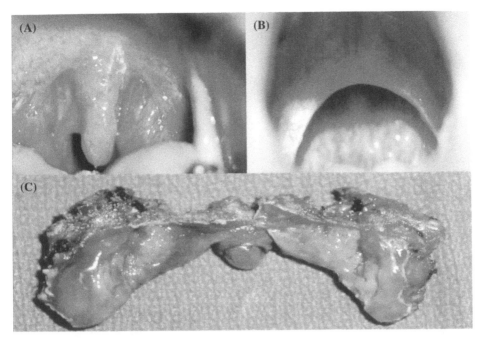

Figure 2 Uvulopalatopharyngoplasty (UPPP). (**A**) Physical exam reveals tonsillar hypertrophy, an elongated uvula, and redundant tissue of the lateral pharyngeal wall resulting in obstruction at the palatal region. (**B**) Postoperative view of the palate following excision of the tonsils, lateral pharyngeal wall mucosa, and soft palate mucosa. Note the markedly widened airway. (**C**) Excised surgical specimen.

obstruction is thought to be the primary reason for such a high failure rate. While capable of improving select patients, UPPP is seldom credited with curing moderate or severe SRBD. In fact, this procedure may be overutilized as an isolated surgical procedure to cure SRBD by those who have failed to identify tongue base obstruction. However, if UPPP is used appropriately or combined with procedures aimed at other anatomical sites of obstruction the results can be much more gratifying.

The indications and rationale for performing the uvulopalatal flap (UPF) are the same as UPPP. However, this flap is contraindicated in patients with excessively long and thick palates. In these patients, the flap created will be too bulky and could potentially eliminate a favorable outcome.

The UPF was introduced by Powell et al. as a modification of the UPPP in 1996 (Figs. 3 and 4). The goal was to reduce the risk of velopharyngeal insufficiency (VPI) and stenosis by using a potentially reversible flap that could be "taken down" early in the recovery period if complications arose. Furthermore, the UPF technique was found to have less postoperative pain on a visual analogue scale, as compared with traditional UPPP. This reduction in pain is due to the fact that no sutures are placed on the free edge of the palate (59). Major complications (myocardial infarction, complete airway obstruction, severe hemorrhage) following UPPP are less than 1.5% (60). Typically, patients complain of postoperative pain and palatal swelling. Voice changes, taste disturbances, and dysphagia have been reported, but are usually transient. Although rare, VPI and nasopharyngeal stenosis are often the result of poor surgical technique. The temptation to maximize results by removing large portions of the palate should be resisted to prevent VPI. Judicious resection of tissue and proper patient selection can aid in preventing these complications.

Mandibular Osteotomy with Genioglossus Advancement

Genioglossus advancement is indicated for patients with documented hypopharyngeal (Table 6) obstruction (Fujita type II–III). Considered part of phase I of the Powell–Riley protocol, it may be used alone or in combination with other procedures depending on the regions of obstruction. The rationale of this surgery is to enlarge the PAS by preventing prolapse of the tongue during sleep.

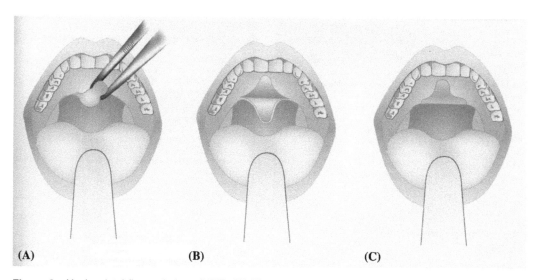

(A)   (B)   (C)

Figure 3 Uvulopalatal flap technique (UPF). (**A**) The mucosal crease is identified by reflecting the uvula. This marks the superior limit of dissection. (**B**) Incision is planned on the lingual aspect of the soft palate. (**C**) Wound is closed with 3-0 Vicryl sutures. These sutures may be removed to release the flap if VPI should occur. *Source:* From Ref. 58.

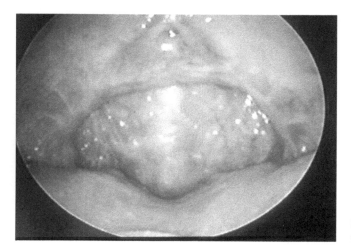

Figure 4 Uvulopalatal flap (UPF). Post-operative view of a UPF.

Essentially, the genial tubercle and the attached genioglossus muscle are advanced anteriorly. This advancement places tension on the tongue musculature and thereby limits posterior displacement during sleep. The degree of advancement is dependent on the thickness of the anterior portion of the mandible and the compliance of the genioglossus muscle. Less muscle compliance will provide a greater degree of tension. Unfortunately, there is no study to determine the compliance of the genioglossus muscle preoperatively. The position of the jaw and dental occlusion remain unchanged. However, a limitation of this surgery is that no additional room is created for the tongue, in contrast to maxillomandibular advancement.

Surgery can be performed under intravenous sedation or general anesthesia. A lateral cephalometric radiograph and a panoramic dental radiograph are required in the preoperative planning. The panoramic radiograph allows the surgeon to identify the genial tubercle and to assess the root length of the mandibular canine and central incisor teeth. Sclerotic bone in the symphyseal region of the mandible aids in locating the genial tubercle. Furthermore, the film should be reviewed for evidence of periodontal disease.

Knowledge of the anatomy is essential to capture the genioglossus muscle fibers within the rectangular osteotomy and to avoid complications. As the muscle's insertion includes the genial tubercle and the lingual surface of the mandible adjacent to the tubercle, the osteotomy must be designed to encompass this region. Thus, the width of the bone fragment should be at least 14 mm and the height about 10 mm (61,62). To avoid injury to the roots of the canine teeth, the vertical osteotomies should be medial to the canine dentition. Careful planning is also required in performing the horizontal osteotomies. The surgeon must be cognizant of the roots of the incisor dentition and the inferior border of the mandible. It is recommended that the superior osteotomy be placed at least 5 mm inferior to the root apices to avoid injury (63). In addition, the inferior osteotomy should be approximately 10 mm above the inferior border of the mandible to prevent a potential fracture.

In 1986, Riley et al. developed the rectangular osteotomy technique (Fig. 5) to advance the genial tubercle for patients with hypopharyngeal obstruction (64). This modification of genioglossus advancement maintained the integrity of the inferior border of the mandible. Subsequently, they evaluated 239 patients who completed phase I surgery and underwent postoperative PSG. Most of these patients had genioglossus advancement with hyoid suspension and UPPP. The overall success rate was 61%. The data was further extrapolated to determine the correlation between disease severity and response rates. Patients with mild disease had a cure rate of 77%, while those with severe disease had a cure rate of 42% (38). Similar results were reported in other studies (43–45,65). In Sher's metaanalysis of patients who only underwent UPPP, the overall responder rate was 39% (46). Thus, it became clear that the addition of genioglossus advancement could substantially increase success rates for treating SRBD.

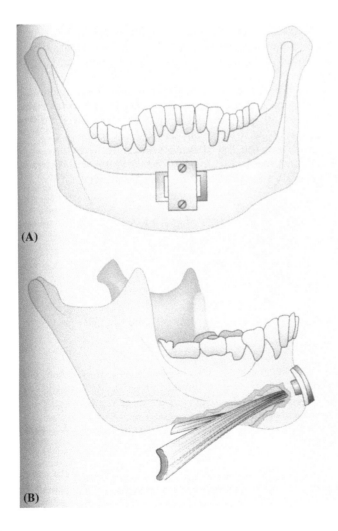

(A)

(B)

Figure 5 Mandibular osteotomy with genioglossus advancement. A rectangular osteotomy is created in the anterior mandible. The genial tubercle and the attached genioglossus muscle are advanced anteriorly. The bony fragment is rotated 90° to overlap the inferior border of the mandible and secured to the mandible with a titanium screw. *Source*: From Ref. 58.

Major complications following genioglossus advancement are uncommon. Obstruction of the airway due to edema or hematoma is the most distressing complication following surgery but it has not been observed in our series. The use of CPAP in the early postoperative period reduces edema and maintains the patency of the airway (66,67). Meticulous hemostasis and aggressive antihypertensive management are critical to prevent hematoma formation. Mild postoperative floor of mouth edema or ecchymosis is common and is usually self-limiting. As previously mentioned, inferior border mandible fractures can occur if the osteotomy is incorrectly designed. This complication has been essentially eliminated by performing a rectangular osteotomy that leaves the inferior border of the mandible intact. Any technique that violates the inferior border increases the risk of a pathologic fracture. Minor complications, such as wound infection, transient anesthesia of the teeth or lower lip, and root injury requiring endodontic therapy have an incidence rate of 2%, 6%, and 1%, respectively, at our center.

Hyoid Myotomy and Suspension

The rationale for hyoid myotomy and suspension is to alleviate hypopharyngeal obstruction by advancing the hyoid complex in an anterior direction. This procedure is considered part of phase I surgery and may be performed as an isolated procedure or in combination with other techniques. The genioglossus and geniohyoid muscles as well as the middle pharyngeal constrictors insert on the hyoid bone. Consequently, the position of the hyoid complex is important in maintaining the integrity of the hypopharyngeal airway. Van de Graaff et al. reported that anterior hyoid advancement improved the PAS in a canine model (68). In 1984, Kaya was the first to demonstrate this concept in human subjects (69).

Currently, we rarely perform hyoid suspension simultaneously with genioglossus advancement. The additional trauma to the hypopharyngeal region can be problematic for the patient to tolerate, and it may prolong recovery. Furthermore, UPPP and genioglossus advancement may have enlarged the PAS, so as to obviate the need for additional surgery. Hyoid myotomy and suspension has become an adjunctive procedure to treat tongue base obstruction for those who previously underwent genioglossus advancement and have evidence of a posteriorly displaced epiglottis.

Originally, this surgery involved suspending the hyoid to the mandible with fascia lata (64). However, this required additional incisions and dissection to harvest the fascia lata and expose the mandible. To reduce the extent of surgery, the technique has been modified to suspend the hyoid bone to the superior border of the thyroid cartilage (42). A single horizontal incision is made at the level of the hyoid. Both the hyoid bone and thyroid cartilage are exposed. The hyoid is advanced anteriorly and secured to the thyroid cartilage with three or four permanent sutures (Fig. 6). Either general or local anesthesia may be utilized (70).

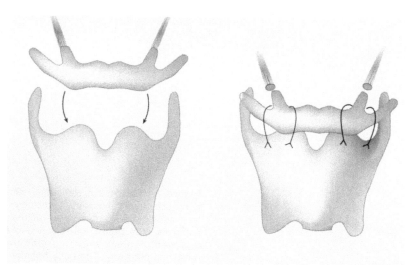

Figure 6 Hyoid myotomy and suspension. The hyoid bone and thyroid cartilage are exposed via a small neck incision. The hyoid bone is advanced anteriorly and secured to the thyroid cartilage with three or four permanent sutures. *Source*: From Ref. 58.

As stated previously, the overall success rate for phase I surgery was 61%. However, the majority of patients underwent genioglossus advancement with hyoid suspension and UPPP (38). Riley and Powell found that hyoid myotomy and suspension improved SRBD and corrected EDS in 75% of consecutively treated patients ($n = 15$) with documented sleep apnea (42). Yet, these patients also had previous genioglossus advancement. Two studies have reviewed the outcomes of patients treated with hyoid suspension alone without concurrent or previous genioglossus advancement for hypopharyngeal obstruction. The success rate from these studies ranged from 17% to 78% (70,71). Our experience has indicated that hyoid suspension is not efficacious as primary treatment for hypopharyngeal obstruction, but rather may be reserved as an adjunctive therapy.

Major complications are exceedingly rare with this surgery. The potential for airway obstruction exists, but this has not been observed at our center. Seroma or hematoma formation are prevented by the insertion of surgical drains for at least 24 hours. Transient aspiration or dysphagia can be observed but usually will resolve within 10 days. If these symptoms persist, removal of the suspension sutures should alleviate this problem (72). Meticulous dissection of the suprahyoid musculature protects vital structures. Specifically, dissection should not extend lateral to the lesser cornu or superior to the upper border of the hyoid to avoid injury to the superior laryngeal nerve and hypoglossal nerve, respectively. Infection can be managed with wound care and antibiotics should it occur.

SURGICAL PROCEDURES—PHASE II

Maxillomandibular Advancement Osteotomy

MMO, also referred to as bimaxillary surgery, is considered phase II of the Powell–Riley two-phase surgical protocol. The rationale for MMO is to ameliorate refractory hypopharyngeal obstruction by advancing the mandible and maxilla forward.

Kuo et al. and Bear and Priest were the first to report the treatment of SRBD with skeletal surgery (73,74). Subjective improvements in SRBD were noted, but there was no postoperative objective data (PSG) to support these claims. Subsequently, our group used PSG to document an improvement in sleep apnea following mandibular advancement (75). Numerous studies have since confirmed these findings (49,76,77).

MMO enlarges both the hypopharyngeal and pharyngeal airway by expanding the skeletal facial framework. It is the only surgery in our protocol that physically creates more space for the tongue in the oral cavity. In addition, it exerts further tension on the velopharyngeal and suprahyoid musculature to prevent their posterior collapse. Advancements of 10 to 15 mm are usually required to adequately clear the PAS of obstruction.

Typically, we reserve MMO for those patients who are incompletely treated with phase I surgery. Some authors have advocated maxillomandibular advancement as primary therapy for hypopharyngeal obstruction, however our experience has demonstrated reasonable response rates with phase I treatment (36,78). Thus, we attempt less invasive surgery prior to MMO surgery.

MMO was originally advocated for patients with maxillomandibular deficiency. However, only approximately 40% of patients with SRBD have contributing craniofacial deficiency (79). Concerns existed that performing MMO in patients without mandibular or maxillary deficiency could create temporomandibular joint dysfunction or unfavorable facial esthetics. Conversely, studies have since proven that MMO is effective in these patients without resulting in these complications. In fact, skeletal facial advancement may impart a more youthful esthetic appearance (80,81).

Maxillomandibular advancement had been used for many years to treat malocclusion. The surgery has undergone several modifications for the treatment of SRBD. The primary modification is a bony advancement of 10 to 15 mm, which tends to be greater than those needed to treat malocclusion. Care must be taken to preserve the descending palatine arteries of the maxilla, and, the dental occlusion should be preserved. This is accomplished by placing arch bars or orthodontic bands prior to the osteotomies. A Le Fort I maxillary osteotomy is performed above the roots of the teeth. The maxilla is down fractured and then advanced anteriorly. Stabilization of the maxilla is accomplished with rigid plate fixation. Mandibular advancement is achieved by a sagittal split osteotomy (Fig. 7). Care is taken to preserve the

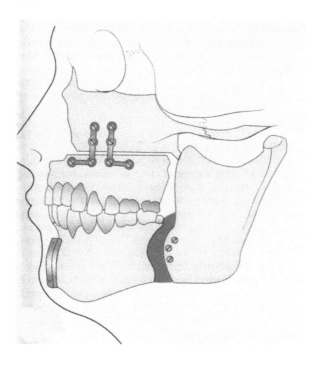

Figure 7 Maxillomandibular advancement osteotomy (MMO). The maxilla and mandible are advanced 10–15 mm. A Lefort I osteotomy and bilateral sagittal split mandibular osteotomy are performed. The advanced segments of bone are stabilized with titanium screws and rigid plate fixation. Note the genioglossus advancement performed prior to MMO. *Source*: From Ref. 58.

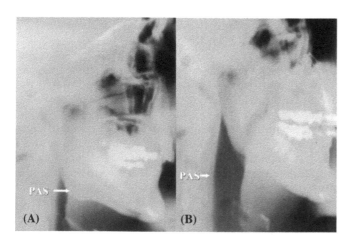

Figure 8 Lateral cephalogram films. This patient underwent both phase I and phase II of the Powell–Riley protocol for SDB. (**A**) Preoperative film. (**B**) Postoperative film—note the markedly widened posterior airway space (PAS).

inferior alveolar nerves. Fixation is maintained by bicortical screws and monocortical plating. Proper alignment of the dental occlusion is needed prior to fixation.

Published data regarding the results of MMO has been well established (47,49,78,82,83). In 1992, we reported 91 patients who underwent bimaxillary surgery. The success rate of phase II therapy was 97% (38). Despite the potential for some skeletal relapse, the long-term success of MMO remains greater than 90% (84). An enlarged PAS can be visualized on postoperative cephalograms (Fig. 8). Ultimately, in order for surgery to be considered efficacious, it must achieve rates of cure similar to CPAP therapy. In 1990, Riley et al. demonstrated no statistical difference between nasal CPAP and surgery in improving sleep architecture and SRBD (85). Consequently, if a logical, stepwise surgical approach is used in treating SRBD patients, cure rates similar to that of medical management can be offered.

As mentioned previously, airway obstruction is the most feared complication following surgery. Risk can be reduced by appropriately utilizing preoperative CPAP and controlling blood pressure (66,67). Necrosis of the palate has been observed as a result of compromised blood supply, although it is quite rare (86). Identifying and protecting the descending palatine vessels can prevent this complication. Skeletal relapse with resulting malocclusion may occur in 15% of patients. This usually does not result in recurrence of SRBD, and can easily be managed with occlusal equilibration. Pain is well controlled with oral analgesics and is not as intense as palatal surgery. Perhaps the most common complaint following MMO surgery is anesthesia or paresthesias of the dentition and perioral region. This symptom is expected in the early recovery period and will resolve within 6 to 12 months for most patients.

ALTERNATIVE TREATMENT OPTIONS FOR PHARYNGEAL RECONSTRUCTION

Temperature-Controlled Radiofrequency of the Palate

Radiofrequency ablation (RF) of tissue has been used extensively in many medical and surgical fields. It has been used to treat Wolfe–Parkinson–White syndrome and benign prostatic hypertrophy (87,88). Powell and Riley adapted this modality to treat redundant tissue of the upper airway in patients with SRBD. Histologic assessments revealed a well-circumscribed lesion with normally healing tissue without damage to peripheral nerves. Volumetric analysis noted an initial inflammatory response that resolved within 48 hours. A 26.3% volumetric reduction of tissue was documented on the tenth postoperative day (89). Based on the positive studies in animal models, RF was attempted on human palates to treat snoring and SRBD. Subsequent trials were then applied to the nasal turbinates and tongue base.

Temperature-controlled radiofrequency (TCRF) has several advantages as compared with traditional techniques when treating SRBD. This procedure is minimally invasive and can be performed on an outpatient basis. Lower temperatures allow for more precise treatment and reduce thermal injury to adjacent tissue. TCRF heats treated tissue from 47°C to 90°C. Electrocautery and laser procedures can heat tissue from 750°C to 900°C. More precise control of thermal energy and limited submucosal tissue injury results in less morbidity without sacrificing efficacy.

Treatment is administered by inserting an electrode probe into the submucosal layer of the tissue to be ablated. Low frequency (465 kHz), low heat electromagnetic energy is administered to denature tissue protein. This region of necrosis is resorbed by the body with resulting volumetric reduction and stiffening of the tissue. By sparing the mucosal layer of tissue, patients experience less postoperative pain.

TCRF treatment of the palate reduced subjective snoring scores by 77% and reduced EDS (90). Multiple studies have demonstrated that TCRF of the palate improves snoring as effectively as other treatment modalities (91–93). Relapse of snoring has been noted at rates similar to those obtained by other treatment protocols (94). However, patients are more likely to undergo repeat RF treatments than more invasive procedures. While outcomes may be similar for different treatment options for snoring, the main advantage RF offers is minimal postoperative pain. Narcotics are usually not required to alleviate pain following TCRF, while they are needed in nearly all patients who undergo UPPP or laser-assisted palatoplasty (95). In fact, ibuprofen is adequate for analgesia after TCRF. Although improvement in SRBD has been documented following TCRF, it is unlikely to cure palatal obstruction as primary therapy. Blumen et al. have demonstrated a significant reduction in RDI following TCRF of the palate in patients with mild to moderate disease (96). It is our experience that, due to the bulk of tissue, which needs to be reduced, TCRF is best utilized as an adjunctive technique to treat palatal obstruction.

TCRF is well tolerated. The incidence of postoperative complications is exceedingly low. A study of the postoperative outcomes demonstrated no major complications and less than a 1% chance of minor complications (97). Mucosal ulceration or sloughing was defined as a minor complication. Airway obstruction, hemorrhage, palatal fistula, and severe dysphagia are potential serious negative outcomes.

PILLAR® PALATAL IMPLANT SYSTEM

The Pillar palatal implant (Restore Medical, Inc., St. Paul, MN) was introduced as a treatment for snoring in 2003. These implants are composed of polyethylene terephthalate (PET). This material is biocompatible and inert resulting in minimal tissue reaction to the implant. The nature of the material allows tissue ingrowth to stabilize the material. Histologic analysis of the implant system indicates that a chronic inflammatory response occurs as a result of PET implantation. Inflammation results in the formation of a fibrous capsule. This process should be complete within four weeks.

The rationale for this procedure is to reduce palatal flutter and snoring by stiffening the soft palate. Implantation of the PET material imparts a degree of rigidity to the palate. Additional stiffening of the palate is achieved by fibrosis and formation of capsule in response to the inflammatory reaction (98).

The procedure is minimally invasive and can be performed in the clinic setting. A handheld applicator is used to insert the PET implants. The palate must have a length >25 mm to be eligible to receive an implant. After the palate is anesthetized, an 18 mm by 1.5 mm implant is placed in the midline above the uvula. The implants should be positioned in the muscular layer of the soft palate. Two additional implants are placed 2 mm lateral to the midline on each side. Postoperative antibiotics are given to prevent infection. Pain can usually be controlled with over-the-counter analgesics (99,100).

The Pillar Implant received U.S. Food and Drug Administration (FDA) clearance for the treatment of snoring and mild to moderate OSA. Initially, this implant was studied to determine its role in eliminating snoring. The outcomes of these studies indicate that the implant system has efficacy and relapse rates similar to other treatment modalities (99–102). However, these studies often excluded patients with OSA and did not always obtain a PSG. More recently, Nordgård evaluated 25 patients with mild to moderate sleep apnea to determine if palatal implants could alleviate SRBD. All patients underwent PSG before and after treatment. Inclusion in the study required an AHI of 10 to 30 and a BMI of ≤30. AHI was reduced from a mean of 16.2 to a mean of 12.1. The AHI was reduced to below 10 in 48% of patients at 90 days postimplant (103).

Mild palatal swelling and pain can occur postoperatively, yet they are transient. Extrusion of the implants is the most common complication. Different rates of extrusion have been noted from 2.7% to 8.8% (99,100). The most feared negative outcome would be aspiration of an extruded implant. This has not been documented in the literature. Surgeon inexperience and short palatal length may increase the incidence of implant extrusion.

Laser-Assisted Uvulopalatoplasty

The rationale and indications for laser-assisted uvulopalatoplasty (LAUP) are the same as for traditional UPPP. However, this surgery was developed as an office-based procedure to treat snoring and SRBD.

The technique attempts to shorten and stiffen the soft palate via a series of carbon dioxide laser incisions. A portion of the uvula is resected and vertical incisions are made lateral to the uvula. Redundant tissue of the lateral pharyngeal may be excised. Local anesthesia is used for this procedure. Walker et al. demonstrated a 48% success rate; however, 21% of patients had worsening of their SRBD following LAUP (104).

LAUP is associated with significant palatal edema and scarring. Furthermore, concerns exist regarding the safety of performing this procedure in the office. Terris et al. noted a fourfold increase in the apnea index and a significant narrowing of the airway at 72 hours following LAUP. These findings prompted them to discourage LAUP in patients with moderate or severe sleep apnea (105). With the advent of less painful techniques, the popularity of LAUP has waned. In fact, a variety of procedures are now available with similar cure rates to treat the palate with less pain and morbidity. Additionally, the American Academy of Sleep Medicine released an evidence-based review in 2000, in which they did not recommend LAUP for the treatment of SRBD (106).

Injection Snoreplasty

Palatal injection sclerotherapy (injection snoreplasty) was introduced as a minimally invasive and inexpensive office procedure that treats palatal flutter snoring. Essentially, a sclerotherapy agent is injected into the submucosal layer of the soft palate to promote fibrosis and scarring (107). Several different sclerotherapy agents have been employed to stiffen the soft palate. The two most commonly used agents are 3% sodium tetradecyl sulfate (sotradecol) and 50% ethanol (108). The average number of injections required to achieve adequate reduction in snoring was 1.2 injections per patient. Exclusion criteria for this modality include comorbid diseases that interfere with wound healing (uncontrolled diabetes, uncontrolled hypothyroidism, and periodontal disease), marked tonsillar hypertrophy, previous surgical procedures for snoring, and significant OSA. Complete cessation or a significant reduction in snoring was reported by 92% of patients or bed partners. However, the rate of snoring relapse was 18% at long-term follow-up (107,109). The success and relapse rates of injection snoreplasty are similar to those of other modalities used to treat snoring (94,110,111).

The primary advantage of injection snoreplasty is the minimal postoperative pain. In fact, most patients experience no interruption in the activities of daily life. This procedure can be performed during a routine office visit. The most common reported complications are palatal swelling and superficial mucosal breakdown. These are managed with observation. Other more serious complications include mucosal ulceration, palatal fistulae, VPI, and anaphylaxis to the agent. This technique has not shown to significantly reduce the RDI (107,109).

ALTERNATIVE TREATMENT OPTIONS FOR HYPOPHARYNGEAL OBSTRUCTION

Genial Bone Advancement Trephine System

The genial bone advancement trephine system (GBAT™) system (Stryker Leibinger Corporation, Kalamazoo, MI) attempts to alleviate tongue base obstruction by advancing the genial tubercle. This system is a modification of the rectangular mandibular osteotomy with genioglossus advancement. The rationale and indications for the GBAT procedure are the same as for traditional genioglossus advancement.

Identification of the genial tubercle is essential to perform the surgery. A circular osteotomy is created in the mandible with the provided trephine (12 mm or 14 mm). The bone segment with the attached genioglossus muscle is advanced and secured to the anterior mandible with a rigid plate (112). The surgeon must ensure that the mandible has sufficient size to accommodate the osteotomy without violating the apices of the tooth roots and the inferior border of the mandible.

As this technique is a simple modification of existing genioglossus advancement, one would expect similar outcomes. Miller et al. studied 35 patients who underwent the GBAT procedure with simultaneous UPPP for SRBD. The RDI and apnea index were reduced by 70%. Furthermore, the lowest oxygen desaturation increased from 80% to 88% and the PAS increased by 4.7 mm. Overall, the cure rate was 67% (112). Studies have demonstrated subjective improvement in SRBD with the GBAT procedure (113). However, long-term objective studies have not documented the success rate of the GBAT technique when used as primary treatment for SRBD.

The GBAT was developed to allow the surgeon to perform an osteotomy with greater ease and speed. While the device is effective in capturing the genial tubercle, there are significant complications (112–114). Major complications have been noted to be as high as 15% (112). These complications include exposure of the hardware, persistent infection, and hematoma of the floor of the mouth requiring drainage. The potential for tooth root injury and pathologic fracture of the mandible exists. Other minor complications noted in traditional genioglossus surgery can occur with the GBAT system. However, the most worrisome complication is avulsion of the genioglossus muscle by the trephine. The circular motion of the trephine places the muscle at greater risk of avulsion as compared with the rectangular osteotomy technique.

While the GBAT system is capable of capturing the genial tubercle and has an acceptable rate of cure, it does not offer a significant advantage versus traditional surgery. Traditional genioglossus osteotomy can be performed in a similar amount of time. Furthermore, the GBAT system lacks the tactile sensation provided by a sagittal saw, which could potentially result in trauma to the floor of the mouth and muscle avulsion. Lastly, once the genioglossus muscle is avulsed, it is exceedingly difficult to salvage the surgery.

Repose™ Genioglossus Advancement Hyoid Myotomy

The Repose (Influent, Inc., San Francisco, California, U.S.) genioglossus advancement hyoid myotomy (GAHM) suspension suture technique is a minimally invasive procedure to treat hypopharyngeal obstruction (115). The concept of the surgery is to place tension on the tissues of the tongue base and/or the hyoid complex by anchoring a suture to the mandible. These sutures are passed through the base of the tongue or the hyoid bone. No tissue is removed and there is minimal dissection. Thus, the procedure can be performed quickly and with less trauma.

The surgery is performed under general anesthesia. A small incision is placed in the floor of the mouth. A screw is then inserted into the lingual surface of the mandible for the tongue procedure. A suture is passed through the base of the tongue and secured to the screw anchored to the mandible. For the hyoid procedure, a screw is inserted into the inferior border of the mandible. A permanent suture attached to the screw is tunneled to the level of the hyoid bone. The suture is passed around the hyoid bone with resulting anterior displacement of the hyoid complex.

The Repose system has been evaluated as primary therapy and in combination with UPPP to treat SRBD. Subjective improvements in snoring and daytime fatigue have been noted. Also, a reduction of the RDI and apnea index with improvement of oxygen saturation was observed. Unfortunately, the overall cure rate was approximately 20% in several studies (116,117).

Mild complications include sialoadenitis (salivary gland inflammation), wound infection, dysphagia, and trauma to the neurovascular bundle of the tongue. In terms of the long-term efficacy of this technique, a significant concern exists whether or not the suture is able to prevent the hypopharyngeal muscles from prolapsing into the PAS.

Temperature-Controlled Radiofrequency of the Tongue

TCRF applied to the tongue has been shown to improve the RDI; however, the results have varied (118,119). While TCRF may have a role as primary therapy for mild SRBD or UARS, we consider this to be an adjunctive therapy for most patients. Similar to the palate and turbinates, TCRF of the tongue can be performed in the office. However, most patients will require multiple treatments. Thus, therapy can be extended over several months. However, this protocol is intended to prevent complications associated with delivering large amounts of energy to the tongue in a single treatment.

Complications are extremely uncommon and are similar to those of other sites treated with TCRF. If performed properly, this procedure is safe and offers promising outcomes for patients.

Midline Glossectomy and Lingualplasty

Midline glossectomy (MLG) has been used for many years to treat macroglossia. However, this procedure is quite invasive and results in significant postoperative pain. In addition, many patients require a tracheotomy to protect their airway as a result of massive tongue edema. Thus, patients are reluctant to undergo this surgery.

A variation of traditional glossectomy surgery is the laser glossectomy and lingualplasty described by Woodson and Fujita (120). They reported a 77% responder rate using the criteria of a postoperative RDI less than 20. Despite these encouraging results, a complication rate of 27% was noted. Other transcervical submucosal approaches have been developed to resect a portion of the tongue base (121). However, these procedures can be complicated and require extensive dissection. Typically, these surgeries require placement of a tracheotomy tube and thus meet patient resistance.

AIRWAY BYPASS SURGERY

Tracheotomy

Tracheotomy was once the only treatment available for SRBD. By creating an external opening in the trachea, the obstructing tissue of the upper airway was bypassed. This provided immediate resolution of airway obstruction during sleep. However, tracheotomy is poorly accepted by patients. This prompted a search for site-specific surgical procedures. In addition, the advent of CPAP provided a nonsurgical method to prevent upper airway obstruction. The efficacy of CPAP has markedly reduced the number of patients needing tracheotomy (51).

Yet, indications still exist for the insertion of a tracheotomy tube. A tracheotomy should be inserted when there is a need to secure an airway prior to a multiphased protocol. Furthermore, it should be considered in morbidly obese patients with severe SRBD and an oxygen desaturation below 70%, especially in those who cannot tolerate CPAP. Patients with significant cardiac disease may not be able to tolerate hypoxemia following surgery; thus a tracheotomy may be warranted. A tracheotomy may be temporary if the upper airway is subsequently reconstructed to alleviate obstruction.

CONCLUSIONS

A multidisciplinary approach is indicated for the optimal management of patients with SRBD. Although CPAP is considered first-line treatment, a referral for a surgical evaluation should be offered to patients, especially in those struggling to tolerate nasal CPAP. It is the obligation of the surgeon to educate a patient regarding complications and expected efficacy. Patients should have a realistic expectation of outcomes. Armed with this knowledge, a patient can make an informed decision regarding their care.

Surgery can achieve long-term cure rates similar to nasal CPAP (85). A systematic evaluation of each patient and a rationale stepwise surgical approach are necessary to produce these outcomes. While not all procedures have similar outcomes, new technology is evolving to offer less invasive options to patients.

REFERENCES

1. Schwab RJ, Kuna ST, Remmers JE. Anatomy and physiology of upper airway obstruction. In: Kryger MH, Roth T, Dement WC, eds. Principles and Practices of Sleep Medicine. 4th ed. Philadelphia: Elsevier Saunders, 2005:983–1000.
2. American Academy of Sleep Medicine. Sleep related breathing disorders in adults: recommendations for syndrome definition and measurement techniques in clinical research. Sleep 1999; 22: 667–689.
3. Kales A, Cadieux RJ, Bixler EO, et al. Severe obstructive sleep apnea. I: onset, clinical course, and characteristics. J Chron Dis 1985; 38(5):419–425.
4. Kuhlo W, Doll E, Franck MD. Erfolgreiche behandlung eines Pickwick syndroms durch eine dauertrachekanuele. Dtsch Med Wochenschr 1969; 94:1286–1290.
5. Harman EM, Wynne JW, Block AJ. The effect of weight loss on sleep-disordered breathing and oxygen saturation in morbidly obese men. Chest 1982; 82(3):291–294.
6. Guilleminault C. Weight loss in sleep apnea. Chest 1989; 96(3):703–704.
7. Rubinstein I, Colapinto N, Rotstein L, et al. Improvement in upper airway function after weight losss in patients with obstructive sleep apnea. Am Rev Respir Dis 1988; 138(5):1192–1195.
8. Cartwright RD, Lloyd S, Lilie J, et al. Sleep position training as treatment for sleep apnea syndrome: a preliminary study. Sleep 1985; 8(2):87–94.
9. Issa FG, Sullivan CE. Alcohol, snoring and sleep apnea. J Neurol Neurosurg Psychiatry 1982; 45(4): 353–359.
10. Sullivan CE, Issa FG, Berthon-Jones M, et al. Reversal of obstructive sleep apnea by continuous positive airway pressure applied through the nares. Lancet 1981; 1(8225):862–865.
11. Ballestar E, Badia JR, Hernandez L, et al. Evidence of the effectiveness of CPAP in the treatment of sleep apnea/hypopnea syndrome. Am J Respir Crit Care Med 1999; 159(5 pt 1):495–501.
12. Sin DD, Mayers I, Man GC, et al. Long-term compliance rates of CPAP in obstructive sleep apnea: a population-based study. Chest 2002; 121(2):430–435.
13. Means MK, Edinger JD, Husain AM. CPAP compliance in sleep apnea patients with and without laboratory CPAP titration. Sleep Breath 2004; 8(1):7–14.
14. He J, Kryger M, Zorick T, et al. Mortality and apnea index in obstructive sleep apnea: experience in 385 male patients. Chest 1998; 94(1):9–14.
15. Dyugovskaya L, Lavie P, Lavie L. Increased adhesion molecules expression and production of reactive oxygen species in leukocytes of sleep apnea patients. Am J Respir Crit Care Med 2002; 165(7): 934–939.
16. Dincer HE, O'Neill W. Deleterious effects of sleep-disordered breathing on the heart and vascular system. Respiration 2006; 73(1):124–130.
17. Yaggi HK, Concato J, Kernan WN, et al. Obstructive sleep apnea as a risk factor for stroke and death. N Engl J Med 2005; 353(19):2034–2041.
18. Powell NB, Riley RW, Guilleminault C. Surgical management of sleep-disordered breathing. In: Kryger MH, Roth T, Dement WC, eds. Principles and Practices of Sleep Medicine. 4th ed. Philadelphia: Elsevier Saunders, 2005:1081–1097.

19. Mickelson SA. Patient selection for surgery. In: Terris DJ, Goode RL, eds. Surgical Management of Sleep Apnea and Snoring. Boca Raton: Taylor & Francis, 2005:223–232.
20. Riley R, Guilleminault C, Powell NB, et al. Palatopharyngoplasty failure, cephalometric roentgenograms, and obstructive sleep apnea. Otolaryngol Head Neck Surg 1985; 93(2):240–244.
21. Shepard J, Gefter W, Guilleminault C, et al. Evaluation of the upper airway in patients with obstructive sleep apnea. Sleep 1991; 14(4):361–371.
22. Rivlin J, Hoffstein V, Kalbfleisch J, et al. Upper airway morphology in patients with idiopathic obstructive sleep apnea. Am Rev Respir Dis 1984; 129(3):355–360.
23. Rojewski TE, Schuller DE, Clark RW, et al. Videoendoscopic determination of the mechanism of obstruction in obstructive sleep apnea. Otolaryngol Head Neck Surg 1984; 92(2):127–131.
24. Remmers JE, DeGrott WJ, Sauerland EK, et al. Pathogenesis of upper airway occlusion during sleep. J Appl Physiol 1978; 44(6):931–938.
25. Olsen K, Kern E, Westbrook P. Sleep and breathing disturbance secondary to nasal obstruction. Otolaryngol Head Neck Surg 1981; 89(5):804–810.
26. Mallampati SR, Gatt SP, Gugino LD, et al. A clinical sign to predict difficult tracheal intubation: a prospective study. Can Anaesth Soc J 1985; 32(4):429–434.
27. Friedman M, Ibrahim H, Joseph NJ. Staging of obstructive sleep apnea/hypopnea syndrome: a guide to appropriate treatment. Laryngoscope 2004; 114(3):454–459.
28. Fujita S. Pharyngeal surgery for obstructive sleep apnea and snoring. In: Fairbanks D, Fujita S, Ikematsu T, et al., eds. Snoring and Obstructive Sleep Apnea. New York: Raven Press, 1987:101–128.
29. Fujita S, Conway W, Zorick F, et al. Surgical correction of anatomical abnormalities in obstructive sleep apnea syndrome: uvulopalatopharyngoplasty. Otolaryngol Head Neck Surg 1981; 89(6):923–934.
30. Sher AE, Thorpy MJ, Shrintzen RJ, et al. Predictive value of Müller maneuver in selection of patient for uvulopalatopharyngoplasty. Laryngoscope 1985; 95(12):1483–1487.
31. Riley R, Guilleminault C, Herran J, et al. Cephalometric analyses and flow volume loops in obstructive sleep apnea patients. Sleep 1983; 6(4):303–311.
32. Ikeda K, Ogura M, Oshima T, et al. Quantitative assessment of the pharyngeal airway by dynamic magnetic resonance imaging in obstructive sleep apnea syndrome. Ann Otol Rhinol Laryngol 2001; 110(2):183–189.
33. Welch KC, Foster GD, Ritter CT, et al. A novel volumetric magnetic resonance imaging paradigm to study upper airway anatomy. Sleep 2002; 25(5):532–542.
34. Shepard JW, Stanson AW, Sheedy PF, et al. Fast-CT evaluation of the upper airway during wakefulness in patients with obstructive sleep apnea. Prog Clin Biol Res 1990; 345:273–279.
35. Riley R, Powell N, Guilleminault C. Cephalometric roentgenograms and computerized tomographic scans in obstructive sleep apnea. Sleep 1986; 9(4):514–515.
36. Riley R, Powell N, Guilleminault C, et al. Obstructive sleep apnea syndrome: a surgical protocol for dynamic upper airway reconstruction. J Oral Maxillofac Surg 1993; 51(7):742–747.
37. Powell NB, Riley RW, Robinson A. Surgical management of obstructive sleep apnea syndrome. Clin Chest Med 1998; 19(1):77–86.
38. Riley R, Powell N, Guilleminault C. Obstructive sleep apnea syndrome: a review of 306 consecutively treated surgical patients. Otolaryngol Head Neck Surg 1993; 108(2):117–125.
39. Riley RW, Powell NB. Maxillofacial surgery and obstructive sleep apnea syndrome. Otolaryngol Clin N Am 1990; 23(4):809–826.
40. Powell NB, Riley RW. A surgical protocol for sleep disordered breathing. Oral Maxillofac Surg Clin North Am 1995; 7(2):345–356.
41. Riley R, Powell N, Guilleminault C. Inferior mandibular osteotomy and hyoid myotomy suspension for obstructive sleep apnea: a review of 55 patients. J Oral Maxillomaxfac Surg 1989; 47(2):159–164.
42. Riley R, Powell N, Guilleminault C. Obstructive sleep apnea and the hyoid: a revised surgical procedure. Otolaryngol Head Neck Surg 1994; 111(6):717–721.
43. Ramirez SG, Loube DI. Inferior sagittal osteotomy with hyoid bone suspension for obese patients with sleep apnea. Arch Otolaryngol Head Neck Surg 1996; 122(9):953–957.
44. Johnson NT, Chinn J. Uvulopalatopharyngoplasty and inferior sagittal mandibular osteotomy with genioglossus advancement for treatment of obstructive sleep apnea. Chest 1994; 105(1):278–283.
45. Lee N, Givens C, Wilson J, et al. Staged surgical treatment of obstructive sleep apnea syndrome: a review of 35 patients. J Oral Maxillofac Surg 1999; 57(4):382–385.
46. Sher AE, Schechtman KB, Piccirillo JF. The efficacy of surgical modifications of the upper airway in adults with obstructive sleep apnea syndrome. Sleep 1996; 19(2):156–177.
47. Waite PD, Wooten V, Lachner J, et al. Maxillomandibular advancement surgery in 23 patients with obstructive sleep apnea syndrome. J Oral Maxillofac Surg 1989; 47(12):1256–1261.
48. Hochban W, Brandenburg U, Hermann PJ. Surgical treatment of obstructive sleep apnea by maxillomandibular advancement. Sleep 1994; 17(7):624–629.
49. Hochban W, Conradt R, Brandenburg U, et al. Surgical maxillofacial treatment of obstructive sleep apnea. Plast Reconstr Surg 1997; 99(3):619–626.

50. McConkey P. Postobstructive pulmonary oedema—a case series and review. Anaesth Intensive Care 2000; 28(1):72–76.
51. Powell N, Riley R, Guilleminault C, et al. Obstructive sleep apnea, continuous positive airway pressure, and surgery. Otolaryngol Head Neck Surg 1988; 99(4):362–369.
52. Olsen K. The role of nasal surgery in the treatment of obstructive sleep apnea. Otolaryngol Head Neck Surg 1991; 2(5):63–68.
53. Hoijer U, Ejnell H, Hedner J, et al. The effects of nasal dilatation on snoring and obstructive sleep apnea. Arch Otolaryngol Head Neck Surg 1992; 118(3):281–284.
54. Powell N, Zonato A, Weaver E, et al. Radiofrequency treatment of turbinate hypertrophy in subjects using continuous positive airway pressure: a randomized, double-blind, placebo-controlled clinical pilot trial. Laryngoscope 2001; 111(10):1783–1790.
55. Utley DS, Goode RL, Hakim I. Radiofrequency energy tissue ablation for the treatment of nasal obstruction secondary to turbinate hypertrophy. Laryngoscope 1999; 109(5):683–686.
56. Passali D, Lauriello M, Anselmi M, et al. Treatment of hypertrophy of the inferior turbinate: long-term results in 382 patients randomly assigned to therapy. Ann Otol Rhinol Laryngol 1999; 108 (6):569–575.
57. Ikematsu T. Study of snoring, 4th report: therapy [in Japanese]. Jpn Otorhinolaryngol 1964; 64:434–435.
58. Troell RJ, Powell NB, Riley RW. Hypopharyngeal airway surgery for obstructive sleep apnea syndrome. Semin Respir Crit Care Med 1998; 19(2):175–183.
59. Powell NB, Riley RW, Guilleminault C, et al. A reversible uvulopalatal flap for snoring and obstructive sleep. Sleep 1996; 19(17):593–599.
60. Kezirian EJ, Weaver EM, Yueh B, et al. Incidence of serious complications after uvulopalatopharyngoplasty. Laryngoscope 2004; 114(3):450–453.
61. Mintz SM, Ettinger AC, Geist JR, et al. Anatomic relationship of the genial tubercles to the dentition as determined by cross-sectional tomography. J Oral Maxillofac Surg 1995; 53(11):1324–1326.
62. Silverstein K, Costello BJ, Giannakpoulos H, et al. Genioglossus muscle attachments: an anatomic analysis and the implications for genioglossus advancement. Oral Surg Oral Med Oral Pathol Oral Radiol Endod 2000; 90(6):686–688.
63. McBride KL, Bell WH. Chin surgery. In: Bell WH, Proffit WR, White RP, eds. Surgical Correction of Dentofacial Deformities. 1st ed. Philadelphia: WB Saunders, 1980:1210–1281.
64. Riley R, Powell N, Guilleminault C. Inferior sagittal osteotomy of the mandible with hyoid myotomy-suspension: a new procedure for obstructive sleep apnea. Otolaryngol Head Neck Surg 1986; 94(5):589–593.
65. Yoa M, Utlet D, Terris D. Cephalometric parameters after multi-level pharyngeal surgery for patients with obstructive sleep apnea. Laryngoscope 1998; 108(6):789–795.
66. Riley RW, Powell NB, Guilleminault C, et al. Obstructive sleep apnea surgery: Risk management and complications. Otolaryngol Head Neck Surg 1997; 117(6):648–652.
67. Li KK, Powell N, Riley R. Postoperative management of the obstructive sleep apnea patient. Oral Maxillofacial Surg Clin N Am 2002; 14:401–404.
68. Van de Graaff W, Gottfried S, Mitra J, et al. Respiratory function of hyoid muscles and hyoid arch. J Appl Physiol 1984; 57(1):197–204.
69. Kaya N. Sectioning the hyoid bone as a therapeutic approach for obstructive sleep apnea. Sleep 1984; 7(1):77–78.
70. Neruntarat C. Hyoid myotomy with suspension under local anesthesia for obstructive sleep apnea syndrome. Eur Arch Otorhinolaryngol 2003; 260(5):286–290.
71. Bowden MT, Kezirian EJ, Utley D, et al. Outcomes of hyoid suspension for the treatment of obstructive sleep apnea. Arch Otolaryngol Head Neck Surg 2005; 131(5):440–445.
72. Li KK, Riley R, Powell N. Complications of obstructive sleep apnea surgery. Oral Maxilllofacial Surg Clin N Am 2003; 15:297–304.
73. Kuo PC, West RA, Bloomquist DS. The effect of mandibular osteotomy in three patients with hypersomnia and sleep apnea. Oral Surg Oral Med Oral Pathol 1979; 48(5):385–392.
74. Bear SE, Priest JH. Sleep apnea syndrome: correction with surgical advancement of the mandible. J Oral Surg 1980; 38(7):543–549.
75. Powell NB, Guilleminault C, Riley RW, et al. Mandibular advancement and obstructive sleep apnea syndrome. Bull Eur Physiopathol Respir 1983; 19(6):607–610.
76. Conradt R, Hochban W, Bradenburg U, et al. Long-term follow-up after surgical treatment of obstructive sleep apnoea by maxillomandibular advancement. Eur Respir J 1997; 10(1):123–128.
77. Smatt Y, Ferri J. Retrospective study of 18 patients treated by maxillomandibular advancement with adjunctive procedures for obstructive sleep apnea syndrome. J Craniofac Surg 2005; 16(5):770–777.
78. Prinsell JR. Maxillomandibular advancement surgery in a site-specific treatment approach for obstructive sleep apnea in 50 consecutive patients. Chest 1999; 116(6):1503–1506.
79. Hochban W, Brandenburg U. Morphology of the viscerocranium in obstructive sleep apnoea syndrome—cephalometric evaluation of 400 patients. J Craniomaxillofac Surg 1994; 22(4):205–213.

80. Li KK, Riley RW, Powell NB, et al. Maxillomandibular advancement for persistent obstructive sleep apnea after phase I surgery in patients without maxillomandibular deficiency. Laryngoscope 2000; 110(10 Pt 1):1684–1688.

81. Li KK, Riley RW, Powell NB, et al. Patient's perception of the facial appearance after maxillomandibular advancement for obstructive sleep apnea syndrome. J Oral Maxillofac Surg 2001; 59(2):377–380.

82. Riley R, Powell N, Guilleminault C. Maxillofacial surgery and obstructive sleep apnea: a review of 80 patients. Otolaryngol Head Neck Surg 1989; 101(3):353–361.

83. Bettega G, Pepin J, Veale D, et al. Obstructive sleep apnea syndrome: fifty-one consecutive patients treated by maxillofacial surgery. Am J Crit Care Med 2000; 162(2 pt 1):641–649.

84. Riley R, Powell N, Li K, et al. Surgery and obstructive sleep apnea: Long-term clinical outcomes. Otolaryngol Head Neck Surg 2000; 122(3):415–421.

85. Riley RW, Powell NB, Guilleminault C. Maxillofacial surgery and nasal CPAP: a comparison of treatment for obstructive sleep apnea syndrome. Chest 1990; 98(6):1421–1425.

86. Lanigan DT, Hey JH, West RA. Aseptic necrosis following maxillary osteotomies: report of 36 cases. J Oral Maxillofac Surg 1990; 48(2):142–156.

87. Issa M, Oesterling J. Transurethral needle ablation (TUNA): an overview of radiofrequency thermal therapy for the treatment of benign prostatic hyperplasia. Curr Opin Urol 1996; 6:20–27.

88. Jackman WM, Wang XZ, Friday KJ, et al. Catheter ablation of accessory atrioventricular pathways (Wolfe–Parkinson–White syndrome) by radiofrequency current. N Engl J Med 1991; 324(23): 1605–1611.

89. Powell NB, Riley RW, Troell RJ, et al. Radiofrequency volumetric reduction of the tongue: a porcine pilot study for the treatment of obstructive sleep apnea syndrome. Chest 1997; 111(5):1348–1355.

90. Powell NB, Riley RW, Troell RJ, et al. Radiofrequency volumetric tissue reduction of the palate in subjects with sleep-disordered breathing. Chest 1998; 113(5):1163–1174.

91. Wedman J, Miljeteig H. Treatment of simple snoring using radiowaves for ablation of uvula and soft palate: a day-case surgery procedure. Laryngoscope 2002; 112(7 pt 1):1256–1259.

92. Johnson J, Pollack G, Wagner R. Transoral radiofrequency treatment of snoring. Otolaryngol Head Neck Surg 2002; 127(3):235–237.

93. Stuck BA, Maurer JT, Hein G, et al. Radiofrequency surgery of the soft palate in the treatment of snoring: a review of the literature. Sleep 2004; 27(3):551–555.

94. Li KK, Powell NB, Riley RW, et al. Radiofrequency volumetric reduction of the palate: an extended follow-up study. Otolaryngol Head Neck Surg 2000; 122(3):410–414.

95. Troell RJ, Powell NB, Riley RW, et al. Comparison of postoperative pain between laser-assisted uvulopalatoplasty, uvulopalatopharyngoplasty, and radiofrequency volumetric tissue reduction of the palate. Otolaryngol Head Neck Surg 2000; 122(3):402–409.

96. Blumen M, Dahan S, Fleury B, et al. Radiofrequency ablation for the treatment of mild to moderate obstructive sleep apnea. Laryngoscope 2002; 112(11):2086–2092.

97. Kezirian EJ, Powell NB, Riley RW, et al. Incidence of complications in radiofrequency of the upper airway. Laryngoscope 2005; 115(7):1298–1304.

98. Friedman M, Ramakrishnan V, Bliznikas D, et al. Patient selection and efficacy of Pillar implant technique for treatment of snoring and obstructive sleep apnea/hypopnea syndrome. Otolaryngol Head Neck Surg 2006; 134(2):187–196.

99. Romanow JH, Catalano PJ. Initial U.S. pilot study: palatal implants for the treatment of snoring. Otolaryngol Head Neck Surg 2006; 134(4):551–557.

100. Nordgård S, Stene BK, Skjøstad KW, et al. Palatal implants for the treatment of snoring: Long-term results. Otolaryngol Head Neck Surg 2006; 134(4):558–564.

101. Ho WK, Wei WI, Chung KF. Managing disturbing snoring with palatal implants. A pilot study. Arch Otolaryngol Head Neck Surg 2004; 130(6):753–758.

102. Nordgård S, Wormdal K, Bugten V, et al. Palatal implants: a new method for the treatment of snoring. Acta Otolaryngol 2004; 124(8):970–975.

103. Nordgård S, Stene BK, Skjøstad KW. Soft palate implants for the treatment of mild to moderate obstructive sleep apnea. Otolaryngol Head Neck Surg 2006; 134(4):565–570.

104. Walker RP, Grigg-Damberger MM, Gopalsami C, et al. Laser-assisted uvulopalatoplasty for snoring and obstructive sleep apnea: results in 170 patients. Laryngoscope 1995; 105(9 pt 1):938–943.

105. Terris DJ, Clerk AA, Norbash AM, et al. Characterization of post-operative edema following laser-assisted uvulopalatoplasty using MRI and polysomnography: implication for the outpatient treatment of obstructive sleep apnea syndrome. Laryngoscope 1996; 106(2 Pt 1):124–128.

106. Littner M, Kushida CA, Hartse K, et al. Practice parameters for the use of laser-assisted uvulopalatoplasty: an update for 2000. Sleep 2001; 24(5):603–619.

107. Brietzke SE, Mair EA. Injection snoreplasty: how to treat snoring without all the pain and expense. Otolaryngol Head Neck Surg 2001; 124(5):503–510.

108. Brietzke SE, Mair EA. Injection snoreplasty: investigation of alternative sclerotherapy agents. Otolaryngol Head Neck Surg 2004; 130(1):47–57.

109. Brietzke SE, Mair EA. Injection snoreplasty: extended follow-up and new objective data. Otolaryngol Head Neck Surg 2003; 128(5):605–615.

110. Levin BC, Becker GD. Uvulopalatopharyngoplasty for snoring: long term results. Laryngoscope 1994; 104(9):1150–1152.

111. Wareing MJ, Callanan VP, Mitchell DB. Laser assisted uvuloplasty: six and eighteen month results. J Laryngol Otol 1998; 112(7):639–641.

112. Miller FR, Watson D, Boseley M. The role of the Genial Bone Advancement Trephine system in conjunction with uvulopalatopharyngoplasty in the multilevel management of obstructive sleep apnea. Otolaryngol Head Neck Surg 2004; 130(1):73–79.

113. Lewis MR, Ducic Y. Genioglossus muscle advancement with the genioglossus bone advancement technique for base of tongue obstruction. J Otolaryngol 2003; 32(3):168–173.

114. Hennessee J, Miller FR. Anatomic analysis of the Genial Bone Advancement Trephine System's effectiveness at capturing the genial tubercle and its muscular attachments. Otolaryngol Head Neck Surg 2005; 133(2):229–233.

115. DeRowe A, Gunther E, Fibbi A, et al. Tongue-base suspension with a soft tissue-to-bone anchor for obstructive sleep apnea: preliminary clinical results of a new minimally invasive technique. Otolaryngol Head Neck Surg 2000; 122(1):100–103.

116. Miller FR, Watson D, Malis D. Role of the tongue base suspension suture with the repose system bone screw in the multilevel surgical management of obstructive sleep apnea. Otolaryngol Head Neck Surg 2002; 126(4):392–398.

117. Woodson BT. A tongue suspension suture for obstructive sleep apnea and snorers. Otolaryngol Head Neck Surg 2001; 124(3):297–303.

118. Li K, Powell N, Riley R, et al. Temperature-controlled radiofrequency tongue base reduction for sleep-disordered breathing: long-term outcomes. Otolaryngol Head Neck Surg 2002; 127(3):230–234.

119. Stuck B, Maurer J, Verse T, et al. Tongue base reduction with temperature controlled radiofrequency volumetric tissue reduction for treatment of obstructive sleep apnea syndrome. Acta Otolaryngol 2002; 122(5):531–536.

120. Woodson BT, Fujita S. Clinical experience with lingualplasty as part of the treatment of severe obstructive sleep apnea. Otolaryngol Head Neck Surg 1992; 107(1):40–48.

121. Chabolle F, Wagner I, Blumen MB, et al. Tongue base reduction with hyoepiglottoplasty: a treatment for severe obstructive sleep apnea. Laryngoscope 1999; 109(8):1273–1280.

33 | Oral Appliance Treatment of Sleep-Related Breathing Disorders

Aarnoud Hoekema

Department of Oral and Maxillofacial Surgery, University Medical Center Groningen, University of Groningen, Groningen, The Netherlands

Marie Marklund

Department of Orthodontics, Faculty of Medicine, Umeå University, Umeå, Sweden

Dental devices represent a common alternative for patients with sleep-related breathing disorders (SRBD), who are unsuitable candidates for treatment with continuous positive airway pressure (CPAP) (1). These intraoral devices, commonly known as oral appliances, aim at relieving upper airway obstruction and snoring by modifying the position of the mandible, tongue, and other oropharyngeal structures. Oral appliance treatment of SRBD has gained considerable popularity because of its simplicity and supposed reversibility. In 1902, the French physician Pierre Robin laid the foundation for oral appliance therapy. With a "monobloc" appliance, Robin treated children who suffered from breathing difficulties and glossoptosis due to hypoplasia of the mandible (2). The first case of an oral appliance that repositioned the mandible in an adult patient with obstructive sleep apnea (OSA) was not reported until 1980 (3). The first patient series of oral appliance therapy for OSA was reported in 1982 and described the effects of an appliance that repositioned the tongue (4). Currently, well over 60 different oral appliances are marketed for the treatment of snoring and OSA (5).

TYPES OF ORAL APPLIANCES

On the basis of their mode of action, oral appliances may be roughly divided into tongue-retaining appliances and mandibular repositioning appliances (MRAs). Palatal lifting devices, tongue posture trainers, and labial shields represent other types of oral appliances for SRBD, although these are rarely used because of poor efficacy and patient discomfort (6–8). Tongue-retaining appliances reposition the tongue in an anterior position by securing it with negative pressure in a soft plastic bulb or with a plastic depressor that directly contacts the base of the tongue. Large-scale application of these appliances is, however, generally hampered by discomfort and poor results (5). MRAs are used most commonly in clinical practice, and the quantity and quality of scientific literature supporting their use are far greater than that for the other types of oral appliances (1,5). This chapter will focus on the application of MRAs as oral appliances for the treatment of SRBD.

MRAs are either of a one-piece ("monobloc") (Fig. 1A) or a two-piece ("bibloc") design (Fig. 1B, C) and may be custom-made or prefabricated (5). A prefabricated MRA requires only individual molding of a thermolabile material, while custom-made appliances necessitate dental impressions, bite registration, and fabrication by a dental laboratory. Retention for an MRA in upper and lower dentition is provided by clasps, acrylic or thermoplastic polymer embedded in the appliance (10). A one-piece MRA rigidly fixes the mandible in an anterior position, whereas a two-piece MRA usually allows for some freedom of mandibular movement (i.e., lateral, vertical, or anterior). This latter feature has been suggested to decrease the chance of temporomandibular disorders and improve comfort (11). Two-piece MRAs are sagittally adjustable, thereby allowing for individual titration of the appliance and a more optimal degree of mandibular advancement (12). Conversely, fixation of the mandible with a one-piece appliance is suggested to prevent suppression of tongue-protruding muscles, resulting in a less collapsible upper airway during sleep (13). Studies comparing different custom-made one-piece and two-piece MRAs in patients with OSA did not demonstrate significant differences in physiological outcomes (5,14). However, one study has shown that a prefabricated one-piece MRA is not as effective as a custom-made MRA in improving physiological outcomes in OSA

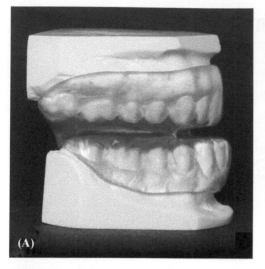

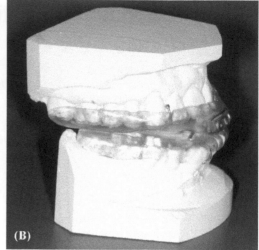

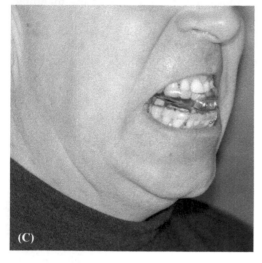

Figure 1 Lateral views of one-piece and two-piece mandibular repositioning appliances. (**A**) One-piece appliance placed on plaster casts. (**B**) Upper and lower parts of two-piece appliance placed on plaster casts. (**C**) Intraoral view of a patient wearing the two-piece appliance. *Source*: Figure 1B, C adapted from Ref. 9.

treatment (15). Another feature in MRA design is the degree of bite opening imposed by the appliance. Fluoroscopic recordings suggest that bite opening should be kept to a minimum since it results in posterior movement of both tongue and soft palate (16). Conversely, bite opening has been suggested to improve upper airway patency by increasing genioglossus muscle activity and stretching the pharyngeal musculature (13,17). One randomised study that evaluated the effect of different degrees of bite opening in MRA therapy could not demonstrate any differences in physiological or subjective outcomes (18). It appears that despite the considerable variations in MRA design, physiological effects of different types of custom-made oral appliances that reposition the mandible are remarkably consistent. Appliance design may, however, influence therapeutic efficacy by affecting the patient's preference or subjective outcomes (5).

MECHANISM OF ACTION

Forward displacement of the mandible in oral appliance therapy appears to prevent snoring and airway obstruction by indirectly moving the suprahyoid and genioglossal muscles anteriorly. It has also been suggested that forward and inferior displacement of the mandible decreases the gravitational effect on the tongue and preserves the velopharyngeal airway by stretching the palatoglossal and palatopharyngeal arches (5). Moreover, stabilization of the mandible and hyoid bone prevents posterior rotation of the mandible and retrolapse of

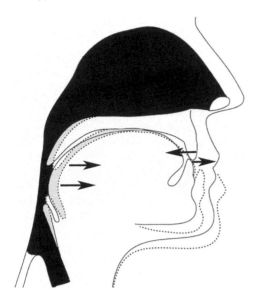

Figure 2 Illustration of the increase in upper airway dimensions following repositioning of the mandible with oral appliance therapy. The arrows on the teeth indicate the reciprocal forces that are generated by holding the mandible in a forward and vertically opened position. These forces transmit in a labial direction against the lower incisors and in a palatal direction against the upper incisors. In the long term, this may change the inclination and position of teeth, affect the position of the mandible, and increase the loading of the craniomandibular complex.

the tongue during sleep (7). Three-dimensional imaging and cephalometric studies have demonstrated that mandibular repositioning increases hypo-, oro-, and velopharyngeal airway dimensions (Fig. 2) (5,19,20). Endoscopic and computerized tomography studies have shown that mandibular advancement results particularly in an increased cross section of the lateral dimensions in the oro- and velopharynx (5,21). It has also been demonstrated that mandibular advancement has a positive effect on airflow dynamics in the upper airway during sleep by diminishing airway curvature in the velopharynx (22). Beside anatomical changes, the mechanism of action in MRA therapy has also been attributed to changes in neuromuscular properties of the upper airway. For example, both mandibular rotation and advancement have been implicated in an increased muscle activity of the upper airway (5,17). Because of conflicting results and the fact that most imaging studies have been performed in the wake state, the precise mechanism of action in oral appliance therapy remains undefined.

Titration Procedures
Controlled studies have demonstrated that an oral appliance derives its therapeutic effect mainly from the amount of mandibular advancement imposed by the appliance (5,23). However, in some OSA patients, the number of upper airway obstructions may increase when the mandible is protruded toward its maximum (7). Determination of the amount of mandibular advancement required to prevent snoring or OSA in a given patient is therefore generally a matter of trial and error. Treatment usually commences with an adaptation period (generally four weeks) that is followed by a titration period (generally two to three months) (1). Titration of the appliance should be aimed at accomplishing the amount of mandibular advancement, which yields a resolution of symptoms with minimum discomfort and side effects. Because a two-piece MRA is in most cases sagittally adjustable, titration is usually more straightforward when compared with a one-piece MRA. However, details of the titration process, including the initial and target degrees of mandibular advancement, are highly variable between different types of appliances and practitioners (1). The need for an acclimatization period is considered a drawback of oral appliance therapy, particularly in situations where rapid initiation of treatment is required (e.g., severe OSA). Studies have reported on the feasibility of a single-night titration of an MRA by using remotely controlled appliances (24,25). This technique may offer the advantage of directly ascertaining the likelihood of treatment success as well as the amount of mandibular advancement required in an individual patient. However, the difficulty of achieving the required mandibular advancement without discomfort on the first night and the laborious character may limit wide-scale application of this technique.

EFFECTIVENESS

On the basis of reports of patients and their bed partners, oral appliance therapy results in an improvement of snoring in a high proportion of patients (9,26). Other reported benefits include substantial improvements in daytime sleepiness, work performance, and sleep quality of both patients and their bed partners (5). Sleep registration generally confirms the patient-perceived benefits by demonstrating improvements in snoring frequency and intensity, apnea-hypopnea index (AHI), oxygen desaturation frequency and intensity, and the number of arousals during sleep (5). Therapy is also associated with significant increases in slow-wave and rapid eye movement sleep. More recent investigations have explored neuropsychological and cardiovascular end points in OSA treatment (27–31). These studies demonstrated significant improvements in vigilance, simulated driving performance, blood pressure, and cardiac function following oral appliance therapy. Despite an unsatisfactory change in the AHI, OSA patients may report fewer symptoms when initiating oral appliance therapy (5). In fact, an increase in the AHI has been reported in approximately 13% of OSA patients following therapy (26).

The overall success rate of oral appliance therapy in OSA patients is reported to be variable and may range from 15% to 88% (1,5,32). Factors including the amount of mandibular advancement and inclusion of OSA patients of different disease severities may account for this variation in reported success (5). Another factor of consideration is that various definitions for treatment success are being used. In OSA patients, oral appliance therapy should be aimed at accomplishing a resolution of symptoms and a normalization of the AHI (i.e., <5) and oxyhemoglobin saturation (33). A literature review published in 2006 identified at least seven different definitions for treatment success in oral appliance therapy (32). To compare different studies, a uniform definition for treatment success is clearly indicated.

Comparison with Other Treatment Modalities

Several studies have compared the effects of an oral appliance with that of an inactive control device in the treatment of OSA. When compared with control devices, oral appliance therapy is clearly more effective in improving the AHI, blood pressure, and other physiological outcomes (5,28,34,35). Variable results are, however, reported in the improvement of symptoms including sleepiness and snoring. These findings have been attributed to factors other than mandibular advancement, such as stimulation of neuromuscular reflexes and changes in the bite relationship, in both oral appliance and control treatment (36). However, one study that used a placebo tablet instead of an inactive control device has demonstrated similar findings (29). These results indicate an important placebo effect when treating patients with oral appliances.

When compared with surgical interventions, oral appliance therapy has been demonstrated to be more effective than uvulopalatopharyngoplasty (UPPP) in patients with mild to moderate OSA (37). Although success rates of both treatments showed a tendency to decrease, oral appliance therapy remained more successful than UPPP after a four-year treatment period (38). However, the number of dropouts in the oral appliance group at the four-year follow-up examination limits the implications of the results from this study. In another study, the effects of an oral appliance of the tongue-retaining type were compared with that of somnoplasty (i.e., radiofrequency tissue reduction) of the soft palate for the treatment of snoring (39). This study did not find any significant difference between these treatments in the percentage of sleep time the patient had loud snoring.

Seven crossover studies have been published that compared the effects of CPAP and oral appliance therapy for the treatment of OSA (5,29). Results from these trials indicate that when considering physiological outcomes like the AHI, CPAP should be preferred over oral appliance therapy. Most of these trials did not observe significant differences in subjective parameters, including the Epworth sleepiness scale, when comparing CPAP and oral appliance therapy. Moreover, changes in sleep quality like the amount of rapid eye movement or slow-wave sleep did not differ between these therapies. Oral appliance therapy is generally more successful in patients with nonsevere OSA (5). Some authors propose oral appliance therapy as a first-line alternative to CPAP in patients with mild to moderate OSA (31,40,41), whereas others obtain superior results with CPAP in this respect (27,42). In most studies, however, patients have a clear preference for oral appliance instead of CPAP therapy (5,29). These results indicate that CPAP therapy is not ideal in the management of all OSA patients.

Long-Term Effects
Studies on the long-term effects of oral appliances in the treatment of OSA suggest high success rates after follow-up periods ranging from two to five years (38,43–45). Approximately 80% of patients who were initially successfully treated also experienced long-term control of their OSA. A slightly lesser percentage of patients also experienced a satisfactory effect on snoring with long-term oral appliance therapy. In the long term, a gradual decline in treatment effect should therefore be anticipated. These numbers, however, also reflect bias, because not all patients originally treated were included in these analyses. Long-term effectiveness of oral appliance therapy in unselected OSA patients is therefore probably lower (1). The main reasons for an attenuation of the treatment effect following an initially successful treatment relate to a failure of maintaining advancement of the mandible in the prescribed position and an increase in body weight during the follow-up period (44,46).

Oral Appliances as Adjuvant Treatment
Although oral appliances have been shown to be effective as sole treatment for SRBD, they may also be used as adjuvants to other therapies. The combined use of CPAP and oral appliance therapy has been suggested as an option in situations where there is a desire to reduce the CPAP pressure to control OSA (1). Oral appliance therapy has also been shown to be highly successful for the treatment of OSA following an unsuccessful UPPP (47). In addition to oral appliances being used in combination with another treatment, they may also be used as predictors for the outcome of other interventions. Oral appliance therapy has been shown to be a good predictor for the outcome of maxillomandibular advancement surgery in OSA patients (48). An MRA may be used to simulate the effects and to allow patients to accustom to the idea of surgical advancement of their mandibular complex. Although there is little evidence that supports the routine use of oral appliances as an adjuvant treatment for SRBD (49), it may offer some potential advantages in selected cases.

Treatment Adherence
Patient-reported adherence with oral appliance therapy is generally high, with studies reporting regular use in 75% to 100% of patients initiating therapy (10). Long-term adherence has been reported to decrease over time. After a four-year period, one study reported appliance use as prescribed in only 32% of patients (49). Others have observed higher therapeutic adherence, ranging from 48% to 76%, after a two- to five-year follow-up period (12,38,44,50). Discontinuation of oral appliance therapy is generally related to side effects, complications, or the lack of perceived benefits (5). Although patient-reported adherence may be an overestimate of actual use, covert adherence monitoring has shown excellent agreement between objective and patient-reported adherence (51). Adherence rates of oral appliance compared with that of CPAP therapy have been reported to be variable. Some studies did not find any difference between these treatments (27,52), whereas others suggest superior adherence with oral appliance therapy (40,42).

ADVERSE EFFECTS AND COMPLICATIONS

Most oral appliances are anchored to the patient's dentition, but may also extend over the oral mucosa to increase the area of retention. Consequently, teeth and surrounding tissues are continuously loaded when the appliance is worn. By holding the mandible in a forward and vertically opened position, reciprocal forces that transmit in a labial direction against the lower incisors and in a palatal direction against the upper incisors are generated (Fig. 2). This may change the inclination and position of teeth, affect the position of the mandible, and increase the loading of the craniomandibular complex (5,53–59). Almost 90% of patients who continue treatment on a regular basis consider that the benefits of treatment outweigh any adverse effect (1).

Short Term
In the initial period of use, patients commonly report tenderness of teeth and jaws, gum irritation, excessive salivation, or xerostomia (1,36,60). Mild complaints of pain and strain of the masticatory muscles and temporomandibular joint also frequently occur when initiating

oral appliance therapy (60). A temporary bite change in the morning after removal of the appliance occurs in almost all patients (10). This phenomenon has been attributed to a partially contracted lateral pterygoid muscle and accumulation of retrodiskal blood in the temporomandibular joint area after full-night mandibular protrusion (13). In more exceptional cases, treatment may be complicated by involuntary removal of the device, an exaggerated gag reflex, periodontal damage, or fractured teeth and fillings (60,61). Problems of discomfort and salivation are usually mild and acceptable, with most symptoms subsiding when treatment is continued. Small adjustments of treatment may, however, enhance the tolerability to the appliance and increase the chance of success.

Long Term

In the long term, oral appliance therapy has been suggested to initiate or aggravate temporomandibular joint disease in individual patients (38), but in the clinical situation, signs or symptoms of temporomandibular joint disorders that result from oral appliance therapy are not commonly reported (5). Two studies that incorporated two- and four-year follow-up periods of MRA treatment demonstrated only few adverse effects of therapy on the masticatory muscles and temporomandibular joints (38,56). These findings suggest that long-term adverse effects of oral appliance therapy on the craniomandibular complex are generally limited.

In contrast to the temporomandibular joints, orthodontic effects on teeth and dentofacial skeleton are observed more frequently with long-term oral appliance therapy (5). Although generally minor, a decreased dental overbite and overjet accompanied by a forward shift of the mandibular first molars relative to the maxillary first molars is reported most uniformly (5,53,54,57,58). Other effects, such as a posterior open bite or reduced anterior mandibular crowding, may accompany these changes in the dental occlusion. Patient-perceived changes in occlusion may be of additional value in detecting changes in dental occlusion. Although not reported uniformly, cephalometric studies suggest a more palatal inclination of the maxillary incisors and a more labial inclination of the mandibular incisors following long-term oral appliance therapy (5,53,54,57). Long-term mandibular advancement may also result in a posterior rotation of the mandible, a change in the vertical position of the mandibular condyles, and an increased anterior face height. The changes in dental occlusion following long-term oral appliance therapy have been attributed to the movement of teeth, myostatic contracture of the lateral pterygoid muscles, and failure of the mandibular condyles to fully reposition following full-night mandibular protrusion (13,60). The available data suggest that dental and skeletal changes with oral appliance therapy may progress by becoming more prominent over time (53,60,62,63). Skeletal changes, which most likely relate to repositioning of the mandibular condyles, have been demonstrated to occur soon after the onset of treatment, whereas changes in the dental occlusion appear to develop as treatment continues (63).

Several features in MRA design have been implicated in the occurrence of side effects. It has been suggested that an MRA with full dental coverage, a minimum degree of bite opening, and both soft elastomeric and rigid acrylic appliances minimize the chance of occlusal changes (5,53,59). Others suggest that occlusal side effects in MRA treatment are not related to the specific design of the oral appliance (60,61). The occurrence of dental side effects may be predicted on the basis of initial characteristics in dental occlusion or dentofacial pattern. A small reduction of the dental overjet has been associated with an initially large overbite and a small overjet (58,59). Changes in dental occlusion following long-term oral appliance use have also been classified as "favorable" and "unfavorable" (58). In this study, 44% of patients were deemed to have unfavorable dental changes after an average of 7.4 years of therapy. The "favorable" dental changes were seen mostly in patients with greater initial overbites and mandibular deficiencies. It should, however, be noted that other factors including periodontal health, patient adherence, and the amount of mandibular protrusion may affect the frequency and severity of side effects with oral appliance therapy (5). Provided there is a good patient follow-up, it is thought reasonable to persist with oral appliance therapy in the presence of acceptable and nonprogressive adverse effects (60,61). However, the likelihood of adverse effects or complications should always be discussed and the patient's written informed consent should be obtained before oral appliance therapy is initiated.

PATIENT SELECTION

Contraindications

When considering oral appliance therapy, several dental exclusion criteria should be taken into account. In upto 34% of cases, an MRA cannot be inserted because of dental contraindications (64). Factors of consideration include (extensive) periodontal disease and dental decay, active temporomandibular joint disorders, and restrictions in mouth opening (i.e., <25 mm) or advancement of the mandible (i.e., <5 mm). In the majority of cases, however, there are an insufficient number of teeth to support and retain the appliance (5,64). Especially, this is the case in edentulous patients. Several types of oral appliances have been described for the treatment of SRBD in edentulous patients (e.g., tongue-retaining appliances) (65). Full-night application of these appliances is generally compromised by discomfort or poor retention. Although some consider a minimum of ten sound teeth in each of the dental arches a requisite in MRA therapy, the location rather than the number of teeth may be more important (i.e., posterior teeth provide more adequate retention) (64). To stabilize and retain an MRA in edentulous patients, osseointegrated dental implants may be used (65). Because this technique requires a longer period before therapy may be initiated, it is generally worth considering only in selected patients. The dental limitations must be considered in overall evaluations of oral appliance therapy.

Predictors of Treatment Outcome

Although oral appliance therapy usually reduces snoring, it is not always effective in OSA patients (5,29,35). Predictors of treatment outcome are therefore of importance for selecting suitable OSA patients who may benefit from therapy. Several clinical and polysomnographic variables have been reported to correlate with increased effectiveness of oral appliance therapy. For example, the outcome of therapy is generally more favorable in patients who have a smaller AHI (5). Treatment may also be more successful in patients who are younger and have a smaller body mass index or neck circumference (36,66) and in patients with a more extended maximum mandibular advancement (31). Others suggest that, possibly because of lower pharyngeal collapsibility, oral appliance therapy is particularly effective in women, and in men with supine-dependent OSA (defined by an AHI <10 in the lateral position) (46). In addition to clinical and polysomnographic predictors, a variety of variables in craniofacial and upper airway morphology have been implicated in a favorable outcome of oral appliance therapy (5,31,67). Variables obtained from these cephalometric and magnetic resonance imaging studies include a cranial position of the hyoid bone, a smaller mandibular plane angle, a reduced anterior face height, a longer anterior cranial base, an increased maxillary length, a larger intermaxillary discrepancy or mandibular deficiency, a more pronounced overjet and overbite, a shorter soft palate, and a relatively "normal" airway diameter or soft palate and tongue proportion.

A significant shortcoming in literature is that most clinical, polysomnographic, and morphological predictors for treatment outcome of oral appliance therapy are not reported uniformly (46). In addition, predictors have not been systematically validated to test their accuracy in a separate population of patients (35). Studies suggest an important role for more sophisticated techniques to predict the outcome of oral appliance therapy in OSA patients. For instance, a remotely controlled mandibular positioner during an overnight sleep study (25) or mimicking the action of an MRA during sleep nasoendoscopy (68) has been shown to be highly predictive for the response to oral appliance therapy. Although these techniques may be of additional value in selecting suitable candidates, they are generally costly, laborious, or sensitive to a specific operator. Therefore, the ability to predict treatment outcome and preselect suitable OSA patients for oral appliance therapy is still limited in clinical practice.

Treatment Guidelines

Since oral appliances generate orthodontic forces, they should generally not be contemplated when treating children or adolescents with SRBD. However, oral appliance therapy has been described as effective for the treatment of OSA in children with malocclusions (69). According to the practice parameters of the American Sleep Disorders Association, oral appliance therapy should be considered in patients with simple snoring who do not respond to or are not appropriate candidates for behavioral measures (e.g., weight loss or modification of sleep position) (33). In mild to moderate OSA, oral appliances are recommended in patients who prefer this treatment to CPAP or in patients who fail treatment attempts with CPAP or behavioral measures. Because in severe OSA oral appliances are generally not as effective as CPAP therapy, these patients should always have an initial trial with CPAP. In patients with severe OSA, oral appliances may be considered when CPAP therapy is not tolerated or refused and when patients are no candidates for or refuse upper airway surgery (e.g., maxillomandibular advancement). It is advised that oral appliances should be fitted by a dental specialist who is trained and experienced in the treatment of patients with SRBD. Following the final adjustments of treatment in OSA patients, effectiveness of therapy should always be evaluated by polysomnography with the appliance in place. Once optimal fit is obtained and efficacy shown, it is recommended that patients have follow-up visits by a dental specialist every six months for the first year and at least annually thereafter. During these consultations, patient adherence, the condition of the appliance, and health and integrity of the dentition should be evaluated and patients can be questioned for worsening of symptomatology and increases in weight. Besides these regular dental follow-up visits, patients should also return for periodic follow-up visits with the referring physician. Should oral appliance therapy cause discomfort or fail during the follow-up period, treatment should be adjusted or patients may discontinue therapy and start with an alternative treatment.

CONCLUSIONS

Since their introduction in the 1980s, oral appliances have been used increasingly for the treatment of SRBD. MRAs are the mainstay in oral appliance treatment. Effectiveness of these oral appliances appears to be related primarily to the degree of mandibular advancement imposed by the appliance. Oral appliances are generally effective for the treatment of snoring and, in a slight majority of cases, effective for the treatment of OSA. However, a placebo effect should always be considered, and a gradual decline in treatment effect may be anticipated in the long term. In OSA patients, effectiveness of therapy should always be evaluated by polysomnography, both in the initial phase of treatment and when relapse is suspected during long-term follow-up examinations. Although usually not serious, oral appliance therapy usually results in transient adverse effects on the craniomandibular and craniofacial complex when therapy is initiated. When continued, long-term adverse effects generally involve changes in the dental occlusion. Although there is convincing evidence that oral appliance therapy is effective for the treatment of OSA, it is generally less effective than CPAP. Nevertheless, many patients prefer an oral appliance to CPAP. Unfortunately, the ability to predict treatment outcome and preselect suitable OSA patients for oral appliance therapy is still limited in clinical practice. On the basis of the current level of evidence, oral appliance therapy is recommended as primary treatment for snoring and mild to moderate OSA besides CPAP therapy. In severe OSA, CPAP therapy should always be considered first. Treatment of patients with oral appliances should be performed by a dental specialist and supervised by a physician, both with experience in the field of SRBD. To guarantee long-term efficacy and safety, follow-up examinations should be conducted on a regular basis.

REFERENCES

1. Cistulli PA, Gotsopoulos H, Marklund M, et al. Treatment of snoring and obstructive sleep apnea with mandibular repositioning appliances. Sleep Med Rev 2004; 8(6):443–457.
2. Robin P. Glossoptosis due to atresia and hypotrophy of the mandible. Am J Dis Child 1994; 48:541–547.
3. Bear SE, Priest JH. Sleep apnea syndrome: correction with surgical advancement of the mandible. J Oral Surg 1980; 38(7):543–549.
4. Cartwright RD, Samelson CF. The effects of a nonsurgical treatment for obstructive sleep apnea. The tongue-retaining device. JAMA 1982; 248(6):705–709.
5. Hoekema A, Stegenga B, de Bont LG. Efficacy and comorbidity of oral appliances in the treatment of obstructive sleep apnea-hypopnea: a systematic review. Crit Rev Oral Biol Med 2004; 15(3):137–155.

6. Marklund M, Franklin KA. Dental appliances in the treatment of snoring. A comparison between an activator, a soft-palate lifter, and a mouth-shield. Swed Dent J 1996; 20(5):183–188.
7. Loube DI. Oral-appliance treatment for obstructive sleep apnea. Clin Pulm Med 1998; 5(2):124–128.
8. Barthlen GM, Brown LK, Wiland MR, et al. Comparison of three oral appliances for treatment of severe obstructive sleep apnea syndrome. Sleep Med 2000; 1(4):299–305.
9. Hoekema A, Wijkstra PJ, Buiter CT, et al. Treatment of the obstructive sleep-apnea syndrome in adults. Ned Tijdschr Geneeskd 2003; 147(49):2407–2412.
10. Lindman R, Bondemark L. A review of oral devices in the treatment of habitual snoring and obstructive sleep apnoea. Swed Dent J 2001; 25(12):39–51.
11. Henke KG, Frantz DE, Kuna ST. An oral elastic mandibular advancement device for obstructive sleep apnea. Am J Respir Crit Care Med 2000; 161(2):420–425.
12. Pancer J, Al-Faifi S, Al-Faifi M, et al. Evaluation of variable mandibular advancement appliance for treatment of snoring and sleep apnea. Chest 1999; 116(6):1511–1518.
13. George PT. Selecting sleep-disordered-breathing appliances. Biomechanical considerations. J Am Dent Assoc 2001; 132(2):339–347.
14. Lawton HM, Battagel JM, Kotecha B. A comparison of the Twin Block and Herbst mandibular advancement splints in the treatment of patients with obstructive sleep apnoea: a prospective study. Eur J Orthod 2005; 27(1):82–90.
15. Vanderveken OM, Devolder A, Marklund M, et al. Comparison of a custom-made and a thermoplastic oral appliance for the treatment of mild sleep apnea. Am J Respir Crit Care Med 2008; 178(2):197–202.
16. L'Estrange PR, Battagel JM, Harkness B, et al. A method of studying adaptive changes of the oropharynx to variation in mandibular position in patients with obstructive sleep apnoea. J Oral Rehabil 1996; 23(10):699–711.
17. Lowe A, Fleetham J, Ryan F, et al. Effects of a mandibular repositioning appliance used in the treatment of obstructive sleep apnea on tongue muscle activity. Prog Clin Biol Res 1990; 345:395–405.
18. Pitsis AJ, Darendeliler MA, Gotsopoulos H, et al. Effect of vertical dimension on efficacy of oral appliance therapy in obstructive sleep apnea. Am J Respir Crit Care Med 2002; 166(6):860–864.
19. Smith AM, Battagel JM. Nonapneic snoring and the orthodontist: radiographic pharyngeal dimension changes with supine posture and mandibular protrusion. J Orthod 2004; 31(2):124–131.
20. Gao X, Otsuka R, Ono T, et al. Effect of titrated mandibular advancement and jaw opening on the upper airway in nonapneic men: a magnetic resonance imaging and cephalometric study. Am J Orthod Dentofacial Orthop 2004; 125(2):191–199.
21. Kyung SH, Park YC, Pae EK. Obstructive sleep apnea patients with the oral appliance experience pharyngeal size and shape changes in three dimensions. Angle Orthod 2005; 75(1):15–22.
22. Tsuiki S, Lowe AA, Almeida FR, et al. Effects of mandibular advancement on airway curvature and obstructive sleep apnoea severity. Eur Respir J 2004; 23(2):263–268.
23. Walker-Engstrom ML, Ringqvist I, Vestling O, et al. A prospective randomized study comparing two different degrees of mandibular advancement with a dental appliance in treatment of severe obstructive sleep apnea. Sleep Breath 2003; 7(3):119–130.
24. Petelle B, Vincent G, Gagnadoux F, et al. One-night mandibular advancement titration for obstructive sleep apnea syndrome: a pilot study. Am J Respir Crit Care Med 2002; 165(8):1150–1153.
25. Tsai WH, Vazquez JC, Oshima T, et al. Remotely controlled mandibular positioner predicts efficacy of oral appliances in sleep apnea. Am J Respir Crit Care Med 2004; 170(4):366–370.
26. Schmidt-Nowara W, Lowe A, Wiegand L, et al. Oral appliances for the treatment of snoring and obstructive sleep apnea: a review. Sleep 1995; 18(6):501–510.
27. Engleman HM, McDonald JP, Graham D, et al. Randomized crossover trial of two treatments for sleep apnea-hypopnea syndrome: continuous positive airway pressure and mandibular repositioning splint. Am J Respir Crit Care Med 2002; 166(6):855–859.
28. Gotsopoulos H, Kelly JJ, Cistulli PA. Oral appliance therapy reduces blood pressure in obstructive sleep apnea: a randomized, controlled trial. Sleep 2004; 27(5):934–941.
29. Barnes M, McEvoy RD, Banks S, et al. Efficacy of positive airway pressure and oral appliance in mild to moderate obstructive sleep apnea. Am J Respir Crit Care Med 2004; 170(6):656–664.
30. Naismith SL, Winter VR, Hickie IB, et al. Effect of oral appliance therapy on neurobehavioural functioning in obstructive sleep apnea: a randomized controlled trial. J Clin Sleep Med 2005; 1(4):374–380.
31. Hoekema A. Oral-Appliance Therapy in Obstructive Sleep Apnea-Hypopnea Syndrome: a Clinical Study on Therapeutic Outcomes [academic thesis]. Groningen, The Netherlands: University of Groningen, 2007.
32. Ferguson KA, Cartwright R, Rogers R, et al. Oral appliances for snoring and obstructive sleep apnea: a review. Sleep 2006; 29(2):244–262.
33. Kushida CA, Morgenthaler TI, Littner MR, et al. Practice parameters for the treatment of snoring and obstructive sleep apnea with oral appliances: an update for 2005. Sleep 2006; 29(2):240–243.

34. Blanco J, Zamarron C, Abeleira Pazos MT, et al. Prospective evaluation of an oral appliance in the treatment of obstructive sleep apnea syndrome. Sleep Breath 2005; 9(1):20–25.
35. Lim J, Lasserson T, Fleetham J, et al. Oral appliances for obstructive sleep apnoea. Cochrane Database Syst Rev 2006; 1:CD004435.
36. Mehta A, Qian J, Petocz P, et al. A randomized, controlled study of a mandibular advancement splint for obstructive sleep apnea. Am J Respir Crit Care Med 2001; 163(6):1457–1461.
37. Wilhelmsson B, Tegelberg A, Walker-Engström ML, et al. A prospective randomized study of a dental appliance compared with uvulopalatopharyngoplasty in the treatment of obstructive sleep apnoea. Acta Otolaryngol 1999; 119(4):503–509.
38. Walker-Engström ML, Tegelberg A, Wilhelmsson B, et al. Four-year follow-up of treatment with dental appliance or uvulopalatopharyngoplasty in patients with obstructive sleep apnea: a randomized study. Chest 2002; 121(3):739–746.
39. Cartwright R, Venkatesan TK, Caldarelli D, et al. Treatments for snoring: a comparison of somnoplasty and an oral appliance. Laryngoscope 2000; 110(10):1680–1683.
40. Ferguson KA, Ono T, Lowe AA, et al. A short-term controlled trial of an adjustable oral appliance for the treatment of mild to moderate obstructive sleep apnea. Thorax 1997; 52(4):362–368.
41. Tan YK, L'Estrange PR, Luo YM, et al. Mandibular advancement splints and continuous positive airway pressure in patients with obstructive sleep apnoea: a randomized crossover trial. Eur J Orthod 2002; 24(3):239–249.
42. Randerath WJ, Heise M, Hinz R, et al. An individually adjustable oral appliance vs. continuous positive airway pressure in mild-to-moderate obstructive sleep apnea syndrome. Chest 2002; 122(2): 569–575.
43. Rose EC, Barthlen GM, Staats R, et al. Therapeutic efficacy of an oral appliance in the treatment of obstructive sleep apnea: a two-year follow-up. Am J Orthod Dentofacial Orthop 2002; 121(3):273–239.
44. Marklund M, Sahlin C, Stenlund H, et al. Mandibular advancement device in patients with obstructive sleep apnea: long-term effects on apnea and sleep. Chest 2001; 120(1):162–169.
45. Fransson AM, Tegelberg A, Leissner L, et al. Effects of a mandibular protruding device on the sleep of patients with obstructive sleep apnea and snoring problems: a two-year follow-up. Sleep Breath 2003; 7(3):131–141.
46. Marklund M, Stenlund H, Franklin KA. Mandibular advancement devices in 630 men and women with obstructive sleep apnea and snoring: tolerability and predictors of treatment success. Chest 2004; 125(4):1270–1278.
47. Millman RP, Rosenberg CL, Carlisle CC, et al. The efficacy of oral appliances in the treatment of persistent sleep apnea after uvulopalatopharyngoplasty. Chest 1998; 113(4):992–996.
48. Hoekema A, de Lange J, Stegenga B, et al. Oral appliances and maxillomandibular advancement surgery: an alternative treatment protocol for the obstructive sleep apnea-hypopnea syndrome. J Oral Maxillofac Surg 2006; 64(6):886–891.
49. Rose E, Staats R, Schulte-Mönting J, et al. Obstruktive schlafatmungsstörung: therapie compliance mit einem intraoralen protrusionsgerät. Dtsch Med Wochenschr 2002; 127(23):1245–1249.
50. Clark GT, Sohn JW, Hong CN. Treating obstructive sleep apnea and snoring: assessment of an anterior mandibular positioning device. J Am Dent Assoc 2000; 131(4):765–771.
51. Lowe AA, Sjöholm TT, Ryan CF, et al. Treatment, airway and compliance effects of a titratable oral appliance. Sleep 2000; 23(4):172S–178S.
52. Ferguson KA, Ono T, Lowe AA, et al. A randomized crossover study of an oral appliance vs. nasal-continuous positive airway pressure in the treatment of mild-moderate obstructive sleep apnea. Chest 1996; 109(5):1269–1275.
53. Robertson C, Herbison P, Harkness M. Dental and occlusal changes during mandibular advancement splint therapy in sleep-disordered patients. Eur J Orthod 2003; 25(4):371–376.
54. Ringqvist M, Walker-Engstrom ML, Tegelberg A, et al. Dental and skeletal changes after four years of obstructive sleep apnea treatment with a mandibular advancement device: a prospective, randomized study. Am J Orthod Dentofacial Orthop 2003; 124(1):53–60.
55. Monteith BD. Altered jaw posture and occlusal disruption patterns following mandibular advancement therapy for sleep apnea: a preliminary study of cephalometric predictors. Int J Prosthodont 2004; 17(3):274–280.
56. Fransson AM, Tegelberg A, Johansson A, et al. Influence on the masticatory system in treatment of obstructive sleep apnea and snoring with a mandibular protruding device: a two-year follow-up. Am J Orthod Dentofacial Orthop 2004; 126(6):687–693.
57. Almeida FR, Lowe AA, Sung JO, et al. Long-term sequellae of oral appliance therapy in obstructive sleep apnea patients: Part 1. Cephalometric analysis. Am J Orthod Dentofacial Orthop 2006; 129(2): 195–204.
58. Almeida FR, Lowe AA, Otsuka R, et al. Long-term sequellae of oral appliance therapy in obstructive sleep apnea patients: Part 2. Study-model analysis. Am J Orthod Dentofacial Orthop 2006; 129(2): 205–213.

59. Marklund M. Predictors of long-term orthodontic side effects from mandibular advancement devices in patients with snoring and obstructive sleep apnea. Am J Orthod Dentofacial Orthop 2006; 129(2): 214–221.

60. Pantin CC, Hillman DR, Tennant M. Dental side effects of an oral device to treat snoring and obstructive sleep apnea. Sleep 1999; 22(2):237–240.

61. Rose EC, Staats R, Virchow C Jr., et al. Occlusal and skeletal effects of an oral appliance in the treatment of obstructive sleep apnea. Chest 2002; 122(3):871–877.

62. Fritsch KM, Iseli A, Russi EW, et al. Side effects of mandibular advancement devices for sleep apnea treatment. Am J Respir Crit Care Med 2001; 164(5):813–818.

63. Robertson CJ. Dental and skeletal changes associated with long-term mandibular advancement. Sleep 2001; 24(5):531–537.

64. Petit FX, Pépin JL, Bettega G, et al. Mandibular advancement devices: rate of contraindications in 100 consecutive obstructive sleep apnea patients. Am J Respir Crit Care Med 2002; 166(3):274–278.

65. Hoekema A, de Vries F, Heydenrijk K, et al. Implant retained oral appliances; a novel treatment for edentulous patients with obstructive sleep apnea-hypopnea syndrome. Clin Oral Implants Res 2007; 18(3):383–387.

66. Liu Y, Lowe AA, Fleetham JA, et al. Cephalometric and physiologic predictors of the efficacy of an adjustable oral appliance for treating obstructive sleep apnea. Am J Orthod Dentofacial Orthop 2001; 120(6):639–647.

67. Horiuchi A, Suzuki M, Ookubo M, et al. Measurement techniques predicting the effectiveness of an oral appliance for obstructive sleep apnea-hypopnea syndrome. Angle Orthod 2005; 75(6):1003–1011.

68. Battagel JM, Johal A, Kotecha BT. Sleep nasendoscopy as a predictor of treatment success in snorers using mandibular advancement splints. J Laryngol Otol 2005; 119(2):106–112.

69. Villa MP, Bernkopf E, Pagani J, et al. Randomized controlled study of an oral jaw-positioning appliance for the treatment of obstructive sleep apnea in children with malocclusion. Am J Respir Crit Care Med 2002; 165(1):123–127.

34 | Adjunctive and Alternative Treatments of Sleep-Related Breathing Disorders

Alan T. Mulgrew and Krista Sigurdson

Sleep Disorders Program, University of British Columbia, Vancouver, British Columbia, Canada

Najib T. Ayas

Sleep Disorders Program, University of British Columbia and Centre Clinical Epidemiology and Evaluation, Vancouver Coastal Health Research Institute, Vancouver, British Columbia, Canada

INTRODUCTION

Obstructive sleep apnea (OSA) is a common disorder (1) characterized by recurrent collapse of the pharyngeal airway during sleep, leading to sleep fragmentation, hypersomnolence, neurocognitive dysfunction, automobile crashes, and possibly cardiovascular sequelae (2–7). Continuous positive airway pressure therapy (CPAP), oral appliances, and upper airway surgery are the most common first-line treatment modalities for this disease, and are described in detail in chapters 30 to 33. This chapter will focus instead on adjunctive and alternative therapies for sleep apnea.

BEHAVIORAL THERAPIES AND AVOIDANCE OF SPECIFIC SUBSTANCES AND MEDICATIONS

A variety of agents and activities (e.g., alcohol, smoking, sedatives, anabolic steroids, sleep deprivation) may potentially worsen sleep apnea.

Alcohol is a respiratory depressant that has a greater effect on upper airway dilator muscle activity than on ventilatory pump muscles (such as the diaphragm), thus predisposing the upper airway to collapse (8,9). Alcohol ingestion prior to bedtime leads to worsening of sleep-disordered breathing (9). It is therefore advisable for untreated patients with OSA to avoid drinking alcohol at least four to five hours prior to bedtime. In patients treated with CPAP, moderate amounts of alcohol ingestion (1.5 mL/kg of vodka, approximately equivalent to a half bottle of wine) seem to have little effect on pressure requirements (10).

Smoking may potentially aggravate OSA by increasing upper airway edema. Wetter et al., for example, demonstrated that current smokers had a threefold greater risk of OSA as compared with nonsmokers (11). In contrast, a report from the Sleep Heart Health Study found an inverse relationship between smoking and sleep apnea (12). Nevertheless, given the multiple adverse cardiovascular and respiratory health effects, we advise all of our patients to stop smoking.

Benzodiazepines decrease the arousal response to hypoxia and hypercapnia leading to increased apnea duration (13). Furthermore, even a small (0.25 mg) dose of triazolam increased the apnea duration and worsened oxygen saturation in patients with severe OSA (14). Zolpidem, a non-benzodiazepine sedative, does not cause an increase in desaturation in patients with mild to moderate chronic obstructive pulmonary disease (COPD). However, the effects of this drug in patients with severe OSA have not been studied, and its potential to adversely affect nocturnal oxygen saturation should be considered (15). In one study of eight patients, zopiclone had no adverse effect on respiratory parameters; however, this study only included patients with upper airway resistance syndrome rather than OSA (10). The effects of sedatives on CPAP pressure are unclear, but there is the potential for the required pressure to be increased. Close clinical monitoring of patients with OSA treated with CPAP and prescribed sedatives is advised.

The effect of narcotics on sleep apnea has been poorly studied. In normal subjects given small doses of oral narcotic analgesics (2–4 mg of hydromorphone), there was no increase in sleep-disordered breathing (16). However, postoperative intravenous narcotic analgesia was associated with more episodes of nocturnal desaturation compared with regional analgesia, suggesting that systemic narcotics may increase sleep apnea severity (17). Patients using methadone chronically may develop significant central sleep apnea that can lead to desaturation and sleep disruption (18).

Exogenous testosterone worsens sleep-disordered breathing in hypogonadal men, predominately through non-anatomic effects (19,20). When possible, we avoid these drugs in patients with OSA; if not possible, careful monitoring of OSA patients after prescription of exogenous androgens is warranted to ensure that no worsening of sleep apnea occurs.

Finally, a single night of sleep deprivation increases the number and length of apneas (21). This is likely because sleep deprivation decreases upper airway muscle tone and thus increases collapsibility of the upper airway. (13,22) Therefore, we believe that all OSA patients should be counseled to obtain adequate amounts of nocturnal sleep.

POSITIONAL THERAPY

Gravity influences pharyngeal structures and lung volumes (23), with the upper airway being less collapsible in the lateral versus the supine position (24). Consequently, sleep apnea is often less severe in the lateral position (25). Positional sleep apnea is defined as a total apnea-hypopnea index (AHI) >5 events per hour, a 50% reduction in the AHI between the supine and non-supine postures, and an AHI that normalizes in the non-supine posture. In a report by Mador and colleagues (15), there was a high prevalence (50%) of positional sleep apnea in patients with overall mild disease (AHI 5–15 events/hr), which decreased to 19.4% in patients with moderate disease (AHI, 15–30) and 6.5% in severe patients (AHI > 30).

Positional therapy can be considered if positional sleep apnea is documented by overnight polysomnography [including a period of rapid eye movement (REM) sleep in the lateral position]. This could include methods to prevent individuals from sleeping in the supine posture; techniques used include sewing a tennis ball into the back of the pajama top, attaching a pillow to the sleeper's back with a belt, or wearing a knapsack. Gravity-activated alarms may also be helpful in maintaining patients in the lateral position during sleep (26). The efficacy of positional therapy, in selected patients, may be similar to CPAP (27). After positional therapy is prescribed, careful follow-up of OSA symptoms is necessary to ensure adequate therapy.

WEIGHT LOSS

The majority of patients with OSA are obese. The mechanism through which obesity increases the propensity for OSA is unclear but may involve fat deposition around the upper airway (28,29). Data from the Sleep Heart Health Study (30) showed that a weight loss of 10 kg or more in men had approximately 5 times the odds of a 15 unit or greater reduction in respiratory disturbance index compared with weight stability, suggesting that all obese patients with sleep apnea should be counseled and encouraged to lose weight.

Three types of therapy have been attempted to promote weight loss: diet and exercise, pharmacological therapy, and bariatric surgery.

No consensus has been reached regarding the optimal weight reduction diet in terms of the proportion of carbohydrates and fat (31). Weight loss with a very low calorie diet was effective in treating OSA with a favorable effect on oxygen desaturation index (32). Maintaining weight loss is, however, a significant barrier to the success of this treatment with the majority of patients regaining weight leading to a recurrence of OSA (33,34). Cognitive behavioral therapy may achieve satisfactory weight loss and may also be of benefit in weight loss maintenance (35).

Drug therapy for obesity is controversial, mainly due to side effects of medications and questionable efficacy. Dexfenfluramine, for instance, has been associated with cardiac valvular abnormalities and pulmonary vascular changes (36,37). Newer agents may be more successful in achieving weight loss while avoiding significant side effects. Orlistat, a lipase inhibitor, is useful in achieving weight loss when used as part of a weight management program (38,39) and maintains weight reduction after dieting (40). Sibutramine, a serotonin reuptake inhibitor, has also been successful in achieving weight loss particularly when used in combination with lifestyle modification (41). Long-term follow-up data is lacking for these agents, and there are no studies examining their effects on OSA parameters. It is likely that trial evidence will soon be available to clarify the role of theses agents in the management of OSA.

Bariatric surgery includes a variety of surgical techniques designed to promote weight reduction. A variety of studies (42–44) have demonstrated the efficacy of these surgical techniques in the treatment of obesity and its complications. A comprehensive meta-analysis outlining the impact of bariatric surgery on weight loss and on four obesity comorbidities (including OSA) was published in 2004 (45). The percentage of patients in the total population ($n = 726$) whose OSA resolved or improved was 83.6% [95% confidence interval (CI), 71.8–95.4%]. The most robust evidence for changes in OSA was available for gastric bypass patients. This was particularly so for the AHI, which decreased by 34 events per hour in patients who underwent gastric bypass surgery (95% CI, 17.5–50.2 per hour). Currently, we consider bariatric surgery for morbidly obese individuals (BMI > 40 kg/m^2) who have failed conservative measures at weight loss.

CORRECTION OF OTHER MEDICAL DISORDERS

Treatment of hypothyroidism, acromegaly, and nasal congestion may improve the severity of OSA.

In patients with OSA, the prevalence of undiagnosed hypothyroidism is in the range of 3.1% to 11.5% (46,47). Treatment of hypothyroidism will help improve daytime fatigue and promote weight loss (48,49), and may lead to an improvement of OSA (50). Whether all patients with OSA should be screened for hypothyroidism is controversial (51); however, at the very least, clinicians should have a low threshold for testing thyroid function in patients with OSA.

Patients with acromegaly, a rare disease characterized by hypersecretion of growth hormone, have a very high prevalence (60–70%) of both obstructive and central sleep apnea (52,53). The increased prevalence of OSA is attributed to both structural abnormalities induced by growth hormone and increased respiratory drive leading to breathing instability (54). Treatment with octreotide may lead to improvement of sleep-disordered breathing (55,56). Consequently, appropriate testing for acromegaly should be performed in patients with suggestive clinical findings.

Nasal pathology may also contribute to OSA (57). This could be secondary to increased nasal resistance leading to increased negative pressure in the pharynx during inspiration, or due to interference with reflexes designed to protect the patency of the upper airway (58). Use of nasal steroids leads to improvement in AHI and nasal resistance (59) in patients with concomitant OSA and seasonal allergic rhinitis. Other nasal decongestants have shown limited success in alleviating OSA (60). External nasal dilators in mild OSA lead to a small increase in nocturnal oxygen saturation, but no change in AHI or sleep architecture (61). Surgical repair of nasal pathology has resulted in dramatic improvements of OSA in a small case series (62), although the majority of patients do not seem to benefit (63). Nevertheless, OSA patients should be examined for symptoms and signs of nasal pathology and consider surgical or medical treatment if abnormalities are identified. Treatment of nasal pathology is important in maximizing tolerance to CPAP therapy.

PHARMACOLOGICAL THERAPY OF OSA

Drugs That Increase Respiratory Drive

While awake, patients with OSA are able to maintain pharyngeal patency through reflex mechanisms that lead to increased upper airway dilator muscle activity keeping the collapsible part of the upper airway open (64,65). With sleep, these reflex mechanisms are lost resulting in a reduction in dilator muscle activity and consequent upper airway collapse in anatomically susceptible patients (65–70). A number of respiratory stimulants have been used to increase upper airway muscle activity to treat patients with sleep apnea. Thus far, the results have been disappointing.

Medroxyprogesterone, a hormone and respiratory stimulant, has been used to treat OSA. An uncontrolled study by Strohl et al. demonstrated improvement in four of nine patients with OSA; however, three of the four subjects who improved were hypercapnic suggesting that they may have had an element of obesity/hypoventilation syndrome in addition to OSA (71). Subsequent studies have demonstrated mild to no improvement of OSA after treatment with progesterone (72,73), even in postmenopausal women (74), and even when combined with estrogen (75). Currently, although progesterone cannot be considered an effective treatment for OSA, it may play an adjunctive role in patients with the obesity hypoventilation syndrome through its stimulation of central respiratory drive. However, we would suggest caution even under these conditions given the potential procoagulant effects of progesterone, and the increased risk of thromboembolic and cardiovascular disease in obese OSA patients (76).

Protriptyline, a tricyclic antidepressant, may modestly decrease the AHI in patients with OSA (77). Though the drug may increase genioglossus tone (perhaps through its anti-cholinergic effect), the predominant mechanism of action is likely its suppression of REM sleep (the stage of sleep when OSA is usually most severe). Although this drug may be a reasonable alternative option in patients with mild predominately REM associated OSA, the drug is often poorly tolerated due to its myriad side effects (including urinary retention, dry mouth, and impotence).

Serotonin is a major neurotransmitter involved in the regulation of upper airway tone. A reduction in serotonergic output to the hypoglossal nucleus occurs during sleep (especially REM sleep), and augmentation of serotonin around the nucleus may increase upper airway tone and improve sleep-disordered breathing (78–80). Selective serotonin reuptake inhibitors (SSRIs) have been used to counter the reduction in upper airway muscle activity that occurs at sleep onset in OSA patients. However, results in patients with OSA have been disappointing. For instance, Berry et al. administered a single dose (40 mg) of paroxetine to eight men with severe OSA. Although peak genioglossus activity increased in this trial, there was no improvement in sleep apnea (75 vs. 74 events/hr for drug vs. placebo, respectively) (81). A placebo-controlled crossover trial of paroxetine (20 mg/day) and placebo in 20 patients with OSA (82) demonstrated a significant difference in AHI in the paroxetine versus the placebo group (36 vs. 30 events/hr) but the overall magnitude was small. There was no significant difference in symptoms.

SSRIs cannot be currently recommended as a treatment option for OSA, especially given their multiple potential toxicities (i.e., insomnia, REM suppression, worsened periodic limb movements, increased appetite, serotonin syndrome, and hypomania). Direct serotonin agonists (or antagonists acting at autoregulatory presynaptic receptors) may be more effective in treating patients with sleep apnea, and we await future studies in this area (83).

Other respiratory stimulants such as nicotine, theophylline, acetazolamide, naloxone, almitrine, and bromocriptine are also not useful in treating OSA (84–86).

Etanercept

Tumor necrosis factor (TNF) is a somnogenic pro-inflammatory cytokine whose levels are increased in patients with OSA (87). Vgontzas et al. (88) administered etanercept, a TNF antagonist, to eight patients with OSA to determine if hypersomolence improves with the drug. In this trial, the use of etanercept resulted in an improvement of objective sleepiness [multiple sleep latency test (MSLT)] reduced by 3 minutes] and a reduction in AHI of 8 events per hour compared with placebo. Limitations of this study included the nonrandom order of the interventions (i.e., all patients received placebo first) and the small sample size. Although interesting from a mechanistic standpoint, anti-TNF therapies are costly and are associated with substantial side effects (e.g., life-threatening infections), making this therapy impractical (89).

Modafinil

Modafinil is a novel wake-promoting agent that is effective in treating patients with residual sleepiness after OSA therapy (90). A 12-week randomized multicentre trial of OSA patients showed residual hypersomnolence in patients despite use of CPAP (i.e., Epworth Sleepiness Scale score ≥ 10). Three hundred and five OSA patients were randomized to placebo, 200 mg modafinil per day, or 400 mg modafinil per day (91). Patients on modafinil had significant improvements in objective daytime sleepiness (maintenance of wakefulness test) and the

Epworth Sleepiness Scale score. Adherence was similar in all three groups. Although the drug was reasonably well tolerated, six patients had to withdraw because of headaches, five for chest pain, and four for dizziness. Although the manuscript was written by the authors, the data were analyzed by the sponsoring company.

One must be aware that modafinil does not treat sleep apnea per se, but only the symptom of sleepiness. Therefore, we believe that treated OSA patients with residual daytime sleepiness should first have other causes of sleepiness excluded; attention should be directed toward verifying CPAP adherence, effectiveness of therapy, and excluding other causes of hypersomnolence (e.g., periodic limb movements of sleep, narcolepsy, depression, medications, inadequate daily sleep, systemic illness). Reduced CPAP adherence may occur with modafinil presumably because of symptom improvement (92). Even though this was not shown in the large randomized trial referenced in the previous paragraph, we would be concerned that adherence may be worse in patients not followed closely as part of a sponsored clinical trial. Furthermore, the long-term health effects of chronic modafinil use are not well understood. Nevertheless, modafinil may be a useful adjunctive therapy in the treatment of patients with persistent sleepiness despite adherence with CPAP, and after a search for other potential causes of sleepiness have been excluded.

CONCLUSIONS

Table 1 summarizes the various adjunctive and alternative therapies discussed in this chapter. We believe that all patients with OSA should be encouraged to lose weight if obese, maintain nasal patency, avoid sleep deprivation, and stop smoking. The negative effects of alcohol, androgens, and sedatives on OSA severity should be kept in mind. Vigilance for signs and symptoms of hypothyroidism and acromegaly are advised, with appropriate diagnostic testing and therapy as indicated. Modafinil may play a role in patients persistently sleepy despite

Table 1 Summary of Alternative and Adjunctive Treatments of OSA

Treatment	Advantages	Disadvantages	Comments
Behavioral			
Lifestyle modification (i.e., avoid smoking and sleep deprivation, maintain nasal patency)	Likely confers other health benefits	Will rarely eliminate OSA	Should be advised in everyone with OSA
Weight loss	Clear-cut overall health benefit	Low success rate and high relapse rate	Should be advised in all obese OSA patients
Positional therapy	Low cost	Effective in only a minority of cases	Consider as a treatment alternative in patients with positional OSA
Pharmacotherapy			
Respiratory stimulants	Easy to use	Inconsistent efficacy Side effects	Not presently recommended for OSA
Etanercept	May reduce sleepiness	Potentially severe side effects Cost Paucity of data	Not recommended
Modafinil	Easy to use		Consider in selected patients with persistent sleepiness despite CPAP
	Reduces sleepiness	Long-term effects unclear, may reduce adherence Side effects Cost	
Correction of other medical disorders (hypothyroidism, acromegaly, severe nasal obstruction)	May improve or eliminate OSA Secondary health benefits	These are rare causes of OSA Treatment does not usually eliminate OSA	These diseases should be considered in the evaluation of all OSA patients

adherence with CPAP therapy. Medications as a single therapy of OSA have not been successful and/or have substantial side effects and are not recommended. Further work to better define the basic neurophysiology of sleep apnea may lead to novel pharmacological therapies that may effectively treat OSA patients.

Dr. Ayas is supported by a Scholar Award from the Michael Smith Foundation for Health Research, a New Investigator Award from the CIHR/BC Lung Association, and a Departmental Scholar Award from the University of British Columbia. Dr. Mulgrew is supported by a BC Lung Fellowship and by the CIHR/HSFC IMPACT training program.

REFERENCES

1. Young T, Palta M, Dempsey J, et al. The occurrence of sleep-disordered breathing among middle-aged adults. N Engl J Med 1993; 328(17):1230–1235.
2. Epstein LJ, Weiss JW. Clinical consequences of obstructive sleep apnea. Semin Respir Crit Care Med 1993; 19:123–132.
3. Teran-Santos J, Jimenez-Gomez A, Cordero-Guevara J. The association between sleep apnea and the risk of traffic accidents. Cooperative Group Burgos-Santander. N Engl J Med 1999; 340(11):847–851.
4. Ayas NT, Epstein LJ. Oral appliances in the treatment of obstructive sleep apnea and snoring. Curr Opin Pulm Med 1998; 4(6):355–360.
5. Sajkov D, Wang T, Saunders NA, et al. Daytime pulmonary hemodynamics in patients with obstructive sleep apnea without lung disease. Am J Respir Crit Care Med 1999; 159(5 pt 1):1518–1526.
6. Marin JM, Carrizo SJ, Vicente E, et al. Long-term cardiovascular outcomes in men with obstructive sleep apnoea-hypopnoea with or without treatment with continuous positive airway pressure: an observational study. Lancet 2005; 365(9464):1046–1053.
7. Yaggi HK, Concato J, Kernan WN, et al. Obstructive sleep apnea as a risk factor for stroke and death. N Engl J Med 2005; 353(19):2034–2041.
8. Krol RC KS, Bartlett D. Selective reduction of genioglossal muscle activity by alcohol in normal human subjects. Am Rev Respir Dis 1984; 132(2):216–219.
9. Issa FG, Sullivan CE. Alcohol, snoring and sleep apnea. J Neurol Neurosurg Psychiatry 1982; 45(4): 353–359.
10. Teschler H, Berthon-Jones M, Wessendorf T, et al. Influence of moderate alcohol consumption on obstructive sleep apnoea with and without AutoSet nasal CPAP therapy. Eur Respir J 1996; 9(11): 2371–2377.
11. Wetter DW, Young TB, Bidwell TR, et al. Smoking as a risk factor for sleep-disordered breathing. Arch Intern Med 1994; 154(19):2219–2224.
12. Newman AB, Nieto FJ, Guidry U, et al. Relation of sleep-disordered breathing to cardiovascular disease risk factors: the sleep heart health study. Am J Epidemiol 2001; 154(1):50–59.
13. Leiter JC, Knuth SL, Bartlett D Jr. The effect of sleep deprivation on activity of the genioglossus muscle. Am Rev Respir Dis 1985; 132(6):1242–1245.
14. Berry RB, Kouchi K, Bower J, et al. Triazolam in patients with obstructive sleep apnea. Am J Respir Crit Care Med 1995; 151(2 pt 1):450–454.
15. Mador MJ, Kufel TJ, Magalang UJ, et al. Prevalence of positional sleep apnea in patients undergoing polysomnography. Chest 2005; 128(4):2130–2137.
16. Robinson RW, Zwillich CW, Bixler EO, et al. Effects of oral narcotics on sleep-disordered breathing in healthy adults. Chest 1987; 91(2):197–203.
17. Catley DM, Thornton C, Jordan C, et al. Pronounced, episodic oxygen desaturation in the postoperative period: its association with ventilatory pattern and analgesic regimen. Anesthesiology 1985; 63(1):20–28.
18. Wang D, Teichtahl H, Drummer O, et al. Central sleep apnea in stable methadone maintenance treatment patients. Chest 2005; 128(3):1348–1356.
19. Liu PY, Yee B, Wishart SM, et al. The short-term effects of high-dose testosterone on sleep, breathing, and function in older men. J Clin Endocrinol Metab 2003; 88(8):3605–3613.
20. Schneider BK, Pickett CK, Zwillich CW, et al. Influence of testosterone on breathing during sleep. J Appl Physiol 1986; 61(2):618–623.
21. Guilleminault C, Rosekind M. The arousal threshold: sleep deprivation, sleep fragmentation, and obstructive sleep apnea syndrome. Bull Eur Physiopathol Respir 1981; 17(3):341–349.
22. Series F, Roy N, Marc I. Effects of sleep deprivation and sleep fragmentation on upper airway collapsibility in normal subjects. Am J Respir Crit Care Med 1994; 150(2):481–485.
23. Pevernagie DA, Stanson AW, Sheedy PF, et al. Effects of body position on the upper airway of patients with obstructive sleep apnea. Am J Respir Crit Care Med 1995; 152(1):179–185.

24. Neill AM, Angus SM, Sajkov D, et al. Effects of sleep posture on upper airway stability in patients with obstructive sleep apnea. Am J Respir Crit Care Med 1997; 155(1):199–204.
25. Oksenberg A, Silverberg DS, Arons E, et al. Positional vs nonpositional obstructive sleep apnea patients: anthropomorphic, nocturnal polysomnographic, and multiple sleep latency test data. Chest 1997; 112(3):629–639.
26. Cartwright RD, Lloyd S, Lilie J, et al. Sleep position training as treatment for sleep apnea syndrome: a preliminary study. Sleep 1985; 8(2):87–94.
27. Jokic R, Klimaszewski A, Crossley M, et al. Positional treatment vs continuous positive airway pressure in patients with positional obstructive sleep apnea syndrome. Chest 1999; 115(3):771–781.
28. Mortimore IL Marshall I, Wraith PK, et al. Neck and total body fat deposition in nonobese and obese patients with sleep apnea compared with that in control subjects. Am J Respir Crit Care Med 1998; 157(1): 280–283.
29. Horner RL, Mohiaddin RH, Lowell DG, et al. Sites and sizes of fat deposits around the pharynx in obese patients with obstructive sleep apnoea and weight matched controls. Eur Respir J 1989; 2(7): 613–622.
30. Newman AB, Foster G, Givelber R, et al. Progression and regression of sleep-disordered breathing with changes in weight: the Sleep Heart Health Study. Arch Intern Med 2005; 165(20):2408–2413.
31. Strychar I. Diet in the management of weight loss. CMAJ 2006; 174(1):56–63.
32. Kansanen M, Vanninen E, Tuunainen A, et al. The effect of a very low-calorie diet-induced weight loss on the severity of obstructive sleep apnoea and autonomic nervous function in obese patients with obstructive sleep apnoea syndrome. Clin Physiol 1998; 18(4):377–385.
33. Sampol G, Munoz X, Sagales MT, et al. Long-term efficacy of dietary weight loss in sleep apnoea/ hypopnoea syndrome. Eur Respir J 1998; 12(5):1156–1159.
34. Wooley SC, Garner DM. Obesity treatment: the high cost of false hope. J Am Diet Assoc 1991; 91(10): 1248–1251.
35. Kajaste S, Brander PE, Telakivi T, et al. A cognitive-behavioral weight reduction program in the treatment of obstructive sleep apnea syndrome with or without initial nasal CPAP: a randomized study. Sleep Med 2004; 5(2):125–131.
36. Connolly HM, Crary JL, McGoon MD, et al. Valvular heart disease associated with fenfluramine-phentermine. N Engl J Med 1997; 337(9):581–588.
37. Abenhaim L, Moride Y, Brenot F, et al. Appetite-suppressant drugs and the risk of primary pulmonary hypertension. International Primary Pulmonary Hypertension Study Group. N Engl J Med 1996; 335(9):609–616.
38. Chanoine JP, Hampl S, Jensen C, et al. Effect of orlistat on weight and body composition in obese adolescents: a randomized controlled trial. JAMA 2005; 293(23):2873–2883.
39. Davidson MH, Hauptman J, DiGirolamo M, et al. Weight control and risk factor reduction in obese subjects treated for 2 years with orlistat: a randomized controlled trial. JAMA 1999; 281(3):235–242.
40. Hill JO, Hauptman J, Anderson JW, et al. Orlistat, a lipase inhibitor, for weight maintenance after conventional dieting: a 1-y study. Am J Clin Nutr 1999; 69(6):1108–1116.
41. Wadden TA, Berkowitz RI, Womble LG, et al. Randomized trial of lifestyle modification and pharmacotherapy for obesity. N Engl J Med 2005; 353(20):2111–2120.
42. Lujan JA, Frutos MD, Hernandez Q, et al. Laparoscopic versus open gastric bypass in the treatment of morbid obesity: a randomized prospective study. Ann Surg 2004; 239(4):433–437.
43. Lee WJ, Huang MT, Yu PJ, et al. Laparoscopic vertical banded gastroplasty and laparoscopic gastric bypass: a comparison. Obes Surg 2004; 14(5):626–634.
44. Hall JC, Watts JM, O'Brien PE, et al. Gastric surgery for morbid obesity. The Adelaide Study. Ann Surg 1990; 211(4):419–427.
45. Buchwald H, Avidor Y, Braunwald E, et al. Bariatric surgery: a systematic review and meta-analysis. JAMA 2004; 292(14):1724–1737.
46. Lin CC, Tsan KW, Chen PJ. The relationship between sleep apnea syndrome and hypothyroidism. Chest 1992; 102(6):1663–1667.
47. Resta O, Pannacciulli N, Di Gioia G, et al. High prevalence of previously unknown subclinical hypothyroidism in obese patients referred to a sleep clinic for sleep disordered breathing. Nutr Metab Cardiovasc Dis 2004; 14(5):248–253.
48. Resta O, Carratu P, Carpagnano GE, et al. Influence of subclinical hypothyroidism and T4 treatment on the prevalence and severity of obstructive sleep apnoea syndrome (OSAS). J Endocrinol Invest 2005; 28(10):893–898.
49. Skjodt NM, Atkar R, Easton PA. Screening for hypothyroidism in sleep apnea. Am J Respir Crit Care Med 1999; 160(2):732–735.
50. Rajagopal KR, Abbrecht PH, Derderian SS, et al. Obstructive sleep apnea in hypothyroidism. Ann Intern Med 1984; 101(4):491–494.
51. Mickelson SA, Lian T, Rosenthal L. Thyroid testing and thyroid hormone replacement in patients with sleep disordered breathing. Ear Nose Throat J 1999; 78(10):768–771, 774–775.

52. Grunstein RR, Ho KY, Sullivan CE. Sleep apnea in acromegaly. Ann Intern Med 1991; 115(7):527–532.
53. Fatti LM, Scacchi M, Pincelli AI, et al. Prevalence and pathogenesis of sleep apnea and lung disease in acromegaly. Pituitary 2001; 4(4):259–262.
54. Wellman A, Jordan AS, Malhotra A, et al. Ventilatory control and airway anatomy in obstructive sleep apnea. Am J Respir Crit Care Med 2004; 170(11):1225–1232.
55. Grunstein RR, Ho KK, Sullivan CE. Effect of octreotide, a somatostatin analog, on sleep apnea in patients with acromegaly. Ann Intern Med 1994; 121(7):478–483.
56. Herrmann BL, Wessendorf TE, Ajaj W, et al. Effects of octreotide on sleep apnoea and tongue volume (magnetic resonance imaging) in patients with acromegaly. Eur J Endocrinol 2004; 151(3):309–315.
57. McNicholas WT, Tarlo S, Cole P, et al. Obstructive apneas during sleep in patients with seasonal allergic rhinitis. Am Rev Respir Dis 1982; 126(4):625–628.
58. Horner RL, Innes JA, Holden HB, et al. Afferent pathway(s) for pharyngeal dilator reflex to negative pressure in man: a study using upper airway anaesthesia. J Physiol 1991; 436:31–44.
59. Kiely JL, Nolan P, McNicholas WT. Intranasal corticosteroid therapy for obstructive sleep apnoea in patients with co-existing rhinitis. Thorax 2004; 59(1):50–55.
60. McLean HA, Urton AM, Driver HS, et al. Effect of treating severe nasal obstruction on the severity of obstructive sleep apnoea. Eur Respir J 2005; 25(3):521–527.
61. Bahammam AS, Tate R, Manfreda J, et al. Upper airway resistance syndrome: effect of nasal dilation, sleep stage, and sleep position. Sleep 1999; 22(5):592–598.
62. Heimer D, Scharf SM, Lieberman A, et al. Sleep apnea syndrome treated by repair of deviated nasal septum. Chest 1983; 84(2):184–185.
63. Series F, St Pierre S, Carrier G. Effects of surgical correction of nasal obstruction in the treatment of obstructive sleep apnea. Am Rev Respir Dis 1992; 146:1261–1265.
64. Mezzanotte WS, Tangel DJ, White DP. Waking genioglossal electromyogram in sleep apnea patients versus normal controls (a neuromuscular compensatory mechanism). J Clin Invest 1992; 89(5):1571–1579.
65. Malhotra A, Edwards JK, Shea SA, et al. Neuromuscular compensatory mechanisms in obstructive sleep apnea: role of upper airway receptor mechanisms. Sleep 1999; 22:S259.
66. White DP. Sleep-related breathing disorder. 2. Pathophysiology of obstructive sleep apnoea. Thorax 1995; 50(7):797–804.
67. Haponik EF, Smith PL, Bohlman ME, et al. Computerized tomography in obstructive sleep apnea. Correlation of airway size with physiology during sleep and wakefulness. Am Rev Respir Dis 1983; 127(2):221–226.
68. Schwab RJ, Gupta KB, Gefter WB, et al. Upper airway and soft tissue anatomy in normal subjects and patients with sleep-disordered breathing. Significance of the lateral pharyngeal walls. Am J Respir Crit Care Med 1995; 152(5 pt 1):1673–1689.
69. Isono S, Remmers JE, Tanaka A, et al. Anatomy of pharynx in patients with obstructive sleep apnea and in normal subjects. J Appl Physiol 1997; 82(4):1319–1326.
70. Malhotra A, Fogel R, Kikinis R, et al. The influence of aging and gender on upper airway structure and function. Am J Respir Crit Care Med 1999; 159:A170.
71. Strohl KP, Hensley MJ, Saunders NA, et al. Progesterone administration and progressive sleep apneas. JAMA 1981; 245(12):1230–1232.
72. Rajagopal KR, Abbrecht PH, Jabbari B. Effects of medroxyprogesterone acetate in obstructive sleep apnea. Chest 1986; 90(6):815–821.
73. Cook WR, Benich JJ, Wooten SA. Indices of severity of obstructive sleep apnea syndrome do not change during medroxyprogesterone acetate therapy. Chest 1989; 96(2):262–266.
74. Saaresranta T, Polo-Kantola P, Rauhala E, et al. Medroxyprogesterone in postmenopausal females with partial upper airway obstruction during sleep. Eur Respir J 2001; 18(6):989–995.
75. Cistulli PA, Barnes DJ, Grunstein RR, et al. Effect of short-term hormone replacement in the treatment of obstructive sleep apnoea in postmenopausal women. Thorax 1994; 49(7):699–702.
76. Herkert O, Kuhl H, Sandow J, et al. Sex steroids used in hormonal treatment increase vascular procoagulant activity by inducing thrombin receptor (PAR-1) expression: role of the glucocorticoid receptor. Circulation 2001; 104(23):2826–2831.
77. Brownell LG, West P, Sweatman P, et al. Protriptyline in obstructive sleep apnea: a double-blind trial. N Engl J Med 1982; 307(17):1037–1042.
78. Horner RL. Motor control of the pharyngeal musculature and implications for the pathogenesis of obstructive sleep apnea. Sleep 1996; 19(10):827–853.
79. Kubin L, Tojima H, Davies RO, et al. Serotonergic excitatory drive to hypoglossal motoneurons in the decerebrate cat. Neurosci Lett 1992; 139(2):243–248.
80. Kubin L, Tojima H, Reignier C, et al. Interaction of serotonergic excitatory drive to hypoglossal motoneurons with carbachol-induced, REM sleep-like atonia. Sleep 1996; 19(3):187–195.
81. Berry RB, Yamaura EM, Gill K, et al. Acute effects of paroxetine on genioglossus activity in obstructive sleep apnea. Sleep 1999; 22(8):1087–1092.

82. Kraiczi H, Hedner J, Dahlof P, et al. Effect of serotonin uptake inhibition on breathing during sleep and daytime symptoms in obstructive sleep apnea. Sleep 1999; 22(1):61–67.

83. Veasey SC. Serotonin agonists and antagonists in obstructive sleep apnea: therapeutic potential. Am J Respir Med 2003; 2(1):21–29.

84. Guilleminault C, Hayes B. Naloxone, theophylline, bromocriptine, and obstructive sleep apnea. Negative results. Bull Eur Physiopathol Respir 1983; 19(6):632–634.

85. Espinoza H, Antic R, Thornton AT, et al. The effects of aminophylline on sleep and sleep-disordered breathing in patients with obstructive sleep apnea syndrome. Am Rev Respir Dis 1987; 136(1):80–84.

86. Tojima H, Kunitomo F, Kimura H, et al. Effects of acetazolamide in patients with the sleep apnoea syndrome. Thorax 1988; 43(2):113–119.

87. Vgontzas AN, Papanicolaou DA, Bixler EO, et al. Sleep apnea and daytime sleepiness and fatigue: relation to visceral obesity, insulin resistance, and hypercytokinemia. J Clin Endocrinol Metab 2000; 85 (3):1151–1158.

88. Vgontzas AN, Zoumakis E, Lin HM, et al. Marked decrease in sleepiness in patients with sleep apnea by etanercept, a tumor necrosis factor-alpha antagonist. J Clin Endocrinol Metab 2004; 89(9):4409–4413.

89. Listing J, Strangfeld A, Kary S, et al. Infections in patients with rheumatoid arthritis treated with biologic agents. Arthritis Rheum 2005; 52(11):3403–3412.

90. Pack AI, Black JE, Schwartz JR, et al. Modafinil as adjunct therapy for daytime sleepiness in obstructive sleep apnea. Am J Respir Crit Care Med 2001; 164(9):1675–1681.

91. Black JE, Hirshkowitz M. Modafinil for treatment of residual excessive sleepiness in nasal continuous positive airway pressure-treated obstructive sleep apnea/hypopnea syndrome. Sleep 2005; 28(4):464–471.

92. Kingshott RN, Vennelle M, Coleman EL, et al. Randomized, double-blind, placebo-controlled crossover trial of modafinil in the treatment of residual excessive daytime sleepiness in the sleep apnea/hypopnea syndrome. Am J Respir Crit Care Med 2001; 163(4):918–923.

35 | Special Considerations for Treatment of Sleep-Related Breathing Disorders

Daniel B. Brown
Greenberg Traurig, LLP, Atlanta, Georgia, U.S.A.

Clete A. Kushida
Division of Sleep Medicine, Department of Psychiatry and Behavioral Sciences, Stanford University School of Medicine, Stanford, California, U.S.A.

SIDE EFFECTS OF TREATMENT

Positive Airway Pressure Therapy
In general, positive airway pressure (PAP) is well tolerated with minimal side effects. Common complaints include dry mouth, claustrophobia, nasal congestion, skin irritation or abrasion, difficulty with exhalation, chest discomfort, aerophagia, claustrophobia, and conjunctivitis due to air leak. The majority of these problems can be resolved by careful evaluation and monitoring of patients on PAP therapy, and should be addressed promptly to avoid decrements in patient's use and adherence to therapy. There are rare reports of serious complications such as pneumocephalus (subsequent to base of skull fracture), pulmonary barotraumas, tympanic membrane rupture, severe epistaxis, subcutaneous emphysema, increased intraocular pressure, and decreased cardiac output at high pressure that have been reported in association with nasal continuous positive airway pressure (CPAP).

Upper Airway Surgery
The side effects of upper airway surgery for sleep-related breathing disorders consist of postoperative pain, infection, swelling, and bleeding in a minority of patients. Voice changes, taste disturbances, and dysphagia have been reported, but are typically transient and are dependent on the type of surgery (see chap. 32).

Oral Appliances
Skeletal and bony changes, dental and temporomandibular joint (TMJ) discomfort, excessive salivation, dry mouth, gum irritation, headaches, and bruxism may occur with oral appliance therapy in the short term; periodontal complications, muscle spasms, otalgia, and displaced, loosened, and broken teeth represent potential long-term side effects (see chap. 33).

Adjunctive and Alternative Treatments
Adjunctive and alternative treatments for sleep-related breathing disorders consist of behavioral and positional therapies, weight loss, correction of other medical disorders, and pharmacological treatment (drugs that increase respiratory drive, etanercept, and modafinil). The side effects of these treatments are discussed in chapter 34.

AGE AND GENDER EFFECTS OF TREATMENT

For children and adolescents, adenotonsillectomy and/or orthodontic expansion treatment are considered the treatment of choice for sleep-related breathing disorders. More extensive upper airway surgery, PAP, and oral appliances are favored for adults; younger adults often have a preference for upper airway surgery to avoid lifelong use of PAP therapy. With respect to gender effects, obstructive sleep-disordered breathing is relatively uncommon in otherwise healthy young women of reproductive age. However, the biochemical and physical changes associated with pregnancy increase the occurrence of sleep-related breathing disorders in women. Similarly, the prevalence and clinical severity of obstructive sleep apnea increase dramatically with menopause. There does not appear to be a consistent trend for adherence to PAP therapy or outcomes of upper airway surgery between men and women. For oral appliances, women with OSA may be more likely to have treatment success compared with men, particularly those with milder forms of obstructive sleep apnea. However, men appear to be more likely to have treatment success when they have predominantly supine-dependent obstructive sleep apnea and are more likely to develop oral appliance treatment failure with even small changes in their body mass indices. Men who appear to have a higher degree of upper airway collapse (as evident by a greater apnea/hypopnea ratio) also have decreased treatment benefit with oral appliances. Weight loss may be a more effective treatment for men compared with women, perhaps because of men's typical pattern of weight loss in their upper body, which may play a role in reducing fat accumulation surrounding the upper airway. By contrast, bariatric surgery is more heavily favored by women, and it has been shown to effectively treat obstructive sleep apnea.

DRIVING RISK AND MEDICOLEGAL ASPECTS

The dangers of dozing and driving are obvious to those who take to the road. In 1996, the National Highway Traffic Safety Administration estimated that 56,000 police-reported crashes are the direct result of driver fatigue each year. These crashes cause over 1550 deaths and 40,000 injuries annually.[a]

American jurisprudence has long examined the risks posed by drowsy driving. Courts have weighed the duties owed to employees, to patients, and to fellow drivers, and have fashioned a variety of remedies for persons damaged by sleep-impaired drivers. State and federal legislatures have adopted laws to deter driving while fatigued altogether. This section discusses the legal duties imposed on drivers, employers, and physicians relative to sleepy driving as well as criminal and regulatory laws applicable to those who drive in a sleep-deprived state.

Legal Obligations of Sleepy Drivers

All persons who get behind the wheel have the legal duty to exercise reasonable care for the protection of others against unreasonable risks.[b] Sleep-deprived persons who know that they are overly fatigued have the heightened duty to get off the road to protect themselves and others against the risk of a foreseeable sleep episode on the road. If a driver senses oncoming sleep or if conditions that the driver knows are likely to induce sleep exist, then the driver has a duty to cease driving until his or her ability to drive unimpaired returns. Otherwise, the fatigued driver will likely be held liable for any damages caused by the driver's subsequent crash.[c]

On the other hand, a driver will not be found negligent if he or she unexpectedly "blacks out" behind the wheel because of the sudden and unexpected onset of sleep or illness.[d] Whether a driver is negligent or not in these cases turns on the foreseeability of the sleep episode. Courts routinely conclude that sleep is foreseeable if persons feel themselves becoming tired behind the wheel.

Employer's Legal Duties Respecting Overtime Scheduling

What about employees whose overtime schedules force them to stay at work for uninterrupted periods of ten, twelve, or more hours? Will courts find the employers liable for their employees' fatigue after work?

---

[a] National Highway Traffic Safety Administration Expert Panel on Driver Fatigue & Sleepiness; "Drowsy Driving and Automobile Crashes," Report H5 808 707, (1998).

[b] Prosser WL. Law of Torts. 4th ed. St. Paul: West Publishing Co., 1980:143.

[c] See, e.g., *McCall v. Wilder*, 913 S.W.2d 150 (Tenn. 1995).

[d] American Law Reports 2d. Physical Defect, Illness, Drowsiness, or Falling Asleep of Motor Vehicle Operator as Affecting Liability for Injury, Section 3, 28 A.L.R.2d 12, 1953 (updated 2006).

Courts typically refuse to extend liability to the employers for acts caused by their employees' sleepiness following working hours. For example, the Illinois Court of Appeals recently determined that Harrah's casino was not liable for its employee's one-car accident following the employee's putting in three consecutive shifts of 13 hours each.[e] The court reasoned that the fatigued driver is in the best position to know of his/her fatigue and to stay off the road. The employer's duty to control the employee's surroundings cease once the employee's workday has ended. Accordingly, the court in this case ruled that an employer has no duty to staff or schedule the workplace or so that employees are guaranteed sufficient time off for their leisure or, if they choose, for their sleep.[f]

A contrary and minority position has been taken by other courts. Thus, in the case of *Escoto v. Estate of Ambriz*, 200 S.W.3d 716 (Tex. App. 2006), the Texas Court of Appeals upheld a jury verdict finding an oil company liable for the death of five persons caused by the crash of a fatigued employee while driving home from work. Over a strong dissent, the Court ruled that the employer knew that the employee's long oil rig shift fatigued the employee, and therefore, the employer failed a duty to adequately train the employee of the dangers of fatigue. An earlier Oregon case likewise found the employer liable when the employee caused a car wreck following a long work shift at McDonald's restaurant. [see *Faverty v. McDonald's Restaurants of Oregon, Inc.*, 133 Or. App. 514, 892 P.2d 703 (1995)]. While theses cases stand for limited authority in their jurisdictions [see, e.g., *Bertram v. Malheur County*, 129 P.3d 222, 204 Or. App. 129 (Or App. 2006)], few other courts have adopted their rulings. [see, e.g., *Black v. William Insulation Co.*, 141 P.3d 123, 2006 WY 106 (WY 2006)].

Employer's Vicarious Liability for Their Employee's Sleepy Driving on the Job

The law treats employers differently if the employee's negligence occurs during work and as part of the driver's employment. The employee's negligence in such cases is imputed to the employer, and the employer will be liable for any damages caused by the employee's negligence.[g] Thus, if a truck driver falls asleep while driving on behalf of his employer and injures a third party, the trucking company will most likely be liable to pay for the injuries suffered by the victim.[h]

Federal and State Sleepy Driving Regulations

Recognizing the public safety risk of fatigued driving, federal and state departments of transportation have adopted strict limits for commercial drivers. Thus, federal driver fitness regulations require that no driver shall operate a commercial motor vehicle while impaired by fatigue or illness.[i] New York has a similar law respecting bus drivers.[j] To safeguard against fatigued driving, federal regulations limit the consecutive hours of service during which commercial drivers may operate a motor vehicle. The basic rule at this time is that no motor carrier shall permit or require a person to drive more than 11 cumulative hours following ten consecutive hours off duty.[k]

Chronic sleep deprivation suffered by commercial truck drivers is given special consideration by highway safety administrators. Thus, in 1991, the Federal Motor Carrier Safety Administration published advisory criteria to assist medical examiners determine a driver's physical qualifications for commercial driving. In part, the guidance provides that

> patients with sleep apnea syndrome having symptoms of excessive daytime somnolence cannot take part in interstate driving, because they likely will be involved in hazardous driving and accidents resulting from sleepiness. Even if

---

[e] *Behrens v. Harrah's Illinois Corp.*, 852 N.E.2d 553, 366 Ill. App. 3d 1154 (Ill. App. 2006).
[f] *Behrens v. Harrah's Illinois Corp.*, 366 Ill. App. 3d at 1158.
[g] See, e.g., *Burlington Industries, Inc. v. Ellerth*, 524 U.S. 742, 756 (1998).
[h] *Dunlap v. W.L. Logan Trucking Co.*, 161 Ohio App. 3d 51 (2005).
[i] 49 CFR § 392.3
[j] Chapter 71 of the New York Consolidated Laws, Vehicle and Traffic, Section 509-k.
[k] 49 CFR § 395.3

these patients do not have the sleep attacks, they suffer from daytime fatigue and tiredness. These symptoms will be compounded by the natural fatigue and monotony associated with the long hours of driving, thus causing increased vulnerability to accidents. Therefore, those patients who are not on any treatment and are suffering from symptoms related to [excessive daytime sleepiness] should not be allowed to participate in interstate driving. Those patients with sleep apnea syndrome whose symptoms (e.g., [excessive daytime sleepiness], fatigue etc.) can be controlled by surgical treatment, e.g., permanent tracheostomy, may be permitted to drive after 3 month period free of symptoms, provided there is constant medical supervision. Laboratory studies (e.g. polysomnographic and multiple sleep latency tests) must be performed to document absence of [excessive daytime sleepiness] and sleep apnea.[l]

Sleepy Driving and Criminal Behavior

Several states have enacted laws to recognize the role of sleep deprivation in cases of criminal vehicular homicide. New Jersey took the lead here with the adoption of "Maggie's Law" in 2003. This law followed upon the 1997 death of college student Margaret "Maggie" McConnell at the hands of a driver who admitted to police that he had smoked crack cocaine hours before his car crashed into Ms. McConnell and that he had not slept for 30 hours leading up to the crash. State prosecutors wanted to use evidence of the driver's fatigue to prove reckless behavior under New Jersey's vehicular homicide law. However, at the time, sleepiness, unlike drunkeness, was not recognized in New Jersey as credible evidence contributing to the crime of vehicular homicide. The judge dismissed the charges and assessed a token $200 penalty against the driver.

The state legislature reacted by enacting "Maggie's Law," which is an evidentiary rule providing that the proof of driving after 24 consecutive hours of sleeplessness "may give rise to an inference that the defendant was driving recklessly."[m] Although a few other states have passed similar laws, legislatures remain skeptical to criminalizing sleepy driving because of concern by law enforcement personnel regarding the lack of an objective test—comparable to the breathalyzer—that can be used to determine whether the driver had reached an unacceptable level of drowsiness. In fact, the New Jersey legislature itself distinguished fatigue from inebriation in Maggie's Law by providing that drunkenness "shall give rise to an inference that the defendant was driving recklessly," whereas sleepiness is a condition that "may" give rise to such an inference.[n]

Physicians' Duty to Warn and Report Fatigued Driving

Physicians who treat patients for hypersomnolence may have legal and ethical duties to the public to inform the patient of the risks of fatigued driving. In appropriate cases, a physician may be required by law to report the patient's condition to applicable state motor vehicle agencies.

As an initial matter, physicians do not generally have a duty to third parties to warn them regarding the dangers that could be caused by their patients' sleepiness. Therefore, a motorist injured by a driver suffering from a sleep disorder is not likely to prevail in a negligence action against the treating physician. Generally, this is because physicians only have duties to third parties when they "take charge" of their patients. Only in this limited instance do the physicians have the duty of reasonable care to prevent the patients from causing harm to others.[o]

---

[l] Federal Motor Carrier Safety Administration, Advisory Criteria; Conference on Neurological Disorders and Commercial Drivers. Available at: http://www.fmcsa.dot.gov/rulesregs/medreports.html. "Seizures, Epilepsy and Interstate Commercial Driving." Available at: http://www.fmcsa.dot.gov/documents/neuro2.pdf
[m] "Maggie's Law," N.J.S.2C:11-5(a).
[n] "Maggie's Law," N.J.S.2C:11-5(a).
[o] *Tarasoff v. Regents of University of California*, 17 Cal 3d 425, 131 Cal. Rptr 14, 551 P.2d 334 (1976).

Thus, the physician is not held responsible if a patient refuses to adopt the healthy sleep treatments, such as nightly CPAP, recommended by the physician. This is because the patient's willingness to follow the treatments is beyond the doctor's control.[p]

Nonetheless, the law does require the physician to warn the patient of the risks flowing from the use or misuse of the treatments.[q] For example, if a doctor prescribes a narcotic to his patient, the doctor has a duty to inform the patient not to drive after taking the drug.[r] In a case where a patient took a strong sedative and crashed while driving in an impaired state, the court ruled that the physician was liable to the victim not because the physician had a duty to prevent the patient from driving but because the physician had the duty to warn the patient not to drive, which the doctor failed to do.[s]

In addition to legal duties under common law negligence, physicians may have a statutory obligation to report impaired driving to the department of motor vehicles. For example, Vermont, Oregon, New Jersey, California, Delaware, Pennsylvania, and Nevada require physicians to report specific disorders of their patients to appropriate state agencies, typically the state department of motor vehicles.[t] Other states permit physicians to report their patients' impaired driving conditions, but do not require reporting. Still other state laws permit the report to be made anonymously, while some laws offer physicians complete immunity from liability if they have reported a patient's condition to the applicable agency prior to the patient's injury.[u]

According to the American Medical Association (AMA) "Physician's Guide to Assessing and Counseling Older Drivers," patients with a diagnosis of narcolepsy should cease driving altogether.[v] In 2000, the AMA adopted Ethical Opinion E-2.24 to address physicians' ethical obligations regarding patients who continue to drive against doctors' orders.[w] According to the Opinion, if clear evidence of substantial driving impairment implies a "strong threat" to patient and public safety and if the patient ignores the advice to discontinue driving, then the AMA believes that it is desirable and ethical for the physician to notify the applicable department of motor vehicles. The Opinion clarifies that physicians must follow state laws and should talk to their patients about the physicians' responsibility to report their patients' insistence to continue driving.

---

[p] *Taylor v. Smith*, 892 So.2d 887, 895 (Ala. 2004).

[q] See, e.g., *McKenzie v. Hawai'i Permanente Med. Group, Inc.*, 98 Hawai'i 296, 309, 47 P.3d 1209, 1222 (2002) (physician "owes a duty to non-patient third parties" to warn patients of possible adverse effects of prescribed medication on patients' driving ability, "where the circumstances are such that the reasonable patient could not have been expected to be aware of the risk without the physician's warning"); *Joy v. Eastern Maine Med. Ctr.*, 529 A.2d 1364 (Me. 1987) (physician who treated a patient by placing a patch over his eye owed a duty to motorists to warn the patient against driving while wearing the patch); *Welke v. Kuzilla*, 144 Mich. App. 245, 252, 375 N.W.2d 403, 406 (1985) (physician who injected a patient with an "unknown substance" owed a duty to motorists "within the scope of foreseeable risk, by virtue of his special relationship with [the patient]"); *Wilschinsky v. Medina*, 108 N.M. 511, 515, 775 P.2d 713, 717 (1989) (physicians owe a duty "to persons injured by patients driving automobiles from a doctor's office when the patient has just been injected with drugs known to affect judgment and driving ability"); *Zavalas v. State Dep't of Corr.*, 124 Ore. App. 166, 171, 861 P.2d 1026, 1028 (1993) (rejecting the argument "that a physician has no duty to third parties ... who claim that the physician's negligent treatment of a patient was the foreseeable cause of their harm"). But see *Kirk v. Michael Reese Hosp. & Med. Ctr.*, 117 Ill.2d 507, 513 N.E.2d 387, 111 Ill. Dec. 944 (1987); *Rebollal v. Payne*, 145 A.D.2d 617, 536 N.Y.S.2d 147 (1988).

[r] *Gooden v. Tips*, 651 S.W.2d 364, 370 (Tex. App. Tyler 1983).

[s] *Gooden v. Tips*, 651 S.W.2d 364 (Tex. App. Tyler 1983).

[t] See, generally, Massachusetts Medical Society, "Medical Perspectives on Impaired Driving" (July, 2003). Available at: http://www.massmed.org/AM/Template.cfm?Section=Home&CONTENTID=5027&TEM-PLATE=/CM/HTMLDisplay.cfm.

[u] American Medical Association, "Physician's Guide to Assessing and Counseling Older Drivers," chapter 8 (May 2003), providing a list of all 51 state laws regarding reporting of impaired drivers. The Guide is available at the American Medical Society: http://www.ama-assn.org/ama/pub/category/10791.html.

[v] See American Medical Association, "Physician's Guide to Assessing and Counseling Older Drivers," chapter 8 (May 2003).

[w] See American Medical Society, Ethics Opinion E-2.24, "Impaired Drivers and Their Physicians," (June 2004). Available at: http://www.ama-assn.org.

Finally, the AMA has adopted Health and Ethics Policy No. H-15.958, "Fatigue, Sleep Disorders, and Motor Vehicle Crashes." Through this policy, the AMA defines sleepy driving as a major public health issue to be studied and deterred. As to physician-patient encounters with sleepy drivers, the Policy recommends that physicians (*i*) become knowledgeable about the diagnosis and management of sleep-related disorders; (*ii*) investigate patient symptoms of drowsiness, wakefulness, and fatigue by inquiring about sleep and work habits and other predisposing factors when compiling patient histories; (*iii*) inform patients about the personal and societal hazards of driving or working while fatigued and advise patients about measures they can take to prevent fatigue-related and other unintended injuries; (*iv*) advise patients about possible medication-related effects that may impair their ability to safely operate a motor vehicle or other machinery; (*v*) inquire whether sleepiness and fatigue could be contributing factors in motor vehicle–related and other unintended injuries; and (*vi*) become familiar with the laws and regulations concerning drivers and highway safety in the state(s) where they practice.

CONCLUSIONS

Treatments for sleep-related breathing disorder are generally well tolerated with minimal side effects. There appears to be a minimal effect of age on treatment; however, gender appears to play a role in oral appliance and weight loss therapy for obstructive sleep apnea. Significant medicolegal ramifications exist for patients with sleep-related breathing disorders, as well as employers and physicians of these patients who have excessive daytime sleepiness as a consequence of these disorders.

36 | Description of Parasomnias

Tore A. Nielsen

Centre d'Etude du Sommeil, Hôpital du Sacré-Coeur de Montréal and Département de Psychiatrie, Université de Montréal, Montréal, Québec, Canada

Dominique Petit

Centre d'Etude du Sommeil, Hôpital du Sacré-Coeur de Montréal, Montréal, Québec, Canada

HISTORY AND NOMENCLATURE

The most recent consensus of the American Academy of Sleep Medicine is that parasomnias are "undesirable physical events or experiences that occur during entry into sleep, within sleep or during arousals from sleep" (1). Parasomnias are often considered to be normal sleep phenomena, especially in children, and do not in general have a serious impact on sleep quality or quantity. However, in some cases, injuries can result, psychological distress can ensue, and sleep disruption can seriously disturb the individual and family members.

Sleep research has demonstrated, and still continues to accumulate evidence, that parasomnias are not homogeneous phenomena, but constitute a diverse group of conditions with different pathophysiologies and responses to treatment. They are currently classified into primary parasomnias (Table 1), which are disorders of sleep states per se, and secondary parasomnias, which are disorders of specific organ systems that manifest preferentially during sleep. Primary parasomnias are further classified into: (*i*) disorders of arousal (or NREM [non-REM] parasomnias), (*ii*) parasomnias associated with REM sleep, and (*iii*) other parasomnias. Disorders of arousal (from NREM sleep) are, in turn, comprised of confusional arousals, somnambulism (or sleepwalking), and sleep terrors. Parasomnias associated with REM sleep consist of nightmare disorder, recurrent isolated sleep paralysis (SP), and REM sleep behavior disorder (RBD). Classification of the other, residual parasomnias includes principally sleep enuresis, sleep-related bruxism, sleep-related rhythmic movement disorder, somniloquy (or sleep talking), and sleep-related groaning. In the following sections, the clinical features, polysomnographic characteristics, incidence, prevalence, and associated factors of each of these primary parasomnias is reviewed.

KEY FEATURES AND CHARACTERISTICS

Disorders of Arousal (From NREM Sleep)
Confusional Arousals
Clinical features. Confusional arousals (or sleep drunkenness) are transitory states of confusional behavior or thought occurring during or following arousals from NREM sleep, typically from slow-wave sleep (SWS) early in the night, but occasionally also upon awakening in the morning (1). Typically, the individual is confused, disoriented, motorically slow, and may display automatic or inappropriate behaviors. Salient sleep mentation is usually not present. Sleep-related abnormal sexual behaviors, such as prolonged or violent masturbation, sexual molestation, initiation of sexual intercourse, and loud sexual vocalizations during sleep, are now considered to be part of the spectrum of confusional arousals (1).

Polysomnographic characteristics. Confusional arousals typically occur during the first two episodes of SWS, but can also occur during other NREM sleep stages later in the night or during naps. Recordings tend to show awakenings from SWS.

Associated factors. Childhood confusional arousals should be considered benign whereas in adults they are often associated with mental disorders or obstructive sleep apnea syndrome. Also, they occur more frequently in night-shift or rotating-shift workers (2). A family history of

Table 1 Primary Parasomnias Classified by Sleep Stage

Disorders associated with NREM sleep (disorders of arousal)	Disorders associated with REM sleep	Other disorders
Confusional arousals	Nightmare disorder	Enuresis
Somnambulism	Recurrent isolated sleep paralysis	Bruxism
Sleep terrors	REM behavior disorder	Rhythmic movement disorder
		Somniloquy
		Nocturnal groaning

confusional arousals is a major precipitating factor although many conditions (sleep deprivation, obstructive sleep apnea, drug/alcohol use) can enable them.

Sleepwalking (Somnambulism)

Clinical features. Sleepwalking is characterized by complex behaviors usually initiated during arousals from SWS; it may begin with simple movements, such as sitting up in bed, and culminate in walking, bolting from the room, or worse (1). Episodes of surprising complexity have been reported: cooking or eating (3), driving a car (4), even homicide (5–9). Accordingly, the duration of episodes may vary from a few seconds to several minutes (3). Related mental activities have not been studied in detail but various reports suggest instances of amnesia, confusion, perceived threat, dreaming, and even pseudohallucination. Although usually considered a benign condition in children, sleepwalking in adults is potentially injurious.

Polysomnographic characteristics. Analyses of sleep architecture reveal no significant differences between adult somnambulistic patients and control subjects (10–15), except for a greater number of arousals selectively out of SWS in sleepwalkers (10,12). As shown in Figure 1, sleepwalkers were found to have lower power in slow-wave activity during the first NREM cycle and a higher number of awakenings during SWS than control subjects (12). Several studies have documented the presence of high-amplitude delta waves, termed "hypersynchronous delta (HSD)" activity, just prior to somnambulistic episodes (10,13,16,17). However, although sleepwalkers have higher ratios of HSD per time in NREM sleep on frontal and central electroencephalographic (EEG) derivations than do controls, the presence of HSD activity prior to somnambulistic episodes was not confirmed in more recent and controlled studies (18). Finally, EEG analyses have produced no evidence of complete awakenings during any laboratory-recorded episodes (19).

Full-blown episodes of somnambulism are rare in the sleep laboratory, but they may be triggered by sleep deprivation. A new method of total sleep deprivation for 38 hours increases the frequency and behavioral complexity of episodes during recovery sleep (18,20). Diagnosis may be substantially aided by such techniques.

Associated factors. There is a strong genetic component to somnambulism (21); it was recently found to be linked to the HLA-DQB1 gene (22). Also, anxiety may increase somnambulistic occurrences in both children and adults (23–25). Based on clinical and research experience, Rosen and colleagues (25) proposed that somnambulism and sleep terrors may be nocturnal expressions of repressed anger concerning major life events such as separation, divorce, marital conflict, or family relocation.

Sleep Terrors

Clinical features. Sleep terrors (also known as night terrors or pavor nocturnus) are "arousals from SWS accompanied by a cry or piercing scream and autonomic nervous system and behavioral manifestations of intense fear" (1). Typically, within 90 minutes after sleep onset, the individual screams loudly and sits up in bed bearing a panic-stricken expression. There is usually intense autonomic activity (sweating, tachycardia, rapid breathing) and, less often, complex behaviors such as leaving the bed, fleeing the room, or thrashing around. Injuries may result in such cases. The distinction between sleep terrors and somnambulism is not clear-cut

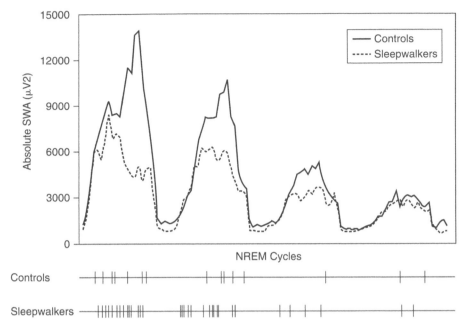

Figure 1 Slow-wave activity (SWA) over four consecutive NREM-REM cycles in 15 sleepwalkers and 15 healthy paired controls. Power is significantly reduced in the second half of the 1st NREM period among sleepwalkers. Awakenings from SWS are indicated on the 2 horizontal lines below the graph. *Source*: From Ref. 12.

although the activity displayed during sleep terrors is usually more rapid and abrupt than it is during somnambulism (26). Inconsolability is a key feature of sleep terrors; attempting to console or awaken an individual during an episode will only unduly prolong or intensify it. As is the case for somnambulism and confusional arousals, an individual suffering sleep terrors usually does not wake up fully and remains amnesic for the event the next day.

Polysomnographic characteristics. As for somnambulism, sudden awakenings from SWS, especially in the second half of the first two SWS sleep episodes, is typical of sleep terrors. However, a normal polysomnogram does not rule out a diagnosis of sleep terrors. Time spent in stages 3 and 4 sleep preceding an episode appears to be positively correlated with severity of the episode (26). Rarely, sleep terrors may arise from stage 2.

Associated factors. Sleep terrors that occur in childhood are usually not associated with a neurological condition, whereas onset in adulthood could indicate a neurological disease. As is true for somnambulism and confusional arousals, genetic factors play a major role. Monozygotic twins are more concordant than dizygotic twins for sleep terrors (27) and terrors are twice as frequent in children for whom one or both parents have a sleepwalking history than in children with nonaffected parents (28).

Parasomnias Associated with REM Sleep
Nightmare Disorder
Clinical features. Nightmare disorder consists of persistent disturbing dreams that arise primarily from REM sleep (more rarely from stage 2 sleep) and that usually awaken the sleeper (1,29). Presence or absence of an awakening is often used to distinguish nightmares from bad dreams and there is typically a much lower level of autonomic activation in nightmares than in sleep terrors. There is also usually an absence of dream-enacting behaviors except in situations of intense emotional stress and sleep disruption such as during the postpartum state (30). Awakenings from nightmares are usually abrupt, not confused and accompanied by recall of a detailed disturbing dream. Idiopathic nightmares, which have no apparent cause, are commonly distinguished from post-traumatic nightmares, which are the result of one or more prior trauma.

Polysomnographic characteristics. Nightmares are associated with fluctuations in heart rate and respiratory activity during REM sleep but often the autonomic arousal appears much less than might be expected from the disturbing dream content (31). Evidence from brain-lesioned patients (32) demonstrates a link between temporo-limbic brain regions and frequent nightmares of both recurring and nonrecurring types. Post-traumatic nightmares are accompanied by heightened physiological reactivity in the form of more frequent awakenings (33), longer wake time after sleep onset (WASO) (33,34), and increased motor and rapid eye movement activity during REM sleep (35–37). PTSD patients with trauma-related nightmare complaints also exhibit higher REM and NREM sleep respiration rates than do non-PTSD controls (38). Both idiopathic and post-traumatic nightmare patients exhibit more periodic leg movements (PLMs) in REM and NREM sleep (33).

Associated factors. A genetic contribution to nightmares has been suggested by one large population study to be 44% for men and 45% for women in the case of childhood nightmares (39). Bad dreams among 29-month-old preschoolers are predicted by mother ratings of difficult temperament as early as 5 months of age and by mother and father ratings of child anxiety as early as 17 months (40). Among adults, nightmares are also associated with psychopathological traits (41–43) and personality variables such as physical and emotional reactivity (41,44,45), fantasy proneness (46,47), and thin boundaries (48–55). Nightmares are more frequent and prevalent in psychiatric populations (56–60) and are associated with pathological symptoms such as anxiety, neuroticism, post-traumatic stress disorder, schizophrenia-spectrum symptoms, suicide risk, dissociative phenomena, problematic health behaviors, and sleep disorders (29,61). Nightmares are also reactive to increased life stress (41,44,62–66). This general pattern of comorbidity between nightmares, pathological symptoms, and stress has been explained as due to an underlying distress-prone personality style (29,61).

Recurrent Isolated Sleep Paralysis
Clinical features. Recurrent isolated SP, previously known as isolated SP or simply SP, is a common, generally benign, parasomnia characterized by brief episodes of motor or vocal paralysis combined with a waking state of consciousness (1). During SP episodes, frightening dreamlike hallucinations often intrude and produce considerable distress. Episodes occur primarily at sleep onset (hypnagogic) and on awakening (hypnopompic). Isolated SP is distinguished from narcolepsy, which is characterized by cataplexy and excessive daytime sleepiness in addition to SP and hypnagogic hallucinations (1). Feelings of fear and terror are the most prevalent emotional reactions accompanying SP experiences (67) and are often linked to the hallucination of *sensed presence*, i.e., a vivid, perception-like, impression that a sentient being is nearby, but frequently without a clear visual image of that being (68,69).

Polysomnographic characteristics. SP episodes most often arise from sleep-onset REM periods (Fig. 2) (70,71), leading to the view that the episodes are bouts of state dissociation during which some REM sleep mechanisms—muscle atonia and vivid dreaming in particular—intrude on the waking state (72,73).

Associated factors. Among the factors associated with SP episodes are stress (71,74,75), shift work, and irregular sleep-wake schedules (75,76). A genetic component has also been reported, e.g., 36% of respondents in a Japanese sample had family members who experienced SP (77).

Several studies link SP to various neurological and psychiatric disorders. It is predicted by bipolar disorder, automatic behavior, and use of anxiolytic medications (78). It is also comorbid with PTSD (79–81), depression symptoms (82–84), anxiety disorder with agoraphobia (85), panic disorder (81,86–89), generalized anxiety disorder, and social anxiety (90,91). This wide comorbidity has recently been attributed to mediation by an affect distress personality style ("SP distress") in a manner analogous to that proposed for nightmare disorder ("nightmare distress") (68).

Associations of SP with psychiatric conditions vary among ethnic groups. Atypically high rates were found in African Americans with panic disorders (88,89), Moroccan patients (92), and Cambodians (79). Some of these differences may stem from cultural interpretations of SP hallucinations, sensed presence in particular, as a form of spiritual entity, e.g., "ghost

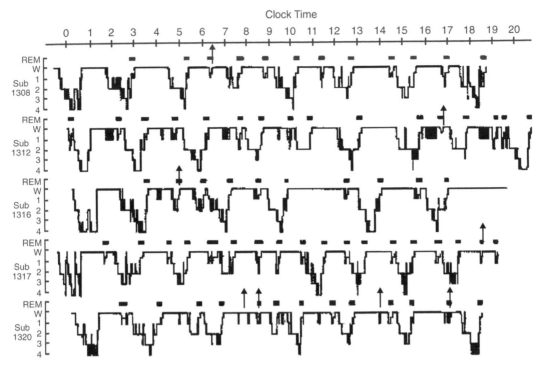

Figure 2 Somnograms of five healthy subjects reporting sleep paralysis (SP) episodes during a multiphasic sleep-wake schedule. Vertical arrows above somnograms indicate awakening points where SP episodes were reported. Out of 184 awakenings, 8 paralysis episodes were reported; 2 immediately prior to impending REM episodes (spontaneous awakenings) and 6 from a sleep-onset REM episode (planned awakenings). *Source*: From Ref. 71.

oppression" in China (75), "Old Hag" in Newfoundland (93), "the ghost that pushes you down" in Cambodia (79), etc.

REM Sleep Behavior Disorder
Clinical features. RBD is characterized by the loss of skeletal muscle atonia normally present during REM sleep and accompanied by complex dream-enacting motor activity. It was first described as a clinical entity in 1986 (94). Diagnostic criteria include: (*i*) complaint of violent or injurious behaviors during sleep, (*ii*) limb or body movements associated with dream mentation, and (*iii*) one of the following: harmful or potentially harmful sleep behaviors, dreams that appear to be acted out, sleep behaviors that disrupt sleep continuity. In addition, the dream process and its content appear altered. Most patients (87%) report that their dreams become more vivid, intense, action-filled, and violent with the onset of RBD (95). Dream themes associated with behaviors are largely stereotyped in structure and emotional content (94,96). Among published reports of dreams for which investigators identified specific behaviors, the most frequent pattern is of vigorous defense against attacks by people (58.8%) and animals (23.5%) (97). Content analyses of recently remembered dreams reveal an elevated proportion of aggressive contents, yet normal levels of daytime aggressiveness (98).

Sleep behaviors produce injuries to the patient or the bedpartner such as ecchymoses, lacerations, fractures, and subdural hematomas. Injuries are a main reason for consultation, being reported by 79% to 96% of consulting cases (99,100).

Polysomnographic characteristics. Polysomnographic recording reveals an intermittent or complete loss of REM sleep muscle atonia and excessive phasic EMG activity during REM sleep (96). The PSG diagnostic criteria are presence of: (*i*) excessive augmentation of chin EMG tone, (*ii*) excessive chin or limb phasic EMG twitching, and (*iii*) one of the following features during REM sleep: excessive limb or body jerking, complex, vigorous, or violent behaviors or absence of epileptic activity.

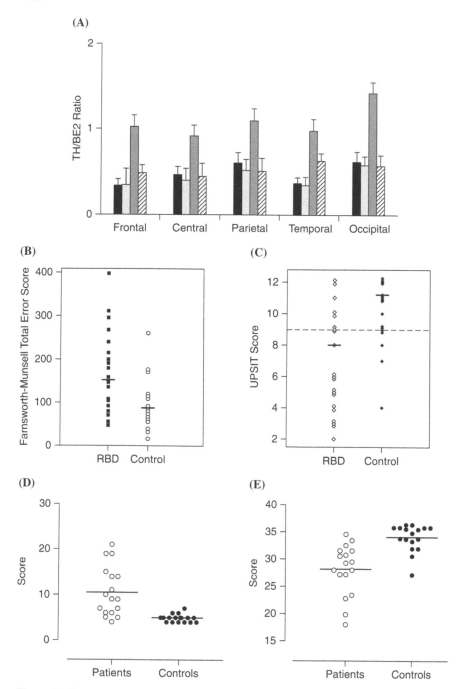

Figure 3 Electroencephalographic changes and sensory and neuropsychological deficits associated with REM sleep behavior disorder (RBD). (**A**) EEG slowing during wakefulness is indicated by a generalized increase in the theta/beta2 ratio in male RBD patients (gray bars) relative to male controls (black bars), female controls (white bars), and female RBD patients (hatched bars). (**B**) Visual discrimination deficits are apparent as higher error scores on the Farnsworth–Munsell 100-Hue Test for RBD patients. (**C**) Olfactory discrimination deficits are apparent as lower average scores on the University of Pennsylvania Brief Smell Identification Test. (**D** and **E**) Neuropsychological deficits are shown by higher error scores on the Corsi Supraspan Learning Test (**D**) and lower scores on the Rey–Osterrieth's Complex Figure (**E**). *Source*: (**A**) From Ref. 103, (**B**) from Ref. 122, (**C**) from Ref. 122, and (**D** and **E**) from Ref. 126.

To quantify the PSG variables in this condition, a method has been proposed (101) that uses only EEG and EOG channels to score REM sleep. Compared with age-matched controls, RBD patients demonstrate a higher percentage of SWS (102), more delta power in NREM sleep (102), lower occipital beta power during REM sleep (103), markedly higher theta power in frontal, temporal, and occipital regions, lower occipital beta power, and lower dominant occipital frequency during wakefulness (103). Other waking state anomalies are described below.

Associated factors. RBD is strongly associated with neurodegenerative diseases, especially the synucleinopathy subtype (104) which include Parkinson's disease (105,106), dementia with Lewy bodies (107–111), and multiple system atrophy (112–118). Recently, RBD has been shown to coexist with two tauopathies: Alzheimer's disease (119) and progressive supranuclear palsy (120). Even patients with idiopathic RBD show some signs of neurodegeneration. For example, FDG-PET brain imaging of cognitively normal patients with dream-enacting behaviors revealed lower metabolic activity in several brain regions known to be affected in dementia with Lewy bodies (121).

Multiple dysfunctions have been described in the last 5 years for RBD patients (see Fig. 3), including olfactory deficits, color identification deficits, and decreased motor speed (122), EEG slowing (103), mild dysautonomia (123,124), and subtle neuropsychological dysfunctions (103,125,126).

RBD has also been associated with narcolepsy and other neurological disorders, such as olivopontocerebellar degeneration, ischemic cerebrovascular disease, multiple sclerosis, Guillain–Barré syndrome, Shy–Drager syndrome, and Arnold–Chiari syndrome (96).

Other Parasomnias

Sleep Enuresis

Clinical features. Sleep enuresis is characterized by recurrent involuntary voiding during sleep at least twice a week among individuals who are at least five years of age (1). It is considered primary if the child has never been constantly dry during sleep and secondary when the child (or adult) had been previously dry for at least six consecutive months and started wetting at least twice a week for at least three months.

Polysomnographic characteristics. Although parents commonly consider sleep enuresis to be caused by sleeping too deeply, consistent changes in sleep depth and sleep architecture have not been demonstrated (127). However, a study using polysomnographic recording has shown that enuretic boys are more difficult to arouse from sleep than are age-matched controls (128). For most children, micturition occurs in the first half of the night and is not associated with a specific sleep stage (127). Tachycardia and short EEG arousals are often seen prior to enuretic events (127).

Associated factors. An association between enuresis and delayed achievement of early childhood developmental milestones such as motor skills (for boys) and language (for girls) has been demonstrated (129). This indicates that bed-wetting may reflect delayed development of the central nervous system. Enuresis is not linked with anxiety in preschoolers (130) but is in older children (131–133). However, anxiety is more likely a consequence than a cause of enuresis. Hereditary factors have been recognized; it is inherited via an autosomal dominant mode of transmission (134). Prevalence is 77% when both parents were enuretic as children and 44% when one parent was enuretic (135).

Sleep-Related Bruxism

Clinical features. Sleep-related bruxism is the grinding or clenching of one's teeth during sleep, usually in association with sleep arousals (1). This activity results in tooth wear, headaches, jaw dysfunction, and pain. Orofacial morphology is not likely a causal factor since it has been shown not to differentiate sleep bruxers from controls (136).

Polysomnographic characteristics. Although abnormal tooth wear is highly indicative of sleep bruxism, a definite diagnosis rests on the presence of rhythmic masticatory muscle

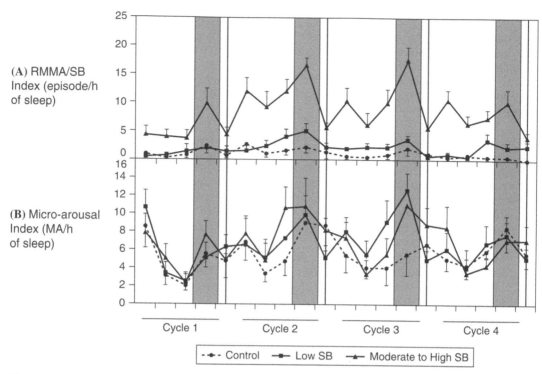

Figure 4 Rhythmic masticatory muscle activity (RMMA) and micro-arousals during four NREM-REM cycles in patients with sleep bruxism and controls. Each NREM sleep cycle is divided into four segments (**A**). RMMA/SB index is significantly higher during the last NREM sleep segment (gray vertical bars) before REM sleep (shown with the vertical line) within each sleep cycle for all SB subjects but not for controls. (**B**). Microarousals per hour of sleep also peaked towards the last NREM sleep segment before REM sleep. *Source*: From Ref. 140.

activity and grinding sounds during all-night polysomnographic recording. Bruxism episodes most frequently occur in stages 1 and 2 but can occur in all stages (137,138). Bruxers have normal sleep architecture and high sleep efficiency, i.e., greater than 90% (137). However, a clear sequence of cortical to cardiac activation preceding jaw motor activity in bruxism patients (139) suggests that sleep bruxism is secondary to microarousals. In fact, both microarousals and rhythmic masticatory muscle activity/sleep bruxism episodes were shown to increase concomitantly just prior to each REM sleep period (Fig. 4) (140).

Associated factors. Anxiety has been reported as an associated factor in children (141), adolescents, and adults (142,143). Smoking also exacerbates bruxism (144). As is the case for many parasomnias, there is a strong genetic influence (145).

Sleep-Related Rhythmic Movement Disorder
Clinical features. Sleep-related rhythmic movement disorder is characterized by the repetitive, stereotyped, and rhythmic activity of large muscle groups that occurs predominantly during drowsiness (sleep onset) or sleep (1). It can involve any body part although the most frequent rhythmic movements are body rocking, head rolling, and head banging. Body rocking may be difficult to distinguish from head banging because the former movement sometimes includes banging of the head into a solid object. It is largely a parasomnia of infancy and early childhood. The frequency of movements ranges between 0.5 and 2.0 Hz but is more typically around 1 Hz (146). Time spent in rhythmic motion can vary from a few seconds to more than an hour (146) but in most cases will occur nightly or almost nightly (147). The majority of episodes (around 80%), at least for head banging, occur at sleep onset (147). When appearing at sleep onset, rhythmic movements are considered to be self-soothing or tension-releasing behaviors linked with pleasurable sensations that have hypnotic properties. However, more violent movements, usually in cases of mental retardation, can cause eye or head injuries (148–150).

Polysomnographic characteristics. Different case reports indicate that rhythmic movement disorder can arise from REM sleep, NREM sleep, or sleep onset with persisting activity in light sleep. Longer movements are usually observed at sleep onset and during stage 1 sleep whereas shorter movements are seen in stages 2, 3, 4, and REM sleep (146). Sleep-related rhythmic movements are not preceded by EEG changes as are nocturnal seizures (146) and do not provoke arousals or interrupt SWS even in older children (147,151).

Associated factors. There are no reports of rhythmic movement disorder in association with other parasomnias or sleep problems except for restless legs syndrome, which is associated with body rocking (152). Cases of adult rhythmic movement disorder are not usually associated with severe psychiatric disorders as previously believed. However, some studies have reported daytime complaints such as attentional difficulties, sleepiness, morning headaches, fatigue, and poor concentration, and even more serious problems such as anxiety, depression, hyperactivity, and irritability (146,153,154). Whether the daytime symptoms result from poor sleep caused by the rhythmic movements remains to be determined.

Somniloquy
Clinical features. Somniloquy, also known as sleep talking, is defined as talking during sleep "with varying degrees of comprehensibility" (1). Somniloquy is such a prevalent phenomenon that it is considered to be a normal sleep behavior, especially in childhood.

Polysomnographic characteristics. Somniloquy can arise from all sleep stages (155). Since there are few systematic polysomnographic studies, no clear profiles have been identified. However, EMG-induced artifact is common and may begin several seconds prior to, and continue for several seconds after, verbalizations (156). Temporary suspension of eye movements and the occurrence of sustained alpha EEG trains during REM sleep somniloquy episodes have also been noted (156) as has suppression of theta and alpha activity prior to the utterances (157). Episodes frequently occur in parallel with sleep mentation, but concordance between verbal utterances and ongoing dreamed speech may vary from isomorphic to completely absent (158). As shown in Figure 5, concordances of any kind are more common in REM (82.6%) than in stage 2 (58.2%) or stage 3–4 (34.4.1%) sleep (156).

Associated factors. Since somniloquy is so prevalent, it is virtually impossible to isolate predisposing factors. Nonetheless, there is a clear genetic influence (159). Somniloquy is also the parasomnia that most often co-occurs with other parasomnias. It often accompanies the behavioral manifestations of either RBD or somnambulism. Stereotyped vocalizations can also be heard during nocturnal seizures. In most cases, however, somniloquy is idiopathic.

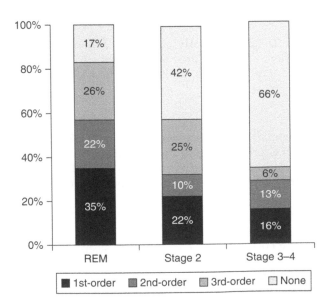

Figure 5 Sleep-speech/mentation-report concordances in relation to associated sleep stage in 122 laboratory speech-mentation pairs. All three types of concordance are more frequent for REM sleep (82.6%) than for either Stage 2 (58.2%) or Stage 3 to 4 (34.4%) sleep reports (*N* = 23, 67, 32 reports respectively; awakenings with no recall removed). 1st-order concordances = same words spoken and dreamed; 2nd-order concordances = conceptually related words spoken and dreamed; 3rd-order concordances = dreamed words referred nonspecifically to spoken words (adapted from Arkin, 1981, p. 120, Table 7.6) (156).

Sleep-Related Groaning
Clinical features. Also known as catathrenia, sleep-related groaning is defined as "a chronic, usually nightly, disorder characterized by expiratory groaning during sleep, particularly during the second half of the night" (1). Groaning or moaning sounds typically begin two to six hours after sleep onset. The sounds produced are usually loud but the pitch and timbre vary among individuals: groaning, loud humming, roaring, and high-pitched sounds have all been observed. By contrast, within individuals the type of sound is usually fairly constant. Catathrenia is not associated with abnormal motor activity and is qualitatively different from somniloquy. Degree of concordance with sleep mentation is unknown. The affected individual is usually unaware of the problem and, apart from occasional complaints of daytime sleepiness, typically has no other sleep complaints. However, production of the sounds may disturb the bed partner. The identification of this disorder is relatively new, with approximately 45 cases in total reported in the literature (160–170).

Polysomnographic characteristics. Catathrenia occurs during either REM or NREM sleep but episodes arise predominantly from REM sleep; only one patient presented groaning exclusively in NREM sleep (164). PSG tracings reveal bradypneic events, often occurring in clusters, with deep inspirations followed by long expirations and monotonous vocalization. There is a high night-to-night consistency of the groaning episodes (165). Although catathrenia is associated with bradypneic events, only one of the reported cases (162) had significant obstructive apneas or hypopneas and had an oxygen saturation remaining above 90% across the night. Body position does not seem to have any influence (164). Whereas the loud sounds of snoring or obstructive sleep apneas occur during the inspiratory phase, the vocalizations of catathrenia occur during expiration. Unlike sleep apnea, sleep architecture for nocturnal groaners is usually preserved. However, a few patients will show either reduced total sleep time combined with reduced sleep efficiency, or a reduction of either slow-wave or REM sleep (164).

Associated factors. Neurological and physical (including otorhinolaryngologic) examination, routine laboratory testing, and medical history show no specific anomaly (164–166). Apart from the fact that a small proportion of patients (7%) present concomitant bruxism, there are no associated conditions or obvious predisposing factors (164). As for many parasomnias, catathrenia seems to be, at least in part, genetically determined. In about 15% of cases, there is at least one family relative also affected, sometimes in a way consistent with an autosomal dominant pattern of inheritance (164).

INCIDENCE AND PREVALENCE

Disorders of Arousal (From NREM Sleep)
Confusional Arousals
The incidence is unknown but episodes are frequent in early childhood and diminish in occurrence after the age of five years (25). Often, young children with persisting confusional arousals become sleepwalkers in adolescence. Prevalence in adults is 3% to 4% (2) and no gender difference has been reported.

Somnambulism
The peak incidence of somnambulism (approximately 17%) is around age 12 (171). For adults, a suggested prevalence of 2% to 2.5% (78,172) is probably an underestimate. Although many studies report no gender difference in older children, adolescents, or adults (141,171), a recent study of two large cohorts of young children (2.5–6 and 4–9 years old) found it to be more common in boys than in girls (130,173).

Sleep Terrors
Reported incidence estimates are wide-ranging (141,174–176). For childhood sleep terrors, the age range studied and the sampling method and definition used affect the estimate. Further, some parents may fail to differentiate nightmares and sleep terrors. When an operational definition is supplied, a high overall prevalence (40%) is seen in preschoolers (130). As for

somnambulism and confusional arousals, sleep terrors tend to resolve during adolescence and do not display a gender difference (130,141). In adults, there is a high degree of overlap among the three principal disorders of arousal.

Parasomnias Associated with REM Sleep

Nightmare Disorder

Nightmare Disorder per se is rarely evaluated in prevalence studies whereas nightmares as a subjective symptom usually are. The prevalence of nightmare symptoms is estimated in tandem with their temporal frequency. Accordingly, nightmares as a symptom occur occasionally in over 85% of the general population, at least once a month in 8% to 29% and at least once a week in 2% to 6% (45,59,172,177,178). A large literature on prevalence is difficult to decipher due to the use of different operational definitions, response scales, age ranges, and study samples (see reviews (29,61,179)). Nonetheless, there is a broad consensus that a frequency of at least one nightmare per week reflects clinical pathology.

Bad dreams are surprisingly infrequent among preschoolers (1.5–3.9% report them *often* or *always*) but may appear as early as 29 months and remain highly stable until age six (40). An internet survey of approximately 24,000 respondents (see also Ref. 180) found that the typical monthly recall of nightmares peaks between the ages of 20 to 29 and declines steadily—a pattern consistent with many previous studies. A gender difference favoring girls appears in adolescence (181,182) and continues throughout the lifespan, as shown in Figure 6 (180).

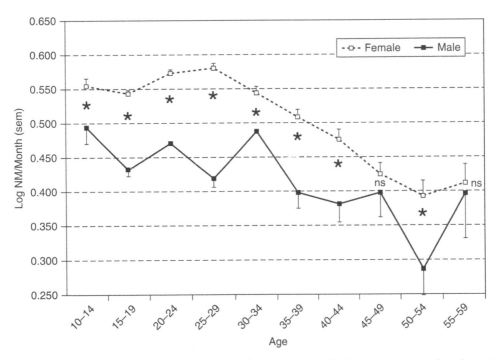

Figure 6 Retrospective estimates of monthly nightmare frequency by five-year age strata in an internet sample of 23,839 respondents (see also Ref. 180). *Significant difference between female and male subjects at that stratum, $p < .05$.

Recurrent Isolated Sleep Paralysis

Variations in prevalence estimates (5–40%) depend on differences in operational definitions, age of subjects, and sociocultural factors (74,76,78). Age of onset is typically 14 to 17 years. Accompanying sensed presence hallucinations occur in 60% to 69% of cases (68,69,183,184).

REM Sleep Behavior Disorder

Overall prevalence of RBD remains largely unknown. A large telephone survey assessing violent behaviors during sleep in the general population (15–100 years) suggested a prevalence of about 0.5% (185). Another study of 1034 individuals (70+ years) in the Hong Kong area found a prevalence of PSG-confirmed RBD of 0.4% (186). There is a male predominance (87%) with primarily men over the age of 50 being affected (95). Milder forms of RBD with less aggressive behaviors that do not lead to clinical consultation have been postulated for women (95).

Other Parasomnias
Sleep Enuresis
Three population-based studies (130,187,188) found that between 20% and 33% of children were bedwetting at the age of five years. A male predominance in prevalence is well-established (130,141,187,188). Adult enuresis is rare, occurring in about 3% of elderly women (65+ years) and 1% of elderly men living at home (189).

Sleep-Related Bruxism
Sleep bruxism is very common in early childhood. A recent longitudinal, population-based study found that the prevalence increases from 10% at 2.5 years to 33% at 6 years of age (130). Another longitudinal study reported a progressive decrease toward adolescence attaining 9% at age 13 (141). An age-related decline in prevalence has also been described throughout adulthood in a population-based study (190). Overall prevalence in adults has been estimated to be around 8% (191). No gender difference has been found for either children (141) or adults (190). The presence of sleep bruxism in childhood and adulthood are highly correlated (145).

Sleep-Related Rhythmic Movement Disorder
In infancy, this parasomnia is quite common but decreases rapidly in prevalence with increasing age. Incidences of 66% at nine months, 26% at 2 years, and 6% at 5 years had been reported using a small sample of children (192) but a recent epidemiological study reported lower incidences of about 6% at 2.5 years, 3% at 4 and 5 years, and 2% at 6 years (130). Body rocking was found present in 3% of children aged 11 to 13 years (141). In rare cases, rhythmic movement disorder persists into adulthood. No gender differences have been demonstrated.

Somniloquy
Although considered the most frequent parasomnia, somniloquy is usually without consequences and thus rarely a reason for consultation. Its prevalence among preschoolers (84% (130)) is much higher than among older children and adolescents. A prevalence of 30% was found for children aged 11 to 13 years using mainly retrospective reports (141) while in adults, an estimate of 24% was found using a telephone sampling method (185). There is no apparent gender difference.

Sleep-Related Groaning
Nocturnal groaning represents less than 1% of the population consulting at a sleep disorder center (164). However, since this parasomnia is without major consequences, there is probably a large number of affected individuals that does not seek medical help. It appears to be three times more prevalent in men than in women although too few cases have been reported so far to be able to determine the gender ratio accurately. Onset is habitually during adolescence or early adulthood and the parasomnia persists for several years (164). The precise time course of the condition is unknown due to lack of follow-up on this recently identified condition.

PHYLOGENY AND ANIMAL MODELS

Whereas animal models have been developed for cataplexy, restless legs syndrome and even sleep apnea syndrome, there are very few animal models for parasomnias, except for RBD and perhaps nightmare disorder.

REM Sleep Behavior Disorder
Using various approaches (electrophysiology, lesions, neuropharmacology), studies with cats suggest that there are two motor systems involved in normal REM sleep: one for generating

muscle atonia and one for suppressing locomotor activity (193–201). To illustrate, lesions to the atonia system alone (coeruleus/subcoeruleus and/or magnocellular reticular formation in the cat and nucleus sublaterodorsal in the rat) produce only REM sleep without atonia (202), a phenomenon frequently encountered in neurodegenerative diseases and thought to be an incomplete form of RBD. To produce full-blown RBD in animals, lesions must also involve the system that normally suppresses brainstem motor generators during REM sleep (202). However, there may be species-specific differences in REM sleep control (203). Further research in humans will be necessary to determine how similar REM sleep control or its dysregulation is between humans and animal models and what the corresponding structures are.

Nightmare Disorder

Although there is no animal model of nightmare disorder per se, the AMPHAC model (short for amygdala, medial prefrontal cortex, hippocampus, and anterior cingulate cortex) was proposed recently as a possible neurophysiological substrate of nightmare formation (29,61). This model is based on a vast literature on animal and human fear learning and the brain correlates of social distress and personality (61,204,205). While there is some redundancy of function in this network, each of the brain regions corresponds roughly to a particular domain of processing in the fear extinction process: the amygdala in emotional activation and control of fear memory acquisition; the hippocampus in the control of memory context; the medial prefrontal cortex in the storage and control of extinction memories; and the anterior cingulate cortex in the regulation of affect distress. Converging findings indicate that the same four brain regions of the network are also implicated in REM sleep, PTSD (206,207), anxiety disorders (208), and some individual state and trait differences in emotion regulation (29). Dysfunction in this network is proposed to underlie nightmares of varying severity.

SOCIAL AND ECONOMIC FACTORS

Sleep is an integral part of health and daily functioning. Yet the full magnitude of the social and economic costs of sleep disorders is only starting to become clear and our ability to directly measure these costs is rapidly improving. The direct and indirect costs of sleep disorders as a whole were estimated to be $7.5 billion for the Australian population (20.1 million people) in 2004; on a per capita basis, this would translate to about $109 billion for the United States (209) and $12.3 billion for Canada. More specific estimates have been calculated for sleep apnea syndrome (210) and insomnia (211,212) but less is known about the economic impact of parasomnias. As for the social consequences of parasomnias, more research is also needed. However, at least two parasomnias, sleepwalking and RBD, warrant more immediate attention because of the injuries they often inflict on patients and their families.

Somnambulism

Adult somnambulism can result in serious injuries to the sleeper or to others or can lead to the destruction of property such as the breaking of walls, doors, windows, and plumbing. Reported behaviors during either somnambulism or agitated sleep terrors include running into walls and furniture, jumping out of windows, driving a car, wandering around streets, climbing ladders, sexual activity, and manipulating weapons—even loaded shotguns.

Moreover, the fact that somnambulistic episodes can include such complex and organized behaviors as suspected suicide, homicide and attempted homicide, raises fundamental medicoforensic questions (4,5,213–220). Indeed, the number of legal cases of sleep-related violence is on the rise (221) and sleepwalking represents one of the leading causes of sleep-related injury (222).

REM Behavior Disorder

In one PSG investigation (14) of 100 consecutive patients consulting for repeated nocturnal injury, more than a third were diagnosed with RBD. Injuries are very frequent in RBD (99,100) and are a main reason for consultation. RBD episodes may also cause severe sleep disruption for the bed partner and lead to major marital discord, mood changes, and even suicide attempts (223). Beyond the injurious consequences of RBD, it has been shown that RBD may be a prodrome for neurodegenerative diseases, especially Parkinson and Lewy body diseases.

Idiopathic RBD has been recently associated with the risk of developing a neurodegenerative disorder and dementia. In fact, 45% of patients with idiopathic RBD developed either Parkinson disease, Lewy body disease or multisystemic atrophy after a follow-up of only five years (224). A longer follow-up (11 years) revealed that 65% of RBD patients developed a neurodegenerative disorder leading to dementia in most cases (225).

CONCLUSIONS

Parasomnias are quite varied in their expression, ranging from simple movements (rocking, grinding, groaning) to very complex and seemingly purposeful behaviors (sleepwalking, REM behavior disorder). Fortunately, most parasomnias are considered benign, especially when they occur during childhood, and as such do not require treatment. In addition, the incidence and prevalence of these undesirable sleep events decreases significantly with the onset of adolescence. However, some parasomnias are very problematic because they give rise to injuries, psychological distress, and sleep disruption on the part of the affected individual and, often, his/her bed partner. In such cases, polysomnographic recordings provide strong supplemental support to the clinical diagnosis. Finally, it is important to note, particularly in legal cases of sleep-related violence when a diagnosis of parasomnia has been established, that parasomnias involve behaviors that are not clearly motivated, are devoid of sound judgment, and are not under conscious deliberate control.

REFERENCES

1. American Academy of Sleep Medicine. ICSD-II. International Classification of Sleep Disorders: Diagnostic and Coding Manual. 2nd ed. Chicago: American Academy of Sleep Medicine, 2005.
2. Ohayon MM, Priest RG, Zulley J, et al. The place of confusional arousals in sleep and mental disorders: findings in a general population sample of 13,057 subjects. J Nerv Ment Dis 2000; 188:340–348.
3. Masand P. Sleepwalking. Am Fam Phys 1995; 51:649–653.
4. Schenck CH, Mahowald MW. A polysomnographically documented case of adult somnambulism with long-distance automobile driving and frequent nocturnal violence: parasomnia with continuing danger as a noninsane automatism? Sleep 1995; 18:765–772.
5. Broughton R, Billings R, Cartwright R, et al. Homicidal somnambulism: a case report. Sleep 1994; 17: 253–264.
6. Howard C, D'Orban P. Violence in sleep: medico-legal issues and two case reports. Psychol Méd 1987; 17:915–925.
7. Ovuga EBL. Murder during sleep-walking. East Afr Med J 1992; 69:533–534.
8. Hartmann E. Two case reports: night terrors with sleepwalking—a potentially lethal disorder. J Nerv Ment Dis 1983; 171:503–505.
9. Gottlieb P, Christensen O, Kramp P. On serious violence during sleepwalking. Br J Psychiatr 1986; 149:120–121.
10. Blatt I, Peled R, Gadoth N, et al. The value of sleep recording in evaluating somnambulism in young adults. Electroencephalogr Clin Neurophysiol 1991; 78:407–412.
11. Denesle R, Nicolas A, Gosselin A, et al. Sleepwalking and aggressive behavior in sleep. Sleep 1998; 21(suppl 1):70.
12. Gaudreau H, Joncas S, Zadra A, et al. Dynamics of slow-wave activity during the NREM sleep of sleepwalkers and control subjects. Sleep 2000; 23:755–760.
13. Guilleminault C, Leger D, Philip P, et al. Nocturnal wandering and violence: review of a sleep clinic population. J Forensic Sci 1998; 43:158–163.
14. Schenck CH, Milner DM, Hurwitz TD, et al. A polysomnographic and clinical report on sleep-related injury in 100 adult patients. Am J Psychiatr 1989; 146:1166–1173.
15. Schenck CH, Pareja JA, Patterson AL, et al. Analysis of polysomnographic events surrounding 252 slow-wave sleep arousals in thirty-eight adults with injurious sleepwalking and sleep terrors. J Clin Neurophysiol 1998; 15:159–166.
16. Jacobson A, Kales A, Lehmann D, et al. Somnambulism: all-night electroencephalographic studies. Science 1965; 148:975–977.
17. Kales A, Soldatos CR, Caldwell AB, et al. Somnambulism: clinical characteristics and personality patterns. Arch Gen Psychiatr 1980; 37:1406–1410.
18. Pilon M, Zadra A, Joncas S, et al. Hypersynchronous delta waves and somnambulism: brain topography and effect of sleep deprivation. Sleep 2006; 29:77–84.

19. Zadra A, Pilon M, Joncas S, et al. Analysis of postarousal EEG activity during somnambulistic episodes. J Sleep Res 2004; 13:279–284.

20. Joncas S, Zadra A, Paquet J, et al. The value of sleep deprivation as a diagnostic tool in adult sleepwalkers. Neurology 2002; 58:936–940.

21. Hublin C, Kaprio J, Heikkila K, et al. Prevalence and genetic of sleepwalking: a population-based twin study. Neurology 1997; 48:177–181.

22. Lecendreux M, Bassetti C, Dauvilliers Y, et al. HLA and genetic susceptibility to sleepwalking. Mol Psychiatry 2003; 8:114–117.

23. Cirignotta F, Zucconi M, Mondini S, et al. Enuresis, sleepwalking, and nightmares: an epidemiological survey in the republic of San Marino. In: Guilleminault C, Lugaresi E, eds. Sleep/Wake Disorder: Natural History, Epidemiology, and Long-Term Evolution. New York: Raven Press, 1983:237–241.

24. Crisp AH, Matthews BM, Oakey M, et al. Sleepwalking, night terrors, and consciousness. Br Med J 1990; 300:360–362.

25. Rosen G, Mahowald MW, Ferber R. Sleepwalking, confusional arousals, and sleep terrors in the child. In: Ferber R, Kryger M, eds. Principles and Practice of Sleep Medicine in the Child. Philadelphia: WB Saunders Company, 1995:99–106.

26. Fisher C, Kahn E, Edwards A, et al. A psychophysiological study of nightmares and night terrors: I. Physiological aspects of the Stage 4 night terror. J Nerv Ment Dis 1973; 157:75–98.

27. Abe K, Oda N, Ikenaga K, et al. Twin study on night terrors, fears and some physiological and behavioral characteristics in childhood. Psychiatr Genet 1993; 3:39–43.

28. Abe K, Amatomi M, Oda N. Sleepwalking and recurrent sleeptalking in children of childhood sleepwalkers. Am J Psychiatr 1984; 141:800–801.

29. Levin R, Nielsen TA. Disturbed dreaming, posttraumatic stress disorder, and affect distress: a review and neurocognitive model. Psychol Bull 2007; 133:482–528.

30. Nielsen T, Paquette T. Dream-associated behaviors affecting pregnant and postpartum women. Sleep 2007; 30:1162–1169.

31. Fisher C, Byrne J, Edwards A, et al. A psychophysiological study of nightmares. J Am Psychoanal Assoc 1970; 18:747–782.

32. Solms M. The Neuropsychology of Dreams. Mahwah, NJ: Lawrence Erlbaum Associates, 1997.

33. Germain A, Nielsen TA. Sleep pathophysiology in PTSD and idiopathic nightmare sufferers. Biol Psychiatry 2003; 54:1092–1098.

34. Woodward SH, Arsenault NJ, Murray C, et al. Laboratory sleep correlates of nightmare complaint in PTSD inpatients. Biol Psychiatry 2000; 48:1081–1087.

35. Harvey AG, Jones C, Schmidt DA. Sleep and posttraumatic stress disorder: a review. Clin Psychol Rev 2003; 23:377–407.

36. Orr SP, Roth WT. Psychophysiological assessment: clinical applications for PTSD. J Affect Disord 2000; 61:225–240.

37. Pitman RK, Orr SP, Shalev AY, et al. Psychophysiological alterations in post-traumatic stress disorder. Semin Clin Neuropsychiatry 1999; 4:234–241.

38. Woodward SH, Leskin GA, Sheikh JI. Sleep respiratory concomitants of comorbid panic and nightmare complaint in post-traumatic stress disorder. Depress Anxiety 2003; 18:198–204.

39. Hublin C, Kaprio J, Partinen M, et al. Nightmares: familial aggregation and association with psychiatric disorders in a nationwide twin cohort. Am J Med Genet 1999; 88:329–336.

40. Simard V, Nielsen TA, Tremblay RE, et al. Longitudinal study of bad dreams in preschool children: prevalence, demographic correlates, risk and protective factors. Sleep 2008; 31:62–70.

41. Kales A, Soldatos CR, Caldwell AB, et al. Nightmares: clinical characteristics and personality patterns. Am J Psychiatr 1980; 137:1197–1201.

42. Levin R, Fireman G. Nightmare prevalence, nightmare distress, and self-reported psychological disturbance. Sleep 2002; 25:205–212.

43. Zadra A, Donderi DC. Nightmares and bad dreams: their prevalence and relationship to well-being. J Abn Psychol 2000; 109:273–281.

44. Kramer M, Schoen LS, Kinney L. Psychological and behavioral features of disturbed dreamers. Psychiatr J U Ottawa 1984; 9:102–106.

45. Levin R. Sleep and dreaming characteristics of frequent nightmare subjects in a university population. Dreaming 1994; 4:127–137.

46. Levin R, Fireman G. The relation of fantasy proneness, psychological absorption, and imaginative involvement to nightmare prevalence and nightmare distress. Imagination Cogn Personality 2001; 21: 111–129.

47. Starker S. Daydreams, nightmares, and insomnia: The relation of waking fantasy to sleep disturbances. Imagination Cogn Personality 1984; 4:237–248.

48. Claridge GK, Clark K, Davis C. Nightmares, dreams, and schizotypy. Br J Clin Psychol 1997; 36: 377–386.

49. Cowen D, Levin R. The use of the Hartmann boundary questionnaire with an adolescent population. Dreaming 1995; 5:105–114.

50. Hartmann E. The Nightmare: The Psychology and the Biology of Terrifying Dreams. New York: Basic Books, 1984.

51. Hartmann E, Elkin R, Garg M. Personality and dreaming: the dreams of people with very thick or very thin boundaries. Dreaming 1991; 1:311–324.

52. Kunzendorf RG, Hartmann E, Cohen R, et al. Bizarreness of the dreams and daydreams reported by individuals with thin and thick boundaries. Dreaming 1997; 7:265–271.

53. Levin R, Gilmartin L, Lamontanaro L. Cognitive style and perception: the relationship of boundary thinness to visual-spatial processing in dreaming and waking thought. Imagination Cogn Personality 1999; 18:25–41.

54. Schredl M, Schafer G, Hofmann F, et al. Dream content and personality: thick vs. thin boundaries. Dreaming 1999; 9:257–263.

55. Pietrowsky R, Köthe M. Personal boundaries and nightmare consequences. Dreaming 2003; 13:245–254.

56. Berlin RM, Litovitz GL, Diaz MA, et al. Sleep disorders on a psychiatric consultation service. Am J Psychiatr 1984; 141:582–584.

57. Cernovsky ZZ. MMPI and nightmare reports in women addicted to alcohol and other drugs. Percept Mot Skills 1986; 62:717–718.

58. Levin R. Nightmares and schizotypy. Psychiatry 1998; 61:206–216.

59. Ohayon MM, Morselli PL, Guilleminault C. Prevalence of nightmares and their relationship to psychopathology and daytime functioning in insomnia subjects. Sleep 1997; 20:340–348.

60. Tanskanen A, Tuomilehto J, Viinamaki H, et al. Nightmares as predictors of suicide. Sleep 2001; 24:845–848.

61. Nielsen T, Levin R. Nightmares: a new neurocognitive model. Sleep Med Rev 2007; 11:295–310.

62. Barrett D. Trauma and Dreams. Cambridge, MA: Harvard University Press, 1996.

63. Berquier A, Ashton R. Characteristics of the frequent nightmare sufferer. J Abn Psychol 1992; 101: 246–250.

64. Cernovsky ZZ. Group nightmares about escape from ex-homeland. J Clin Psychol 1990; 46:581–588.

65. Dunn KK, Barrett D. Characteristics of nightmare subjects and their nightmares. Psychiatr J U Ottawa 1988; 13:91–93.

66. Husni M, Cernovsky ZZ, Koye N, et al. Nightmares of refugees from Kurdistan. J Nerv Ment Dis 2001; 189:557–558.

67. Cheyne JA, Rueffer SD, Newby-Clark IR. Hypnagogic and hypnopompic hallucinations during sleep paralysis: neurological and cultural construction of the night-mare. Conscious Cogn 1999; 8:319–337.

68. Solomonova E, Nielsen T, Stenstrom P, et al. Sensed presence as a correlate of sleep paralysis distress, social anxiety and waking state social imagery. Conscious Cogn 2008; 17:49–63.

69. Cheyne JA. The ominous numinous. J Consciousness Stud 2001; 8:133–150.

70. Hishikawa Y, Shimizu T. Physiology of REM sleep, cataplexy, and sleep paralysis. In: Fahn S, Hallett M, Luders HO, et al., eds. Negative Motor Phenomena. Advances in Neurology, Vol. 67. Philadelphia: Lippincott-Raven, 1995:245–271.

71. Takeuchi T, Fukuda K, Sasaki Y, et al. Factors related to the occurrence of isolated sleep paralysis elicited during a multi-phasic sleep-wake schedule. Sleep 2002; 25:89–96.

72. Giaquinto S, Pompeiano O, Somogyi I. Supraspinal modulation of heteronymous monosynaptic and of polysynaptic reflexes during natural sleep and wakefulness. Archives Italiennes de Biologie 1964; 102:230–244.

73. Cheyne JA. Sleep paralysis episode frequency and number, types, and structure of associated hallucinations. J Sleep Res 2005; 14:319–324.

74. Fukuda K, Miyasita A, Inugami M, et al. High prevalence of isolated sleep paralysis: *Kanashibari* phenomenon in Japan. Sleep 1987; 10:279–286.

75. Wing YK, Lee ST, Chen CN. Sleep paralysis in Chinese: ghost oppression phenomenon in Hong Kong. Sleep 1994; 17:609–613.

76. Kotorii T, Uchimura N, Hashizume Y, et al. Questionnaire relating to sleep paralysis. Psychiatr Clin Neurosci 2001; 55:265–266.

77. Arikawa H, Templer DI, Brown R, et al. The structure and correlates of Kanashibari. J Psychol 1999; 133:369–375.

78. Ohayon MM, Guilleminault C, Priest RG. Night terrors, sleepwalking, and confusional arousals in the general population: their frequency and relationship to other sleep and mental disorders. J Clin Psychiatr 1999; 60:268–276.

79. Hinton DE, Pich V, Chhean D, et al. Sleep paralysis among Cambodian refugees: association with PTSD diagnosis and severity. Depress Anxiety 2005; 22:47–51.

80. Ohayon MM, Shapiro CM. Sleep disturbances and psychiatric disorders associated with posttraumatic stress disorder in the general population. Compr Psychiatr 2000; 41:469–478.

81. Yeung A, Xu Y, Chang DF. Prevalence and illness beliefs of sleep paralysis among Chinese psychiatric patients in China and the United States. Transcult Psychiatry 2005; 42:135–145.

82. McNally RJ, Clancy SA. Sleep paralysis in adults reporting repressed, recovered, or continuous memories of childhood sexual abuse. J Anxiety Disord 2005; 19:595–602.

83. McNally RJ, Clancy SA. Sleep paralysis, sexual abuse, and space alien abduction. Transcult Psychiatry 2005; 42:113–122.

84. Szklo-Coxe M, Young T, Finn L, et al. Depression: relationships to sleep paralysis and other sleep disturbances in a community sample. J Sleep Res 2007; 16:297–312.

85. Alfonso SS. Isolated sleep paralysis in patients with disorders due to anxiety crisis. Actas Luso Esp Neurol Psiquiatr Cienc Afines 1991; 19:58–61.

86. Bell CC, Dixie-Bell DD, Thompson B. Further studies on the prevalence of isolated sleep paralysis in black subjects. J Natl Med Assoc 1986; 78:649–659.

87. Bell CC, Hildreth CJ, Jenkins EJ, et al. The relationship of isolated sleep paralysis and panic disorder to hypertension. J Natl Med Assoc 1988; 80:289–294.

88. Paradis CM, Friedman S. Sleep paralysis in African Americans with panic disorder. Transcult Psychiatry 2005; 42:123–134.

89. Friedman S, Paradis C. Panic disorder in African-Americans: symptomatology and isolated sleep paralysis. Cult Med Psychiatr 2002; 26:179–198.

90. Simard V, Nielsen TA. Sensed presence as a possible manifestation of social anxiety. Dreaming 2005; 15:245–260.

91. Otto MW, Simon NM, Powers M, et al. Rates of isolated sleep paralysis in outpatients with anxiety disorders. J. Anxiety Disord 2006; 20:687–693.

92. de Jong JT. Cultural variation in the clinical presentation of sleep paralysis. Transcult Psychiatry 2005; 42:78–92.

93. Hufford DJ. The Terror that Comes in the Night: An Experience-Centered Study of Supernatural Assault Traditions. Philadelphia: University of Pennsylvania Press, 1982.

94. Schenck CH, Bundlie SR, Ettinger MG, et al. Chronic behavioral disorders of human REM sleep: a new category of parasomnia. Sleep 1986; 9:293–308.

95. Schenck CH, Mahowald MW. REM sleep behavior disorder: clinical, developmental, and neuroscience perspectives 16 years after its formal identification in SLEEP. Sleep 2002; 25:120–138.

96. Mahowald MW, Schenck CH. REM sleep parasomnias. In: Kryger MH, Roth T, Dement WC, eds. Principles and Practice of Sleep Medicine. 4th ed. Philadelphia: Elsevier Saunders, 2005:897–916.

97. Nielsen TA. Disturbed dreaming in medical conditions. In: Kryger M, Roth N, Dement WC, eds. Principles and Practice of Sleep Medicine. 4th ed. Philadelphia: Elsevier Saunders, 2005:936–945.

98. Fantini ML, Corona A, Clerici S, et al. Aggressive dream content without daytime aggressiveness in REM sleep behavior disorder. Neurology 2005; 65:1010–1015.

99. Schenck CH, Hurwitz TD, Mahowald MW. Normal and abnormal REM sleep regulation: REM sleep behaviour disorder: an update on a series of 96 patients and a review of the world literature. J Sleep Res 1993; 2:224–231.

100. Olson EJ, Boeve BF, Silber MH. Rapid eye movement sleep behaviour disorder: demographic, clinical and laboratory findings in 93 cases. Brain 2000; 123:331–339.

101. Lapierre O, Montplaisir J. Polysomnographic features of REM sleep behavior disorder: development of a scoring method. Neurology 1992; 42:1371–1374.

102. Massicotte-Marquez J, Carrier J, Decary A, et al. Slow-wave sleep and delta power in rapid eye movement sleep behavior disorder. Ann Neurol 2005; 57:277–282.

103. Fantini ML, Gagnon JF, Petit D, et al. Slowing of electroencephalogram in rapid eye movement sleep behavior disorder. Ann Neurol 2003; 53:774–780.

104. Boeve BF, Silber MH, Ferman TJ, et al. Association of REM sleep behavior disorder and neurodegenerative disease may reflect an underlying synucleinopathy. Mov Dis 2001; 16:622–630.

105. Comella CL, Nardine TM, Diederich NJ, et al. Sleep-related violence, injury, and REM sleep behavior disorder in Parkinson's disease. Neurology 1998; 51:526–529.

106. Gagnon JF, Bedard MA, Fantini ML, et al. REM sleep behavior disorder and REM sleep without atonia in Parkinson's disease. Neurology 2002; 59:585–589.

107. Schenck CH, Bundlie SR, Mahowald MW. Delayed emergence of a Parkinsonian disorder in 38% of 29 older men initially diagnosed with idiopathic rapid eye movement sleep behaviour disorder. Neurology 1996; 46:388–393.

108. Mckeith IG, Perry EK, Perry RH. Report of the second dementia with Lewy body international workshop: diagnosis and treatment. Consortium on dementia with Lewy bodies. Neurology 1999; 53:902–905.

109. Boeve BF, Silber MH, Ferman TJ, et al. REM sleep behavior disorder and degenerative dementia: an association likely reflecting Lewy body disease. Neurology 1998; 51:363–370.

110. Ferman TJ, Boeve BF, Smith GE, et al. REM sleep behavior disorder and dementia: cognitive differences when compared with AD. Neurology 1999; 52:951–957.

111. Turner RS, Chervin RD, Frey KA, et al. Probable diffuse Lewy body disease presenting as REM sleep behavior disorder. Neurology 1997; 49:523–527.

112. Tison F, Wenning GK, Quinn NP, et al. REM sleep behaviour disorder as the presenting symptom of multiple system atrophy. J Neurol Neurosurg Psychiatr 1995; 58:379–385.

113. Plazzi G, Corsini R, Provini F, et al. REM sleep behavior disorders in multiple system atrophy. Neurology 1997; 48:1094–1097.

114. Tachibana N, Kimura K, Kitajima K, et al. REM sleep motor dysfunction in multiple system atrophy: with special emphasis on sleep talk as its early clinical manifestation. J Neurol Neurosurg Psychiatr 1997; 63:678–681.

115. Sforza E, Zucconi M, Petronelli R, et al. REM sleep behavioral disorders. Eur Neurol 1988; 28: 295–300.

116. Quera-Salva MA, Guilleminault C. Olivopontocerebellar degeneration, abnormal sleep, and REM sleep without atonia. Neurology 1986; 36:576–577.

117. Manni R, Morini R, Martignoni E, et al. Nocturnal sleep in multisystem atrophy with autonomic failure: polygraphic findings in ten patients. J Neurol 1993; 240:249–250.

118. Wetter TC, Collado-Seidel V, Pollmacher T, et al. Sleep and periodic leg movement patterns in drug-free patients with Parkinson's disease and multiple system atrophy. Sleep 2000; 23:361–367.

119. Gagnon JF, Petit D, Fantini ML, et al. REM behavior disorder and REM sleep without atonia in probable Alzheimer disease. Sleep 2006; 29:1309–1313.

120. Arnulf I, Merino-Andreu M, Bloch F, et al. REM sleep behavior disorder and REM sleep without atonia in patients with progressive supranuclear palsy. Sleep 2005; 28:349–354.

121. Caselli RJ, Chen K, Bandy D, et al. A preliminary fluorodeoxyglucose positron emission tomography study in healthy adults reporting dream-enactment behavior. Sleep 2006; 29:927–933.

122. Postuma RB, Lang AE, Massicotte-Marquez J, et al. Potential early markers of Parkinson disease in idiopathic REM sleep behavior disorder. Neurology 2006; 66:845–851.

123. Fantini ML, Michaud M, Gosselin N, et al. Periodic leg movements in REM sleep behavior disorder and related autonomic and EEG activation. Neurology 2002; 59:1889–1894.

124. Ferini-Strambi L, Zucconi M. REM sleep behavior disorder. Clin Neurophysiol 2000; 111(suppl 2): S136–S140.

125. Fantini ML, Ferini-Strambi L, Montplaisir J. Idiopathic REM sleep behavior disorder: toward a better nosologic definition. Neurology 2005; 64:780–786.

126. Ferini-Strambi L, Di Gioia MR, Castronovo V, et al. Neuropsychological assessment in idiopathic REM sleep behavior disorder (RBD): does the idiopathic form of RBD really exist? Neurology 2004; 62:41–45.

127. Bader G, Neveus T, Kruse S, et al. Sleep of primary enuretic children and controls. Sleep 2002; 25:579–583.

128. Wolfish NM, Pivik RT, Busby KA. Elevated sleep arousal thresholds in enuretic boys: clinical implications. Acta Paediatrica 1997; 86:381–384.

129. Touchette E, Petit D, Paquet J, et al. Bedwetting and its association with developmental milestones in early childhood. Arch Pediatr Adolesc Med 2005; 159:1129–1134.

130. Petit D, Touchette E, Tremblay RE, et al. Dyssomnias and parasomnias in early childhood. Pediatrics 2007; 119:e1016–e1025.

131. van Hoecke E, Hoebeke P, Braet C, et al. An assessment of internalizing problems in children with enuresis. J Urol 2004; 171:2580–2583.

132. Verduin TL, Kendall PC. Differential occurrence of comorbidity within childhood anxiety disorders. J Clin Child Adolesc Psychol 2003; 32:290–295.

133. Fergusson DM, Horwood LJ. Nocturnal enuresis and behavioral problems in adolescence: a 15-year longitudinal study. Pediatrics 1994; 94:662–668.

134. von Gontard A, Schaumburg H, Hollmann E, et al. The genetics of enuresis: a review. J Urol 2001; 166:2438–2443.

135. Bakwin H. The genetics of enuresis. In: Kolvin I, MacKeith RC, Meadow SR, eds. Bladder Control and Enuresis. London: Spastics International Medical Publications, 1973:73–77.

136. Lobbezoo F, Rompre PH, Soucy JP, et al. Lack of associations between occlusal and cephalometric measures, side imbalance in striatal D2 receptor binding, and sleep-related oromotor activities. J Orofac Pain 2001; 15:64–71.

137. Lavigne GJ, Rompre PH, Montplaisir JY. Sleep bruxism: validity of clinical research diagnostic criteria in a controlled polysomnographic study. J Dent Res 1996; 75:546–552.

138. Macaluso GM, Guerra P, Di Giovanni G, et al. Sleep bruxism is a disorder related to periodic arousals during sleep. J Dent Res 1998; 77:565–573.

139. Kato T, Rompre P, Montplaisir JY, et al. Sleep bruxism: an oromotor activity secondary to micro-arousal. J Dent Res 2001; 80:1940–1944.

140. Huynh N, Kato T, Rompre PH, et al. Sleep bruxism is associated to micro-arousals and an increase in cardiac sympathetic activity. J Sleep Res 2006; 15:339–346.

141. Laberge L, Tremblay RE, Vitaro F, et al. Development of parasomnias from childhood to early adolescence. Pediatrics 2000; 106:67–74.
142. Manfredini D, Landi N, Fantoni F, et al. Anxiety symptoms in clinically diagnosed bruxers. J Oral Rehabil 2005; 32:584–588.
143. Casanova-Rosado JF, Medina-Solis CE, Vallejos-Sanchez AA, et al. Prevalence and associated factors for temporomandibular disorders in a group of Mexican adolescents and youth adults. Clin Oral Investig 2006; 10:42–49.
144. Lavigne GJ, Lobbezoo F, Rompré PH, et al. Cigarette smoking as a risk factor or an exacerbating factor for restless legs syndrome and sleep bruxism. Sleep 1997; 20:290–293.
145. Hublin C, Kaprio J, Partinen M, et al. Sleep bruxism based on self-report in a nationwide twin cohort. J Sleep Res 1998; 7:61–67.
146. Stepanova I, Nevsimalova S, Hanosova J. Rhythmic movement disorder in sleep persisting into childhood and adulthood. Sleep 2005; 28:851–857.
147. de Lissovoy V. Headbanging in early childhood. Child Dev 1962; 33:43–56.
148. Mackenzie JM. "Headbanging" and fatal subdural haemorrhage. Lancet 1991; 338:1457–1458.
149. Noel LP, Clarke WN. Self-inflicted ocular injuries in children. Am J Ophtalmol 1982; 94:630–633.
150. Spalter HF, Bemporad JR, Sours JA. Cataracts following chronic headbanging. Arch Ophtalmol 1970; 83:182–186.
151. Thorpy MJ. Rhythmical body movements during sleep. In: Segawa M, ed. Body Movements During Sleep. Tokyo: Sanposha, 1987:47–52.
152. Walters AS, Hening WA, Chokroverty S. Frequent occurrence of myoclonus while awake and at rest, body rocking and marching in place in a subpopulation of patients with restless legs syndrome. Acta Neurologica Scandinavica 1988; 77:418–421.
153. Chisholm T, Morehouse RL. Adult headbanging: sleep studies and treatment. Sleep 1996; 19:343–346.
154. Mayer G, Tracik F, Wilde J. Rhythmic movement disorder revisited. J Sleep Res 2000; 9:127.
155. Arkin AM, Toth MF, Baker J, et al. The frequency of sleep talking in the laboratory among chronic sleep talkers and good dream recallers. J Nerv Ment Dis 1970; 151:369–374.
156. Arkin AM. Sleep-talking: Psychology and Psychophysiology. Hillsdale, NJ: Lawrence Erlbaum, 1981.
157. Tani K, Yoshu N, Yoshino I, et al. Electroencephalographic study of parasomnia: sleep-talking, enuresis and bruxism. Physiol Behav 1966; 1:241–243.
158. Arkin AM, Toth MF, Baker J, et al. The degree of concordance between the content of sleep talking and mentation recalled in wakefulness. J Nerv Ment Dis 1970; 151:373–393.
159. Hublin C, Kaprio J, Partinen M, et al. Sleeptalking in twins: epidemiology and psychiatric comorbidity. Behavior Genet 1998; 28:289–298.
160. Brunner DP, Gonzalez HL. Catathrenia: a rare parasomnia with prolonged groaning during clusters of central or mixed apneas. J Sleep Res 2004; 13:107.
161. DeRoek J, VanHoof E, Cluydts R. Sleep-related expiratory groaning. A case report. Sleep Res 1983; 12:237.
162. Grigg-Damberger M, Brown LK, Casey KR. A cry in the night: nocturnal moaning in a 12-year-old boy. J Clin Sleep Med 2006; 2:354–357.
163. Iriarte J, Alegre M, Urrestarazu E, et al. Continuous positive pressure as treatment of catathrenia (nocturnal groaning). Neurology 2006; 66:609.
164. Oldani A, Manconi M, Zucconi M, et al. "Nocturnal groaning": just a sound or parasomnia? J Sleep Res 2005; 14:305–310.
165. Pevernagie DA, Boon PA, Mariman AN, et al. Vocalization during episodes of prolonged expiration: a parasomnia related to REM sleep. Sleep Med 2001; 2:19–30.
166. Vetrugno R, Provini F, Plazzi G, et al. Catathrenia (nocturnal groaning): a new type of parasomnia. Neurology 2001; 56:681–683.
167. Guilleminault C, Hagen CC, Khaja AM. Catathrenia: parasomnia or uncommon feature of sleep disordered breathing? Sleep 2008; 31:132–139.
168. Vetrugno R, Lugaresi E, Plazzi G, et al. Catathrenia (nocturnal groaning): an abnormal respiratory pattern during sleep. Eur J Neurol 2007; 14:1236–1243.
169. Siddiqui F, Walters AS, Chokroverty S. Catathrenia: a rare parasomnia which may mimic central sleep apnea on polysomnogram. Sleep Med 2008; 9:460–461.
170. Steinig J, Lanz M, Krugel R, et al. Breath holding—a rapid eye movement (REM) sleep parasomnia (catathrenia or expiratory groaning). Sleep Med 2008; 9:455–456.
171. Klackenberg G. Somnambulism in childhood—prevalence, course and behavioral correlations: a prospective longitudinal study (6–16 years). Acta Paediatrica Scandinavica 1982; 71:495–499.
172. Bixler EO, Kales A, Soldatos CR, et al. Prevalence of sleep disorders in the Los Angeles metropolitan area. Am J Psychiatr 1979; 136:1257–1262.
173. Shang CY, Gau SS, Soong WT. Association between childhood sleep problems and perinatal factors, parental mental distress and behavioral problems. J Sleep Res 2006; 15:63–73.

174. Fisher BE, Pauley C, McGuire K. Children's sleep behavior scale: normative data on 870 children in grades 1 to 6. Percept Mot Skills 1989; 68:227–236.

175. Simonds JF, Parraga H. The parasomnias: prevalence and relationships to each other and to positive family histories. Hillside J Clin Psychiatry 1982; 4:25–38.

176. Vela-Bueno A, Bixler EO, Dobladez-Blanco B, et al. Prevalence of night terrors and nightmares in elementary school children: a pilot study. Res Commun Psychol Psychiatr Behav 1985; 10:177–188.

177. Belicki D, Belicki K. Nightmares in a university population. Sleep Res 1982; 11:116.

178. Haynes SN, Mooney DK. Nightmares: etiological, theoretical, and behavioral treatment considerations. Psychol Rec 1975; 25:225–236.

179. Spoormaker VI, Schredl M, Bout JV. Nightmares: from anxiety symptom to sleep disorder. Sleep Med Rev 2005; 10:19–31.

180. Nielsen TA, Stenstrom P, Levin R. Nightmare frequency as a function of age, gender and September 11, 2001: Findings from an internet questionnaire. Dreaming 2006; 16:145–158.

181. Nielsen TA, Laberge L, Tremblay R, et al. Development of disturbing dreams during adolescence and their relationship to anxiety symptoms. Sleep 2000; 23:727–736.

182. Schredl M, Pallmer R. Geschlechtsspezifische Unterschiede in Angsttraumen von Schulerinnen und Schulern [Gender differences in anxiety dreams of school-aged children]. Praxis der Kinderpsychologie und Kinderpsychiatrie 1998; 47:463–476.

183. Spanos NP, DuBreuil C, McNulty SA, et al. The frequency and correlates of sleep paralysis in a university sample. J Res Pers 1995; 29:285–305.

184. Hufford D. Awakening paralyzed in the presence of a "strange visitor". In: Pritchard A, Pritchard DE, Mack JE, Kasey P, Yapp C, eds. Alien Discussions: Proceedings of the Abduction Study Conference, Massachusetts Institute of Technology, June 1992. Cambridge, MA: North Cambridge Press, 1995:348–353.

185. Ohayon MM, Caulet M, Priest RG. Violent behavior during sleep. J Clin Psychiatr 1997; 58:369–376.

186. Chiu HF, Wing YK, Lam LC, et al. Sleep-related injury in the elderly—an epidemiological study in Hong Kong. Sleep 2000; 15:513–517.

187. Fergusson DM, Hons BA, Horwood LJ, et al. Factors related to the age of attainment of nocturnal bladder control: an 8-year longitudinal study. Pediatrics 1986; 78:884–890.

188. Byrd RS, Weitzman M, Lanphear NE, et al. Bed-wetting in US children: epidemiology and related behavior problems. Pediatrics 1996; 98:414–419.

189. Burgio KL, Locher JL, Ives DG, et al. Nocturnal enuresis in community-dwelling older adults. J Am Geriatr Soc. 1996; 44:139–143.

190. Lavigne GJ, Montplaisir JY. Restless legs syndrome and sleep bruxism: prevalence and association among Canadians. Sleep 1994; 17:739–743.

191. Lavigne GJ, Manzini C, Kato T. Sleep bruxism. In: Kryger MH, Roth T, Dement WC, eds. Principles and Practice of Sleep Medicine. 4th ed. Philadelphia: Elsevier Saunders, 2005:946–959.

192. Klackenberg G. A prospective longitudinal study of children. Data on psychic health and development up to 8 years of age. Acta Paediatrica Scandinavica Suppl 1971; 224:1–239.

193. Jouvet M, Delorme F. Locus coerulus et sommeil paradoxal. CR Soc Biol 1965; 159:895–899.

194. Hendricks JC, Morrison AR, Mann GL. Different behaviors during paradoxical sleep without atonia depend on pontine lesion site. Brain Res 1982; 239:81–105.

195. Lai YY, Siegel JM. Medullary regions mediating atonia. J Neurosci 1988; 8:4790–4796.

196. Lai YY, Siegel JM. Muscle tone suppression and stepping produced by stimulation of midbrain and rostral pontine reticular formation. J Neurosci 1990; 10:2727–2734.

197. Shouse MN, Siegel JM. Pontine regulation of REM sleep components in cats: integrity of the pedunculopontine tegmentum (PPT) is important for phasic events but unnecessary for atonia during REM sleep. Brain Res 1992; 571:50–63.

198. Lai YY, Siegel JM. Brainstem-mediated locomotion and myoclonic jerks. I. Neural substrates. Brain Res 1997; 745:257–264.

199. Lai YY, Siegel JM. Brainstem-mediated locomotion and myoclonic jerks. II Pharmacological effects. Brain Res 1997; 745:265–270.

200. Morrison AR. The pathophysiology of REM-sleep behavior disorder. Sleep 1998; 21:446–449.

201. Rye D. The pathophysiology of REM-sleep behavior disorder. Sleep 1998; 21:446–449.

202. Boeve BF, Silber MH, Saper CB, et al. Pathophysiology of REM sleep behaviour disorder and relevance to neurodegenerative disease. Brain 2007; 130:2770–2788.

203. Siegel JM. The stuff dreams are made of: anatomical substrates of REM sleep. Nat Neurosci 2006; 9:721–722.

204. Kim JJ, Jung MW. Neural circuits and mechanisms involved in Pavlovian fear conditioning: a critical review. Neurosci Biobehav Rev 2006; 30:188–202.

205. Davis M, Myers KM, Chhatwal J, et al. Pharmacological treatments that facilitate extinction of fear: relevance to psychotherapy. NeuroRx 2006; 3:82–96.

206. Nutt DJ, Malizia AL. Structural and functional brain changes in posttraumatic stress disorder. J Clin Psychiatr 2004; 65(suppl 1):11–17.
207. Nemeroff CB, Bremner JD, Foa EB, et al. Posttraumatic stress disorder: a state-of-the-science review. J Psychiatry Res 2006; 40:1–21.
208. Rauch SL, Shin LM, Wright CI. Neuroimaging studies of amygdala function in anxiety disorders. Ann NY Acad Sci 2003; 985:389–410.
209. Hillman DR, Murphy AS, Pezzullo L. The economic cost of sleep disorders. Sleep 2006; 29:299–305.
210. Alghanim N, Comondore VR, Fleetham J, et al. The economic impact of obstructive sleep apnea. Lung 2008; 186:7–12.
211. Fullerton DS. The economic impact of insomnia in managed care: a clearer picture emerges. Am J Manag Care 2006; 12:S246–S252.
212. Ozminkowski RJ, Wang S, Walsh JK. The direct and indirect costs of untreated insomnia in adults in the United States. Sleep 2007; 30:263–273.
213. Kayumov L, Pandi-Perumal SR, Fedoroff P, et al. Diagnostic values of polysomnography in forensic medicine. J Forensic Sci 2000; 45:191–194.
214. Mahowald MW, Bundlie SR, Hurwitz TD, et al. Sleep violence—forensic science implications: polygraphic and video documentation. J Forensic Sci 1990; 35:413–432.
215. Mahowald MW, Schenck CH. Violent parasomnias: forensic medicine issues. In: Kryger MH, Roth T, Dement WC, eds. Principles and Practice of Sleep Medicine. 4th ed. Philadelphia: Elsevier Saunders, 2005:960–968.
216. Mahowald MW, Schenck CH, Goldner M, et al. Parasomnia pseudo-suicide. J Forensic Sci 2003; 48:1158–1162.
217. Mahowald MW, Schenck CH, Cramer Bornemann MA. Sleep-related violence. Curr Neurol Neurosci Rep 2005; 5:153–158.
218. Oswald I, Evans J. On serious violence during sleep-walking. Br J Psychiatr 1985; 147:688–691.
219. Rosenfeld DS, Elhajjar AJ. Sleepsex: a variant of sleepwalking. Arch Sex Behav 1998; 27:269–278.
220. Shapiro CM, Trajanovic NN, Fedoroff JP. Sexsomnia—a new parasomnia? Can J Psychiatry 2003; 48: 311–317.
221. Cartwright R. Sleep-related violence: does the polysomnogram help establish the diagnosis? Sleep Med 2000; 1:331–335.
222. Pareja JA, Schenck CH, Mahowald MW. Current perspectives on sleep-related injury, its updated differential diagnosis and its treatment. Sleep Hypnosis 2000; 2:8–21.
223. Yeh SB, Schenck CH. A case of marital discord and secondary depression with attempted suicide resulting from REM sleep behavior disorder in a 35-year-old woman. Sleep Med 2004; 5:151–154.
224. Iranzo A, Molinuevo JL, Santamaria J, et al. Rapid-eye-movement sleep behaviour disorder as an early marker for a neurodegenerative disorder: a descriptive study. Lancet Neurol 2006; 5:572–577.
225. Schenck CH, Bundlie SR, Mahowald MW. REM behavior disorder (RBD): delayed emergence of Parkinsonism and/or dementia in 65% of older men initially diagnosed with idiopathic RBD, and an analysis of the minimum & maximum tonic and/or phasic electromyographic abnormalities found during REM sleep. Sleep. 2003; 26:A316[Abstract].

37 | Pathophysiology, Associations, and Consequences of Parasomnias

Maria Livia Fantini

Sleep Disorders Center, Department of Clinical Neurosciences, San Raffaele Hospital-Turro, Milan, Italy

INTRODUCTION

Parasomnias are abnormal behavioral or physiological events that intrude into the sleep process, disrupting its continuity. Parasomnias are classified according to the type of sleep in which they occur, namely non–rapid eye movement (NREM) and rapid eye movement (REM) sleep parasomnias (1). The first includes disorders of arousals, namely confusional arousals (and their recently identified variants of sleep-related abnormal sexual behaviors), sleep terrors, and sleepwalking. REM sleep parasomnias include REM sleep behavior disorder, recurrent isolated sleep paralysis, and nightmare disorders. Other parasomnias include sleep enuresis, sleep-related groaning, exploding head syndrome, sleep-related hallucinations, and sleep-related eating disorder. The latter shares many features with the disorders of arousals, being frequently associated to sleepwalking. Hence, parasomnias comprise a variety of abnormal sleep-related movements, behaviors, emotions, dreaming, and autonomic phenomena that emerge from sleep as an expression of an anomalous central nervous system activation during sleep.

NREM PARASOMNIAS

Etiology, Pathophysiology, and Pathogenesis

Disordered arousal mechanisms, with a failure of the brain to fully awaken from slow-wave sleep (SWS), are thought to lead to motor, behavioral, or autonomic automatisms. A conceptual framework to understand parasomnias is the notion of dissociated states (2): the three main states of being, namely, wakefulness, NREM sleep, and REM sleep, that usually occur in a cyclic fashion, are not mutually exclusive, and show various degrees of overlap between themselves, especially during transitions among states. In the case of NREM parasomnia, a combination of wakefulness and NREM SWS would explain confusional arousals, automatic motor behaviors, and the amnesia of episodes. Recent works have focused on increased sleep state instability during NREM sleep as a causal factor for the occurrence of the parasomnia. Indeed, somnambulistic individuals were found to have a higher number of arousals [as defined by the American Sleep Disorders Association (ASDA), now named the American Academy of Sleep Medicine (AASM)] (3) and an increase in cyclic alternating pattern (CAP) rate, which is a measure of arousal oscillation, as compared with controls (4). In particular, an increase in the phase A2 and A3 subtypes of CAP [arousals with electroencephalographic (EEG) desynchronization] and either a decrease or an increase in the A1 subtype (arousals with EEG synchronization) were observed (3,5). Also, the presence of hypersynchronous delta activity (HSD) before arousals has been reported in the sleep EEG of sleepwalkers since the first polysomnographic (PSG) observations (3,6–8), but other studies failed to find it and there is controversy about its clinical significance (9,10). Some researchers argue that HSD is analogous to phase A1 and partly to phase A2 subtypes of CAP, representing, therefore, a further expression of a NREM instability (11), and a recent work showed that HSD is not specific of sleepwalking, being a common finding in patients with sleep-disordered breathing (SDB) (12). The finding of a reduced level of slow-wave activity (SWA) in the first cycles of the night (3,13), as well as an increased number of awakenings in SWS (13), also supports the notion of deep sleep instability and suggests an impaired homeostatic mechanism in sleepwalking. It is therefore believed that the increased arousals oscillation observed in sleepwalker individuals may be able to trigger motor behavioral episodes during SWS, through the activation of subcortical motor pattern generators (MPGs). Those are multiple neural substrates at supraspinal and spinal levels that, in animals, account for the possibility of performing automatic complex motor behavior, including locomotion, fighting, and fleeing, in the absence of cortical inputs, as observed in experimental model of decerebrated cats (14–16). The activation of these MPGs in humans during SWS may thus explain the complex behaviors enacted during sleepwalking and sleep terror episodes, without the involvement of the consciousness.

A study with single photon emission computed tomography (SPECT), performed during a sleepwalking episode, provided new insights on the brain functioning in this state: the study revealed both a selective activation of thalamocingulate circuits, in contrast with the profound deactivation of these brain structures during normal SWS, and a persisting deactivation of prefrontal cortices (17). The cingulate cortex is part of a functional network that modulates behaviors involved in emotional processes. Seizures and stimulations of the cingulate cortex in human beings elicit several motor, autonomic, and emotional responses that are similar to those seen in sleepwalking and sleep terrors. The inhibition of prefrontal cortex, observed also during normal sleep, explains the lack of self-related awareness, insight, and recall that characterize both sleep and sleepwalking.

Predisposing and Precipitating Factors, Associations with Medical Conditions

Epidemiological surveys including familial and twin studies have suggested a strong genetic relationship in sleepwalking (18). Many of the NREM parasomnias are known to run in families (19) and the prevalence of sleepwalking in first-degree relatives of an affected individual is estimated at least 10 times greater than that in the general population (20). The presence of specific human leukocyte antigens (HLA) alleles, namely DQB1*05 and *04, would confer a genetic susceptibility for sleepwalking, being found in 35% of sleepwalkers compared with 13.3% of normal controls (21), but its sensitivity and specificity are low. On a predisposing genetic background, factors precipitating the NREM parasomnias are all conditions that promote both an increase of SWS and NREM sleep instability. These include sleep deprivation, fever, alcohol, emotional stress, and medications (22). Experimental sleep deprivation was found to induce a significant increase in the frequency and complexity of the somnambulistic episodes in the recovery night (23). The role of alcohol in precipitating NREM parasomnia should be regarded cautiously (24,25), since it is usually found to reduce, instead of increasing, SWS and the automatic behaviors may result from a direct effect of intoxication rather than the parasomnia.

Morbidity and Mortality, Consequences, and Psychological/Psychiatric Associations

NREM parasomnias may lead to sleep disruption, sleep deprivation, and excessive daytime sleepiness, social embarrassment with avoidance of sleeping with other persons, and significant impact on a couple's life. Although more often benign, NREM parasomnias may imply violent behaviors and result in serious injuries for self or others. Survey on about 5000 adults found that 2% reported violent behaviors arising from sleep, most likely related to disorders of arousals or REM sleep behavior disorder (26). Another survey of over 13,000 found that confusional arousals occurred in 3% of the adult population, and that 13.5% of these cases were characterized by violent or injurious behaviors (25). In a series of 100 injurious cases of sleepwalking reported by Schenck et al., dangerous behaviors included falling out of bed or running into walls or furniture (54%), jumping out of windows (19%), leaving home and driving vehicles or wandering around streets (19%), and having wielded weapons such as loaded shotguns (7%) (27). In one series of 32 patients with "parasomnia overlap" (a condition with clinical and PSG features of both disorders of arousals and REM sleep behavior disorder), 50% had either jumped or punched through window and 91% had repeated injuries to self or bedpartner including multiple ecchymoses, lacerations, and fractures (28). The actual possibility of harmful behaviors performed to others during sleep, without conscious awareness, brings obvious important forensic implications. There are well-documented cases of somnambulistic homicide of relatives (wives, parents-in-law), filicide (murder of a son or daughter), attempted homicide and suicide, as well as murders or sexual assaults during confusional arousals (29). The possibility that some apparent "suicides" are the unintentional consequence of sleep-related complex behaviors and are therefore without premeditation or conscious awareness may have obvious profound social, religious, and insurance implications for surviving family members and friends (30).

Associations, Complications, and Consequences with Conditions/Disorders of Organ Systems

Conditions resulting in frequent arousals, such as SDB, periodic leg movements, and acoustic (31) or tactile stimuli (32), may play as a trigger factor for NREM parasomnia. In particular, an increased prevalence of SDB, mostly of the type of upper airway resistance syndrome (UARS), was found in both adults and children with disorder of arousals compared with normal subjects (33–35). SWS rebound is probably responsible to precipitate both sleepwalking and night terrors during first-night nasal continuous positive airway pressure (CPAP) treatment for obstructive sleep apnea (OSA) (36,37), although CPAP represents an effective treatment in SDB-related parasomnias. Hormonal factors may play a role in promoting NREM parasomnias, since occurrence or exacerbation of sleepwalking and sleep terrors have been described during premenstrual period and during pregnancy (38–40). However, the overall frequency of NREM parasomnias was found to decline across pregnancy (41). A variety of medications have been reported to precipitate episodes of sleepwalking, night terrors, or confusional arousals, namely hypnotics (especially zolpidem), neuroleptics, lithium, tricyclic antidepressants, selective serotonin reuptake inhibitors (SSRIs), antiepileptics, and antibiotics (22). A strong association between somnambulism and migraine has been found in children (42–44), perhaps suggesting a common serotoninergic mechanism. The high prevalence of sleepwalking in migrainous children has led to propose somnambulism as a minor criterion for the diagnosis of migrainous disease, but some studies did not confirm such association (45). Somnambulism is also highly prevalent in some neurological disorders such as Tourette syndrome (46), Angelman syndrome (47) and in neurofibromatosis type 1 (NF1) (48), and it was also found to be associated with hyperthyroidism (49).

Psychological/Psychiatric Associations, Complications, and Consequences

There is not agreement on the extent of psychological factors or psychopathology associated with disorders of arousal. Early reports indicated significant prevalence of psychiatric diagnosis, especially personality disorders, in adults currently suffering from sleepwalking, in contrast to adults who had outgrown the disorder and had more normal psychological patterns (50,51). Adults with sleep terrors showed more severe psychopathology than sleepwalkers, with higher level of anxiety, obsessive-compulsive traits, phobias, and depression (52). Early works also emphasize the role of psychological trauma, even suggesting that sleepwalking/sleep terrors would be, in some cases, a reenactment of a repressed traumatic experience (53), but later studies rejected the hypothesis of sleepwalking/sleep terrors as a dissociative process, finding a history of psychological trauma only in a minority of adults suffering from NREM parasomnia (54). Although a large epidemiological survey found an increased prevalence of concurrent mood and anxiety disorders in subjects with sleepwalking and sleep terrors compared with controls (55), most recent studies indicate that the majority of patients have normal personality profiles and never had a past or current psychiatric diagnosis (46,56,57). Therefore, the role of concomitant psychopathology has been currently largely downsized, and the decreased stigmatization around sleepwalkers/night terrors sufferers may have resulted in a decrease in their stress reactions, as those observed in early studies (58).

REM PARASOMNIAS

REM Sleep Behavior Disorder

REM sleep behavior disorder (RBD) is a disorder of motor control during REM sleep characterized by complex and often violent motor behaviors usually accompanied by vivid dreams. Polysomnography reveals a complete or intermittent loss of physiological muscle atonia and an excessive electromyographic (EMG) phasic activity during REM sleep.

Etiology, Pathophysiology, and Pathogenesis

RBD can occur in two main clinical forms, acute and chronic. The acute form has been observed during drug abuse (particularly with tricyclic antidepressants, monoamine inhibitors, or serotonin-selective reuptake inhibitors) (59,60) as well as during withdrawal from several substances (namely alcohol, meprobamate, nitrazepam, and pentazocine) (59).

The chronic form may be either idiopathic or secondary to various neurological disorders. Secondary RBD may be triggered by any lesions involving the structures responsible for REM sleep atonia, mainly located in the brain stem, that can be either vascular, infectious, neoplastic, traumatic, or degenerative. RBD has been actually observed in association with cerebrovascular lesions (61,62), brain stem tumors (63), Guillain–Barré syndrome (64), multiple sclerosis (65), and Machado–Joseph disease (66,67). A few cases of RBD have been described in close association with limbic encephalitis (68) and in association with Morvan's syndrome (69), two disorders not related to brain stem impairment. However, the most frequent association of RBD is that with neurodegenerative diseases, particularly α-synucleinopathies, which include Parkinson's disease (PD), dementia with Lewy bodies (DLB), and multiple system atrophy (MSA) (70). In PD, the reported prevalence of PSG and/or behavioral manifestations of RBD in PD ranges from 15% to 33%, depending on the method used to assess the parasomnia (questionnaire versus PSG) (71,72). Interestingly, simple loss of muscle atonia, regardless to the history of behavioral manifestations, was found in 58% of PD patients (72). RBD may also be associated to a dementia that is clinically and neuropsychologically indistinguishable from DLB (73,74). In one study including patients with RBD and dementia, the clinical diagnosis of DLB was confirmed in patients submitted to postmortem examination (75). On the basis of these evidences, RBD has been included within the diagnostic criteria for DLB, as a suggestive feature of the disorder (76). RBD is also frequent in patients with MSA (59,77): one study performed on 39 consecutive patients with diagnosis of MSA found a prevalence of PSG-confirmed RBD of about 90% (78).

RBD may co-occur with other NREM parasomnias, such as sleepwalking or sleep terrors, and this condition has been called "parasomnia overlap" (47). A close association of RBD with narcolepsy has been described in various reports (79–81). In both cases, the age of onset of RBD is significantly earlier and the proportion of females seems to be higher. RBD is often accompanied by an elevated index of periodic leg movement during sleep (PLMS) (82).

When no neurological signs or central nervous system (CNS) lesions are found, RBD is currently defined as "idiopathic." This form accounts for up to 60% of the observed cases in the three large series of RBD patients reported in the literature (83). However, one prospective study performed on idiopathic RBD showed that 11 out of 29 (38%) male RBD patients developed a Parkinsonian syndrome within four years from the RBD diagnosis (84). This study has been updated, showing that 65.4% idiopathic RBD patients originally enrolled and eventually developed a Parkinsonian disorder and/or a dementia without Parkinsonism, after an average interval of 13 years from RBD onset (85). In another study, 45% of 44 patients previously diagnosed with idiopathic RBD developed a neurological disorder (that was either PD, DLB, MSA with predominant cerebellar syndrome, or a mild cognitive impairment with prominent visuospatial dysfunction) after a mean of 11.5 years from the reported onset of RBD and a mean of 5.1 years from the diagnosis (86).

Studies have detected several subtle neurophysiological and neuropsychological abnormalities, besides the known motor dyscontrol during REM sleep, in so-called idiopathic RBD (83). These include a cortical slowing in waking EEG (87), deficits in visuospatial constructional performances and visuospatial learning (88), signs of autonomic impairment during wakefulness and sleep (82,89), olfactory impairment (90,91), deficit in color vision and in quantitative test of motor and gait speed (92). All these abnormalities point at idiopathic RBD as a marker of an underlying widespread degenerative process, probably of α-synucleinopathy type.

Pathophysiology of RBD is still not completely understood. On the basis of animal studies, a multitude of neural substrates, located mainly in the brain stem, participate in the mechanism of REM sleep atonia and may be involved in the pathogenesis of RBD. These include the ventral mesopontine junction, the laterodorsal and pedunculopontine tegmental nuclei (LTD-PPN), the locus coeruleus (LC), and the peri-LC area [with the sublaterodorsal nucleus (SLD)] in the pons and the magnocellularis (NMC), gigantocellularis (NGC), and paramedianus (NPM) nuclei in the medial medulla (93). An experimental animal model of RBD has been obtained in cats after dorsal pontine lesion, and a variety of behavioral manifestations have been found to be dependent on specific sites of pontine lesions (94,95). Meso-striatal dopaminergic neurons might also be implicated (96), and brain imaging studies, performed in small groups of idiopathic RBD patients using positron emission tomography (PET) or SPECT, showed a decreased striatal dopaminergic innervation (97) and a reduced presynaptic striatal DA transporter binding, respectively, in RBD (98). Lesional studies in humans (a total of five reported cases of RBD secondary to brain stem involvement) point at lesions within or near the mesencephalic and pontine tegmentum, but the specific nuclei, projections, and neurochemical systems involved in human RBD pathophysiology are not adequately characterized. The controversial effects of various substances on RBD, namely cholinergic and dopaminergic agents (60), account for the complexity of the pathophysiological mechanisms involved in RBD. On the other hand, the few available neuropathological data in idiopathic RBD led to conflicting results: while severe neuronal loss and gliosis in the substantia nigra (SN) and LC-subcoeruleus was found in one case (99), only mild degeneration was found in another case (100), challenging the role played by these structures in the pathogenesis of RBD. As for cholinergic mesopontine neurons (LTD-PPN), one study found an increased density of these neurons, interpreted as a possible disinhibition resulting from the concomitant reduced number of LC neurons. In this case, the hyperactivity of cholinergic neurons would possibly lead to an increased REM sleep drive and RBD (101). However, the observation of severe depletion of the cholinergic neurons in both the LTD/PPN and LC neurons in patients with MSA associated to RBD (102) seems to contradict the latter pathophysiological mechanisms.

RBD is a disorder of both motor control and dream synthesis. Patients display a relatively stereotypic and repetitive set of dreams associated to motor behaviors (violent activity toward others in response to an aggression). According to the activation synthesis model of dream generation (103), phasic discharges from brain stem generators simultaneously activate motor, perceptual, affective and cognitive pathways and these impulses are synthesized into dreams by the forebrain. In RBD, both the lack of REM sleep atonia and the increased phasic motor activity may allow the release of actual motor behaviors associated to dreams, otherwise inhibited. As for NREM parasomnia, the abnormal activation of brain stem MPGs during sleep is also postulated to explain RBD. In particular, the particular involvement of those MPGs that generate not only locomotor behaviors but automatic responses to an aggression such as fighting or fleeing behaviors may be hypothesized. Such outburst of activity occurring during REM sleep would be translated by the cortical imagery generators in dreams that are rich of actions such as fighting or running, rather than more static ones (104).

Predisposing and Precipitating Factors
The main predisposing factors are male gender and age of 50 years or more, the presence of an underlying neurodegenerative disorder, particularly of α-synucleinopathy type, and narcolepsy. Drugs can precipitate RBD, particularly antidepressants (tricyclics and SSRIs), and noradrenergic antagonists (60). Chocolate has also been reported to exacerbate RBD (105). Familial cases of RBD are very rare. Increased positivity to a specific HLA (DQB1*05) has been found in REM sleep behavior disorder (106), but this finding has not been replicated.

Complications and Consequences
REM sleep behavior disorder represents a potentially harmful condition, and this is usually the main reason for patients to seek medical attention. Injuries during sleep are reported by more than 75% of patients (59), and they may include ecchymoses, lacerations, bone fractures, and even subdural hematomas (77,107). Unintentional injuries to the bedpartners raise important medicolegal issues (48). Furthermore, the disorder may have a significant impact on a couple's life, since spouses often choose to sleep in separate rooms for obvious safety reasons. Sometimes a psychiatric condition may be erroneously suspected and inappropriate treatments may be initiated, with an obvious burden for the patient and his or her family. Besides motor enactment, patients with RBD experience frequent vivid dreams, which tend to be stereotypical, action filled and unpleasant. The dreamer is usually attacked by unfamiliar people or threatened by animals, and he or she would either fight back in self-defense or attempt to flee. Fear and anger are the most common associated emotions, and indicators of aggressiveness in dreams are markedly increased compared with normal controls (108). However, no evidence of psychopathology has been described in patients with RBD and they were found to show normal or even reduced daytime aggressivenes (108).

The increased risk of developing a neurodegenerative disease carried by idiopathic RBD poses the ethical dilemma whether the patient should or should not be told about this risk, especially in view of the current lack of effective neuroprotective strategies. It should be noted that the exact extent of this risk, e.g., the relative risk and risk factors, for a patient newly diagnosed with idiopathic RBD, is not known at the moment, given the lack of large-cohort longitudinal studies. Diagnosis of idiopathic RBD might therefore bring a significant psychological burden for the patient and his or her family. Specialists' attitudes are various, reflecting individual sensibility and experience, but most agree in carefully following these patients over the years, to detect as soon as possible the eventual occurrence of neurological disease.

Nightmare Disorder

According to the second edition of *International Classification of Sleep Disorders* (ICSD-2) (1), nightmares are disturbing mental experiences that generally occur during REM sleep and that often result in awakening. Emotions usually involve anxiety, fear, or terror, but frequently also anger, sadness, embarrassment, disgust, and other negative feelings. Dream content is often represented by imminent physical danger to the individual, but it may also involve distressing themes. Upon awakening, full alertness is commonly observed, and the subject is usually able to detail nightmare content. Nightmares typically, but not exclusively, arise during REM sleep; multiple nightmares within a single night may occur and may bear similar themes.

Etiology, Pathophysiology, and Pathogenesis

The pathophysiology of nightmares is largely unknown. PSG patterns in nightmare disorder have been poorly characterized, also because of the difficulty in eliciting nightmares in the sleep laboratory environment. One study assessed the sleep pattern of patients suffering from idiopathic nightmares and posttraumatic stress disorder (PTSD) nightmares, and healthy controls, finding no difference in the main PSG variables, particularly those pertaining to REM sleep (namely REM latency, REM efficiency, REM density, REM sleep percentage, and the number of microarousals), but only longer and more frequent nocturnal awakenings, with a lower sleep efficiency, in subjects with PTSD nightmares compared with idiopathic nightmare sufferers and healthy controls. However, both types of nightmares were associated with an increased number of PLMS compared with controls (109). Results on autonomic activation associated with the nightmare are conflicting, but a moderate level of sympathetic arousal in the REM period seems to be associated with a nightmare. A significant acceleration of the heart rate was observed in the three minutes of REM sleep before the awakening associated to the nightmare, while no acceleration was observed in the absence of nightmare (110). Respiration rate, however, appears to be only slightly increased during the nightmare.

Predisposing and Precipitating Factors

Nightmares can be idiopathic or can be precipitated by a trauma. It may develop in the immediate period following the trauma [as acute stress disorder (ASD)] or one month or more after it (PTSD). Posttraumatic nightmares may take the form of a realistic rehearsal of a traumatic event or depict only some of its elements. A multitude of drugs have also been associated with a complaint of nightmares, virtually all those affecting the acetylcholine, serotonin, norepinephrine, and dopamine systems, during either chronic intake or withdrawal (111). Among them there are many antidepressant, antihypertensive, amphetamine, antipsychotic, and anti-Parkinsonian medications. Withdrawal from γ-aminobutyric acid (GABA)ergic agents, such as benzodiazepines, barbiturates, and alcohol, may also induce nightmares. Anesthetics, antiinfectives, and immunosuppressants have also been associated to a complaint of nightmares, although the mechanism is not well understood.

Associations, Complications, and Consequences with Conditions/Disorders of Organ Systems

Nightmares may disrupt sleep continuity, causing awakening, although this is not a rule. Indeed, the presence of awakening, this was formerly considered an essential criterion for the definition of a nightmare, seems not to be correlated with the level of nightmare distress (ND). One study suggested that the frequency of dreams with negative effect (bad dreams, which do not awaken the subject) is a better index of low well-being than nightmare frequency (112). Nightmares lead to important cognitive and behavioral consequences. Post-awakening anxiety and difficulty returning to sleep are often present. Nightmare disorder can lead to sleep avoidance and sleep deprivation, and, therefore, to more intense nightmares, which can produce insomnia and daytime sleepiness. Individuals with PTSD are at risk for developing mood disorder and depression, social and employment consequences, self-destructive and impulsive behavior, and substance abuse; it is not clear to what extent the nightmare symptomatic of PTSD contributes to these complications.

Psychological/Psychiatric Associations, Complications, and Consequences
Nightmares have been correlated with various measures of psychopathology, namely neuroticism (112–114), anxiety (113,115,116), and depression (116,117), but not all studies support this relationship and results are controversial (118). Methods of measurement (e.g., retrospective vs. prospective recall of nightmares) may explain some discrepancies in results, since subjects scoring high on neuroticism are more likely to remember their nightmares when asked to report them retrospectively than do subjects who are not neurotic (119). State anxiety, which represents an indicator of current levels of stress, may be a mediating variable between neuroticism and nightmares, since persons with high scores on neuroticism experience more stress and stress is known to increase the frequency of bad dreams (120). Frequency of nightmares have been shown to be only moderately correlated to general waking distress (116,121). Therefore, the measure of ND (e.g., the impact of nightmares on daily functioning), rather than frequency, seems to be more significantly related to psychological complaints and would represent a mediating factor between nightmares and psychopathology. ND is currently measured by the ND scale (121) and is a trait-like variable that correlates with several psychopathological indicators such as trait anxiety, neuroticism, physical complaints, and stress-related symptoms (118). Coping style, e.g., the personal ability to cope with stress, is also considered a mediating factor in the occurrence of nightmares. Dysfunctional coping strategy has been reported in nightmare sufferers compared with non-nightmare subjects (111), and they may exacerbate both nightmare frequency and distress.

Recurrent Isolated Sleep Paralysis
Etiology, Pathophysiology, and Pathogenesis
Sleep paralysis is an example of state dissociation, with elements of REM sleep (muscle atonia, dream imaging) persisting into wakefulness. Sleep paralysis occurs during sleep onset REM periods (SOREMP) when experimentally elicited by nocturnal sleep interruption schedules (122). Familial patterns of sleep paralysis have been described.

Predisposing and Precipitating Factors
Precipitating factors are sleep deprivation and irregular sleep-wake schedule, as well as psychological stress. Body position also seems to influence the occurrence of sleep paralysis, since it was found to occur mostly in the supine position (123). In light of this, some episodes of sleep paralysis might arise from brief microarousals during REM sleep, possibly induced by positional sleep apnea (124). Time of night seems to influence the intensity of the episodes, since fear was found to be significantly less intense at the end of sleep than at the beginning or middle of sleep (124).

Psychological/Psychiatric Associations, Complications, and Consequences
Especially during first episodes, this parasomnia is usually accompanied by intense anxiety. Sleep paralysis may be associated to hallucinatory experiences in up to 75% of cases, including auditory, visual, tactile, vestibular-motor, or a sense of presence (125,126), markedly increasing the levels of anxiety. Fear of having a psychiatric disturbance and worries of negative reactions may prevent telling others about this phenomenon, and considerable relief is brought generally by discovering that this is a relatively common phenomenon (125).

Some studies found an increased prevalence of panic disorder among sleep paralysis sufferers (127). Sleep paralysis accompanied by sensed presence has been associated with higher levels of social anxiety (128). In one study, isolated sleep paralysis sufferers were found to score higher on the paranoia scale at the Minnesota Multiphasic Personality Inventory (MMPI) than healthy controls, but this difference was considered too small to play a major role and it could have resulted from possible overestimation of behavior and experiences concerning delusions and hallucinations (129).

OTHER PARASOMNIAS

Sleep Enuresis

The disorder is heterogeneous and its etiology is multifactorial, involving biological, genetic, environmental, and behavioral factors. Genetic factors play an important role, since approximately two-thirds of cases are familiar and one-third sporadic. Four gene loci associated with nocturnal enuresis have been identified, and the existence of others is presumed (130). Somatic and psychosocial environmental factors have a major modulatory effect. Among the firsts, there are developmental delay or immaturity in the attainment of the central control of bladder function, abnormalities in the bladder size or reactivity, a lack of the normal increase of vasopressin during sleep, and a failure in the arousal system in response to the sensation of full bladder. All these factors are likely to play a role in primary enuresis. On the other hand, psychological stress, such as parental divorce or child neglect or abuse may often precipitate the onset of secondary enuresis (131). However, most children with enuresis show no symptoms of emotional or behavioral disturbance. Wherever they are present, the fact that psychological improvement often occurs after successful treatment of enuresis suggests that, at least in some cases, the psychological disturbance is in reaction to the symptom. Stress and/or anxiety at critical developmental periods may in turn delay the attainment of dryness, as for other developmental milestones. Enuresis is encountered more frequently in children with snoring (132) and sleep apnea (133), and in children with attention-deficit hyperactivity disorder (ADHD) (134). In adults, enuresis may be a symptom of congestive heart failure, OSA, and dementia. Several drugs are reported to induce nocturnal enuresis. Although some SSRIs have been used successfully to treat enuresis, cases of de novo enuresis were reported in children and adult patients taking SSRIs, especially paroxetine (135,136), as well as antipsychotics (137) such as thioridazine, clozapine, and risperidone (138).

Family embarrassment, parental anger, and derision by peers may significantly impact the life of a child with enuresis, with severe impairment in his self-esteem (139). Persistently wet bedding or clothes may actually precipitate episodes of physical or emotional abuse from adults lacking appropriate control (140). Chronic anxiety and delayed developmental steps, such as avoiding activities implying sleeping out of home, may occur as secondary problems. Hence, the psychological and developmental consequences may actually be more significant and devastating to the child than the symptom of enuresis itself.

Sleep-Related Eating Disorder

Sleep-related eating disorder (SRED) is a parasomnia characterized by recurrent episodes of involuntary eating and drinking during incomplete arousals from sleep, with partial recall of the episode. Episodes more frequently follow a confusional arousal from SWS, but occasional SRED can be observed during other stages of NREM sleep and REM sleep.

A family history of SRED was recently described in 26% of affected individuals (141), suggesting a genetic predisposition. SRED can be idiopathic, but is often associated to other sleep disorders or clinical conditions. Sleepwalking is the most commonly associated, and a history of NREM parasomnias in childhood appears to be a predisposing factor. Frequent comorbidity is observed between SRED and restless legs syndrome and periodic limb movement disorder, as well as OSA (141–144). As for NREM parasomnias, with whom SRED shares many features, all conditions implying increased arousals and NREM sleep instability may act as precipitating factors triggering the behavioral episodes. These also include acute psychological stress, cessation of smoking, cessation of alcohol, or substance abuse (142). Daytime dieting or a history of eating disorders may be present. Several drugs can precipitate SRED, many of these also precipitating somnambulism, namely hypnotics (especially zolpidem) (145), lithium, risperidone (146), and olanzapine (147).

Consequences of SRED may include insomnia from sleep disruption, avoiding sleeping in unfamiliar places and social embarrassment, possible sleep-related injuries, morning anorexia, and more serious health-related consequences such as undesired weight gain with problematic control of body weight.

Sleep-Related Groaning

Sleep-related groaning is characterized by bradypneic episodes in which prolonged expiration produces a monotonous, often loud vocalization that resembles a groaning. Episodes tend to cluster and occur mainly during REM sleep.

Pathophysiology is largely unknown. Neurological and neuroradiological examination are usually unremarkable (148), and otolaryngological examination including static and dynamic vocal cord fibroscopy during wakefulness (149) reveal no functional obstruction of the upper airways during expiration. The protracted phase of bradypnea associated to groaning was found to be accompanied by a slight decrease in heart rate and systemic arterial blood pressure and a moderately positive intraesophageal pressure. Hemoglobin oxygen saturation always remains normal, and the end of the episode is often marked by an EEG arousal, with a rebound in heart rate and arterial pressure (149).

There are no known precipitating factors. Genetic predisposition may be present. In one series of cases, a positive familiar history of sleep-related groaning was found in 29% of patients, while the presence of various parasomnias (including bruxism, sleepwalking, sleep talking, sleep terrors) was observed in 43% of the patients (150).

Patients are usually unaware of their disorder. The groaning tends to occur every night, apparently not associated with relevant sleep problems. However, daytime fatigue or somnolence may be reported by half of the patients, although it was found to be not related to the duration or intensity of the groaning episodes (150). Interpersonal problems may be the most relevant consequences, including social embarrassment whenever patients have to sleep with other persons, sleep disruption, and noise-related distress in the bedpartner.

CONCLUSIONS

The etiology of NREM parasomnias is unknown, but a study using SPECT found a selective activation of thalamocingulate circuits and a persistent deactivation of prefrontal cortices. Many of the NREM parasomnias are known to run in families and may lead to sleep disruption, sleep deprivation and excessive daytime sleepiness, social embarrassment with avoidance of sleeping with other persons, and significant impact on a couple's life. Conditions resulting in frequent arousals, hormonal factors, and medications may trigger NREM parasomnias. There does not appear to be agreement on the extent of psychological factors or psychopathology associated with disorders of arousal. REM sleep behavior disorder has been associated with neurodegenerative diseases, but the pathophysiology of it is still not completely understood. Antidepressants and noradrenergic antagonists can precipitate RBD, and injuries are reported by more than 75% of patients. The pathophysiology of nightmares is largely unknown, and it can be idiopathic or precipitated by a trauma. Nightmare disorder can lead to sleep avoidance and sleep deprivation and, consequently, to more intense nightmares, which can produce insomnia and daytime sleepiness, and have been correlated with various measures of psychopathology, although not all studies support this relationship. Recurrent isolated sleep paralysis is precipitated by sleep deprivation and irregular sleep-wake schedule, as well as psychological stress; sleep enuresis, sleep-related eating disorder, and sleep-related groaning are conditions that often result in interpersonal problems.

REFERENCES

1. American Academy of Sleep Medicine. International Classification of Sleep Disorders. 2nd ed. Diagnostic & Coding Manual. Westchester: American Academy of Sleep Medicine, 2005.
2. Mahowald MW, Schenck CH. Dissociated states of wakefulness and sleep. Neurology 1992; 42(suppl 6): 44–51.
3. Guilleminault C, Poyares D, Abat F, et al. Sleep and Wakefulness in somnambulism, a spectral analysis study. J Psychosom Res 2001; 51:411–416.
4. Guilleminault C, Kirisoglu C, da Rosa AC, et al. Sleepwalking, a disorder of NREM sleep instability. Sleep Med 2006; 7(2):163–170.
5. Zucconi M, Oldani A, Ferini-Strambi L, et al. Arousal fluctuation in non rapid-eye-movement parasomnia: the role of the cyclic alternating pattern as a measure of sleep instability. J Clin Neurophysiol 1995; 12:147–154.

6. Jacobson A, Kales A, Lehmann D, et al. Somnambulism: all-night electroencephalographic studies. Science 1965; 148:975–977.
7. Blatt I, Peled R, Gadoth N, et al. The value of sleep recording in evaluating somnambulism in young adults. Electroencephalogr Clin Neurophysiol 1991; 78(6):407–412.
8. Espa F, Ondze B, Deglise P, et al. Sleep architecture, slow wave activity, and sleep spindles in adult patients with sleepwalking and sleep terrors. Clin Neurophysiol 2000; 111(5):929–939.
9. Schenck CH, Pareja JA, Patterson AL, et al. Analysis of polysomnographic events surrounding 252 slow-wave sleep arousals in thirty-eight adults with injurious sleepwalking and sleep terrors. J Clin Neurophysiol 1998; 15(2):159–166.
10. Pilon M, Zadra A, Joncas S, et al. Hypersynchronous delta waves and somnambulism: brain topography and effect of sleep deprivation. Sleep 2006; 29(1):77–84.
11. Guilleminault C. Hypersynchronous slow delta, cyclic alternating pattern and sleepwalking. Sleep 2006; 29(1):14–15.
12. Pressman MR. Hypersynchronous delta sleep EEG activity and sudden arousals from slow-wave sleep in adults without a history of parasomnias: clinical and forensic implications. Sleep 2004; 27(4): 706–710.
13. Gaudreau H, Joncas S, Zadra A, et al. Dynamics of slow-wave activity during the NREM sleep of sleepwalkers and control subjects. Sleep 2000; 23:755–760.
14. Mori S, Nishimura H, Aoki M. Brainstem activation of the spinal stepping generator. In: Hobson JA, Brazier MAB, eds. The Reticular Formation Revisited. New York, Raven Press: 1980:241–259.
15. Lai YY, Siegel JM. Brainstem-mediated locomotion and myoclonic jerks. I. Neural substrates. Brain Res 1997; 745:257–264.
16. Lai YY, Siegel JM. Brainstem-mediated locomotion and myoclonic jerks. II Pharmacological effects. Brain Res 1997; 745:265–270.
17. Bassetti C, Vella S, Donati F, et al. SPECT during sleepwalking. Lancet 2000; 356(9228):484–485.
18. Hublin C, Kaprio J, Partinen M. Prevalence and genetics of sleepwalking: a population-based twin study. Neurology 1997; 48:177–181.
19. Hublin C, Kaprio J, Partinen M, et al. Parasomnias: co-occurrence and genetics. Psychiatr Genet 2001; 11(2):65–70.
20. Kales A, Soldatos CR, Bixler EO, et al. Hereditary factors in sleepwalking and night terrors. Br J Psychiatry 1980; 137:111–118.
21. Lecendreux M, Bassetti C, Dauvilliers Y. HLA and genetic susceptibility to sleepwalking. Mol Psychiatry 2003; 8:114–117.
22. Pressman MR. Factors that predispose, prime and precipitate NREM parasomnias in adults: clinical and forensic implications. Sleep Med Rev 2007; 11(1):5–30.
23. Joncas S, Zadra A, Paquet J, et al. The value of sleep deprivation as a diagnostic tool in adult sleepwalkers. Neurology 2002; 58(6):936–940.
24. Pressman MR, Mahowald MW, Schenck CH, et al. Alcohol-induced sleepwalking or confusional arousal as a defense to criminal behavior: a review of scientific evidence, methods and forensic considerations. J Sleep Res 2007; 16(2):198–212.
25. Ohayon MM, Priest RG, Zulley J, et al. The place of confusional arousals in sleep and mental disorders: findings in a general population sample of 13,057 subjects. J Nerv Ment Dis 2000; 188(6): 340–348.
26. Ohayon MM, Caulet M, Priest RG. Violent behavior during sleep. J Clin Psychiatry 1997; 58:369–376.
27. Schenck CH, Milner DM, Hurwitz TD, et al. A polysomnographic and clinical report on sleep-related injury in 100 adult patients. Am J Psychiatry 1989; 146(9):1166–1173.
28. Schenck CH, Boyd JL, Mahowald MW. A parasomnia overlap disorder involving sleepwalking, sleep terrors, and REM sleep behavior disorder in 33 polysomnographically confirmed cases. Sleep 1997; 20(11):972–981.
29. Mahowald MW, Schenck CH. Parasomnias: sleepwalking and the law. Sleep Med Rev 2000; 4:321–339.
30. Mahowald MW, Schenck CH, Goldner M, et al. Parasomnia pseudo-suicide. J Forensic Sci 2003; 48: 1158–1162.
31. Pilon M, Zadra A, Gosselin N, et al. Experimentally induced somnambulistic episodes in adult sleepwalkers: effects of forced arousal and sleep deprivation. Sleep 2005; 28:258.
32. Kales A, Jacobson A, Paulson MJ, et al. Somnambulism: psychophysiological correlates. I All-night EEG studies. Arch Gen Psychiatry 1966; 14:586–594.
33. Espa F, Dauvilliers Y, Ondze B, et al. Arousal reactions in sleepwalking and night terrors in adults: the role of respiratory events. Sleep 2002; 25(8):32–25.
34. Guilleminault C, Palombini L, Pelayo R. Sleepwalking and sleep terrors in prepubertal children: what triggers them? Pediatrics 2003; 111:e17–e25.
35. Guilleminault C, Lee JH, Chan A, et al. Non-REM-sleep instability in recurrent sleepwalking in prepubertal children. Sleep Med 2005; 6(6):515–521.

36. Millman RP, Kipp GJ, Carskadon MA. Sleepwalking precipitated by treatment of sleep apnea with nasal CPAP. Chest 1991; 99:750–751.
37. Pressmann MR, Meyer TJ, Kendick-Mohamed J. Night terror in an adult precipitated by sleep apnea. Sleep 1995; 18(9):773–775.
38. Shenck CH, Mahowald MW. Two cases of premenstrual sleep terrors and injurious sleepwalking. J Psychosom Obstet Gynaecol 1995; 16:79–84.
39. Berlin MR. Sleepwalking disorder during pregnancy. A case report. Sleep 1988; 11(3):298–300.
40. Snyder S. Unusual case of sleep terror in a pregnant patient. Am J Psychiatry 1986; 143(3):391.
41. Hedman C, Pohjasvaara T, Tolonen U, et al. Parasomnias decline during pregnancy. Acta Neurol Scand 2002:105:209–214.
42. Barabas G, Ferrari M, Matthews WS. Childhood migraine and somnambulism. Neurology 1983; 33 (7):948–949.
43. Giroud M, Nivelon JL, Dumas R. Somnambulism and migraine in children. A non-fortuitous association. Arch Fr Pediatr 1987; 44(4):263–265.
44. Bruni O, Fabrizi P, Ottaviano S. Prevalence of sleep disorders in childhood and adolescence with headache: a case-control study. Cephalalgia 1997; 17(4):492–498.
45. Luc ME, Gupta A, Birnberg JM. Characterization of symptoms of sleep disorders in children with headache. Pediatr Neurol 2006; 34(1):7–12.
46. Barabas G, Matthews WS, Ferrari M. Somnambulism in children with Tourette syndrome. Dev Med Child Neurol 1984; 26(4):457–460.
47. Bruni O, Ferri R, D'Agostino G. Sleep disturbances in Angelman syndrome: a questionnaire study. Brain Dev 2004; 26:233–240.
48. Johnson H, Wiggs L, Stores G. Psychological disturbance and sleep disorders in children with neurofibromatosis type 1. Dev Med Child Neurol 2005; 47:237–242.
49. Ajlouni KM, Ahmad AT, El-Zaheri MM. Sleepwalking associated with hyperthyroidism. Endocr Pract 2005; 11(1):5–10.
50. Kales A, Soldatos CR, Caldwell AB, et al. Somnambulism. Clinical characteristics and personality patterns. Arch Gen Psychiatry 1980; 37(12):1406–1410.
51. Soldatos CR, Kales A. Sleep disorders: research in psychopathology and its practical implications. Acta Psychiatr Scand 1982; 65(6):381–387.
52. Kales JD, Kales A, Soldatos CR, et al. Night terrors. Clinical characteristics and personality patterns. Arch Gen Psychiatry 1980; 37(12):1413–1417.
53. Calogeras RC. Sleepwalking ad the traumatic experience. Int J Psychoanal 1982; 63:483–489.
54. Hartman D, Crisp AH, Sedgwick P, et al. Is there a dissociative process in sleepwalking and night terrors? Postgrad Med J 2001; 77(906):244–249.
55. Ohayon MM, Guillelminault C, Priest RG. Night terrors, sleepwalking, and confusional arousals in the general population: their frequency and relationship to other sleep and mental disorders. J Clin Psychiatry 1999; 60(4):268–276.
56. Hartmann E, Greenwald D, Brune P. Night terrors-sleepwalking: personality characteristics. Sleep Res 1982; 11:121.
57. Llorente MD, Currier MB, Norman SE, et al. Night terrors in adults: phenomenology and relationship to psychopathology. J Clin Psychiatry 1992; 53(11):392–394.
58. Szelenberger W, Niemcewicz S, Dabrowska AJ. Sleepwalking and night terrors: psychopathological and psychophysiological correlates. Int Rev Psychiatry 2005; 17(4):263–270.
59. Schenck CH, Mahowald MW. REM sleep behavior disorder: clinical, developmental, and neuroscience perspectives 16 years after its formal identification in SLEEP. Sleep 2002; 25:120–138.
60. Gagnon JF, Postuma RB, Montplaisir J. Update on the pharmacology of REM sleep behavior disorder. Neurology 2006; 67(5):742–747.
61. Culebras A, Moore JT. Magnetic resonance findings in REM sleep behavior disorder. Neurology 1989; 39:1519–1523.
62. Kimura K, Tachibana N, Kohyama J, et al. A discrete pontine ischemic lesion could cause REM sleep behavior disorder. Neurology 2000; 55:894–895.
63. Schenck CH, Bundlie SR, Smith SA, et al. REM behavior disorder in a 10 years old girl and periodic and aperiodic REM and NREM sleep movements in a 8 years old brother. Sleep Res 1986; 15:162.
64. Cochen V, Arnulf I, Demeret S, et al. Vivid dreams, hallucinations, psychosis and REM sleep in Guillain-Barre syndrome. Brain 2005; 128:2535–2545.
65. Plazzi G, Montagna P. Remitting REM sleep behavior disorder as the initial sign of multiple sclerosis. Sleep Med 2002; 3(5):437–439.
66. Fukutake T, Shinotoh H, Nishino H, et al. Homozygous Machado-Joseph disease presenting as REM sleep behaviour disorder and prominent psychiatric symptoms. Eur J Neurol 2002; 9:97–100.
67. Iranzo A, Munoz E, Santamaria J, et al. REM sleep behavior disorder and vocal cord paralysis in Machado-Joseph disease. Mov Disord 2003; 18(10):1179–1183.

68. Iranzo A, Graus F, Clover L, et al. Rapid eye movement sleep behavior disorder and potassium channel antibody-associated limbic encephalitis. Ann Neurol 2006; 59(1):178–181.

69. Liguori R, Vincent A, Clover L, et al. Morvan's syndrome: peripheral and central nervous system and cardiac involvement with antibodies to voltage-gated potassium channels. Brain 2001; 124:2417–2426.

70. Boeve BF, Silber MH, Ferman TJ, et al. Association of REM sleep behavior disorder and neurodegenerative disease may reflect an underlying synucleinopathy. Mov Disord 2001; 16:622–630.

71. Comella CL, Nardine TM, Diederich NJ, et al. Sleep-related violence, injury, and REM sleep behavior disorder in Parkinson's disease. Neurology 1998; 51:526–529.

72. Gagnon JF, Bédard MA, Fantini ML, et al. REM sleep behavior disorder and REM sleep without atonia in Parkinson's disease. Neurology 2002; 59:585–589.

73. Boeve BF, Silber MH, Ferman TJ, et al. REM sleep behavior disorder and degenerative dementia: an association likely reflecting Lewy body disease. Neurology 1998; 51:363–370.

74. Ferman TJ, Boeve BF, Smith GE, et al. REM sleep behavior and dementia: cognitive difference when compared with AD. Neurology 1999; 52(5):951–957.

75. Turner RS, Chervin RD, Frey KA, et al. Probable diffuse Lewy body disease presenting as REM sleep behavior disorder. Neurology 1997; 49:523–527.

76. McKeith IG, Dickson DW, Lowe J, et al. Diagnosis and management of dementia with Lewy bodies: third report of the DLB Consortium. Neurology 2005; 65(12):1863–1872.

77. Sforza E, Krieger J, Petiau C. REM sleep behavior disorder: clinical and physiopathological findings. Sleep Med Rev 1997; 1:57–69.

78. Plazzi G, Corsini R, Provini F, et al. REM sleep behavior disorders in multiple system atrophy. Neurology 1997; 48:1094–1097.

79. Schenck CH, Mahowald MW. Motor dyscontrol in narcolepsy: rapid-eye-movement (REM) sleep without atonia and REM sleep behavior disorder. Ann Neurol 1992; 32:3–10.

80. Nightingale S, Orgill JC, Ebrahim IO, et al. The association between narcolepsy and REM behavior disorder (RBD). Sleep Med 2005; 6(3):253–258.

81. Mathis J, Hess CW, Bassetti C. Isolated mediotegmental lesion causing narcolepsy and rapid eye movement sleep behaviour disorder: a case evidencing a common pathway in narcolepsy and rapid eye movement sleep behaviour disorder. J Neurol Neurosurg Psychiatry 2007; 78(4):427–479.

82. Fantini ML, Michaud M, Gosselin N, et al. Periodic leg movements in REM sleep behavior disorder and related autonomic and EEG activation. Neurology 2002; 59:1889–1894.

83. Fantini MIL, Ferini-Strambi L, Montplaisir J. Idiopathic REM sleep behavior disorder: toward a better nosological definition. Neurology 2005; 64:780–786.

84. Schenck CH, Bundlie SR, Mahowald MW. Delayed emergence of a parkinsonian disorder in 38% of 29 older men initially diagnosed with idiopathic rapid eye movement sleep behavior disorder. Neurology 1996a; 46:388–393.

85. Schenck CH, Bundlie SR, Mahowald MW. REM behavior disorder (RBD): delayed emergence of parkinsonism and/or dementia in 65% of older men initially diagnosed with idiopathic RBD, and analysis of the minimum and maximum tonic and/or phasic electromyographic abnormalities found during REM sleep. Sleep 2003; 26(suppl):A316.

86. Iranzo A, Molinuevo JL, Santamaría J, et al. Rapid-eye-movement sleep behaviour disorder as an early marker for a neurodegenerative disorder: a descriptive study. Lancet Neurol 2006; 5:572–577.

87. Fantini ML, Gagnon JF, Petit D, et al. Slowing of electroencephalogram in rapid eye movement sleep behavior disorder. Ann Neurol 2003; 53:774–780.

88. Ferini-Strambi L, Di Gioia MS, Castronovo V, et al. Neuropsychological assessment in idiopathic REM sleep behavior disorder (RBD). Does the idiopathic form of RBD really exist? Neurology 2004; 62:41–45.

89. Ferini-Strambi L, Oldani A, Zucconi M, et al. Cardiac autonomic activity during wakefulness and sleep in REM sleep behavior disorder. Sleep 1996; 19:367–369.

90. Stiasny-Kolster K, Doerr Y, Moller JC, et al. Combination of 'idiopathic' REM sleep behaviour disorder and olfactory dysfunction as possible indicator for alpha-synucleinopathy demonstrated by dopamine transporter FP-CIT-SPECT. Brain 2005; 128:126–137.

91. Fantini ML, Postuma RB, Montplaisir J, et al. Olfactory deficit in idiopathic REM sleep behavior disorder. Brain Res Bull 2006; 70:386–390.

92. Postuma RB, Lang AE, Massicotte-Marquez J. Potential early markers of Parkinson disease in idiopathic REM sleep behavior disorder. Neurology 2006; 66:845–851.

93. Boeve BF, Silber MH, Saper CB, et al. Pathophysiology of REM sleep behaviour disorder and relevance to neurodegenerative disease. Brain 2007; 130(pt 11):2770–2788.

94. Jouvet M, Delorme F. Locus coeruleus et sommeil paradoxal. C R Soc Biol 1965; 159:895–899.

95. Hendricks JC, Morrison AR, Mann GL. Different behaviors during paradoxical sleep without atonia depend on pontine lesion site. Brain Res 1982; 239:81–105.

96. Rye DB. Contributions of the pedunculopontine region to normal and altered REM sleep. Sleep 1997; 20(9):757–788.

97. Albin RL, Koeppe RD, Chervin RD, et al. Decreased striatal dopaminergic innervation in REM sleep behavior disorder. Neurology 2000; 55:1410–1412.

98. Eisensehr I, Linke R, Noachtar S, et al. Reduced striatal dopamine transporters in idiopathic rapid eye movement sleep behaviour disorder. Comparison with Parkinson's disease and controls. Brain 2000; 123:1155–1160.

99. Uchiyama M, Isse K, Tanaka K, et al. Incidental Lewy body disease in a patient with REM sleep behavior disorder. Neurology 1995; 45:709–712.

100. Boeve B, Dickson D, Olson E, et al. Insights into REM sleep behavior disorder pathophysiology in brainstem predominant Lewy body disease. Sleep Med 2007; 8:60–64.

101. Schenck CH, Mahowald MW, Anderson ML, et al. Lewy body variant of Alzheimer's disease (AD) identified by postmortem ubiquitin staining in a previously reported case of AD associated with REM sleep behavior disorder [letter]. Biol Psychiatry 1997; 42:527–528.

102. Benarroch EE, Schmeichel AM. Depletion of cholinergic mesopontine neurons in multiple system atrophy: a substrate for REM behavior disorder? Neurology 2002; 58(suppl 3):A345.

103. Hobson JA, McCarley RW. The brain as a dream state generator: an activation-synthesis hypothesis of the dream process. Am J Psychiatry 1977; 134:1335–1348.

104. Fantini ML, Ferini-Strambi L. REM-related dreams in REM sleep behavior disorder. In: McNamara P and Barrett D, eds. The New Science of Dreaming. Vol. 1. Westport: Praeger Publishers, 2007:185–200.

105. Vorona RD, Ware JC. Exacerbation of REM sleep behavior disorder by chocolate ingestion: a case report. Sleep Med 2002; 3(4):365–367.

106. Schenck CH, Garcia-Rill E, Segall M, et al. HLA class II genes associated with REM sleep behavior disorder. Ann Neurol 1996; 39(2):261–263.

107. Olson EJ, Boeve BF, Silber MH. Rapid eye movement sleep behaviour disorder: demographic, clinical and laboratory findings in 93 cases. Brain 2000; 123:331–339.

108. Fantini ML, Corona A, Clerici S, et al. Aggressive dream content without daytime aggressiveness in REM sleep behaviour disorder. Neurology 2005; 65(7):1010–1015.

109. Germain A, Nielsen TA. Sleep pathophysiology in posttraumatic stress disorder and idiopathic nightmare sufferers. Biol Psychiatry 2003; 54:1092–1098.

110. Nielsen TA, Zadra AL. Nightmare and other common dream disturbances. In: Kryger MH, Roth T, Dement C, eds. Principles and Practice of Sleep Medicine. 4th ed. Philadelphia: W.B. Saunders, 2005:926–935.

111. Pagel JF, Helfter P. Drug induced nightmares–an etiology based review. Hum Psychopharmacol 2003; 18(1):59–67.

112. Blagrove M, Farmer L, Williams E. The relationship of nightmare frequency and nightmare distress to well-being. J Sleep Res 2004; 13:129–136.

113. Zadra AL, Donderi DC. Nightmares and bad dreams: their prevalence and relationship to well-being. J Abnorm Psychol 2000; 109:273–281.

114. Berquier A, Ashton R. Characteristics of the frequent nightmare sufferer. J Abnorm Psychol 1992; 101:246–250.

115. Nielsen TA, Laberge L, Paquet J, et al. Development of disturbing dreams during adolescence and their relationship to anxiety symptoms. Sleep 2000; 23:727–736.

116. Levin R, Fireman G. Nightmare prevalence, nightmare distress, and self-reported psychological disturbance. Sleep 2002; 25:205–212.

117. Tanskanen A, Tuomilehto J, Viinamäki H, et al. Nightmares as predictors of suicide. Sleep 2001; 24:844–847.

118. Spoomaker VI, Schredl M, van den Bout J. Nightmares: from anxiety symptom to sleep disorder. Sleep Med Rev 2006; 10:19–31.

119. Bernstein DM, Belicki K. On the psychometric properties of retrospective dream questionnaires. Imag Cogn Pers 1995–96; 15:351–364.

120. Schredl M. Effects of state and trait factors on nightmare frequency. Eur Arch Psychiatry Clin Neurosci 2003; 253:241–247.

121. Belicki K. Nightmare frequency versus nightmare distress: relations to psychopathology and cognitive style. J Abnorm Psychol 1992; 101:592–597.

122. Takeuchi T, Miyasita A, Sasaki Y, et al. Isolated sleep paralysis elicited by sleep interruption. Sleep 1992; 15(3):217–225.

123. Spanos NP, McNulty SA, DuBreuil SC, et al. The frequency and correlates of sleep paralysis in a University sample. J Res Pers 1995; 29:285–305.

124. Cheyne JA. Situational factors affecting sleep paralysis and associated hallucinations: position and timing effects. J Sleep Res 2002; 11(2):169–177.

125. Cheyne JA, Newby-Clark IR, Rueffer SD. Relations among hypnagogic and hypnopompic experiences associated with sleep paralysis. J Sleep Res 1999; 8(4):313–317.

126. Cheyne JA. Sleep paralysis episode frequency and number, types, and structure of associated hallucinations. J Sleep Res 2005; 14(3):319–324.

127. Bell CC, Dixie-Bell DD, Thompson B. Panic attacks: relationship to isolated sleep paralysis. Am J Psychiatry 1986; 143(11):1484.

128. Simard V, Nielsen TA. Sleep paralysis–associated sensed presence as a possible manifestation of social anxiety. Dreaming 2005; 15(4):245–260.

129. Fukuda K, Inamatsu N, Kuroiwa M, et al. Personality of healthy young adults with sleep paralysis. Percept Mot Skills 1991; 73(3 pt 1):955–962.

130. von Gontard A, Schaumburg H, Hollmann E, et al. The genetics of enuresis: a review. J Urol 2001; 166(6):2438–2443.

131. Fritz G, Rockney R, Bernet W, et al. Practice parameter for the assessment and treatment of children and adolescents with enuresis. J Am Acad Child Adolesc Psychiatry 2004; 43(12):1540–1550.

132. Alexopoulos EI, Kostadima E, Pagonari I. Association between primary nocturnal enuresis and habitual snoring in children. Urology 2006; 68(2):406–409.

133. Brooks LJ, Topol HI. Enuresis in children with sleep apnea. J Pediatr 2003; 142:515–518.

134. Baeyens D, Roeyers H, Demeyere I, et al. Attention-deficit/hyperactivity disorder (ADHD) as a risk factor for persistent nocturnal enuresis in children: a two-year follow-up study. Acta Paediatr 2005; 94(11):1619–1925.

135. Toros F, Erdogan K. Paroxetine-induced enuresis. Eur Psychiatry 2003; 18:43–44.

136. Monji A, Yanagimoto K, Yoshida I, et al. SSRI-induced enuresis: a case report. J Clin Psychopharmacol 2004; 24(5):564–565.

137. Cheng LY. Nocturnal enuresis and psychotropic drugs. Am J Psychiatry 1981; 138:538–539.

138. Took KJ, Buck BJ. Enuresis with combined risperidone and SSRI use. J Am Acad Child Adolesc Psychiatry 1996; 35:840–841.

139. Schulpen TW. The burden of nocturnal enuresis. Acta Paediatr 1997; 86:981–984.

140. Can G, Topbas M, Okten A, et al. Child abuse as a result of enuresis. Pediatr Int 2004; 46(1):64–66.

141. Winkelman J. Clinical and polysomnographic features of sleep-related eating disorder. J Clin Psychiatry 1998; 59:14–19.

142. Schenck CH, Hurwitz TD, Bundlie SR, et al. Sleep-related eating disorders: polysomnographic correlates of a heterogeneous syndrome distinct from daytime eating disorders. Sleep 1991; 14(5): 419–431.

143. Schenck CH, Hurwitz TD, O'Connor KA, et al. Additional categories of sleep-related eating disorders and the current status of treatment. Sleep 1993; 16(5):457–466.

144. Schenck CH, Mahowald MW. Review of nocturnal sleep-related eating disorders. Int J Eat Disord 1994; 15(4):343–356.

145. Morgenthaler TI, Silber MH. Amnestic sleep-related eating disorder associated with zolpidem. Sleep Med 2002; 3(4):323–327.

146. Lu ML, Shen WW. Sleep-related eating disorder induced by risperidone. J Clin Psychiatry 2002; 63(7): 597.

147. Paquet V, Strul J, Servais L, et al. Sleep-related eating disorder induced by olanzapine. J Clin Psychiatry 2004; 65(2):273–274.

148. Pevernagie DA, Boon PA, Mariman AN, et al. Vocalization during episodes of prolonged expiration: a parasomnia related to REM sleep. Sleep Med 2001; 2(1):19–30.

149. Vetrugno R, Provini F, Plazzi G, et al. Catathrenia (nocturnal groaning): a new type of parasomnia. Neurology 2001; 56(6):681–683.

150. Oldani A, Manconi M, Zucconi M. 'Nocturnal groaning': just a sound or parasomnia? J Sleep Res 2005; 14(3):305–310.

38 | Types of Parasomnias

Meredith Broderick

University Hospitals of Cleveland Case Medical Center, Cleveland, Ohio, U.S.A.

INTRODUCTION

Parasomnias are characterized by the presence of unpleasant motor activity and activation of cognitive systems, with or without autonomic activation during sleep. Parasomnias are generally separated into two categories, primary and secondary parasomnias. Primary parasomnias are a group of sleep disorders classified in the *International Classification of Sleep Disorders*, second edition, (*ICSD-2*) (1) into three broad subtypes based on the respective sleep states in which they arise. They include disorders of arousal from non–rapid eye movement (NREM) sleep, disorders of arousal from rapid eye movement (REM) sleep, and other parasomnias. Secondary parasomnias manifest in the sleep period as events from another organ system.

As awareness for sleep disorders evolves, an increasing overlap of parasomnias within subtypes as well as with other sleep disorders is becoming recognized. Continuing pursuit with time is also bringing about descriptions of newer parasomnias.

DISORDERS OF AROUSAL FROM NREM SLEEP

Disorders of arousal from NREM sleep tend to arise in stage N3 sleep and therefore occur most often in the first third of the sleep cycle. They are common in children. This subclass of parasomnias includes confusional arousals, sleepwalking, and sleep terrors. In these conditions, there is a dissociation in the activation patterns of the brain in the transitions between the waking and NREM states.

CONFUSIONAL AROUSALS

Demographics
Ohayon et al. surveyed 4972 subjects between 15 and 100 years of age and found a prevalence of 4.2%, which was comparable for females and males (2). Prevalence was highest (8.9%) in the age subgroup from 15 to 24 years. Prevalence diminished with age, decreasing to 4.8% in the age subgroup 25 to 44 years, to 2.5% in the 45 to 64 years age subgroup, and to 1.4% in patients older than 65 years.

Key Symptoms and Signs
The key feature of confusional arousals is an agitated awakening associated with a combination of motor activity such as moaning, crying, thrashing, or staring. This subtype of parasomnia also encompasses sleep drunkenness or sleep inertia, which are also characterized by mental confusion upon awakenings. The *ICSD-2* (1) diagnostic criteria requires recurrent mental confusion or confusional behaviors occurring during awakening from nocturnal sleep or a daytime nap that is not better explained by medication use, or sleep, medical, neurological, mental, or substance abuse disorders. Episodes usually occur in the first third of the night because of their association with NREM sleep, but may very well occur upon awakening at the end of the sleep period.

Individuals with confusional arousals typically exhibit inappropriate behavior that can range from simple to complex. They may appear partially awake, with eyes open or closed. Children may have a confused expression as if they are staring through the observer (usually a parent) during the arousal. Attempts to console the child may result in worsening agitation. Episodes usually last 5 to 15 minutes but may last as long as 30 to 40 minutes. Patients are usually amnestic for the event. There is no reported difference in frequency of occurrence between females and males.

Onset, Ontogeny, and Clinical Course
As described earlier, the highest prevalence for this condition is in the late teens to young adulthood. Over time, confusional arousals in children may evolve into sleepwalking or resolve spontaneously.

Risk Factors
Precipitating factors for the confusional arousals include sleep deprivation, alcohol consumption, obstructive sleep apnea (OSA), periodic limb movement disorder (PLMD), psychotropic medication use, drug abuse, or forced awakenings. Abnormal sleep-related sexual behavior, so-called sexsomnia or sleepsex, is a more recently described disorder, which also falls into the category of confusional arousals. Complications include sleep-related injury, violence, poor school or job attendance, or other interpersonal difficulties.

SLEEPWALKING

Demographics
Sleepwalking can occur at any age, but has been reported by Ohayon et al. (2) to have a prevalence of 2.0%. The prevalence was highest (4.9%) in the subgroup from 15 to 24 years of age with a trend of decreasing with increasing age. The prevalence was reported to be 2.1%, in the subgroup from 25 to 44 years of age, 1.1% in the subgroup of patients from 45 to 64 years of age, and 0.5% in the subgroup of patients over 65 years of age. There was no sex difference reported in this study. The Finnish Twin Cohort consisting of 11,220 subjects aged 33 to 60 years and including 1045 monozygotic and 1899 dizygotic twins published by Hublin et al. (3) demonstrated genetic effects in sleepwalking. They reported a concordance rate of 0.55 for monozygotic and 0.35 for dizygotic pairs for sleepwalking in childhood. For adults, the concordance rate was 0.32 for monozygotic and 0.06 for dizygotic pairs. Kales et al. (4) postulated hereditary factors in sleepwalking after examining the families of 25 proband, proposing a two threshold multifactorial role. Bakwin et al. (5) conducted a twin study consisting of 199 monozygotic and 124 dizygotic twin pairs and concordance for sleepwalking was six times greater in monozygotic pairs than in dizygotic pairs.

Key Symptoms and Signs
Sleepwalking or somnambulism is defined by the *ICSD-2* (1) as ambulation occurring during sleep, persistence of sleep in an altered state of consciousness, or impaired judgment during ambulation, which is not better explained by medication use or medical, neurological, mental, or substance abuse disorders. The altered state of consciousness manifests as difficulty arousing the person during an event, complete or partial amnesia for the event, routine behaviors at inappropriate times, nonsensical behaviors, or dangerous behaviors. It usually occurs in the first third of the sleep period, which consists of a part of the sleep period with increased density of slow-wave sleep. The patient may describe sitting up in bed, followed by ambulation. If an attempt is made to awaken the patient during an event, one will appear confused or report details of dream content. Alternatively, the patient may awaken spontaneously during an event while ambulating or return to bed spontaneously. Sleepwalking can be calm, violent, or part of a more complex behavior in an inappropriate place such as urinating in the corner or moving furniture. In extreme cases it may result in physical harm or assault against a bed partner or family member.

Onset, Ontogeny, and Clinical Course
As described earlier it can occur at any age; however, it is most common in children. The disorder often resolves with puberty, although if it is precipitated by another underlying sleep disorder, it may persist or worsen with age.

Risk Factors
Conditions or disorders that can fragment sleep (e.g., obstructive sleep apnea), sleep deprivation, and stress can precipitate sleepwalking episodes in predisposed individuals.

SLEEP TERRORS

Demographics
Ohayon et al. (2) reported sleep terrors as having an overall prevalence of 2.2%. The highest prevalence was seen in the age group of 15- to 24-year-olds, which was 2.6%. The prevalence decreased with age. It was reported as 2.5% in the subgroup 25 to 44 years of age, 2.3% in the subgroup 45 to 64 years of age, and 1% in the subgroup of patients greater than 65 years of age.

Key Symptoms and Signs
Sleep terrors or night terrors consist of an abrupt awakening from sleep, often with a vocalization. According to the *ICSD-2* (1), sleep terrors are a sudden episode of terror during sleep, beginning with a loud vocalization, autonomic activation, and fearful behavioral manifestations. Episodes are analogous to sleepwalking, there is difficulty arousing the person, mental confusion upon awakening from an episode, presence of complete or partial amnesia, and potentially dangerous behaviors. Events are not better explained by medication use or sleep, medical, neurological, mental, or substance abuse disorder. Night terrors may occur several times per sleep period or with weeks to months between occurrences.

Onset, Ontogeny, and Clinical Course
In the majority of cases, it spontaneously resolves in adolescence but may also evolve into sleepwalking.

Risk Factors
Conditions or disorders that can fragment sleep (e.g., obstructive sleep apnea), sleep deprivation, and stress can precipitate sleepwalking episodes in predisposed individuals.

PARASOMNIAS ASSOCIATED WITH REM SLEEP

Parasomnias occurring out of REM sleep tend to occur in the second half of the sleep period due to the high density of REM sleep during this part of the sleep cycle. The parasomnias associated with REM sleep as classified by the *ICSD-2* includes REM sleep behavior disorder, recurrent isolated sleep paralysis, and nightmare disorder.

REM SLEEP BEHAVIOR DISORDER

Demographics
Prevalence of REM sleep behavior disorder (RBD) is estimated as 0.38% in the general population, although no large scale demographic studies have been done. Idiopathic RBD, in which no neurological or medical cause can be found, is thought to account for 60% of cases (6,7). RBD is predominant in patients over 50 years of age, 80% to 90% of those being men (8,9).

Key Symptoms and Signs
RBD is a sleep disruption due to the presence of abnormal behaviors in REM sleep. Patients usually visit the physician's office due to injury to self or a bed partner, especially if episodes are violent in nature. *ICSD-2* criteria for RBD has four main components: presence of REM sleep without atonia, disruptive or injurious behaviors, absence of EEG epileptiform activity during REM sleep, and no better explanation by medications or sleep, medical, mental, neurological, or substance abuse disorders. At the end of episodes, individuals may be able to associate sleep behaviors with dreaming or it may be inferred by a spouse. Schenck et al. described the initial case reports of five patients whose REM sleep was characterized by jerky movements and complex and inappropriate behaviors (10).

RBD may be difficult to distinguish from sleepwalking, although there are several distinguishing clinical features. Patients with RBD are more likely to have their eyes closed during an episode, rarely ambulate, and almost never leave the bedroom. Episodes are more likely to consist of swearing, shouting, grasping, flailing, punching, or kicking. RBD is also more likely to occur at least 90 minutes after sleep onset, in the second half of the sleep period, and only rarely during naps (11). Episodes may occur several times per night or at intervals as long as months. Olson et al. (8) studied trends in frequency of episodes in 49 patients. In 26 of the cases, frequency remained unchanged over time, in 16 frequency increased over time, and in seven patients frequency decreased with time. In their patient series, 64% of patients had assaulted spouses, 13% caused injury, 32% caused injury to self, and in 93% of cases actions were associated with dream content. Injuries to self included bruises, lacerations, fires, and in rare cases severe head injuries such as subdural hematomas were documented (12).

Onset, Ontogeny, and Clinical Course
Reported mean age of onset ranges from 53.4 to 60.9 years of age (8,10). Prior to diagnosis of RBD, patients or their bed partners may describe many preceding years of somniloquy, vivid, or violent dreams.

Risk Factors
It is estimated that one third of patients diagnosed with Parkinson's disease (PD) and 90% of patients with multiple systems atrophy (MSA) have RBD (13). Due to its strong association with dementia with Lewy bodies, it has been added as one of the suggestive criteria for the diagnosis (14). Iranzo et al. showed that 45% of patients with RBD developed a neurological disorder in a mean of 11.5 years from reported symptoms onset and 5.1 years from diagnosis of idiopathic RBD (15). Schenck et al. studied 29 male patients over the age of 50 diagnosed with idiopathic RBD and found 38% were eventually diagnosed with PD at a mean of 3.7 ± 1.4 years after diagnosis of idiopathic RBD and 12.7 ± 7.3 years after onset of symptoms. RBD retains its sex predisposition for men. However, this finding is weaker in patients with RBD and MSA (16).

RBD has a similar pathophysiology as narcolepsy in the dissociation between REM and wake states, and therefore, investigators have studied and found that the prevalence of narcolepsy is 13% in patients with RBD. RBD may also be present in the setting of narcolepsy, precipitated by treatment for cataplexy with tricyclic depressants, monoamine oxidase inhibitors, or tricyclic antidepressants.

Other disorders associated with RBD includes obstructive sleep apnea (17), periodic limb movement disorder (8), stroke (18), multiple sclerosis (19), Tourette's syndrome (20) brainstem tumors, spinocerebellar ataxia type 3 (21), olivopontocerebellar degeneration (22), psychiatric disorders (17), and autism (23). Certain medications such as tricyclic antidepressants (24,25), mirtazpine (26), and selective serotonin reuptake inhibitors (SSRIs) have also been reported in association with RBD. RBD can also be seen in withdrawal states from alcohol or barbiturate use due to a REM rebound phenomenon (17). There is some evidence RBD is familial but no definitive genetic linkage has been revealed. RBD is usually a progressive disease, especially in the setting of a neurodegenerative disease.

RECURRENT ISOLATED SLEEP PARALYSIS

Demographics
Ohayon et al. (27) surveyed 8085 individuals and found a reported lifetime prevalence of 6.2% for sleep paralysis. Although many sources report the most common age of onset in the second to third decade, Ohayon et al. (27) found that the onset of sleep paralysis was as likely to occur at any age. Studies have not shown evidence of a sex predisposition.

Key Symptoms and Signs
Recurrent Isolated Sleep Paralysis is defined by the *ICSD-2* as an inability to move the trunk and limbs at transition periods from wake to sleep (hypnagogic) or in transition from sleep to wakefulness (hypnopompic). To meet the criteria for recurrent isolated sleep paralysis, patients must not carry the diagnosis of narcolepsy. Usually consciousness, breathing, and memory for the events are unaffected. The episodes are not better explained by medications or another sleep, medical, neurological, mental, or substance abuse disorder. Sleep paralysis usually resolves on its own within seconds to minutes and may include an auditory, visual, or tactile hallucination (28). Some patients have observed that sensory or auditory stimuli abort

the episodes. There are no known long-term effects of the episodes other than the possible anxiety a person may experience as an after effect of the experience.

Onset, Ontogeny, and Clinical Course
The onset of this condition can occur at any age. Frequency of episodes ranges from once in a person's lifetime to several times per year.

Risk Factors
Predisposing factors for episodes include sleep deprivation, stress, fatigue, shift work, supine position, alcohol use, and irregular sleep-wake schedules (28). Associations with hypnagogic hallucinations, moderate daytime sleepiness, early morning awakenings, nonrestorative sleep, confusional arousals, nocturnal leg cramps, sleep starts, sleep talking, anxiety, and depression have also been reported (27). Bell et al. published studies showing a possible relationship between panic attacks (29) and hypertension (30) with sleep paralysis. Sleep paralysis has been postulated as transmitted via a maternal inheritance, with studies showing a familial pattern (31), but no large scale confirmatory study has been done.

NIGHTMARE DISORDER

Demographics
Prevalence of nightmares in the general population is reported from 5% to 11% (32,33). About 20% to 39% of children from the age 5 to 12 have nightmares (34).

Key Symptoms and Signs
Nightmare disorder consists of nightmares characterized by disturbing mental experiences that generally occur during REM sleep and result in awakenings (28). The *ICSD-2* criteria for a diagnosis of nightmare disorder has three components: recurrent episodes of awakenings from sleep with recollection of dream content that may involve any combination of dysphoric emotions, full awareness upon awakening, and either delayed return to sleep after an event or recurrence of nightmares in the second half of the typical sleep period. Consciousness of dream content is retained and therefore distressing to individuals as it often contains a physical threat such as being pursued, falling, or death. Nightmares may also have a recurrent theme. Nightmares may make it difficult for individuals to fall back to sleep after an event, leading to avoidance of sleep, insomnia, and daytime sleepiness.

Onset, Ontogeny, and Clinical Course
Nightmares can arise at any age, but often appear from 3 to 6 years of age, peaking at 6 to 10 years of age and then decreasing.

Risk Factors
Hublin et al. (35) conducted a twin study including 1298 monozygotic twins and 2419 dizygotic twins. They found a genetic predisposition to nightmares stable from childhood to adulthood. They also reported a linear relationship between nightmare frequency and presence of psychiatric disorders. Nightmares have a strong association with Post Traumatic Stress Disorder, certain personality characteristics, and psychopathology. Being female, lower socioeconomic status, and lower education level are predisposing factors for nightmare disorder (33). Medications acting through neurotransmitters can also be associated with nightmares. Conditions such as a febrile illness or delirium may also precipitate nightmares.

OTHER PARASOMNIAS

This category encompasses several parasomnias that do not have a strong association with NREM or REM sleep. This includes sleep-related dissociative disorders, nocturnal enuresis, sleep-related groaning, exploding head syndrome, sleep-related hallucinations, and sleep-related eating disorder (SRED).

SLEEP-RELATED DISSOCIATIVE DISORDERS

Demographics
One study reported a prevalence of 7% in patients presenting to the sleep clinic (1). These disorders are thought to be more prevalent in women.

Key Symptoms and Signs
Sleep-related dissociative disorders are a distinct but related variant of dissociative disorders. Episodes are typically elaborate behaviors occurring at transitions from wakefulness to sleep or within minutes from an awakening from stage N1, stage N2, or REM sleep. The *ICSD-2* diagnostic criteria are threefold: a dissociative disorder fulfilling the *Diagnostic and Statistical Manual of Mental Disorders*, fourth edition, emerging in close association with main sleep period, polysomnographic evidence that episodes emerge during sustained wakefulness in transition from wakefulness to sleep or after an awakening from NREM or REM sleep, or a history by observers supporting the diagnosis. The sleep disorder is not better explained by another sleep, medical, neurological, medication, or substance abuse disorder. Dissociation can manifest as a dissociative fugue, dissociative identity disorder, or dissociative disorder not otherwise specified. Associated behaviors may include yelling, ambulation, running, or even self-mutilation lasting minutes to hours. Frequency of events is variable and the occurrences may be several times per night or at weekly intervals. Cases associated with history of sexual or physical abuse may include reenactments of those events. Episodes of driving, taking a flight to another city, and binge eating have been reported. Dissociative episodes often have daytime correlates. Often individuals are amnestic for the behaviors.

Onset, Ontogeny, and Clinical Course
The typical age of onset of this condition is from childhood to middle adulthood, and the clinical course varies between individuals.

Risk Factors
Predisposing factors include a prior history of abuse or psychiatric disorders. There is no known familial transmission. The disease course is usually chronic in nature. Individuals may experience complications such as bruises, lacerations, burns, or cuts from self-mutilation.

SLEEP ENURESIS

Demographics
Primary sleep enuresis is present in 15% to 25% of 5-year-olds (36), 10% of 6-year-olds, 7% of 7-year-olds, 5% of 10-year-olds, 3% of 12-year-olds, and 1% to 2% of 18-year-olds (1). It has been reported in 2.1% of adults. Hublin et al. found enuresis occurring weekly in 0.3% of females and 0.1% of males (37), which may be associated with neurological conditions such as multiple sclerosis, epilepsy, and mental retardation of cerebral palsy. It is more common in younger children than older, boys than girls, and in whites than in other races (38).

Key Symptoms and Signs
Sleep enuresis, also known as nocturnal bedwetting, is divided into two categories, primary and secondary enuresis. According to the *ICSD-2* diagnostic criteria, the individual must be older than five years old with recurrent involuntary voiding during sleep occurring twice per week for at least three months. In primary sleep enuresis, the patient has no history of being consistently dry throughout the night, whereas in secondary sleep enuresis, the patient will have a history of being consistently dry during sleep for at least a six-month period. In children, enuresis can be related to physiological or a psychosocial problem. If episodes occur during the daytime, they are more likely due to physiological problems such as diabetes mellitus, obstructive sleep apnea, urinary tract infection, or epilepsy. In cases of secondary enuresis, psychosocial causes may be related to a stressor such as a parental divorce or abuse.

Onset, Ontogeny, and Clinical Course

As discussed earlier, it appears in children, and it spontaneously resolves in about 15% of cases per year (1).

Risk Factors

Children experiencing any kind of physical illness or psychological distress are at increased risk. Prevalence increases for each parent who had enuresis as a child. Children of two parents who both had enuresis have a 77% chance of having enuresis, 43% with one parent, and 15% if neither parent had enuresis (39). Hublin et al. reported a genetic predisposition to enuresis (37). Several studies have postulated an autosomal dominant inheritance with a suggested linkage to chromosome 12q (40,41).

Nocturnal enuresis has a known association with sleep-disordered breathing (42). It may also occur in the setting of sexual abuse or excessive liquid intake. In benign cases, the main complications of sleep enuresis are damage to a patient's self-esteem due to embarrassment. Thus, the family's reactions to the disorder will impact the degree to which self-esteem is affected. In cases associated with an underlying physical abnormality such as obstruction, neurogenic bladder, ectopic ureter, or posterior urethral valves, complications such as urinary tract infections may be present.

SLEEP-RELATED GROANING

Demographics

Prevalence is probably less than 1% of the population (43). Despite the paucity of cases reported in the literature, it is consistently reported as three times more common in women. Oldani et al. (43) published a cases series of 21 patients, with a mean age of onset at 21.7±7.0 years of age and a literature review of 27 patients with a mean age of onset at 19.6 years. Nine of the 21 patients (43%) had a family history of another parasomnia such as sleepwalking, sleep talking, or night terrors and 14.8% had a family history of catathrenia. In addition, 92.6% of patients had episodes exclusively or predominantly during REM sleep. None of the patients in their sample had associated pulmonary or neurological disease. Another case series of four patients ranging in age from 5 to 16 years had no family histories of sleep-related groaning or other parasomnias (44). All four of the patients in their series had normal otorhinolaryngologic examinations.

Key Symptoms and Signs

Sleep-related groaning or catathrenia is a rare disorder consisting of bradypneic, expiratory, and monotonous groaning after a prolonged inspiration. Its classic descriptions consist of a deep inspiration followed by a short expiration, then a longer expiration associated with noise production. The nature of the groaning is described as morose, lasting 2 to 20 seconds and occurs in clusters. Most patients present to the physician because of the negative social consequences of the noise production and are usually unaware of it unless alerted of it by an observer.

The *ICSD-2* diagnostic criteria require a history consistent with monotonous vocalization during sleep or polysomnographic evidence of respiratory-related sound production. Vocalizations occur within two to six hours of onset of sleep, occur every night, and are strongly associated with REM sleep, although some cases report episodes out of both REM and NREM sleep. The pitch of the noise varies between patients but is consistent for individual patients. Vocalizations may be short ten second episodes or repetitive sounds over 4 minutes (43). It is not position dependent.

Onset, Ontogeny, and Clinical Course

Cases of sleep-related groaning are usually chronic in nature and may occur every night for years. Patients may have symptoms for over 10 years before visiting a physician. Long-term prognosis is unknown. With the exception of the select cases described previously that responded to CPAP, no other successful drug treatment such as clonazepam, gabapentin, pramipexole, carbamazepine, paroxetine, trazodone, and dosulpine have been successful. Complications are predominantly related to the disrupted sleep of a bed partner or the patient's perceived embarrassment given the unusual nature of the symptoms including the morose connotation or sexual connotation to the vocalization.

Risk Factors

Guilleminault et al. (45) published a case series of seven young women ranging in age from 20 to 34 years of age, body mass index (BMI) less than 25, and mean respiratory disturbance index (RDI) of 13.1 who experienced a remission in catathrenia with treatment of sleep disordered breathing. Their findings suggested a possible relationship between catathrenia and sleep disordered breathing in a specific subset of patients, although arguments have been made that their cases might have actually represented expiratory snoring (46). Guilleminault et al. (45) and Iriarte et al. (47) reported catathrenic patients with slightly different characteristics in that there was a clinical response to CPAP, a slight improvement in REM sleep, and presence of groaning through all stages of sleep. The differences point to the possibility of various subtypes of catathrenia or the possible need to evaluate its classification (48).

EXPLODING HEAD SYNDROME

Demographics

The syndrome is rare and therefore the prevalence is unknown.

Key Symptoms and Signs

Exploding head syndrome is often described as a "snapping in the brain," which awakens an individual from sleep, lasting a few seconds. Other descriptions of the syndrome include loud bang, shotgun, or bomb like explosion. In 10% of cases, snapping may be associated with a flash of light (49). The *ICSD-2* criterion for exploding head syndrome has three main components. Patients complain of a sudden loud noise or sense of explosion in the head during wake to sleep transition or upon waking from sleep. Although there is no pain with the episode, many patients may become frightened by the symptoms and seek medical attention with fear of a serious underlying cause. The key feature of exploding head syndrome to distinguish it from other sudden onset headache syndromes is its painless nature. In contrast to paroxysmal hemicrania and cluster headaches, there are no associated autonomic features or lateralization of symptoms. Episodes occur during wakefulness and usually resolve on their own without any intervention (50).

Onset, Ontogeny, and Clinical Course

Age of onset of exploding head syndrome is usually in middle age (51), typically after age 50, although it may begin at any age. Episodes may occur several times per night for days or weeks at a time in clusters, with periods of remission in between.

Risk Factors

Exploding headache syndrome has been studied with polysomnography and has been documented as arising out of any stage of sleep, including REM sleep as well as in transition from wakefulness to sleep (49). Since this parasomnia is thought to be related to emotional stress during wakefulness, reassurances about the benign nature of the headache can help in its resolution (50).

SLEEP-RELATED HALLUCINATIONS

Demographics

Prevalence of sleep-related hallucinations is not known. They are thought to be slightly more common in women (52) and in younger persons.

Key Symptoms and Signs

Sleep-related hallucinations are defined by the *ICSD-2* criteria as hallucinations occurring just prior to sleep (hypnagogic) or upon awakening (hypnopompic), predominantly visual, and not better explained by another sleep, neurological, medical, mental health disorder, or medication. Although the hallucinations are predominantly visual in nature, tactile or auditory hallucinations may also occur. Patients typically describe complex, vivid, immobile images of people or animals. The images may persist for minutes and frequently disappear with increasing illumination. One of the key features of sleep-related hallucinations is that patients are clearly awake during the episodes. The perceived images are felt to be real and may even be frightening.

Onset, Ontogeny, and Clinical Course
The onset of sleep-related hallucinations is more common in youth, and the clinical course is variable between affected individuals.

Risk Factors
Sleep-related hallucinations are more common in the setting of drug and alcohol use, anxiety, mood disorders, insomnia, and insufficient sleep (1). There is no known familial pattern. Complications involve reactions to the hallucinations such as fear responses in which the individual may injure oneself.

SLEEP-RELATED EATING DISORDER

Demographics of Sleep-Related Eating Disorder
The prevalence has been reported to be 1.5% in the general population (53). Vetrugno et al. (54) reported a cases series of 35 patients with a mean age of onset at 39.6 ± 13.9 years. Of the 35 patients, 21 (60%) were women, suggesting a predominance in women. Schenck et al. (55) published an earlier study consisting of 19 patients with a slightly younger mean age of onset at 24.7±12.9. The latter study also showed a predominance of SRED in women.

Key Symptoms and Signs
Sleep-related eating disorder (SRED) is defined in the *ICSD-2* as recurrent episodes of involuntary eating and drinking in the main sleep period associated with consumption of unusual forms or combinations of food. The majority of patients present to the physician because of unwanted weight gain (56). After falling asleep, they typically awaken with a compulsive desire to eat but without hunger. Substances ingested may include inedible or toxic substances such as cigarette butts, oils, or raw food. Recurrent episodes of eating, sleep-related injury, dangerous behaviors while in pursuit of food or cooking, or adverse health-related consequences from recurrent binge eating are present. The disturbance is not better explained by another sleep, neurological, medical, mental health, or substance abuse disorder. Episodes may occur once or several times per night and is usually associated with daytime hyporexia.

Onset, Ontogeny, and Clinical Course
The onset of SRED is in young-to-middle aged adults and the clinical course, although variable among affected individuals, appears to be a chronic condition.

Risk Factors
In the *ICSD-2*, SRED is inclusive of nocturnal eating syndrome (NES) (56). There is controversy as to whether the nocturnal eating syndrome is a distinct disorder from SRED and if these two disorders can be distinguished based on whether an individual retains memory of the events of ingestion. Some studies have suggested SRED can be distinguished from NES in that there is partial or no awareness of the events in SRED while in NES, the patient recalls the episode clearly (55,57). Other research suggests memory of events is impaired only when a medication, substance abuse, or psychiatric disease is present. Studies including patients with partial or total amnesia for nocturnal eating also tended to have a greater association with confusional arousals and sleepwalking, raising the question of whether the sleep state dissociation was secondary to another parasomnia rather than the nocturnal eating disorder (58).

Episodes of eating are characterized by an EEG pattern of wakefulness and usually occur out of NREM sleep. Arousals do not have a relationship to periodic limb movements or respiratory-related events. Vetrugno et al. studied 35 patients with SRED. They observed

45 episodes in 26 different patients. Of those 45 episodes of sleep-related eating, all with the exception of one occurred out of NREM sleep (54). They also reported an associated PLMD in 22 patients, restless leg syndrome (RLS) in 5 patients, and recurring chewing and swallowing in 29 patients. SRED is more common in the setting of other sleep disorders such as somniloquy, sleepwalking, PLMD, OSA, and RLS. Mean length of the episodes of eating has been reported from 3.5 (58) to 6.2 minutes with a range of 0.41 to 20 minutes (54). All of the patients in this study were able to clearly recall the episodes of sleep-related eating on the following day. There is no proven association with other metabolic or daytime eating disorders such as daytime binge eating, anorexia, or bulimia.

SRED is usually a chronic disorder, although it may occur in an idiopathic form when associated with medication use such as zolpidem, triazolam, lithium carbonate, or anticholinergic agents. SRED can be exacerbated by acute stress, nicotine withdrawal, autoimmune disease, narcolepsy, or hepatitis (59). Complications include insomnia due to the nighttime arousals, weight gain, poor glucose control, allergic reactions, accidents, fires, and embarrassment. Physical injury is less common in this parasomnia compared to sleepwalking and confusional arousals.

MISCELLANEOUS

Parasomnia, unspecified parasomnia due to a drug or substance, and parasomnia due to a medical condition are used as the diagnosis when suspected psychiatric diagnoses, association with a medication, or medical condition are responsible for the parasomnia. Medications commonly associated with parasomnias include selective SSRIs, venlafaxine, tricyclic antidepressants, monoamine oxidase inhibitors, mirtazapine, bisoprolol, selegiline, or cholinergics. Medical conditions associated with parasomnias include delirium tremens, Morvan's fibrillary chorea, fatal familial insomnia, Parkinson's disease, and dementia with Lewy bodies.

Secondary parasomnias are generally classified based on their organ system of origin. The three main organ systems responsible for common parasomnias include the central nervous system, cardiopulmonary, gastrointestinal, and psychiatric parasomnias. Central nervous system parasomnias include vascular and nonvascular headaches, nocturnal seizures, and tinnitus. Cardiopulmonary parasomnias include nocturnal angina pectoris, nocturnal asthma, and sleep coughing. Gastrointestinal parasomnias include gastroesophageal reflux and esophageal spasm. Psychiatric parasomnias include nocturnal panic attacks, post-traumatic stress disorder, psychogenic dissociative disorder, and malingering. Other miscellaneous disorders may present as secondary parasomnias including nocturnal muscle cramps, nocturnal pruritus, night sweats, nocturnal tongue biting, and benign alternating hemiplegia of childhood.

CONCLUSIONS

Types of parasomnias are distinguished based on clinical features. Current evidence is limited due to relative rarity of many of the parasomnias or also because of the benign nature of the condition. Further exploration of the parasomnias with increasing awareness of sleep disorders will allow larger studies, and provide more insight into the genetics, familial patterns, relationship to other sleep disorders, and medical condition.

REFERENCES

1. American Academy of Sleep Medicine. International Classification of Sleep Disorders, 2nd ed. Diagnostic and Coding Manual. Westchester, Il: American Academy of Sleep Medicine, 2005.
2. Ohayon MM, Guilleminault C, Priest RG. Night terrors, sleepwalking, and confusional arousals in the general population: their frequency and relationship to other sleep and mental disorders. J Clin Psychiatry 1999; 60(4):268–276; quiz 277.
3. Hublin C, Kaprio J, Partinen M, et al. Prevalence and genetics of sleepwalking: a population-based twin study. Neurology 1997; 48(1):177–181.

4. Kales A, Soldatos CR, Bixler EO, et al. Hereditary factors in sleepwalking and night terrors. Br J Psychiatry 1980; 137:111–118.
5. Bakwin H. Sleep-walking in twins. Lancet 1970; 2(7670):446–447.
6. Fantini ML, Corona A, Clerici S, et al. Aggressive dream content without daytime aggressiveness in REM sleep behavior disorder. Neurology 2005; 65(7):1010–1015.
7. Fantini ML, Ferini-Strambi L, Montplaisir J. Idiopathic REM sleep behavior disorder: toward a better nosologic definition. Neurology 2005; 64(5):780–786.
8. Olson EJ, Boeve BF, Silber MH. Rapid eye movement sleep behaviour disorder: demographic, clinical and laboratory findings in 93 cases. Brain 2000; 123(pt 2):331–339.
9. Montagna P. Sleep-related non epileptic motor disorders. J Neurol 2004; 251(7):781–794.
10. Schenck CH, Hurwitz TD, Mahowald MW. Symposium: normal and abnormal REM sleep regulation: REM sleep behaviour disorder: an update on a series of 96 patients and a review of the world literature. J Sleep Res 1993; 2(4):224–231.
11. Schenck CH, Bundlie SR, Ettinger MG, et al. Chronic behavioral disorders of human REM sleep: a new category of parasomnia. Sleep 1986; 9(2):293–308.
12. Dyken ME, Lin-Dyken DC, Seaba P, et al. Violent sleep-related behavior leading to subdural hemorrhage. Arch Neurol 1995; 52(3):318–321.
13. Gagnon JF, Bedard MA, Fantini ML, et al. REM sleep behavior disorder and REM sleep without atonia in Parkinson's disease. Neurology 2002; 59(4):585–589.
14. McKeith IG, Dickson DW, Lowe J, et al. Diagnosis and management of dementia with Lewy bodies: third report of the DLB Consortium. Neurology 2005; 65(12):1863–1872.
15. Iranzo A, Molinuevo JL, Santamaría J, et al. Rapid-eye-movement sleep behaviour disorder as an early marker for a neurodegenerative disorder: a descriptive study. Lancet Neurol 2006; 5(7): 572–577.
16. Plazzi G, Corsini R, Provini F, et al. REM sleep behavior disorders in multiple system atrophy. Neurology 1997; 48(4):1094–1097.
17. Iranzo A, Santamaria J. Severe obstructive sleep apnea/hypopnea mimicking REM sleep behavior disorder. Sleep 2005; 28(2):203–206.
18. Kimura K, Tachibana N, Kohyama J, et al. A discrete pontine ischemic lesion could cause REM sleep behavior disorder. Neurology 2000; 55(6):894–895.
19. Plazzi G, Montagna P. Remitting REM sleep behavior disorder as the initial sign of multiple sclerosis. Sleep Med 2002; 3(5):437–439.
20. Trajanovic NN, Voloh I, Shapiro CM, et al. REM sleep behaviour disorder in a child with Tourette's syndrome. Can J Neurol Sci 2004; 31(4):572–575.
21. Syed BH, Rye DB, Singh G. REM sleep behavior disorder and SCA-3 (Machado-Joseph disease). Neurology 2003; 60(1):148.
22. Salva MA, Guilleminault C, Olivopontocerebellar degeneration, abnormal sleep, and REM sleep without atonia. Neurology 1986; 36(4):576–577.
23. Thirumalai SS, Shubin RA, Robinson R. Rapid eye movement sleep behavior disorder in children with autism. J Child Neurol 2002; 17(3):173–178.
24. Bental E, Lavie P, Sharf B. Severe hypermotility during sleep in treatment of cataplexy with clomipramine. Isr J Med Sci 1979; 15(7):607–609.
25. Besset A. Effect of antidepressants on human sleep. Adv Biosci 1978; 21:141–148.
26. Nash JR, Wilson SJ, Potokar JP, et al. Mirtazapine induces REM sleep behavior disorder (RBD) in parkinsonism. Neurology 2003; 61(8):1161; author reply 1161.
27. Ohayon MM, Zulley J, Guilleminault C, et al. Prevalence and pathologic associations of sleep paralysis in the general population. Neurology 1999; 52(6):1194–1200.
28. Mason TB II, Pack AI. Pediatric parasomnias. Sleep 2007; 30(2):141–151.
29. Bell CC, Dixie-Bell DD, Thompson B. Panic attacks: relationship to isolated sleep paralysis. Am J Psychiatry 1986; 143(11):1484.
30. Bell CC, Hildreth CJ, Jenkins EJ, et al. The relationship of isolated sleep paralysis and panic disorder to hypertension. J Natl Med Assoc 1988; 80(3):289–294.
31. Dahlitz M, Parkes JD. Sleep paralysis. Lancet 1993; 341(8842):406–407.
32. Bixler EO, Kales A, Soldatos CR, et al. Prevalence of sleep disorders in the Los Angeles metropolitan area. Am J Psychiatry 1979; 136(10):1257–1262.
33. Ohayon MM, Morselli PL, Guilleminault C. Prevalence of nightmares and their relationship to psychopathology and daytime functioning in insomnia subjects. Sleep 1997; 20(5):340–348.
34. Pagel JF. Nightmares and disorders of dreaming. Am Fam Physician 2000; 61(7):2037–2042, 2044.
35. Hublin C, Kaprio J, Partinen M, et al. Nightmares: familial aggregation and association with psychiatric disorders in a nationwide twin cohort. Am J Med Genet 1999; 88(4):329–336.
36. Thiedke CC. Nocturnal enuresis. Am Fam Physician 2003; 67(7):1499–1506.
37. Hublin C, Kaprio J, Partinen M, et al. Nocturnal enuresis in a nationwide twin cohort. Sleep 1998; 21(6): 579–585.

38. Foxman B, Valdez RB, Brook RH. Childhood enuresis: prevalence, perceived impact, and prescribed treatments. Pediatrics 1986; 77(4):482–487.

39. Norgaard JP, Djurhuus JC, Watanabe H, et al. Experience and current status of research into the pathophysiology of nocturnal enuresis. Br J Urol 1997; 79(6):825–835.

40. Arnell H, Hjälmås K, Jägervall M, et al. The genetics of primary nocturnal enuresis: inheritance and suggestion of a second major gene on chromosome 12q. J Med Genet 1997; 34(5):360–365.

41. Eiberg H. Nocturnal enuresis is linked to a specific gene. Scand J Urol Nephrol Suppl 1995; 173:15–16; discussion 17.

42. Weissbach A, Leiberman A, Tarasiuk A, et al. Adenotonsilectomy improves enuresis in children with obstructive sleep apnea syndrome. Int J Pediatr Otorhinolaryngol 2006; 70(8):1351–1356.

43. Oldani A, Manconi M, Zucconi M, et al. 'Nocturnal groaning': just a sound or parasomnia? J Sleep Res 2005; 14(3):305–310.

44. Vetrugno R, Provini F, Plazzi G, et al. Catathrenia (nocturnal groaning): a new type of parasomnia. Neurology 2001; 56(5):681–683.

45. Guilleminault C, Hagen CC, Khaja AM. Catathrenia: parasomnia or uncommon feature of sleep disordered breathing? Sleep 2008; 31(1):132–139.

46. Vetrugno R, Lugaresi E, Ferini-Strambi L, et al. Catathrenia (nocturnal groaning): what is it? Sleep 2008; 31(3):308–309.

47. Iriarte J, Alegre M, Urrestarazu E, et al. Continuous positive airway pressure as treatment for catathrenia (nocturnal groaning). Neurology 2006; 66(4):609–610.

48. Ortega-Albas JJ, Diaz JR, Serrano AL, et al. Continuous positive airway pressure as treatment for catathrenia (nocturnal groaning). Neurology 2006; 67(6):1103; author reply 1103.

49. Pearce JM. Clinical features of the exploding head syndrome. J Neurol Neurosurg Psychiatry 1989; 52(7): 907–910.

50. Sachs C, Svanborg E. The exploding head syndrome: polysomnographic recordings and therapeutic suggestions. Sleep 1991; 14(3):263–266.

51. Evans RW, Pearce JM. Exploding head syndrome. Headache 2001; 41(6):602–603.

52. Silber MH, Hansen MR, Girish M. Complex nocturnal visual hallucinations. Sleep Med 2005; 6(4): 363–366.

53. Rand CS, Macgregor AM, Stunkard AJ. The night eating syndrome in the general population and among postoperative obesity surgery patients. Int J Eat Disord 1997; 22(1):65–69.

54. Vetrugno R, Manconi M, Ferini-Strambi L, et al. Nocturnal eating: sleep-related eating disorder or night eating syndrome? A videopolysomnographic study. Sleep 2006; 29(7):949–954.

55. Schenck CH, Hurwitz TD, O'Connor KA, et al. Additional categories of sleep-related eating disorders and the current status of treatment. Sleep 1993; 16(5):457–466.

56. Stunkard AJ, Grace WJ, Wolff HG. The night-eating syndrome; a pattern of food intake among certain obese patients. Am J Med 1955; 19(1):78–86.

57. Winkelman JW. Sleep-related eating disorder and night eating syndrome: sleep disorders, eating disorders, or both? Sleep 2006; 29(7):876–877.

58. Spaggiari MC, Granella F, Parrino L, et al. Nocturnal eating syndrome in adults. Sleep 1994; 17(4): 339–344.

59. Schenck CH, Hurwitz TD, Bundlie SR, et al. Sleep-related eating disorders: polysomnographic correlates of a heterogeneous syndrome distinct from daytime eating disorders. Sleep 1991; 14(5): 419–431.

39 | Diagnostic Tools for Parasomnias

Mark R. Pressman

Sleep Medicine Services, The Lankenau Hospital, Wynnewood; Paoli Hospital, Paoli; and Department of Medicine, Jefferson Medical College, Philadelphia, Pennsylvania, U.S.A.

INTRODUCTION

Primary parasomnias are reported to occur during both rapid eye movement (REM) and non–rapid eye movement (NREM) sleep. The most common examples of NREM parasomnias are the disorders of arousal—confusional arousal, sleep terrors, and sleepwalking (1) (see chaps. 36 and 38). The most common REM sleep parasomnia is REM sleep behavior disorder (see chaps. 36 and 38) (2,3). The diagnostic evaluation and tools differ between these two types of parasomnias. This chapter will discuss the differing approaches and tools available for their diagnosis.

HISTORY AND PHYSICAL EXAMINATION

Description of Behavior
The evaluation of both NREM and REM parasomnias should start with a detailed history and description of behaviors that occurred. This should include not just the recent behaviors that resulted in the patient's referral for diagnosis and treatment, but other behaviors in the past. Most often behaviors that resulted in injury to the patient and others or behaviors that were dangerous or potentially dangerous will result in a referral to a doctor. However, other behaviors that might have been thought of as amusing or unimportant may also be useful to the clinician. Family members, friends, and anyone else who has directly observed the patient "in the act" should attend the initial evaluation or provide written descriptions of observed behaviors. Additionally, any other evidence of the patient's behavior such as broken items, disarray in the kitchen, etc. should be documented.

Age
The patient's age when the undesirable behaviors began is an important piece of the clinical history. Disorders of arousal are most common in childhood with the frequency declining rapidly into the early teenage years. The overall frequency of disorders of arousal is up to 15% in childhood and 1% to 4% in adulthood (4–6). Disorders of arousal may appear for the first time in adults. However, unrecognized episodes may have occurred in childhood. Additionally, it is not uncommon for disorders of arousal to recur in adults with a history of childhood disorders of arousal after being symptom free for many years. It is relatively rare for adults with a complaint consistent with disorders of arousal not to have a history of some type of disorders of arousal in childhood.

On the other hand, REM behavior disorder rarely, if ever, occurs in childhood. It most often occurs in individual who are 50 years or older (3). However, disorders of arousal and REM behavior disorder may occur together in the same patient as part of an overlap disorder (7).

Sex
Both disorders of arousal and REM behavior disorder are more common in adult males than females. In REM behavior disorder, the male predominance is 80% to 90% (3). In children, disorders of arousal are slightly more common in females (8).

Family History
Disorders of arousal are reported to have a genetic basis and to run in families while REM behavior disorder is not reported to run in families (5). A history of disorders of arousal in first-degree relatives indicates a significantly higher likelihood of disorders of arousal in the patient under evaluation.

Personal History

As noted above, adult patients who also provide a childhood history of sleep-related behaviors are common. Approximately 25% of children who had frequent disorders of arousal will also experience disorders of arousal as adults (8). For REM behavior disorder, clinical histories are most likely to begin in middle age with episodes of sleep talking, minor motor behaviors, or leg movements.

Medical History

Disorders of arousal are generally not associated with any particular medical disorder. However, a history of recent medications may be of interest (see below). The occurrence of REM behavior disorder–related behaviors may be preceded by a history of many years including sleep talking, less severe complex behaviors, and limb movements in sleep as well as a variety of neurological symptoms. In older patients, a variety of neurological disorders may be present.

Sleep History

Time of Night

Disorders of arousal typically occur during periods of deep sleep that are most often found in the first two hours of the usual sleep period. However, disorders of arousals more rarely have been reported to occur during intermediate NREM stage N2 and later during the sleep period.

REM behavior disorder typically does not occur in the first two hours of the sleep period unless there is some reason for REM sleep to occur earlier than is expected. REM behavior disorder occurs more frequently in the second half of the sleep period during times when an increased quantity and percentage of REM sleep is likely to occur.

Memory

Patients with disorders of arousal most frequently have little or no memory for their behaviors. However, patients with sleep terrors may recall a particularly frightening image at the beginning of their episodes. However, this image differs from typical REM sleep–related dreams in that it lacks plot and actions. Frightening images may be of a house on fire or an attacker in the bedroom, but typically are described as static. REM behavior disorder patients most often can recall in detail the content of the dreams and what their role in the dream was. It is often possible to correlate observed behaviors to dream content.

Type of Behavior

Patients with disorders of arousal may perform a wide variety of complex motor behaviors including walking, talking, eating, sex, and driving. Sleepwalkers may leave their beds and bedrooms and navigate to other rooms of the house. On rare occasions sleepwalkers may actually leave the house. Sleepwalkers have a rudimentary awareness of their surroundings, and especially in areas they are familiar with may navigate successfully to other areas. Sleepwalkers are reported to move about with their eyes open. However, accidents and injuries are common as higher cognitive functions such as planning are absent.

Patients with REM behavior disorder rarely leave their bed and bedroom unless some action occurring during the dream causes them to throw themselves accidentally out the door of the bedroom. REM behavior disorder patients are not aware of their surroundings as they are within the ongoing environment of their "dream world." They are not able to navigate to other locations and are not aware of bed partners or others in the same room. Bed partners who are injured during REM behavior disorder episodes are most likely in the wrong place at the wrong time within arms reach of the dream enacting individual. During REM behavior disorder episodes, patients are reported to act out their dreams with their eyes closed.

Prior Sleep Deprivation

Adult patients with disorders of arousal report that their behaviors frequently follow periods of acute sleep deprivation. The frequent clinical reports of sleep deprivation have been empirically tested and confirmed in the sleep laboratory (9–11). REM behavior disorder does not follow prior sleep deprivation. However, REM sleep deprivation, typically by drugs, medication, and alcohol can result in rebound REM sleep when discontinued and in the acute form of REM behavior disorder (3).

Situational Stress

The presence of situational stresses is commonly present in addition to sleep deprivation prior to the occurrence of behaviors in disorders of arousal (12). There are no reports of stress involved in the occurrence of REM sleep–related behaviors.

Medications

A long list of medications has been reported to be associated with the sudden onset of NREM sleep–related behaviors. The majority of these medications are sedative/hypnotics, although many other central nervous system (CNS) depressants and other drug types have been implicated (13). Most presumed episodes of medication-induced NREM parasomnia occur with medications that are relatively short acting and following the first day or two of administration. Additionally, some cases have been reported closely following an increase in dosage.

Alcohol has been classically associated with the onset of disorders of arousal. However, recent reviews have noted that this theory is not based on empirical research, but appears to be incorrectly extrapolated from research on the effects of alcohol on deep sleep (14). No studies of the effect of alcohol on clinically diagnosed sleepwalkers have ever been conducted. Instead, this theory appears to be based on some early reports that alcohol may increase the quantity of deep sleep. An increase in deep sleep following sleep deprivation has been confirmed empirically in the sleep laboratory to increase complex behaviors in NREM sleep. However, a detailed examination of the alcohol and sleep literature has found that only 6 of 19 studies of alcohol use by social drinkers resulted in a small but significant increase in deep sleep while alcohol abuse almost always resulted in a significant decrease or absence of deep sleep. Thus, the classic wisdom that alcohol can induce sleepwalking rests on extremely weak scientific grounds.

The acute and chronic forms of REM behavior disorder have been reported to follow administration of or withdrawal from a variety of medications and substances. Sudden withdrawal from alcohol and meprobamate has been associated with significant increases in total REM sleep percentages and the appearance of tonic electromyographic (EMG) activity and dream enacting behaviors. Tricyclic antidepressants, monoamine oxidase inhibitors (MAOIs), and selective serotonin reuptake inhibitors (SSRIs), including the widely prescribed drugs venlafaxine and fluoxetine, have been reported to result in tonic EMG activity during REM sleep (15). Certain patients with diagnosed narcolepsy and Parkinsonism may also demonstrate tonic EMG activity during REM sleep.

SUBJECTIVE ASSESSMENT TOOLS

Disorders of arousal and REM behavior disorder have no specific findings on questionnaires or rating scales. However, psychological tests such as the Minnesota Multiphasic Personality Inventory (MMPI) may be useful to identify or rule out other disorders with a similar presentation. Several recent studies have reported that patients diagnosed with disorders of arousal do not have significant psychopathology indicating that psychological testing is not required as part of the primary evaluation (16). However, in forensic situation, these tests may be valuable in order to identify malingering individuals (13,17).

OBJECTIVE ASSESSMENT TOOLS

Polysomnography

Other than the occurrence of a complex behavior during a diagnostic sleep study, there are no valid and reliable diagnostic signs to support a diagnosis of confusional arousal, sleep terrors, or sleepwalking. Unfortunately, disorders of arousal are rarely manifested during a diagnostic polysomnography (PSG). It seems likely that sleeping in the sleep laboratory with all the accompanying changes in environment as well as the disturbance of numerous electrodes, sensors, and wires may disrupt the usual sleep patterns. Additionally, any factor that might prime or trigger disorders of arousal in the home environment such as prior sleep deprivation, stress, noise, etc. are not likely to be present during the sleep laboratory study.

There are no pathognomonic PSG features for disorders of arousals. This is a change from classically held beliefs that a number of findings on the PSG were consistent and even pathognomonic for disorders of arousals. These factors included the following observations.

High Quantity or Percentage of Naturally Occurring Deep Sleep

The high incidence of disorders of arousals in children compared to adults is often attributed to the higher percentage of deep sleep found in children compared to adults. This hypothesis is further supported by the effects of sleep deprivation. Generally, the end of sleep deprivation is followed by rebound deep sleep and a significantly elevated percentage of deep sleep. However, studies of sleepwalkers under normal conditions have not found deep sleep to be elevated. In fact, frequency analysis of deep sleep has found less slow wave activity (SWA) in sleepwalkers than in matched controls, and other studies have not found deep sleep to be elevated. Some researchers have suggested that the increased number of arousals in deep sleep is responsible for the reduction in the deep sleep percentages in these patients.

Frequent Arousals from Deep Sleep

The number of arousals from deep sleep has been frequently reported to be higher than in matched normal controls (18). However, there is significant variability in these findings and no clear cutoff value. Additionally, several recent studies have noted that arousals from deep sleep are common findings in patients with sleep diagnoses other than disorders of arousal (19–21). In particular, a high percentage of patients diagnosed with obstructive sleep apnea (OSA) and periodic leg movements in sleep (PLMS), and who had some scored deep sleep also have arousals from deep sleep. The presence of arousals in deep sleep in patients who do not carry the clinical diagnosis of sleepwalking or other disorders of arousals indicate a low specificity for this finding.

Hypersynchronous Delta Waves

Hypersynchronous delta waves (HSD) consist of two or more high amplitude delta frequency waves often preceding an arousal from deep sleep or an episode of complex behavior. As with arousals from deep sleep, HSD has also been noted to occur frequently in patients with OSA only (20). Additionally, HSD may not be present in patients with clinical histories of sleepwalking or even during PSG recording during which sleepwalking occurred (22,23).

Thus, arousals from deep sleep and HSD are associated with both low sensitivity and low specificity. As a result these classic finding are no longer considered typical or diagnostic of disorders of arousal. However, diagnostic PSG may assist in ruling out other disorders in the differential diagnosis or identifying potential triggers for disorders of arousal (13).

Several recent studies have identified sleep-disordered breathing as the proximal trigger of disorders of arousal in both children and adults (24–26). Successful treatment of the sleep-disordered breathing with continuous positive airway pressure (CPAP) or surgery is reported to significantly reduce or eliminate the occurrence of disorders of arousal. However, the presence of sleep-disordered breathing in a diagnostic polysomnography (DPSG) is not in and of itself evidence for the diagnosis of a disorder of arousal.

Of the 12 primary parasomnias described in the *International Classification of Sleep Disorders* only REM behavior disorder requires a positive finding during a PSG for the diagnosis (27). As opposed to patients with disorders of arousal, the PSG of patients with REM behavior disorder shows a highly typical if not pathognomonic pattern of phasic and tonic EMG activity during otherwise clear REM sleep. This may be associated with sudden arousals from sleep and movements of the arms, legs, torso, and head. Additionally, more complex behaviors may occur, including behaviors and movements that are related to the content of current dreams. Technical staff may be able to correlate the observed behavior with dream content by asking the patient to describe the dream in detail.

OTHER SCREENING OR ADJUNCTIVE TOOLS

Brain imaging may be indicated in REM behavior disorder if neurological disorders are present or suspected.

NEW DIAGNOSTIC TOOLS

The general failure to induce and capture episodes of disorders of arousal during a sleep study has resulted in several recent attempts to improve the chances of inducing an episode in the sleep laboratory.

Sleep Deprivation

Total sleep deprivation lasting 25 to 38 hours has been performed on clinically proven sleepwalkers and matched normal controls in a number of sleep laboratory–based studies (10,11,21,28). Total sleep deprivation of about 25 hours has been proven to significantly increase the number of complex behaviors in sleepwalkers while no increase in similar behaviors was noted in matched normal controls. However, administration of 38 hours of sleep deprivation was reported to decrease the number of complex behaviors in a group of clinically proven sleepwalkers. This suggests there may be the equivalent of a dose-response curve for the effects of sleep deprivation in provoking disorders of arousal with the likelihood of the occurrence of behaviors during sleep being lowest during normal sleep and extreme sleep deprivation states and highest with approximately one day of total sleep deprivation.

Use of this technique in clinical settings increases the chances of inducing and capturing an episode of a disorder of arousal in the sleep laboratory. However, it falls short of the requirements for a diagnostic test. This test appears to have 100% sensitivity in a well-selected and screened group of young adult sleepwalkers. Its specificity is also 100% in a similar well-selected and screened group of normal controls. However, the sensitivity and specificity of this technique in the typical group of mixed sleep disorder center patients with complicated presenting symptoms, medications, sleep schedules, and medical/psychological disorders are unknown. Additionally, it has recently been established in the sleep laboratory that the individual response to sleep deprivation is quite variable (29). Thus, it is possible that the duration of prior sleep deprivation required to induce sleepwalking or other behaviors may vary between individuals. Thus, negative finding may reflect some trait and not the absence of a disorder of arousal. This test's reliability and replicability also remain to be determined.

A variation on this method has paired sleep deprivation with audio stimulation (9). Forced arousals to provoke NREM parasomnias have been attempted in the past with mixed results. This study demonstrated that forced arousals alone are not as effective in inducing complex behaviors as a combination of the sleep deprivation described above and acoustic stimulation. As noted above, this technique will require further studies before it can be labeled as diagnostic for disorders of arousal.

Other techniques have been shown to have significant research interest and with further development may have diagnostic utility.

Brain Imaging

There have been several attempts to use sophisticated imaging techniques to capture NREM parasomnia episodes and describe its pathophysiology and other functional neurophysiology (30). Bassetti and colleagues were successful in capturing an episode of sleep terrors during a single photon emission computed tomography (SPECT) test of a single patient. They noted an activation of thalamocingulate pathways and persisting deactivation of other thalamocortical arousal systems that differs from that noted in normals.

Frequency Analysis

A number of researchers have subjected the sleep electroencephalogram (EEG) of clinically diagnosed sleepwalkers to EEG frequency analysis and correlation with arousals (18,31). All have reported essentially the same findings, a reduced quantity of SWA in the first sleep period associated with an increased number of arousals. They have suggested that this finding is characteristic of sleepwalkers, but note that this finding is not sufficient to stand alone in the diagnosis of a sleepwalker or to use in medicolegal settings. As with the sleep deprivation techniques discussed above, this technique's sensitivity, specificity, and reliability are unknown. Its use as a diagnostic test will await further studies.

Genetic Analysis
Specific DQB1 genes have been implicated in disorders of arousal and REM behavior disorder along with narcolepsy (5,8,12,32). However, these findings are not yet specific enough to allow for a genetic test for parasomnias.

Alcohol Induction
One technique to avoid has been proposed as useful for forensic purposes is Alcohol Induction. It has been suggested that alcohol might be useful to induce sleepwalking episodes in individuals who purportedly suffer from alcohol-induced sleepwalking (33,34). As noted below, there is no scientific evidence that alcohol primes or induces sleepwalking or any related disorder (14). Secondly, this method is completely unvalidated without any data on sensitivity, specificity, reliability, or reproducibility (14). It has never been tested with clinically diagnosed sleepwalkers or any other patient group making interpretation of any results impossible.

FORENSIC CONSIDERATIONS

Criminal behavior requires the ability to form an intent to commit the criminal act. An individual committing a criminal act without intent is said to be suffering from an automatism and cannot be found guilty of a crime. Disorders of arousal are characterized by complex motor behaviors but lack of conscious awareness of their actions. Someone who commits an otherwise criminal act during a sleepwalking episode can be found innocent as they should not have been able to form the required criminal intent. For this reason, sleepwalking defenses have been increasing in popularity in recent years (33,35–37). Often the defense attorneys attempting to make the case that their client was sleepwalking during commission of crime and is a bona fide sleepwalker will send him to the sleep laboratory to hopefully generate objective evidence for this condition and defense.

The use of sleep studies as part of a sleepwalking defense lacks a basis in sleep science for the following reasons.

1. Generally, forensic sleep studies are performed months or years after the date of the criminal act. This assumes that a study performed much later can retroactively prove that the defendant was in a sleepwalking state on the night of the criminal act. There is no scientific evidence to suggest that certain features in the brain of a defendant noted during the sleep study were present on the night of the criminal act. The sleep study is most likely to represent only the defendant's current sleep patterns and habits (13).
2. It is impossible to recreate these circumstances present on the night of the criminal act in the sleep laboratory. Indeed, most major sleepwalking episodes appear to be a "perfect storm" of (*i*) genetic predisposition, (*ii*) priming factors such as sleep deprivation and/or situation stress, (*iii*) triggering factors, and (*iv*) close proximity or contact with the victim. None of these factors other than the hypothetical genetic predisposition can be present in the sleep laboratory.
3. As noted above there are no "objective" signs of sleepwalking or other disorders of arousals to be found in the forensic sleep evaluation (19–21). Further, these signs may not be present even in patients who are clinically diagnosed as sleepwalkers. Thus, sleep studies lack both statistical sensitivity and specificity and are invalid and unreliable measures for the diagnosis of sleepwalking.
4. With this said, sleep studies can also not be used to prove that a defendant is not a sleepwalker. They simply have no diagnostic value.

CONCLUSIONS

Disorders of arousal remains primarily a diagnosis based on clinical history. However, these disorders can be easily distinguished from REM behavior disorder using the techniques described above.

REFERENCES

1. Broughton RJ. Sleep disorders: disorders of arousal? Enuresis, somnambulism, and nightmares occur in confusional states of arousal, not in "dreaming sleep". Science 1968; 159(819):1070–1078.
2. Schenck CH, Bundlie SR, Ettinger MG, et al. Chronic behavioral disorders of human REM sleep: a new category of parasomnia. Sleep 1986; 9(2):293–308.
3. Mahowald MW, Schenck CS. REM sleep parasomnias. In: Kryger MH, Roth T, Dement WC, eds. Principles and Practice of Sleep Medicine. 4th ed. Philadelphia: Elsevier Saunders, 2005:897–916.
4. Wills L, Garcia J. Parasomnias: epidemiology and management. CNS Drugs 2002; 16(12):803–810.
5. Hublin C, Kaprio J. Genetic aspects and genetic epidemiology of parasomnias. Sleep Med Rev 2003; 7(5): 413–421.
6. Ohayon MM, Guilleminault C, Priest RG. Night terrors, sleepwalking, and confusional arousals in the general population: their frequency and relationship to other sleep and mental disorders. J Clin Psychiatry 1999; 60(4):268–276.
7. Schenck CH, Boyd JL, Mahowald MW. A parasomnia overlap disorder involving sleepwalking, sleep terrors, and REM sleep behavior disorder in 33 polysomnographically confirmed cases. Sleep 1997; 20 (11):972–281.
8. Hublin C, Kaprio J, Partinen M, et al. Prevalence and genetics of sleepwalking: a population-based twin study. Neurology 1997; 48(1):177–181.
9. Pilon M, Montplaisir J, Zadra A. Precipitating factors of somnambulism: impact of sleep deprivation and forced arousals. Neurology 2008; 70:2284–2290.
10. Pilon M, Zadra A, Adam B, et al. 25 hours of sleep deprivation increases the frequency and complexity of somnambulistic episodes in adult sleepwalkers. Sleep 2005; 28:A257.
11. Joncas S, Zadra A, Paquet J, et al. The value of sleep deprivation as a diagnostic tool in adult sleepwalkers. Neurology 2002; 58(6):936–940.
12. Lecendreux M, Bassetti C, Dauvilliers Y, et al. HLA and genetic susceptibility to sleepwalking. Mol Psychiatry 2003; 8(1):114–117.
13. Pressman MR. Factors that predispose, prime and precipitate NREM parasomnias in adults: clinical and forensic implications. Sleep Med Rev 2007; 11(1):5–30.
14. Pressman MR, Mahowald MW, Schenck CS, et al. Alcohol induced sleepwalking or confusional arousals as a defense to criminal behavior: review of scientific evidence, methods and forensic considerations. J Sleep Res 2007; 16:1–15.
15. Mahowald MW, Schenck CH. NREM sleep parasomnias. Neurol Clin 1996; 14(4):675–696.
16. Schenck CH, Milner DM, Hurwitz TD, et al. A polysomnographic and clinical report on sleep-related injury in 100 adult patients. Am J Psychiatry 1989; 146(9):1166–1173.
17. Schenck CH, Mahowald MW. On the reported association of psychopathology with sleep terrors in adults [comment]. Sleep 2000; 23(4):448–449.
18. Gaudreau H, Joncas S, Zadra A, et al. Dynamics of slow-wave activity during the NREM sleep of sleepwalkers and control subjects. Sleep 2000; 23(6):755–760.
19. Brozman B, Foldvary NR, Dinner D, et al. The value of the unexplained polysomnographic arousals from slow-wave sleep in predicting sleepwalking and sleep terrors in a sleep laboratory patient population. Sleep 2003; 26:A325.
20. Pressman MR. Hypersynchronous delta sleep EEG activity and sudden arousals from slow-wave sleep in adults without a history of parasomnias: clinical and forensic implications. Sleep 2004; 27(4): 706–710.
21. Pilon M, Zadra A, Joncas S, et al. Hypersynchronous delta waves and somnambulism: brain topography and effect of sleep deprivation [see comment]. Sleep 2006; 29(1):77–84.
22. Kavey NB, Whyte J, Resor SR Jr., et al. Somnambulism in adults. Neurology 1990; 40(5):749–752.
23. Schenck CH, Pareja JA, Patterson AL, et al. Analysis of polysomnographic events surrounding 252 slow-wave sleep arousals in thirty-eight adults with injurious sleepwalking and sleep terrors. J Clin Neurophysiol 1998; 15(2):159–166.
24. Guilleminault C, Palombini L, Pelayo R, et al. Sleepwalking and sleep terrors in prepubertal children: what triggers them? Pediatrics 2003; 111(1):e17–e25.
25. Guilleminault C, Kirisoglu C, Bao G, et al. Adult chronic sleepwalking and its treatment based on polysomnography. Brain 2005; 128(pt 5):1062–1069.

26. Espa F, Dauvilliers Y, Ondze B, et al. Arousal reactions in sleepwalking and night terrors in adults: the role of respiratory events. Sleep 2002; 25(8):871–875.

27. American Academy of Sleep Medicine. ICSD-2—International Classification of Sleep Disorders: Diagnostic and Coding Manual. 2nd ed. Westchester, IL: American Academy of Sleep Medicine, 2005.

28. Mayer G, Neissner V, Schwarzmayr P, et al. [Sleep deprivation in somnambulism. Effect of arousal, deep sleep and sleep stage changes]. Nervenarzt 1998; 69(6):495–501.

29. Van Dongen HPA, Baynard MD, Maislin G, et al. Systematic interindividual differences in neurobehavioral impairment from sleep loss: evidence of trait-like differential vulnerability. Sleep 2004; 27(3):423–433.

30. Bassetti C, Vella S, Donati F, et al. SPECT during sleepwalking. Lancet 2000; 356(9228):484–485.

31. Guilleminault C, Poyares D, Aftab FA, et al. Sleep and wakefulness in somnambulism: a spectral analysis study. J Psychosom Res 2001; 51(2):411–416.

32. Hublin C, Kaprio J, Partinen M, et al. Parasomnias: co-occurrence and genetics. Psychiatr Genet 2001; 11(2):65–70.

33. R. v. Lowe, 2003.

34. R. v. Calting, 2005.

35. Arizona v. Scott Falater, 1999.

36. R. v. James Bilton, 2005.

37. R. v. Parks [1992] 2 S.C.C.R. 871; 95 D.L.R.(4th) 27.

40 | Diagnostic Algorithm for Parasomnias

Michael H. Silber

Center for Sleep Medicine, Mayo Clinic College of Medicine, Rochester, Minnesota, U.S.A.

INTRODUCTION

Parasomnias are undesirable events or experiences occurring at sleep onset, during sleep, or after partial arousals from sleep. *The International Classification of Sleep Disorders*, second edition, classifies parasomnias into disorders of arousal [from non–rapid eye movement (NREM) sleep] such as sleepwalking; parasomnias usually associated with rapid eye movement (REM) sleep such as REM sleep behavior disorder; and other parasomnias, such as sleep-related eating disorder (SRED) (1). Simpler movements during sleep that appear nonpurposeful, such as periodic limb movements, bruxism, and rhythmic movement disorder are classified separately under sleep-related movement disorders (see chaps. 43–49). Some abnormal behaviors at night are not generally classified under the parasomnias but need to be considered in their differential diagnosis. These include nocturnal seizures, abnormal behavior associated with arousals from sleep-disordered breathing, and nocturnal wanderings by patients with dementia. While these various groupings are helpful in classifying the disorders and understanding their pathogenesis, they are not particularly useful for the clinician faced with the problem of a patient with unusual behavior or experiences at night. This chapter will propose practical approaches for diagnosing specific parasomnias and distinguishing them from other disorders that mimic them. The clinical vignettes that follow are examples of the types of diagnostic problems to which such approaches can be applied.

CLINICAL VIGNETTES

Patient 1

A seven-year-old girl presented with a three-year history of nocturnal behavior characterized by waking about one hour after sleep onset, screaming unintelligibly, and flailing her arms while sitting up in bed. The events lasted about one to two minutes and were followed by a period of unresponsiveness to her mother. She would then return to sleep. At three years of age, she had experienced a single generalized tonic-clonic seizure associated with a high fever from otitis media. A first cousin was said to have a seizure disorder. Neurological examination was normal. An electroencephalogram (EEG) awake and asleep was normal. A magnetic resonance imaging (MRI) scan of the head was normal. Are the events nocturnal seizures or sleep terrors?

Patient 2

A 65-year-old man presented with a one-year history of nocturnal events characterized by shouting, flailing of the arms, and kicking, usually occurring after 2 a.m. He had no recollection of the events in the morning. He snored heavily, and his wife noticed instances when he seemed not to be breathing during sleep. He was overweight. Neurological examination was normal apart from some difficulty with short-term memory on mental status testing. Are the events due to REM sleep behavior disorder (RBD) or arousals associated with obstructive sleep apnea (OSA)?

KEY STEPS IN THE DIAGNOSIS OF PARASOMNIAS

Step 1: A Complete History

The most important step in the diagnosis of the parasomnias is a careful history from the patient and, more importantly, collateral history from a bed partner, parent, or caregiver (Table 1). Both the background history and a detailed description of events are essential. In some

Table 1 Important Features in the History of a Patient with a Suspected Parasomnia

Background history
  Age of onset
  Gender
  Family history
  Medications and substance use
  Medical, neurological, or psychiatric disorders
Description of events
  Frequency
  Time of night
  Duration
  Sensory and experiential symptoms
  Motor behaviors
  Vocalization
  Autonomic features
  Injuries and degree of aggression
  Associated snoring or apneas
  Location of behaviors (in or out of bed)
  Stereotyped nature of behaviors
  Patient responsiveness during and after the event
  Patient recall

circumstances, such as classic sleepwalking or sleep terrors in children, the diagnosis becomes obvious, whereas in other situations the history may give important clues to the diagnosis but may not be definitive.

The background history may be extremely useful. Disorders of arousal, rhythmic movement disorders, and many seizure disorders commence in childhood, while RBD usually commences after the age of 50 (2). Ninety percent of patients with RBD are men, while SRED, dissociative disorder, and complex nocturnal visual hallucinations are more common in women (2–4). A family history of a sibling or parent with sleepwalking or sleep terrors is commonly elicited in patients with disorders of arousal. Sleepwalking and SRED can occur with the use of short-acting hypnotics (5,6) and sleepwalking is also associated with use of multiple psychotropic agents including neuroleptics and lithium (7). Most antidepressants can induce RBD (8), while β-blockers can cause nightmares and complex nocturnal visual hallucinations (4). RBD is associated with Parkinson's disease, dementia with Lewy bodies and multiple system atrophy (9), while nocturnal confusional wanderings can occur with any cause of dementia, including Alzheimer's disease (10). Patients with daytime panic disorder or dissociative disorder may also manifest similar symptoms at night (1).

Descriptions of the actual event are usually obtained from a bed partner or parent who may often be too sleepy to observe accurately. Thus collateral histories may range from detailed recollections sufficient to reach a definitive diagnosis to vague recollections of nonspecific movements. Some events, such as nocturnal frontal lobe seizures, may occur at least nightly and sometimes several times a night (11). Disorders of arousal tend to occur earlier in the night when slow wave sleep predominates, while RBD occurs later during periods of more intense REM sleep. Episodes of RBD last minutes, while nocturnal wanderings in patients with dementia can last hours. Behaviors associated with RBD are usually described by an observer as the patient acting out dreams while clearly asleep; while in nocturnal wanderings associated with dementia, the patient may appear to be awake but unresponsive or confused. A description of the motor activity may in some cases help differentiate between seizures, RBD, and sleep terrors.

Sensory and experiential symptoms may range from vivid frightening dreams in nightmares, through vague images of danger in some cases of sleep terrors, to complex nocturnal hallucinations during definite wakefulness after arousal. Vocalization of various types may be the predominant or an accompanying feature of some disorders, such a sleep terrors, RBD, and sleep-related groaning (catathrenia) (12,13). Heightened autonomic activity usually accompanies sleep terrors and nocturnal panic attacks. Injuries to the patient and bed partner are common in RBD and may occur in disorders of arousal (14). Nocturnal seizures usually show consistent, stereotypical behavior, while RBD activity varies from episode to episode. As discussed below, it is useful to distinguish activities occurring predominately in bed from those that are associated with ambulation. Arousals from sleep apnea or snoring may precipitate sleepwalking or cause motor activity that mimics the events of RBD (15). Patients are generally unresponsive during episodes of sleep terrors with little later recall in contrast to nocturnal panic attacks. While most nocturnal seizures are associated with lack of response to the environment or later recollection, nocturnal frontal lobe seizures are sometimes exceptions (11). Nightmares and complex nocturnal hallucinations are recalled, while episodes of RBD are not. SRED occurs with partial or complete amnesia (3), while nocturnal eating syndrome consists of night eating in full consciousness (16).

Step 2: Physical Examination

The physical examination is normal in most patients with parasomnias. However, evidence for Parkinsonism or dysautonomia may suggest that RBD is a likely cause for the nocturnal disturbances (17) and a finding of cognitive impairment may lead one to consider either RBD or nocturnal wanderings in dementia. Focal neurological signs might suggest the presence of a structural brain lesion causing seizures. Physical findings on examination of the head and neck, such as a narrowed oropharyngeal diameter or an overbite, might predict the presence of OSA.

Step 3: Neurological Investigations

If a seizure disorder is suspected, a routine wake and sleep EEG should be performed to search for interictal or ictal discharges. An MRI scan of the head is indicated if a structural lesion is suspected, but is not routinely needed.

Step 4: Video-EEG Polysomnography

Polysomnography is indicated for suspected parasomnias when the diagnosis is not clear after the clinical evaluation or when the behavior is violent or potentially injurious to the patient or others (18). Examples of an unclear diagnosis are difficulty differentiating a seizure disorder from a disorder of arousal in a child, or difficulty distinguishing RBD from arousals associated with OSA in an older adult. Depending on the available expertise and facilities, a decision should be made whether it is most appropriate to study the patient in a sleep laboratory or an epilepsy monitoring unit. In general, if a seizure disorder is considered more likely than a parasomnia, then an initial evaluation in an epilepsy monitoring unit is preferable, and vice versa. In complex cases, with sometimes more than one diagnosis, monitoring in both environments may be necessary. It is essential that parasomnia studies be performed in sleep laboratories with time synchronized video recordings available to record actual behaviors. Most parasomnia studies also require the addition of 16 extra EEG derivations beyond the routine sleep montage and at least one additional arm electromyogram (EMG) derivation. Interpreters should have sufficient knowledge and experience in EEG interpretation to be able to detect epileptiform discharges. Even if the technologist and the patient report no events during the night, it is essential to review the entire study, as findings such as REM sleep without atonia, interictal spikes, or confusional arousals may still be present.

IMPORTANT DIAGNOSTIC FEATURES AND CRITERIA TO DISTINGUISH DISORDER TYPES

Predominantly Sensory or Experiential Phenomena (Table 2)

Nightmares are vivid, frightening, emotionally-charged dreams from which patients wake. They are associated with excellent recall, at least initially, and patients are usually aware they have been dreaming. In contrast to RBD, patients usually remain still in bed, despite dreaming of locomotion. Hypnagogic hallucinations are dreamlike visual and sometimes auditory phenomena occurring at or around sleep onset (1). Often patients are unsure whether they are awake or asleep. Complex nocturnal hallucinations are vivid, often distorted, images of people or animals occurring after waking from sleep during the night (4). They disappear when the room light is switched on. They do not usually follow dreaming and are associated with full recall. Simple partial seizures can be characterized by visual hallucinations, which are usually brief and less complex (19). Exploding head syndrome consists of a sudden, loud,

Table 2 Predominantly Sensory or Experiential Phenomena

Nightmare disorder
Sleep-related hallucinations
  Hypnagogic hallucinations
  Complex nocturnal hallucinations
Exploding head syndrome
Simple partial seizures

Table 3 Behaviors Characterized Predominantly by Vocalization

Sleep talking
REM sleep behavior disorder
Confusional arousals
Sleep-related groaning (catathrenia)

Table 4 Motor Behaviors Occurring Predominantly in Bed

REM sleep behavior disorder
Confusional arousals
Sleep terrors
Nocturnal panic attacks
Arousals associated with obstructive sleep apnea
Dissociative disorder
Sleep starts
Rhythmic movement disorder
Periodic limb movements of sleep
Nocturnal seizures

usually painless, hallucinatory noise or sense of a violent explosion in the head at sleep onset (20). With the exception of seizures, these phenomena can usually be diagnosed by history alone.

Behaviors Characterized Predominantly by Vocalization (Table 3)

In some patients, the parasomnia may be predominantly characterized by vocalizations. If intelligible or unintelligible speech is accompanied by flailing of the arms and kicking of the legs, RBD is likely. When mumbled speech is accompanied by the patient briefly sitting up in bed, confusional arousals should be considered. Talking during sleep without other motor manifestations is common and usually a benign phenomenon. Sudden screaming is most often a manifestation of sleep terrors, especially if accompanied by autonomic manifestations such as tachycardia, tachypnea, and diaphoresis (1). However, complex partial seizures may sometimes produce similar manifestations and epilepsy should be especially considered if the episodes are stereotyped and associated with orofacial automatisms or reproducible posturing of the limbs (11). Prolonged expiratory nocturnal groaning may indicate catathrenia but should be differentiated from inspiratory stridor. Video-EEG polysomnography may be needed to differentiate these conditions if the diagnosis is not clinically obvious.

Motor Behaviors Occurring Predominantly in Bed (Table 4)

Many parasomnias are characterized by motor activity of the trunk or limbs that occurs predominantly in bed rather than while ambulating. While this distinction is not a rigid one, it provides a useful framework for differential diagnosis. Confusional arousals, sleep terrors, nocturnal panic attacks, and arousals associated with OSA all occur after sudden, partial, or complete arousal from sleep. Arousal disorders (confusional arousals and sleep terrors) and arousals from OSA are associated with reduced responsiveness and little later recall. In contrast, nocturnal panic attacks occur during full wakefulness with extreme fear and retained memory of the events. A history or observation of heavy snoring, apneas, and a snort at the time of arousal suggests that the behavior is due to upper airway obstruction. RBD behaviors

Table 5 Motor Behaviors Occurring Predominantly Outside the Bed

Sleepwalking
Nocturnal confusional wanderings
Dissociative disorder
Nocturnal seizures
Sleep-related eating disorder
Night eating syndrome

Table 6 Behaviors Characterized Predominantly by Episodes of Paralysis

Recurrent isolated sleep paralysis
Sleep paralysis associated with narcolepsy
Compression neuropathies
Hypokalemic periodic paralysis
Dissociative disorder

are typically described as arm flailing or punching and leg kicking, often but not always, associated with vocalization. Sleep starts are sudden jerks of the trunk or limbs at sleep onset (1). Periodic limb movements are most often described as repetitive, quasi-rhythmic leg jerks. Rhythmic movement disorder may manifest as head banging, body rocking, or other large amplitude rhythmic jerks of head, limbs, or trunk. Nocturnal seizures have different manifestations depending on type and localization, but the stereotyped nature of the events is a characteristic feature. Generalized tonic-clonic seizures are characterized by a phase of stiffness of the body followed by repetitive generalized jerks. Tongue biting and urination are common and the seizure is followed by obstructive breathing, a period of loss of consciousness, and amnesia. Nocturnal frontal lobe seizures may manifest as episodes of stereotyped dystonic posturing, often unaccompanied by scalp EEG seizure discharges (11). Dissociative phenomena (pseudoseizures) may be difficult to distinguish from seizures by history alone and generally need video observation by an experienced neurologist for a definitive diagnosis. They often manifest as repetitive bizarre pelvic thrusting movements and occur during full EEG wakefulness, commencing 15 to 60 seconds after arousal (21). A history of prior sexual abuse is common (22).

Motor Behaviors Occurring Predominantly Outside the Bed (Table 5)
The most frequent abnormal behavior occurring out of bed is sleepwalking. Most often this takes the form of quiet walking, although patients may bump into obstacles and are unresponsive to stimuli. Occasionally sleepwalkers may behave violently, leaping out of bed, running and even throwing themselves through windows (14). In contrast, patients with RBD may sometimes jump or fall out of bed, but far less commonly walk. SRED is probably a variant of sleepwalking in which patients eat in their sleep, consuming often strange combinations of food (3). This is associated with complete or partial amnesia, which differentiates the condition from night eating syndrome in which patients consume a high proportion of their daily calories at night but with full awareness and recollection (16). The nocturnal wanderings of confused patients with dementia are often recognizable by their clinical setting, prolonged duration (often an hour or more), the partial responsiveness of patients to questions, and the overall impression that they are awake and confused rather than walking while asleep. In the borderlands of epilepsy and parasomnias lies the condition of episodic nocturnal wanderings which probably represent a form of nocturnal frontal lobe epilepsy (23). Dissociative disorders can take place out of bed and may be hard to diagnose with certainty (21). Video-EEG studies are needed to assist in these diagnoses.

Behaviors Characterized Predominantly by Episodes of Paralysis (Table 6)
Episodes of generalized paralysis at sleep onset or after waking are usually due to sleep paralysis. Sometimes associated with hypnagogic or hypnopompic hallucinations, they may be very frightening (1). They can often be aborted by an observer touching the patient. They are

usually isolated benign phenomena unless accompanied by daytime sleepiness or cataplexy, in which case narcolepsy should be considered. They should not be confused with transient compression neuropathies that result in weakness, numbness, and tingling of a single limb. Episodes of hypokalemic periodic paralysis can occur at rest and after waking from sleep, but usually last hours, are associated with carbohydrate consumption and are generally diagnosable by the presence of hypokalemia. Dissociative disorder can also manifest by paralysis at night but the clinical features usually differ sufficiently from those of organic conditions to make diagnosis relatively easy, especially if the spell is observed. Sleep studies are rarely needed to differentiate these conditions.

DIFFERENTIAL DIAGNOSIS

Only certain undesirable nocturnal events are classified as parasomnias, although other disorders may closely resemble them. Conditions which may mimic parasomnias include nocturnal seizure disorders, arousals from sleep-disordered breathing, nocturnal movement disorders such as periodic limb movements of sleep and rhythmic movement disorder, nocturnal wanderings of confused patients with dementia, dissociative disorders, malingering, night eating syndrome, hypokalemic periodic paralysis, and transient compression neuropathies. For the sake of clarity, the features that distinguish these disorders from parasomnias are discussed in the section "Important Diagnostic Features and Criteria to Distinguish Disorder Types."

Occasionally, toxic-metabolic encephalopathies, cerebral infections, and structural brain lesions may result in behaviors resembling parasomnias, but can usually be distinguished by the clinical setting. Substance abuse and psychoses, including schizophrenia, may need to be considered but manifestations while awake generally predominate. When considered clinically relevant, toxicology screens, blood tests for metabolic dysfunction, MRI scans of the head, EEG, nerve conduction studies and electromyography, and cerebrospinal fluid analysis may be needed. A psychiatric consultation may sometimes be helpful.

SUMMARY

Important steps in the diagnosis of the parasomnias include a complete history (including a collateral history from a bed partner, parent, or caregiver); physical examination (especially a neurologic assessment and upper airway evaluation); neurological investigations if a seizure disorder is suspected (e.g., EEG, MRI); and EEG-video polysomnography (for an unclear diagnosis or if the behavior is violent or potentially injurious to the patient or others). A clinical classification system for grouping parasomnias on the basis of similar symptoms and signs is proposed; the five major groups are predominantly sensory or experiential phenomena, behaviors characterized predominantly by vocalization, motor behaviors occurring predominantly in bed, motor behaviors occurring predominantly outside the bed, and behaviors characterized predominantly by episodes of paralysis. Further testing may occasionally be needed to screen for other conditions and disorders in the differential diagnosis of parasomnias, including imaging procedures, toxicology screens, or psychiatric evaluation.

REFERENCES

1. American Academy of Sleep Medicine. International Classification of Sleep Disorders. 2nd ed. Diagnostic and Coding Manual. Westchester, Illinois: American Academy of Sleep Medicine, 2005.
2. Olson EJ, Boeve BF, Silber MH. Rapid eye movement sleep behavior disorder: demographic, clinical and laboratory findings in 93 cases. Brain 2000; 123:331–339.
3. Schenck CH, Hurwitz TD, O'Connor KA, et al. Additional categories of sleep-related eating disorders and the current status of treatment. Sleep 1993; 16:457–466.
4. Silber MH, Hansen MR, Girish M. Complex nocturnal visual hallucinations. Sleep Med 2005; 6:363–366.
5. Mendelson WB. Sleepwalking associated with zolpidem. J Clin Psychopharmacol 1994; 14:150.
6. Morgenthaler TI, Silber MH. Amnestic sleep related eating disorder associated with zolpidem. Sleep Med 2002; 3:323–328.

7. Mahowald MW, Cramer-Bornemann MA. NREM sleep-arousal parasomnias. In: Kryger MH, Roth T, Dement WC, eds. Principles and Practice of Sleep Medicine. 4th ed. Philadelphia: Elsevier Saunders, 2005:889–896.

8. Winkelman JW, James L. Serotonergic antidepressants are associated with REM sleep without atonia. Sleep 2004; 27:317–321.

9. Boeve B, Silber MH, Parisi JE, et al. Synucleinopathy pathology and REM sleep behavior disorder plus dementia or parkinsonism. Neurology 2003; 61:40–45.

10. Petit D, Montplaisir J, Boeve BF. Alzheimer's disease and other dementias. In: Kryger MH, Roth T, Dement WC, eds. Principles and Practice of Sleep Medicine. 4th ed. Philadelphia: Elsevier Saunders, 2005:853–862.

11. Provini F, Plazzi G, Tinuper P, et al. Nocturnal frontal lobe epilepsy, a clinical and polygraphic review of 100 consecutive cases. Brain 1999; 122:1017–1031.

12. Vertrugno R, Provini F, Plazzi G, et al. Catathrenia (nocturnal groaning): a new type of parasomnia. Neurology 2001; 56:681–683.

13. Pevernagie DA, Boon PA, Mariman AN, et al. Vocalization during episodes of prolonged expiration: a parasomnia related to REM sleep. Sleep Med 2001; 2:19–30.

14. Schenck CH, Milner DM, Hurwitz TD, et al. A polysomnographic and clinical report on sleep-related injury in 100 adult patients. Am J Psychiatry 1989; 146:1166–1173.

15. Iranzo A, Santamaria J. Severe obstructive sleep apnea/hyponea mimicking REM sleep bahavior disorder. Sleep 2005; 28:203–206.

16. Birketvedt GS, Florholmen J, Sundsfjord J, et al. Behavioral and neuroendocrine characteristics of the night-eating syndrome. JAMA 1999; 282:657–663.

17. Boeve BF, Silber MH, Ferman TJ, et al. REM sleep behavior disorder and degenerative dementia: an association likely reflecting Lewy body disease. Neurology 1998; 51:363–370.

18. Kushida CA, Littner MR, Morgentaler T, et al. Practice parameters for the indications for polysomnography and related procedures: an update for 2005. Sleep 2005; 28:499–521.

19. Manford M, Andermann F. Complex visual hallucinations. Clinical and neurobiological insights. Brain 1998; 121:1819–1840.

20. Pierce JMS. Clinical features of the exploding head syndrome. J Neurol Neurosurg Psychiatr 1989; 52:907–910.

21. Schenck CH, Milner DM, Hurwitz TD, et al. Dissociative disorders presenting as somnambulism: video and clinical documentation (8 cases). Dissociation 1989; 2:194–204.

22. Shen W, Bowman ES, Markand ON. Presenting the diagnosis of pseudoseizure. Neurology 1990; 40:756–759.

23. Plazzi G, Tinuper P, Montagna P et al. Epileptic nocturnal wanderings. Sleep 1995; 18:749–756.

41 | Treatment of Parasomnias

J. F. Pagel

Department of Family Practice, University of Colorado School of Medicine, Southern Colorado Residency Program, Pueblo; Sleep Disorders Center of Southern Colorado, Pueblo; and Sleepworks Sleep Laboratory, Colorado Springs, Colorado, U.S.A.

INTRODUCTION

Parasomnias are defined as undesirable physical events or experiences that occur during entry into sleep, within sleep, or during arousals from sleep. Parasomnias encompass a diverse group of diagnoses involving sleep-related movements, autonomic motor system functioning, behaviors, perceptions, emotions, and dreaming. These sleep-related behaviors are experiences over which the patient has no conscious deliberate control. Parasomnias are classified based on sleep stage of origin into the disorders of arousal occurring out of deep sleep [stage N3, formerly non–rapid eye movement sleep (NREM) stages 3 and 4], those associated with rapid eye movement (REM) sleep, and a grouping including less well-defined diagnoses with unclear sleep stage association (Table 1). In the most recent diagnostic classification schemata, *International Classification of Sleep Disorders*, second edition (*ICSD-2*), the sleep-related movement disorders that had been classified as parasomnias were moved into their own diagnostic category (1).

Parasomnias become clinical diagnoses when associated with sleep disruption, nocturnal injuries, waking psychosocial effects, and adverse health effects. In the elderly, parasomnias are among the sleep disorders that have been associated with an increase risk of falls (2). If a parasomnia is not associated with adverse affects on waking function or nocturnal injury, no treatment of the parasomnia may be required beyond diagnosis and reassurance. In general, treatment of a parasomnia should be based on diminishing or eliminating the adverse waking effects of the diagnosis (Table 2).

PARASOMNIA ASSOCIATIONS WITH UNDERLYING DISEASE

Parasomnia complaints can develop as a symptom of an underlying medical or sleep disorder. REM sleep behavior disorder (RBD), nightmare disorder, sleep-related groaning (catathrenia), night terrors, enuresis, sleep-related eating disorder (SRED), and confusional arousals can occur or increase in frequency as obstructive sleep apnea (OSA) becomes symptomatic. In one study, sleep-disordered breathing was found in greater than 50% of children with parasomnia diagnoses, primarily somnambulism and sleep terrors (3). The same study suggested a possible association of parasomnia complaints with periodic limb movement disorder (PLMD). Treatment of underlying OSA will often lead to a decrease or elimination of the parasomnia complaint (4,5). Sleep paralysis and hypnagogic hallucinations occur in individuals with narcolepsy. RBD is associated with PLMD and neurological disorders, of which the Parkinsonian disorders are the most common. Underlying neurological abnormalities such as lacunar infarcts and other central nervous system (CNS) pathology are associated with RBD and parasomnia overlap disorder (6,7). The treatment of the parasomnia in many cases is treatment of the underlying or precipitating disorder, particularly in individuals presenting with OSA with the complaint of a parasomnia.

Parasomnia complaints can also develop as a symptom of an underlying psychiatric disorder. The sleep-related dissociative disorders occur only in individuals meeting *Diagnostic and Statistical Manual of Mental Disorders, Fourth Edition* (*DSM-IV*) criteria for those diagnoses 'while awake' including dissociative identity disorder (formerly called multiple personality disorder) and dissociative fugue (8). It is important clinically to establish whether nightmares are associated with posttraumatic stress disorder (PTSD) or acute stress disorder (ASD) because the evaluation, course, complications, and treatment differ significantly for these groups. Individuals with PTSD are at risk for mood disorder/depression, marital conflict/divorce, loss of job, self-destructive and impulsive behavior, dissociative symptoms, somatic

Table 1   Parasomnias

Disorders of arousal (from NREM sleep)
  1. Confusional arousal
  2. Sleepwalking
  3. Sleep terrors
Parasomnias usually associated with REM sleep
  1. REM sleep behavioral disorder
  2. Recurrent isolated sleep paralysis
  3. Nightmare disorder
Other parasomnias
  1. Sleep-related dissociative disorders
  2. Sleep enuresis
  3. Sleep-related groaning
  4. Exploding head syndrome
  5. Sleep-related hallucinations
  6. Sleep-related eating disorder
  7. Parasomnias unspecified
  8. Parasomnias due to drug or substance
  9. Parasomnias due to medical condition

Source: From Ref. 1.

Table 2   Treatment of Parasomnias: General Approaches

Treatment of underlying disease
  1. Sleep associated diagnoses
  2. Medical diagnoses
  3. Psychiatric illness
  4. Eliminating precipitating medications
Environmental protection and reassurance
Sleep hygiene
Specific parasomnia treatments
  1. Behavioral treatments
  2. Medications
    a. Sleep state manipulation
    b. Parasomnia-specific medications

complaints, hostility, social withdrawal, substance abuse and nightmares after withdrawal from substance abuse, survivor guilt, and despair or hopelessness. In adults, sleep terrors occur in higher frequency in individuals with bipolar disorder, nonpsychotic depressive disorders, and anxiety disorders. Parasomnia complaints may increase during periods of stress or decompensation in patients with psychiatric disease.

NONPHARMACOLOGICAL TREATMENT

Environmental Protection and Reassurance
Parental and child reassurance is often the treatment for parasomnias in which there are minimal effects on waking behavior and no history of nocturnal injury. The arousal disorders of childhood decline in frequency as the child enters adolescence. The overall prevalence of enuresis decreases at a rate of 15% until the adult incidence of 1% is reached (9,10). For many children, reassurance can help alleviate nightmares (even those attributed to PTSD). Adults with nightmares respond positively to the knowledge that non-trauma-associated nightmares do not indicate abuse or psychiatric illness and are often associated with creative personality characteristics.

Safety precautions in the home useful in protecting patients with somnambulism can include baby gates across stairs, window and door locks, and electric eyes at the bedroom door that will sound an alarm. Individuals with parasomnias should be protected from the capability of getting outside the house unobserved while sleepwalking. Sleeping in bunk beds should be avoided. The use of ground floor bedrooms should be considered. In RBD, basic measures to create a safe bedroom environment are of utmost importance. These include removal of all furniture from the bedside and sharp objects from the bedroom floor, padding or mattresses on the floor next to the bed, pillow barriers to protect bed partners, and even creative self-containment devices. The treatment of SRED should include the deliberate placement of food to avoid indiscriminate wandering.

Sleep Hygiene

Sleep deprivation, psychological distress, and changes in sleep schedule are known to increase the chances that parasomnia events will occur. Irregular schedules and sleep deprivation can trigger arousal disorder events. Parasomnias are likely to increase during vacations in which sleep environments change and episodic sleep deprivation is likely to occur. With changes in normal sleep patterns such events tend to increase in frequency. Relaxing activity easing the transition to sleep and hypnosis have proven useful in the treatment of arousal disorders (11).

Sodas containing caffeine have been noted to precipitate arousal parasomnias (12). Fluid loading before bedtime can increase the chance for bedwetting, but has also been used to precipitate somnambulism in the laboratory setting (13).

Psychotherapy

There is a long tradition of treating patients with parasomnias with supportive psychotherapy; however, there is little data supporting the efficacy of such an approach. In childhood the only clear association of a parasomnia with psychiatric illness is in the association of nightmares with PTSD. Nightmares respond much better to behavioral approaches to therapy. In adults when a psychiatric diagnosis is associated with a parasomnia, therapy should be based on the specific underlying diagnosis. It is important for a therapist involved in the treatment of these disorders to remember that these sleep-related behaviors are experiences over which the patient has no conscious deliberate control.

PHARMACOLOGICAL TREATMENT

The arousal disorders can occur or increase in intensity secondary to medications that increase the amount of deep sleep. Such medications include lithium, γ-hydroxybutyrate, and the opiates (14). Nicotine, caffeine, and alcohol have been implicated as well in somnambulism (15).

The clinical use of pharmacological agents affecting the neurotransmitters norepinephrine, serotonin, and dopamine are associated with the complaint of nightmares (Table 3). A majority of these agents are antidepressants [primarily selective serotonin reuptake inhibitors (SSRIs), and tricyclic antidepressants], antihypertensives (β-blockers and α-agonists), and dopamine agonists. Agents affecting the immunological response to infectious disease are likely to induce nightmares in some patients. A possible association exists between reports of nightmares and agents affecting the neurotransmitters acetylcholine, γ-aminobutyric acid (GABA), and histamine, as well as for some anesthetics, antipsychotics, and antiepileptic agents (16,17). The withdrawal of REM sleep suppressive agents such as ethanol, antidepressants, barbiturates, and benzodiazepines can also be associated with increases in the complaint of nightmares.

RBD can be triggered by a variety of antidepressant medications as well as dopamine agonists and cholinergics used to treat Alzheimer's disease. Acute RBD has been noted to occur during the withdrawal from cocaine, amphetamines, ethanol, barbiturate, and meprobamate abuse. Caffeine may unmask RBD.

SRED is often associated with the use of zolpidem, triazolam, and other psychotropic agents, including lithium carbonate, amitriptyline, olanzapine, and risperidone (18). SRED can also develop in individuals withdrawing from ethanol or other substance abuse.

Psychoactive medications and those with CNS side effects are known to alter CNS electrophysiology, particularly the background CNS rhythms of the electroencephalogram (EEG) utilized by protocols to divide sleep into stages. The more common parasomnias, the arousal disorders of deep sleep and the REM-associated parasomnias, are sleep stage specific. Medications are known to induce parasomnias based on their effects on sleep stages. Most of the medications with historic clinical use for treatment of the specific parasomnias have effects on specific sleep stages. This combination of factors suggest that one facet of medication treatment of parasomnias can be sleep stage manipulation (Table 4). REM suppressive

Table 3 Medications Reported to Induce Nightmares

Affected neuroreceptor drug	Patient reports of nightmares—evidence-based clinical trials (CT) and case reports (CR)	Probability assessment of drug effect
Acetylcholine–cholinergic agonists		
Donepezil	CT (3/747 report disordered dreaming)	Possible
Norepinephrine—β-blockers		
Atenolol	CT (3/20 patients)	Probable
Bisoprolol	CT (3/68 patients): CR [1]—dechallenge	Probable
Labetalol	CT (5/175 patients)	Probable
Oxprenolol	CT (11/130 patients)	Probable
Propranolol	CT (8/107 patients)	Probable
Norepinephrine affecting agents		
Guanethidine	CT (4/48 patients)	Probable
Serotonin—SSRI		
Fluoxetine	CT (1–5%—greater frequency in OCD and bulemic trials: CR (4)—de- & rechallenge	Probable
Escitalopram oxylate	CT (abnormal dreaming—1% of 999 patients)	Probable
Nefazodone	CT [3% (372) vs. 2% control]	Probable
Paroxetine	CT [4% (392) vs. 1% control]	Significant
Agents affecting serotonin and norepinephrine		
Risperidone	CT (1% increased dream activity—2607 patients)	Probable
Venlafaxine	CT [4% (1033) vs. 3% control]	Probable
Dopamine—agonists		
Amantadine	CT (5% report abnormal dreams): CR (1)	Probable
Levodopa	CT (2/9 patients)	Probable
Ropinirole	CT [3% (208) report abnormal dreaming vs. 2% placebo]	Probable
Selegiline	CT [2/49 reporting vivid dreams]	Probable
Amphetamine-like agents		
Bethanidine	CT (2/44 patients)	Probable
Fenfluramine	CT (7/28 patients): CR (1) de- & rechallenge	Probable
Phenmetrazine	CT (3/81 patients)	Probable
GABA		
γ-Hydroxybutyrate	CT (nightmares >1% 473 patients)	Probable
Triazolam	CT (7/21 patients)	Probable
Zopiclone	CT (3–5/83 patients)	Probable
Nicotine agonists		
Varenicline	CT (Abnormal Dreams 14/821 patients)	Probable
Nicotine patches	CT (Disturbed dreaming in up to 12% of patients)	Probable
Anti-infectives and immunosupressants		
Amantadine	CT (5% reporting abnormal dreams): CR (1)	Probable
Fleroxacin	CT (7/84 patients)	Probable
Ganciclovir	CR (1)—de & rechallenge	Probable
Gusperimus	CT (13/36 patient)	Probable
Antipsychotics		
Clozapine	CT (4%)	Probable
Antihistamine		
Chlorpheniramine	CT (4/80 patients)	Probable
Ace inhibitors		
Enalapril	CT (0.5–1% abnormal dreaming—2987 patients)	Probable
Losartan potassium	CT (>1% dream abnormality—858 patients)	Probable
Quinapril	CT (>3%)	Probable
Other agents—no proposed mechanism		
Digoxin	CR (1)—de & rechallenge	Probable
Naproxen	CR (1)—de & rechallenge	Probable
Verapamil	CR (1)—de & rechallenge	Probable

Medications included in each class are those considered most likely to induce nightmares based on meta-analysis of clinical trials and case reports.

Key: CR, case reports: probable association of nightmares based on dechallenge and rechallenge with medication; CT, clinical trials: probable association based on >1% incidence of nightmares compared with control groups, or >3% incidence of nightmares in trials without controls. Older medications >15 years in use are not included since subjects were not queried for nightmares as a side effect in clinical trials.

Source: From Refs. 11 and 12.

Table 4 Medication Classes Known to Alter Sleep Stages

Medication classes suppressing REM sleep	Medication classes suppressing deep sleep [N3 (stages 3 and 4)]	Medication classes increasing deep sleep [N3 (stages 3 and 4)]
Antidepressants:	Antidepressants:	Lithium (+)
Tricyclic (++)	Tricyclic (+)	
MAOI (+++)	SSRI (+) frequency changes	
SSRI (+)		
Others (+)		
Barbiturates (++)	Amphetamines (++)	γ-Hydroxybutyrate (+)
Barbiturate-like agents (++)		
Benzodiazepines (+)	Benzodiazepines—amplitude changes	Opiates (+)

Key: (+, ++, +++) degree of effect.
Source: From Ref. 20.

medications may prove useful in the treatment of REM-associated parasomnias. Medications that alter or suppress stage N3 sleep have proven useful in the treatment of the arousal disorders. This approach to treating parasomnias has an apparently sound theoretical basis; however, there have been no investigational studies supporting this general approach to treatment (19,20).

TREATMENT OF SPECIFIC PARASOMNIAS

Disorders of Arousal

The disorders of arousal constitute a continuum of overlapping disorders, all of which respond to the same general therapeutic manipulations. The disorders of arousal are most generally treated with environmental protection of the patient and family reassurance, particularly in children since the parasomnia most often decreases and disappears as the individual enters into adolescence. A familial and genetic basis for the arousal disorders is well established (21). These parasomnias can recur in adulthood secondary to the development of OSA or PLMD in the patient or the use of medications increasing N3 sleep. In individuals with known or suspected epilepsy, an evaluation for nocturnal seizures may be indicated. These disorders tend to increase in frequency when the individual is exposed to change or stress. There is little evidence, however, that behavioral or psychotherapy is particularly useful in the treatment of these disorders. One study has sown the positive benefit of self-hypnosis in the treatment of sleep terrors in children (22).

Medications used in the treatment of the arousal disorders include benzodiazepines, particularly clonazepam (Klonopin) (23). Both sleep terrors and somnambulism have been successfully treated with SSRI antidepressants, particularly paroxetine (24). Alprazolam (Xanax), diazepam (Valium), and imipramine hydrochloride (Tofranil) have also been utilized in treatment regimens (21).

Disorders Usually Associated with REM Sleep

REM Sleep Behavioral Disorder

It is important in RBD to preserve environmental safety for both the patient and sleeping partner. Underlying associated illnesses such as OSA and PLMD should be addressed. Neurological evaluation or a brain magnetic resonance imaging (MRI) scan may be indicated because of the known association or RBD with CNS lesions and progressive degenerative neurological disorders—most commonly Parkinson's disease. RBD can develop or worsen following significant psychological trauma or stress (25).

Clonazepam is the medication most commonly utilized in the treatment of RBD and can be remarkably effective in treating the behavioral and dream-disordered components of RBD on a long-term basis with few reports of tolerance or abuse (21,25). Positive responses have also been noted for both SSRI and tricylic antidepressants (imipramine and desipramine), other benzodiazepines, such as alprazolam and triazolam, and for antiepileptic medications, such as carbamazepine (6,7). Anecdotal and case reports suggest positive effects for melatonin, tryptophan, monoamine oxidase inhibitors (MAOIs), valproic acid, gabapentin, clonidine, levodopa/carbidopa, and clozapine in specific cases (26).

Nightmares

Nightmares and insomnia are associated complaints. Frequent nightmares can be associated with decreased sleep quality and sleep disruption, and this sleep disruption has been shown to affect daytime functioning and induce psychological distress (27,28). Disruption of sleep associated with nightmares can produce conditioning patterns similar to those found in association with psychophysiological insomnia where the individual develops a fear of going to sleep (29). Since nightmares can be associated with psychiatric disorders such as PTSD, depression, and anxiety disorders, a common perspective has been that remission occurs only through treatment of an underlying psychiatric disorder (30). Studies have also suggested that undiagnosed sleep-disordered breathing is common in patients presenting with symptoms of PTSD (31). There is a growing body of evidence, however, that the targeted therapy of nightmares can lead to improvements in sleep disturbance, psychological distress, and severity of associated psychiatric conditions (30,32).

Behavioral approaches to the treatment of nightmares include desensitization and imagery rehearsal. Currently, the best data demonstrate significant improvement in nightmares for cognitive-based imagery therapy (31,33). This approach deemphasizes discussion of the traumatic association of nightmares emphasizing instead the habitual pattern of recurrent nightmares. The nightmare sufferer is asked to change one of his or her nightmares "in any way you wish" (34). The sufferer is then advised to rehearse the "new" dream while awake. This approach is coupled with cognitive insomnia therapy including sleep hygiene, stimulus control, and sleep restriction. Significant improvements have been obtained utilizing this approach in nightmare frequency, sleep quality, anxiety, and depression (27,30).

PTSD Nightmares

PTSD nightmares are often treated with prolonged exposure therapy that includes focusing and reliving the traumatic experience. This approach, coupled with medication (typically SSRI antidepressants) has shown evidence for improved outcomes compared with individuals treated with medication (31). Some studies have suggested the possibility that acute debriefing without further support is likely to worsen symptoms of PTSD (32). Such critical incidence stress debriefing (CISD) approaches to the treatment of PTSD are currently in general utilization in both the military and civilian first response units. There is little evidence that any of the early behavioral approaches to the treatment of acute trauma leads to improved outcomes or a lower incidence of chronic PTSD (33).

In our modern world, PTSD is common and psychological services have limited availability. The practice of psychodynamic psychotherapy remains commonplace in clinical settings with little evidence to support its clinical use (32). There is better evidence supporting the use of postal self-exposure (home self-treatment using a manual mailed to the patient); positive benefits have been shown in one study (35). There is little evidence, however, that exposure approaches are more beneficial than therapies in which there is no exposure to the main traumatic event (36). Cognitive behavioral therapy that does not include traumatic reexposure has shown positive benefit in the treatment of PTSD-associated nightmares (37,38). This approach has proved useful in children (39). Eye movement desensitization reprocessing (EMDR) has shown effectiveness for some patients, as have newer approaches including memory restructuring intervention, dialectical behavioral therapy and interpersonal psychotherapy (32).

The following conclusions were reached based on a meta-analysis of psychological treatments for PTSD:

1. Psychological treatment can reduce traumatic stress symptoms (including nightmares) in individuals with PTSD.
2. Trauma-based cognitive therapy has the best evidence for efficacy at present.
3. Limited evidence suggests that stress management is effective.
4. Limited evidence supports the efficacy of other non-trauma-focused psychological treatments.
5. Dropout from treatment is a major issue with currently available psychological treatments (40).

Medications for the treatment of PTSD run the gamut of the psychoactive pharmacopoeia. The current medications of choice for the treatment of PTSD are the SSRI antidepressants (27,41,42). Medications that have shown positive efficacy include antianxiety agents, nonbenzodiazepine hypnotics, antidepressants, mood stabilizers, anticonvulsants, and antipsychotics (43–47). The acute use of hypnotics after trauma does not prevent the development of PTSD (48). These mediations are in general use for the treatment of PTSD in children and adolescents with partial responders to pharmacological treatment often requiring the addition of a second class of medication. (40). The effects of these agents on nightmare frequency in PTSD have not been addressed for most of these agents, except for antidepressants such as trazodone, nefazodone, and fluvoxamine, which has been shown to improve both the nightmare frequency and insomnia associated with chronic PTSD (27,49).

It has been postulated that some patients with PTSD exhibit abnormalities in noradrenergic function (50). Antihypertensive agents in general use affect noradrenergic CNS receptors. These drugs have been shown to affect both REM sleep and reports of dreaming. The reported effects of these agents on both dreams and nightmares are often opposite to the drugs' known pharmacological effects on REM sleep (16,17). Decreases in dream recall occur with use of both α-agonists (REM suppressant) and β-blockers (NREM suppressant) (51). An agent's effect on REM sleep may or may not be associated with an associated change on reported dreaming. β-Blockers depress REM sleep percentages yet can result in reports of increased dreaming, nightmares, and hallucinations (52). β-Blockers (propranolol) have shown positive results in the treatment of PTSD (53). Prazosin is the α-agonist most commonly used for the treatment of recurrent nightmares in PTSD patients. Significant decreases in disturbing dreams and improvement in both sleep onset and maintenance insomnia have been achieved in PTSD patients (54).

A meta-analysis of the literature on the pharmacotherapy of PTSD reached the conclusion that medication treatments can be useful in the treatment of PTSD and should be considered as part of the treatment of this disorder. Although there was limited evidence showing that one class of medications is more effective than any other, the greatest number of trials showing efficacy to date had been with the SSRIs. In contrast, there had been negative studies of benzodiazepines, MAOIs, antipsychotics, lamotrigine, and inositol. Maximizing treatment outcomes appeared to require psychotherapy in addition to medication use. Maintenance trials also suggested that long-term interventions increase the efficacy of medications and prevent relapse (55).

Recurrent Isolated Sleep Paralysis
Sleep paralysis is present in 17% to 40% of narcoleptics, but also occurs as an independent diagnosis (56). Acute anxiety is commonly seen with the attacks and often resolves with diagnosis and medical explanation of the events. Avoidance of stress and shift work, and supine sleep, as well as maintaining good sleep hygiene are the cornerstones of therapy. In severe, frequent, and chronic cases, several different kinds of antidepressants and sedatives have been used, including SSRIs, tricyclic antidepressants, MAOIs, and benzodiazepines. Only anecdotal reports are cited in the literature as to the efficacy of these drugs (56).

Sleep Enuresis
Nocturnal enuresis can occur secondary to urinary tract infection, diabetes, and structural abnormalities of the urinary tract. In patients with purely nocturnal bedwetting, a normal urinalysis, normal development, and no known or suspected anatomic or neurological disorder, no further workup is indicated. Enuresis is familial; in families where both parents were enuretic, 77% of the children have enuresis, or 44% if one parent was enuretic (10). There is a high prevalence of enuresis in children with sleep-disordered breathing (57).

Enuresis responds well to behavioral treatments with success rates in excess of 90% obtained with combination therapies that include alarms, rewards, and responsibility training (58). Responsibility training includes hand washing and bed cleanup after the enuretic event. Positive reinforcement may include a star chart in which the child is rewarded for dry nights. Visual imagery and self-hypnosis are useful adjuncts to therapy. The child can be taught to visualize a urinary gate that she or he closes mentally. Positive results have been reported for bladder and sphincter training in which the child is instructed to stop and start urine flow and hold onto urine before elimination. If the child has a usual time for enuresis, awakening the child to urinate can be helpful. Systems are available with a sensor in the bed or underpants that sound an alarm with a few drops of urine, awakening the child and training him to void on his own (58,59).

Patients with nocturnal enuresis may not demonstrate the normal nocturnal decrease in antidiuretic hormone (60). Desmopressin (DDAVP) pills or nasal sprays are effective and in general use for the treatment of nocturnal enuresis. Imipramine has a long history of use in children for the treatment of functional enuresis; however, children are more sensitive than adults to acute overdosage, and electrocardiac abnormalities have been noted with routine use. The goal of medication therapy for enuresis is the maintenance of dry nights pending the eventual urological neurogenic maturity that comes with increasing patient age.

Sleep-Related Eating Disorder

Treatment of SRED should in general be directed toward treating the underlying sleep disorder. In cases associated with sleepwalking and restless legs syndrome, monotherapy or combined therapy with dopamine agonists such as pramipexole or ropinirole, benzodiazepines (clonazepam), and opiates (codeine) can be effective. Fluoxetine hydrochloride (Prozac) and bupropion hydrochloride (Wellbutrin) can be useful as adjunctive therapies. Psychological and behavioral treatments are usually ineffective (21).

Sleep-Related Dissociative Disorders

The dissociative disorders and their associated psychiatric disorders require long-term therapy of the underlying disorder. Treatment is usually initialized in a specialized inpatient setting. Nocturnal utilization of benzodiazepine agents may aggravate a nocturnal dissociative disorder (21).

Sleep-Related Hallucinations

Hypnagogic and hypnopompic hallucinations can be seen in patients with narcolepsy. Patients are clearly awake, but often initially perceive these primarily visual hallucinations as real and frightening. Patients with hallucinations as a symptom of underlying psychiatric disease such as schizophrenia may also have nocturnal hallucinations as part of their presentation. Treatment of the hallucinations relates to treatment of the associated illness for these individuals.

Sleep-Related Groaning

Sleep-related groaning may occur in association with OSA. Treatments attempted to this point, however, including continuous positive airway pressure (CPAP) and several medications have not been shown to demonstrate treatment efficacy (61,62).

Exploding Head Syndrome

This is a rare disorder with a characteristic presentation. Patients have shown a good response to the behavioral approach of diagnosis and reassurance. Anecdotal treatment success with medications has been obtained with indomethacin, nifedipine, and clomipramine (63,64).

CONCLUSIONS AND FUTURE RESEARCH

Nightmares are the most commonly experienced parasomnia, and the parasomnia most likely is associated with waking impairment. It is not surprising, therefore, that both the diagnostic differential and treatment modalities for this diagnosis is best delineated and available to serve as a model for the future development of the least common parasomnia diagnoses.

Some of the parasomnias can be specifically associated with REM and/or deep sleep. However, even if these parasomnias are classified by their association with a particular sleep stage, sleep stage association remains somewhat problematic for several of the parasomnia diagnoses, specifically PTSD nightmares and parasomnia overlap disorder. The sleep stage association of the grouping classified as "other parasomnias" remains unclear. This lack of sleep stage correlation affects the ability to utilize medications to treat parasomnias by manipulating the parasomnia-associated sleep stage. Specific medications are available to treat the more common parasomnias such as REM behavior disorder. The medications used to treat the rarer parasomnias encompass the spectrum of psychoactive medications and others known to have applicable CNS side effects. Current approaches to behavioral and pharmacological treatment of the parasomnias are largely anecdotal. There are almost no clinical trial studies utilizing placebo controls. The pharmacological treatment construct of sleep stage manipulation exists as a model but has not been systematically studied as an approach to the treatment of the sleep stage–specific parasomnias (20,65).

General treatment modalities for all parasomnias include sleep hygiene and environmental protection. Diagnosis and reassurance are particularly important in the childhood parasomnias that tend to decrease as the child transitions to adulthood. Behavioral treatments have shown excellent efficacy in the treatment of specific parasomnias such as nightmares and enuresis. Future treatment protocols need to compare behavioral to pharmacological therapies.

Parasomnias often become symptomatic secondary to precipitating diagnoses, such as OSA, PLMD, trauma, and psychiatric illness. Multiple medications are known to induce parasomnias. The more recently described parasomnias such as sleep-related hallucinations and dissociative disorders are found in patients with known psychiatric and sleep disorders. The effects of the treatment of these underlying disorders on parasomnia symptomatology need to be clarified.

These parasomnias are sleep-related behaviors in which the patient has no conscious deliberate control. In general, treatment of a parasomnia is based on diminishing or eliminating the adverse waking effects of the diagnosis. The treatment of parasomnias requires a baseline principle of training medical providers to utilize the parasomnia diagnostic criteria, including an awareness of associated underlying disorders. This approach makes it possible for the provider to clarify the diagnosis and educate the symptomatic patient and family. If the parasomnia is not associated with adverse affects on waking function or nocturnal injury, no treatment of the parasomnia may be required beyond diagnosis and reassurance.

REFERENCES

1. Hauri PJ. The International Classification of Sleep Disorders: Diagnostic and Coding Manual. 2nd ed. Westchester, IL: American Academy of Sleep Medicine, 2005:155–158.
2. Brassington GS, King AC, Bliwise DL. Sleep problems as a risk factor for falls in a sample of community-dwelling adults aged 64–99 years. J Am Geriatr Soc 2000; 48(10):1234–1240.
3. Guilleminault C, Palombini L, Pelayo R, et al. Sleepwalking and sleep terrors in prepubertal children: what triggers them? Pediatrics 2003; 111(1):e17–e25.
4. Schenck CH, Hurwitz TD, Mahowald MW. Symposium: normal and abnormal REM sleep regulation: REM sleep behaviour disorder: an update on a series of 96 patients and a review of the world literature. J Sleep Res 1993; 2(4):224–231.
5. Auger RR, Morgenthaler TI. Sleep-related eating disorders. In: Lee-Chiong T, ed. Sleep: A Comprehensive Handbook. Hoboken, NJ: John Wiley and Sons, 2006:457–462.
6. Bahro M, Katzmann KJ, Guckel F, et al. [REM sleep parasomnia]. Nervenarzt 1994; 65(8):568–571.
7. Schenck CH, Boyd JL, Mahowald MW. A parasomnia overlap disorder involving sleepwalking, sleep terrors, and REM sleep behavior disorder in 33 polysomnographically confirmed cases. Sleep 1997; 20 (11):972–981.
8. Francis A. Diagnostic and Statistical Manual of Mental Disorders. 4th ed. Washington D.C.: American Psychiatric Association, 1994.
9. Brooks LJ. Enuresis and sleep apnea. Pediatrics 2005; 116(3):799–800.
10. Rushton HG. Nocturnal enuresis: epidemiology, evaluation, and currently available treatment options. J Pediatr 1989; 114(4 pt 2):691–696.
11. Reid WH, Ahmed I, Levie CA. Treatment of sleepwalking: a controlled study. Am J Psychother 1981; 35(1):27–37.
12. Huritz TD, Mahowald MW, Schenck CH, et al. A retrospective outcome study and review of hypnosis as treatment of adults with sleep walking and sleep terror. J Nerv Ment Dis 1991; 179:228–233.
13. Cartwright RD. Sleepwalking. In: Lee-Chiong T, ed. Sleep: A Comprehensive Handbook. Hoboken, NJ: John Wiley and Sons, 2006:429–433.
14. Broughton R. Sleep disorders: disorders of arousal? Science 1968; 159:1070–1077.
15. Moldofsky H, Gilbert R, Lue f, et al. Sleep related violence. Sleep 1995; 18:731–739.
16. Pagel JF, Helfter P. Drug induced nightmares—an etiology based review. Hum Psychopharmacol 2003; 18(1):59–67.

17. Pagel JF. The neuropharmacology of nightmares. In: Pandi-Perumal SR, Cardinali DP, Lander M, eds. Sleep and Sleep Disorders: Neuropsychopharmacologic Approach. Georgetown, TX: Landes Bioscience, 2006:241–250.

18. Morgenthaler T, Silber M. Amnestic sleep-related eating disorder associated with zolpidem. Sleep Med 2002; 3:323–327.

19. Pagel JF. Modeling drug actions on electrophysiologic effects produced by EEG modulated potentials. Hum Psychopharmacol 1993; 8:211–216.

20. Pagel J. Disease, psychoactive medication, and Sleep States. Prim Psychiatry 1996; 3(3):47–51.

21. Schenck CH, Mahowald MW. Parasomnias. Managing bizarre sleep-related behavior disorders. Postgrad Med 2000; 107(3):145–156.

22. Kohen DP, Mahowald MW, Rosen GM. Sleep-terror disorder in children: the role of self-hypnosis in management. Am J Clin Hypn 1992; 34(4):233–244.

23. Schenck CH, Mahowald MW. Long term nightly benzodiazepine treatment of injurous parasomnias and other disorders with disrupted nocturnal sleep in 170 adults. Am J Med 1996; 100(3):333–337.

24. Lillywhite AR, Wilson SJ, Nutt DJ. Successful treatment of night terrors and somnambulism with paroxitine. Br J Psychiatry 1994; 164(4):551–554.

25. Chiu HF, Wing YK. REM sleep behaviour disorder: an overview. Int J Clin Pract 1997; 51(7):451–454.

26. Wills L, Garcia J. Parasomnias: epidemiology and management. CNS Drugs 2002; 16(12):803–810.

27. Singareddy RK, Balon R. Sleep in posttraumatic stress disorder. Ann Clin Psychiatry 2002; 14(3): 183–190.

28. Nielsen TA, Zadra A. Dreaming disorders. In: Kryger M, Roth T, Dement W, eds. Principles and Practice of Sleep Medicine. 3rd ed. Philadelphia: W. B. Saunders, 2000:753–772.

29. Kales A, Soldatos CR, Caldwell AB, et al. Nightmares: clinical characteristics and personality patterns. Am J Psychiatry 1980; 187(10):1197–1201.

30. Krakow B, Melendrez D, Johnston L, et al. Sleep-disordered breathing, psychiatric distress, and quality of life impairment in sexual assault survivors. J Nerv Ment Dis 2002; 190(7):442–452.

31. Krakow B, Melendrez D, Pedersen B, et al. Complex insomnia: insomnia and sleep-disordered breathing in a consecutive series of crime victims with nightmares and PTSD. Biol Psychiatry 2001; 49(11): 948–953.

32. Krakow B, Kellner R, Pathak D, et al. Imagery rehearsal treatment for chronic nightmares. Behav Res Ther 1995; 33(7):837–843.

33. Robertson M, Humphreys L, Ray R. Psychological treatments for posttraumatic stress disorder: recommendations for the clinician based on a review of the literature. J Psychiatr Pract 2004; 10(2): 106–118.

34. Krakow B, Niedhardt J. Conquering bad dreams and nightmares. New York: Berkley Books, 1992.

35. Burgess M, Gill M, Marks I. Postal self-exposure treatment of recurrent nightmares. Randomised controlled trial. Br J Psychiatry 1998; 172:257–262.

36. Hinton DE, Chhean D, Pich V, et al. A randomized controlled trial of cognitive-behavior therapy for Cambodian refugees with treatment-resistant PTSD and panic attacks: a cross-over design. J Trauma Stress 2005; 18(6):617–629.

37. Germain A, Nielsen T. Impact of imagery rehearsal treatment on distressing dreams, psychological distress, and sleep parameters in nightmare patients. Behav Sleep Med 2003; 1(3):140–154.

38. Hinton DE, Pham T, Tran M, et al. CBT for Vietnamese refugees with treatment-resistant PTSD and panic attacks: a pilot study. J Trauma Stress 2004; 17(5):429–433.

39. Brown EJ. Clinical characteristics and efficacious treatment of posttraumatic stress disorder in children and adolescents. Pediatr Ann 2005; 34(2):138–146.

40. Bisson J, Andrew M. Psychological treatment of post-traumatic stress disorder (PTSD). Cochrane Database Syst Rev 2005; (2):CD003388.

41. Putnam FW, Hulsmann JE. Pharmacotherapy for survivors of childhood trauma. Semin Clin Neuropsychiatry 2002; 7(2):129–136.

42. Rapaport MH, Endicott J, Clary CM. Posttraumatic stress disorder and quality of life: results across 64 weeks of sertraline treatment. J Clin Psychiatry 2002; 63(1):59–65.

43. Bartzokis G, Lu PH, Turner J, et al. Adjunctive risperidone in the treatment of chronic combat-related posttraumatic stress disorder. Biol Psychiatry 2005; 57(5):474–479.

44. Douglas Bremner J, Mletzko T, Welter S, et al. Treatment of posttraumatic stress disorder with phenytoin: an open-label pilot study. J Clin Psychiatry 2004; 65(11):1559–1564.

45. Hamner MB, Brodrick PS, Labbate LA. Gabapentin in PTSD: a retrospective, clinical series of adjunctive therapy. Ann Clin Psychiatry 2001; 13(3):141–146.

46. Wheatley M, Plant J, Reader H, et al. Clozapine treatment of adolescents with posttraumatic stress disorder and psychotic symptoms. J Clin Psychopharmacol 2004; 24(2):167–173.

47. Davidson JR, Weisler RH, Butterfield MI, et al. Mirtazapine vs. placebo in posttraumatic stress disorder: a pilot trial. Biol Psychiatry 2003; 53(2):188–191.

48. Mellman TA, Bustamante V, David D, et al. Hypnotic medication in the aftermath of trauma. J Clin Psychiatry 2002; 63(12):1183–1184.
49. Warner MD, Dorn MR, Peabody CA. Survey on the usefulness of trazodone in patients with PTSD with insomnia or nightmares. Pharmacopsychiatry 2001; 34(4):128–131.
50. Southwick SM, Krystal JH, Morgan CA, et al. Abnormal noradrenergic function in posttraumatic stress disorder. Arch Gen Psychiatry 1993; 50(4):266–274.
51. Danchin N, Genton P, Atlas P, et al. Comparative effects of atenolol and clonidine on polygraphically recorded sleep in hypertensive men: a randomized, double-blind, crossover study. Int J Clin Pharmacol Ther 1995; 33(1):52–55.
52. Dimsdale J, Newton R. Cognitive effects of beta-blockers. J Psychosom Res 1991; 36(3):229–236.
53. Schoenfeld FB, Marmar CR, Neylan TC. Current concepts in pharmacotherapy for posttraumatic stress disorder. Psychiatr Serv 2004; 55(5):519–531.
54. Raskind MA, Peskind ER, Kanter ED, et al. Reduction of nightmares and other PTSD symptoms in combat veterans by prazosin: a placebo-controlled study. Am J Psychiatry 2003; 160(2):371–373.
55. Stein DJ, Ipser JC, Seedat S. Pharmacotherapy for post traumatic stress disorder (PTSD). Cochrane Database Syst Rev 2006; (1):CD002795.
56. Queshi A. Other parasomnias. In: Lee-Chiong T, ed. Sleep: A Comprehensive Handbook. Hoboken, NJ: John Wiley and Sons, 2006:463–470.
57. Brooks LJ, Topol HI. Enuresis in children with sleep apnea. J Pediatr 2003; 142(5):515–518.
58. Challamel MJ, Cochat P. Nocturnal enuresis in children. In: Lee-Chiong T, ed. Sleep: A Comprehensive Handbook. Hoboken, NJ: John Wiley and Sons, 2006:443–448.
59. Geffken G, Johnson SB, Walker D. Behavioral interventions for childhood nocturnal enuresis: the differential effect of bladder capacity on treatment progress and outcome. Health Psychol 1986; 5(3):261–272.
60. Norgaard JP, Rittig S, Djurhuus JC. Nocturnal enuresis: an approach to treatment based on pathogenesis. J Pediatr 1989; 114(4 pt 2):705–710.
61. Vetrugno R, Provini F, Plazzi G, et al. Catathrenia (nocturnal groaning): a new type of parasomnia. Neurology 2001; 56(5):681–683.
62. Oldani A, Manconi M, Zucconi M, et al. 'Nocturnal groaning': just a sound or parasomnia? J Sleep Res 2005; 14(3):305–310.
63. Jacome DE. Exploding head syndrome and idiopathic stabbing headache relieved by nifedipine. Cephalalgia 2001; 21(5):617–618.
64. Casucci G, d'Onofrio F, Torelli P. Rare primary headaches: clinical insights. Neurol Sci 2004; 25(suppl 3): S77–S83.
65. Pagel JF. Pharmachologic alterations of sleep and dream: a clinical framework for utilizing the electrophysiological and sleep stage effects of psychoactive medications. Hum Psychopharmachol 1996; 11:217–223.

42 | Special Considerations for Treatment of Parasomnias

Mehran Farid

Peninsula Sleep Center, Inc., Burlingame, California, U.S.A.

SIDE EFFECTS OF TREATMENT

In addition to safety measures, treatment of parasomnias includes pharmacotherapeutic agents and nonpharmacotherapy options as well as behavior modification and hypnosis. Non-pharmacotherapy options do not have significant or well-known adverse effects. The adverse effects of pharmacotherapeutic agents are discussed here.

1. Medications that are used for sleep-stage manipulation
   - Medications that suppress slow-wave sleep stages.
   - Medications that suppress rapid eye movement (REM) sleep.

   Slow-wave sleep-suppressing agents are mainly benzodiazepine medications, including diazepam (1), midazolam (2), oxazepam, clonazepam, and the most commonly used REM sleep-suppressing agents are tricyclic antidepressants including clomipramine, desipramine, and imipramine (3). Other medications include paroxetine and trazodone.

2. Adjunctive or alternative medications
   - Clonidine, carbidopa/L-dopa, L-tryptophan, gabapentin, melatonin, and prami-pexole.

The major side effects of the above medications, including effects on sleep architecture are summarized here.

Tricyclic Antidepressants
These medications include imipramine, amitryptyline, nortryptyline, clomipramine, desipr-amine, and doxepin. They affect a wide variety of brain receptors that account for their effects and side effects. Their overdosage can cause cardiac toxicity as well as seizures. Their anticholinergic effects, including a dry mouth and orthostatic hypotension, are dose dependent. These medications are reported to be associated with a higher chance of myocardial infarction and sudden cardiac death at higher doses (4). Moreover, due to a higher chance of suicidal attempts and suicidal ideation, the Food and Drug Administration (FDA) has issued public health advisories regarding the effects of antidepressants on adults and children (5). Sleep-related side effects of these medications mainly include increasing REM sleep latency and suppression of time in REM sleep (6). Withdrawal from tricyclic antidepressants causes a transient increase in REM sleep time.

Selective Serotonin Reuptake Inhibitors
Selective serotonin reuptake inhibitors (SSRIs) include fluoxetine, sertraline, paroxetine, fluvoxamine, citalopram, and escitalopram. These medications have good tolerability with a mild side effect profile. Additionally, overdosage is safer than with tricyclic antidepressants. The most common side effects are nausea and anxiety. Among the sleep-related side effects, insomnia is the most common. These medications decrease sleep quality and quantity, and suppress REM sleep.

Benzodiazepines
This class of medications includes clonazepam, alprazolam, diazepam, and many more medications that are used in the treatment of parasomnias especially in REM sleep behavior disorder (RBD) and sleepwalking (3,7,8). Clonazepam is the most extensively used

benzodiazepine in the treatment of RBD and disorders of arousal (8). It is a potent benzodiazepine with a long half-life of 19 to 50 hours that may cause mild drowsiness the next day. Benzodiazepines are known to induce some degree of amnesia associated with their hypnotic effect. Benzodiazepines are effective hypnotic agents that increase non-REM (NREM) stages N1 and N2 sleep, and they generally decrease slow-wave and REM sleep (9,10). Clonazepam increases slow-wave sleep duration. It is relatively contraindicated in patients with significant liver disease and narrow angle glaucoma.

Zolpidem and the other medications in its category are not typically used in the management of parasomnias. This is due to the fact that a higher chance of having episodes of sleepwalking and sleep eating disorder are reported with these medications.

Clonidine

An α2-adrenergic agonist, widely used for the treatment of hypertension, has also been used for sleep bruxism (11), but due to its main side effects, orthostatic hypotension and hypotension, no further studies have been carried out. It may also cause sedation, drowsiness, and insomnia. It increases slow-wave sleep and decreases REM sleep.

Gabapentin

This anticonvulsant has been tried for the management of certain parasomnias including bruxism (12). It may cause fatigue, drowsiness, and sedation on the following day.

Melatonin

This over-the-counter preparation is successfully used for the treatment of RBD (13–15). It should be taken at a relatively higher dosage, i.e., around 3 mg, and at a fixed time every night. The FDA in the United States does not regulate melatonin, which is considered a "natural drug." No significant toxicity has been reported.

AGE AND GENDER EFFECTS OF TREATMENT

Tricyclic Antidepressants

This class of medication may be used in all age groups with a lower dose in elderly individuals due to side effects in this age group. The FDA has issued a public health advisory for both adults and children on all antidepressants with regard to the risk of suicide (5). These medications are considered category D for pregnant women and are not recommended in breast-feeding mothers.

Selective Serotonin Reuptake Inhibitors

These medications are used in all age groups and both genders. The FDA advisory in regard to antidepressants is applicable to this class of medication as well as to tricyclic antidepressants (5). Medications in this class are category D for pregnant women. The risks and benefits of using SSRIs in pregnancy should be carefully considered. These medications enter breast milk.

Benzodiazepines

This class of medication is used in all ages and both genders. Clonazepam, which is the most often used benzodiazepine in parasomnias, is a category D medication in pregnancy and is not recommended in breast-feeding mothers.

Clonidine

This medication is used in both genders, and it is also used in both adults and the pediatric population. It should not be stopped abruptly, especially if the patient is taking a β-blocker at the same time. It is a category C medication in pregnancy. It crosses the placenta and enters breast milk; therefore, it is not recommended in lactation.

Gabapentin

This anticonvulsant may be used in the pediatric population. Due to lower clearance of this drug in the elderly, the dose should be adjusted. Gabapentin has been teratogenic in animal studies and is considered a category C medication in pregnancy. It enters breast milk and the risk and benefits of this medication should be evaluated in lactating mothers.

Melatonin
This preparation is considered a natural drug, and its effects on extreme age groups and in pregnancy are not known.

DRIVING RISK AND MEDICOLEGAL ASPECTS

Patients with certain parasomnias may be at a higher risk of injuring themselves or injuring others. Patients with sleepwalking disorder and RBD may cause injuries to themselves or others. Additionally, injuries may occur due to the side effects of the medications that are used for the treatment of parasomnias, or medications that are used to improve sleep consolidation. Similarly, driving may be affected by the side effect of the medications or rarely a sleepwalker may drive an automobile and be exposed to the risks associated with driving.

Medication Side Effects as the Cause of Injuries
Benzodiazepines may increase the risk of falls in the elderly population (16–18). Zolpidem may increase the risk of sleepwalking (19,20), sleep-related eating disorder (21), and may have adverse effects on psychomotor vigilance and driving ability the next morning after use (22) if it is taken close to the morning awakening time.

Sleepwalking
Sleepwalking, its associated violence (23), and occasionally, sleep-related sexual behavior (24) have been the subject of criminal trials (25–29). A sleepwalker may be engaged in complex motor activities including driving. Special precautions should be taken to minimize or eliminate the risks associated with sleepwalking. These include using special locks on doors, heavy drapes on glass doors and windows, and using special alarms to alert other family members when the sleepwalker is about to leave the bedroom. To avoid agitation, resistance, and possibly violence, the sleepwalker should be gently guided back to his or her bed with no attempt to awaken the person. Moreover, the physician should discuss the risks associated with sleepwalking and should advise the patient against keeping weapons at home.

REM Sleep Behavior Disorder
Similarly, patients with RBD may injure themselves or their bed partners (30–32). However, patients with RBD often do not leave the bedroom and do not engage in complex motor activities including driving. RBD-related activities are related to dream enactment and are limited to the bed or around the bed. However, they may violently attack their bed partner and cause serious injuries. A patient with violent RBD should be treated as soon as possible, safety measures including precautions regarding falling out of the bed and, if needed, a short period of sleeping in a separate room from his or her bed partner should be considered.

SUMMARY

A higher chance of suicidal attempts and suicidal ideation has been observed in patients on antidepressants. The sleep-related side effects of tricyclic antidepressants include increasing REM sleep latency and suppressing REM sleep time, while SSRIs have been associated with insomnia. Benzodiazepines tend to increase NREM stages N1 and N2 sleep and generally decrease slow-wave and REM sleep, and clonidine is associated with an increase in slow-wave sleep and a decrease in REM sleep. Tricyclic antidepressants and SSRIs are considered category D for pregnant women, while clonidine and gabapentin are considered category C. Zolpidem has been associated with increasing the risk of sleepwalking, and both sleepwalking and RBD independently are associated with a risk of injury to the patients themselves or their bed partners.

REFERENCES

1. Fisher C, Kahn E, Edwards A, et al. A psychophysiological study of nightmares and night terrors. The suppression of stage 4 night terrors with diazepam. Arch Gen Psychiatry 1973; 28(2):252–259.
2. Popoviciu L, Corfariu O. Efficacy and safety of midazolam in the treatment of night terrors in children. Br J Clin Pharmacol 1983; 16(suppl 1):97S–102S.
3. Cooper AJ. Treatment of coexistent night terrors and somnambulism in adults with imipramine and diazepam. J Clin Psychiatry 1987; 48(5):209–210.
4. Ray WA, Meredith S, Thapa PB, et al. Cyclic antidepressants and the risk of sudden cardiac death. Clin Pharmacol Ther 2004; 75(3):234–241.
5. FDA. Antidepressant, FDA's Public Health Advisory. 10-21-0004.
6. Vogel GW, Buffenstein A, Minter K, et al. Drug effects on REM sleep and on endogenous depression. Neurosci Biobehav Rev 1990; 14(1):49–63.
7. Reid WH, Haffke EA, Chu CC. Diazepam in intractable sleepwalking: a pilot study. Hillside J Clin Psychiatry 1984; 6(1):49–55.
8. Schenck CH, Mahowald MW. Long-term nightly benzodiazepine treatment of injurious parasomnias and other disorders of disrupted nocturnal sleep in 170 adults. Am J Med 1996; 100(3):333–337.
9. Obermeyer WH, Benca RM. Effects of drugs on sleep. Neurol Clin 1996; 14(4):827–840.
10. Hemmeter U, Muller M, Bischof R, et al. Effect of zopiclone and temazepam on sleep EEG parameters, psychomotor and memory functions in healthy elderly volunteers. Psychopharmacology (Berl) 2000; 147(4):384–396.
11. Huynh N, Lavigne GJ, Lanfranchi PA, et al. The effect of 2 sympatholytic medications—propranolol and clonidine—on sleep bruxism: experimental randomized controlled studies. Sleep 2006; 29(3):307–316.
12. Brown ES, Hong SC. Antidepressant-induced bruxism successfully treated with gabapentin. J Am Dent Assoc 1999; 130(10):1467–1469.
13. Takeuchi N, Uchimura N, Hashizume Y, et al. Melatonin therapy for REM sleep behavior disorder. Psychiatry Clin Neurosci 2001; 55(3):267–269.
14. Kunz D, Bes F. Melatonin effects in a patient with severe REM sleep behavior disorder: case report and theoretical considerations. Neuropsychobiology 1997; 36(4):211–214.
15. Kunz D, Bes F. Melatonin as a therapy in REM sleep behavior disorder patients: an open-labeled pilot study on the possible influence of melatonin on REM-sleep regulation. Mov Disord 1999; 14(3):507–511.
16. Wang PS, Bohn RL, Glynn RJ, et al. Zolpidem use and hip fractures in older people. J Am Geriatr Soc 2001; 49(12):1685–1690.
17. Herings RM, Stricker BH, de Boer A, et al. Benzodiazepines and the risk of falling leading to femur fractures. Dosage more important than elimination half-life. Arch Intern Med 1995; 155(16):1801–1807.
18. Ray WA, Griffin MR, Downey W. Benzodiazepines of long and short elimination half-life and the risk of hip fracture. JAMA 1989; 262(23):3303–3307.
19. Yang W, Dollear M, Muthukrishnan SR. One rare side effect of zolpidem—sleepwalking: a case report. Arch Phys Med Rehabil 2005; 86(6):1265–1266.
20. Barrett J, Underwood A. Perchance to . . . eat? Newsweek 2006; 147(13):54.
21. Morgenthaler TI, Silber MH. Amnestic sleep-related eating disorder associated with zolpidem. Sleep Med 2002; 3(4):323–327.
22. Verster JC, Veldhuijzen DS, Volkerts ER. Residual effects of sleep medication on driving ability. Sleep Med Rev 2004; 8(4):309–325.
23. Ohayon MM, Caulet M, Priest RG. Violent behavior during sleep. J Clin Psychiatry 1997; 58(8):369–376.
24. Guilleminault C, Moscovitch A, Yuen K, et al. Atypical sexual behavior during sleep. Psychosom Med 2002; 64(2):328–336.
25. On serious violence during sleep-walking. Br J Psychiatry 1986; 148:476–477.
26. Howard C, D'Orban PT. Violence in sleep: medico-legal issues and two case reports. Psychol Med 1987; 17(4):915–925.
27. Oswald I, Evans J. On serious violence during sleep-walking. Br J Psychiatry 1985; 147:688–691.
28. Schenck CH, Mahowald MW. A polysomnographically documented case of adult somnambulism with long-distance automobile driving and frequent nocturnal violence: parasomnia with continuing danger as a noninsane automatism? Sleep 1995; 18(9):765–772.
29. Cartwright R. Sleepwalking violence: a sleep disorder, a legal dilemma, and a psychological challenge. Am J Psychiatry 2004; 161(7):1149–1158.
30. Comella CL, Nardine TM, Diederich NJ, et al. Sleep-related violence, injury, and REM sleep behavior disorder in Parkinson's disease. Neurology 1998; 51(2):526–529.
31. Olson EJ, Boeve BF, Silber MH. Rapid eye movement sleep behaviour disorder: demographic, clinical, and laboratory findings in 93 cases. Brain 2000; 123(Pt 2):331–339.
32. Yeh SB, Schenck CH. A case of marital discord and secondary depression with attempted suicide resulting from REM sleep behavior disorder in a 35-year-old woman. Sleep Med 2004; 5(2):151–154.

43 | Description of Sleep-Related Movement Disorders

Thomas C. Wetter and Stephany Fulda
Max Planck Institute of Psychiatry, Munich, Germany

HISTORY AND NOMENCLATURE

Movement disorders have been recognized for centuries; however, rigorous scientific studies were mostly initiated in the middle of the last century. Indeed, the category of "sleep-related movement disorders" (SRMD) (Table 1) is a very recent one, introduced in 2006 in the 2nd edition of the *International Classification of Sleep Disorders* (ICSD-2) (1). Figure 1 shows key milestones in the history of SRMD.

The first description of restless legs associated with severe sleep disturbances dates back to the 17th century and was reported by the English physician Sir Thomas Willis. Originally published in Latin in 1672 (2) it was later published in English in *The London Practice of Physick* (3)

> Wherefore to some, when being a Bed they betake themselves to sleep, presently in the Arms and Legs Leapings and Contractions to the Tendons, and so great a Restlessness and Tossing of their Members ensue, that the diseased are no more able to sleep, than if they were in a Place of the greatest Torture (p. 404).

In the 19th and 20th century the disorder was given other names, such as *anxietas tibiarum* by Wittmaack (4) and *leg jitters* by Allison (5). The Swede Karl Axel Ekbom was the first to provide a detailed description of the clinical features of the disorder (6) and first named it *asthenia crurum paraesthetica*. In 1945 (7) he coined the term *restless legs syndrome* (RLS) to distinguish it from other similar conditions and also reported that the syndrome may cluster in families and that there might be a secondary form of RLS in anemia or pregnancy. In recognition of Ekbom's major contribution to the understanding of this condition, it has also been referred to as *Ekbom syndrome*. Alternate names include *focal akathisia* of the legs (1), although this term is used very infrequently. Scientific interest was slow to respond to RLS in earlier years but picked up considerably during the 1980s when Akpinar reported that RLS was treated successfully with levodopa (8), which remained to be the first line of treatment for nearly two decades. Scientific developments were further helped along by the foundation of the International RLS Study Group (IRLSSG) that in 1995 defined uniform and internationally accepted criteria for the diagnosis of RLS (9) which were updated in 2003 (10).

Involuntary leg movements during sleep were first described 1953 by Symonds (11) as *nocturnal myoclonus*, a term that was used until the 1980s. It is generally attributed to Oswald (12) to be the first to record leg movements during sleep in 1959. He recorded mostly *hypnic jerks*, leg movements that occurred at the transition of sleep and wakefulness and during light sleep. The first recording of periodic leg movements during sleep have been performed in patients with RLS by Lugaresi et al., reported in 1965 (13). They were also the first to record periodic leg movements in the absence of RLS (14). In the early 1980s, Coleman (15) introduced the term *periodic movements in sleep* and later *periodic leg movements*, and was the first to propose standardized scoring criteria. In 1993, this scoring criteria were modified by the Atlas Task Force of the American Sleep Disorders Association (now the American Academy of Sleep Medicine) (16), which remained the international standard until 2006 when the World Association of Sleep Medicine (WASM) together with a task force of the IRLSSG modified the criteria for scoring periodic leg movements during sleep and proposed the first criteria for periodic leg movements during wakefulness (17).

Table 1 Some Common Abbreviations Used with Sleep-Related Movement Disorders

Abbreviations	Description
SRMD	Sleep-related movement disorders
RLS	Restless legs syndrome
PLM	Periodic limb movement—one or more movement(s) which meet the criteria for repetitive periodic movements, but not restricted to sleep state
PLMS	Periodic limb movement(s) in sleep—one or more PLM occurring in sleep
PLMW	Periodic limb movement(s) during wake—one or more PLM occurring during wakefulness
PLMD	Periodic limb movement disorder
PLMI	Periodic limb movement index—number of PLM per hour
PLMAI	Periodic limb movement arousal index—number of PLMS per hour of sleep associated with an arousal on polysomnography
SB	Sleep bruxism
RMMA	Rhythmical masticatory muscle activity—three masseter muscle rhythmical contractions in the absence of tooth grinding
RMD	Rhythmic movement disorder

Sleep-related leg cramps are a universal phenomenon and it is estimated that almost everyone will experience at least one leg cramp during a lifetime. In the American English–speaking regions these also go by the name *charley horse*. The most helpful remedy for leg cramps—the stretching of the affected muscle—has already been described by the English physician Thomas Sydenham in 1669 (18). Early medical descriptions date back to the turn of the beginning of the last century when prominent French and German neurologists were of the opinion that muscle cramps might be caused by different medical conditions such as irritability and neurotic states, and fatigue (19). Féré[1] in 1900 (20) thought that the musculature would be irritated by action of chemical fatigue products of unknown composition and that accumulation of fatigue products during daytime would explain nocturnal muscle cramps. The German neurologist Vold, in the same year, even suggested that in nervous individuals musculocutaneous irritation from calf muscles could give rise to psychopathological phenomena like visual hallucinations of cramped calves, both during daytime and during dreams at night (21). Näcke, in 1901, suggested an inverse relationship between dreams and nocturnal muscle cramps, pointing out that accidental leg movements such as the extension of the foot during terrifying dreams may cause muscle cramps (20). Throughout the following decades several other theories regarding the etiology of leg cramps were brought forward that ascribed the phenomenon to vascular origin, with vascular insufficiency as the prime cause [brought forward by Erben in 1928 (22)], to muscular origin as advocated by Bittdorf in 1910 (23), or to neuronal origin as favored by Wernicke in 1904 (24). The first electromyographic (EMG) recording of a leg cramp in the musculus soleus was performed by Dennig in 1926 (25) and later by Denny-Brown and Pennybacker in 1938 (26). Lambert, in 1969, was the first to demonstrate the neurogenic origin of the cramp by verifying that it was impossible to elicit cramps in curarized muscles (27). The first to try quinine with good success in the treatment of leg cramps were Moss and Herrmann in 1940 (28).

Bruxism is another disorder that has been recognized for a long time and the first medical description of the grinding of teeth during sleep is ascribed to Parmele in 1881 (29). Marie and Pietkiewicz introduced the French term *la bruxomania* in 1907 (30) to designate habitual teeth grinding and regarded it as a manifestation of cerebral organic lesions showing familial occurrence in some cases. Not until 1931 was the term *bruxism* introduced into the English language by Frohman (31). Another French term *brycose*—from the Greek word *brycho* for movement with teeth contact—has been used to describe a severe form of bruxism. Diurnal and nocturnal tooth grinding were not clearly differentiated until the middle of the last century, and it has more recently been recognized that there are several differences between the two manifestations. The first polysomnographic recording of sleep-related bruxism was performed by Takahama in 1961 (32). During the night, the jaw contractions can take two forms: sustained jaw clenching, termed tonic contractions, and a series of repetitive muscle contractions termed *rhythmic masticatory muscle activity* (RMMA) (33).

---

[1] Féré C. Les crampes et les paralysies nocturnes. Medicine Moderne.

1672 — **Willis:** first medical description of RLS

Wepfer: first medical description of rhythmic head — **1727**
movement activity occurring at night

1861 — **Wittmaack:** medical description of RLS as
anxietas tibiarum

Putnam–Jacobi: first medical description of rhythmic
body rolling at night as *nocturnal rotary spasm* — **1880**
Parmele: first medical description of grinding of — **1881**
teeth during sleep

Zappert: introduced the term *jactatio capitis nocturna*
for sleep related head banging — **1905**
Marie & Pietkiewicz: introduced the term — **1907**
la bruxomania

1923 — **Oppenheim:** first description of familial RLS

Frohman: introduced the term *bruxism* into the — **1931**
English language

Ekbom: publishes his first description of RLS
1944 — as *Asthenia crurum paraesthetica* (irritable legs)
1945 — **Ekbom:** publishes seminal monograph on
RLS as *Restless Legs*

1953 — **Symonds:** first medical description of leg
movements during sleep as *nocturnal myoclonus*

Oswald: first polysomnographic recording
Takahama: first polysomnographic recording   1959 — of leg movements during sleep
of sleep related bruxism — **1961**

Lugaresi: first polysomnographic recording
Oswald: first polysomnographic recording — **1965** — of PLMS in RLS
of body rocking during sleep   1966 — **Lugaresi:** first polysomnographic recording
of PLMS without RLS

Coleman: first scoring criteria for PLMS and
1980 — introduction of the term *periodic movements
in sleep*
1982 — **Akpinar:** first treatment of RLS with levodopa

1993 — **ASDA:** updated scoring criteria for PLMS
1995 — **IRLSSG:** first diagnostic criteria for RLS

2003 — **IRLSSG:** updated diagnostic criteria for RLS

2006 — **WASM & IRLSSG:** updated scoring criteria
for PLMS, first scoring criteria for PLMW

Figure 1   Key milestones in the history of sleep-related movement disorders.

Sleep-related rhythmic movement disorder (RMD) may present in different forms, which consequently have given rise to different names throughout the years. The first medical description of rhythmic head movement activity during the night is ascribed to Wepfer[2] in 1727 [as cited by Cruchet (34)]. More than 150 years later in 1880 Putnam-Jacobi (35) gave a detailed medical description of rhythmic body rolling occurring at night.

> A few weeks later I had an opportunity of observing a nocturnal paroxysm. This began punctually at 9, the child having fallen asleep at 7. At first the rotation was confined to the head [...]. But a little later after some interruption, the movement changed. With the left hand over the left ear, the child began rotating the entire upper half of his body, softly, rhythmically, about seventy times a minute. The head moved with the shoulders and trunk: the lower limbs remained quiescent. A little later in the evening, this rotation was accompanied by a crooning cry, also rhythmical. The child had the air of rocking himself to sleep to his own lullaby (p. 393).

The author described this behavior as *nocturnal rotary spasm*, which at that time was used to describe nocturnal epileptic seizures, but was of the opinion that the disorder was not of epileptic origin. The first term, still common today, was coined by Zappert in 1905 (36), who described nocturnal head banging as *jactatio capitis nocturna*. At the same time Cruchet described various forms of nocturnal rhythmic movements first as *tics du sommeil* (1905) (37) and later as *rhythmies du sommeil* (1912) (38). One of the most detailed descriptions of the different forms of rhythmic movements, namely head banging, head rolling, and body rolling was given by de Lissovoy in 1962 (39). Oswald was the first in 1965 to perform a polysomnographic recording of head and body rocking during sleep that occurred during all sleep stages but with the majority occurring during rapid eye movement (REM) sleep (40). Rhythmic movements restricted solely to REM sleep were first reported in 1977 by Regestein who presented a report on a 25-year-old woman with head movement activity occurring nightly (41). In the scientific literature until now, less than 100 polysomnographically documented cases of sleep-related RMDs have been reported (42).

KEY FEATURES AND CHARACTERISTICS

SRMD are relatively simple, stereotyped movements or monophasic movement disorders such as sleep-related leg cramps that disturb sleep. An exception is RLS, which has been included into this diagnostic category due to its close association with periodic limb movements during sleep (PLMS). Common to all SRMD are complaints of disturbed sleep, daytime sleepiness, and/or fatigue, which are a prerequisite for the diagnosis, as opposed to mere incidental findings during nocturnal polysomnography.

RLS is characterized by an imperative desire to move the extremities associated with paresthesias, motor restlessness, worsening of symptoms at rest and in the evening or at night and, as a consequence, sleep disturbances (Table 2). In 1995, the IRLSSG developed standardized criteria for the diagnosis of RLS (9), which have been recently modified (10), and are included in the ICSD-2 criteria. Supportive clinical features for RLS are a positive family history for RLS, an initial response to dopaminergic therapy and the presence of PLMS. The clinical course of the disorder varies considerably and in some patients RLS can be intermittent and may spontaneously remit for many years. To diagnose RLS in pediatric patients, the child meets four essential adult criteria for RLS and is in addition either able to relate an indicative description in his or her own words or at least two of the following criteria are met: a sleep disturbance, a biological sibling or parent with definite RLS, or more than five periodic leg movements per hour of sleep, documented by polysomnography. Diagnostic criteria in other special populations such as the cognitively impaired elderly have also been proposed (10).

The presence of PLMS is the key feature of the periodic limb movement disorder (PLMD). Periodic limb movements (PLM), which may also occur during relaxed wakefulness (PLMW, periodic limb movement(s) during wake), are highly regular, jerky, stereotyped, unilateral or bilateral movements, and are characterized by involuntary repetitive extensions

---

[2] Wepfer JJ. Observationes medico-practicae, de affectibus capitis internis & externis. Schaffhausen: Joh. Adam Ziegler, 1727

Table 2 Key Features of Sleep-Related Movement Disorders

Key features of all SRMDs
1 Complaint of sleep disturbances, daytime sleepiness, or fatigue
2 The disorders are not better explained by another current sleep disorder, medical or neurological disorder, mental disorder, medication use, or substance use disorder

Key features of RLS (adults)
1 An urge to move the legs, usually accompanied or caused by uncomfortable and unpleasant sensations in the legs
2 The urge to move or unpleasant sensations begin or worsen during periods of rest or inactivity such as lying or sitting
3 The urge to move or unpleasant sensations are partially or totally relieved by movement such as walking or stretching, at least as long as the activity continues
4 The urge to move or unpleasant sensations are worse in the evening or night than during the day or only occur in the evening or night

Key features of PLMD
1 Repetitive, highly stereotyped limb movements (PLMS) during nocturnal polysomnography
2 PLMS index >15 in adults, PLMS index >5 in children

Key features of sleep-related leg cramps
1 Strong muscle contraction associated with a painful sensation in the leg or foot and sudden muscle hardness or tightness
2 The leg cramp occurs during the sleep period although it may arise from either sleep or wakefulness
3 The pain is relieved by forceful stretching of the affected muscles

Key features of sleep-related bruxism
1 Teeth-grinding sounds or teeth clenching during sleep
2 Abnormal wear of teeth OR discomfort, fatigue or pain of the jaw muscle and jaw lock upon awakening OR masseter muscle hypertrophy upon voluntary forceful clenching

Key features of sleep-related rhythmic movement disorder
1 Repetitive, stereotyped, and rhythmic motor behaviors
2 Movements involve large muscle groups and occur predominantly during sleep, near bedtime or naptime or when the subject is drowsy or sleepy
3 Movements interfere with normal sleep OR significant impairment in daytime functioning OR self-inflicted bodily injury that requires medical treatment

---

of the big toe, often accompanied by flexions of the hip, knees, and ankles. In some cases, the arms may be affected as well. For a limb movement to be considered a periodic limb movement, its amplitude must exceed an 8-microvolt increase in EMG voltage above resting EMG, the duration is between 0.5 and 10 seconds, and the intermovement interval measured from onset to onset lies between 5 and 90 seconds. Only movements that occur in a sequence of at least four movements are considered. Refined standards for recording and scoring periodic leg movements have been proposed by the WASM in collaboration with a task force of the IRLSSG (17). The PLMS index refers to the number of PLMS per hour of sleep. Sleep-related breathing disorders should be excluded as a direct cause of the PLMS since repetitive breathing pauses and the associated arousals may in turn lead to repetitive body movements including the limbs that may mimic PLMS. PLMS may be associated with an arousal or a brief awakening. Typically, the patient is unaware of the limb movements or the frequent sleep disruptions, and it is the observation of the bed partner that suggests the presence of PLMS. Indeed, PLMS can be significantly disruptive to the bed partner's sleep. Because PLMS are a frequent finding in non-complaining subjects, especially in the elderly (see next section on prevalence), the clinical significance has to be carefully evaluated, taking the sleep-related and daytime functioning–related complaints into account.

Sleep-related leg cramps are painful sensations caused by sudden and intense involuntary contractions of muscles usually in the calf or foot. They occur during the sleep period but may arise from either sleep or wakefulness. Sometimes the leg cramps may be preceded by a less painful warning sensation. The cramp may last up to several minutes and remits spontaneously; it can be relieved by a strong stretching of the affected muscle or sometimes movement, massage, or the application of heat. Discomfort and tenderness in the muscle may persist for several hours after the cramp. The sleep-related leg cramp causes pain and also reduces sleep due to the activities used to reduce the pain but also due to the persisting discomfort after the cramp. The frequency of sleep-related leg cramps varies widely from less than yearly to repeated episodes every night. Leg cramps may occur primarily during the daytime, primarily during sleep, or during both day and night. Only when they occur primarily during sleep and are associated with disturbed sleep are they considered sleep-related leg cramps.

Sleep-related bruxism is characterized by forceful rhythmical grinding or clenching of the teeth during sleep. Jaw contractions during sleep may present as tonic contractions (isolated sustained jaw clenching) or as a series of repetitive phasic muscle contractions (RMMA). Most patients are completely unaware of these nocturnal contractions, but their bed partners may complain of disturbance from the clicking or grating sound. Sleep-related bruxism may be associated with brief arousals from sleep but rarely with awakenings. The repetitive nocturnal clenching may lead to the complaint of morning jaw discomfort, which usually improves over the course of the day. Bruxism can lead to significant tooth damage, dental thermal hypersensitivity, hypermobility, hypercementosis, or the need for dental restoration. Sleep-related bruxism may also be associated with headaches. There is considerable variability in the duration and intensity of sleep-related bruxism. Bruxism may also occur during daytime but is characterized more by tooth clenching and jaw bracing without tooth contact. In contrast to sleep-related bruxism, tooth grinding is rarely noted during the daytime.

RMDs mostly occur during sleep onset but may emerge also at other times during the night and even during quiet wakeful activities. RMD is typically seen in infants and children and includes several subtypes of movements. Sleep-related RMD is characterized by repetitive, stereotyped, rhythmic motor behaviors that occur predominantly during drowsiness or sleep involving large muscle groups. Body rocking may occur either when the child is on the hands and knees (with the whole body thrust in an anterior-posterior direction) or when sitting (rocking of the torso). Head banging often occurs with the child prone, involving violent moving of the head in an anterior-posterior direction. Typically, the head is banged into a pillow, occasionally into a wall or the side of a crib. Because of the forceful nature of the head movements this form of RMD is often the most injurious. Head rolling is associated with the head being rotated from side to side, usually in a supine position. Less common rhythmic movement forms include body rolling, leg banging, or leg rolling. Rhythmic humming or sounds—sometimes quite loud—may accompany the body, head, or limb movements. The duration of RMD episodes is variable and so is their frequency. However, most episodes last less than 15 minutes and the typical frequency of the rhythmic movements is between 0.5 and 2 seconds.

INCIDENCE AND PREVALENCE

SRMD differ in terms of their overall and gender- and age-dependent prevalence (Table 3). Prevalence estimates are well established for RLS, largely unknown for sleep-related RMD and difficult to assess for sleep bruxism and PLMD due to the considerable day-to-day variability of these disorders and due to the reliance on the observation of a bed partner who might be missing, especially in the older population. Prevalence estimates for RLS symptoms of any severity range from 5% to 15% in the U.S. and European population studies (43). About 2% to 4% of the population is expected to exhibit RLS symptoms that occur at least weekly and are associated with sleep disturbances and/or daytime dysfunction (44). The prevalence of RLS increases linearly with age (44) and women are twice as likely to experience RLS (45). Most notably, about 20% to 30% of women will experience RLS in varying severity during pregnancy (74).

The finding of an increased PLMS index ($\geq$5/hr of sleep) with nocturnal polysomnography increases with age. A PLMS index above 5 can be found in up to 40% to 60% of subjects older than 60 years (53–55). In middle-aged healthy populations (mean age 40–50 years) polysomnographically verified prevalence estimates between 5% (50) and 18% (51) have been reported, while in a study using actigraphy, 52% of men and 22% of women had a PLM index $\geq$5/hr of time in bed (52). Prevalence estimates in healthy children are lacking but in two studies the prevalence of PLMS >5/hr was between 5% and 23% in children referred to a sleep laboratory (48,49). In both studies, however, the occurrence of an elevated PLMS index without any other sleep relevant finding was substantially lower (0.08% and 1.2%). The mere occurrence of increased PLMS, however, must be distinguished from PLMD, which includes some daytime complaint that accompanies the nocturnal disturbances. One very large-scale epidemiological study, using a detailed telephone interview and the ICSD criteria from 1990,

Table 3 Prevalence of Sleep-Related Movement Disorders

		Prevalence (%)	Relation to age and gender	References
Restless legs syndrome				
Symptoms		5–10	Women ↑; Age ↑	43–46
Diagnosis[a]		2–6	Women ↑; Age ↑	44,46,47
Periodic limb movement disorder				
PLMS	Children	0–1		48,49
	Adults	6–37	Women ↑↓; Age ↑↓	50–52
	Elderly >65 yr	40–60	Age ↑	53–55
PLMD diagnosis[a]		4	Women ↑	47[b]
Sleep-related leg cramps				
Symptoms	Children	7	Age ↑	56
	Adults	12–25	Women ↑; Age ↑	57–59
	Elderly	30–60	Age ↑	60–62
Diagnosis[a]		0.2		63[b]
Sleep-related bruxism				
Symptoms	Children	12–28	Age ↓	64–67
	Adults	5–10	Age ↓	68–70
Diagnosis[a]		4	Age ↓	69[b]
Sleep-related rhythmic movement disorder				
Symptoms	Children <3 yr	5–30	Age ↓	66,71–73
	Children >3 yr	3–5	Age ↓	66,71
	Adults	?		
Diagnosis[a]		?		

[a]The term "diagnosis" refers to complaints that are associated with daytime consequences and of at least moderate frequency.
[b]Diagnosis made with Sleep-EVAL system.

established prevalence rates of 3.9% in a random multinational population sample of 18,980 subjects (47). In this study no increase with age was found and PLMD was more frequent in women than in men (4.6% vs. 3.1%).

Leg cramps are a common condition with reported prevalence rates of 7.3% in children (56), 15% in young adults (57), 20% to 30% in middle-aged adults (58), and up to 60% in the elderly (60,61). Incidence rates in the elderly are considerably lower and range between 14% [4 weeks incidence (75)] and 30% [two months incidence (62)]. In one study, frequent awakenings due to leg cramps were reported by 8.7% of men and 12.1% of women in the Sleep Heart Health Study comprising 6440 men and women aged 40 years or older (59). There seems to be a slightly higher prevalence in women as evidenced by significant differences only emerging in very large-scale studies (58,59).

Bruxism is another very common condition with nocturnal teeth grinding reported in about 14% to 30% in children (64–66), 5% to 15% in young adults (68,69), 8% of adults (69,70), and only 3% of individuals aged 60 years or older (70). In general, no major gender difference in nocturnal bruxism has been observed (69,70).

Rhythmic movements during bedtime or sleep are a frequent finding during childhood. Incidence rates of around 30% have been reported for any rhythmic behavior below the age of 1 year decreasing rapidly with age (71), with prevalence of body rocking being around 18% in children up to 10 years (66,72) and around 5% for head banging (72,73). After the age of 10 years, prevalence rates decrease to around 3% (66). In older children, stereotypic movements may be associated with mental retardation, autism, and pervasive developmental disorder. Case reports indicate that RMDs may persist into adulthood (76) but prevalence rates are unknown.

PHYLOGENY AND ANIMAL MODELS

There are only a few animal models for SRMD. Those for RLS are facing a serious challenge since the clinical diagnosis of this disorder relies exclusively on the description of the patient. Nevertheless, behavioral observations of the latency to sleep and episodes of standing upright in rats with 6-hydroxydopamine (6-OHDA) lesions into the A11 nucleus (77) and computer-based analysis of polysomnographic sleep stages during the dark period in iron-deprived mice (78) have been used as proxies for restless legs symptoms in animals. The direct injection of 6-OHDA in the A11 was based on the hypothesis that lesioning of the diencephalic-spinal dopaminergic nucleus could potentially induce behavioral correlates to the clinical symptoms of RLS. In a small number of animals Ondo et al. (77) found that the lesioned animals showed an increased number and duration of standing episodes, although total sleep time was unchanged. In addition, the number and duration of standing episodes was reduced after administration of pramipexole. However, PLM or similar correlates were not observed in the animals and sleep evaluation was based solely on behavioral observation. Based on the role of iron in the pathophysiology of RLS, Dean et al. (78) obtained polysomnograms of young adult, nutritionally iron deprived, C57BL-6J mice. In accordance with their hypothesis, an increased wake time and consequently decreased sleep time were observed selectively at the end of the dark period (the period of activity). So far, it remains a challenge to the field of animal models for RLS to find the adequate correlate to the primary feature of RLS: the sensation. Other approaches, such as a forced-choice paradigm between environments with restricted mobility but no punishment on the one hand, and unrestricted mobility but some punishment on the other hand, have been proposed (79) but not realized so far.

An animal model for PLM (found in 80% to 90% of RLS patients) seems another promising approach. Okura et al. (80) were the first to describe spontaneous PLM in narcoleptic Doberman dogs. The movements were characterized by repetitive dorsiflexions of the ankle, lasting 0.5 to 1.5 seconds that occurred in intervals of 3 to 20 seconds, similar to those found in humans. An increased number of PLMS is also found in human narcoleptic subjects (81,82). In a more detailed study of PLM in rats, Baier et al. (83) recorded hind limb movements using subcutaneously implanted magnets and magneto-inductive device, which were scored according to criteria similar to those applied in humans. Periodic hind limb movements (PHLM) were observed in 4 of 10 old rats but in none of the young rats, which is in accordance with the increased prevalence of PLMS in elderly subjects. However, administration of the classical dopamine antagonist haloperidol affected neither the sleep patterns nor the number of PHLM in the old rats. Overall, Baier et al. (83) were able to set up a reliable method for detecting PHLM in rats in relation to a sleep recording. The development of a behavioral condition that captures the primary feature of RLS as a disorder of sensation rather than movement remains an important goal for animal RLS models.

Several attempts have been made to develop animal models of bruxism, although none of these have been totally accepted as valid (84). Animal models for bruxism were introduced in the 1960s by Kawamura et al. (85) who produced grinding of teeth in rabbits by using high-frequency electrical stimulation in the cortical jaw motor area of the brain while monitoring masseter and digastric muscle activity with a kymograph and teeth contact noise with a tape recorder. They concluded that teeth grinding resulted from abnormal excitation of cerebral cells in some parts of the cortical jaw motor areas. These findings were extended in a later work by this group (86), again on rabbits, but this time using intraoral radiotransmitters to record tooth contacts and stimulation of various areas of the central nervous system (CNS) including the amygdala and the lateral hypothalamic area. Teeth contacts were regularly recorded with amygdala stimulation. Since then a variety of other paradigms have been used such as sound recording of bruxism episodes in the rat (87), high-resolution optoelectronic mandibular tracking and EMG of the anterior temporalis muscle (88), behavioral rating of nonfunctional masticatory activity and the measurement of incisal attrition (84), and behavioral observation and radiographic examination of teeth in Macaca monkeys (89).

Two different approaches to the pathophysiology of bruxism were developed and have by now merged: one concentrating on the involvement of the central catecholaminergic system and its relationship to stress, and a second line focusing on occlusal disharmonies as a trigger for bruxism. The placement of caps on the upper incisors of the rat causes cyclic EMG bursts in masseter muscles during nonfunctional activity, which resemble those recorded for bruxism (90). On the other side, activation of central dopaminergic receptors by apomorphine induces oral stereotyped behavior and in high doses also chattering and scraping of the teeth, considered as a form of drug-induced experimental bruxism (91). In addition, the degree of bruxism induced by high doses of apomorphine is greater after placement of incisal caps (84,87). Overall, diverse studies have pointed to alterations in central neurotransmission, particularly dopaminergic neurotransmission, as the principal cause of bruxism. However, the evidence also suggests that in animals, alterations in occlusion, which result in modified oral sensory inputs to the CNS, influence central dopaminergic neurotransmission. It must be pointed out, however, that animal studies have made no specific attempt to distinguish between daytime and nocturnal bruxism and thus the applicability to the sleep disorder bruxism has yet to be established.

There are no specific animal models for sleep-related RMDs. However, animal models have been developed to study stereotypies, i.e., repetitive, invariant behavior patterns with no obvious goal or function, which may also include head banging, head rolling, or body rocking but without reference to the time of day of their occurrence. Stereotypic behavior has been studied in the context of drug-induced paradigms, environmental restriction, learning or conditioning settings, and genetic studies. For example, head banging in pigeons (92) and monkeys (93) has been brought under experimental control, and reinforced, extinguished, and reestablished based on learning paradigms. This corresponds to hypotheses regarding the potential rewarding or reinforcing nature of SRMD itself and the successful application of the learning paradigm to extinguish head banging in retarded children (94–96). Pharmacological animal models typically use dopaminergic agonists [e.g., levodopa (97), dopamine agonists (98), amphetamine (99), cocaine (100), apomorphine (101)] to induce motor stereotypic behavior in animals. Stereotypic behavior due to restricted environments can be found in a broad range of animal species (102). The forms of stereotyped behavior depend on the species and the specific environmental constraints and among others include jumping, bar chewing, head swinging, and pacing. More recent approaches focus on establishing a genetic basis for stereotypic behavior and used a mouse model of human trisomy 21 in which an increased rate of spontaneous stereotypy compared to the control animals was observed (103). However, as with bruxism, it must be stressed that none of animal models focused on stereotypic behavior occurring during sleep and that generalizations to sleep-related RMD, therefore, are questionable.

To the best of our knowledge, no animal models for sleep-related leg cramps have been developed.

SOCIAL AND ECONOMIC FACTORS

So far, detailed analyses of the impact of SRMD on economics and society are largely lacking in terms of concrete costs. A significant burden of SRMD to the individual has to be assumed in entirety, because by definition the nocturnal movements and complaints have to be associated with sleepiness, daytime sleepiness or fatigue. However, there is a striking omission of quality of life research with respect to PLMD, leg cramps, bruxism, and RMD. The exception is RLS where several large-scale studies have shown that in subjects with RLS quality of life is significantly impaired both on general measures such as the Medical Outcomes Study Short Form-36 (SF-36) (46,104) as well as in disease-specific instruments such as the American (105) and German Restless Legs Syndrome Quality of Life Questionnaires (106). The areas most often impaired in RLS subjects relate to vitality and fatigue dimensions. In addition, a detailed analysis using structural equation modeling showed that the impact of RLS on decreased functional alertness and emotional distress was almost completely mediated by the sleep disturbances (107). As for PLMD, there is only one study on quality of life; the investigators found no difference in quality of life between 30 PLMD subjects and 30 matched controls (108). Studies assessing quality of life in sufferers of nocturnal leg cramps are lacking so far. For sleep bruxism, there is one study showing that quality of life was reduced in 19 individuals with nocturnal bruxism, in particular, those who reported pain (109). For RMD, again systematic studies are lacking; however, from the published case reports (42) it seems that the persistence of RMD into adulthood is associated with significant distress for the individual.

Costs for sleep disorders divide into direct (e.g., hospitalization, medication, therapy) and indirect costs (e.g., missed income, reduced work performance) (110). Detailed analyses have shown that the economic costs for sleep disorders in general (111,112), for insomnia (113,114), and for daytime sleepiness (115–117) are enormous, but to which extent this applies to SRMD as disorders associated with either insomnia or daytime sleepiness is unclear.

Increased direct or indirect costs for RLS, PLMD, and sleep bruxism could be inferred from the few available studies. In the 2005 National Sleep Foundation Poll, individuals with restless legs symptoms reported to be more often late to work, missing work because of sleepiness, and making errors at work (118). In addition, they reported missing events and driving drowsy more frequently than subjects without restless legs symptoms (118). In a group of 26 patients with PLMS or restless legs, four patients had been involved in traffic accidents (119). Accident rates are not available for any other SRMD, but two population studies (69,120) have reported that subjects with sleep bruxism not only consulted a dentist more often and needed dental work but also consulted a physician more often than subjects without bruxism.

OTHER SLEEP-RELATED MOVEMENT DISORDERS

A clinician may encounter other SRMD that do not belong to the diagnosed conditions described above. The ICSD-2 lists three additional diagnoses within the class of SRMD. *Sleep-related movement disorder due to drug or substance* refers to those SRMD in which the movement is due to a drug or substance. This may include dependence, abuse, poisoning, adverse effects, or underdosing of a drug. The diagnosis *sleep-related movement disorder due to medical condition* is intended for a sleep-related movement disorder for which there is a clinical suspicion that an underlying medical or neurological condition may cause the sleep disorder. *Sleep-related movement disorder, unspecified* is assigned when the sleep-related movement disorder cannot be classified elsewhere or is suspected to be associated with an underlying psychiatric condition that causes the movement disorder. All three diagnoses can serve as a temporary diagnosis and often will be in the case where an association with a medical or psychiatric condition or a drug is suspected. For example, once a medical condition is established that caused the movement disorder, this condition becomes the sole diagnosis unless the sleep complaint is unusually severe, the complaint needs the specialized skills of a sleep specialist, or the relationship between sleep disruption and the supposed underlying condition is questionable.

CONCLUSIONS

Movement disorders have been observed for centuries; however, the term "sleep-related movement disorders" is relatively new and this category of sleep disorders includes RLS, PLMD, sleep-related leg cramps, sleep-related bruxism, and sleep-related RMD. Each SRMD has separate key features and characteristics, yet they share common complaints of disturbed sleep, daytime sleepiness, and/or fatigue. SRMD also vary considerably in their overall as well as gender- and age-dependent prevalence, and some of the disorders in this category do not have prevalence estimates. There are a few animal models that have been proposed for SRMD; a challenge to the field is to find adequate animal preparations that can serve as a model of the sensory symptoms that are key characteristics of the human disorders. Extensive or detailed analyses of the impact of SRMD on economics and society are largely lacking, although there are studies that explore the impact of some SRMD on quality of life and direct or indirect costs can be inferred from other studies that evaluated the work performance, health utilization, or accident rates of patients with SRMD.

REFERENCES

1. American Academy of Sleep Medicine. The international classification of sleep disorders: diagnostic and coding manual. Westchester, Illinois: American Academy of Sleep Medicine, 2005.
2. Willis T. De Animae Brutorum. London: Wells and Scott, 1672.
3. Willis T. The London practice of physick: or the whole practical part of physick contained in the works of Dr. Willis. Faithfully made English, and printed together for the publick good. London: Basset and Crooke, 1685.
4. Wittmaack T. Pathologie und Therapie der Sensibilität-Neurosen. Leipzig: E. Schäfer, 1861.
5. Allison FG. Obscure pains in the chest, back or limbs. Can Med Assoc J 1943; 48:36–38.

6. Ekbom KA. Asthenia crurum paraesthetica ('irritable legs'). New syndrome consisting of weakness, sensation of cold and nocturnal paresthesia in legs, responding to certain extent to treatment with Priscol and Doryl; note on paresthesia in general. Acta Med Scand 1944; 118:197–209.
7. Ekbom KA. Restless legs: clinical study of hitherto overlooked disease in legs characterized by peculiar paresthesia ('anxietas tibiarum'), pain and weakness and occurring in two main forms, asthenia crurum paresthetica and asthenia crurum dolorosa; short review of paresthesias in general. Acta Med Scand 1945; 158:1–123.
8. Akpinar S. Treatment of restless legs syndrome with levodopa plus benserazide. Arch Neurol 1982; 39:739.
9. Walters AS. Toward a better definition of the restless legs syndrome. The International Restless Legs Syndrome Study Group. Mov Disord 1995; 10:634–642.
10. Allen RP, Picchietti D, Hening WA, et al. Restless legs syndrome: diagnostic criteria, special considerations, and epidemiology. A report from the restless legs syndrome diagnosis and epidemiology workshop at the National Institutes of Health. Sleep Med 2003; 4:101–119.
11. Symonds CP. Nocturnal myoclonus. J Neurol Neurosurg Psychiatry 1953; 16:166–171.
12. Oswald I. Sudden bodily jerks on falling asleep. Brain 1959; 81:92–103.
13. Lugaresi E, Coccagna G, Tassinari CA, et al. Rilievi poligrafici sui fenomeni motori nella sindrome delle gambe senza riposo. Riv Neurol 1965; 35:550–561.
14. Lugaresi E, Coccagna G, Gambi D, et al. [Apropos of some nocturnal myoclonic manifestations. (Symond's nocturnal myoclonus)]. Rev Neurol 1966; 115:547–555.
15. Coleman RM, Pollak CP, Weitzman ED. Periodic movements in sleep (nocturnal myoclonus): relation to sleep disorders. Ann Neurol 1980; 8:416–421.
16. American Sleep Disorders Association. Recording and scoring leg movements. The Atlas Task Force. Sleep 1993; 16:748–759.
17. Zucconi M, Ferri R, Allen R, et al. The official World Association of Sleep Medicine (WASM) standards for recording and scoring periodic leg movements in sleep (PLMS) and wakefulness (PLMW) developed in collaboration with a task force from the International Restless Legs Syndrome Study Group (IRLSSG). Sleep Med 2006; 7:175–183.
18. Sydenham T. Epistolae responsoriae, I, 7, 1669. In: Latham RG, ed. The works of Thomas Sydenham, Vol 11. London: Sydenham Society, 1848.
19. Jansen PHP, Joosten EMG, Vingerhoets HM. Muscle cramp: main theories as to aetiology. Eur Arch Psychiatry Clin Neurosci 1990; 239:337–342.
20. Näcke P. Zur Pathogenese und Klinik der Wadenkrämpfe. Neurol Zentralbl 1901; 7:290–296.
21. Vold E. Ueber "Hallucinationen" vorzüglich "Gesichtshallucinationen". Allg Z Psychiatr 1900; 17:654.
22. Erben S. Ueber den Crampus und seine Bekämpfung. Wien Klin Wochenschr 1928; 43:1499–1501.
23. Bittorf A. Zu Kenntnis der Muskelkrämpfe peripheren Ursprungs und verwandter Erscheinungen. Dtsch Z Nervenheilk 1910; 39:208–227.
24. Wernicke C. Ein Fall von Crampus-Neurose. Berl Klin Wochenschr 1904; 43:1121–1124.
25. Dennig H. Über den Muskelcrampus. Dtsch Z Nervenheilk 1926; 93:96–104.
26. Denny-Brown D, Pennybacker JB. Fibrillation and fasciculation in voluntary muscle. Brain 1938; 61:311–334.
27. Lambert EH. Electromyography in amyotrophic lateral sclerosis. In: Norris FH, Kurland LT, eds. Motor neuron diseases and related disorders. New York: Gruner & Stratton, 1969:135–153.
28. Moss HK, Herrmann LG. Quinine for relief of night cramps in the extremities. JAMA 1940; 115:1358–1359.
29. Parmele GL. The grinding of teeth during sleep. Dent Cosmos 1881; 23:668.
30. Pietkiewicz M, Marie MM. La bruxomania: memoires originaux. Revue Stomatol 1907; 14:107–116.
31. Frohman BS. The application of psychotherapy to dental problems. Dent Cosmos 1931; 73:1117–1122.
32. Takahama Y. Bruxism. J Dent Res 1961; 40:227.
33. Lavigne GJ, Lobbezoo F, Montplaisir J. The genesis of rhythmic masticatory muscle activity and bruxism during sleep. In: Morimoto T, Matsuya T, Takada T, eds. Brain and Oral Functions. Amsterdam: Elsevier, 1995:249–255.
34. Cruchet R. Traité des Torticolis Spasmodiques, Spasmes, Tics, Rhythmies Du Cou, Torticolis Mental, etc. Paris: Masson et Cie, 1907.
35. Putnam-Jacobi M. Case of nocturnal rotary spasm. J Nerv Ment Dis 1880; 7:390–402.
36. Zappert J. Über nächtliche Kopfbewegungen bei Kindern (Jactatio capitis nocturna). Jahrb Kinderheilkd 1905; 62:70–83.
37. Cruchet R. Tics et sommeil. Presse Med 1905; 13:33–36.
38. Cruchet R. Six nouveaux cas de rhythmies du sommeil (les rhythmies a la caserne). Gaz Hebd Sci Med 1912; 33:303–308.
39. de Lissovoy V. Head banging in early childhood. Child Dev 1962; 33:43–56.
40. Oswald I. The mechanism of sleep disorders: some recent advances. Int J Neurology 1965; 5:187–195.

41. Regestein QR, Hartmann E, Reich P. A head movement disorder occurring in dreaming sleep. J Neurol Nerv Ment Dis 1977; 164:432–436.
42. Kohyama J, Matsukura F, Kimura K, et al. Rhythmic movement disorder: polysomnographic study and summary of reported cases. Brain Dev 2002; 24:33–38.
43. Masood A, Phillips B. Epidemiology of restless legs syndrome. In: Chokroverty S, Hening WA, Walters AS, eds. Sleep and Movement Disorders. Philadelphia: Butterworth Heinemann, 2003: 316–321.
44. Allen RP, Walters AS, Montplaisir J, et al. Restless legs syndrome prevalence and impact. REST general population study. Arch Int Med 2005; 165:1286–1292.
45. Berger K, Luedemann J, Trenkwalder C, et al. Sex and the risk of restless legs syndrome in the general population. Arch Int Med 2004; 164:196–202.
46. Hening W, Walters AS, Allen RP, et al. Impact, diagnosis and treatment of restless legs syndrome (RLS) in a primary care population: the REST (RLS epidemiology, symptoms, and treatment) primary care study. Sleep Med 2004; 5:237–246.
47. Ohayon MM, Roth T. Prevalence of restless legs syndrome and periodic limb movement disorder in the general population. J Psychosom Res 2002; 53:547–554.
48. Kirk VG, Bohn S. Periodic limb movements in children: prevalence in a referred population. Sleep 2004; 27:313–315.
49. Martinez S, Guilleminault C. Periodic leg movements in prepubertal children with sleep disturbances. Dev Med Child Neurol 2004; 46:765–770.
50. Bixler EO, Kales A, Vela-Bueno A, et al. Nocturnal myoclonus and nocturnal myoclonic activity in the normal population. Res Commun Chem Pathol Pharmacol 1982; 36:129–140.
51. Schiavi RC, Stimmel BB, Mandeli J, et al. Diabetes, sleep disorders, and male sexual function. Biol Psychiatry 1993; 34:171–177.
52. Morrish E, King MA, Pilsworth SN, et al. Periodic limb movement in a community population detected by a new actigraphy technique. Sleep Med 2002; 3:489–495.
53. Ancoli-Israel S, Kripke DF, Klauber MR, et al. Periodic limb movements in sleep in community-dwelling elderly. Sleep 1991; 14:496–500.
54. Dickel MJ, Mosko SS. Morbidity cut-offs for sleep apnea and periodic leg movements in predicting subjective complaints in seniors. Sleep 1990; 13:155–166.
55. Claman DM, Redline S, Blackwell T, et al. Prevalence and correlates of periodic limb movements in older women. J Clin Sleep Med 2006; 2:438–445.
56. Leung AK, Wong BE, Chan PY, et al. Nocturnal leg cramps in children: incidence and clinical characteristics. J Natl Med Assoc 1999; 91:329–332.
57. Norris FH, Gasteiger EL, Chatfield PO. An elctromyographic study of induced and spontaneous muscle cramps. Electroencephalogr Clin Neurophysiol 1957; 9:139–147.
58. Gulich M, Heil P, Zeitler HP. Epidemiology and determinants of nocturnal calf cramps. Eur J Gen Pract 1998; 4:109–113.
59. Baldwin CM, Kapur VK, Holberg CJ, et al. Associations between gender and measures of daytime somnolence in the Sleep Heart Health Study. Sleep 2004; 27:305–311.
60. Hall AJ. Cramp and salt balance in ordinary life. Lancet 1947; 3:231–233.
61. Oboler SK, Prochazka AV, Meyer TJ. Leg symptoms in outpatient veterans. West J Med 1991; 155:256–259.
62. Naylor JR, Young JB. A general population survey of rest cramps. Age Ageing 1994; 23:418–420.
63. Ohayon MM, Ferini-Strambi L, Plazzi G, et al. Frequency of narcolepsy symptoms and other sleep disorders in narcoleptic patients and their first-degree relatives. J Sleep Res 2005; 14:437–445.
64. Abe K, Shimakawa M. Genetic and developmental aspects of sleeptalking and teethgrinding. Acta Paedopsychiatr 1966; 33:339–344.
65. Widmalm SE, Christiansen RL, Gunn SM. Oral parafunctions as temporomandibular disorder risk factors in children. Cranio 1995; 13:242–246.
66. Laberge L, Tremblay RE, Vitaro F, et al. Development of parasomnias from childhood to early adolescence. Pediatrics 2000; 106:67–74.
67. Reding GR, Rubright WC, Zimmerman SO. Incidence of Bruxism. J Dent Res 1966; 45:1198–1204.
68. Glaros AG. Incidence of diurnal and nocturnal bruxism. J Prosthet Dent 1981; 45:545–549.
69. Ohayon MM, Li KK, Guilleminault C. Risk factors for sleep bruxism in the general population. Chest 2001; 119:53–61.
70. Lavigne GJ, Montplaisir JY. Restless legs syndrome and sleep bruxism: prevalence and association among Canadians. Sleep 1994; 17:739–743.
71. Klackenberg G. Rhythmic movements in infancy and early childhood. Acta Paediatr Scand 1971; 224 (suppl):74–82.
72. Sallustro F, Atwell CW. Body rocking, head banging, and head rolling in normal children. J Pediatr 1978; 93:704–708.

73. Kravitz H, Rosenthal V, Teplitz Z, et al. A study of head-banging in infants and children. Dis Nerv Syst 1960; 21:203–208.

74. Manconi M, Govoni V, De Vito A, et al. Restless legs syndrome and pregnancy. Neurology 2004; 63:1065–1069.

75. Gentili A, Weiner DK, Kuchibhatla M, et al. Factors that disturb sleep in nursing home residents. Aging Clin Exp Res 1997; 9:207–213.

76. Stepanova I, Nevsimalova S, Hanusova J. Rhythmic movement disorder in sleep persisting into childhood and adulthood. Sleep 2005; 28:851–857.

77. Ondo WG, He Y, Rajasekaran S, et al. Clinical correlates of 6-hydroxydopamine injections into A11 dopaminergic neurons in rats: a possible model for restless legs syndrome. Mov Disord 2000; 15: 154–158.

78. Dean T, Allen RP, O'Donnell CP, et al. The effects of dietary iron deprivation on murine circadian sleep architecture. Sleep Med 2006; 7:634–640.

79. Earley CJ, Allen RP, Beard JL, et al. Insight into the pathophysiology of restless legs syndrome. J Neurosci Res 2000; 62:623–628.

80. Okura M, Fujiki N, Ripley B, et al. Narcoleptic canines display periodic leg movements during sleep. Psychiatry Clin Neurosci 2001; 55:243–244.

81. Bédard MA, Montplaisir J, Godbout R. Effect of L-dopa on periodic movements in sleep in narcolepsy. Eur Neurol 1987; 27:35–38.

82. Boivin DB, Montplaisir J, Poirier G. The effects of L-dopa on periodic leg movements and sleep organization in narcolepsy. Clin Neuropharmacol 1989; 12:339–345.

83. Baier PC, Winkelmann J, Höhne A, et al. Assessment of spontaneously occurring periodic limb movements in sleep in the rat. J Neurol Sci 2002; 198:71–77.

84. Gómez FM, Areso MP, Giralt B, et al. Effects of dopaminergic drugs, occlusal disharmonies, and chronic stress on non-functional masticatory activity in the rat, assessed by incisal attrition. J Dent Res 1998; 77:1454–1464.

85. Kawamura Y, Tsukamoto S, Miyoshi K. Experimental studies in neural mechanisms of bruxism. J Dent Res 1961; 40:217.

86. Scharer P, Kasahara Y, Kawamura Y. Tooth contact patterns during stimulation of the rabbit brain. Arch Oral Biol 1967; 12:1041–1051.

87. Pohto P. Experimental aggression and bruxism in rats. Acta Odontol Scand 1979; 37:117–126.

88. Byrd KE. Characterization of brux-like movements in the laboratory rat by optoelectronic mandibular tracking and electromyographic techniques. Arch Oral Biol 1997; 42:33–43.

89. Budtz-Jorgensen E. Bruxism and trauma from occlusion. An experimental model in Macaca monkeys. J Clin Periodontol 1980; 7:149–162.

90. Shoji Y, Bruce IC, Siu LYL. Electromyographic assessment on non-functional masseter muscle in an awake animal model. J Craniomandibular Pract 1994; 12:110–113.

91. Pohto P. A neuropharmacological approach to experimental bruxism. Proc Finn Dent Soc 1977; 73:1–13.

92. Layng TVJ, Andronis PT, Goldiamond I. Animal model of psychopathology: the establishment, maintenance, attenuation, and persistence of head-banging in pigeons. J Behav Ther Exp Psychiatry 1999; 30:45–61.

93. Schaefer HH. Self-injurious behavior: shaping "head-banging" in monkeys. J Appl Behav Anal 1970; 3:111–116.

94. Wolf M, Risley T, Johnston M, et al. Application of operant conditioning procedures to the behavior problems of an autistic child: a follow-up and extension. Behav Res Ther 1967; 5:103–111.

95. Wolf M, Risley T, Mees H. Application of operant conditioning procedures to the behavior of an autistic child. Behav Res Ther 1963; 1:305–312.

96. Prochaska J, Smith N, Marzilli R, et al. Remote-control aversive stimulation in the treatment of head-banging in a retarded child. J Behav Ther Exp Psychiatry 1974; 5:285–289.

97. Kakazato T, Akiyama A. Behavioral activity and stereotypy in rats induced by L-DOPA metabolites: a possible role in the adverse effects of chronic L-DOPA treatment of Parkinson's disease. Brain Res 2002; 930:134–142.

98. Ben-Pazi A, Szechtman H, Eilam D. The morphogenesis of motor rituals in rats treated chronically with the dopamine agonist quinpirole. Behav Neurosci 2001; 115:1301–1317.

99. Randrup A, Munkvad I. Stereotyped activities produced by amphetamine in several animal species and man. Psychopharmacologia 1967; 11:300–310.

100. Kuczenski R, Segal DS, Aizenstein ML. Amphetamine, cocaine, and fencamfamine: relationship between locomotor and stereotypy response profiles and caudate and accumbens dopamine dynamics. J Neurosci 1991; 11:2703–2712.

101. Vandebroek I, Ödberg FO. Effect of apomorphine on the conflict-induced jumping stereotypy in bank voles. Pharmacol Biochem Behav 1997; 57:863–868.

102. Mason GJ. Stereotypies: a critical review. Anim Behav 1991; 41:1015–1037.

103. Turner CA, Presti MF, Newman HA, et al. Spontaneous stereotypy in an animal model of down syndrome: Ts65Dn mice. Behav Genet 2001; 31:393–400.
104. Abetz L, Allen R, Follet A, et al. Evaluating the quality of life of patients with restless legs syndrome. Clin Ther 2004; 26:925–835.
105. Abetz L, Vallow SM, Kirsch J, et al. Validation of the Restless Legs Syndrome Quality of Life Questionnaire. Value Health 2005; 8:157–167.
106. Kohnen R, Beneš H, Heinrich CR, et al. Development of the disease-specific Restless Legs Syndrome Quality of Life (RLS-QoL) questionnaire. Mov Disord 2002; 17(suppl 5):P743 (abstr).
107. Kushida CA, Allen RP, Atkinson MJ. Modeling the causal relationships between symptoms associated with restless legs syndrome and the patient-reported impact of RLS. Sleep Med 2004; 5:485–488.
108. Saletu B, Anderer P, Saletu M, et al. EEG mapping, psychometric, and polysomnographic studies in restless legs syndrome (RLS) and periodic limb movement disorder (PLMD) patients as compared with normal controls. Sleep Med 2002; 3(suppl):S35–S42.
109. Dao TT, Lund JP, Lavigne GJ. Comparison of pain and quality of life in bruxers and patients with myofascial pain of the masticatory muscles. J Orofac Pain 1994; 8:350–356.
110. Crawford B. Clinical economics and sleep disorders. Sleep 1997; 20:829–834.
111. Chilcott LA, Shapiro CM. The socioeconomic impact of insomnia. An overview. Pharmacoeconomics 1996; 10(suppl 1):1–14.
112. Hillman DR, Murphy DL, Antic R, et al. The economic cost of sleep disorders. Sleep 2006; 29: 299–305.
113. Martin SA, Aikens JE, Chervin RD. Toward cost-effectiveness analysis in the diagnosis and treatment of insomnia. Sleep Med Rev 2004; 8:63–72.
114. Metlaine A, Leger D, Choudat D. Socioeconomic impact of insomnia in working populations. Ind Health 2005; 43:11–19.
115. Leger D. The cost of sleep-related accidents: a report for the National Commission on Sleep Disorders Research. Sleep 1994; 17:84–93.
116. Philip P, Taillard J, Niedhammer I, et al. Is there a link between subjective daytime somnolence and sickness absenteeism? A study in a working population. J Sleep Res 2001; 10:111–115.
117. Philip P, Åkerstedt T. Transport and industrial safety, how are they affected by sleepiness and sleep restriction? Sleep Med Rev 2006; 10:347–356.
118. Phillips B, Hening W, Britz P, et al. Prevalence and correlates of restless legs syndrome. Results from the 2005 National Sleep Foundation Poll. Chest 2006; 129:76–80.
119. Aldrich MS. Automobile accidents in patients with sleep disorders. Sleep 1987; 12:487–494.
120. Ahlberg J, Rantala M, Savolainen A, et al. Reported bruxism and stress experience. Community Dent Oral Epidemiol 2002; 30:405–408.

44 | Pathophysiology, Associations, and Consequences of Sleep-Related Movement Disorders

William G. Ondo

Department of Neurology, Baylor College of Medicine, Houston, Texas, U.S.A.

RESTLESS LEGS SYNDROME

Etiology, Pathophysiology, and Pathogenesis

A National Institutes of Health (NIH) consensus panel defined restless legs syndrome (RLS) as: (*i*) an urge to move the limbs with or without sensations, (*ii*) worsening at rest, (*iii*) improving with activity, and (*iv*) worsening in the evening or night (1). The diagnosis of RLS is exclusively based on these criteria. A validated diagnostic phone interview (2), rating scale (3), and quality of life scale (4) have all been developed based on these features.

Patients, however, seldom quote the RLS inclusion criteria at presentation, and often have difficulty describing the sensory component of their RLS. The descriptions are quite varied and tend to be suggestible and education dependent. The sensation is always unpleasant but not necessarily painful. It is usually deep within the legs. Patients usually deny the "burning" or "pins and needles" sensations that are commonly experienced in neuropathies or nerve entrapments, although neuropathic pain and RLS can coexist. Other clinical features typical of RLS include the tendency for symptoms to gradually worsen with age, improvement with dopaminergic treatments, a positive family history of RLS, and periodic limb movements of sleep (PLMS).

RLS in children can be difficult to diagnose. Although some children report classic RLS symptoms that meet inclusion criteria, others complain of "growing pains" (5,6), and some appear to present with an attention deficit hyperactivity disorder (ADHD) phenotype. Kotagal et al. reported that children with RLS have lower-than-expected serum ferritin levels and in most cases appear to inherit the disorder from their mother (7). NIH diagnostic criteria for RLS in children is less well validated but emphasizes supportive features such as a family history of RLS, sleep disturbances, and the presence of PLMS, which is uncommon in pediatric controls (1). The exact relationship between RLS and ADHD is not known. Children diagnosed with ADHD, however, often have PLMS (8–11) and meet criteria for RLS (8). Children with ADHD also have a higher prevalence of a parent with RLS (12) and children diagnosed with PLMS often have ADHD (13). Dopaminergic treatment of RLS/PLMS in children also improves ADHD symptoms (14). Therefore, there is clearly some association between RLS and ADHD.

Historically, epidemiologic studies of RLS were limited by the subjective nature of the disease, the lack of standardized diagnostic criteria, and the indolent onset of the condition. Ekbom initially estimated a 5% prevalence of RLS in the general population (15). Subsequent general population prevalence surveys varied from 1% to 29% (Table 1) (16–18).

The largest epidemiological study of RLS involved more than 23,000 persons from five countries (19). Similar to smaller reports, 9.6% of all people met criteria for RLS. In general, northern European countries demonstrated higher prevalence compared to Mediterranean countries. The vast majority of these subjects were not previously diagnosed, despite frequently reporting symptoms to their physicians.

RLS can occur in all ethnic backgrounds; however most feel that Caucasians are mainly affected. While most Caucasian surveys demonstrate an approximate 10% prevalence, two surveys in Asian populations report much lower prevalence. Tan et al., in a door-to-door survey of 1,000 people over age 21 in Singapore, found only one person (0.1%) who met the International Restless Legs Study Group (IRLSSG) criteria for RLS (20). Kageyama et al. distributed a written questionnaire asking "if you ever experience sleep disturbances due to

Table 1 Epidemiology of RLS in General Population since 1995

Author (reference) (Year)	N	RLS diagnostic criteria	Population	Location	RLS(%)
Henning (19) (2004)	23,052	NIH written	adults	Europe/United States	9.6
Garbarino (166) (2002)	2,560	written	police shift workers	Genoa Italy	8.5: shift workers
					4.2: day workers
Ohayan (167) 2002	18,980	ICSD phone interview	15–100	Europe	5.5
Berger (168), 2004	4,310	IRLSSG interview	20–79	Northeast Germany	10.6
Rothdach (169) 2000	369	IRLSSG interview	65–83	Ausberg, Germany	9.8
Nichols (170) 2003	2,099	IRLSSG	adults	Idaho (single PCP)	24.0
Ulfberg (171) 2001	200	IRLSSG written	women 18–64	Sweden	11.4
Ulfberg (172) 2001	4,000	IRLSSG written	men 18–64	Sweden	5.8
Phillips (18) 2000	1,803	single phone question	>18	Kentucky, U.S.A.	10.0
Lavigne (154) 1997	2,019	two written questions	adults	Quebec Canada	10–15
Sevim, (173) 2002	3,234	IRLSSG interview	adults, no secondary RLS	Turkey	3.2
Tan (20) 2001	1,000	IRLSSG interview	>21	Singapore	0.1
Kageyama (21) 2000	3,600 (females)	single written question	adults	Japan	1.5
	1,012 (males)				

Abbreviations: RLS, restless legs syndrome; NIH, National Institute of Health RLS diagnostic criteria; ICSD, International Classification of Sleep Disorders; IRLSSG, International Restless Legs Study Group diagnostic criteria; PCP, Primary Care Physician.

creeping sensations or hot feeling in your legs" to 3,600 women and 1,012 men (21). They reported that approximately 5% responded affirmatively to that single question but far fewer would meet all criteria for RLS. People from African descent have never been specifically studied but anecdotally African Americans only rarely present with RLS. It is unclear whether this represents a true lower prevalence, or rather differences in medical sophistication and referral patterns.

In roughly 60% of the cases, a family history of RLS can be found, although this is often not initially reported by the patient (22). Twin studies also show a very high concordance rate (23). Most pedigrees suggest an autosomal dominant pattern (24), although an autosomal recessive pattern with a very high carrier rate is possible. A complex segregation analysis performed in German families revealed a single gene autosomal pattern in subjects with a young onset of RLS (<30 years), but no clear pattern in subjects with older onset of RLS (24). To date, several gene linkages have been demonstrated, although specific causative proteins remain elusive. Given the wide distribution of RLS, however, it is likely that additional specific genetic etiologies are yet to be discovered.

Desaultels first reported a linkage using an autosomal recessive pattern with a very high penetrance on chromosome (12q) in a large French Canadian family (25). Multipoint linkage calculations yielded a logarithm (base 10) of odds (LOD score) of 3.59. Haplotype analysis refined the genetic interval, positioning the RLS-predisposing gene in a 14.71-cM region between D12S1044 and D12S78. This linkage site has been corroborated in Iceland (Rye, personal communication).

Bonati et al. next identified an autosomal dominant linkage in a single Italian family on chromosome 14q13-21 region. The maximum two-point log of odds ratio score value of 3.23 at theta = 0.0, was obtained for marker D14S288 (26).

Chen et al. characterized 15 large and extended multiplex pedigrees, consisting of 453 subjects (134 affected with RLS). Model-free linkage analysis identified one novel significant susceptibility locus for RLS on chromosomal 9p24.2-22.3 with a multipoint nonparametric linkage (NPL) score 3.22. Model-based linkage analysis assuming an autosomal dominant mode of inheritance validated the 9p24.2-22.3 linkage to RLS in two families (two-point LOD score of 3.77; multipoint LOD score of 3.91). This site has been independently corroborated in a separate German family (Winkelmann, personal communication).

Two additional linkage sites have been recently reported, and it is likely that others will be identified in the future. A gene variant located on chromosome 6 in an intron of a gene known as BTBD9 has been recently identified, and the frequency of this gene variant is correlated in a dose-dependent fashion to periodic limb movements (PLM) of sleep (which are present in nearly all patients with restless legs) and to the different prevalence rates for RLS noted across different population groups, but inversely correlated with serum iron status.

Pathological research suggests that the pathophysiology of RLS involves central nervous system (CNS) iron homeostatic dysregulation. Cerebrospinal fluid (CSF) ferritin is lower in RLS cases (27), and specially sequenced magnetic resonance imaging (MRI) studies show reduced iron stores in the striatum and red nucleus (28). CNS ultrasonography was also able to identify RLS based on reduced iron echogenicity in the substantia nigra (29). Most importantly, pathologic data in RLS autopsied brains show not only reduced ferritin staining, iron staining, and increased transferrin, but also reduced staining for transferrin receptors. Thy-1 expression, which is activated by iron, is also reduced (30). The reduced transferrin receptor finding is important because globally reduced iron stores would normally upregulate transferrin receptors. Therefore, it appears that primary RLS has reduced intracellular iron indices secondary to a perturbation of homeostatic mechanisms that regulate iron influx or efflux from the cell. Intracellular iron regulation is very complex; however, subsequent staining of RLS brains has shown reduced levels of iron regulatory protein-type 1 (IRB-1) (31). This potentiates or inhibits (depending on feedback mechanisms involving iron atoms themselves) the production of ferritin molecules, which are the main iron storage proteins in the CNS, and transferrin receptors, which facilitate intracellular iron transport.

CNS dopaminergic systems are strongly implicated in RLS. Most researchers agree that dopamine agonists (DA) most robustly treat RLS, and dopaminergic functional brain imaging studies inconsistently show modest abnormalities (32–35). Normal circadian dopaminergic variation is also augmented in patients with RLS (36). There is, however, no evidence to suggest reduced dopamine in the brains of RLS patients. Substantia nigra dopaminergic cells are not reduced in number, nor are there any markers associated with neurodegenerative diseases, such as tau or alpha-synuclein abnormalities (37,38).

There are several potential interactions between iron and dopamine systems. First, iron is a co-factor for tyrosine-hydroxylase, which is the rate-limiting step in the production of dopamine. Iron chelation reduces dopamine transporter (DAT) protein expression and activity in mice (39). Human CSF studies, however, have failed to demonstrate reduced dopaminergic metabolites (40,41). Second, iron is a component of the dopamine type-2 (D2) receptor. Iron deprivation in rats results in a 40% to 60% reduction of D2 post-synaptic receptors (42,43). The effect is quite specific, as other neurotransmitter systems including D1 receptors are not affected. Third, iron is necessary for Thy1 protein regulation. This cell adhesion molecule, which is robustly expressed on dopaminergic neurons, is reduced in brain homogenates in iron-deprived mice (44) and in brains of patients with RLS (30). Thy1 regulates vesicular release of monoamines, including dopamine (45). It also stabilizes synapses and suppresses dendritic growth (46).

Another puzzle that remains is the identification of a specific neuroanatomy culpable for RLS. There are multiple dopaminergic systems in the brain, but RLS patients do not have symptoms consistent with dysfunction seen in most known dopaminergic systems, such as Parkinsonism or olfactory loss (47). Involvement of the seldom-studied diencephalospinal dopaminergic tract, originating from the A11–A14 nuclei might explain some RLS features. It is involved in anti-nociception, is near circadian control centers, and would explain why legs are involved more than arms. A preliminary animal model with A11 lesions demonstrated increased standing episodes, which improved after the administration of pramipexole, a dopamine agonist (48). Subsequent studies of this model in mice, with and without dietary iron deprivation, also demonstrate increased movement, as measured in laser-marker cages, in the lesioned animals. This hyperkinesia is normalized by D2 agonists such as ropinirole and pramipexole, but not by the D1 agonist SKF.

Associations, Complications, and Consequences

Despite the appropriate attention given to RLS genetics, between 2% and 6% of the population probably suffer from RLS without any identifiable highly penetrant genetic pattern. It is not known whether some "genetic" forms of RLS could express low penetrance and mimic a sporadic pattern of onset. Currently, however, there is no evidence to support this pattern (24). Therefore, patients without a positive family history are classified as either primary RLS, if no other explanation is found, or secondary RLS, if they concurrently posses a condition known to be associated with RLS.

The most common associations with RLS include renal failure, iron deficiency, neuropathy, myelinopathy, pregnancy, and possibly Parkinson's disease and essential tremor. There is some evidence to support an association of RLS with some genetic ataxias (49–51), fibromyalgia (52,53), and rheumatological diseases (54–56). A variety of other associations are at best tenuous. Finally, several medications are known to exacerbate existing RLS or possible precipitate RLS themselves. The most notable of these include antihistamines, dopamine antagonists, including many antinausea medications, mirtazapine, and possibly tricyclic antidepressants and serotonergic reuptake inhibitors.

Neuropathy

Numerous forms of neuropathy, including diabetic, alcoholic, amyloid, motor neuron disease, poliomyelitis, and radiculopathy, have been seen at higher than expected frequency in patients presenting with RLS (22,57–67).

For example, our series reported that 37/98 (36.6%) of RLS patients demonstrated electrophysiologic evidence of neuropathy using standard electromyographic/nerve conduction velocity (EMG/NCV) techniques. The exact etiologies varied. Many of these patients demonstrated no evidence of neuropathy on clinical examination. The presence of neuropathy was much higher in patients who did not have a family history of RLS, compared to those who did have a family history, 22/31 (71%) versus15/67 (24%), $p < 0.001$. Small fiber neuropathy, which is only detectable with biopsy, is also found in a large number of patients presenting with RLS (61).

Specific forms of neuropathy may incur different risks for the development of RLS. Gemignani et al. reported that 10/27 (37%) of patients with Charcot Marie Tooth type II (CMT II), an axonal neuropathy, had RLS, whereas RLS was not seen in any of the 17 patients with CMT I, a demyelinating neuropathy (57).

The phenotype of neuropathic RLS may be slightly different from idiopathic RLS (22,61). In our population, neuropathic RLS symptoms initially presented more acutely and at an older age, and then progressed much more rapidly. A large number of patients with neuropathic RLS reached maximum symptom intensity within one year from the initial symptom onset, which is unusual in idiopathic cases. Neuropathic RLS may also have accompanying neuropathic pain, which is often burning and more superficial. The painful component and the urge to move, however, are seldom differentiated by the patient.

In contrast, series evaluating RLS in populations presenting with neuropathy have not shown a particularly high prevalence of RLS, usually ranging from 5% to 10%, similar to the general population (63,64). Hogl et al. published the only large population-based study on neuropathy and RLS (68). RLS was diagnosed in personal interviews according to standard criteria, and polyneuropathy according to clinical and electrodiagnostic criteria. Peripheral neuropathy was present in 2.7% of the subjects with, and 2.4% of the subjects without RLS. There was no significant difference. In short, the relationship between neuropathy and RLS is not clear.

Spinal Lesions

Spinal cord lesions (69,70) including neoplastic spinal lesions (71), demyelinating or post-infectious lesions (72–74), and syringomyelia (75)can all precipitate RLS and PLMS. Spinal cord blocks used for anesthesia also frequently cause or exacerbate RLS (76,77). Hogl et al. systematically evaluated RLS following spinal anesthesia (76). Of 161 subjects without any history of RLS, 8.7% developed RLS immediately after the procedure.

Uremia

Uremia, secondary to renal failure, is strongly associated with RLS symptoms. Multiple series report a 20% to 57% prevalence of RLS in renal dialysis patients (Table 2); however, only a minority of uremic patients volunteer RLS symptoms unless specifically queried (78–97). The prevalence of RLS in mild to moderate renal failure that does not require dialysis is unknown.

The RLS seen in dialysis patients is often severe. Wetter et al. compared clinical and polysomnographic features of idiopathic RLS and uremic RLS in a large clinical series (93). They reported no differences in sensory symptoms but noted increased wakeful leg movements (78% vs. 51%) and significantly greater numbers of PLMS in uremic RLS patients. Both RLS and PLMS have also been associated with increased mortality in the dialysis population (94,98).

Overall, dialysis does not improve RLS. In fact, one study suggested that RLS correlated with greater dialysis frequency (85). However, patients who receive a successful, but not unsuccessful, kidney transplant usually experience dramatic improvement in RLS within days to weeks (99,100). The degree of symptom alleviation appears to correlate with improved kidney function.

Iron Deficiency

Reduced CNS iron is implicated in all cases of RLS. It is intuitive to suggest that reduced body stores of iron could also result in low CNS intracellular iron and also cause RLS symptoms. A series of reports have associated low serum ferritin levels with RLS (27,28,101–105). Anemia has not been independently associated with RLS; however, blood donors do frequently develop RLS symptoms (103,106).

Low serum iron stores are only associated with certain demographics of RLS patients. We have reported that serum ferritin is lower in patients with RLS who lack a family history compared to those with familial RLS (101–107). Earley et al. have made the same general observation but segregated the groups based upon age of RLS onset (108). The patients with an older age of RLS onset had lower serum ferritin levels compared to patients with a younger

Table 2 Studies Evaluating RLS in Renal Failure

Author (reference) (year)	Cohort	RLS diagnosis	Number and % with RLS	RLS predictors
Unruh (174) (2004)	HD United States	Single question for "severe" RLS	15% of 894	Associated with increased mortality
Mucsi (175) (2004)	HD/PD Hungary		15%	NR
Gigli (176) (2004)	HD/PD Italy	written IRLSSG	21.5% of 601	greater duration of dialysis
Bhowmik (177) (2004)	India		1.5% of 65	NR
Takaki (178) (2003)	HD Japan	IRLSSG (4/4) IRLSSG ($\geq$2/4)	60 / 490 (12.2%) 112 / 490 (22.9%)	Hyperphosphatemia Stress
Goffredo (179) (2003)	HD Brazil	IRLSSG interview	/176 (14.8%)	Caucasian>Non-Caucasian
Bhatia (78) (2003)	HD India		6.6%	NR
Kutner (180) (2002)	HD United States	IRLSSG interview	308 68% Caucasion 48% African	Caucasian>African American, no other significant predictors
Cirignotta (181) (2002)	HD Italy	written questionnaire IRLSSG interview	/127 (50%) /127 (33.3%)	NR
Sabbatini (89) (2002)	HD Italy	RLS question	257/694 (37%)	None
Miranda (182) (2001)	HD Chile	Interview	43/166 (26%)	None
Hui (83) (2000)	PD Hong Kong	written question	124/201 (62%)	Insomnia
Virga (92) (1998)	HD	"RLS"	(27.4%)	None
Collado-Seidel (80) (1998)	HD Germany	IRLSSG (4/4) IRLSSG ($\geq$3/4)	32/138 (23%) 44/138 (32%)	Increased parathyroid hormone
Winkelmann (94) (1996)	HD United States	IRLSSG (3/4)	/204 (20%)	None Decreased Hct poor sleep
Walker (183) (1995)	HD Canada	ICSD	31/54 (57%)	Increased BUN, $p = 0.04$ Increased Cr, $p = 0.08$
Stepanski (90) (1995)	PD	"Leg twitching"	26/81 (32%)	NR
Holley (82) (1992)	HD/PD	"RLS"	30/70 (42%)	NR
Roger (88) (1991)	HD/PD United Kingdom	"RLS"	22/55 (40%)	Hct, $p = 0.03$ female
Bastani (184) (1987)	HD	"RLS"	6/42 (17%)	NR
Nielson (97) (1971)	None	"RLS"	43/109 (39%)	NR

Abbreviations: RLS, restless legs syndrome; HD, hemodialysis; PD, peritoneal dialysis; NR, not reported; IRLSSG, International Restless Legs Study Group diagnostic criteria; ICSD, International Classification of Sleep Disorders; Hct, hematocrit; BUN, blood urea nitrogen; Cr, creatinine.

age of onset. These groups, however, generally represent the same dichotomy as do genetic-based segregations since there is a very strong correlation between a younger age of onset of RLS and the presence of a family history of RLS.

Pregnancy

The development of RLS during pregnancy has long been recognized (15,109,110). Manconi et al. evaluated risk factors for RLS in 606 pregnancies (111). They reported that 26% of these women suffered from RLS, usually in the last trimester. The authors could find no significant differences in age, pregnancy duration, mode of delivery, tobacco use, the woman's body mass index, baby weight, or iron/folate supplementation in those with RLS. Hemoglobin, however, was significantly lower in the RLS group, and plasmatic iron tended to be lower, compared to those without RLS. Lee et al. reported that 23% of 29 third-trimester women developed RLS during pregnancy (112). The RLS resolved shortly post-partum in all but one subject. Women with RLS in their population demonstrated lower preconception levels of ferritin but were similar to women without RLS during pregnancy. Since the RLS usually resolves within days of delivery, the etiology may be hormonal, possibly increased estradiol; however, there is no data to support any definitive etiology.

Parkinson's Disease

RLS and Parkinson's disease (PD) both respond to dopaminergic treatments, both show dopaminergic abnormalities on functional imaging (34,113), and both are associated with PLMS (114). However, we now know that the pathology of the two dopaminergically treated diseases are very different and wih regard to iron accumulation, are actually quite opposite (38).

In a survey of 303 consecutive PD patients, we found that 20.8% of patients with PD met the diagnostic criteria for RLS. Only lower serum ferritin was associated with RLS (101). Similar epidemiological findings are reported by other groups evaluating Caucasian populations (115) (Chaudhuri, personal communication) but not Asian populations (116,117). Despite this high number of cases, there are several caveats that tend to lessen its clinical significance. The RLS symptoms in PD patients are often ephemeral, usually not severe, and can be confused with other PD symptoms such as wearing off dystonia, akathisia, or internal tremor. Furthermore, most patients in our group were not previously diagnosed with RLS, and few recognized that this was separate from other PD symptoms. Most importantly, the PD preceded the RLS in most cases. There is no evidence to suggest that RLS evolves into PD.

Essential Tremor

We prospectively evaluated for an association between essential tremor (ET) and RLS (118). Of 100 consecutive patients presenting to our clinic with ET (60 female, and 75 with a family history of ET), the age was 65.2±16.3 years, and the age at tremor onset was 37.8±19.9 years. Concurrent dystonia was seen in 19 patients: neck (6), arm/hand (5), voice (5), and cranial (3). Thirty-three met all criteria for RLS, of which 25 had never been previously diagnosed. A family history of RLS was reported in 57.6% of these 33 patients and was the only significant predictor of RLS in the ET population. The onset of ET preceded the onset of RLS in 19, RLS preceded ET in 10, and 4 reported a simultaneous onset. Their International Restless Legs Syndrome Study Group Rating Scale (IRLSRS) score was 16.6±8.1, (scale range: 0–40), which is generally less severe than those presenting to us for RLS.

We also examined 68 consecutively seen RLS patients (63.2% female, and 54.4% with a family history of RLS) for the presence of tremor. Their age was 55.8±14.4 years and the age at RLS onset was 33.7 ± 19.5 years. No RLS patient demonstrated any rest tremor. No patient demonstrated a postural tremor of greater than 1, and only a single patient demonstrated a kinetic tremor of 2. Mild tremor; however, was very common. Clinically, we felt that these very low amplitude tremors represented an "enhanced physiological tremor" rather than ET. The tremor did not cause any subjective disability in any case. We concluded that there is a familial phenotype of combined ET/RLS that usually presents with ET.

Mild RLS may have relatively few consequences; however, severe RLS can result in a marked reduction in quality of life. Sleep deprivation greatly contributes to this as does the learned helplessness and frustration derived from the sensations themselves.

Abetz et al. demonstrated a selected group of RLS subjects who sought treatment at a tertiary referral center and had quality of life score (Medical Outcomes Study Short Form-36 [SF-36]) as bad or worse to those in-patients with congestive heart failure, diabetes mellitus, and osteoarthritis (119).

PERIODIC LIMB MOVEMENTS

PLMS are defined by the American Academy of Sleep Medicine as "periodic episodes of repetitive and highly stereotyped limb movements that occur during sleep". Greater than 5 per hour are required to be considered abnormal. Periodic limb movement disorder (PLMD) refers to an idiopathic form not associated with other sleep disorders.

PLMS can occur simultaneously in both legs, alternate between legs, or occur unilaterally. The duration of movement is typically between 1.5 and 2.5 seconds and varies in intensity from slight extension of the great toe to a triple flexion response. Other tonic and myoclonic patterns are less frequently observed, and arms are involved in a minority of cases. Patients frequently demonstrate a movement periodicity of between 20 and 40 seconds, although wide ranges of frequencies have been reported (120). Movements are most pronounced in Stage I (N1) and Stage II (N2) of non-rapid eye movement (NREM) sleep. PLMS intensity and frequency lessen as sleep deepens. They may persist during rapid eye movement (REM) sleep but both their amplitude and frequency are significantly reduced.

Etiology, Pathophysiology, and Pathogenesis

The exact pathophysiology of PLM is not known. From their initial description, similarities with the Babinski sign lead to speculation that they result from cortical disinhibition. Subsequent research has generally supported this. First, back-averaging techniques triggered from the movements do not elicit any cortical potentials, suggesting that they are not generated from the cortex (121). Second, functional MRI demonstrates increased pontine and red nucleus activity during PLM in RLS patients (122). The cortex was not abnormal. The spinal cord is implicated by the phenomenology of the movements, the fact that spinal cord injury often causes PLM, and evidence of spinal cord disinhibition and spatial spread (69,123).

PLM are also associated with other rhythmic, often autonomic activities. They are often accompanied by K-complexes, and by increases in pulse and blood pressure (121). The K-complexes usually precede the PLMS and may persist even if PLMS are reduced with L-dopa (124). PLM may also correlate with the cyclic alternating pattern seen in electroencephalogram (125).

Dopamine systems are strongly suggested by the response to dopaminergic treatments. Inhibition of dopaminergic tracts that descend to the spinal cord (see RLS pathophysiology) may be involved. These are reciprocally inhibited by descending serotonergic systems, which may explain why serotonergic reuptake inhibitors precipitate PLM (126,127). Imaging of dopamine-receptor occupancy in the striatum is also abnormal in patients with PLM (32).

The incidence in the general population increases with age and is reported to occur in as many as 57% of elderly people (128–130). Bixler reported that 29% of people over the age of 50 had PLMS, whereas only 5% of those aged between 30 and 50 and almost none under 30 were affected (131). PLMS in normal children are uncommon.

Associations, Complications, and Consequences

PLM are strongly associated with RLS. The largest single study, employing a cut off of 5 PLMS/hour, reported that 81% of RLS patients showed pathologic PLMS (132). The prevalence increased to 87% if two nights were recorded. Although PLMS accompany most cases of RLS, the only data evaluating RLS prevalence in the setting of polysomnographically documented PLMS found that only 9 of 53 (17%) PLMS patients complained of RLS symptoms (133). The degree of diligence with which RLS symptoms were queried, however, is unclear. Therefore, most people with RLS have PLMS, but many patients with isolated PLMS do not have RLS.

PLMS counts generally correlate with RLS severity; however, the exact relationship between the two phenotypes is unclear (132).

Several other sleep disorders are associated with PLM. The majority of narcolepsy patients have PLM (134). This prevalence increases with greater age but PLM does not correlate with the sleep dysfunction. A large number of REM sleep behavior disorder (RBD) patients have PLM. Sleep apnea episode often precipitate a PLM, frequently associated with an arousal. These improve, but do not disappear with successful continuous positive airway pressure (CPAP) treatment (135,136).

Medical problems associated with RLS (uremia, iron deficiency, and pregnancy) are also associated with PLM. Finally, Parkinson's disease has higher rates of PLMS (114).

The consequences of isolated PLM are debated. In most cases, there are no frank arousals and therefore no overt sleep dysfunction. Microarousals are relatively common, but there is little consensus on their diagnosis or implications. When severe, isolated PLMS may result in overt arousals, but overall, they generally do not cause insomnia (131,137), are not associated with daytime sleepiness or abnormalities on sleep latency tests (138). Therefore, it is not clear that PLMD requires treatment unless it worsens sleep.

BRUXISM

Sleep bruxism (SB) is a parasomnia characterized by stereotyped activity of the jaw musculature together with tooth grinding or clenching during sleep. Bruxism is involuntary, and in awake individuals, it is manifested by jaw clenching (so-called awake bruxism). During SB, both clenching and tooth-grinding are observed (139). It is definitively diagnosed by polysomnographic study with electromyographic or pressure recording. Some researchers report SB during all sleep stages, while others observe the majority of bruxing during light sleep and REM (139). Bruxism epochs generally accompany physiologic arousals that recur at 20- to 40-second intervals, often along with PLMS. Patients with bruxism have more frequent, and more intense, arousal periods; however, the cause and effect status is not known (140).

Sleep bruxism is common in the general population. The prevalence of awake bruxism in the general population is approximately 20%, while the prevalence of SB is about 8% (16,141). The prevalence peaks in late childhood and gradually decreases with greater age. Up to 20% of children are reported to have SB by their parents (142,143). Gender does not overtly affect prevalence.

Bruxism is generally associated with anxious high achieving personality types; however, not all formal studies have objectively corroborated this (144). One detailed evaluation failed to correlate nocturnal bruxism intensity with any daytime events, concentrating mostly on stress (145).

Etiology, Pathophysiology, and Pathogenesis

The pathophysiology of sleep bruxism is not known and is likely multifactorial. Older theories that bruxism resulted from jaw misalignment or other anatomic features have been largely abandoned, as the majority of data supports a CNS genesis. In fact, a large number of "normal" subjects demonstrate rhythmic masticatory muscle activity without actual tooth grinding. SB may be an exaggeration of this probably physiologic occurrence, postulated by some to lubricate the airway (146).

Increased subcortical CNS excitability, or disinhibition, is shown by transcranial magnetic stimulation of the masseter reflex (147). With paired stimuli, the degree of suppression of the late silent period was significantly lower ($p < 0.01$) in bruxism patients compared to controls. Dopamine systems have been implicated by associations with bruxism and several disease states and medications, and possibly by physiologic studies. One D2 receptor antagonist radioligand study did not reveal overall differences in dopamine receptor availability between bruxers and controls, but did show greater side-to-side asymmetry in the bruxers (148). A genetic component is suggested by the high rates reported in monozygotic twins but specific gene linkages are lacking (149).

Associations, Complications, and Consequences

Bruxism is termed secondary when it occurs in the presence of a neurological or psychiatric disorder. The most common associations include parkinsonism, depression, Huntington's disease, cranial dystonia, oral tardive dyskinesia, and REM sleep behavior disorder. Temporomandibular joint (TMJ) syndrome is also strongly associated with bruxism but it is not clear whether the TMJ pain is simply the bruxism. No specific polysomnographic features differentiate bruxism patients who meet diagnostic criteria for TMJ versus those who do not (150). However, TMJ patients have higher depression and somatization levels (151). Certain medications are also associated with bruxism. The most associated are serotonin specific reuptake inhibitors and dopamine antagonists (152,153). A variety of other prescription and recreational drugs (L-dopa, amphetamines, cocaine, alcohol, or smoking) have also been implicated (154). Patients with sleep-disordered breathing and tinnitus may also have a higher risk for sleep bruxism (141,155).

SB can cause tooth destruction, temporomandibular dysfunction (e.g., jaw pain or movement limitation), headaches, and the disruption of the bed partner's sleep because of the grinding sounds. Interestingly, total sleep and sleep macrostructure are grossly normal, although one group reported decreased numbers of K-complexes (156).

NOCTURNAL LEG CRAMPS

Nocturnal leg cramps, often referred to as "charley-horse" are a common, multi-factorial disorder manifested by paroxysmal, disorganized spasms that usually involve the legs. The calves (gastrocnemius and soleus muscles) are most commonly affected. Cramps in the feet (usually toe flexion) and thighs (hamstrings more than quadriceps) also occur (157,158). Arm cramps are much less common. The muscle contractions usually last seconds to minutes but are occasionally longer. They are usually unilateral and may be initiated by plantar flexion of the foot.

Detailed epidemiologic studies of nocturnal cramps are rare. One study reported that 16% of adults have nocturnal cramps (159). Incidence probably increases with older age. Children can also cramp, the prevalence increasing in late teens (160).

Etiology, Pathophysiology, and Pathogenesis

The exact pathophysiology of nocturnal cramps is not known, and is likely heterogeneous. A variety of metabolic and electrolyte disorders have been proposed. One study of U.S. veterans found that peripheral vascular disease and neuropathy were more common in subjects with cramps (161). Cramps may also be familial, although no specific gene has been identified (162,163).

Electrophysiology studies demonstrate very high frequency discharges from anterior horn cells that subsequently contract several motor units. Therefore, most cramps likely originate cephalad to the muscle along the neuromuscular axis. No CNS abnormalities have been found.

Associations, Complications, and Consequences

Cramps are very common during pregnancy, in dialysis patients, and in patients with thyroid abnormalities. Electrolyte abnormalities, especially hypokalemia, hypocalcemia, and hypomagnesemia are associated with cramps. A variety of neuromuscular diseases (both myopathies and neuropathies) are associated with cramps; however, the clinical features of those conditions are usually obvious (157,158). Medications reported to be associated with cramps include diuretics, steroids, morphine, cimetidine, statins, penicillamine, and lithium (164).

Cramps in themselves are usually benign but may cause sleep disturbance and, of course, pain. Cramps as part of muscle disease may be more severe.

RHYTHMIC MOVEMENT DISORDER

Rhythmic movement disorder (also known as head banging, headrolling, bodyrocking, and jactatito capitus nocturnus) is usually a benign condition of late infancy and early childhood. It may occur to some extent in the majority of all children younger than 18 months (165). The pathophysiology is not known and most consider it normal in infants. Polysomnography is unremarkable aside from 0.5 to 2 Hz muscle artifact. Rhythmic movements may be seen at a later age in patients with brain injury or developmental delay, but formal epidemiology is lacking. Although speculated to be a stress relief mechanism, there is no data to demonstrable any psychological comorbidities. Head banging may occasionally result in head injury. Serious injuries including subdural hematoma and carotid dissection have been reported. Usually there are no consequences.

SUMMARY

Studies have implicated CNS iron homeostatic dysregulation in the pathophysiology of RLS, and there are several potential interactions between the iron and dopamine systems. There are known associations of RLS with neuropathy, spinal lesions, uremia, iron deficiency, pregnancy, Parkinson's disease, and essential tremor. The exact pathophysiology of periodic limb movements is unknown, but they are strongly associated with RLS and other sleep disorders such as narcolepsy, REM sleep behavior disorder, and obstructive sleep apnea. It is believed that the pathophysiology of bruxism is multifactorial, and common associations of this condition include Parkinsonism, depression, Huntington's disease, cranial dystonia, oral tardive dyskinesia, and REM sleep behavior disorder. The pathophysiology of nocturnal leg cramps is not known but is likely heterogeneous, and this condition is associated with pregnancy, dialysis, thyroid, electrolyte abnormalities, and various medications and neuromuscular diseases. Rhythmic movement disorder is considered to be normal in infants, its pathophysiology is unknown, and head banging may occasionally result in head injury.

REFERENCES

1. Allen RP, Picchietti D, Hening WA, et al. Restless legs syndrome: diagnostic criteria, special considerations, and epidemiology. A report from the restless legs syndrome diagnosis and epidemiology workshop at the National Institutes of Health. Sleep Med 2003; 4(2):101–119.
2. Hening WA, Allen RP, Thanner S, et al. The Johns Hopkins telephone diagnostic interview for the restless legs syndrome: preliminary investigation for validation in a multi-center patient and control population. Sleep Med 2003; 4(2):137–141.
3. Walters AS, LeBrocq C, Dhar A, et al. Validation of the International Restless Legs Syndrome Study Group rating scale for restless legs syndrome. Sleep Med 2003; 4(2):121–132.
4. Atkinson MJ, Allen RP, DuChane J, et al. Validation of the Restless Legs Syndrome Quality of Life Instrument (RLS-QLI): findings of a consortium of national experts and the RLS Foundation. Qual Life Res 2004; 13(3):679–693.
5. Ekbom KA. Growing pains and restless legs. Acta Paediatr Scand 1975; 64(2):264–266.
6. Rajaram SS, Walters AS, England SJ, et al. Some children with growing pains may actually have restless legs syndrome. Sleep 2004; 27(4):767–773.
7. Kotagal S, Silber MH. Childhood-onset restless legs syndrome. Ann Neurol 2004; 56(6):803–807.
8. Chervin RD, Archbold KH, Dillon JE, et al. Associations between symptoms of inattention, hyperactivity, restless legs, and periodic leg movements. Sleep 2002; 25(2):213–218.
9. Picchietti DL, England SJ, Walters AS, et al. Periodic limb movement disorder and restless legs syndrome in children with attention-deficit hyperactivity disorder. J Child Neurol 1998; 13(12):588–594.
10. Chervin RD, Dillon JE, Archbold KH, et al. Conduct problems and symptoms of sleep disorders in children. J Am Acad Child Adolesc Psychiatry 2003; 42(2):201–208.
11. Konofal E, Lecendreux M, Bouvard MP, et al. High levels of nocturnal activity in children with attention-deficit hyperactivity disorder: a video analysis. Psychiatry Clin Neurosci 2001; 55(2):97–103.
12. Picchietti DL, Underwood DJ, Farris WA, et al. Further studies on periodic limb movement disorder and restless legs syndrome in children with attention-deficit hyperactivity disorder. Mov Disord 1999; 14(6):1000–1007.
13. Picchietti DL, Walters AS. Moderate to severe periodic limb movement disorder in childhood and adolescence. Sleep 1999; 22(3):297–300.
14. Walters AS, Mandelbaum DE, Lewin DS, et al. Dopaminergic therapy in children with restless legs/periodic limb movements in sleep and ADHD. Dopaminergic Therapy Study Group. Pediatr Neurol 2000; 22(3):182–186.

15. Ekbom KA. Restless legs syndrome. Neurology 1960; 10:868–873.
16. Lavigne GJ, Montplaisir JY. Restless legs syndrome and sleep bruxism: prevalence and association among Canadians. Sleep 1994; 17(8):739–743.
17. Oboler SK, Prochazka AV, Meyer TJ. Leg symptoms in outpatient veterans. West J Med 1991; 155 (3):256–259.
18. Phillips B, Young T, Finn L, et al. Epidemiology of restless legs symptoms in adults. Arch Intern Med 2000; 160(14):2137–2141.
19. Hening W, Walters AS, Allen RP, et al. Impact, diagnosis and treatment of restless legs syndrome (RLS) in a primary care population: the REST (RLS epidemiology, symptoms, and treatment) primary care study. Sleep Med 2004; 5(3):237–246.
20. Tan EK, Seah A, See SJ, et al. Restless legs syndrome in an Asian population: a study in Singapore. Mov Disord 2001; 16(3):577–579.
21. Kageyama T, Kabuto M, Nitta H, et al. Prevalences of periodic limb movement-like and restless legs-like symptoms among Japanese adults. Psychiatry Clin Neurosci 2000; 54(3):296–298.
22. Ondo W, Jankovic J. Restless legs syndrome: clinicoetiologic correlates. Neurology 1996; 47(6): 1435–1441.
23. Ondo WG, Vuong KD, Wang Q. Restless legs syndrome in monozygotic twins: clinical correlates. Neurology 2000; 55(9):1404–1406.
24. Winkelmann J, Muller-Myhsok B, Wittchen HU, et al. Complex segregation analysis of restless legs syndrome provides evidence for an autosomal dominant mode of inheritance in early age at onset families. Ann Neurol 2002; 52(3):297–302.
25. Desautels A, Turecki G, Montplaisir J, et al. Identification of a major susceptibility locus for restless legs syndrome on chromosome 12q. Am J Hum Genetics 2001; 69(6):1266–1270.
26. Bonati MT, Ferini-Strambi L, Aridon P, et al. Autosomal dominant restless legs syndrome maps on chromosome 14q. Brain 2003; 126(pt 6):1485–1492.
27. Earley CJ, Connor JR, Beard JL, et al. Abnormalities in CSF concentrations of ferritin and transferrin in restless legs syndrome. Neurology 2000; 54(8):1698–1700.
28. Allen RP, Barker PB, Wehrl F, et al. MRI measurement of brain iron in patients with restless legs syndrome. Neurology 2001; 56(2):263–265.
29. Schmidauer C, Sojer M, Stocckner H, et al. Brain parenchyma sonography differentiates RLS patients from normal controls and patients with Parkinson's disease. Mov Disord 2005; 20(suppl10):S43.
30. Wang X, Wiesinger J, Beard J, et al. Thy1 expression in the brain is affected by iron and is decreased in Restless Legs Syndrome. J Neurol Sci 2004; 220(1–2):59–66.
31. Connor JR, Wang XS, Patton SM, et al. Decreased transferrin receptor expression by neuromelanin cells in restless legs syndrome. Neurology 2004; 62(9):1563–1567.
32. Staedt J, Stoppe G, Kogler A, et al. Nocturnal myoclonus syndrome (periodic movements in sleep) related to central dopamine D2-receptor alteration. Eur Arch Psychiatry Clin Neurosci 1995; 245(1): 8–10.
33. Trenkwalder C, Walters AS, Hening WA, et al. Positron emission tomographic studies in restless legs syndrome. Mov Disord 1999; 14(1):141–145.
34. Turjanski N, Lees AJ, Brooks DJ. Striatal dopaminergic function in restless legs syndrome: 18F-dopa and 11C-raclopride PET studies. Neurology 1999; 52(5):932–937.
35. Tribl GG, Asenbaum S, Happe S, et al. Normal striatal D2 receptor binding in idiopathic restless legs syndrome with periodic leg movements in sleep. Nucl Med Commun 2004; 25(1):55–60.
36. Garcia-Borreguero D, Larrosa O, Granizo JJ, et al. Circadian variation in neuroendocrine response to L-dopa in patients with restless legs syndrome. Sleep 2004; 27(4):669–673.
37. Pittock SJ, Parrett T, Adler CH, et al. Neuropathology of primary restless leg syndrome: absence of specific tau- and alpha-synuclein pathology. Mov Disord 2004; 19(6):695–699.
38. Connor JR, Boyer PJ, Menzies SL, et al. Neuropathological examination suggests impaired brain iron acquisition in restless legs syndrome. Neurology 2003; 61(3):304–309.
39. Nelson C, Erikson K, Pinero DJ, et al. In vivo dopamine metabolism is altered in iron-deficient anemic rats. J Nutr 1997; 127(12):2282–2288.
40. Stiasny-Kolster K, Moller JC, Zschocke J, et al. Normal dopaminergic and serotonergic metabolites in cerebrospinal fluid and blood of restless legs syndrome patients. Mov Disord 2004; 19(2):192–196.
41. Earley CJ, Hyland K, Allen RP. CSF dopamine, serotonin, and biopterin metabolites in patients with restless legs syndrome. Mov Disord 2001; 16(1):144–149.
42. Ben-Shachar D, Finberg JP, Youdim MB. Effect of iron chelators on dopamine D2 receptors. J Neurochem 1985; 45(4):999–1005.
43. Ashkenazi R, Ben-Shachar D, Youdim MB. Nutritional iron and dopamine binding sites in the rat brain. Pharmacol Biochem Behav 1982; 17(suppl 1):43–47.
44. Ye Z, Connor JR. Identification of iron responsive genes by screening cDNA libraries from suppression subtractive hybridization with antisense probes from three iron conditions. Nucleic Acids Res 2000; 28(8):1802–1807.

45. Jeng CJ, McCarroll SA, Martin TF, et al. Thy-1 is a component common to multiple populations of synaptic vesicles. J Cell Biol 1998; 140(3):685–698.
46. Shults CW, Kimber TA. Thy-1 immunoreactivity distinguishes patches/striosomes from matrix in the early postnatal striatum of the rat. Brain Res Dev Brain Res 1993; 75(1):136–140.
47. Adler CH, Gwinn KA, Newman S. Olfactory function in restless legs syndrome. Mov Disord 1998; 13 (3):563–565.
48. Ondo WG, He Y, Rajasekaran S, et al. Clinical correlates of 6-hydroxydopamine injections into A11 dopaminergic neurons in rats: a possible model for restless legs syndrome. Mov Disord 2000; 15 (1):154–158.
49. Abele M, Burk K, Laccone F, et al. Restless legs syndrome in spinocerebellar ataxia types 1, 2, and 3. J Neurol 2001; 248(4):311–314.
50. Schols L, Haan J, Riess O, et al. Sleep disturbance in spinocerebellar ataxias: is the SCA3 mutation a cause of restless legs syndrome? Neurology 1998; 51(6):1603–1607.
51. Van Alfen N, Sinke RJ, Zwarts MJ, et al. Intermediate CAG repeat lengths (53,54) for MJD/SCA3 are associated with an abnormal phenotype. Annals of Neurology 2001; 49(6):805–807.
52. Yunus MB, Aldag JC. Restless legs syndrome and leg cramps in fibromyalgia syndrome: a controlled study. BMJ 1996; 312(7042):1339.
53. Moldofsky H. Management of sleep disorders in fibromyalgia. Rheum Dis Clin North Am 2002; 28 (2):353–365.
54. Reynolds G, Blake DR, Pall HS, et al. Restless leg syndrome and rheumatoid arthritis. BMJ (Clin Res Ed) 1986; 292(6521):659–660.
55. Salih AM, Gray RE, Mills KR, et al. A clinical, serological and neurophysiological study of restless legs syndrome in rheumatoid arthritis. Br J Rheumatol 1994; 33(1):60–63.
56. Gudbjornsson B, Broman JE, Hetta J, et al. Sleep disturbances in patients with primary Sjogren's syndrome. Br J Rheumatol 1993; 32(12):1072–1076.
57. Gemignani F, Marbini A, Di Giovanni G, et al. Charcot-Marie-Tooth disease type 2 with restless legs syndrome. Neurology 1999; 52(5):1064–1066.
58. Gemignani F, Marbini A, Di Giovanni G, et al. Cryoglobulinaemic neuropathy manifesting with restless legs syndrome. J Neurol Sci 1997; 152(2):218–223.
59. Frankel BL, Patten BM, Gillin JC. Restless legs syndrome. Sleep-electroencephalographic and neurologic findings. JAMA 1974; 230(9):1302–1303.
60. Iannaccone S, Zucconi M, Marchettini P, et al. Evidence of peripheral axonal neuropathy in primary restless legs syndrome. Mov Disord 1995; 10(1):2–9.
61. Polydefkis M, Allen RP, Hauer P, et al. Subclinical sensory neuropathy in late-onset restless legs syndrome. Neurology 2000; 55(8):1115–1121.
62. Salvi F, Montagna P, Plasmati R, et al. Restless legs syndrome and nocturnal myoclonus: initial clinical manifestation of familial amyloid polyneuropathy. J Neurol Neurosurg Psychiatry 1990; 53 (6):522–525.
63. O'Hare JA, Abuaisha F, Geoghegan M. Prevalence and forms of neuropathic morbidity in 800 diabetics. Ir J Med Sci 1994; 163(3):132–135.
64. Rutkove SB, Matheson JK, Logigian EL. Restless legs syndrome in patients with polyneuropathy. Muscle Nerve 1996; 19(5):670–672.
65. Harriman DG, Taverner D, Woolf AL. Ekbom's syndrome and burning paresthesiae: a biopsy study by vital staining and electron microscopy of the intramuscular innervation with a note on age changes in motor nerve endings. Brain 1970; 93:393–406.
66. Gorman CA, Dyck PJ, Pearson JS. Symptom of restless legs. Arch Intern Med 1965; 115:155–160.
67. Walters AS, Wagner M, Hening WA. Periodic limb movements as the initial manifestation of restless legs syndrome triggered by lumbosacral radiculopathy [letter]. Sleep 1996; 19(10):825–826.
68. Hogl B, Kiechl S, Willeit J, et al. Restless legs syndrome: a community-based study of prevalence, severity, and risk factors. Neurology 2005; 64(11):1920–1924.
69. De Mello MT, Lauro FA, Silva AC, Tufik S. Incidence of periodic leg movements and of the restless legs syndrome during sleep following acute physical activity in spinal cord injury subjects. Spinal Cord 1996; 34(5):294–296.
70. Hartmann M, Pfister R, Pfadenhauer K. Restless legs syndrome associated with spinal cord lesions. J Neurol Neurosurg Psychiatry 1999; 66(5):688–689.
71. Lee MS, Choi YC, Lee SH, Lee SB. Sleep-related periodic leg movements associated with spinal cord lesions. Mov Disord 1996; 11(6):719–722.
72. Brown LK, Heffner JE, Obbens EA. Transverse myelitis associated with restless legs syndrome and periodic movements of sleep responsive to an oral dopaminergic agent but not to intrathecal baclofen. Sleep 2000; 23(5):591–594.
73. Bruno RL. Abnormal movements in sleep as a post-polio sequelae. Am J Phys Med Rehabil 1998; 77 (4):339–343.

74. Hemmer B, Riemann D, Glocker FX, et al. Restless legs syndrome after a borrelia-induced myelitis. Mov Disord 1995; 10(4):521–522.
75. Winkelmann J, Wetter TC, Trenkwalder C, et al. Periodic limb movements in syringomyelia and syringobulbia. Mov Disord 2000; 15(4):752–753.
76. Hogl B, Frauscher B, Seppi K, et al. Transient restless legs syndrome after spinal anesthesia: a prospective study. Neurology 2002; 59(11):1705–1707.
77. Moorthy SS, Dierdorf SF. Restless legs during recovery from spinal anesthesia. Anesth Analg 1990; 70(3):337.
78. Bhatia M, Bhowmik D. Restless legs syndrome in maintenance haemodialysis patients. Nephrol Dial Transplant 2003; 18(1):217.
79. Callaghan N. Restless legs syndrome in uremic neuropathy. Neurology 1966; 16(4):359–361.
80. Collado-Seidel V, Kohnen R, Samtleben W, et al. Clinical and biochemical findings in uremic patients with and without restless legs syndrome. Am J Kidney Dis 1998; 31(2):324–328.
81. Fukunishi I, Kitaoka T, Shirai T, et al. Facial paresthesias resembling restless legs syndrome in a patient on hemodialysis [letter]. Nephron 1998; 79(4):485.
82. Holley JL, Nespor S, Rault R. Characterizing sleep disorders in chronic hemodialysis patients. ASAIO Transactions 1991; 37(3):M456–M457.
83. Hui DS, Wong TY, Ko FW, et al. Prevalence of sleep disturbances in Chinese patients with end-stage renal failure on continuous ambulatory peritoneal dialysis. Am J Kidney Dis [computer file] 2000; 36 (4):783–788.
84. Hui DS, Wong TY, Li TS, et al. Prevalence of sleep disturbances in Chinese patients with end stage renal failure on maintenance hemodialysis. Med Sci Monit 2002; 8(5):CR331–C336.
85. Huiqi Q, Shan L, Mingcai Q. Restless legs syndrome (RLS) in uremic patients is related to the frequency of hemodialysis sessions. Nephron 2000; 86(4):540.
86. Parker KP. Sleep disturbances in dialysis patients. Sleep Med Rev 2003; 7(2):131–143.
87. Pieta J, Millar T, Zacharias J, et al. Effect of pergolide on restless legs and leg movements in sleep in uremic patients. Sleep 1998; 21(6):617–622.
88. Roger SD, Harris DC, Stewart JH. Possible relation between restless legs and anaemia in renal dialysis patients [letter]. Lancet 1991; 337(8756):1551.
89. Sabbatini M, Minale B, Crispo A, et al. Insomnia in maintenance haemodialysis patients. Nephrol Dial Transplant 2002; 17(5):852–856.
90. Stepanski E, Faber M, Zorick F, et al. Sleep disorders in patients on continuous ambulatory peritoneal dialysis. J Am Soc Nephrol 1995; 6(2):192–197.
91. Walker SL, Fine A, Kryger MH. L-DOPA/carbidopa for nocturnal movement disorders in uremia. Sleep 1996; 19(3):214–218.
92. Virga G, Mastrosimone S, Amici G, et al. Symptoms in hemodialysis patients and their relationship with biochemical and demographic parameters. Int J Artif Organs 1998; 21(12):788–793.
93. Wetter TC, Stiasny K, Kohnen R, et al. Polysomnographic sleep measures in patients with uremic and idiopathic restless legs syndrome. Mov Disord 1998; 13(5):820–824.
94. Winkelman JW, Chertow GM, Lazarus JM. Restless legs syndrome in end-stage renal disease. Am J Kidney Dis 1996; 28(3):372–378.
95. Read DJ, Feest TG, Nassim MA. Clonazepam: effective treatment for restless legs syndrome in uraemia. BMJ (Clin Res Ed) 1981; 283(6296):885–886.
96. Tanaka K, Morimoto N, Tashiro N, et al. The features of psychological problems and their significance in patients on hemodialysis—with reference to social and somatic factors. Clin Nephrol 1999; 51(3):161–176.
97. Nielsen V. The peripheral nerve function in chronic renal failure. Acta Med Scand 1971; 190:105–111.
98. Benz RL, Pressman MR, Peterson DD. Periodic limb movements of sleep index (PLMSI): a sensitive predictor of mortality in dialysis patients. J Am Soc Nephrol 1994; 5:433.
99. Yasuda T, Nishimura A, Katsuki Y, Tsuji Y. Restless legs syndrome treated successfully by kidney transplantation—a case report. Clinical Transplants 1986:138.
100. Winkelmann J, Stautner A, Samtleben W, et al. Long-term course of restless legs syndrome in dialysis patients after kidney transplantation. Mov Disord 2002; 17(5):1072–1076.
101. Ondo WG, Vuong KD, Jankovic J. Exploring the relationship between Parkinson disease and restless legs syndrome. Arch Neurol 2002; 59(3):421–424.
102. O'Keeffe ST, Gavin K, Lavan JN. Iron status and restless legs syndrome in the elderly. Age Ageing 1994; 23(3):200–203.
103. Silber MH, Richardson JW. Multiple blood donations associated with iron deficiency in patients with restless legs syndrome. Mayo Clin Proc 2003; 78(1):52–54.
104. Sun ER, Chen CA, Ho G, et al. Iron and the restless legs syndrome. Sleep 1998; 21(4):371–377.
105. Aul EA, Davis BJ, Rodnitzky RL. The importance of formal serum iron studies in the assessment of restless legs syndrome. Neurology 1998; 51(3):912.
106. Ulfberg J, Nystrom B. Restless legs syndrome in blood donors. Sleep Med 2004; 5(2):115–118.

107. Ondo W, Tan EK, Mansoor J. Rheumatologic serologies in secondary restless legs syndrome. Mov Disord 2000; 15(2):321–323.
108. Earley CJ, Allen RP, Beard JL, et al. Insight into the pathophysiology of restless legs syndrome. J Neurosci Res 2000; 62(5):623–628.
109. Goodman JD, Brodie C, Ayida GA. Restless leg syndrome in pregnancy. BMJ 1988; 297(6656):1101–1102.
110. Botez MI, Lambert B. Folate deficiency and restless-legs syndrome in pregnancy [letter]. N Engl J Med 1977; 297(12):670.
111. Manconi M, Govoni V, Cesnik E, et al. Epidemiology of restless legs syndrome in a population of 606 pregnant women. Sleep 2003; 26(Abstract Supplement):A300–A301.
112. Lee KA, Zaffke ME, Baratte-Beebe K. Restless legs syndrome and sleep disturbance during pregnancy: the role of folate and iron. J Womens Health Gend Based Med 2001; 10(4):335–341.
113. Ruottinen HM, Partinen M, Hublin C, et al. An FDOPA PET study in patients with periodic limb movement disorder and restless legs syndrome. Neurology 2000; 54(2):502–504.
114. Wetter TC, Collado-Seidel V, Pollmacher T, et al. Sleep and periodic leg movement patterns in drug-free patients with Parkinson's disease and multiple system atrophy. Sleep 2000; 23(3):361–367.
115. Braga-Neto P, Da Silva FP, Jr., Sueli Monte F, et al. Snoring and excessive daytime sleepiness in Parkinson's disease. J Neurol Sci 2004; 217(1):41–45.
116. Krishnan PR, Bhatia M, Behari M. Restless legs syndrome in Parkinson's disease: a case-controlled study. Mov Disord 2003; 18(2):181–185.
117. Tan EK, Lum SY, Wong MC. Restless legs syndrome in Parkinson's disease. J Neurol Sci 2002; 196 (1–2):33–36.
118. Ondo WG, Lai D. Association between restless legs syndrome and essential tremor. Mov Disord 2006; 21(4):515–518.
119. Abetz L, Allen R, Follet A, et al. Evaluating the quality of life of patients with restless legs syndrome. Clin Ther 2004; 26(6):925–935.
120. Smith RC. The Babinski response and periodic limb movement disorder. J Neuropsychiatry Clin Neurosci 1992; 4(2):233–234.
121. Lugaresi E, Coccagna G, Mantovani M, et al. Some periodic phenomena arising during drowsiness and sleep in man. Electroencephalogr Clin Neurophysiol 1972; 32(6):701–705.
122. Wetter TC, Eisensehr I, Trenkwalder C. Functional neuroimaging studies in restless legs syndrome. Sleep Med 2004; 5(4):401–406.
123. Bara-Jimenez W, Aksu M, Graham B, et al. Periodic limb movements in sleep: state-dependent excitability of the spinal flexor reflex. Neurology 2000; 54(8):1609–1616.
124. Montplaisir J, Boucher S, Gosselin A, et al. Persistence of repetitive EEG arousals (K-alpha complexes) in RLS patients treated with L-DOPA. Sleep 1996; 19(3):196–199.
125. Terzano MG, Mancia D, Salati MR, et al. The cyclic alternating pattern as a physiologic component of normal NREM sleep. Sleep 1985; 8(2):137–145.
126. Clemens S, Rye D, Hochman S. Restless legs syndrome: revisiting the dopamine hypothesis from the spinal cord perspective. Neurology 2006; 67(1):125–130.
127. Yang C, White DP, Winkelman JW. Antidepressants and periodic leg movements of sleep. Biol Psychiatry 2005; 58(6):510–514.
128. Ancoli-Israel S, Kripke DF, Klauber MR, et al. Periodic limb movements in sleep in community-dwelling elderly. Sleep 1991; 14(6):496–500.
129. Mosko SS, Dickel MJ, Paul T, et al. Sleep apnea and sleep-related periodic leg movements in community resident seniors. J Am Geriatr Soc 1988; 3 6(6):502–508.
130. Roehrs T, Zorick F, Sicklesteel J, et al. Age-related sleep-wake disorders at a sleep disorder center. J Am Geriatr Soc 1983; 31(6):364–370.
131. Bixler EO, Kales A, Vela-Bueno A. Nocturnal myoclonus and nocturnal myoclonic activity in a normal population. Res Commun Chem Pathol Pharmacol 1982; 36:129–140.
132. Montplaisir J, Boucher S, Poirier G, et al. Clinical, polysomnographic, and genetic characteristics of restless legs syndrome: a study of 133 patients diagnosed with new standard criteria. Mov Disord 1997; 12(1):61–65.
133. Coleman RM, Miles LE, Guilleminault CC, et al. Sleep-wake disorders in the elderly: polysomnographic analysis. J Am Geriatr Soc 1981; 29(7):289–296.
134. Montplaisir J, Michaud M, Denesle R, et al. Periodic leg movements are not more prevalent in insomnia or hypersomnia but are specifically associated with sleep disorders involving a dopaminergic impairment. Sleep Med 2000; 1(2):163–167.
135. Morisson F, Decary A, Petit D, et al. Daytime sleepiness and EEG spectral analysis in apneic patients before and after treatment with continuous positive airway pressure. Chest 2001; 119(1):45–52.
136. Fry JM, DiPhillipo MA, Pressman MR. Periodic leg movements in sleep following treatment of obstructive sleep apnea with nasal continuous positive airway pressure. Chest 1989; 96(1):89–91.
137. Wiegand M, Schacht-Muller W, Starke C. [Psychophysiologic insomnia and periodic leg movements in sleep syndrome]. Wien Med Wochenschr 1995; 145(17–18):527–528.

138. Nicolas A, Lesperance P, Montplaisir J. Is excessive daytime sleepiness with periodic leg movements during sleep a specific diagnostic category? Eur Neurol 1998; 40(1):22–26.

139. Bader G, Lavigne G. Sleep bruxism: an overview of an oromandibular sleep movement disorder. Review Article. Sleep Med Rev 2000; 4(1):27–43.

140. Macaluso GM, Guerra P, Di Giovanni G, et al. Sleep bruxism is a disorder related to periodic arousals during sleep. J Dent Res 1998; 77(4):565–573.

141. Ohayon MM, Li KK, Guilleminault C. Risk factors for sleep bruxism in the general population. Chest 2001; 119(1):53–61.

142. Laberge L, Tremblay RE, Vitaro F, et al. Development of parasomnias from childhood to early adolescence. Pediatrics 2000; 106(1 pt 1):67–74.

143. Kieser JA, Groeneveld HT. Relationship between juvenile bruxing and craniomandibular dysfunction. J Oral Rehabil 1998; 25(9):662–665.

144. Pierce CJ, Chrisman K, Bennett ME, et al. Stress, anticipatory stress, and psychologic measures related to sleep bruxism. J Orofac Pain 1995; 9(1):51–56.

145. Watanabe T, Ichikawa K, Clark GT. Bruxism levels and daily behaviors: 3 weeks of measurement and correlation. J Orofac Pain 2003; 17(1):65–73.

146. Lavigne GJ, Rompre PH, Poirier G, et al. Rhythmic masticatory muscle activity during sleep in humans. J Dent Res 2001; 80(2):443–448.

147. Gastaldo E, Quatrale R, Graziani A, et al. The excitability of the trigeminal motor system in sleep bruxism: a transcranial magnetic stimulation and brainstem reflex study. J Orofac Pain 2006; 20 (2):145–155.

148. Lobbezoo F, Soucy JP, Montplaisir JY, et al. Striatal D2 receptor binding in sleep bruxism: a controlled study with iodine-123-iodobenzamide and single-photon-emission computed tomography. J Dent Res 1996; 75(10):1804–1810.

149. Hublin C, Kaprio J, Partinen M, Koskenvuo M. Sleep bruxism based on self-report in a nationwide twin cohort. J Sleep Res 1998; 7(1):61–67.

150. Camparis CM, Formigoni G, Teixeira MJ, et al. Sleep bruxism and temporomandibular disorder: clinical and polysomnographic evaluation. Arch Oral Biol 2006.

151. Camparis CM, Siqueira JT. Sleep bruxism: clinical aspects and characteristics in patients with and without chronic orofacial pain. Oral Surg Oral Med Oral Pathol Oral Radiol Endod 2006; 101(2): 188–193.

152. Ellison JM, Stanziani P. SSRI-associated nocturnal bruxism in four patients. J Clin Psychiatry 1993; 54 (11):432–434.

153. Micheli F, Fernandez Pardal M, Gatto M, et al. Bruxism secondary to chronic antidopaminergic drug exposure. Clin Neuropharmacol 1993; 16(4):315–323.

154. Lavigne GL, Lobbezoo F, Rompre PH, et al. Cigarette smoking as a risk factor or an exacerbating factor for restless legs syndrome and sleep bruxism. Sleep 1997; 20(4):290–293.

155. Camparis CM, Formigoni G, Teixeira MJ, et al. Clinical evaluation of tinnitus in patients with sleep bruxism: prevalence and characteristics. J Oral Rehabil 2005; 32(11):808–814.

156. Lavigne GJ, Rompre PH, Guitard F, et al. Lower number of K-complexes and K-alphas in sleep bruxism: a controlled quantitative study. Clin Neurophysiol 2002; 113(5):686–693.

157. Cutler P. Cramps in the legs and feet. JAMA 1984; 252:98.

158. Weiner IH, Weiner HL. Nocturnl leg cramps. JAMA 1980; 244:2332.

159. Norris FH. An electomyographic study of induced and spontaeous muscle cramps. Electroencep Clin Neurophysiol 1957; 9:139.

160. Leung AK, Wong BE, Chan PY, et al. Nocturnal leg cramps in children: incidence and clinical characteristics. J Natl Med Assoc 1999; 91(6):329–332.

161. Haskell SG, Fiebach NH. Clinical epidemiology of nocturnal leg cramps in male veterans. Am J Med Sci 1997; 313(4):210–214.

162. Jacobsen JH, Rosenberg RS, Huttenlocher PR, et al. Familial nocturnal cramping. Sleep 1986; 9(1):54–60.

163. Ricker K, Moxley RT, 3rd. Autosomal dominant cramping disease. Arch Neurol 1990; 47(7):810–812.

164. Butler JV, Mulkerrin EC, O'Keeffe ST. Nocturnal leg cramps in older people. Postgrad Med J 2002; 78 (924):596–598.

165. Hoban TF. Rhythmic movement disorder in children. CNS Spectr 2003; 8(2):135–138.

166. Garbarino S, De Carli F, Nobili L, et al. Sleepiness and sleep disorders in shift workers: a study on a group of Italian police officers. Sleep 2002; 25(6):648–653.

167. Ohayon MM, Roth T. Prevalence of restless legs syndrome and periodic limb movement disorder in the general population. J Psychosom Res 2002; 53(1):547–554.

168. Berger K, Luedemann J, Trenkwalder C, et al. Sex and the risk of restless legs syndrome in the general population. Arch Intern Med 2004; 164(2):196–202.

169. Rothdach AJ, Trenkwalder C, Haberstock J, et al. Prevalence and risk factors of RLS in an elderly population: the MEMO study. Memory and morbidity in Augsburg elderly. Neurology 2000; 54(5): 1064–1068.

170. Nichols DA, Allen RP, Grauke JH, et al. Restless legs syndrome symptoms in primary care: a prevalence study. Arch Intern Med 2003; 163(19):2323–2329.
171. Ulfberg J, Nystrom B, Carter N, et al. Restless Legs Syndrome among working-aged women. Eur Neurol 2001; 46(1):17–19.
172. Ulfberg J, Nystrom B, Carter N, et al. Prevalence of restless legs syndrome among men aged 18 to 64 years: an association with somatic disease and neuropsychiatric symptoms. Mov Disord 2001; 16(6):1159–1163.
173. Sevim S, Dogu O, Camdeviren H, et al. Unexpectedly low prevalence and unusual characteristics of RLS in Mersin, Turkey. Neurology 2003; 61(11):1562–1569.
174. Unruh ML, Levey AS, D'Ambrosio C, et al. Restless legs symptoms among incident dialysis patients: association with lower quality of life and shorter survival. Am J Kidney Dis 2004; 43(5):900–909.
175. Mucsi I, Molnar MZ, Rethelyi J, et al. Sleep disorders and illness intrusiveness in patients on chronic dialysis. Nephrol Dial Transplant 2004; 19(7):1815–1822.
176. Gigli GL, Adorati M, Dolso P, et al. Restless legs syndrome in end-stage renal disease. Sleep Med 2004; 5(3):309–315.
177. Bhowmik D, Bhatia M, Tiwari S, et al. Low prevalence of restless legs syndrome in patients with advanced chronic renal failure in the Indian population: a case controlled study. Ren Fail 2004; 26(1):69–72.
178. Takaki J, Nishi T, Nangaku M, et al. Clinical and psychological aspects of restless legs syndrome in uremic patients on hemodialysis. Am J Kidney Dis 2003; 41(4):833–839.
179. Goffredo Filho GS, Gorini CC, Purysko AS, et al. Restless legs syndrome in patients on chronic hemodialysis in a Brazilian city: frequency, biochemical findings and comorbidities. Arq Neuropsiquiatr 2003; 61(3B):723–727.
180. Kutner NG, Bliwise DL. Restless legs complaint in African-American and Caucasian hemodialysis patients. Sleep Med 2002; 3(6):497–500.
181. Cirignotta F, Mondini S, Santoro A, et al. Reliability of a questionnaire screening restless legs syndrome in patients on chronic dialysis. Am J Kidney Dis 2002; 40(2):302–306.
182. Miranda M, Araya F, Castillo JL, et al. [Restless legs syndrome: a clinical study in adult general population and in uremic patients]. Rev Med Chil 2001; 129(2):179–186.
183. Walker S, Fine A, Kryger MH. Sleep complaints are common in a dialysis unit. Am J Kidney Dis 1995; 26(5):751–756.
184. Bastani B, Westervelt FB. Effectiveness of clonidine in alleviating the symptoms of "restless legs" [letter]. Am J Kidney Dis 1987; 10(4):326.

45 | Types of Sleep-Related Movement Disorders

Chang-Kook Yang
Sleep Disorders Clinic, Busan Sleep Center, Busan, Korea

John Winkelman
Division of Sleep Medicine, Brigham & Women's Hospital, Harvard Medical School, Boston, Massachusetts, U.S.A.

INTRODUCTION

Although sleep is popularly conceptualized as a quiet state without movement, a variety of motor phenomena can occur during this time. With the aid of video-polysomnographic electroencephalographic (EEG) and electromyographic (EMG) monitoring, sleep-related movements can be directly observed. Movements can be described based on duration, amplitude, periodicity, and most importantly their predilection to disturb sleep or produce other undesirable consequences. Sleep-related movement disorders (SRMD) constitute a class of movements that are simple and usually stereotyped, and are associated with undesirable effects such as impaired sleep quantity or quality, and/or impairment in daytime functioning. Unlike parasomnias, they are not associated with sleep-related mentation and are not goal-directed. They may occur during the transition between sleep and waking, and vice versa, or during any sleep stages.

In the revised International Classification of Sleep Disorders (ICSD-2) [American Academy of Sleep Medicine (AASM), 2005], SRMD comprise restless legs syndrome, periodic limb movement disorder (PLMD), sleep-related leg cramps (SRLC), sleep-related bruxism, and sleep-related rhythmic movement disorder (SRRMD). In addition, several conditions involving abnormal movements during sleep are listed under section "Isolated Symptoms, Apparently Normal Variants, and Unresolved Issues" in the revised ICSD-2 (AASM, 2005), such as sleep starts, benign sleep myoclonus of infancy, hypnagogic foot tremor (HFT), and alternating leg muscle activation (ALMA) during sleep, propriospinal myoclonus at sleep onset, and excessive fragmentary myoclonus. However, among these conditions, only HFT and ALMA during sleep will be described in this chapter, because the remaining conditions are relatively rare. This chapter addresses SRMD described in the revised ICSD-2 (AASM, 2005) and HFT and ALMA during sleep, with an emphasis on the key symptoms and signs, demographic, onset, clinical course, and risk factors of each condition.

RESTLESS LEGS SYNDROME

Demographics
Age of Onset
Restless legs syndrome (RLS) has generally been considered a condition of adulthood, but studies of adults with RLS have shown that a substantial portion report their symptoms as starting from childhood or adolescence (Walters et al., 1994, 1996; Montplaisir et al., 1997). Similarly, recent clinical case series and one epidemiologic study of children demonstrate that RLS does exist in a pediatric context. Walters et al. (1996) conducted an age of onset survey among 138 adults with RLS: 12% to 20% had experienced the onset of RLS before the age of 10 and 25% had experienced it between the age of 11 and 20. Most respondents stated that their symptoms were mild at onset and then became progressively more severe. Montplaisir et al. (1997) also studied age of onset of 133 patients by questionnaire and found that RLS started at a mean age of 27.2 years, and before 20 in 38.5% of patients. Among 551 RLS sufferers identified by a questionnaire survey of 23,051 patients in primary care offices in the United States and four European countries, those who reported at least twice weekly symptoms with appreciable negative impact on quality of life, and likely warranting treatment for RLS, the mean age of

onset of the symptoms was 48.5 years for males and 44.5 years for females. Overall, 53.4% of males and 64.8% of females (61.1% overall) reported onset at 50 years of age or younger (Hening et al., 2004).

Descriptions of RLS in children demonstrate an identical phenotype as adult RLS, suggesting that it is the same disorder with an early onset. One case series reported onset of symptoms at age 7 to 10, with a family history of RLS in 60% of definite cases, and ferritin levels below the fifth percentile of age and weight in one-third of cases. Thus, it may be seen from these studies that RLS can set in at any age, from early childhood to late adult life.

Racial Variation

There have been some reports suggesting marked ethnic and geographic differences in the prevalence of RLS. Three studies from Asian countries have shown much lower prevalence of RLS than has been reported in studies from North American or Europe: 0.1% (in 1000 individuals aged 21 years and older) to 0.6% (in 157 individuals aged 55 years and older) in Singapore (Tan et al., 2001), 1.1% (Mizuno et al., 2005) and 1.5% (Kageyama et al., 2000) in Japan, and 3.2% in Turkey (Sevim et al., 2003). In a direct interview survey of 308 chronic renal failure patients on hemodialysis aged 60 to 87 in Georgia, patients of African-American descent showed lower prevalence of RLS compared with those of Caucasian descent (68% vs. 48%) (Kutner and Bliwise, 2002).

Sex

All large cohort studies using accepted RLS diagnostic criteria, whether questionnaire based or from direct interviews, have shown a female preponderance in the prevalence of RLS regardless of ethnic background (Rothdach et al., 2000; Nichols et al., 2003; Sevim et al., 2003; Hening et al., 2004; Bjorvatn et al., 2005; Mizuno et al., 2005; Tison et al., 2005; Hogl et al., 2005; Allen et al., 2005). In a study of the general adult population in two Scandinavian countries, employing the International Restless Legs Syndrome Study Group (IRLSSG) criteria, prevalence was higher in females than in males (13.4% vs. 9.4%) (Bjorvatn et al., 2005). A study based on face-to-face interviews of 369 elderly people aged 65 to 83 in Germany, employing the IRLSSG criteria, found that the prevalence of RLS in females is twice that of males (13.9% vs. 6.1%) (Rothdach et al., 2000). A similar study of 701 people aged 50 to 89 in northern Italy also employed IRLSSG criteria, and also found that females were suffering RLS more than twice as much as males (14.2% vs. 6.6%) (Hogl et al., 2005). Similarly, in the REST (RLS Epidemiology, Symptoms, and Treatment) population study performed in four European countries and the U.S., females were roughly twice as commonly affected by RLS when symptoms at any frequency were included (9.0% vs. 5.4%) or when only those with symptoms at least twice per week associated with moderate distress were counted (3.7% vs. 1.7%). This was true in all age groups (Hening et al., 2004).

Key Symptoms and Signs

RLS is a sensorimotor disorder characterized by complaints of a compelling, nearly irresistible, urge to move the legs (AASM, 2005). According to criteria for developed by the IRLSSG (Allen et al., 2003), RLS is diagnosed by the following four cardinal features: (*i*) an urge to move the legs, usually accompanied or caused by uncomfortable and unpleasant sensations in the legs, (*ii*) the urge to move, or unpleasant sensations either begin or worsen during periods of rest or inactivity such as lying or sitting, (*iii*) the urge to move, or unpleasant sensations are partially or totally relieved by movement such as walking or stretching, at least as long as the activity continues, and (*iv*) the urge to move, or unpleasant sensations either become worse in the evening or night than during the day, or occur only in the evening or night.

Diagnostically, an urge to move the legs (or arms) while awake at rest is the predominant feature of RLS. This compulsion becomes greater if this urge is suppressed, and may then evolve into an involuntary movement of the affected limb(s). At times, it may be difficult for patients to distinguish the voluntary movements produced by the urge to move from such involuntary movements. Such movements may be recognized to be periodic when recorded with electromyography (EMG), and under such conditions have been called dyskinesias when awake (Hening et al., 1986), or more recently, periodic limb movements during wakefulness (PLMW) (Montplaisir et al., 1998).

Although an urge to move is the defining feature of RLS, it is referred to as a sensorimotor disorder because of the common presence of sensory symptoms, which are variously described as creepy-crawly, tension, ants crawling, jittery, pulling, electric current, pain, burning, numb, and growing pains. Ekbom (1960), who was responsible for naming RLS, and its first modern description, reported the symptoms typically as creeping sensations felt at greater than skin depth, in the muscles or bones, but not in the joints. The symptoms are typically bilateral, but may be asymmetrical, and occasionally may alternate between the right and left legs. The majority of patients describe their symptoms as occurring predominantly between the ankle and knee, and the shin may be more affected than the calf (Morgan, 1967). Besides the legs, the sensations may also affect the thighs or feet, and less often the buttocks and lower back. Sometimes, they may be limited to one region such as the thighs, or feet. The arms may also be affected, particularly in patients with severe RLS, though the symptoms in the arms are often mild (Michaud et al., 2000).

One of the defining characteristics of RLS is that it follows a circadian rhythm, with a worsening of symptoms during the evening and the night. Studies using a constant routine protocol in which RLS patients remain lying down over a 24-hour period demonstrate that this evening/nighttime worsening of symptoms is a true circadian rhythm rather than simply due to a propensity to be less active, physically or mentally at this time of day (Michaud et al., 2005; Hening et al., 1999). As a result of the difficulty remaining still at night, sleep-related problems are rated by patients with RLS as their most troublesome symptom (Hening et al., 2004). In a study of 133 patients with RLS (Montplaisir et al., 1997), employing the IRLSSG diagnostic criteria (Walters, 1995), 84.7% reported difficulty falling asleep at night because of RLS symptoms, while 86% reported that symptoms woke them up frequently during the night. Female patients with RLS report more complaints of sleep-related symptoms (difficulty in falling asleep, difficulty in staying asleep, and involuntary movements while awake) than males (Bentley et al., 2006).

Onset, Ontogeny, and Clinical Course

The natural history of RLS has been poorly characterized, as it is predominantly understood through the study of patients who present for clinical attention. In the clinical context, RLS appears to be slowly progressive, with frequency, intensity, latency, and time of day of symptom onset gradually worsening over time. However, it is believed that the course of RLS may show marked variation, as either progressive, staying the same, waxing and waning, or even resolving (Trenkwalder et al., 1996). What complicates matters is that for many patients, symptoms vary considerably from day to day depending on a variety of factors, but particularly by the extent and timing of sedentary activities, such as a long flight or car rides, attending long meetings or performances, or by attempting to fall asleep. The symptoms may occur several times a day, while they may be totally absent on other days. Sudden remissions may also be experienced, lasting for months or even years, without apparent reason.

Some insight into clinical course may be gleaned from studies of RLS prevalence within different age groups. The majority of studies have reported increasing rates of RLS with advancing age, with a decline in RLS prevalence in the very elderly (Sevim, et al., 2003; Nichols et al., 2003; Allen et al., 2005; Rothdach et al., 2000). The REST population-based study found a linear increase in RLS prevalence (among those with symptoms at least twice per week, associated with at least moderate distress) across each decade from 20 to 80 years of age, with a decline in those over 80 years (Allen et al., 2005). Ulfberg et al.'s study (2001) of men living in central Sweden, employing IRLSSG criteria, also showed that the prevalence of RLS increased linearly with age, affecting 1.2% of participants aged 18 to 24 years, 4.0% of those aged 25 to 34 years, 6.2% of those aged 35 to 44 years, 8.0% of those aged 45 to 54 years, and 10.5% of those aged 55 to 64 years.

On the other hand, studies have shown that the clinical course of RLS may vary as a function of age of onset. Earlier onset RLS (before age 45) may be slowly progressive while later onset RLS may show more rapid progression (Allen and Earley, 2000, 2001). The IRLSSG (Allen et al., 2003) has also described a similar clinical course as previous studies for associated features of RLS

> The clinical course of RLS varies considerably. When the age of onset of RLS symptoms is less than 50 years, the onset is more insidious; when the age of onset is

greater than 50 years, the symptoms often occur more abruptly and more severely. In some patients, RLS can be intermittent and may spontaneously remit for many years.

Risk Factors

The only established risk factors for RLS are female gender, older age, and family history of RLS. No biochemical marker for RLS exists and thus RLS remains a clinical diagnosis. However, RLS is observed more commonly in several distinct conditions than it is in the general population, and usually disappears when such conditions resolve, and in such cases it is called "secondary RLS."

Pregnancy has long been considered as an important risk factor for causing or worsening RLS. Epidemiologic studies have shown that the risk of RLS for a pregnant woman is at least two or three times higher than for other women (Phillips et al., 2000). Manconi et al. (2004a) performed a structural interview including IRLSSG criteria to 642 pregnant women at the time of delivery and found 26.6% of participants (61.7% of them never had experienced RLS in their life) were affected by RLS. RLS associated with pregnancy appears most frequently during the last trimester, and those with pre-existing RLS usually become worse at this time. Pregnancy-related RLS is usually mild, and symptoms generally begin to improve in the four weeks preceding delivery and disappear afterwards (Goodman et al., 1988; Manconi et al., 2004a). Three main hypotheses as the underlying mechanism of the association between RLS and pregnancy have been suggested (Manconi et al., 2004b): hormonal (e.g., estrogen, progesterone, and prolactin), psychomotor behavioral (e.g., anxiety, stress, and motor habits), and metabolic hypotheses (serum folate, iron, and other iron indicators). Current pathophysiologic models for RLS focus on the central dopaminergic system, central iron pathways, and endogenous opioid system dysfunction (Allen, 2004). On the other hand, serotonergic, noradrenergic, and GABAergic systems may also be implicated, at least in part, in RLS (Wetter and Pollmacher 1997; Trenkwalder and Paulus, 2004). Thus, it is plausible that drugs that affect these neurotransmitter systems may influence the expression of RLS. Some evidence from published case reports suggest that RLS symptoms may be caused or worsened by several medications. Among them, the association of RLS with antidepressants has been most frequently reported, though some studies failed to find an association (Leubtgeb and Martus, 2002; Brown et al., 2005; Hogl et al., 2005). Antidepressant medications such as selective serotonin reuptake inhibitors (SSRIs) (Bakshi, 1996; Sanz-Fuentenebro et al., 1996; Hargrave and Beckley, 1998; Ohayon and Roth, 2002), mirtazapine (Pae et al., 2004), mianserine (Markkula and Lauerma, 1997), and tricyclic antidepressants (Morgan, 1967) have been reported to cause or worsen RLS. Besides antidepressants, antihistamines (Ondo, 2004), lithium (Terao et al., 1991), antipsychotic agents such as phenothiazine derivatives (Blom and Ekbom, 1961), olanzapine (Kraus et al., 1999), and risperidone (Wetter et al., 2002), zonisamide (Chen et al., 2003), and nonopioid analgesics (Leubtgeb and Martus, 2002) also have been reported to cause or worsen RLS. All of these drugs share some common pharmacologic characteristics, namely, significant antidopaminergic, antiserotonergic, antiadrenergic, anticholinergic, and antihistaminergic effects.

Several substances have also been reported as risk factors for RLS. Three recent epidemiologic studies found a significant correlation between smoking and RLS (Phillips et al., 2000; Ohayon and Roth, 2002; Sevim et al., 2003). On the other hand, a Canadian population-based study failed to find a significant association of smoking with RLS (Lavigne et al., 1997). Caffeine has long been implicated in worsening of RLS symptoms (Missak, 1987; Jeddy and Berridge, 1994). On the basis of therapeutic experience with 62 patients over an 11-year period, Lutz (1978) observed that the occurrence of RLS in some patients coincided with their initial consumption of caffeine-containing beverages, while in others it followed their increased consumption. Alcohol also has been considered to be a risk factor. The general population telephone survey in five European countries found that individuals drinking at least three alcoholic beverages a day were more likely to have RLS [odds ratio (OR) 1.47] (Ohayon and Roth, 2002). Among a sample from a general sleep disorders clinic, women who consumed two or more drinks a day were more likely to report RLS symptoms and to be diagnosed with RLS (Aldrich and Shipley, 1993). On the other hand, one epidemiologic study revealed that RLS was associated with alcohol abstinence (Phillips et al., 2000).

It has been reported that depression, stress, and anxiety may aggravate the symptoms and distress of RLS (Gorman et al., 1965). However, this finding does not necessarily indicate an involvement of psychologic factors in RLS. There is a possibility that the higher frequency of psychologic distresses in patients with RLS may be a consequence of the RLS symptoms themselves.

Other factors, such as shift work, engaging in strenuous physical activity close to bedtime, fatigue, insufficient exercise, a very warm environment, and prolonged exposure to cold may also exacerbate RLS symptoms.

PERIODIC LIMB MOVEMENT DISORDER

Demographics
Age of Onset
The typical age of onset of PLMD is not known. Like RLS, periodic limb movements in sleep (PLMS) have also been identified among children, even though the prevalence of isolated PLMS is low (Kirk and Bohn, 2004; Traeger et al., 2005). In a study of children referred to a pediatric sleep laboratory for any reason, only 1.2% of the 591 children studied had evidence of PLMS index greater than 5 with no other comorbidity (Kirk and Bohn, 2004). This result shows that PLMS is an uncommon disorder of childhood, even in a select population at increased risk for having a sleep disorder. PLMS in children have been reported mostly to be associated with attention deficit hyperactivity disorder (ADHD) (Chervin et al., 2002; Crabtree et al., 2003) and obstructive sleep apnea (OSA) (Kirk and Bohn, 2004; Martinez and Guilleminault, 2004). Researchers have proposed that PLMS may directly lead to symptoms of ADHD through the mechanisms of sleep disruption and/or PLMS and ADHD may share a common dopaminergic deficit (Picchietti et al., 1998; Walters et al., 2000).

Sex
Results of studies for a difference in prevalence of PLMS between sexes are mixed. In a study of 100 people aged 18 to 74 using polysomnography, Bixler et al. (1982) did not find any sex difference. A study of 100 people aged 60 and above, using three nights' polysomnography, also showed no gender relationship with PLMD (Dickel and Mosko, 1990). On the other hand, there are studies reporting a male preponderance. One such study of 427 people aged 65 and older, using leg EMG measurements recorded at home, found that males had significantly higher PLM indices than females (Ancoli-Israel et al., 1991) and in a study of 111 people aged 21.2 to 70.9, using bilateral foot actigraphy, males had significantly higher PLM indices than females, and a greater proportion of males (52%) than females (22%) had a PLM index greater than five events per hour (Morrish et al., 2002).

Key Symptoms and Signs
PLMS is a sleep-related phenomenon, consisting of extension of the great toe followed by partial flexions of the remaining toes (similar to the Babinski reflex), the ankle, the knee, and sometimes the hip, lasting 0.5 to 5 seconds and recurring periodically at intervals of 5 to 90 seconds during sleep. PLMS occur most frequently in the lower limbs, although similar movements may occur in the upper limbs in which the affected arm repetitively flexes at the elbow. The movements can be unilateral or bilateral, and sometimes they alternate from one extremity to the other. The movements vary, from one sustained tonic contraction to a polyclonic burst (AASM, 2005).

PLMD is defined by the presence of a PLMS index greater than 15 in adults (greater than 5 in children), which is associated with a complaint of sleep disturbance or daytime fatigue that can not be accounted for by other means (AASM, 2005). Thus, in contrast to a diagnosis of RLS, which is based on a patient's report, a diagnosis of PLMD is only confirmed by polysomnography. The causal association between PLMS and sleep disturbance is hotly debated (Mahowald, 2001, 2007; Walters, 2001; Hogl, 2007). Nevertheless, the revised ICSD-2 (AASM, 2005) recommends that the diagnosis of PLMD should be made in cases where there is either clinical sleep disturbance or a description of daytime fatigue without other concurrent conditions or disorders accounting for these complaints. PLMD is thus a diagnosis of exclusion. PLMD is explicitly disallowed in patients with RLS, narcolepsy, and REM sleep behavior disorder where PLMS are commonly observed and considered to be ancillary symptoms of the disorder. Although there is substantial information regarding the physiology of PLMS, little is known about the clinical characteristics of PLMD.

PLMS appear more frequently during light sleep stages N1 and N2, although they may also occur in sleep stages N3 and in REM sleep. Microarousals associated with PLM, are more prevalent in sleep stages N1 and N2 than in sleep stage N3 and REM (Sforza et al., 2003). PLMS may be related to the cyclic alternating pattern (CAP), which is a physiologic component of non-REM (NREM) sleep and a measure of NREM instability. Parrino et al. (1996) investigated the relationship of PLMS and CAP and found that of all the PLMS detected in NREM sleep, 92% occurred in CAP, with the great majority of limb movements (96%) associated with phase A. PLM can also occur during waking (PLMW), especially in patients with RLS. In RLS, it has been proposed that PLMW bursts can be longer lasting (up to 10 seconds), perhaps due to a voluntary prolongation of an initial involuntary movement (Michaud et al., 2001). Pollmacher and Schulz (1993) investigated the relationship of the characteristic features of PLM to the duration of movements, their sleep stage distribution, and their arousing effects on sleep. They observed that relative frequency of movements, their duration, and their arousing effect decreased along the NREM stages, whereas the intermovement interval increased. During REM sleep, the duration of movements was shortest and the intermovement interval was longest. They also found that the PLM index did not differ among stages wake, N1 and N2, and the duration of movements was longest during stage wake. It has been suggested to score PLMW separately because excluding PLMW from scoring may lead to an underestimation of the relative frequency of PLM (Pollmacher and Schulz, 1993), and PLMW provide a better diagnostic index for RLS (Michaud et al., 2002). Like RLS, PLMS are influenced by a circadian rhythm with PLMS index progressively declining from the first to the last sleep cycle (Trenkwalder et al., 1999; Sforza et al., 2003).

The clinical significance of PLMS is still being debated. Intense PLMs may be an important causal factor of poor sleep quality and nonrestorative sleep by provoking EEG arousals or awakenings. Patients who are unaware of sleep disruptions may complain of daytime sleepiness (Bastuji and Garcia-Larrea, 1999; Montplaisir et al., 2000). On the other hand, clinical presentations among children with PLMS are somewhat different. They may present with nonspecific symptoms such as leg pains at morning awakening, growing pains, restless sleep, inattention, and hyperactivity (Chervin and Hedger, 2001; Martinez and Guilleminault, 2004). Other studies have also shown that cerebral and cardiac activations occur in association with PLMS even without EEG microarousal (Winkelman, 1999; Sforza et al., 2002; Ferrillo et al., 2004; Pennestri et al., 2007). These findings indicate that PLMS may have clinical significance in terms of sleep continuity (insomnia), daytime functioning (sleepiness), as well as cardiovascular consequences. However, substantial numbers of studies published have failed to find any correlation between PLMS and clinical symptoms such as insomnia or daytime sleepiness (Mendelson, 1996; Nicolas et al., 1998; Karadeniz et al., 2000; Hornyak et al., 2004; Haba-Rubio et al., 2005). Thus, it has been suggested that PLMS represent a phenomenon associated with an underlying arousal disorder (Karadenia et al., 2000; Montplaisir et al., 2000) or may even simply reflect a general aging process because of its extremely common occurrence in the elderly (Carrier et al., 2005). PLMS also may be an epiphenomenon accompanying conditions with diminished dopaminergic function such as Parkinson's disease. However, the influence of other factors, such as sleep stages, sleep duration of prior nights, and amount of physical activity during the day may have confounded studies examining the correlation of PLMS and clinical outcomes.

Onset, Ontogeny, and Clinical Course

Studies have shown that the prevalence of PLMS increases with advancing age: 29% of people aged 50 and older had PLMS, whereas only 5% of those aged 30 to 50 and almost none under 30 were affected (Bixler et al., 1982). Other community-based PLM studies have also shown a correlation between age and PLMS (Dickel and Mosko, 1990; Ancoli-Israel et al., 1991). However, Morrish et al. (2002) failed to find such a correlation between PLM index and age. The natural clinical course is not known (AASM, 2005).

Risk Factors

Since PLMD and RLS may share the same pathophysiology, they may also share risk factors. There have also been reported associations between PLMD and use of medications, such as antidepressant agents (Ware et al., 1984; Hussain et al., 1997; Salin-Pascual et al., 1997; Yang et al., 2005), and antipsychotics (Cohrs et al., 2004). Interestingly, bupropion has been reported as the only antidepressant not to cause or worsen PLMD. In a retrospective case series, Nofzinger et al. (2000) found that bupropion was not associated with drug-induced PLMD; rather, its administration reduced objective measures of PLMD in five depressed patients with the disorder. Yang et al.'s study (2005) also showed that the mean PLM index of patients with bupropion was similar to that of a control group, and was significantly lowered compared with those of patients treated with SSRIs and venlafaxine.

In an epidemiologic study of 18,980 adults aged 15 to 100 in the general population using ICSD criteria for PLMD, Ohayon and Roth (2002) identified several factors associated with PLMD, such as female gender (OR 1.47), shift work (OR 1.41), engaging in strenuous physical activity close to bedtime (OR 1.43), drinking more than six cups of coffee a day (OR 2.32), and high life stress (OR 2.01).

SLEEP-RELATED LEG CRAMPS

Demographics
Age of Onset
SRLC affect all age groups, but they tend to occur more in middle-aged and older populations. In one study, the mean age of onset of cramps was 60 years; for both males and females (Naylor and Young, 1994). Leung et al. (1999) found that no SRLC were reported in children younger than 8 years, and the incidence increased sharply from the age of 12, with a majority of the affected children experiencing leg cramps one to four times per year. A majority of studies suggest that the peak period of onset of SRLC is usually in adulthood, and both the prevalence and the frequency of their occurrence increases with age (Hall, 1947; Oboler et al., 1991; Naylor and Young, 1994; Abdulla et al., 1999; Leung et al., 1999; Young, 2004; Giglio et al., 2005). Hall (1947) observed that 56% of 200 adults aged 15 to 80 had cramps and the incidence increased to 70% in individuals aged 50 and older. Naylor and Young (1994) also found that 27% of their subjects aged 50 to 59, and 54% of those aged 80 and older had rest cramps, indicating a significant increase with age.

Sex
The results on sex differences for SRLC are mixed. Leung et al. (1999) found no sex differences in children and adolescents aged 3 to 18. There was also no significant sex difference in adults (Naylor and Young, 1994). However, Jansen et al. (1991) reported a female preponderance in cases of muscle cramps (3:2), even though the authors did not specify whether the cramps were nocturnal. Abdulla et al. (1999) also reported that SRLC was more common in females (56%) than in males (40%) (OR 1.96).

Key Symptoms and Signs
SRLC are painful sensations caused by sudden and intense involuntary contractions of muscles or muscle groups, usually in the calf or small muscles of the foot, occurring during any sleep stage (AASM, 2005). During the cramps, the muscles involved become firm and tender, and feet and toes are held in extreme plantar flexion. When the cramps occur, sufferers may try to relieve the symptoms by flexion of the foot of the affected limb or by massaging the calf muscle. Individuals who experience SRLC are awakened by painful spasms or tightening of the muscles of the calf or foot, and sometimes the affected individuals get out of bed and walk to cope with the cramps, which may cause distress or difficulty in sleeping. One study reported that 6% of nursing home residents experienced sleep difficulty because of SRLC (Gentili et al., 1997). Symptoms vary from very mild to very severe and the frequency varies considerably, from less than yearly to multiple episodes every night (Oboler et al., 1991; Naylor and Young, 1994; Abdulla et al., 1999; Leung et al., 1999).

The following two studies, involving children and adults, respectively, show a characteristic outline of SRLC. In a study of 2527 healthy children aged 3 to 18 seen in an ambulatory care clinic, SRLC was reported in 7.3% of them, 73% experienced leg cramps while asleep, with the mean duration of episodes being 1.7 minutes; the episodes usually occurred unilaterally, and approximately 1/3 of the affected children had residual tenderness that usually lasted for half an hour (Leung et al., 1999). In a general practice based study of 233 people aged 50 and older, 37% of subjects had had rest cramps during the preceding two months, the cramps usually occurring only, or mostly, at night (73%). The most frequently affected sites were leg, foot, or thigh muscles. The mean duration of the episodes was nine minutes, though symptoms experienced in the thigh muscle lasted longer than those from muscles of the foot or leg. Only 37% of sufferers had reported their symptoms to their primary physician, and over a third of those who described their symptoms as very distressing had not reported them (Naylor and Young, 1994).

Onset, Ontogeny, and Clinical Course

In many patients, SRLC shows a fluctuating course of many years' duration, although it has been believed that most leg cramps are benign and self-limited (Weiner and Weiner, 1980). One study reported that 20% of SRLC sufferers had been suffering for more than 10 years (Abdulla et al., 1999). There was a significant increase in the mean age of subjects self-rating their cramps to be very distressing (Naylor and Young, 1994). These studies suggest that SRLC is a chronic condition and symptoms tend to be worse with age.

Risk Factors

Epidemiologic data describing SRLC in the general population are limited and little is known about risk factors. A majority of cases of SRLC are idiopathic, but several medications reported to be associated with the condition include diuretics, purgatives, calcium channel blockers (nifedipine), phenothiazines, selective estrogen receptor modulators (raloxifene), vincristine, clofibrate. beta-agonists (salbutamol, terbutaline), steroids, morphine withdrawal, cimetidine, penicillamine, statins, lithium, and cholinesterase inhibitors, analgesic (Keidar et al., 1982; Eaton, 1989; McGee, 1990; Mandal et al., 1995; Riley and Antony, 1995; Haskell and Fiebach, 1997; Abdulla et al., 1999; Leung et al., 1999; Kanaan and Sawaya, 2001). Fluid and electrolyte disturbances such as hypoglycemia, hyponatremia, and hypovolemia may cause SRLC (Layzer, 1994; Riley and Antony, 1995; Young, 2004). Profuse sweating without sodium replacement and strenuous exercise per se also may be a cause (Leung et al., 1997; Young, 2004).

SLEEP-RELATED BRUXISM

Demographics

Age of Onset

The onset of sleep-related bruxism (SRB) is at about one year of age, soon after the eruption of the deciduous incisors (AASM, 2005). SRB is believed to show a high night-to-night fluctuation, with none occurring on some nights and severe SRB on others (Lavigne et al., 2001).

Sex

The sex ratio of SRB prevalence remains controversial, with various reports of no difference (Reding et al., 1966; Glaros, 1981; Lavigne and Montplaisir, 1994; Baba et al., 2004), a preponderance of girls in childhood (Bayardo et al., 1996; Hublin et al., 1998), a male preponderance (Watanabe et al., 2003), and a female preponderance (Ahlberg et al., 2002; Johansson et al., 2004).

Key Symptoms and Signs

SRB is an oral activity characterized by grinding or clenching of the teeth during sleep, usually associated with sleep arousals (AASM, 2005). There are three clinical expression of SRB: tooth grinding, tooth clenching, and tapping or jaw bracing (Lavigne and Montplaisir, 1994). SRB episodes can occur during all sleep stages, primarily in sleep stage 2 (Reding et al., 1968; Lavigne et al., 1996; Bader et al., 1997; Tosun et al., 2003). SRB also may occur during REM sleep, although the prevalence here is low (Bader et al., 1997; Tosun et al., 2003). Bader et al.

(1997) reported that the duration of the bruxing episode significantly increased with the deepening of sleep (i.e., stage N1 < N2 < N), and was significantly shorter in REM sleep compared with stage N2 sleep. The EMG during bruxing episodes shows a phasic pattern of activity at 1 Hz frequency lasting from one to five seconds (Reding et al., 1968; Hartmann et al., 1987). Most studies have demonstrated that SRB is strongly related to cerebral and autonomic nervous system activation (e.g., microarousals) (Bader et al., 1997; Macaluso et al., 1998; Kato et al., 2001), although negative results have been reported (Tosun et al., 2003). Shifts in sleep stages can also be seen before or after bruxism episodes (Bader et al., 1997). Polysomnographic data of six patients with SRB and six healthy age matched controls showed that 88% of bruxism episodes were associated with a CAP and always occurred during transient arousals (Macaluso et al., 1998).

Onset, Ontogeny, and Clinical Course

Several studies have shown that SRB is a persistent trait. In a large retrospective Finnish twin cohort questionnaire study of adults aged 33 to 60, Hublin et al. (1998) evaluated the persistence of SRB childhood to adulthood. They found that those who had SRB weekly or monthly as adults had reported it often or sometimes in childhood in 86.9% of males and 90.1% of females. Lavigne et al. (2001) analyzed night-to-night variability over time in nine patients with moderate to severe SRB, with a recording interval varying from 2 months to 7.5 years. This study also demonstrated that the frequency of SRB remained constant over time for each subject. Carlsson et al. (2003) reported a prospective 20-year follow-up study aimed at analyzing predictors of bruxism (originally with 402 randomly selected 7-, 11-, and 15-year-old subjects) and found that 100% who had reported frequent bruxism and 75% of those with occasional bruxism 20 years earlier reported they still had SRB. All of the aforementioned studies suggest that SRB might be a chronic disorder. However, SRB has been reported to gradually decrease with age; in an interview study of 2019 Canadians aged 18 and older, SRB showed a linear decrease with age, from 13% of subjects aged 18 to 29 to 3% of those aged 60 and older (Lavigne and Montplaisir, 1994).

Risk Factors

A variety of risk factors for SRB have been proposed. A history of childhood bruxism appears to predict its presence in adulthood. Carlsson et al. (2003) observed that subjective reports of bruxism in childhood were predictors of SRB 20 years later in adulthood (OR 3.1). It has been supposed that SRB is triggered by psychological factors (Funch and Gale, 1980; Ahlberg et al., 2002; Antonio et al., 2006), and bruxers are reported to have greater anxiety or vulnerability to stress (Bader et al., 1997; Bader and Lavigne, 2000). However, the association between SRB and psychological factors still remains uncertain. In a study, which used sleep recordings made at night for at least three weeks on 12 subjects (six females and six males), SRB was not found to be significantly related to daytime behaviors, such as stress, physical activity, and anger (Watanabe et al., 2003). These data are consistent with previous studies (Da Sliva et al., 1995; Pierce et al., 1995). Many epidemiologic studies have indicated smoking as a risk factor for SRB. In an epidemiologic study of 8888 Swedish 50-year-old subjects, there was a significant correlation between smoking and SRB (Johansson et al., 2004). In a study of 205 subjects randomly selected from an original cohort of 1339 Finns (Ahlberg et al., 2004), frequent smokers were more than twice as likely to report frequent SRB as nonfrequent smokers (OR 2.4). Furthermore, in a nationwide survey of 2019 Canadian adults aged 18 and older (Lavigne et al., 1997), cigarette smokers were almost twice as likely to report SRB (OR 1.9). In a cross-sectional telephone survey across three European countries, OSA, snoring, moderate daytime sleepiness, heavy caffeine or alcohol drinking, and stress and anxiety were found to be significant risk factors for sleep bruxism (Maurice et al., 2001). It has been reported that SRB was common in patients with OSA (Sjoholm et al., 2000; DiFrancesco et al., 2004) and in an epidemiologic study, OSA was the highest risk factor for SRB in the general population (Ohayon et al., 2001). The effect of continuous positive airway pressure in adults (Oksenberg and Arons, 2002) and adenotonsillectomy in children (DiFrancesco et al., 2004) on the elimination of SRB has been reported in patients who had both OSA and SRB. SRB may also be induced by medications, such as SSRIs (Ellison and Stanziani, 1993; Por et al., 1996; Romanelli et al., 1996) and antipsychotic agents (Amir et al. 1997).

SLEEP-RELATED RHYTHMIC MOVEMENT DISORDER

Demographics
Age of Onset
Age of onset of SRRMD generally is between 8 and 18 months. Spontaneous onset in adolescence or adulthood is very rare (AASM, 2005). In a study of 525 healthy children aged three months to six years, body rocking appeared first at the age of about six months, followed then, some three months later, by head banging and head rolling (Sallustro and Atwell, 1978). Kravitz et al. (1960) and de Lissovoy (1962) also reported that the average age of onset of headbanging was nine months.

Sex
Most types of SRRMD do not show significant difference in prevalence between the sexes. However, headbanging has been reported to occur three times more frequently in males than females (de Lissovoy, 1962; Sallustro and Atwell, 1978).

Key Symptoms and Signs
SRRMD, formerly termed jactatio capitis nocturna, is characterized by repetitive, stereotyped, and rhythmic motor behaviors of head, neck, or large muscle groups, often associated with rhythmic vocalizations. SRRMD comprises several subtypes: body rocking, head banging, head rolling, body rolling, leg banging, and leg rolling. Of the subtypes of SRRMD, body rocking is the earliest to appear and the most prevalent. It is associated with anteroposterior whole-body movements in the sitting, prone, or supine position. Head banging refers to repeated, rhythmic striking of the head and neck caused by anteroposterior head and neck movements that generally occur while the patient is in a supine or prone position. Alternately, the patient may sit with the back of the head against a headboard or wall, repeatedly banging the occiput. Head rolling usually occurs while the patient is in a supine position, with side-to-side head movements. Body rolling, leg banging, and leg rolling are less common forms (Sallustro and Atwell, 1978; Hoban, 2003; AASM, 2005).

Movements usually occur during the transition from wakefulness to sleep and persist or recur during stages N1 and N2, and less frequently during REM sleep and slow wave sleep (Chisholm and Morehouse, 1996; Dyken et al., 1997; Hoban, 2003; AASM, 2005), although a group exhibiting SRRMD exclusively during REM sleep has been described (Kempenaers et al., 1994; Kohyama et al., 2002; Anderson et al., 2006). In older patients, head and body rocking have been reported with increased frequency in REM sleep (Kavey et al., 1981; Thorpy and Spielman, 1984). SRRMD may occur with or without evidence of arousal from sleep (Happe et al., 2000) and it may show close association with the CAP A phases (Manni et al. 2004).

The frequency of rhythmic movements can vary, but they typically occur at a frequency of 0.5 to 2 Hz (Dyken et al., 1997; Stepanova et al., 2005). Their duration varies, generally lasting from several seconds up to approximately 20 minutes (Sallustro and Atwell, 1978; Dyken et al., 1997); however, they can persist for up to four hours (de Lissovoy, 1962). Rhythmic episodes appear to last longer in wakefulness and stage N1 sleep compared with those in stages N2, N3, and REM sleep (Stepanova et al., 2005). Patients are usually unresponsive during and amnestic for the events (Dyken et al., 1997), but cessation of movements may occur following environmental disturbance or being spoken to (AASM, 2005).

The majority of patients with SRRMD are normal infants and toddlers, where the behavior is usually not associated with injury. The ICSD-2 (AASM, 2005) recommends that SRRMD should be considered as pathologic only if the behaviors markedly interfere with normal sleep, cause significant impairment in daytime function, or result in self-inflicted bodily injury that requires medical treatment. A patient with persistent and problematic symptoms may disrupt the sleep of family members and pose a possible risk of serious injury. There have been case reports of cataracts (Bemporad, 1968), carotid dissection (Jackson et al., 1983), and fatal subdural hemorrhage (Mackenzie, 1991) resulting from headbanging.

Onset, Ontogeny, and Clinical Course
Most studies agree that SRRMD in its typical form is considered to be a benign and self-limited condition, which generally resolves in preschool. However, reports show that some cases

persist beyond childhood long into adolescence or adulthood (Chisholm and Morehouse, 1996; Happe et al. 2000; Stepanova et al., 2005; Anderson et al., 2006). In a longitudinal follow-up study of 212 normal Swedish infants, elements of rhythmic activity declined from 66% at the age of 9 months to 6% at the age of 5 years (Klackenberg, 1971). Kravitz et al. (1960) and de Lissovoy (1962) also reported that headbanging usually resolves before the fourth year and it is rarely present at the age of 10. Larberge et al. (2000) found persistent body rocking in 3% of 1353 children at the age of 13. Persistence of SRRMD into older childhood can lead to psychosocial problems (Klackenberg, 1971; Walsh et al., 1981). It has been reported that when SRRMD persists beyond childhood, it is more often associated with mental retardation, autism, or attention-deficit hyperactivity disorder (Stepanova et al., 2005).

Risk Factors
There has been little study of risk factors for SRRMD, but stimulus deprivation and environmental stressors have been proposed (Levy, 1944). Laberge et al. (2000) identified high anxiety scores among 42 children with bodyrocking compared with 1296 healthy children. Self-stimulation has been suggested as a factor, particularly in retarded, autistic, and emotionally disturbed children.

HYPNAGOGIC FOOT TREMOR AND ALTERNATING LEG MUSCLE ACTIVATION

Demographics
Age of Onset
Most studies have reported that HFT and alternating leg muscle activation (ALMA) are prevalent among middle-aged people. However, the fact should be taken into account that these results were obtained from patients who were having polysomnography performed mainly for evaluating sleep-disordered breathing, which is itself prevalent in middle aged and older people.

Sex
RFT and HFLM have been reported to affect males and females equally (Wichniak et al., 2001; Yang and Winkelman, 2005), but ALMA showed a male preponderance (3:1) (Chervin et al., 2003).

Key Symptoms and Signs
HFT and ALMA (see below) have been recently described in the literature. They are classified as "Isolated Symptoms, Apparently Normal Variants and Unresolved Issues" in the ICSD-2 (AASM, 2005). According to the ICSD-2 (AASM, 2005), HFT is defined as "rhythmic movement of the feet or toes that occurs at the transition between wake and sleep or during light NREM sleep stages 1 and 2." On the other hand, ALMA is defined as "brief activation of the anterior tibialis in one leg in alternation with similar activation in the other leg during sleep or arousals from sleep." In the ICSD-2 (AASM, 2005), these two phenomena are considered together because the frequency and duration of muscle activations and occurrence primarily with arousals suggest that these may be the same phenomena, or that ALMA represents an EMG manifestation of a subtype of HFT episodes. Yang and Winkelman (2005) also have described similar movements, with the proposed term high frequency leg movements (HFLM) rather than HFT or ALMA because their frequency is slower than tremor (tremor is usually faster than 3 Hz), they appear during all sleep stages including slow wave and REM sleep as well as at the transitional stage from wakefulness to sleep, and they usually tend to appear unilaterally, although sometimes they exhibit a bilateral alternating pattern. HFLM descriptively is very similar to HFT and ALMA.

HFT was first reported by Broughton (1988) in two patients who had suffered severe head injury and subsequently complained of insomnia. A coarse tremor of one or both feet occurred associated with sleep onset and resulted in sleep maintenance insomnia. As described by Broughton, the frequency of HFT varied between 0.5 and 1.5 Hz, and it tended to occur during presleep wakefulness, usually persisting in stages N1 and N2, but absent in stage N3 and REM sleep.

Wichniak et al. (2001) also described similar phenomena in 355 consecutive sleep-disordered patients (79.1% of them presented with sleep-related breathing problems) and 20 healthy controls, and found a prevalence of 7.5%. They proposed the term "rhythmic feet movements (RFM) while falling asleep" for these movements. In most cases the RFM occurred in a single short series generally lasting 10 to 15 seconds but sometimes persisting for up to 1 to 2 minutes. Movements were rhythmic, oscillating movements of the whole foot or toes. The frequency of the RFM was usually 1 to 2 Hz. The individual muscle bursts usually varied from 300 to 700 milliseconds in duration. The amplitude of the bursts was variable and ranged between 60 and 650 microvolts. The RFM at highest intensity occurred during presleep wakefulness and during arousals, mostly from stages N1 and N2 but also from REM sleep. They did not occur during stage N3. Most subjects were unaware of the presence of these movements. Wichniak et al. (2001) suggested that, considering its high prevalence and the lack of a major sleep-disturbing effect, short series of RFM could be considered a quasiphysiologic phenomenon, although in more severe cases with evidence of a sleep-disturbing effect, they should be considered abnormal.

Chervin et al. (2003) reported similar movements, but noted that they alternated from one leg to another, and coined the term ALMA. They identified the records of 16 patients with ALMA among 1500 polysomnographic records performed for other reasons, usually for sleep-disordered breathing. ALMA was defined as more than four discrete and alternating muscle activations with less than two seconds between activations. The frequency of the contractions was approximately 1 to 2 Hz (range 0.5–3.0 Hz) with burst duration of 100 to 500 milliseconds. The sequence of movements usually lasted between several and 20 seconds (range 1.4–22.2 seconds). ALMA occurred primarily in stages N1, N2 and REM sleep but particularly during arousals, and was at times associated with PLMS. Similarly with HFT, ALMA was observed in otherwise asymptomatic patients. Cosentino et al. (2006) precisely described a 33-year-old male patient with ALMA who had been complaining of non-restorative sleep and excessive daytime sleepiness. They found that CAP subtypes, especially A3 subtype, almost always preceded the occurrence of ALMA sequences. They also suggested that ALMA might be considered as an additional phenomenon correlated with NREM sleep instability.

In Yang and Winkelman's study (2005), among 486 consecutive patients referred for overnight polysomnography (PSG), mainly to rule out sleep-disordered breathing, 37 patients demonstrated HFLM: 19 males (8.2% of PSGs) and 18 females (7.1% of PSGs), thus showing a similar sex distribution. Two-thirds (64.3%) of all HFLM occurred during waking and 35.7% occurred during sleep. Of those HFLM episodes occurring during sleep, 44.8% occurred during stage N1, 45.0% during stage N2, 0.5% during stage N3, and 9.5% during the REM stage. The mean frequency was 1.6 Hz (range 0.4–3.7 Hz), the mean number of episodes of HFLM per subject per night was 26.5 (range 2–111), and the mean duration was 17.6 seconds (range 1.5 seconds to 6.1 minutes). Among HFLM, which occurred during sleep stages, 10.0% developed independently of American Academy of Sleep Medicine [formerly American Sleep Disorder Association (ASDA)] defined EEG arousal, 8.7% developed during arousal, and 17.0% preceded ASDA-defined EEG arousal.

Onset, Ontogeny, and Clinical Course
Only a small number of studies have reported HFT or ALMA. Furthermore, they were cross-sectional rather than longitudinal so the onset and clinical course of these phenomena have yet to be determined.

Risk Factors
There is no report in the literature of risk factors for HFT and ALMA. However, 75% of Chervin et al.'s (2003) subjects were taking antidepressant medication. The authors speculated that antidepressant therapy may provoke ALMA, but Yang and Winkelman (2005) could not find any correlation between HFLM and antidepressant medication in their subjects.

Most previous studies have reported HFT and ALMA in patients with other sleep disorders, such as sleep-related breathing disorder, RLS or PLMD, not among the general population. Large cohort epidemiologic studies are needed to establish the general characteristics, such as demographics, time of onset, natural clinical course, and risk factors of HFT and ALMA and to determine whether they are normal physiologic epiphenomena or pathologic conditions. In addition, as mentioned above, different terminologies have been used to describe similar phenomena, and some agreement on this issue will also move this field forward.

CONCLUSIONS

SRMD are common disturbances of sleep. Until the consequences, if any, of SRMD are better established, the motivation for clinicians to diagnose and treat these disorders will be limited. In addition, in many SRMD, information on gender difference, ethnic associations, age of onset, clinical courses, and risk factors are insufficient. Thus, further studies are definitely desirable. In addition, many case reports and epidemiologic studies indicate that various medications or substances, either through intake or withdrawal, may contribute to developing or worsening of SRMD. However, since the majority of associations are based on case reports, and the prevalence of SRMD in the general population is relatively high, any causal interpretations should be made with extreme caution. Well-designed prospective studies may help with clarification regarding the prevalence and pathophysiology of drug-induced SRMD.

REFERENCES

Abdulla AJJ, Jones PW, Pearce VR. Leg cramps in the elderly: prevalence, drug and disease associations. Int J Clin Pract 1999; 53:494–496.

Ahlberg J, Rantala M, Savolainen A, et al. Reported bruxism and stress experience. Community Dent Oral Epidemiol 2002; 30:405–408.

Ahlberg J, Savolainen A, Rantala M, et al. Reported bruxism and biopsychosocial symptoms: a longitudinal study. Community Dent Oral Epidemiol 2004; 32:307–311.

Aldrich MS, Shipley JE. Alcohol use and periodic limb movements of sleep. Alcohol Clin Exp Res 1993; 17:192–119.

Allen R. Dopamine and iron in the pathophysiology of restless legs syndrome (RLS). Sleep Med 2004; 5:385–391.

Allen RP, Earley CJ. Defining the phenotype of the restless legs syndrome (RLS) using age-of-symptom-onset. Sleep Med 2000; 1:11–19.

Allen RP, Earley CJ. Restless legs syndrome: a review of clinical and pathophysiologic features. J Clin Neurophysiol 2001; 18:128–147.

Allen RP, Picchietti D, Hening WA, et al. Restless legs syndrome: diagnostic criteria, special considerations, and epidemiology: a report from the restless legs syndrome diagnosis and epidemiology workshop at the National Institutes of Health. Sleep Med 2003; 4:101–109.

Allen RP, Walters AS, Montplaisir J, et al. Restless legs syndrome prevalence and impact: REST general population study. Arch Intern Med 2005; 165:1286–1292.

American Academy of Sleep Medicine. The International Classification of Sleep Disorders. Diagnostic and Coding Manual. Second Edition. American Academy of Sleep Medicine. Sleep Related Movement Disorders, Westchester, IL, 2005.

Amir I, Hermesh H, Gavish A. Bruxism secondary to antipsychotic drug exposure: a positive response to propranolol. Clin Neuropharmacol. 1997; 20:86–89.

Ancoli-Israel S, Kripke DF, Klauber MR, et al. Periodic limb movements in sleep in community-dwelling elderly. Sleep 1991; 14:496–500.

Anderson KN, Smith IE, Shneerson JM. Rhythmic movement disorder (head banging) in an adult during rapid eye movement sleep. Mov Disord 2006; 21:866–867.

Antonio AG, da Silva Pierro VS, Maia LC. Bruxism in children: a warning sign for psychological problems. J Can Dent Assoc 2006; 72:155–160.

Baba K, Haketa T, Clark GT, et al. Does tooth wear status predict ongoing sleep bruxism in 30-year-old Japanese subjects? Int J Prothodont 2004; 17:39–44.

Bader GG, Kampe T, Tagdae T, et al. Descriptive physiological data on a sleep bruxism population. Sleep 1997; 20:982–990.

Bader G, Lavigne G. Sleep bruxism; an overview of an oromandibular sleep movement disorder. Sleep Med Rev 2000; 4:27–43.

Bakshi R. Fluoxetine and restless legs syndrome. J Neurol Sci 1996; 142:151–152.

Bastuji H, Garcia-Larrea L. Sleep/wake abnormalities in patients with periodic leg movements during sleep: factor analysis on data from 24-h ambulatory polygraphy. J Sleep Res 1999; 8:217–223.

Bayardo RE, Mejia JJ, Orozco S, et al. Etiology of oral habits. ASDC J Dent Child 1996; 63:350–353.

Bemporad JR. Cataracts following chronic head banging: a report of two cases. Am J Psychiatry 1968; 125:245–249.

Bentley AJ, Rosman KD, Mitchell D. Gender differences in the presentation of subjects with restless legs syndrome. Sleep Med 2006; 7:37–41.

Bixler EO, Kales A, Vela-Bueno A, et al. Nocturnal myoclonus and nocturnal myoclonic activity in the normal population. Res Commun Chem Pathol Pharmacol 1982; 36:129–140.

Bjorvatn B, Leissner L, Ulfberg J, et al. Prevalence, severity and risk factors of restless legs syndrome in the general adult population in two Scandinavian countries. Sleep Med 2005; 6:307–312.

Blom S, Ekbom KA. Comparison between akathisia developing on treatment with phenothiazine derivatives and the restless legs syndrome. Acta Medica Scandinavica 1961; 170:689–694.

Broughton R. Pathological fragmentary myoclonus, intensified hypnic jerks and HFT: three unusual sleep-related movement disorders. In: Koella WP, Obal F, Schulz H, Visser P, eds. Sleep 86 Symposium 10. Stutgart, New York: Gustav Fischer Verlag, 1988:240–243.

Brown LK, Dedrick DL, Doggett JW, et al. Antidepressant medication use and restless legs syndrome in patients presenting with insomnia. Sleep Med 2005; 6:443–450.

Carlsson GE, Egermark I, Magnusson T. Predictors of bruxism, other oral parafunctions, and tooth wear over a 20-year follow-up period. J Orofac Pain 2003; 17:50–57.

Carrier J, Frenette S, Montplaisir J, et al. Effects of periodic leg movements during sleep in middle-aged subjects without sleep complaints. Mov Disord 2005; 20:1127–1132.

Chen JT, Garcia PA, Alldredge BK. Zonisamide-induced restless legs syndrome. Neurology 2003; 60:147.

Chervin RD, Archbold KH, Dillon JE, et al. Association between symptoms of inattention, hyperactivity, restless legs, and periodic leg movements. Sleep 2002; 25:213–218.

Chervin RD, Consens FB, Kutluay E. Alternating leg muscle activation during sleep and arousals: a new sleep-related motor phenomenon? Mov Disord 2003; 18:551–559.

Chervin RD, Hedger KM. Clinical prediction of periodic leg movements during sleep in children. Sleep Med 2001; 2:501–510.

Chisholm T, Morehouse RL. Adult headbanging: sleep studies and treatment. Sleep 1996; 19:343–346.

Cohrs S, Rodenbeck A, Guan Z, et al. Sleep promoting properties of quetiapine in healthy subjects. Psychopharmacol. (Berl) 2004; 174:421–429.

Cosentino FII, Iero I, Lanuzza B, et al. The neurophysiology of the alternating leg muscle activation (ALMA) during sleep: study of one patient before and after treatment with pramipexole. Sleep Med 2006; 7:63–71.

Crabtree VM, Ivanenko A, O'Brien LM, et al. Periodic limb movement disorder of sleep in children. J Sleep Res 2003; 12:73–81.

Dickel MJ, Mosko SS. Morbidity cut-offs for sleep apnea and periodic leg movements in predicting subjective complaints in seniors. Sleep 1990; 13:155–166.

DiFrancesco RC, Junqueira PAS, Trezza PM, et al. Improvement of bruxism after T & A surgery. Int J Pediatr Otorhinolaryngol 2004; 68:441–445.

de Lissovoy V. Head banging in early childhood. Child Dev 1962; 33:43–56.

Dyken ME, Lin-Dyken DC, Yamada T. Diagnosing rhythmic movement disorder with video-polysomnography. Pediatr Neurol 1997; 16:37–41.

Eaton JM. Is this really a muscle cramp? Postgrad Med J 1989; 86:227–232.

Ekbom KA. Restless legs syndrome. Neurology 1960; 10:868–873.

Ellison JM, Stanziani P. SSRI-associated nocturnal bruxism in four patients. J Clin Psychiatry 1993; 54: 432–434.

Ferrillo F, Beelke M, Canovaro P, et al. Changes in cerebral and autonomic activity heralding periodic limb movements in sleep. Sleep Med 2004; 5:407–412.

Funch DP, Gale EN. Factors associated with nocturnal bruxism and its treatment. J Behav Med 1980; 3:385–387.

Gentili A, Weiner DK, Kuchibhatil M, et al. Factors that disturb sleep in nursing home residents. Aging (Milano) 1997; 9:207–213.

Giglio P, Undevia N, Spire J-P. The primary parasomnias: a review for neurologists. Neurologist 2005; 11:90–97.

Glaros AG. Incidence of diurnal and nocturnal bruxism. J Prosthet Dent 1981; 45:545–549.

Goodman JDS, Brodie C, Ayida GA. Restless leg syndrome in pregnancy. Br Med J 1988; 297:1101–1102.

Gorman CA, Dyck PJ, Pearson JS. Symptoms of restless legs. Arch Int Med 1965; 115:155–160.

Haba-Rubio J, Staner L, Krieger J, et al. Periodic limb movements and sleepiness in obstructive sleep apnea patients. Sleep Med 2005; 6:225–229.

Hall AJ. Cramp and salt balance in ordinary life. Lancet 1947; ii:231–233.

Happe S, Ludemann P, Ringelstein EB. Persistence of rhythmic movement disorder beyond childhood: a videotape demonstration. Mov Disord 2000; 15:1296–1298.

Hargrave R, Beckley DF. Restless legs syndrome exacerbated by sertraline (letter). Psychosomatics 1998; 39:177–178.

Hartmann E, Mehta N, Forgione A, et al. Bruxism: effects of alcohol. Sleep Res 1987; 16:351.

Haskell SG, Fiebach NH. Clinical epidemiology of nocturnal leg cramps in male veterans. Am J Med Sci 1997; 313:210–214.

Hening W, Walters AS, Allen RP, et al. Impact, diagnosis and treatment of restless legs syndrome (RLS) in a primary care population: the REST (RLS epidemiology, symptoms, and treatment) primary care study. Sleep Med 2004; 5:237–246.

Hening WA, Walters AS, Wagner M, et al. Circadian rhythm of motor restlessness and sensory symptoms in the idiopathic restless legs syndrome. Sleep 1999; 22:901–912.

Hoban TF. Rhythmic movement disorder in children. CNS Spectrums 2003; 8:135–138.

Hogl B. Periodic leg movements are associated with disturbed sleep. J Clin Sleep Med 2007; 3:12–14.

Hogl B, Kiechl S, Willeit J, et al. Restless legs syndrome: a community-based study of prevalence, severity, and risk factors. Neurology 2005; 64:1920–1924.

Hornyak M, Riemann D, Voderholzer U. Do periodic leg movements influence patients' perception of sleep quality? Sleep Med 2004; 5:597–600.

Hublin C, Kaprio J, Partinen M, et al. Sleep bruxism based on self-report in a nationwide twin cohort. J Sleep Res 1998; 7:61–67.

Hussain MRG, Novak M, Jindal R, et al. Periodic leg movements in patients on different antidepressants therapies. Sleep Res 1997; 26:380.

Jackson MA, Hughes RC, Ward SP. "Headbanging" and carotid dissection. Br Med J 1983; 287:1262.

Jansen PHP, Joosten EMG, VanDiyck JAAM, et al. The incidence of muscle cramps. J Neurol Neurosurg Psychiatry 1991; 54:1124–1125.

Jeddy TA, Berridge DC. Restless leg syndrome. Br J Surg 1994; 81:49–45.

Johansson A, Unell L, Carlsson G, et al. Associations between social and general health factors and symptoms related to temporomandibular disorders and bruxism in a population of 50-year-old subjects. Acta Odontol Scand 2004; 62:231–237.

Kageyama T, Kabuto M, Nitta H, et al. Prevalence of periodic limb movement-like and restless legs-like symptoms among Japanese adults. Psychiatry Clin Neurosci 2000; 54:296–298.

Kanaan N, Sawaya R. Nocturnal leg cramps. Clinically mysterious and painful—but manageable. Geriatrics 2001; 56:34, 39–42.

Karadeniz D, Ondze B, Besset A, et al. Are periodic leg movements during sleep (PLMS) responsible for sleep disruption in insomnia patients? Eur J Neurol 2000; 7:331–336.

Kato T, Rompre P, Montplaisir JY, et al. Sleep bruxism: an oromotor activity secondary to micro-arousal. J Dent Res 2001; 80:1940–1944.

Kavey NB, Sewitch DE, Bloomingdale E, et al. Jactatio capitis nocturna: a longitudinal study of a boy with familial history. Sleep Res 1981; 10:208.

Keidar S, Binenboim C, Palant A. Muscle cramps during treatment with nifedipine. Br Med J 1982; 285:1241–1242.

Kempenaers C, Bouillon E, Mendlewicz J. A rhythmic movement disorder in REM sleep: a case report. Sleep 1994; 17:274–279.

Kirk VG, Bohn S. Periodic limb movements in children: prevalence in a referred population. Sleep 2004; 27:313–315.

Klackenberg G. Rhythmic movements in infancy and early childhood. Acta Paediatr Scand 1971; 224 (suppl 1):74–82.

Kohyama J, Matsukura F, Kimura K, et al. Rhythmic movement disorder: polysomnographic study and summary of reported cases. Brain Dev 2002; 24:33–38.

Kravitz H, Rosenthal V, Teplitz Z, et al. A study of headbanging in infants and children. Dis Nerv Syst 1960; 21:203–208.

Kraus T, Schuld A, Pollmacher T. Periodic leg movements in sleep and restless legs syndrome probably caused olanzapine. J Clin Psychopharmacol 1999; 19:478–479.

Kutner NG, Bliwise DL. Restless legs complaint in African-American and Caucasian hemodialysis patients. Sleep Med. 2002; 3:497–500.

Laberge L, Tremblay RE, Vitaro F, et al. Development of parasomnias from childhood to early adolescence. Pediatrics 2000; 106(1 pt 1):67–74.

Lavigne GJ, Guitard F, Rompre PH, et al. Variability in sleep bruxism activity over time. J Sleep Res 2001; 10:237–244.

Lavigne GJ, Lobbezoo F, Rompre PH, et al. Cigarette smoking as a risk factor or an exacerbating factor for restless legs syndrome and sleep bruxism. Sleep 1997; 20:290–293.

Lavigne GJ, Montplaisir JY. Restless legs syndrome and sleep bruxism: prevalence and association among Canadians. Sleep 1994; 17:739–743.

Lavigne GJ, Rompre PH, Montplaisir JV. Sleep bruxism: validity of clinical research diagnostic criteria in a controlled polysomnographic study. J Dent Res 1996; 75:546–552.

Layzer RB. The origin of muscle fasciculations and cramps. Muscle Nerve 1994; 17:1243–1249.

Leubtgeb U, Martus P. Regular intake of non-opioid analgesics is associated with an increased risk of restless legs syndrome in patients maintained on antidepressants. Eur J Med Res 2002; 7:368–378.

Leung AKC, Wong BE, Cho HYH, et al. Leg cramps in children. Clin Pediatr 1997; 32:69–73.

Leung AKC, Wong BE, Chan PYH, et al. Nocturnal leg cramps in children: incidence and clinical characteristics. J Natl Med Assoc 1999; 91:329–332.

Levy DM. On the problem of movement restraint (tics, stereotyped movements, hyperactivity). Am J Orthopsychiatry 1944; 14:644–671.

Lutz E. Restless legs, anxiety and caffeinism. J Clin Psychiatry 1978; 39:693–698.

Macaluso GM, Guerra P, Di Giovanni E, et al. Sleep bruxism is a disorders related to periodic arousals during sleep. J Dent Res 1998; 77:565–573.

Mackenzie JM. "Headbanging" and fatal subdural haemorrhage. Lancet 1991; 338:1457–1458.

Mahowald MW. Assessment of periodic leg movements is not an essential component of an overnight sleep study. Am J Respir Crit Care Med 2001; 164:1340–1341.

Mahowald MW. Periodic leg movements are NOT associated with disturbed sleep. J Clin. Sleep Med 2007; 3:15–17.

Manconi M, Govoni V, De Vito A, et al. Restless legs syndrome and pregnancy. Neurology 2004a; 63: 1065–1069.

Manconi M, Govoni V, De Vito A, et al. Pregnancy as a risk factor for restless legs syndrome. Sleep Med 2004b; 5:305–308.

Mandal AK, Abernathy T, Nelluri SN, et al. Is quinine effective and safe in leg cramps? J Clin Pharmacol 1995; 35:588–593.

Manni R, Terzaghi M, Sartori I, et al. Rhythmic movement disorder and cyclic alternating pattern during sleep: a video-polysomnographic study in a 9-year old boy. Mov Disord 2004; 19:1186–1190.

Markkula J, Lauerma H. Mianserin and restless legs. Int Clin Psychopharmacol 1997; 12:53–58.

Martinez S, Guilleminault C. Periodic leg movements in prepubertal children with sleep disturbances. Dev Med Child Neurol 2004; 46:765–770.

Maurice M, Ohayon KK, Guilleminault LC. Risk factors for sleep bruxism in the general population. Chest 2001; 119:53–61.

McGee SR. Muscle cramps. Arch Intern Med 1990; 150:511–518.

Mendelson WB. Are periodic leg movements associated with clinical sleep disturbances? Sleep 1996; 19:219–223.

Michaud M, Chabli A, Lavigne G, et al. Are restlessness in patients with restless legs syndrome. Mov Disord 2000; 15:289–293.

Michaud M, Dumont M, Paquet J, et al. Circadian variation of the effects of immobility on symptoms of restless legs syndrome. Sleep 2005; 28:843–846.

Michaud M, Paquet J, Lavigne G, et al. Sleep laboratory diagnosis of restless legs syndrome. Eur Neurol 2002; 48:108–113.

Missak SS. Does the human body produce a substance similar to caffeine? Med Hypotheses 1987; 24: 161–165.

Mizuno S, Miyaoka T, Inagaki T, et al. Prevalence of restless legs syndrome in non-institutionalized Japanese elderly. Psychiatr Clin Neurosci 2005; 59:461–465.

Montplaisir J, Boucher S, Nicolas A, et al. Immobilization tests and periodic leg movements in sleep for the diagnosis of restless legs syndrome. Mov Disord 1998; 13:324–329.

Montplaisir J, Boucher S, Poirier G, et al. Clinical, polysomnographic, and genetic characteristics of restless legs syndrome: a study of 133 patients diagnosed with the new standard criteria. Mov Disord 1997; 12:61–65.

Montplaisir J, Michaud M, Denesle R, et al. Periodic leg movements are not more prevalent in insomnia or hypersomnia but are specifically associated with sleep disorders involving a dopaminergic impairment. Sleep Med 2000; 1:163–167.

Morgan LK. Restless limbs: a commonly overlooked symptom controlled 'Valium'. Med J Aust 1967; 2:589–594.

Morrish E, King MA, Pilsworth SN, et al. Periodic limb movement in a community population detected by a new actigraphy technique. Sleep Med 2002; 3:489–495.

Naylor JR, Young JB. A general population survey of rest cramps. Age Ageing 1994; 23:418–420.

Nichols DA, Allen RP, Grauke JH, et al. Restless legs syndrome symptoms in primary care: a prevalence study. Arch Intern Med 2003; 163:2323–2329.

Nicolas A, Lesperance P, Montplaisir J. Is excessive daytime sleepiness with periodic leg movements during sleep a specific diagnostic category? Eur Neurol 1998; 40:22–26.

Nofzinger EA, Fasiczka A, Berman S, et al. Bupropion SR reduces periodic limb movements associated with arousals from sleep in depressed patients with periodic limb movement disorder. J Clin Psychiatry 2000; 61:858–862.

Oboler SK, Prochazka AV, Meyer TJ. Leg symptoms in outpatient veterans. West J Med 1991; 155:256–259.

Ohayon MM, Li KK, Guilleminault C. Risk factors for sleep bruxism in the general population. Chest 2001; 119:53–61.

Ohayon MM, Roth T. Prevalence of restless legs syndrome and periodic limb movement disorder in the general population. J Psychosom Res 2002; 53:547–554.

Oksenberg A, Arons E. Sleep bruxism related to obstructive sleep apnea: the effect of continuous positive airway pressure. Sleep Med 2002; 3:513–515.

Ondo W. Secondary restless legs syndrome. In: Chaudhuri KR, Odin P, Olanow CW, eds. Restless Legs Syndrome. London and New York: Taylor & Francis, 2004:57–84.

Pae CU, Kim TS, Kim JJ, et al. Re-administration of mirtazapine could overcome previous mirtazapine-associated restless legs syndrome? Psychiatr Clin Neurosci 2004; 58:669–670.

Parrino L, Boselli M, Buccino GP, et al. The cyclic alternating pattern plays a gate-control on periodic limb movements during non-rapid eye movement sleep. J Clin Neurophysiol 1996; 13:314–323.

Pennestri MH, Montplaisir J, Colombo R, et al. Nocturnal blood pressure changes in patients with restless legs syndrome. Neurology 2007; 68:1213–1218.

Phillips B, Young T, Finn L, et al. Epidemiology of restless legs syndrome in adults. Arch Intern Med 2000; 160:2137–2141.

Picchietti DL, England SJ, Walters AS, et al. Periodic limb movement disorder and restless legs syndrome in children with attention-deficit hyperactivity disorder. J Child Neurol 1998; 13:589–594.

Pierce CJ, Chrisman K, Bennett ME, et al. Stress, anticipatory stress, and psychological measures related to sleep bruxism. J Orofac Pain 1995; 9:51–56.

Pollmacher T, Schulz H. Periodic leg movements (PLM): their relationship to sleep stages. Sleep 1993; 16:572–577.

Por CH, Watson L, Doucetter D, et al. Sertraline-associated bruxism. Can J Clin Pharmacol 1996; 3: 123–125.

Reding GR, Rubright WC, Zimmerman SO. Incidence of bruxism. J Dent Res 1966; 45:1198–1204.

Reding GR, Zepelin H, Robinson JE, et al. Nocturnal teeth grinding. All-night psychophysiologic studies. J Dent Res 1968; 47:796–797.

Riley JD, Antony SJ. Leg cramps: differential diagnosis and management. Am Fam Physcian 1995; 52:1794–1798.

Romanelli F, Adler DA, Bungay KM. Possible paroxetine-induced bruxism. Ann Pharmacother 1996; 30:1246–1248.

Rothdach AJ. Trenkwalder C, Haberstock J, et al. Prevalence and risk factors of RLS in an elderly population: the MEMO study. Neurology 2000; 54:1064–1068.

Salin-Pascual RJ, Galicia-Polo L, Drucker-Colin R. Sleep changes after 4 consecutive days of venlafaxine administration in normal volunteers. J Clin Psychiatry 1997; 58:348–350.

Sallustro F, Atwell CW. Body rocking, head banging, and head rolling in normal children. J Pediatr 1978; 93:704–708.

Sanz-Fuentenebro FJ, Huidobro A, Tejadas-Rivas A. Restless legs syndrome and paroxetine. Acta Psychiatr Scand 1996; 94:482–484.

Sevim S, Dogu O, Camdeviren H, et al. Unexpectedly low prevalence and unusual characteristics of RLS in Mersin, Turkey. Neurology 2003; 61:1562–1569.

Sforza E, Jouny C, Ibanez V. Time-dependent variation in cerebral and autonomic activity during periodic leg movements in sleep: implications for arousal mechanisms. Clin Neurophysiol 2002; 113:883–891.

Sforza E, Jouny C, Ibanez V. Time course of arousal response during periodic leg movements in patients with periodic leg movements and restless legs syndrome. Clin Neurophysiol 2003; 114: 1116–1124.

Sjoholm T, Lowe AA, Miyamoto K, et al. Sleep bruxism in patients with sleep-disordered breathing. Arch Oral Biol 2000; 45:889–896.

Stepanova I, Nevsimalova S, Hanusova J. Rhythmic movement disorder in sleep persisting into childhood and adulthood. Sleep 2005; 28:851–857.

Tan EK, Seah A, See SJ, et al. Restless legs syndrome in an Asian population: a study in Singapore. Mov Disord 2001; 16:577–579.

Terao T, Terao M, Yohimura R, et al. Restless legs syndrome induced by lithium. Biol Psychiatry 1991; 30:1167–1170.

Thorpy MJ, Spielman AJ. Persistent jactatio nocturna. Neurology 1984; 34(suppl 1):208–209.

Tison F, Crochard A, Leger D, et al. Epidemiology of restless legs syndrome in French adults: a nationwide survey: the INSTANT study. Neurology 2005; 65:239–246.

Tosun T, Karabuda C, Cuhadaroglu C. Evaluation of sleep bruxism by polysomnographic analysis in patients with dental implants. Int J Oral Maxillofac Implants 2003; 18:286–292.

Traeger N, Schultz B, Pollock AN, et al. Polysomnographic values in children 2–9 years old: additional data and review of the literature. Pediatr Pulmonol 2005; 40:22–30.

Trenkwalder C, Hening WA, Walters AS, et al. Circadian rhythm of periodic limb movements and sensory symptoms of restless legs syndrome. Mov Disord 1999; 14:102–110.

Trenkwalder C, Paulus W. Why do restless legs occur at rest?—pathophysiology of neuronal structures in RLS. Neurophysiology of RLS (part 2). Clin Neurophysiol 2004; 115:1975–1988.

Trenkwalder C, Walters AS, Hening W, et al. Periodic limb movements and restless legs syndrome. Neurol Clin 1996; 14:629–649.

Ulfberg J, Nystrom B, Carter N, et al. Prevalence of restless legs syndrome among men aged 18 to 64 years: an association with somatic disease and neuropsychiatric symptoms. Mov Disord 2001; 16:1159–1163.

Walsh JK, Kramer M, Skinner JE. A case report of jactatio capitis nocturna. Am J Psychiatry 1981; 138: 524–526.

Walters AS. International restless legs syndrome study group. Towards a better definition of restless legs syndrome. Mov Disord 1995; 10:34–42.

Walters AS. Assessment of periodic leg movements is an essential component of an overnight sleep study. Am J Respir Crit Care Med 2001; 164:1339–1340.

Walters AS, Hickey K, Maltzmann J, et al. A questionnaire study of 138 patients with restless legs syndrome: the 'night-walkers' survey. Neurology 1996; 46:92–95.

Walters AS, Mandelbaum ED, Lewin DS, et al. Dopaminergic therapy in children with restless legs syndrome/periodic limb movements in sleep and attention deficit hyperactivity disorder. Pediatr Neurol 2000; 22:182–186.

Walters AS, Picchietti DL, Ehrenberg BL, et al. Restless legs syndrome in childhood and adolescence. Pediatr neurol 1994; 11:241–245.

Ware JC, Brown FW, Moorad PJ, et al. Nocturnal myoclonus and tricyclic antidepressants. Sleep Res 1984; 13:72 (abstr).

Watanabe T, Ichikawa K, Clark GT. Bruxism levels and daily behaviors: 3 weeks of measurement and correlation. J Orofac Pain 2003; 17:65–73.

Weiner IH, Weiner HL. Nocturnal leg muscle cramps. JAMA 1980; 244:2332–2333.

Wetter TC, Brunner J, Bronisch T. Restless legs syndrome probably induced by risperidone treatment. Pharmacopsychiatry 2002; 35:109–111.

Wetter TC, Pollmacher T. Restless legs and periodic leg movements in sleep syndromes. J Neurol 1997; 244(4 suppl):S37–S45.

Wichniak A, Tracik F, Geisler P et al. Rhythmic feet movements while falling asleep. Mov Disord 2001; 16:1164–1170.

Winkelman JW. The evoked heart rate response to periodic leg movements of sleep. Sleep 1999; 22: 575–580.

Yang C, White DP, Winkelman JW. Antidepressants and periodic leg movements of sleep. Biol Psychiatry 2005a; 58:510–514.

Yang C, Winkelman J. Clinical and polysomnographic characteristics of high frequency leg movements. Sleep 2005b; 28:A267 (abstr).

Young G. Leg cramps. Clin Evid 2004; 12:1637–1642.

46 | Diagnostic Tools for Sleep-Related Movement Disorders

Luigi Ferini-Strambi and Mauro Manconi

Sleep Disorders Center, University Vita-Salute San Raffaele, Milan, Italy

INTRODUCTION

Sleep-related movement disorders are conditions that are primarily characterized by relatively simple, usually stereotyped, movements that may disturb sleep or by other sleep-related monophasic movement disorders such as nocturnal cramps.

Nocturnal sleep disturbances or complaints of daytime sleepiness or fatigue are mandatory for a diagnosis of a sleep-related movement disorder. The history may be usually telling; however, polysomnography may be necessary to make a firm diagnosis of sleep-related movement disorders. Since body movements that disturb sleep are also seen in other sleep disorder categories, e.g., in non–rapid eye movement (NREM) and in rapid eye movement (REM) parasomnias, in some cases it may be necessary to perform a video-polysomnography for the differential diagnosis.

HISTORY AND PHYSICAL EXAMINATION

Restless Legs Syndrome

Restless legs syndrome (RLS) is a sensorimotor disorder characterized by an unpleasant and uncomfortable feeling in the legs that leads to an urge to move. The diagnosis of RLS is largely based on the patient's report of clinical symptoms (1). Individuals often have difficulty describing the unpleasant sensations experienced with RLS. Some of the terms used include "creepy crawling," "jittery," "soda bubbling in the veins," "worms moving," and "itching bones." A common thread appears to be the sensation of movement deep within the leg rather than superficially or on the surface of the leg. In some patients, RLS symptoms may also involve the arms. With increasing severity, symptoms may spread to the trunk and face. However, by definition, RLS must involve the legs. The need to move the legs and the unpleasant sensations are exclusively present or worsen during periods of rest or inactivity such as lying or sitting. Physical stimulation (e.g., rubbing the legs, walking) or intense, concentrated mental activity appears to reduce the symptoms. Factors that lead to a reduced arousal (e.g., restricted or confined activity, drowsiness) tend to exacerbate or precipitate the symptoms. Another important clinical feature is the circadian variation of symptoms, which are worse in the evening and at night. In addition to the four essential criteria for an RLS diagnosis (Table 1), there are supportive clinical features that can help resolve diagnostic uncertainty and avoid misdiagnosis (2). These include a positive family history of RLS and a positive therapeutic response to dopaminergic compounds. Both these features may strongly help in the differential diagnosis. More than 50% of patients with primary RLS report a familial pattern, and early onset of RLS symptoms (before the age of 45 years) indicates an increased risk of RLS occurrence in the family. Indeed, family history and age at onset appear to differentiate two phenotypes of RLS. Early-onset RLS, in which symptoms occur before the age of 45, has an autosomal dominant mode of inheritance. Patients with earlier- rather than later-onset RLS generally have much slower progression of symptoms with age, have milder symptoms, and tend to have less relation between body iron stores and severity of disease.

In people with later onset of RLS symptoms (>45 years of age), symptoms progress more rapidly with advancing age. For this reason, the most severely affected individuals tend to be middle aged or elderly (3).

RLS can be divided into primary and secondary forms. Primary, or idiopathic, RLS refers to patients without associated conditions that may explain the symptoms. Secondary causes of

Table 1 The Four Minimal Criteria for the Diagnosis of RLS

1. A desire to move legs associated with a sensory discomfort
2. A motor restlessness that consists of moving
3. Leg discomfort occurring predominantly at rest with at least temporary relief of discomfort occurring with movement
4. Leg discomfort that is worse in the evening and at night. RLS can lead to severe sleep disruption, with daytime fatigue and other functional consequences

Abbreviation: RLS, restless legs syndrome.

RLS include pregnancy and iron deficiency. RLS occurs more commonly in subjects that present with these conditions; however, only approximately one-third to one-half of patients with these conditions develop RLS. Symptoms also resolve with resolution of the condition. For example, RLS occurs in approximately 20% of pregnant women, but symptoms usually resolve within one to four weeks after delivery. Successful kidney transplantation and treatment of iron deficiency anemia have also resulted in resolution of RLS symptoms (4).

RLS appears to be a chronic condition; however, little is known about the pattern of expression of mild or intermittent RLS because most patients with this subtype typically do not seek treatment. It is also unknown whether this group experiences periods of remission. The clinical course varies according to the age of onset. For those with more severe disease who seek medical attention, the severity and frequency of exacerbations usually increase over time. For those with late-onset RLS, there generally is a more rapid development of symptoms. In patients with early-onset RLS, symptoms develop more insidiously over many years and may not become persistent until the patient is 40 to 60 years of age. Although secondary RLS appears to remit with correction of the secondary condition, long-term studies are lacking (5).

In most of the cases the patients are not aware of periodic limb movements (PLM), but occasionally they can refer to sudden involuntary movements or shakes of the limbs, usually involving the legs and occurring during the night especially in the transition from relaxed wakefulness to sleep. When PLM occur during sleep, the patient complaining of frequent awakenings or bed partner observations may help in the clinical suspect of PLM. Patients with PLM may report some generic associated symptoms such as unrefreshing sleep, insomnia, excessive daytime sleepiness, or weakness. However, the medical history is usually insufficient in sensitivity or specificity to supplant instrumental investigations in the diagnosis of PLM.

Sleep-Related Leg Cramps

A detailed medical history is fundamental in the diagnosis of nocturnal leg cramps. In these cases the patients usually complain of abrupt involuntary and sustained contractions of one or a group of muscles associated with painful sensations and relieved by stretching the affected region (6). Leg cramps arise during night period either in wake or sleep and remit spontaneously after seconds or few minutes. Possible persistent leg discomfort after the cramp may delay the following return to sleep. Massages or heat applications may be other possible strategies used by the patients to improve the symptoms. Leg cramps occur more often in elderly people and in patients with neuromuscular, metabolic, endocrine, and peripheral vascular disorders; in young subjects, leg cramps occur after prolonged and intense exercise.

Bruxism

Bruxism is a sleep-related movement disorder, characterized by grinding or clenching of the teeth during sleep, provoked by a tonic or repetitive masticatory muscles activity (7). The characteristic noise is often reported by the bed partner, while the patient may complain of morning temporomandibular discomfort, orofacial discomfort, headache, pain, fatigue, muscular tension, limitation of jaw movements, and teeth hypersensitivity to cold food or beverages. In severe cases, sleep disruption may be a consequence of bruxism. Abnormal wear of the teeth are frequently present at oral inspection. Risk factors to be considered during the historical assessment are young age, anxiety, and the use of cigarettes and caffeine before sleep; the role of occlusal defects remains uncertain.

SUBJECTIVE ASSESSMENT TOOLS

Restless Legs Syndrome

Assessing the most bothersome symptoms and quantifying the severity of RLS are important because not all patients require medical therapy. Furthermore, therapy may vary depending on which symptom is the major problem.

Three validated scales are used to quantify RLS symptom severity. One was developed by the International Restless Legs Syndrome Study Group (IRLSSG) (8). It is a 10-question scale; the questionnaire typically is completed by a person trained in administering the scale, who records the patient's responses during an interview. The scale is divided into five questions that ask about symptom frequency and intensity and five questions that address the impact of symptoms on daily life and sleeping. Each item is rated on a 5-point scale; higher scores represent greater RLS severity. Therefore, the sum score ranges from 0 (no RLS symptoms present) to 40 (maximum severity in all symptoms).

The second scale was developed by the Johns Hopkins RLS Research Group (9). It focuses on the circadian characteristics or the time of onset of symptoms. It is easier to use and has only four ratings (from 0 = none to 3 = severe). A 0 score means the patient has no symptoms. A score of 3 means the symptoms begin in early afternoon or may be present all day.

The third scale is the RLS-6 that consists of six subscales (10). The subscales assess severity of symptoms at the following times of the day/evening: falling asleep, during the night, during the day at rest, and during the day when engaged in daytime activities. In addition, the subscales assess satisfaction with sleep and severity of daytime tiredness/sleepiness. Scores for each subscale range from 0 (completely satisfied) to 10 (completely dissatisfied).

The RLS-QoL is used to evaluate changes in quality of life due to RLS symptoms (11). This disease-specific instrument consists of 12 items. In general, the items address the effects of RLS symptoms on sleep, activities of daily living, mood, social interactions, and coping behaviors. Scores for each item range from 0 (not at all) to 5 (extremely). The RLS Quality-of-Life Instrument (RLS-QLI) represents another questionnaire used to assess the impact of RLS on patients.

OBJECTIVE ASSESSMENT TOOLS

Restless Legs Syndrome and Periodic Limb Movements

Given that the four essential criteria for the diagnosis of RLS are ascertainable by an accurate clinical approach, objective investigations are not really mandatory to verify the presence of RLS (5,12). However, instrumental evaluations may be useful in several situations such as in doubtful RLS cases, differential diagnosis, distinction between primary and secondary RLS forms, sleep impact estimation, diagnosis and quantification of PLM, and valuation of treatment efficacy on sleep and PLM. In particular, because of their high frequency of occurrence in RLS patients, the positive response to dopaminergic treatment, together with the presence of PLM and sleep disruption, is included among the supportive criteria for the diagnosis of RLS, and their assessment is often helpful for a better definition of the RLS phenotype (5). Specifically, as suggested by the IRLSSG guidelines, in patients with a diagnosis of possible RLS who satisfy only three of the four essential diagnostic criteria, the PLM documentation confirms the RLS diagnosis (5). The gold standard in documenting the above-mentioned RLS features is considered the full-night polysomnographic (PSG) study, which should always include the monitoring of both tibialis anterior (TA) muscles for the PLM detection. Actigraphy, the suggested and the forced immobilization tests (FITs), has been proposed as possible cost-effective substitute of PSG.

Other neurophysiological techniques, such as electromyography- and motor/somatosensory-evoked potentials, or neuroimaging investigations, such as computed tomography (CT) and magnetic resonance imaging (MRI) of the cerebrospinal structures, represent second-line instrumental tools helpful in identifying neurological symptomatic RLS forms (13).

Table 2 Suggested PSG Montages for Each Sleep-Related Movement Disorders

	RLS	PLM	Bruxism	Leg cramps
EEG	▲	▲	▲	▲
EOG	▲	▲	▲	▲
Oronasal flow		•	•	
Respiratory effort		•	•	
Microphone			▲	
VIDEO	•	•	•	
EMG				
Submental	▲	▲	▲	▲
Deltoid	•	•		•
Masseter			▲	
Temporalis			•	▲
Tibialis anterior	▲	▲	•	

▲, mandatory; •, desirable.

Polysomnography

At least two of the associated RLS features, such as sleep disruption and PLM, need the full-night PSG study to be described in detail. PLM occur in around 80% to 90% of patients affected by RLS and represent the only one real objective diagnostic marker of the syndrome (14). Although there are reliable portable multichannel devices, which allow a good quality home recording, the laboratory PSG may better define parameters as the time in bed, sleep efficiency, or sleep latency and may associate an audio-video recording to improve the chance of a correct differential diagnosis. As shown in Table 2, the diagnostic PSG in RLS should always include central electroencephalogram (EEG), electrooculogram (EOG), and electromyogram (EMG) of the chin and of both TA muscles. Since in about 30% of RLS patients the restlessness extends to the arms, additional electrodes might be positioned on both deltoid muscles for upper limb movement detection (15). Since PLM should not be scored if they occur together with an abnormal breathing event, supplementary channels for the oronasal flow and for the thoracic-abdominal effort may be integrated if a sleep breathing disorder has not been already ruled out (16).

Regarding the sleep consequences of RLS and PLM, the PSG can give information about sleep macro- and microstructure alterations. Sleep disturbances in RLS patients overall affect the first part of night and are mainly associated with difficulty in initiating and maintaining sleep in the context of a so-called sleep-onset insomnia (17). If on one side, sleep problems may be the only symptoms that the patients refer to because some of them do not realize about sensory symptoms, on the other side, insomnia may be almost absent in patients with mild RLS. The typical hypnogram of a patient with RLS complicated by insomnia (Fig. 1) usually shows an increase in sleep latency and in the number of awakenings in addition to a reduction in total sleep time and sleep efficiency. Percentages of single sleep stages may be preserved or may change to an increase in S1 (N1) and S2 (N2) NREM sleep to the disadvantage of slow-wave sleep. Microstructure instability is due to a rising of the number of arousals. Although a direct relationship between PLM and sleep disruption has never been clearly demonstrated (18), PLM are often associated with cerebral cortical arousals, and when they are found together with insomnia or excessive daytime sleepiness of unknown causes, they constitute the nosological entity of the so-called periodic limb movement disorder (PLMD) (19,20). Despite the fact that the real pathogenetic meaning of PLM is still unclear, their detection is a very important standard procedure in all accredited sleep laboratories, and the scoring of PLM events to ascertain their effect have evolved considerably. The clinical importance of periodic limb movements during sleep (PLMS) was also demonstrated by the finding of a significant correlation between the PLMS index (number of PLMS per hour of sleep) and subjective RLS severity (21), assessed by using the IRLSSG rating scale (8).

How to record and score PLM. Methods for recording and scoring PLM was first established by Coleman et al. (22) accepted by the American Sleep Disorders Association [ASDA, now the

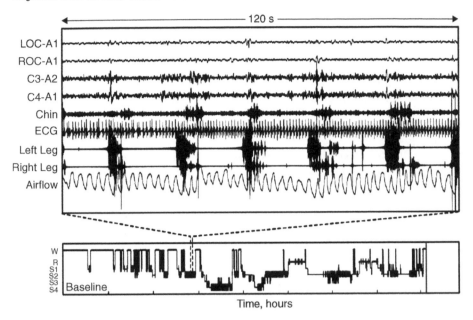

Figure 1 Examples of the hypnogram (*bottom panel*) in a patient affected by RLS/PLM; a short PSG segment is shown in the top panel, as an example. *Abbreviations*: RLS/PLM, restless legs syndrome/periodic limb movements; PSG, polysomnography; LOC, ROC, left and right electrooculogram; A1, A2, left and right reference electrodes placed on the earlobes; chin, electromyogram; ECG, electrocardiogram; W, wakefulness; R, REM sleep; S1, S2, S3 and S4, NREM sleep stages 1, 2, 3, and 4.

American Academy of Sleep Medicine (AASM)] in 1993 (23), and recently revised (16). For the TA EMG activity, two surface electrodes have to be placed, longitudinally and symmetrically, around the middle (2–3 cm apart) of the belly of each muscle. Impedance should be ≤ 10 KΩ for clinical studies, but ≤ 5 KΩ is recommended for research studies. Two channels, one for each leg, are strongly recommended to distinguish between mono and bilateral movements. Filters should be no more restrictive than 10 to 100 Hz for clinical use and 10 to 200 Hz for research studies. Use of 60 Hz (notch) filters should be avoided. Sensitivity limits of -100 and 100 μV (upper/lower) are preferred. Digital sampling rates should be no less than 200 Hz. The signal from the TA muscles has to be carefully calibrated before the starting of the study. Therefore, baseline resting EMG amplitude with a relaxed muscle should be lower than ± 5 μV (for a nonrectified signal), and it should be compared with the maximum dorsiflexion at the ankle without resistance. A single leg movement (LM) was first defined when the EMG signal of one of the TA muscles increased over 25% in amplitude of the maximum of the previous calibrated contraction (24). This amplitude criterion has been considered to be vague at least for research investigations (25). More precise rules have been accepted, stating that an LM is defined when the EMG signal increases in amplitude over 8 μV with respect to the resting voltage, and remains over this threshold for a duration longer than 0.5 seconds (16). The duration for an LM event should range between 0.5 and 10 seconds. The timing of the ending of an LM event is defined as the start of a period lasting at least 0.5 seconds during which the EMG does not exceed 2 μV above resting EMG. LM have to be scored as PLM if they are included in a series of at least four consecutive events, and if the interval between the end of an LM and the onset of the following consecutive one ranges from 5 to 90 seconds. LM movements on two different legs separated by less than five seconds between movement onsets are counted as a single bilateral movement; if they are separated by five seconds or more, they are counted as two different monolateral events.

An LM should not be scored if it occurs during a period from 0.5 seconds preceding an apnea or hypopnea to 0.5 seconds following an apnea or hypopnea. An arousal should be considered as LM associated when it occurs together or when there is less than 0.5 seconds between the end of one event and the onset of another event regardless of which is first.

PLM parameters. The final polysomnographic report usually includes the absolute number of PLM and the PLM index (number of PLM per hour of sleep); both these parameters may be considered separately for wakefulness and sleep time and also for each sleep stage. PLM arousal index stands for the number of PLM associated with an arousal per hour of sleep. A PLM index greater than 5 for the entire night is usually considered pathological, despite data supporting this feature are very limited. When a PLMS index of 15 or greater in adults is associated with an otherwise unexplained sleep-wake complaint, the diagnosis of the PLMD can be defined. Indeed, PLM also occur in several other sleep disorders and in healthy subjects, especially in the elderly (14).

Recently, especially for research reasons, several other parameters, in particular concerning the time structure of PLM, have been considered for outcome analysis. For these purposes, reliable automatic computed methods have replaced manual detection (26). The morphological features of the single LM can be illustrated by its duration, amplitude, and area under the curve. These parameters are better calculated after a rectification of the EMG signal. The side (right or left) of each LM should be also considered, together with its classification as mono or bilateral. Two types of interval between two consecutive movements may be calculated: (*i*) the separation interval, defined as the time between the end of one LM and the onset of the following LM (currently used in clinical practice in PLM scoring), used for the separation of different LM intervening in the same leg on or the contralateral leg and (*ii*) the interval to calculate the periodicity, defined as the time between the end of one LM and the onset of the following LM, used for the separation of different LM intervening in the same leg on or the contralateral leg (mostly used for research purposes) (25,26). The distribution of the intervals between LM usually ranges from 10 to 30 seconds, with a double peak at 1 to 2 seconds (LM not scored as PLM for criteria reasons) and at 15 to 20 seconds. It is not discriminating the first peak because it occurs in both subjects with and without PLM, while the second peak occurs in patients affected by RLS or in general by PLM. Therefore, one of the most characteristic features of PLM is represented by their periodic occurrence. This feature can be quantified calculating the so-called periodicity index, which stands for the number of intervals belonging to sequences of at least three inter-LM intervals $10 < i \leq 90$ seconds per total number of inter-LM intervals (26). This index can vary between 0 (absence of periodicity) to 1 (all intervals with length $10 < i \leq 90$ seconds) and is independent of the absolute number of LM recorded. PLM sequences highly organized in cyclic occurrence result in low levels of entropy and high levels of periodicity.

Suggested and Forced Immobilization Tests

The suggested immobilization test (SIT) and the FIT were validated in 1998 as two polysomnographic tests able to identify and score PLM during wakefulness (PLMW) (27). During the SIT, the patients are asked to sit at a 45° angle in bed with their legs outstretched, and are instructed not to move. During the FIT, the patient sits at a 45° angle in bed with the legs immobilized in a stretcher. In both tests the polysomnographic montage includes central EEG, EOG, and EMG of the chin and both TA muscles. Sleep is scored by the standard method; if any patient falls asleep, he or she should be awakened after 20 seconds of any stage of sleep. Standard criteria are used to score PLMW (criteria for duration includes LM from 0.5 to 10 seconds) (16). The PLMW index (number of PLMW per hour) represents the main outcome measure. If a patient, because of the RLS symptoms, is unable to maintain the rest position till the end of the test, the movement index has to be calculated as the number of the PLMW multiplied for 60 minutes and divided for the duration in minutes of the test until that moment. Patients affected by RLS present significantly more LM than normal controls during the immobilization tests. These movements are periodic and usually occur at a frequency of approximately 1 every 12 seconds (28). According to Montplaisir et al. (27), a SIT movement index greater than 40 is considered abnormal, while it should be greater than 25 in the case of the FIT. Using these pathological thresholds, the clinical RLS diagnosis is correctly predicted in 81% of subjects (28). SIT has been used more than FIT, probably because it does not need any special equipment to hold the legs. The low cost and the possibility to repeat the tests more time during the day are the two major advantages associated with SIT and FIT.

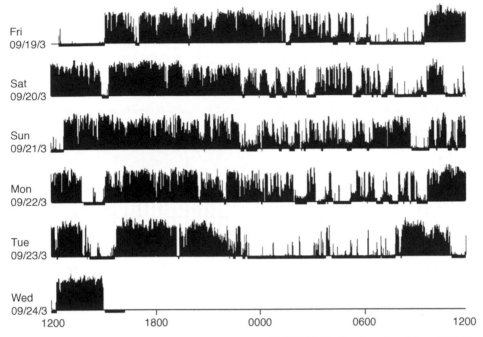

Figure 2 Actigraphic pattern of a patient affected by RLS/PLM (device placed on right ankle). The decrease in motor activity during the last night of recording is due to a single administration of an evening dose of a dopamine agonist. *Abbreviation:* RLS/PLM, restless legs syndrome/periodic limb movements.

Actigraphy

General evidence for eventual RLS- or PLM-related insomnia may come from ordinary actigraphic monitoring by placing the device on the nondominant wrist of the patient (29). This analysis usually shows an increase of the mean motor activity during the first part of the night usually proportional with severity of the symptoms. By attaching the accelerometer to one, or better, to both ankles (or to both of the big toes for particular versions), PLM can be reliably diagnosed (30). This method has a few advantages, such as the low cost, portability, and the possibility to record for long period, but does not collect any other information regarding sleep. At the beginning, the actimeter method showed lower sensitivity in measuring PLM compared with the classic polysomnographic techniques. In particular the short and small amplitude leg jerks could be underestimated. The development of new hardware with an increase in the sampling rate and of more accurate scoring algorithms has improved reasonably the sensitivity of this instrumental tool in PLM detection. Comparing with traditional polysomnographic method, the actigraphic way of PLMS detection showed a specificity of 90% and a sensitivity of 60% for the PLM diagnosis (PLM index > 5), with a close correlation of the PLM index (31). There are several brands of devices specifically created for PLM assessment (32). Nowadays, actigraphy is considered to be a suitable method for PLMS diagnosis for the epidemiological screening of a large population or for the assessment of therapeutic effects (Fig. 2) (33).

Tibialis Anterior Activities Other Than PLM

Analyzing the EMG signal during routine PSG studies for other typical patterns of movement, different from PLM, have been described. The pathogenetic meaning of this leg activity is still debated and likely depends on their frequency of occurrence during the night and their hypothetical causal role in sleep disruption. At the moment, there are no clear reported clinical consequences of these motor phenomena. PLM may associate with this particular TA activity. In all of the following cases the diagnosis needs a full-night PSG study including the EMG recording of both TA muscles with the above-mentioned rules.

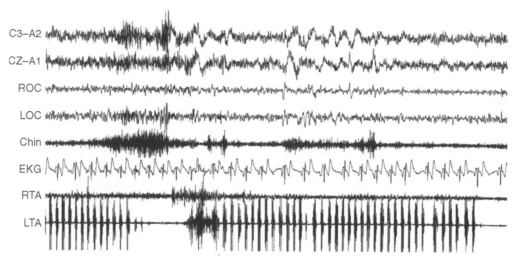

Figure 3 Polysomnographic example of hypnagogic foot tremor in the left leg. *Abbreviations:* LOC, ROC, left and right electrooculogram; A1, A2, left and right reference electrodes placed on the earlobes; chin, electromyogram; EKG, electrocardiogram; RTA, LTA, right and left tibialis anterior.

Alternating leg muscle activation (ALMA) is defined as a repetition of at least four TA alternating bursts between legs, with a minimum frequency of EMG jerks of 0.5 Hz to a maximum of 3.0 Hz. Usually a single EMG burst in the context of an ALMA sequence ranges from 100 to 500 milliseconds in duration (16,34).

Following the ASDA (now AASM) criteria, the excessive fragmentary myoclonus (EFM) is characterized by repetitive EMG bursts shorter than 150 milliseconds in duration, occurring with a frequency higher than 5 per minute and for a period longer than 20 minutes of NREM sleep. Usually EFM occurs without visible limb movements, but minor movements of the fingers or feet may be observed (16,35–37).

Hypnagogic foot tremor (HFT) is classified as a series of at least four EMG bursts with a minimum frequency of 0.3 Hz and a maximum of 4.0 Hz. The duration of a single EMG burst usually ranges between 250 and 1000 milliseconds (Fig. 3) (16).

Sleep-Related Leg Cramps

Leg cramps during sleep has been accepted as an individual nosological disorder characterized by a painful sensation in the leg or foot associated with sudden and strong muscle contraction, which occurs during sleep and is relieved by forceful stretching of the affected muscles (6,38). Sleep-related leg cramps may coexist with other sleep disorders, especially in the elderly and may be confused with RLS/PLM (6,39,40). Only in cases of difficult differential diagnoses with other sleep-related movement disorders, a full-night PSG including EMG of both TA to document the affected movements, together with the video recording, is indicated. The typical cramp lasts usually from one to several minutes and appear as tonic stereotyped EMG activity.

Bruxism

In most of the cases, clinicians can diagnose sleep bruxism by an accurate medical history supported by a visual inspection of orofacial structures (7,38). The typical teeth grinding or tapping is usually noted by the patient's partner or family members. Orofacial discomfort, such as pain, fatigue, muscular tension, and teeth hypersensitivity to cold food or beverages are often reported by the patient (41,42). Clinicians can corroborate the suspicion of bruxism by observing teeth wear, tongue indentation, masseter and temporalis muscles hypertrophy, and temporomandibular joint sound during chewing.

Instrumental techniques are recommended only in specific cases: confirmation of diagnosis in uncertain patients; severe bruxism; differential diagnosis, especially with other sleep disorders; scoring of bruxism episodes for a better severity quantification or for research purposes; and documentation of teeth and oromandibular damage.

The first level of instrumental diagnosis is represented by the ambulatory assessment of bruxism by the detection of sound, EMG activity of masticatory muscles, or pressure exerted by jaw movements. Self-made audio-video recordings may be useful in confirming bruxism and in verifying its frequency of occurrence. Ambulatory polygraphic monitoring is available with different levels of complexity: from a single-channel EMG recording of masseter muscles to full multichannel polysomnography, which can include EEG, EOG, EMG, and respiratory effort. Ambulatory polygraphy may provide a good quality signal, and depending on the number of recorded parameters, a high reliable diagnosis. Moreover, ambulatory techniques allow a low-cost monitoring of even more than one night in the habitual environment of the patient. The lower specificity of ambulatory compared with laboratory polysomnography in differentiating bruxism from other orofacial physiological (talking, yawning, coughing, and swallowing) or pathological (oromandibular myoclonus, nocturnal groaning, and epileptic bursts) activities mainly depends on the absence of the audio-video recording during the ambulatory studies (43).

How to Detect and Score Sleep Bruxism
Table 2 shows the suggested montage for a correct assessment of bruxism during a full-night laboratory polysomnography study. Beside the standard parameters for sleep scoring (EEG, EOG, and chin EMG) and respiratory analysis (oronasal flow, thoracic effort, microphone, and oxygen saturation), two surface electrodes for each masseter muscle should be placed. In specific cases and for research purpose, further electrodes on the temporalis or other facial muscles may be positioned. Before starting the sleep recordings, patients should produce a few voluntary lateral, protrusive, and occlusive jaw movements to allow the signal EMG calibration. The interelectrode impedances should be under 5 KΩ for masseter electrodes. For the EMG amplification, the high cutoff filter should be set around 100 to 200 Hz and the low cutoff filter around 10 Hz (16). Sampling rates should be at least 200 Hz. The typical polysomnographic pattern of bruxism (Fig. 4) is characterized by rhythmic bursts of masticatory muscle activity, usually at 1 Hz of frequency, with a duration ranging between 0.25 and 2 seconds, accompanied by muscular artifacts on EEG channels. When the single burst of masseter exceeds two seconds in duration, generally it is classified as tonic bruxism, while shorter contractions as phasic. For scoring purposes, a bruxism episode is classified when at least three masseter contractions with

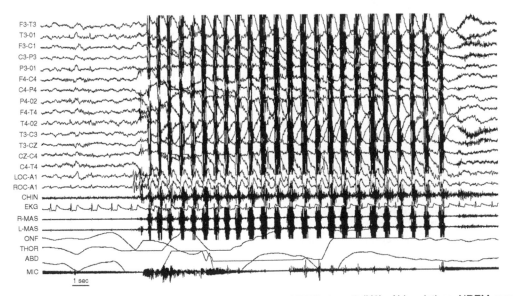

Figure 4 Polysomnographic example of bruxism during NREM stage 2 (N2). *Abbreviations:* NREM, non–rapid eye movement; LOC, ROC, left and right electrooculogram; A1, A2, left and right reference electrodes placed on the earlobes; chin, electromyogram; EKG, electrocardiogram, R-MAS, L-MAS, right and left masseter muscles; ONF, oronasal flow; THOR, thoracic movements; ABD, abdominal movements; MIC, microphone.

the above-mentioned features and with an amplitude of at least twice the amplitude of background EMG are detected (16). A period of at least three seconds of stable background chin EMG must occur before a new episode of bruxism can be scored. Bruxism can be scored reliably by audio in combination with polysomnography by a minimum of two audible tooth grinding episodes/night of polysomnography in the absence of epilepsy. Possible scoring parameters, overall for research reasons, are the number of bruxism episodes or bruxism bursts per sleep stages and per hour of sleep. The audio recording of the characteristic sound produced by the teeth grinding allows a better differentiation of bruxism from other orofacial motor activity such as swallowing, cough, talking, and irregular breathing patterns (44).

NEW DIAGNOSTIC TOOLS

A study tried to validate the use of a single standard question for the rapid screening of RLS (45). The question is the following: "When you try to relax in the evening or sleep at night, do you ever have unpleasant restless feelings in your legs that can be relieved by walking or movement?" The authors found that, in comparison to the four standard criteria, the single question had 100% sensitivity and 96.8% specificity for the diagnosis of RLS. This study represents the effort to simplify both the clinical and the epidemiological approaches to the diagnosis of RLS.

New reliable methods for the computed automatic detection of PLM have been developed (26). Moreover, a more sophisticated analysis of PLM features, such as duration, amplitude, area under the curve, and periodicity and distribution across the night, have demonstrated some interesting differences in the PLM phenotype of RLS compared with those of narcolepsy (46) and REM behavior disorder (47). The traditional method used to analyze PLMS is insufficient to capture these detailed differences in the EMG signal. Under this point of view, the presence of PLM is not specific for a particular disorder, but their time structure and qualitative pattern might be disease related.

CONCLUSIONS

During the history and physical examination, the diagnoses of RLS, sleep-related leg cramps, and bruxism are largely based on the patient's report of clinical symptoms; however, the PLMD diagnosis requires objective measures. There are three validated scales for assessing RLS symptom severity and two questionnaires for evaluating the impact of RLS on a patient's quality of life. Polysomnography is used to confirm the diagnosis of RLS and for documenting PLMS, and the suggested and forced immobilization tests can be used to identify and score PLMW. Polysomnography may also be useful for evaluating motor phenomena other than PLM and difficult cases of sleep-related leg cramps or bruxism. Actigraphy may be used for the PLMS diagnosis for the epidemiological screening of a large population or for the assessment of therapeutic effects. New diagnostic tools for sleep-related movement disorders include a single standard question for the rapid screening of RLS and new reliable methods for the computed automatic detection of PLM and a more sophisticated analysis of PLM features have been developed.

GLOSSARY

ALMA   alternative leg muscle activation
EEG   electroencephalogram
EFM   excessive fragmentary myoclonus
EMG   electromyography
EOG   electrooculogram
FIT   forced immobilization test
HFT   hypnagogic foot tremor
LM   leg movement
PLM   periodic limb movements
PLMD   periodic limb movement disorder

PLMS PLM during sleep
PLMW PLM during wakefulness
PSG polysomnography
RLS restless legs syndrome
SIT suggested immobilization test
TA tibialis anterior

REFERENCES

1. Allen RP, Earley CJ. Restless legs syndrome: a review of clinical and pathophysiologic features. J Clin Neurophysiol 2001; 18(2):128–147.
2. Ferini-Strambi L. RLS-like symptoms: differential diagnosis by history and clinical assessment. Sleep Med 2007; 8(suppl 2):S3–S6.
3. Milligan SA, Chesson AL. Restless legs syndrome in the older adult: diagnosis and management. Drugs Aging 2002; 19(10):741–751.
4. Kushida CA. Clinical presentation, diagnosis, and quality of life issues in restless legs syndrome. Am J Med 2007; 120(1 suppl 1):S4–S12.
5. Allen RP, Picchietti D, Hening WA, et al. Restless legs syndrome: diagnostic criteria, special considerations, and epidemiology. A report from the restless legs syndrome diagnosis and epidemiology workshop at the National Institutes of Health. Sleep Med 2003; 4(2):101–119.
6. Riley JD, Antony SJ. Leg cramps: differential diagnosis and management. Am Fam Physician 1995; 52 (6):1794–1798.
7. Bader G, Lavigne G. Sleep bruxism; an overview of an oromandibular sleep movement disorder (review article). Sleep Med Rev 2000; 4(1):27–43.
8. Walters AS, LeBrocq C, Dhar A, et al. Validation of the International Restless Legs Syndrome Study Group rating scale for restless legs syndrome. Sleep Med 2003; 4(2):121–132.
9. Allen RP, Earley CJ. Validation of the Johns Hopkins restless legs severity scale. Sleep Med 2001; 2(3): 239–242.
10. Kohnen R, Oertel WH, Stiasny-Kolster K. Severity rating of RLS: review of 10 years experienced with the RLS-6 scale in clinical trialsSleep 2003; 26 (abstr).
11. Kohnen R, Benes H, Heinrich B, et al. Development of the disease-specific restless legs syndrome quality of life (RLS-QoL) questionnaireMov Disord 2002; 232(5):743 (abstr).
12. Walters AS. Toward a better definition of the restless legs syndrome. The international restless legs syndrome study group. Mov Disord 1995; 10(5):634–642.
13. Radtke R. Sleep disorders in neurology. J Clin Neurophysiol 2001; 18(2):77.
14. Hornyak M, Feige B, Riemann D, et al. Periodic leg movements in sleep and periodic limb movement disorder: prevalence, clinical significance and treatment. Sleep Med Rev 2006; 10(3):169–177.
15. Chabli A, Michaud M, Montplaisir J. Periodic arm movements in patients with the restless legs syndrome. Eur Neurol 2000; 44(3):133–138.
16. Iber C, Ancoli-Israel S, Chesson A Jr., et al. The AASM Manual for the Scoring of Sleep and Associated Events. Rules, Terminology and Technical Specifications. 1st ed. Westchester, IL: American Academy of Sleep Medicine, 2007.
17. Montplaisir J, Boucher S, Poirier G, et al. Clinical, polysomnographic, and genetic characteristics of restless legs syndrome: a study of 133 patients diagnosed with new standard criteria. Mov Disord 1997; 12(1):61–65.
18. Carrier J, Frenette S, Montplaisir J, et al. Effects of periodic leg movements during sleep in middle-aged subjects without sleep complaints. Mov Disord 2005; 20(9):1127–1132.
19. Hornyak M, Riemann D, Voderholzer U. Do periodic leg movements influence patients' perception of sleep quality? Sleep Med 2004; 5(6):597–600.
20. Nicolas A, Lesperance P, Montplaisir J. Is excessive daytime sleepiness with periodic leg movements during sleep a specific diagnostic category? Eur Neurol 1998; 40(1):22–26.
21. Garcia-Borreguero D, Larrosa O, de la LY, et al. Correlation between rating scales and sleep laboratory measurements in restless legs syndrome. Sleep Med 2004; 5(6):561–565.
22. Coleman RM. Periodic movements in sleep (nocturnal myoclonus) and restless legs syndrome. In: Guilleminault C, ed. Sleeping and Waking Disorders: Indications and Techniques. Menlo Park, CA: Addison-Wesley, 1982:265–295.
23. Recording and scoring leg movements. The Atlas Task Force. Sleep 1993; 16(8):748–759.
24. Practice parameters for the indications for polysomnography and related procedures. Polysomnography Task Force, American Sleep Disorders Association Standards of Practice Committee. Sleep 1997; 20(6):406–422.

25. Ferri R, Zucconi M, Manconi M, et al. Computer-assisted detection of nocturnal leg motor activity in patients with restless legs syndrome and periodic leg movements during sleep. Sleep 2005; 28(8): 998–1004.

26. Ferri R, Zucconi M, Manconi M, et al. New approaches to the study of periodic leg movements during sleep in restless legs syndrome. Sleep 2006; 29(6):759–769.

27. Montplaisir J, Boucher S, Nicolas A, et al. Immobilization tests and periodic leg movements in sleep for the diagnosis of restless leg syndrome. Mov Disord 1998; 13(2):324–329.

28. Michaud M, Poirier G, Lavigne G, et al. Restless legs syndrome: scoring criteria for leg movements recorded during the suggested immobilization test. Sleep Med 2001; 2(4):317–321.

29. Littner M, Kushida CA, Anderson WM, et al. Practice parameters for the role of actigraphy in the study of sleep and circadian rhythms: an update for 2002. Sleep 2003; 26(3):337–341.

30. Kazenwadel J, Pollmacher T, Trenkwalder C, et al. New actigraphic assessment method for periodic leg movements (PLM). Sleep 1995; 18(8):689–697.

31. Kemlink D, Pretl M, Kelemen J, et al. [Periodic limb movements in sleep: polysomnographic and actigraphic methods for their detection]. Cas Lek Cesk 2005; 144(10):689–691.

32. Sforza E, Johannes M, Claudio B. The PAM-RL ambulatory device for detection of periodic leg movements: a validation study. Sleep Med 2005; 6(5):407–413.

33. Zucconi M, Oldani A, Castronovo C, et al. Cabergoline is an effective single-drug treatment for restless legs syndrome: clinical and actigraphic evaluation. Sleep 2003; 26(7):815–818.

34. Chervin RD, Consens FB, Kutluay E. Alternating leg muscle activation during sleep and arousals: a new sleep-related motor phenomenon? Mov Disord 2003; 18(5):551–559.

35. Walters AS. Clinical identification of the simple sleep-related movement disorders. Chest 2007; 131(4): 1260–1266.

36. Lins O, Castonguay M, Dunham W, et al. Excessive fragmentary myoclonus: time of night and sleep stage distributions. Can J Neurol Sci 1993; 20(2):142–146.

37. Broughton R, Tolentino MA, Krelina M. Excessive fragmentary myoclonus in NREM sleep: a report of 38 cases. Electroencephalogr Clin Neurophysiol 1985; 61(2):123–133.

38. American Academy of Sleep Medicine, . International Classification of Sleep Disorders: Diagnostic and Coding Manual. 2nd ed. Westchester, IL: American Academy of Sleep Medicine, 2005.

39. Lagerlof H. [Nocturnal leg cramp is a common and painful symptom in the elderly. Underlying causes and treatment]. Lakartidningen 1999; 96(20):2505–2506.

40. Whiteley AM. Cramps, stiffness and restless legs. Practitioner 1982; 226(1368):1085–1087.

41. Ahlgren J, Omnell KA, Sonesson B, et al. Bruxism and hypertrophy of the masseter muscle. A clinical, morphological and functional investigation. Pract Otorhinolaryngol (Basel) 1969; 31(1):22–29.

42. Lavigne GJ, Rompre PH, Montplaisir JY, et al. Motor activity in sleep bruxism with concomitant jaw muscle pain. A retrospective pilot study. Eur J Oral Sci 1997; 105(1):92–95.

43. Kato T, Thie NM, Montplaisir JY, et al. Bruxism and orofacial movements during sleep. Dent Clin North Am 2001; 45(4):657–684.

44. Kato T, Montplaisir JY, Blanchet PJ, et al. Idiopathic myoclonus in the oromandibular region during sleep: a possible source of confusion in sleep bruxism diagnosis. Mov Disord 1999; 14(5):865–871.

45. Ferri R, Lanuzza B, Cosentino FI, et al. A single question for the rapid screening of restless legs syndrome in the neurological clinical practice. Eur J Neurol 2007; 14(9):1016–1021.

46. Ferri R, Zucconi M, Manconi M, et al. Different periodicity and time structure of leg movements during sleep in narcolepsy/cataplexy and restless legs syndrome. Sleep 2006; 29(12):1587–1594.

47. Manconi M, Ferri R, Zucconi M, et al. Time structure analysis of leg movements during sleep in REM sleep behavior disorder. Sleep 2007; 30(12):1779–1785.

47 | Diagnostic Algorithm for Sleep-Related Movement Disorders

Stephany Fulda and Thomas C. Wetter

Max Planck Institute of Psychiatry, Munich, Germany

CLINICAL VIGNETTE

Mr. H is a 57-year-old male with a history of severe recurrent depression. After several trials with different antidepressant drugs, a series of electroconvulsive treatments (ECT) had been started with good success and continued during his treatment in a day clinic. After several ECT treatments without complications, the patient developed aspiration pneumonia, making a transfer to an intensive care unit necessary. Interviews revealed that Mr. H had ingested food during the night before ECT, although he had been instructed to refrain from eating for 12 hours before ECT. Mr. H reported that he had noticed food or signs of nocturnal eating in the morning for several weeks. At times, he had found a half-eaten bowl of cornflakes in the morning in the kitchen without having any recollection of getting up and eating it in the night. Also, crumbs and food remains were found in the kitchen and other rooms. After remission of pneumonia, the patient was admitted to the sleep laboratory for a detailed evaluation with the suspicion of a sleep-related eating disorder.

Sleep Laboratory Evaluation

The nocturnal video-polysomnography revealed severe sleep disturbances with sleep onset only in early morning hours and severe periodic leg movements during wake and sleep (Fig. 1). Total sleep time was around three hours, and consequently, sleep efficiency was below 40%. The total number of periodic leg movements exceeded 900 per night. In addition, Mr. H left the bed frequently to walk beside the bed or exhibited several unusual movements such as cycling the legs while lying on the back. A detailed sleep history revealed that the patient had been experiencing an irresistible urge to move the legs, accompanied by extremely unpleasant sensations in both legs as well as involuntary leg movements. These symptoms forced him to stay awake for a long time, resulting in a sleep duration of only three to four hours every night.

The patient reported that these symptoms coincided with the beginning of starting venlafaxine, a combined serotonin and noradrenaline reuptake inhibitor. The urge to move and unpleasant sensations had gradually increased over time, leading to significant sleep disruption and sleep curtailment. As the sleep disturbances worsened, he began to notice signs of nocturnal wanderings and eating. Although he sometimes had a vague recollection of walking during the night, he was amnesic for nocturnal eating. Because the patient had no bed partner, no additional information was available. The patient had experienced episodes of insomnia before, mostly at times when depressive symptoms worsened. However, he denied to have had paresthesias of the limbs or the urge to move before the current episode. The neurological examination was normal, and all routine laboratory findings including ferritin and iron were within the normal range. Magnetic resonance imaging, electroencephalography, and neurophysiological studies revealed no abnormalities.

Interpretation and Clinical Course

Because of the close temporal association with the onset of antidepressant treatment with venlafaxine, a drug-induced restless legs syndrome (RLS) was suspected. Subsequently, venlafaxine treatment was stopped and a trial with pramipexole, a dopamine agonist with antidepressant properties, was initiated. After medication change, the symptoms—both

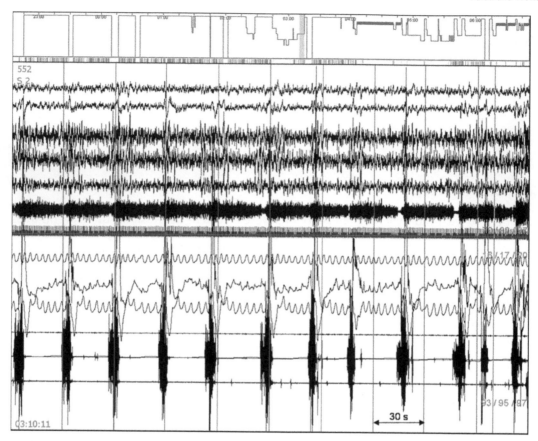

Figure 1 A five-minute section of the nocturnal polysomnography of a patient. From top to bottom, the features are: the hypnogram (*top*) shows wake and sleep stages across the night, with the black line moving downward from wake through sleep stages N1, N2, and slow-wave sleep (N3, stages 3 and 4). The broad black horizontal lines denote REM sleep. The hypnogram showed that severe sleep onset disturbances and consolidated sleep for more than 10 minutes occurred only in the second half of the night. Even then, longer and shorter awakenings were frequent. Below the hypnogram, the distribution of leg movements during the night is shown in gray. Each light gray (left leg) or dark gray (right leg) vertical line denotes one leg movement. The leg movements ceased only during REM sleep, slow-wave sleep, and the later part of the night. The five-minute section of the polysomnographic recording shows, from top to bottom, two electrooculography channels, three EEG channels, one chin EMG channel, electrocardiography, airflow, respiratory movements of the thorax and abdomen, snoring sound recording, and left and right leg EMG (tibialis anterior muscle). The section was taken from sleep stage N2 shortly before the patient awoke again. The strong repetitive leg movements were prominent and occurred every 30 seconds during sleep stage N2. Each leg movement was associated with an EEG arousal and, because the leg movements were quite forceful, they affected the respiratory channels as well. *Abbreviations*: REM, rapid eye movement; EEG, electroencephalography; EMG, electromyography.

restless legs symptoms and nocturnal eating—gradually declined, corroborating the diagnosis of venlafaxine-induced RLS. Whether the nocturnal eating episodes were due to automatic behavior because of the severe sleep deprivation or whether they were an independent substance-induced sleep-related eating disorder could not be clarified since no such episode was recorded in the sleep laboratory.

DIAGNOSTIC ALGORITHM FOR SLEEP-RELATED MOVEMENT DISORDERS

Sleep-related movement disorders (SRMDs) encompass a group of relatively simple, stereotyped movements or monophasic movement disorders such as periodic limb movement disorder (PLMD), sleep-related leg cramps, sleep-related bruxism, and sleep-related rhythmic movement disorder (RMD) that disturb sleep (1). In addition, RLS has been included into this diagnostic category because of its close association with periodic limb movements during sleep

(PLMS). Common to all SRMDs is a complaint of disturbed sleep, and daytime sleepiness or fatigue, which is a prerequisite for the diagnosis as opposed to a mere accidental finding during a nocturnal polysomnography (PSG).

In general, the diagnostic process in case of suspected SRMD follows a general algorithm whereby the clinician seeks out four types of information: (*i*) type of complaints (e.g., disturbed sleep, daytime sleepiness), (*ii*) specific nighttime symptoms and observations (e.g., urge to move, leg kicking), (*iii*) history of current or previous medical, neurological, or psychiatric illnesses, and (4) drug history.

1. Type of complaint: Nocturnal sleep disturbances or complaints of daytime sleepiness or fatigue are a prerequisite for the diagnosis of SRMD. For example, many normal sleepers exhibit some episodes of periodic limb movements (PLMs) (2–4) or rhythmic jaw contractions. However, if they have no complaints of sleep disturbances or impaired daytime functioning or show no significant objective disturbances of their sleep, they would not be classified as having SRMD. The complaints are assessed with a detailed clinical interview that is comprehensive and includes the types of complaints being manifested, and the chronology and course and any success or failure of prior treatment interventions. To assist the clinician in conducting such an interview, various diagnostic tools are available (see chap. 46). Often it is useful to supplement this information with standardized questionnaires that assess the patient-perceived daytime sleepiness and the degree of sleep disturbances or quality-of-life impact. In selected cases, the multiple sleep latency test (MSLT), the maintenance of wakefulness test (MWT) (5), vigilance tasks, or neuropsychological testing (6) may be used to quantify daytime sleepiness or daytime dysfunction or to rule out other suspected sleep disorders such as narcolepsy.

2. Specific nighttime symptoms and observations: While disturbed sleep or impaired daytime functioning is present in all cases with SRMD, each sleep disorder is characterized by specific nighttime symptoms. In some cases, the patient is able to describe the symptoms, such as an urge to move or painful nocturnal leg cramps; in other cases, the bed partner is the primary source of information describing, for example, nocturnal teeth-grinding sounds or repetitive leg movements. Therefore, the reports of the bed partner should be sought, and when possible, the partner should be invited along with the patient for the interview or the patient should be alerted beforehand to seek out this information. Depending on the type of SRMD, additional diagnostic procedures may be needed to document or quantify nocturnal motor activity. These may include home-based monitoring, such as actigraphy or video recording, or overnight PSG recording with video documentation.

3. History of current or previous medical, neurological, or psychiatric illnesses: SRMD may be associated with a broad range of disorders. It is especially important to go into the details of the neurological history as certain abnormal movements during sleep may be the manifestations of an underlying neurological disorder. Also, many daytime movement disorders may persist during sleep or reemerge during stage shifts, underlining the importance of a neurological evaluation. A detailed physical examination may uncover various medical disorders that might be responsible for the abnormal behavior during sleep or might mimic the symptoms of specific SRMDs and are thus part of the differential diagnosis. Specific laboratory tests such as blood serum evaluation and neurophysiological and vascular investigations may be indicated for the same purpose. In the vast majority of patients with suspected SRMD, other techniques such as long-term EEG monitoring or neuroimaging are not required.

4. Drug history: In the diagnosis of SRMD, it often pays to suspect possible drug-induced causes early in the diagnostic process. The physician should inquire about drugs that may induce or exacerbate the symptoms of SRMD. At the same time, the physician should also elicit from the history any causal relationship between medications and abnormal behavior or movements. In particular, psychiatric medications such as selective serotonin reuptake inhibitors (SSRIs) or selective serotonin-noradrenalin reuptake inhibitors (SNRIs) and typical and atypical anti-psychotics are prime suspects (see the section on SRMD due to drug or substance).

RESTLESS LEGS SYNDROME

Key Steps in the Diagnosis of the Disorder

Subjects with RLS typically complain about disturbed sleep and in particular about disturbed sleep onset due to the restless legs symptoms occurring in the evening and at times of inactivity. Most RLS patients are be able to describe clearly the urge to move and the associated paresthesias, although the clinician is bound to hear a broad range of creative descriptions of the symptomatology. Typical examples are "crawling ants," "jittery legs," "moving worms," or "soda bubbling in the veins" (7). For children and cognitively impaired elderly, additional diagnostic criteria have been proposed (7). In unclear cases, the suggested immobilization test (SIT), which may elicit and quantify the motor symptoms (involuntary leg movements) of RLS, may be helpful (Ref. 8, chap. 46). Improvement of symptoms with a single dose of levodopa has a high sensitivity and specificity in subjects with RLS and might be considered as a supportive feature (9).

A laboratory evaluation including serum ferritin, electrolytes, and renal parameters can rule out potentially secondary forms of RLS such as iron deficiency anemia (10,11) or renal failure (12). In an atypical presentation or when symptoms resemble peripheral neuropathy, nerve conduction velocities and electromyogram should be performed. PSG is generally reserved for patients in whom other or additional sleep disorders are suspected or the degree of sleep disturbances needs to be quantified, for example, for judicial purposes. In addition, because opioids can worsen preexistent sleep-related breathing disorders (SRBDs), PSG may be warranted to rule out SRBD before treatment with opioids is initiated (13,14).

Important Diagnostic Features and Criteria to Distinguish Types

RLS is characterized by: (*i*) an imperative desire to move the extremities, which is (*ii*) at least temporarily relieved with movement and (*iii*) worse or exclusively present at rest and (*iv*) in the evening or at night. These standard diagnostic criteria (7) are included in the second edition of *International Classification of Sleep Disorders* (ICSD-2) (1). A positive family history for RLS, an initial response to dopaminergic therapy, and the presence of PLMS are supportive clinical features for RLS (7). The clinical course of the disorder varies considerably, and in some patients, RLS can be intermittent and may spontaneously remit for many years (15,16).

Differential Diagnosis

A number of conditions other than RLS must be considered in the differential diagnosis of altered sensations in the legs (Table 1). These include disorders of the peripheral nervous system such as peripheral neuropathies and syndromes owing to irritation of the nerve root or compression of peripheral nerves, and vascular conditions such as peripheral arterial disease. Altered sensations in the legs and motor restlessness are also reported in patients with antipsychotic-induced akathisia, anxiety disorders, and attention-deficit hyperactivity disorder. Table 1 lists the conditions, their distinguishing features, and diagnostic procedures that might be considered in the differential diagnosis for RLS. In addition, several drugs can induce RLS, and a careful examination of the patient's drug history is recommended in all cases (Table 2).

PERIODIC LIMB MOVEMENT DISORDER

Key Steps in the Diagnosis of the Disorder

Typically, the patient is unaware of the limb movements or the frequent sleep disruptions and it is the observation of the bed partner that suggests the presence of PLMS. Indeed, PLMS can be significantly disruptive to the bed partner's sleep. The diagnosis of PLMD requires objective measurement of the PLMs either by actigraphy or by nocturnal PSG. Actigraphy has the advantage of being cheaper and therefore more feasible to measurements spanning over several nights. This might be especially important because of the high night-to-night variability of PLMs (60,61). On the other hand, PLMs are often found in other sleep disorders such as narcolepsy (62,63), REM sleep behavior disorder (64,65), and SRBD (66,67). In addition, PLMS may be associated with repetitive respiratory events such as the breath ending of an apnea/hypopnea event. PLMS and sleep apnea may coexist, but it should be attempted to treat the

Table 1 Differential Diagnosis for Restless Legs Syndrome

Differential diagnosis	Common features	Distinguishing features	Diagnostic procedures
Polyneuropathy (17,18)	Paresthesias focusing on foot and leg, can be worse at night	No urge to move, no relief with movement, no clear circadian pattern	Nerve conduction studies, EMG, surealis biopsy
Leg compartment syndromes	Paresthesias	No urge to move, no circadian pattern	Nerve conduction studies
Lumbosacral radiculopathy (19)	Paresthesias	No urge to move, no circadian pattern	EMG, imaging
Neuroleptic-induced akathisia (20)	Urge to move	No circadian pattern, no relief with movement	Medication history, polysomnography
Venous diseases of the leg	Paresthesias, can be worse at night	No urge to move	Doppler sonography, angiography
Painful legs and moving toes (21,22)	Paresthesias and pain, urge to move	No circadian pattern, unusual movements	EMG
Muscular pain fasciculation syndromes	Paresthesia and pain	No urge to move, no circadian rhythm	EMG
Sleep-related leg cramps (23)	Paresthesia and pain, need to stretch the leg	No urge to move, residual pain after the cramp, restricted to single muscles, muscle hardness	History
Erythromelalgia	Paresthesia and pain, worse in the evening, fluctuating	No urge to move, no clear circadian pattern	History

Abbreviation: EMG, electromyogram.

Table 2 Some Medications Associated with Sleep-Related Movement Disorders

RLS (24)	PLMS	Bruxism (25,26)
SSRI (27,28)	**SSRI** (33)	**SSRI** (36)
Fluoxetine (29,30)	Fluoxetine (33,34)	Fluoxetine (37)
Sertraline (31)	Venlafaxine (33,35)	Sertraline (37)
Paroxetine (32)	Citalopram (33)	Paroxetine (38)
		Citalopram (39)
	Other Antidepressants	
Venlafaxine (35)	Clomipramine (47)	
Mirtazapine (40–44)		
Mianserin (45,46)		
	Antipsychotics, first generation	
Haloperidol (48)	Haloperidol (48)	Haloperidol (49)
Chlorpromazine (24)		Chlorpromazine (25)
Pimozide (24)		Perphenazine (49)
	Antipsychotics, second generation	
Olanzapine (50)	Quetiapine (53)	
Risperidone (51)		
Clozapine (52)		
Lithium (54,55)	**Lithium** (54)	**Lithium** (25)
Anticonvulsant drugs		**Amphetamines**
Methsuximide (56)		Methylphenidate (25)
Phenytoin (56)		
Zonisamide (57)		**Cardioactive calcium blockers**
γ-**Hydroxybutyrate** (58)		Flunarizine (25)
Histamine receptor antagonists (59)		**Antiarrhythmic drugs**
		Flecainide (25)

Abbreviations: RLS, restless legs syndrome; PLMS, periodic limb movements during sleep; SSRI, selective serotonin reuptake inhibitor.

SRBD first to unmask the possible independent limb movements (68). Also, PLMS may be associated with arousals or a brief awakening, and these can be quantified only with the use of PSG. For a limb movement to be considered a PLM, its amplitude must exceed 25% of toe dorsiflexion during calibration, the duration must be between 0.5 and 5 seconds, and the intermovement interval measured from onset to onset should lie between 5 and 90 seconds

Table 3 Differential Diagnosis for Periodic Limb Movement Disorder

Differential diagnosis	Common features	Distinguishing features	Diagnostic procedures
Sleep starts (76,77)	Involuntary movements during sleep	Onset during drowsiness, non-periodic	PSG
Fragmentary myoclonus (72,78)	Frequent EMG activity	EMG activity shorter than 0.5 sec	PSG
Propriospinal myoclonus (73,79)	Quasiperiodic, involuntary movements at sleep onset	Only at sleep onset or sleep-wake transitions, EMG activity usually shorter than 0.5 sec	Video PSG
Nocturnal epileptic seizures, myoclonic epilepsy	Involuntary movements during sleep	Non-periodic, epileptic EEG activity	Video PSG
Myoclonus, other	Involuntary movements during sleep	EMG activity shorter than 0.5 sec	PSG
SRBD	Involuntary, sometimes periodic movements during sleep	Associated with breathing abnormalities during sleep	PSG, reevaluation after treatment of SRBD

Abbreviations: EMG, electromyogram; PSG, polysomnogram; EEG, electroencephalography; SRBD, sleep-related breathing disorder.

(69). Only movements that occur in a sequence of at least four movements are considered. Recently, refined standards for recording and scoring PLMs have been proposed by the World Association of Sleep Medicine (WASM) in collaboration with a task force of the International Restless Legs Syndrome Study Group (IRLSSG) (68).

Important Diagnostic Features and Criteria to Distinguish Types

The key features of PLMD are stereotyped, repetitive, brief movements during sleep that are most often observed for the legs but can also occur in the arms. PLMS are quantified by the PLMS index, which refers to the number of PLMs per hour of sleep. As a general rule, a PLMS index of 15 is considered as the lower limit to diagnose PLMD (1). However, an increased PLMS index can also be found in a substantial number of asymptomatic subjects, especially in the elderly (2,70,71). A significant complaint of sleep disturbances or daytime functioning is therefore a mandatory symptom of PLMD.

Differential Diagnosis

The differential diagnosis of PLMD includes other involuntary movements that occur during sleep such as normal phenomena (e.g., hypnic jerks), as well as sleep-related epilepsy, excessive fragmentary myoclonus (72), propriospinal myoclonus (73), REM sleep behavior disorder (74), or nocturnal paroxysmal dystonia (75). In addition, SRBDs may mimic PLMD (Table 3). For differentiation, PSG and videotaping may be helpful; other procedures are listed in Table 3.

SLEEP-RELATED BRUXISM

Key Steps in the Diagnosis of the Disorder

The clinical diagnosis of sleep-related bruxism is based on the patient's history and orofacial examination. Most patients are completely unaware of these nocturnal teeth-grinding or tapping sounds, but their bed partners may complain of disturbance from the clicking or grating sound. The repetitive nocturnal clenching may lead to the complaint of morning jaw discomfort, which usually improves over the course of the day. Bruxism can lead to significant tooth damage, dental thermal hypersensitivity, hypermobility, hypercementosis, or the need for dental restoration. Sleep-related bruxism may also be associated with headaches. Nocturnal PSG shows jaw contractions during sleep that may present as tonic contractions (isolated sustained jaw clenching) or as a series of repetitive phasic muscle contractions rhythmical masticatory muscle activity (RMMA) (80). Sleep-related bruxism may be associated with brief arousals from sleep but rarely with awakenings. There is considerable variability in the duration and intensity of sleep-related bruxism (81). Bruxism may also occur during daytime but is characterized more by teeth clenching and jaw bracing without teeth contact. In contrast to sleep-related bruxism, teeth grinding is rarely noted during the daytime.

Important Diagnostic Features and Criteria to Distinguish Types

Sleep-related bruxism is characterized by forceful rhythmical grinding or clenching of the teeth during sleep. A complaint of jaw muscle discomfort, fatigue or stiffness, and occasional headaches may be reported by the patient. In addition, the presence of tooth wear, teeth that are sensitive to hot or cold, and muscle hypertrophy may be found (1).

Differential Diagnosis

The clinical diagnosis of sleep bruxism based on the patient's history and orofacial examination seldom poses diagnostic problems; however, the clinician should be aware of other phenomena that can mimic the features of bruxism (25). Facio-mandibular activities during sleep can occur with facio-mandibular myoclonus (82), which may coexist with sleep bruxism in up to 10% of frequent teeth grinders (83). Natural ongoing rhythmical masticatory muscle activity or chewing automatisms have to be differentiated from sleep bruxism. Daytime orofacial/cervical myoclonia as in dystonia, tremor, chorea, or dyskinesia may persist in sleep. Orofacial movements may also be associated with sighs, sleep-talking (somniloqui), and swallowing or coughing during sleep. In rare cases, epileptic motor activities, in particular partial complex seizure disorders, need to be considered in the differential diagnosis. The teeth-grinding sounds may at times be confused with other nocturnal sounds such as snoring, throat clearing, or temporal mandibular joint sounds. Repetitive and periodically occurring jaw muscle activity may also be observed in the context of SRBDs, which is an important differential diagnosis to consider in case of impaired daytime functioning and nonresponse to the management of sleep-related bruxism.

SLEEP-RELATED RHYTHMIC MOVEMENT DISORDER

Key Steps in the Diagnosis of the Disorder

The clinical diagnosis of sleep-related rhythmic movement disorder (RMD) rests on the observation of the typical repetitive stereotyped and rhythmic behaviors occurring during sleep, near nap, or bedtime, or when the individual appears drowsy or asleep. Since RMDs are predominantly found in children, the diagnosis relies on the reports of the parents. Sleep-related rhythmic movements, however, are common in normal infants and children, and without evidence for significant consequences, the movements alone should not be considered a disorder. In particular, a marked interference with normal sleep, a significant impairment in daytime functioning, and self-inflicted bodily injury that requires medical treatment are considered significant consequences and must be explored. RMD in adults or with a new occurrence after the age of three should often provoke the exploration of potential differential diagnoses described below.

Important Diagnostic Features and Criteria to Distinguish Types

Sleep-related RMD is characterized by repetitive, stereotyped, rhythmic motor behaviors that occur predominantly during drowsiness or sleep involving large muscle groups (1). RMD can occur during all stages of sleep or even during quiet wakefulness, but mostly occur during sleep onset (84). RMD is typically seen in infants and children and includes several subtypes of movements (75). Head banging involves the violent moving of the head in an anteroposterior direction. Typically, the head is banged into a pillow, occasionally into a wall or the side of a crib. Because of the forceful nature of the head movements, this form of RMD is often the most injurious (84). Body rocking may occur either when the child is on the hands and knees (with the whole body thrust in an anteroposterior direction) or when he or she is sitting (rocking of the torso). Head rolling is associated with the head being rotated from side to side, usually in a supine position. Less common rhythmic movement form includes body rolling, leg banging, or leg rolling. Rhythmic humming or sounds—sometimes quite loud—may accompany the body, head, or limb movements. The duration of RMD episodes is variable, and so is their frequency. However, most episodes last less than 15 minutes, and the typical frequency of the rhythmic movements is between 0.5 and 2 seconds (85).

Differential Diagnosis
Diagnosing RMD by history alone can be difficult, and the video-PSG is the gold standard to distinguish RMD from epileptic disorders, REM sleep behavior disorder, or sleep terrors (86). Although an epileptic etiology has been rarely reported, it should be considered in cases of new onset of RMD after the age of three (75). In addition, RMD must also be distinguished from repetitive movements involving restricted small muscle groups such as sleep-related bruxism, thumb-sucking, rhythmic sucking of a pacifier or the lips. Hypnagogic foot tremor is another frequent rhythmic movement of restricted small muscle groups (87). Children with autism or pervasive developmental disorders often exhibit repetitive behaviors, but these are typically in wakefulness. Indeed, in children with these disorders, the additional diagnosis of RMD should only be made if the movements are predominantly sleep related. Autoerotic or masturbatory behaviors may also involve repetitive body movements, but the primary focus here is the genital stimulation. It is worth mentioning that many adults with RLS employ rhythmic movements as a conscious strategy to suppress restless legs symptoms.

LEG CRAMPS

Key Steps in the Diagnosis of the Disorder
The diagnosis of leg cramps is a clinical diagnosis based on the distinctive symptoms brought forward by the patient. In uncomplicated cases, an interview that assesses the severity of symptoms and elucidates potential secondary causes or risk factors (such as substances, see substance-induced SRMD) for this disorder suffices. However, many, if not most, sleep-related leg cramps appear to be idiopathic, unrelated to any other disorder (88).

Important Diagnostic Features and Criteria to Distinguish Types
Sleep-related leg cramps are painful sensations caused by sudden and intense involuntary contractions of muscles usually in the calf or foot (1). Leg cramps occurring during the sleep period may arise from either sleep or wakefulness. The cramp may last up to several minutes and may remit spontaneously. In many cases, it can be relieved by a strong stretching of the affected muscle or sometimes movement and massage. Discomfort and tenderness in the muscle may persist for several hours after the cramp. Sleep disturbances are the result of the pain caused by the leg cramp but also of the activities used to reduce the pain and the persisting discomfort after the cramp. The frequency of sleep-related leg cramps varies widely from less than once a year to repeated episodes every night. Leg cramps may occur primarily during the daytime, primarily during sleep, or during both day and night. Only when they occur primarily during sleep and are associated with disturbed sleep, they are considered sleep-related leg cramps.

Differential Diagnosis
Sleep-related leg cramps can be differentiated from other disorders involving pain or increased muscle tone such as chronic myelopathy, peripheral neuropathy, claudication, akathisia, muscular pain fasciculation syndrome, and disorders of calcium metabolism by clinical history and physical examination (89). Sleep-related leg cramps and RLS share the presence of leg pains and the urge to move the legs during the sleep period. However, relieving the pain from leg cramps requires both more time and more vigorous stretching of the muscle. Also, RLS does not usually involve a sensation of pain, but when reported, the pain is at least partially relieved by any movement of the leg, not necessarily the stretching that relieves muscle cramps. Sleep-related leg cramps may also coexist with other sleep disorders such as PLMD or SRBDs.

SLEEP-RELATED MOVEMENT DISORDER DUE TO DRUG OR SUBSTANCE

SRMDs due to drug or substance refer to those SRMDs in which the movement is due to a drug or substance. This may include dependence, abuse, poisoning, adverse effects, or underdosing of a drug. Medications associated with RLS (24), PLMS (90), or bruxism (80) are listed in

Table 2. Psychoactive drugs such as antidepressants and antipsychotics have been repeatedly associated with these movement disorders. Particularly prominent is the relationship between SSRIs and both RLS and PLMS. In addition, antipsychotic agents can affect SRMD presumably by their anti-dopaminergic activity. To the best of our knowledge, no specific substances have been reported to trigger sleep-related RMDs. Leg cramps have been associated with a wide range of substances (89,91,92) including calcium channel blockers [e.g., nifedipine (93,94)], selective estrogen receptor modulators [e.g., ralofixene (95)], acetylcholinesterase (AChE) inhibitors [e.g., donepezil (96)], β-agonists [terbutaline (97), salbutamol (98)], and lipid-lowering agents [clofibrate (99)]. Diuretics are frequently mentioned as being related to leg cramps, however, the clinical evidence is scarce (100,101). A suspicion of substance-induced SRMD is always warranted when the movement disorder appears in close temporal association with a specific drug. If the movement disorder disappears or improves markedly once the drug is discontinued, a causative mechanism is generally assumed.

CONCLUSIONS

The diagnostic process in the case of suspected SRMD involves the type of complaints; the specific nighttime symptoms and observations; the history of current or previous medical, neurological, or psychiatric illnesses; and a drug history. For RLS, a clear description of the symptoms is important; a SIT, levodopa trial, a laboratory evaluation to rule out potentially secondary forms of RLS, nerve conduction velocities and electromyogram, and PSG may be considered in the discrimination of difficult cases. The diagnosis of PLMD requires documenting PLMs either by actigraphy or by PSG, since the patient is typically unaware of the limb movements or the frequent sleep disruptions. Sleep-related bruxism is based on the patient's history and orofacial examination, and may be documented by PSG. Sleep-related RMD relies on observations of the characteristic repetitive stereotyped and rhythmic behaviors occurring during sleep, particularly by the reports of parents, since this disorder is predominantly found in children. Leg cramps and SRMD due to drug or substance are typically diagnosed during clinical evaluation.

REFERENCES

1. American Academy of Sleep Medicine. The International Classification of Sleep Disorders: Diagnostic and Coding Manual. Westchester: American Academy of Sleep Medicine, 2005.
2. Ancoli-Israel S, Kripke DF, Klauber MR, et al. Periodic limb movements in sleep in community-dwelling elderly. Sleep 1991; 14:496–500.
3. Dickel MJ, Mosko SS. Morbidity cut-offs for sleep apnea and periodic leg movements in predicting subjective complaints in seniors. Sleep 1990; 13:155–166.
4. Claman DM, Redline S, Blackwell T, et al. Prevalence and correlates of periodic limb movments in older women. J Clin Sleep Med 2006; 2:438–445.
5. Arand D, Bonnet M, Hurwitz T, et al. The clinical use of the MSLT and MWT. Review by the MSLT and MWT Task Force of the Standards of Practive Commitee of the American Academy of Sleep Medicine. Sleep 2005; 28:123–144.
6. Lezak MD. Neuropsychological Assessment. New York: Oxford University Press, 1995.
7. Allen RP, Picchietti D, Hening WA, et al. Restless legs syndrome: diagnostic criteria, special considerations, and epidemiology. A report from the restless legs syndrome diagnosis and epidemiology workshop at the National Institutes of Health. Sleep Med 2003; 4:101–119.
8. Michaud M, Paquet J, Lavigne G, et al. Sleep laboratory diagnosis of restless legs syndrome. Eur Neurol 2002; 48:108–113.
9. Stiasny-Kolster K, Kohnen R, Möller JC, et al. Validation of the "L-DOPA test" for diagnosis of restless legs syndrome. Mov Disord 2006; 21:1333–1339.
10. Nordlander NB. Therapy in restless legs. Acta Med Scand 1953; 145:453–457.
11. O'Keeffe ST, Gavin K, Lavan JN. Iron status and restless legs syndrome in the elderly. Age Ageing 1994; 23:200–203.
12. Collado-Seidel V, Kohnen R, Samtleben W, et al. Clinical and biochemical findings in uremic patients with and without restless legs syndrome. Am J Kidney Dis 1998; 31:324–328.
13. Wang D, Teichtahl H. Opioids, sleep architecture and sleep-disordered breathing. Sleep Med Rev 2007; 11:35–46.

14. Walters AS, Winkelmann J, Trenkwalder C, et al. Long-term follow-up on restless legs syndrome patients treated with opioids. Mov Disord 2001; 16:1105–1109.
15. Walters AS, Hickey K, Maltzman J, et al. A questionnaire study of 138 patients with restless legs syndrome: the 'Night-Walkers' survey. Neurology 1996; 46:92–95.
16. Ondo W, Jankovic J. Restless legs syndrome: clinicoetiologic correlates. Neurology 1996; 47:1435–1441.
17. Gemignani F, Brindani F, Negrotti A, et al. Restless legs syndrome and polyneuropathy. Mov Disord 2006; 21:1254–1257.
18. Gemignani F, Marbini A, Di Giovanni G, et al. Cryoglobulinaemic neuropathy manifesting with restless legs syndrome. J Neurol Sci 1997; 152:218–223.
19. Walters AS, Wagner M, Hening WA. Periodic limb movements as the initial manifestation of restless legs syndrome triggered by lumbosacral radiculopathy. Sleep 1996; 19:825–826.
20. Walters AS, Hening W, Rubinstein M, et al. A clinical and polysomnographic comparison of neuroleptic-induced akathisia and the idiopathic restless legs syndrome. Sleep 1991; 14:339–345.
21. Spillane JD, Nathan PW, Kelly RE, et al. Painful legs and moving toes. Brain 1971; 94:541–556.
22. Dressler D, Thompson PD, Gledhill RF, et al. The syndrome of painful legs and moving toes. Mov Disord 1994; 9:13–21.
23. Yunus MB, Aldag JC. Restless legs syndrome and leg cramps in fibromyalgia syndrome: a controlled study. Br Med J 1996; 312:1339.
24. Yang C, Winkelman JW. Iatrogenic restless legs syndrome. In: Ondo WG, ed. Restless Legs Syndrome. Diagnosis and Treatment. New York: Informa Healthcare USA, Inc., 2007:255–267.
25. Lavigne GJ, Manzini C, Kato T. Sleep bruxism. In: Kryger MH, Roth T, Dement WC, eds. Principles and Practice of Sleep Medicine. 4th ed. Philadelphia: Elsevier Saunders, 2005:946–959.
26. Winocur E, Gavish A, Voikovitch M, et al. Drugs and bruxism: a critical review. J Orofac Pain 2003; 17:99–111.
27. Dimmitt SB, Riley GJ. Selective serotonin receptor uptake inhibitors can reduce restless legs symptoms. Arch Intern Med 2000; 160:712.
28. Ohayon MM, Roth T. Prevalence of restless legs syndrome and periodic limb movement disorder in the general population. J Psychosom Res 2002; 53:547–554.
29. Maany I, Dhopesh V. Akathisia and fluoxetine. J Clin Psychiatry 1990; 51:210–212.
30. Bakshi R. Fluoxetine and restless legs syndrome. J Neurol Sci 1996; 142:151–152.
31. Hargrave R, Beckley DJ. Restless leg syndrome exacerbated by sertraline. Psychosomatics 1998; 39:177–178.
32. Sanz-Fuentenebro FJ, Huidobro A, Tejadas-Rivas A. Restless legs syndrome and paroxetine. Acta Psychiatr Scand 1996; 94:482–484.
33. Yang C, White DP, Winkelman JW. Antidepressants and periodic leg movements of sleep. Biol Psychiatry 2005; 58:510–514.
34. Dorsey CM, Lukas SE, Cunningham SL. Fluoxetine-induced sleep disturbance in depressed patients. Neuropsychopharmacology 1996; 14:437–442.
35. Salin-Pascual R, Galicia-Polo L, Drucker-Colin R. Sleep changes after 4 consecutive days of venlafaxine administration in normal volunteers. J Clin Psychiatry 1997; 58:348–350.
36. Gerber PE, Lynd LD. Selective serotonin-reuptake inhibitor-induced movement disorders. Ann Pharmacother 1998; 32:692–698.
37. Ellison JM, Stanziani P. SSRI-associated nocturnal bruxism in four patients. J Clin Psychiatry 1993; 54:432–444.
38. Romanelli F, Adler DA, Bungay KM. Possible paroxetine-induced bruxism. Ann Pharmacother 1996; 30:1246–1248.
39. Wise M. Citalopram-induced bruxism. Br J Psychiatry 2001; 178:182.
40. Markkula J, Lauerma H. Mirtazapine-induced restless legs. Hum Psychopharmacol 1997; 12:497–499.
41. Bonin B, Vandel P, Kantelip JP. Mirtazapine and restless leg syndrome: a case report. Therapie 2000; 55:649–656.
42. Agargün MY, Kara H, Özbek H, et al. Restless legs syndrome induced by mirtazapine. J Clin Psychiatry 2002; 63:1179.
43. Teive HA, de Quadros A, Barros FC, et al. Worsening of autosomal dominant restless legs syndrome after use of mirtazapine: case report (Portuguese). Arq Neuropsiquiatr 2002; 60(4):1025–1029.
44. Bahk WM, Pae CU, Chae JH, et al. Mirtazapine may have the propensity for developing a restless legs syndrome? A case report. Psychiatry Clin Neurosci 2002; 56:209–210.
45. Paik IH, Lee C, Choi BM, et al. Mianserin-induced restless legs syndrome. Br J Psychiatry 1989; 155:415–417.
46. Markkula J, Lauerma H. Mianserin and restless legs. Int Clin Psychopharmacol 1997; 12:53–58.
47. Casas M, Garcia-Ribera C, Alvarez E, et al. Myoclonic movements as a side-effect of treatment with therapeutic doses of clomipramine. Int Clin Psychopharmacol 1987; 2:333–336.
48. Horiguchi J, Yamashita H, Mizuno S, et al. Nocturnal eating/drinking syndrome and neuroleptic-induced restless legs syndrome. Int Clin Psychopharmacol 1999; 14:33–36.

49. Amir I, Hermesh H, Gavish A. Bruxism secondary to antipsychotic drug exposure: a positive response to propranolol. Clin Neuropharmacol 1997; 20:86–89.
50. Kraus T, Schuld A, Pollmächer T. Periodic leg movements in sleep and restless legs syndrome probably caused by olanzapine. J Clin Psychopharmacol 1999; 19:478–479.
51. Wetter TC, Brunner J, Bronisch T. Restless legs syndrome probably induced by risperidone treatment. Pharmacopsychiatry 2002; 35:109–111.
52. Duggal HS, Mendhekar DN. Clozapine-associated restless legs syndrome. J Clin Psychopharmacol 2007; 27:89–90.
53. Cohrs S, Rodenbeck A, Guan Z, et al. Sleep-promoting properties of quetiapine in healthy subjects. Psychopharmacology (Berl) 2004; 174:421–429.
54. Heiman EM, Christie M. Lithium-aggravated nocturnal myoclonus and restless legs syndrome. Am J Psychiatry 1986; 143:1191–1192.
55. Terao T, Terao M, Yoshimura R, et al. Restless legs syndrome induced by lithium. Biol Psychiatry 1991; 30:1167–1170.
56. Drake ME. Restless legs with antiepileptic drug therapy. Clin Neurol Neurosurg 1988; 90:151–154.
57. Chen JT, Garcia PA, Alldredge BK. Zonisamide-induced restless legs syndrome. Neurology 2003; 60: 147.
58. Abril B, Carlander B, Touchon J, et al. Restless legs syndrome in narcolepsy: a side effect of sodium oxybate? Sleep Med 2007; 8:181–183.
59. O'Sullivan RL, Greenberg DB. H2 antagonists, restless legs syndrome, and movement disorders. Psychosomatics 1993; 34:530–532.
60. Hornyak M, Kopasz M, Feige B, et al. Variability of periodic leg movements in various sleep disorders: implications for clinical and pathophysiologic studies. Sleep 2005; 28:331–335.
61. Sforza E, Haba-Rubio J. Night-to-night variability in periodic leg movements in patients with restless legs syndrome. Sleep Med 2005; 6:259–267.
62. Bédard MA, Montplaisir J, Godbout R. Effect of L-dopa on periodic movements in sleep in narcolepsy. Eur Neurol 1987; 27:35–38.
63. Boivin DB, Montplaisir J, Poirier G. The effects of L-dopa on periodic leg movements and sleep organization in narcolepsy. Clin Neuropharmacol 1989; 12:339–345.
64. Lapierre O, Montplaisir J. Polysomnographic features of REM sleep behavior disorder: development of a scoring method. Neurology 1992; 42:1371–1374.
65. Fantini ML, Michaud M, Gosselin N, et al. Periodic leg movements in REM sleep behavior disorder and related autonomic and EEG activation. Neurology 2002; 59:1889–1894.
66. Fry JM, DiPhillipo MA, Pressman MR. Periodic leg movements in sleep following treatment of obstructive sleep apnea with nasal continuous positive airway pressure. Chest 1989; 96:89–91.
67. Briellmann RS, Mathis J, Bassetti C, et al. Patterns of muscle activity in legs in sleep apnea patients before and during nCPAP therapy. Eur Neurol 1997; 38:113–118.
68. Zucconi M, Ferri R, Allen R, et al. The official World Association of Sleep Medicine (WASM) standards for recording and scoring periodic leg movements in sleep (PLMS) and wakefulness (PLMW) developed in collaboration with a task force from the International Restless Legs Syndrome Study Group (IRLSSG). Sleep Med 2006; 7:175–183.
69. American Sleep Disorders Association. Recording and scoring leg movements. The Atlas Task Force. Sleep 1993; 16:748–759.
70. Bixler EO, Kales A, Vela-Bueno A, et al. Nocturnal myoclonus and nocturnal myoclonic activity in the normal population. Res Commun Chem Pathol Pharmacol 1982; 36:129–140.
71. Wetter TC, Collado-Seidel V, Pollmächer T, et al. Sleep and periodic leg movement patterns in drug-free patients with Parkinson's disease and multiple system atrophy. Sleep 2000; 23:361–367.
72. Broughton R, Tolentino MA, Krelina M. Excessive fragmentary myoclonus in NREM sleep: a report of 38 cases. Electroencephalogr Clin Neurophysiol 1985; 61:123–133.
73. Montagna P, Provini F, Vetrugno R. Propriospinal myoclonus at sleep onset. Neurophysiol Clin 2006; 36:351–355.
74. Schenck CH, Mahowald MW. REM sleep behavior disorder: clinical, developmental, and neuroscience perspectives 16 years after its formal identification in SLEEP. Sleep 2002; 25:120–138.
75. Derry CP, Duncan JS, Berkovic SF. Paroxysmal motor disorders of sleep: the clinical spectrum and differentiation from epilepsy. Epilepsia 2006; 47:1775–1791.
76. Oswald I. Sudden bodily jerks on falling asleep. Brain 1959; 81:92–103.
77. Sander HW, Geisse H, Quinto C, et al. Sensory sleep starts. J Neurol Neurosurg Psychiatry 1998; 64:690.
78. Vetrugno R, Plazzi G, Provini F, et al. Excessive fragmentary hypnic myoclonus: clinical and neurophysiological findings. Sleep Med 2002; 3:73–76.
79. Vetrugno R, Provini F, Meletti S, et al. Propriospinal myoclonus at the sleep-wake transition: a new type of parasomnia. Sleep 2001; 24:835–843.

80. Lavigne GJ, Kato T, Kolta A, et al. Neurobiological mechanisms involved in sleep bruxism. Crit Rev Oral Biol Med 2003; 14:30–46.

81. Lavigne GJ, Guitard F, Rompré PH, et al. Variability in sleep bruxism activity over time. J Sleep Res 2001; 10:237–244.

82. Vetrugno R, Provini F, Plazzi G, et al. Familial nocturnal facio-mandibular myoclonus mimicking sleep bruxism. Neurology 2002; 58:644–647.

83. Kato T, Montplaisir JY, Blanchet PJ, et al. Idiopathic myoclonus in the oromandibular region during sleep: a possible source of confusion in sleep bruxism diagnosis. Mov Disord 1999; 14:865–871.

84. Montagna P. Sleep-related non epileptic motor disorders. J Neurol 2004; 251:781–794.

85. Manni R, Terzaghi M. Rhythmic movements during sleep: a physiological and pathological profile. Neurol Sci 2005; 26:s181–s185.

86. Dyken ME, Lin-Dyken DC, Yamada T. Diagnosing rhythmic movement disorder with video-polysomnography. Pediatr Neurol 1997; 16:37–41.

87. Wichniak A, Tracik F, Geisler P, et al. Rhythmic feet movements while falling asleep. Mov Disord 2001; 16(6):1164–1170.

88. McGee SR. Muscle cramps. Arch Intern Med 1990; 150:511–518.

89. Eaton JM. Is this really a muscle cramp? Postgrad Med J 1989; 86:227–232.

90. Hornyak M, Feige B, Riemann D, et al. Periodic leg movements in sleep and periodic limb movement disorder: prevalence, clinical significance and treatment. Sleep Med Rev 2006; 10:169–177.

91. Kanaan N, Sawaya R. Nocturnal leg cramps. Clinically mysterious and painful—but manageable. Geriatrics 2001; 56:39–42.

92. Butler JV, Mulkerrin EC, O'Keeffe ST. Nocturnal leg cramps in older people. Postgrad Med J 2002; 78:596–598.

93. Keidar S, Binenboin C, Palant A. Muscle cramps during treatment with nifedipine. Br Med J 1982; 285:1241–1242.

94. Poole-Wilson PA, Kirwan BA, Vokó Z, et al. Safety of nifedipine GITS in stable angina: the ACTION trial. Cardiovasc Drugs Ther 2006; 20:45–54.

95. Cranney A, Adachi JD. Benefit-ris assessment of raloxifene in postmenopausal osteoporosis. Drug Saf 2006; 28:721–730.

96. Birks J, Flicker L. Donezepil for mild cognitive impairment. Cochrane Database Syst Rev 2006; 3: CD006104.

97. Zelman S. Terbutaline and muscular symptoms. JAMA 1978; 239:930.

98. Palmer KNV. Muscle cramp and oral salbutamol. Br Med J 1978; 2:833.

99. Langer T, Levy RI. Acute muscular syndrome associated with administration of clofrimate. N Engl J Med 1968; 279:856–858.

100. Haskell SG, Fiebach NH. Clinical epidemiology of nocturnal leg cramps in male veterans. Am J Med Sci 1997; 313:210–214.

101. Abdulla AJ, Jones PW, Pearce VM. Leg cramps in the elderly: prevalence, drug and disease associations. Int J Clin Pract 1999; 53:494–496.

48 | Treatment of Sleep-Related Movement Disorders

Pasquale Montagna
Department of Neurological Sciences, University of Bologna, Bologna, Italy

Wayne A. Hening
UMDNJ-RW Johnson Medical School, New Brunswick, New Jersey, U.S.A.

INTRODUCTION

Sleep-related movement disorders represent a newly established category of sleep disorders in the new *International Classification of Sleep Disorders*, second edition (*ICSD-2*), recently published (2005). This category includes restless legs syndrome (RLS), periodic limb movement disorder (PLMD), sleep-related leg cramps, sleep-related bruxism, sleep-related rhythmic movement disorders (RMDs), sleep-related movement disorder due to a drug or substance, and sleep-related movement disorder due to a medical condition; finally sleep-related movement disorder, unspecified when the disturbance does not fit into any of the above disorders. Some of these entities were previously categorized within the parasomnias or the wake-sleep transition disorders. Mostly, they involve simple, stereotyped movements during sleep or at the transition between waking and sleeping. RLS is a more complex disease with sensory disturbances occurring at rest and in the evening, and in which the motor accompaniment is mainly represented by the periodic limb movements in sleep (PLMS). All of these sleep-related movement disorders may cause fragmented sleep, insomnia, and/or excessive daytime sleepiness (EDS).

MANAGEMENT OF RESTLESS LEGS SYNDROME

Background

RLS is a sensorimotor disorder characterized by a complaint of a strong, nearly irresistible urge to move the legs. The urge is often accompanied by unconfortable paresthesia felt deep in the legs, and such paresthesia and urge only occur or are worsened by rest and at the evening, while being at least in part relieved by walking and moving the legs. Symptoms of RLS may greatly distress patients impeding falling asleep or causing awakenings or arousals, and are frequently associated with jerking or twitching movements of the legs and, especially during light sleep but sometimes also during relaxed wakefulness, by periodic limb movements in sleep (PLMS) or while awake (PLMW). RLS may occur secondary to other medical and neurological conditions, in particular during pregnancy and associated with uremia, but in most of the cases occurs as a primary condition, often familial. Five to 10% of the general population may be affected with RLS of various degrees of severity. RLS occurs more frequently in women.

The pathogenesis of the disease is still unclear, but an important genetic determination is indicated by familial linkage and association studies that have disclosed several linkage loci and three variants in different genes that associated with RLS (1). Aside from genetic factors, there is circumstantial evidence that RLS is associated to some defect in the dopaminergic system and in iron regulation at the level of the central nervous system (CNS). The clearest evidence for dopamine system involvement is the pharmacological evidence acquired after the clinical observation of Akpinar (2) of the beneficial effects of levodopa in RLS. Evidence for an abnormality of iron metabolism also originated from clinical observations (3,4), and was substantiated by pathological and metabolic studies suggesting a deficient regulation of iron stores at the CNS level (5–7). These considerations are relevant to the treatment of RLS, since the absence of a clear and unambiguous rationale for the pathogenesis of the disease had led to the proposal and adoption of haphazard treatment strategies. Following the establishment of international diagnostic criteria for RLS and of validated scales of clinical severity; however, large controlled trials have been made possible. Consequently, practice parameters and guidelines for treatment of primary RLS based on proofs of evidence have been formed and, as such, they will form the basis of our considerations for the treatment of RLS here (8–11). All of these guidelines concur that dopaminergic agents are the drugs having the best evidence for activity in RLS.

Nonpharmacological Treatment

Primarily opinion evidence has been presented concerning nonpharmacological treatment in RLS. Behavioral options, including sleep hygiene, have been recommended by various authorities and included within the RLS Foundation Medical Advisory Board treatment algorithm (12). Two modalities have undergone formal study: leg counter-pulsation and exercise. Enhanced external counter-pulsation was found to be effective in a small open series (13), but a tiny controlled trial was unable to confirm any benefit (14) (ongoing studies may help resolve this conflict). An aerobic and leg strengthening exercise routine was found to be of benefit in a controlled trial (15), consistent with opinion that moderate levels of exercise may benefit RLS. A small pilot study in hemodialysis patients also found benefit from a 16-week aerobic exercise program (16).

Surgical interventions [deep brain stimulation (DBS) for Parkinson's disease, venous sclerotherapy, kidney transplant in RLS secondary to uremia] have been reported for cases of secondary RLS. The effect of DBS has not been consistent; kidney transplantation seems to greatly benefit RLS induced by uremia (17,18). Sclerotherapy and the association of RLS and venous disease remain controversial.

Pharmacological Treatment

Dopaminergic Agents

Levodopa was the first dopaminergic agent found effective in RLS (2) and has since shown evidence of efficacy in controlled trials. Benes et al. (19) found improved quality of sleep, reduced sleep latency, and better quality of life with levodopa/benserazide given in a single bedtime dose (mean 159/40 mg) versus placebo in primary RLS patients. Curiously, however, RLS symptoms were not considered as an outcome here. Other trials (20–23) also concurred that levodopa/benserazide in a single 100 to 200 mg bedtime dose without or with an extra 100 mg dose three hours after bedtime significantly reduced RLS symptoms. A comparison of rapid release levodopa/benserazide (100/25 to 200/50 mg) with rapid release levodopa/benserazide + slow release levodopa/benserazide (100/25 mg) at bedtime showed that the latter was better at reducing symptoms in the second half of the night and improved subjective sleep quality (24). Open phase studies of long-term (2–24 months) levodopa use suggest that the drug is effective in up to 70% of patients. On long-term use, however, dropouts ranged from 30% to 70% of the patients. Levodopa (in single bedtime doses of 100–200 mg plus benserazide or carbidopa) was effective also in RLS secondary to uremia (21,25). Levodopa caused several side effects typical of dopaminergic drugs: diarrhea, nausea, dyspepsia, somnolence, and headache. One particularly troubling adverse event with levodopa (and with all the dopaminergic agents) is, however, worsening or *augmentation* of RLS. Described for the first time by Allen and Earley (26), augmentation consists of worsening of the sensory and motor symptoms of RLS, which tend to appear earlier and earlier in time and to spread, involving previously unaffected regions of the body (27–30). This is different from the rebound of symptoms into the day that sometimes occurs when levodopa is given in the evening or night. Augmentation may set in after a few weeks or months of drug use, and may be progressive, leading to severe disruption of the quality of life. Immediate attention is warranted and a reduction of the dosage or outright withdrawal of the medication is needed. The mechanisms of augmentation are still speculative but seem unrelated to the kinetic properties of levodopa (31). Augmentation was found in 17% to 27% of patients on levodopa and up to 82% of those on long-term treatment. In a validation study of the Augmentation Severity Rating Scale (ASRS), 60% of patients given up to 500 mg of levodopa daily developed augmentation (29).

Ergot Derivatives

Ergot derivatives used in RLS include α-dihydroergocryptine, bromocriptine, cabergoline, lisuride, pergolide, and terguride. Some evidence for efficacy was given by bromocriptine at a dose of 7.5 mg (32). Controlled trials document that cabergoline, at 0.5, 1, and 2 mg once daily, in 86 patients (33) improved symptoms on the International RLS scale score and remained effective at one year, albeit in an open-label treatment. During such long-term treatment augmentation was reported by 11% of patients. Pergolide also was clearly effective in controlled trials at dosages from 0.05 upwards to 1.5 mg (mean dose of 0.4–0.55 mg) daily (34). Upon long-term use for one year, pergolide was still effective at a mean dosage of 0.52 mg daily. The adverse events typical of dopaminergic drugs (nausea, headache, nasal congestion, dizziness, orthostatic hypotension) were reported as mild with pergolide, but often had to be controlled with domperidone. Pergolide 0.125 mg daily was found better than levodopa 250 mg (35), giving total relief in 82% versus 9% of patients on levodopa. Pergolide 0.05 to 0.25 mg did not, however, improve sleep quality in patients with RLS secondary to uremia undergoing dialysis. Cabergoline has been found to be quite efficacious in several trials (33,36), including a 30-week head-to-head comparison with levodopa (37). Cabergoline has been found to have low levels of augmentation compared to levodopa (4.0% of cabergoline patients dropped out due to augmentation compared to 9.8% of levodopa patients). Some small studies of transdermal (38) or oral (39) lisuride have supported benefit; it is suggested by some that differential serotonin receptor binding may make lisuride less likely to cause fibrotic complications.

A recent problem with the use of ergot-derived dopaminergic agents is the possibility that patients may develop severe multivalvular heart problems and constrictive pericarditis and pleuropulmonary fibrosis. This adverse effect was first noticed in Parkinson's disease patients treated with cabergoline, pergolide, and bromocriptine with daily dosages equivalent to at least 4 mg pergolide for several months. Clinical and echocardiographic improvement seems to occur spontaneously after withdrawal of the ergot dopaminergic agents, but for this serious adverse event the recommendation is to avoid high doses and to monitor patients clinically and possibly echocardiographically at regular intervals of three to six months (40–42). Such fibrotic side effects have not yet been reported with levodopa or other non-ergot-derived dopaminergic agents. Such side effects led to the removal of pergolide from the US market.

Non-Ergot Derivatives

Non-ergot-derived dopaminergic agents include pramipexole, ropinirole, and rotigotine. All of them were effective in controlled trials (involving hundreds of patients for ropinirole and pramipexole). Ropinirole was effective in reducing IRLSS scores and improving quality of life at a mean dose of 1.9 mg/daily (43), and similar results were reported with ropinirole at 1.5 (44) and 4.6 mg daily (45). The usual dopaminergic side effects (nausea, headache, fatigue, and dizziness) were mild and transient. Worsening of RLS (possibly related to augmentation, but the latter was not checked specifically) was found in 7% of the patients. Ropinirole 1.45 mg/day was better than levodopa in 11 patients with RLS secondary to uremia undergoing dialysis (46).

Pramipexole too has recently received controlled trials (47–49) demonstrating that at dosages from 0.25 to 0.75 mg/day it significantly reduces RLS paresthesia (maximally at 0.5 mg) and ameliorates RLS symptoms, sleep quality, and quality of life. Again, the most common side effects were nausea and somnolence, however mild and transient. Pramipexole was also effective on long-term use, but in open-label studies. Rotigotine has been shown effective in several controlled trials when given by continuous transdermal patch delivery, with doses of 1 to 3 mg/24 hr stimated drug delivery most efficatious (50,51). Tolerability was good and comparable to placebo.

Opioids

Opioids used in the treatment of RLS included codeine, dihydrocodeine, dextrometorphan, methadone, morphine, oxycodone, propoxyphene, tilidine, and tramadol. Only for oxycodone (52) has there been a controlled trial that, at a mean dose of 15.9 mg daily, reduced subjective ratings of RLS symptoms (by 52%) and significantly improved PLMS and sleep efficiency, with minimal adverse events and no addiction, at least on short-term use. Though not based on clear proofs of evidence, experts' opinion suggests that opioids should be used only in RLS of moderate to severe degree. In patients who have proven refractory to the usual treatments, methadone has been found to provide continued relief (53). Tramadol, a mixed action drug with both opioidergic and serotoninergic properties, is the only non-dopaminergic drug reported to cause augmentation (54).

Benzodiazepines/Hypnotics

Benzodiazepines were among the first drugs used in the treatment of RLS, on the basis of their sleep-inducing effects. Alprazolam, clonazepam, diazepam, nitrazepam, oxazepam, temazepam, triazolam, and zolpidem were the principal sedative/hypnotic drugs that have been used, but the overall evidence is not adequate for their use to be considered established as effective. Clonazepam is the most widely used benzodiazepine, yet it has conflicting evidence for efficacy (55,56): it ameliorated symptoms of RLS and improved sleep quality when given at 1 mg/bedtime, but it was ineffective when given in four doses of 0.5 to 2 mg throughout the day. Adverse events with clonazepam were mild, consisting mainly of morning sedation, memory dysfunction, and daytime somnolence.

Antiepileptic Drugs

Antiepileptic drugs have been used in the treatment of RLS, based on a rationale of reducing CNS hyperexcitability or abnormally generated sensory inputs. The drugs used comprised carbamazepine, gabapentin, lamotrigine, topiramate, and valproate. Only for gabapentin there is definite proof of efficacy, though still in a small number trial: at the dose of 1800 mg daily (one-third at 12 a.m. and two-thirds at 8 p.m.), it significantly reduced RLS symptoms on the IRLS Rating Scale, improved sleep efficiency, and reduced PLMS (57). Adverse events included malaise, somnolence, and gastrointestinal disturbances. There is also open-label evidence that long-term (6–18 months) use of gabapentin is effective; pregabalin also has potential as an RLS treatment (58). The evidence is minor for carbamazepine at 100 to 300 mg/bedtime, for valproate slow release at 600 mg, and also for gabapentin in patients with RLS secondary to uremia undergoing hemodialyis (200/300 mg after each haemodialysis session).

Adrenergic Agents

The use of this class of drugs was based on the rationale that the autonomic system is involved in the pathogenesis of RLS, possibly through its effects on the limb vasculature. Clonidine, phenoxybenzamine, propranolol, and talipexole were the drugs used, but only for clonidine (mean dose 0.5 mg 2 hours before onset of symptoms) is there some proof of efficacy. PLMS and sleep efficiency were, however, left unaffected, and clonidine caused several, even though, tolerated adverse events (dry mouth, decreased cognition and libido, lightheadedness, sleepiness, headache).

Other Treatments

These include various treatments with myorelaxants, minerals, vitamins, hormones, and antidepressants. Overall, the evidence for these interventions remains anecdotal. In view of the studies demonstrating its involvement in the pathogenesis of RLS, iron has received several therapeutic trials of variable quality; however, the evidence is still inadequate to recommend it as an effective treatment. Iron dextran given intravenously in a single dose of 1000 mg (59) in a clinical series improved RLS severity. A controlled trial of intravenous iron sucrose, however, showed only modest benefit and surprisingly minimal changes in brain iron concentrations (60). Intravenous iron dextran 1000 mg improved RLS symptoms in RLS secondary to uremia (61); its efficacy, however, was no more evident four weeks after the treatment. Finally, while causing relevant adverse events (nausea, constipation, tooth discoloration, RLS worsening), iron sulfate 325 mg by mouth (concurrently with other treatments) was demonstrated ineffective in a population of non-iron-deficient RLS patients (62), although benefit had been shown earlier in patients with low iron stores (4).

Summary

On the basis of the findings to date, the *final recommendations* for treatment of RLS are that dopaminergic agents have the best evidence for efficacy and, considering the issue of the fibrotic side effects of ergot derivatives, non-ergot derivatives have probably the best safety profile: pramipexole (0.25–0.75 mg), ropinirole (0.5–4 mg), and rotigotine (transdermal delivery 1–3 mg) all have clear proofs of efficacy in large sample studies. Pergolide (0.4–0.55 mg) and cabergoline (0.5–2 mg) are also definitely effective, but their use should be monitored for eventual multivalvular heart disease and pleuropericarditis. Levodopa/benserazide (mean dosage 159/40 mg at bedtime) is also definitely effective, but its use may be jeopardized by the frequency of the augmentation adverse effect, which greatly limits its long-term administration. Among all of the other interventions, only gabapentin (800–1800 mg/day) has definite proof of efficacy, albeit in a small sample of patients.

Adjunctive and Alternative Therapy

There has been minimal study and no reports of any complementary or alternative medicine (CAM) therapies in RLS. One patient advocate, Jill Gunzel, has developed a Web site (http:// members.cox.net/gunzel/rls.html) and published a book (63) recommending a variety of techniques for managing RLS with medications. There is one funded study ongoing at the University of Pennsylvania using valerian to treat RLS (Norma Cuellar, personal communication, June, 2008, ncuellar@nursing.upenn.edu).

An important aspect of adjunctive treatment is patient support. There are now a number of worldwide patient support and advocacy groups that have developed support networks and educational materials. The Restless Legs Syndrome Foundation (RLSF) was founded in 1993 and has an excellent Web site with both lay and professional materials free to download (www.rls.org).

MANAGEMENT OF PERIODIC LIMB MOVEMENT DISORDER

PLMS represent a habitual motor accompaniment of RLS, found in over 80% of the cases on polysomnography. The recent finding that genes associated with RLS are highly associated with PLMS also indicates the close, but poorly understood relationship between the two. PLMS, however, may also occur in normal individuals as a quasi-physiological age-related phenomenon, and associated to several other medical and neurological conditions. Therefore, their pathological relevance is still discussed (64–66). PLMS are considered pathological by some authors only when they induce arousals and sleep fragmentation. The *ICSD-2* (67) allows a diagnosis of PLMD only when PLMS occur associated with a clinical sleep disturbance or a complaint of daytime fatigue. In such cases, the PLMS index (number of PLMS per hour of sleep recording) should exceed 5 in children and 15 in adult cases. The decision to treat PLMD should consequently be based on the presence of clinical signs of disturbed sleep or its daytime consequences, and on polysomnographic evidence of a relevant PLMS index.

Nonpharmacological Treatment

In a small study, vibration was found to have only nonsignificant benefits, less than clonazepam (55). In another controlled comparative study, cognitive behavioral therapy benefited sleep satisfaction as well as clonazepam, but did not reduce PLMS (68).

In patients with spinal cord injuries, PLM were reduced by exercise of the arms (69,70). A head to head comparison with levodopa in a sequential paradigm found equal benefit for the two modalities (71).

Pharmacological Treatment

Most of the therapeutic trials in PLMD using medication have considered PLMS associated with RLS. Therefore, the best evidence comes from trials performed in primary RLS patients undergoing polysomnographic recordings, and as such it largely overlaps with RLS therapy. A few trials have, however, been conduced specifically in PLMD. Dopaminergic agents come again as the drugs that have the best proofs of efficacy for suppressing PLMS, often at low dosages and after only a few days of use. Levodopa (+ benserazide, mean dose 159/40 mg) in primary RLS reduced PLMS index by 27.8 events, and also reduced PLMS (at 200 mg/bedtime or 100 mg 5 times/day + benserazide or carbidopa) in PLMD not associated to RLS or associated to narcolepsy or complete spinal lesions. Bromocriptine 7.5 mg and pergolide at dosages from 0.05 upwards to 1.5 mg also significantly decreased PLMS in primary RLS patients: pergolide caused a 79% reduction in PLMS index compared to 45% with levodopa (35). Efficacy in reducing PLMS index in RLS patients was shown also with ropinirole (a mean dose 1.8 mg/day significantly improved PLMS index by 76.2% versus 14% on placebo) (72) and with pramipexole (significant reductions in PLMS index even at the initial dose of 0.125 mg, maximal effect at 0.5 mg) (47). As concerns the other drugs used for treating RLS, oxycodone significantly reduced PLMS index by 34% in primary RLS (52), while short-term propoxyphene (at 100–200 mg before bedtime) reduced the number of arousals associated with the PLMS in PLMD, but not the PLMS index itself. Several trials showed that clonazepam 0.5 to 2 mg/bedtime decreased the PLMS index and sometimes the arousals associated to the PLMS, but the evidence comes all from uncontrolled trials and remains conflicting for the other benzodiazepines: triazolam 0.125 to 0.50 mg was ineffective while temazepam 30 mg and nitrazepam 2.5 to 10 mg were effective in reducing the PLMS index. Neither clonidine 0.5 mg nor valproate slow release 600 mg reduced PLMS index or the arousals associated with the PLMS, while gabapentin 1800 mg daily curtailed the PLMS index by 9.8 events. In a double-blind study, baclofen 20 to 40 mg suppressed the amplitude but not the total number of PLMS. Finally, in PLMD transdermal estradiol 2.5 g/day gel was ineffective either on PLMS index or on the number of the associated arousals (73).

The conclusive evidence for the PLMS is similar to that available for RLS, dopaminergic drugs appearing as the therapeutic agents best efficacious in reducing the PLMS. Remarkably, the dosages effective for PLMS are lower than those effective for RLS, and often act more quickly. Whether dopaminergic treatment may lead to augmentation of PLMS too is still unknown, but there is evidence that such treatment may unmask RLS symptoms (26,74).

Adjunctive and Alternative Therapy
There are no published reports in the medical literature on the use of adjunctive or CAM therapy for PLMD.

MANAGEMENT OF RHYTHMIC MOVEMENT DISORDER

Sleep-related RMD is characterized by repetitive, stereotyped, and rhythmic motor behaviors (such as body rocking, head banging, head rolling, etc.) that occur predominantly during drowsiness and sleep and that involve large muscle groups (67). RMD also occur in developmentally abnormal patients, especially children with mental retardation and autism, but in such cases movements prevail during wakefulness and lead to significant clinical consequences such as face and skull injuries, retinal detachment, and even brain hemorrhage. Sleep-related RMD may be considered quite common in normal children and normal infants: at nine months of age, nearly 60% of all infants exhibit some kind of RMD, but the percentage drops considerably in older children, declining to 33% at 18 months and to only 5% at 5 years of age. Occasionally, sleep-related RMD may persist into adolescence and adulthood even in normal subjects.

The most troublesome type of RMD is head banging, whereby the patients forcibly bang the head into the bed frame, wall, or floor, with substantial risk for self-injuries. However, this consideration usually applies to RMD present during wakefulness and in developmentally abnormal children, since sleep-related RMD in normal infants only rarely results in injury. Thus, when infants or young children are affected with sleep-related RMD in the absence of any neurological impairment, RMD does not require treatment, and only reassurance of parents is needed that the condition will most probably resolve spontaneously (75).

Nonpharmacological Treatment
The first line of intervention in RMD is to provide a safe environment to the child and to avoid all potentially injurious situations; this can include padding the crib or bed or even use of a helmet to prevent injuries that have included fractures. A common theme in trials of RMD is the confusion between RMD leading to self-injurious behavior and sleep-related RMD proper. On the whole, behavioral therapies, either simple ones such as verbal prompting, contingent light signals, audible alarms or more complex interventions such as teaching replacement behaviors, or rewarding alternative motor patterns and sleep initiation behaviors, seem to

afford substantial improvement with more durable and lasting effects than pharmacological treatments (76). Among the nonpharmacological interventions available, behavioral treatments, such as overpracticing the motor activity performed during the RMD during wakefulness, may be helpful. Hypnosis has also been reported as successful in single case reports (77). Sleep restriction, after an initial course of sedative-hypnotics, was reported useful in one case series (78).

Pharmacological Treatment

If RMD persists into adolescence or adulthood and may lead to potential self-injuries, treatment is warranted, though it remains difficult and in the absence of clear evidence for efficacy. Indeed, controlled trials are lacking in sleep-related RMD. Several pharmacological treatments have been reported as useful: short-acting and long-acting benzodiazepines, including clonazepam (79–82), citalopram (83), and imipramine. Among the atypical neuroleptics, risperidone seems effective for stereotypic movement disorders in autistic children and has been employed usefully in the treatment of RMD (84). A recent review of the main therapies suggested for children with sleep-related complaints is now available (76). These authors compared trials of pharmacological interventions versus behavioral therapies, noting that the evidence in favor of pharmacological treatment was weak and based on anecdotal evidence only in RMD.

Adjunctive and Alternative Therapy

There are no published reports in the medical literature on the use of adjunctive or CAM therapy for RMD.

MANAGEMENT OF SLEEP-RELATED BRUXISM

Sleep-related bruxism is an oral activity characterized by grinding or clenching of the teeth during sleep, usually associated with sleep arousals (67,85). Sleep-related bruxism is due to contraction of the jaw muscles and may occur in two forms, isolated sustained tonic contractions, or as series of repetitive phasic muscle contractions called rhythmic masticatory muscle activity. Sleep-related bruxism should be clearly differentiated from bruxism occurring during the daytime, which is often a manifestation of anxiety: the form of jaw muscle contractions and the medical consequences are clearly different. Sleep-related bruxism leads, in the long term, to abnormal wear of the teeth, in particular their coronal surfaces, to temporomandibular joint disturbances, and to mouth mucosal injury, jaw pain, and headache. Since patients are usually unaware of sleep-related bruxism, the disorder is brought to attention either by a bed partner or parent, or when tooth damage is noticed. Sleep-related bruxism is usually a primary disorder, affecting all ages and both sexes and sometimes with a familial recurrence; it is, however, most prevalent in childhood and among teenagers, where it can reach prevalence rates of 12% to 17%. Sleep-related bruxism declines in the mature age and in the elderly. Bruxism may be idiopathic but can also be precipitated by drugs. Instances are known when bruxism developed with the use of psychoactive medications, in particular neuroleptic drugs (86,87) and antidepressants, particularly selective serotonin reuptake inhibitors (SSRIs) (88) or recreational drugs (89). However, use of SSRIs, neuroleptics, and other anti-dopaminergic medications trigger tooth grinding particularly while awake, and no tooth grinding during sleep has been reported with such medications (89). Caffeine and tobacco smoking have been considered as triggering factors of sleep-related bruxism (90). The pathophysiology of sleep-related bruxism is still debated but may be related to arousals and the cyclic alternating pattern (91,92). The role of tooth occlusal deficiency is still unclear. Sleep-related bruxism is currently classified as a sleep-related movement disorder in the *ICSD-2* (67), and pathogenic theories implicate the dopaminergic system, among others, in its mechanisms.

Recently, an oromandibular myoclonus during sleep mimicking bruxism has been reported that may account for up to 10% of all bruxism cases (93), but its relation to sleep-related bruxism proper is still unclear. In such patients, treatment with clonazepam was only partially effective (94).

Nonpharmacological Treatment

Sleep-related bruxism in a child is usually noticed by parents and, since children usually outgrow it by their teens, no therapeutic measure may be necessary if no tooth wear has yet occurred. When sleep-related bruxism is ascertained as a cause of dental wear however, or when temporomandibular joint damage has occurred or the patient complains of headache or facial pain, then the patient should be followed by a dentist in order to monitor the wear and to obtain appropriate interventions, such as crowning of the teeth if excessively worn. Dental interventions said to be beneficial include protective nightguards, adapted to either the maxillary or mandibular arches whereby the occlusal bite splints protect the teeth against excessive wear and damage. Damage to the teeth is thereby avoided, but the splints do not curtail sleep-related bruxism, since most patients continue to have jaw muscle contractions even with the splint. Moreover, compliance of patients is low for night splints, about 50% of the patients still using the device after one year (95). Dental splints are also contraindicated in patients with concomitant sleep apnea.

Among the nonpharmacological interventions, psychological counseling has been advocated on the basis of the hypothesis that sleep-related bruxism represents a marker for anxiety and somatization. No definite evidence, however, is available that nocturnal bruxers have psychopathological traits, and that psychiatric interventions are effective in curtailing the disorder. However, in a study comparing cognitive behavioral therapy to an occlusal splint, both treatments provided a similar but modest benefit (96). Muscle biofeedback under the form of nocturnal EMG biofeedback therapy has been reported as of limited value in the treatment of sleep-related bruxism (97,98); the same applies to hypnosis (98).

Pharmacological Treatment

No intervention, pharmacological or not, has been demonstrated to definitively curtail sleep-related bruxism. Moreover, there are no controlled trials of medications for sleep-related bruxism, and most of the studies are open-label trials or case reports. Medications used for the treatment of sleep-related bruxism include dopaminergics such as bromocriptine and levodopa, on the basis of the rationale of abnormal striatal D2 receptor binding found upon brain single-photon emission computed tomography (SPECT) in patients with bruxism (99). However, bromocriptine proved ineffective when studied in controlled trials (100), while a controlled study revealed that levodopa reduced sleep bruxism motor activity by about 30% (101). Amitryptiline proved ineffective over a time period of four weeks in a controlled trial (102). Beneficial effects have been reported in selected cases with propranolol (103) and, in patients with iatrogenic bruxism related to SSRI or neuroleptic medications, buspirone (104), gabapentin (105), and propranolol (87) administration has been reported as effective. For short-term use, benzodiazepines such as diazepam [5 mg before bedtime or clonazepam 1 mg at bedtime (106)] and muscle relaxants may be beneficial, but long-term use of benzodiazepines appears not to be warranted (107). In an acute sleep laboratory study comparing clonidine and propranolol, clonidine was effective, but at a dose of 0.3 mg caused morning hypotension (108). Propranolol did not decrease bruxism. Finally, patients with severe sleep-related bruxism, primary or secondary to brain injury, may gain some benefit from botulinum toxin administration to the jaw muscles (109,110). However, no controlled trials exist for such an intervention.

Adjunctive and Alternative Therapy

There are no published reports in the medical literature on the use of adjunctive or CAM therapy for sleep bruxism.

Comparative Overview of Treatments

In a recent review of all treatments available for sleep-related bruxism, Huynh and colleagues (111) reported that the numbers needed to treat [i.e., the number of patients needed to treat (NNT) with a specific treatment in order for one patient to receive a benefit] estimated from reported trials was best for mandibular advancement devices (2.2) and occlusal splint (3.8) among oral devices. Among pharmacological agents, clonidine did best (NNT = 3.2), while an NNT could not be calculated for clonazepam, but the studies had a large effect size (0.9). Less effective medications included levodopa, bromocriptine, and tryptophan. Because mandibular advancement devices and clonidine have a higher risk of side effects, the Montreal group concluded that occlusal splints were the optimal therapy (112). However, a subsequent evidentiary analysis found that there was still insufficient evidence to strongly support this conclusion (113).

MANAGEMENT OF SLEEP-RELATED LEG CRAMPS

Sleep-related leg cramps consist of a painful sensation in the leg or foot associated with a strong muscle contraction. The painful muscle contractions occur during sleep, and the pain is usually relieved by forceful stretching of the affected muscles.

Sleep-related leg cramps represent a common complaint in the general population at all ages, but especially affect the elderly and in particular women. Particularly affected with sleep-related leg cramps are pregnant women (up to 81% of pregnant women suffer leg cramps, especially in the last trimester of pregnancy), and patients with lower limb venous insufficiency, liver cirrhosis, diabetes mellitus, cancer, electrolyte disturbances (especially hypokalemia and hypocalcemia), thyroid and parathyroid dysfunction, uremia and hemodialysis, and gout. Several neurological conditions such as Parkinson's disease, motor neuron disease, polyneuropathy and radiculopathy, myotonia, and the myokymia-cramp-fasciculation syndrome are associated with sleep-related leg cramps, which may also complicate therapy with vincristine, β2 agonists, statins and diuretics. Sleep-related leg cramps may finally occur as an idiopathic condition, sometimes hereditary with an autosomal dominant transmission (114).

Nonpharmacological Treatment

Given the wide prevalence of leg cramps in the general population and their varied pathophysiology, the basis for a rational management consists of a preliminary diagnostic approach aimed at recognizing the primary disturbance. Therefore, correction of the primary disturbance and treatment of the underlying condition or drug withdrawal represent the first line of therapy. Treatment should be considered when sleep-related leg cramps severely disrupt sleep and affect quality of life. Both pharmacological and nonpharmacological options are available for treatment. Patients quickly learn to terminate the cramp by forcefully stretching the contracted, in particular the calf muscles. Nonpharmacological therapy under the form of exercises of passive stretching of the affected muscles, in particular forcible dorsal flexion of the feet and toes, has been therefore advocated, but regular calf-stretching exercises proved ineffective as preventative measures for night cramps (115).

Pharmacological Treatment

Among the pharmacological interventions, quinine sulfate, an antimalarial drug, probably represents the drug with the best evidence for efficacy. Quinine efficacy has been related to the drug capability in decreasing excitability of muscle fibers by an action on the neuromuscular transmission. Several controlled trials and meta-analyses have demonstrated the efficacy of quinine given orally at variable dosages (200–325 mg) before bedtime in reducing the numbers of nights with cramps or the number of cramps (116–120). Response to quinine is quick, usually seen within three days (117). There are nonetheless controlled trials that concluded for the inefficacy of quinine when given at 200 mg at bedtime (121). Quinine has a bitter taste and is contained in commercially available beverages such as tonic water or bitter lemon. These commercial preparations are sometimes suggested as home remedies for leg cramps, but their use may be risky in the absence of precise dosing instructions and should be discouraged. Quinine has indeed several untoward effects and may cause serious adverse events, especially in the elderly and in patients with hepatic or renal failure. It also inhibits acetylcholinesterase and is therefore contraindicated in myasthenia and myasthenic syndromes. Quinine may cause tinnitus and loss of hearing, blindness, and serious reactions such as thrombocytopenia, hepatic failure, and vasculitis; the most frequent adverse events are hypersensitivity reactions (122,123). Quinine intoxication causes coma and epileptic seizures and is potentially fatal (124). Quinine should be avoided altogether during pregnancy. The Food and Drug Administration has decided that prescription of quinine drug products should not be used in the treatment of muscle cramps. Butler et al. (116) recommend that in any case, quinine treatment should be given as a trial of four to six weeks, starting with low incremental dosages, and carefully followed up especially in older people.

In addition to quinine, several other drugs have been indicated as efficacious in the treatment of the leg cramps. The evidence for efficacy is however limited, most papers being open-label studies or case reports. In a controlled trial in hemodialysis patients, vitamins E, C, their combination, and placebo gave cramp reductions of 54%, 61%, 97%, and 7%, respectively (125). In idiopathic leg cramps however, vitamin E at a dosage of 800 U at bedtime was shown to be not effective in reducing leg cramp frequency, severity, or sleep disturbance compared to placebo (121). Other pharmacological treatments reported as effective are naftidrofuryl, verapamil hydrochloride 120 mg orally at bedtime, gabapentin, diltiazem, a calcium-channel antagonist, and low-dose aspirin.

Other interventions contemplate injections of xylocaine in calf muscles, reported as more effective than quinine, and botulinum toxin injections (126). Remarkably, chronic release levodopa formulations were effective for sleep-related leg cramps in patients with Parkinson's disease (127), begging the question whether the dopaminergic system is involved and dopaminergic drugs could be active in sleep-related leg cramps.

As regards the particular case of leg cramps in pregnancy, in a controlled trial, oral magnesium supplementation was effective for nocturnal leg cramps both in pregnant women and in nonpregnant individuals (128). Young and Jewell (129) evaluated three controlled trials for leg cramps in pregnancy and found best evidence for magnesium in the treatment of leg cramps in pregnancy; both calcium and sodium chloride appeared to reduce cramps in pregnancy but with weaker evidence.

Adjunctive and Alternative Therapy

A number of CAM treatments have been recommended for leg cramps: jackyakamcho-tang (shaoyaogancao-tang, a Chinese herbal preparation), rutosides for nocturnal leg cramps in chronic venous insufficiency, L-carnitine and extracts of peony and licorice roots for muscle cramps associated with maintenance hemodialysis, and branched-chain amino acids supplements in the late evening for muscle cramps with advanced hepatic cirrhosis.

MANAGEMENT OF ALTERNATING LEG MUSCLE ACTIVATION (HYPNAGOGIC FOOT TREMOR; RHYTHMIC FEET MOVEMENTS WHILE FALLING ASLEEP)

Hypnagogic foot tremor is a sleep-related movement disorder originally described by Broughton (130) as rhythmic foot/leg movements during sleep or at the wake-sleep transition. Recently, ALMA and RFM while falling asleep have been reported (131,132), but the relations between these latter entities and the hypnagogic foot tremor of Broughton are still unclear. All may indeed represent normal variants of sleep and as such they are classified in the *ICSD-2* section VII: isolated symptoms, apparently normal variants, and unresolved issues (67). RFM occurred in 7.5% of polysomnographic recordings in a sleep disorder center as single, short series of leg muscle bursts with a duration of between 10 and 15 seconds especially during pre-hypnic wakefulness and light sleep. RFM did not have any major sleep-disturbing effect in any of the affected subjects, and it was therefore concluded that RFM could be considered a quasi-physiological phenomenon. However, in more severe forms of RFM with evidence of a sleep-disturbing effect, RFM was considered abnormal (132), but no indication was given concerning management. ALMA was described by Chervin et al. (131) as a quickly alternating pattern of anterior tibialis activation in 16 patients examined for sleep-disordered breathing and also showing PLMS. Brief activations of the tibialis anterior in one leg alternated with similar activation in the other leg, with a frequency of about 1 to 2 Hz. Remarkably, 12 of the 16 patients were undergoing treatment with antidepressants, suggesting a pharmacological effect. ALMA has been reported in RLS (133), and Cosentino et al. (134) described a patient with ALMA associated with insomnia and daytime sleepiness, in whom pramipexole was effective in curtailing the leg movements and in improving insomnia and EDS. This suggested that ALMA may be related to dysfunction in dopaminergic systems.

FUTURE RESEARCH

Studies of RLS treatment have been particularly robust and include some with the highest evidentiary quality. Nevertheless, there has been a substantial imbalance in the treatment areas investigated. First, studies have concentrated on treatments of daily RLS and have not provided much evidence for on-demand treatment of intermittent RLS. Second, almost all large-scale trials have employed dopamine agonists as treatment. While there is evidence for other drug classes, this is generally of lower quality. The efficacy and safety of anticonvulsants, opioids, and sedative-hypnotics as well as iron supplements and infusions needs much more investigation. Recent investigations of a gabapentin prodrug that have not yet been published begin to reduce this lack. Third, there are limited studies of special populations (children, pregnant women, patiens with kidney failure) who may also have clinically significant RLS. Fourth, there have been few comparative trials or studies looking into combination treatment. Fifth, nonpharmacological, adjunctive, and CAM treatments have received scant investigation. Sixth, the almost complete reliance on oral medications has just begun to subside with the studies of the rotigotine patch. Other formulations also need to be investigated.

The study of RLS treatments has clearly benefited from the development of diagnostic standards (135) and a severity scale (136). However, the diagnostic standards can fail in specific cases (137), and the total reliance on subjective report is a weakness of the diagnosis. Similarly, the severity scale (International RLS Rating Scale, IRLS), which has often been a primary outcome variable of studies, has been critiqued for failure to include key elements as well as deficiencies in its structure that may promote greater placebo effects (138). A focus on the PLM frequently found in RLS may enhance diagnosis and assessment, but eliminates those who do not have increased PLM and may only modestly reflect the impact of the illness on individuals (139). In the future, it can be hoped that better assessment tools may be developed. Potential tools include sleep and wake diaries (140), with potential for use of electronic ones, the suggested immobilization test (141), and actigraphy to record both sleep and PLM (142).

A rather immediate question is how important augmentation is as a consequence of dopaminergic treatment. Several series suggest that this is a frequent, but manageable complication of dopamine agonist treatment (143,144), but these studies have been limited to several years, while RLS may require long-term management. It seems well established that levodopa is more likely to cause augmentation than the agonists, but whether this is due to half-life remains unclear. There is also need for better instruments for detecting and assessing augmentation: the current state of the art requires an expert panel to review individual cases. An objective measure of augmentation would be particularly welcome (28). This may be particularly important for those drugs with very long half-life (cabergoline) or continuous release (rotigotine), which provide round the clock treatment. It may also be important to determine the distinctions between augmentation, tolerance, and disease progression.

Recent genetic studies (145,146) have suggested new paths for understanding RLS pathophysiology (147) and underscore the close connection between RLS and PLM (148). The full implications of these studies may lead to new and rational therapeutic approaches, going beyond the current medications that have in general been discovered serendipitously and based on clinical considerations. The future of treatment of PLMD, on the other hand, may depend on the resolution of serious issues about the clinical significance of these movements. Like many of the other sleep-related movement disorders, it may be only the rare patient who has a clinically significant condition: this is based on the understanding that PLMD can only be diagnosed when another sleep disorder does not account for its symptoms, including RLS (149). On the other hand, if PLMD does turn out to be a "forme fruste" of RLS (145), it may turn out that treatment is clinically justified. Some recent studies suggest that, beyond psychiatric impairment (150), RLS may be an important risk factor for cardiovascular disease (151,152). Since a potential mechanism may be the autonomic arousal associated with PLMS (153), this may provide a rationale for treating both RLS and PLMD to reduce future risk of cardiovascular disease.

The other sleep-related movement disorders, RMD, sleep bruxism, and nocturnal cramps are far behind RLS in therapeutic investigation. As specific reviews suggest (154), the major need may be for better designed, controlled trials. Definitions of clinical significance, specific diagnostic criteria, and a consensus on how to evaluate improvement are needed to advance the field beyond the current reliance, for the most part, on case reports and small clinical series.

The field might benefit if there were better demonstration that these conditions are clinically significant and that there is a substantial unmet need for treatment. The importance of ALMA or HFT seems to be marginal and these phenomena may merely be part of the RMD spectrum. It seems less likely that good evidentiary studies can be expected.

CONCLUSIONS

The best-studied sleep-related movement disorder, RLS, has seen significant advances in treatment, with specific reliance on the dopaminergics, especially dopamine agonists. The agonists represent all the regulatory approved agents and are first-line treatment. However, to provide relief to all patients, better tools, different agents, alternate formulations, and studies in specific populations are needed. The future of treatment of PLM or PLMD seems more highly tied than in the past to developments concerning the relation between RLS and PLM and their perhaps mutual risk for subsequent medical problems.

The other sleep-related movement disorders remain at a much earlier stage of development. In most cases, there is no clearly established treatment that can be unequivocally endorsed as both safe and effective. Whether there can be better studies to delineate effective treatments may depend on the clinical significance of these conditions and the efficacy of tools to diagnose them and evaluate their treatment response.

REFERENCES

1. Winkelmann J. Genetics of restless legs syndrome. Curr Neurol Neurosci Rep 2008; 8:211–216.
2. Akpinar S. Treatment of restless legs syndrome with levodopa plus benserazide. Arch Neurol 1982; 39:739.
3. Ekbom KA. Restless legs. Acta Med Scand Suppl 1945; 158:5–123.
4. O'Keeffe ST, Gavin K, Lavan JN. Iron status and restless legs syndrome in the elderly. Age Ageing 1994; 23:200–203.
5. Allen R, Barker PB, Werhl F, et al. MRI measurement of brain iron in patients with restless legs syndrome. Neurology 2001; 56:263–265.
6. Connor JR, Boyer PJ, Menzies SL, et al. Neuropathological examination suggests impaired brain iron acquisition in restless legs syndrome. Neurology 2003; 61:304–309.
7. Connnor JR, Wang XS, Patton SM, et al. Decreased transferring receptor express by neuromelanin cells in restless legs syndrome. Neurology 2004; 62:1563–1567.
8. Chesson AL Jr., Wise M, Davila D, et al. Practice parameters for the treatment of restless legs syndrome and periodic limb movement disorder. An American Academy of Sleep Medicine Report. Standards of Practice Committee of the American Academy of Sleep Medicine. Sleep 1999; 22:961–968.
9. Hening WA, Allen R, Earley C, et al. The treatment of restless legs syndrome and periodic limb movement disorder. An American Academy of Sleep Medicine Review. Sleep 1999; 22:970–999.
10. Vignatelli L, Billiard M, Clarenbach P, et al. EFNS guidelines on management of restless legs syndrome and periodic limb movement disorder in sleep. Eur J Neurol 2006; 13(10):1049–1065.
11. Trenkwalder C, Hening WA, Montagna P, et al. Treatment of restless legs syndrome: an evidence-based review and implications for clinical practice. Mov Disord 2008, in press.
12. Silber MH, Ehrenberg BL, Allen RP, et al. An algorithm for the management of restless legs syndrome. Mayo Clin Proc 2004; 79:916–922.
13. Rajaram SS, Shanahan J, Ash C, et al. Enhanced external counter pulsation (EECP) as a novel treatment for restless legs syndrome (RLS): a preliminary test of the vascular neurologic hypothesis for RLS. Sleep Med 2005; 6:101–106.
14. Rajaram SS, Rudzinskiy P, Walters AS. Enhanced external counter pulsation (EECP) for restless legs syndrome (RLS): preliminary negative results in a parallel double-blind study. Sleep Med 2006; 7: 390–391.
15. Aukerman MM, Aukerman D, Bayard M, et al. Exercise and restless legs syndrome: a randomized controlled trial. J Am Board Fam Med 2006; 19:487–493.
16. Sakkas GK, Hadjigeorgiou GM, Karatzaferi C, et al. Intradialytic aerobic exercise training ameliorates symptoms of restless legs syndrome and improves functional capacity in patients on hemodialysis: a pilot study. ASAIO J 2008; 54:185–190.
17. Molnar MZ, Novak M, Ambrus C, et al. Restless legs syndrome in patients after renal transplantation. Am J Kidney Dis 2005; 45:388–396.

18. Azar SA, Hatefi R, Talebi M. Evaluation of effect of renal transplantation in treatment of restless legs syndrome. Transplant Proc 2007; 39:1132–1133.
19. Benes H, Kurella B, Kummer J, et al. Rapid onset of action of levodopa in restless legs syndrome: a double-blind, randomized, multicenter, crossover trial. Sleep 1999; 22:1073–1081.
20. Brodeur C, Montplaisir J, Godbout R, et al. Treatment of restless legs syndrome and periodic movements during sleep with L-dopa: a double-blind, controlled study. Neurology 1988; 38:1845–1848.
21. Trenkwalder C, Stiasny K, Pollmacher T, et al. L-dopa therapy of uremic and idiopathic restless legs syndrome: a double-blind, crossover trial. Sleep 1995; 18:681–688.
22. Montplaisir J, Boucher S, Gosselin A, et al. Persistence of repetitive EEG arousals (K-alpha complexes) in RLS patients treated with L-DOPA. Sleep 1996; 19:196–199.
23. Saletu M, Anderer P, Hogl B, et al. Acute double-blind, placebo-controlled sleep laboratory and clinical followup studies with a combination treatment of rr-L-dopa and sr-L-dopa in restless legs syndrome. J Neural Transm 2003; 110:611–626.
24. Collado-Seidel V, Kazenwadel J, Wetter TC, et al. A controlled study of additional sr-dopa in L-dopa-responsive restless legs syndrome with late-night symptoms. Neurology 1999; 52:285–290.
25. Walker SL, Fine A, Kryger MH. L-DOPA/carbidopa for nocturnal movement disorders in uremia. Sleep 1996; 19:214–218.
26. Allen RP, Earley CJ. Augmentation of the restless legs syndrome with carbidopa/levodopa. Sleep 1996; 19:205–213.
27. Garcia-Borreguero D, Allen RP, Benes H, et al. Augmentation as a treatment complication of restless legs syndrome: concept and management. Mov Disord 2007; 22(suppl 18):S476–S484.
28. Garcia-Borreguero D, Allen RP, Kohnen R, et al. Diagnostic standards for dopaminergic augmentation of restless legs syndrome: report from a World Association of Sleep Medicine-International Restless Legs Syndrome Study Group consensus conference at the Max Planck Institute. Sleep Med 2007; 8:520–530.
29. Garcia-Borreguero D, Kohnen R, Hogl B, et al. Validation of the Augmentation Severity Rating Scale (ASRS): a multicentric, prospective study with levodopa on restless legs syndrome. Sleep Med 2007; 8:455–463.
30. Trenkwalder C, Hogl B, Benes H, et al. Augmentation in restless legs syndrome is associated with low ferritin. Sleep Med 2008; 9(5):572–574.
31. Vetrugno R, Contin M, Baruzzi A, et al. Polysomnographic and pharmacokinetic findings in levodopa-induced augmentation of restless legs syndrome. Mov Disord 2006; 21:254–258.
32. Walters AS, Hening WA, Kavey N, et al. A double-blind randomized crossover trial of bromocriptine and placebo in restless legs syndrome. Ann Neurol 1988; 24:455–458.
33. Stiasny-Kolster K, Benes H, Peglau I, et al. Effective cabergoline treatment in idiopathic restless legs syndrome. Neurology 2004; 63:2272–2279.
34. Trenkwalder C, Hundemer HP, Lledo A, et al. Efficacy of pergolide in treatment of restless legs syndrome: the PEARLS Study. Neurology 2004; 62:1391–1397.
35. Staedt J, Wassmuth F, Ziemann U, et al. Pergolide: treatment of choice in restless legs syndrome (RLS) and nocturnal myoclonus syndrome (NMS). A double-blind randomized crossover trial of pergolide versus L-Dopa. J Neural Transm 1997; 104:461–468.
36. Oertel WH, Benes H, Bodenschatz R, et al. Efficacy of cabergoline in restless legs syndrome: a placebo-controlled study with polysomnography (CATOR). Neurology 2006; 67:1040–1046.
37. Trenkwalder C, Benes H, Grote L, et al. Cabergoline compared to levodopa in the treatment of patients with severe restless legs syndrome: results from a multi-center, randomized, active controlled trial. Mov Disord 2007; 22:696–703.
38. Benes H. Transdermal lisuride: short-term efficacy and tolerability study in patients with severe restless legs syndrome. Sleep Med 2006; 7:31–35.
39. Benes H, Deissler A, Rodenbeck A, et al. Lisuride treatment of restless legs syndrome: first studies with monotherapy in de novo patients and in combination with levodopa in advanced disease. J Neural Transm 2006; 113:87–92.
40. Danoff SK, Grasso ME, Terry PB, et al. Pleuropulmonary disease due to pergolide use for restless legs syndrome. Chest 2001; 120:313–316.
41. Horvath J, Fross RD, Kleiner-Fisman G, et al. Severe multivalvular heart disease: a new complication of the ergot derivative dopamine agonists. Mov Disord 2004; 19:656–662.
42. Schade R, Andersohn F, Suissa S, et al. Dopamine agonists and the risk of cardiac-valve regurgitation. N Engl J Med 2007; 356:29–38.
43. Trenkwalder C, Garcia-Borreguero D, Montagna P, et al. Ropinirole in the treatment of restless legs syndrome: results from the TREAT RLS 1 study, a 12 week, randomised, placebo controlled study in 10 European countries. J Neurol, Neurosurg Psychiatry 2004; 75:92–97.

44. Walters AS, Ondo W, Dreykluft T, et al. TREAT RLS 2 Study Group. Ropinirole is effective in the treatment of restless legs syndrome. TREAT RLS 2: a 12-week, double-blind, randomized, parallel-group, placebo-controlled study. Mov Disord 2004; 19:1414–1423.

45. Adler CH, Hauser RA, Sethi K, et al. Ropinirole for restless legs syndrome: a placebo-controlled crossover trial. Neurology 2004; 62:1405–1407.

46. Pellecchia MT, Vitale C, Sabatini M, et al. Ropinirole as a treatment of restless legs syndrome in patients on chronic hemodialysis: an open randomized crossover trial versus levodopa sustained release. Clin Neuropharmacol 2004 27(4):178–181.

47. Partinen M, Hirvonen K, Jama L, et al. Efficacy and safety of pramipexole in idiopathic restless legs syndrome: a polysomnographic dose-finding study—the PRELUDE study. Sleep Med 2006; 7: 407–417 [Epub July 3, 2006].

48. Winkelman JW, Sethi KD, Kushida CA, et al. Efficacy and safety of pramipexole in restless legs syndrome. Neurology 2006; 67:1034–1039.

49. Oertel WH, Stiasny-Kolster K, Bergtholdt B, et al. Efficacy of pramipexole in restless legs syndrome: a six-week, multicenter, randomized, double-blind study (effect-RLS study). Mov Disord 2007; 22:213–219.

50. Oertel WH, Benes H, Garcia-Borreguero D, et al. Efficacy of rotigotine transdermal system in severe restless legs syndrome: a randomized, double-blind, placebo-controlled, six-week dose-finding trial in Europe. Sleep Med 2008; 9(3):228–239.

51. Oertel WH, Benes H, Garcia-Borreguero D, et al. One year open label safety and efficacy trial with rotigotine transdermal path in moderate to severe idiopathic restless legs syndrome. Sleep Med 2008; Aug 25, in press.

52. Walters AS, Wagner ML, Hening WA, et al. Successful treatment of the idiopathic restless legs syndrome in a randomized double-blind trial of oxycodone versus placebo. Sleep 1993; 16:327–332.

53. Ondo WG. Methadone for refractory restless legs syndrome. Mov Disord 2005; 20:345–348.

54. Earley CJ, Allen RP. Restless legs syndrome augmentation associated with tramadol. Sleep Med 2006; 7:592–593.

55. Montagna P, Sassoli-de-Bianchi L, Zucconi M, et al. Clonazepam and vibration in restless legs syndrome. Acta Neurol Scand 1984; 69:428–430.

56. Boghen D, Lamothe L, Elie R, et al. The treatment of the restless legs syndrome with clonazepam: a prospective controlled study. Can J Neurol Sci 1986; 13: 245–247.

57. Garcia-Borreguero D, Larrosa O, de la Llave Y, et al. Treatment of restless legs syndrome with gabapentin: a double-blind, crossover study. Neurology 2002; 59:1573–1579.

58. Sommer M, Bachmann CG, Liebetanz KM, et al. Pregabalin in restless legs syndrome with and without neuropathic pain. Acta Neurol Scand 2007; 115:347–350.

59. Earley CJ, Heckler D, Allen RP. The treatment of restless legs syndrome with intravenous iron dextran. Sleep Med 2004; 5:231–235.

60. Earley CJ, Horska A, Mohamed MA, et al. A randomized, double-blind, placebo-controlled trial of intravenous iron sucrose in restless legs syndrome. Sleep Med 2008; Feb 13, in press.

61. Sloand JA, Shelly MA, Feigin A, et al. A double-blind, placebo-controlled trial of intravenous iron dextran therapy in patients with ESRD and restless legs syndrome. Am J Kidney Dis 2004; 43: 663–670.

62. Davis BJ, Rajput A, Rajput ML, et al. A randomized, double-blind placebo-controlled trial of iron in restless legs syndrome. Eur Neurol 2000; 43:70–75.

63. Gunzel J. Restless Legs Syndrome: The RLS Rebel's Survival Guide. Wheatmark: Tucson, AZ, 2006.

64. Mendelson WB. Are periodic leg movements associated with clinical sleep disturbance? Sleep 1996; 19:219–223.

65. Hogl B. Periodic limb movements are associated with disturbed sleep. Pro J Clin Sleep Med 2007; 3: 12–14.

66. Mahowald MW. Periodic limb movements are NOT associated with disturbed sleep. Con J Clin Sleep Med 2007; 3:15–17.

67. American Academy of Sleep Medicine. The International Classification of Sleep Disorders Diagnostic and Coding Manual. 2nd ed. Westchester: American Academy of Sleep Medicine, 2005:193–195.

68. Edinger JD, Fins AI, Sullivan RJ, et al. Comparison of cognitive-behavioral therapy and clonazepam for treating periodic limb movement disorder. Sleep 1996; 19:442–444.

69. de Mello MT, da Silva AC, Tufik S. Sleep study after acute physical activity in spinal cord injury. Sleep Res 1995; 24A:391.

70. De Mello MT, Silva AC, Esteves AM, et al. Reduction of periodic leg movement in individuals with paraplegia following aerobic physical exercise. Spinal Cord 2002; 40:646–649.

71. De Mello MT, Esteves AM, Tufik S. Comparison between dopaminergic agents and physical exercise as treatment for periodic limb movements in patients with spinal cord injury. Spinal Cord 2004; 42: 218–221.

72. Allen R, Becker PM, Bogan R, et al. Ropinirole decreases periodic leg movements and improves sleep parameters in patients with restless legs syndrome. Sleep 2004; 27:907–914.
73. Polo-Kantola P, Rauhala E, Erkkola R, et al. Estrogen replacement therapy and nocturnal periodic limb movements: a randomized controlled trial. Obstet Gynecol 2001; 97:548–554.
74. Santamaria J, Iranzo A, Tolosa E. Development of restless legs syndrome after dopaminergic treatment in a patient with periodic leg movements in sleep. Sleep Med 2003; 4:153–155.
75. Khan A, Auger RR, Kushida CA, et al. Rhythmic movement disorder. Sleep Med 2008; 9:329–330.
76. Kuhn BR, Elliott AJ. Treatment efficacy in behavioral pediatric sleep medicine. J Psychosom Res 2003; 54(6):587–597.
77. Rosenberg C. Elimination of a rhythmic movement disorder with hypnosis—a case report. Sleep 1995; 18:608–609.
78. Etzioni T, Katz N, Hering E, et al. Controlled sleep restriction for rhythmic movement disorder. J Pediatr 2005; 147:393–395.
79. Chisholm T, Morehouse RL. Adult headbanging: sleep studies and treatment. Sleep 1996; 19:343–346.
80. Hashizume Y, Yoshijima H, Uchimura N, et al. Case of head banging that continued to adolescence. Psychiatry Clin Neurosci 2002; 56:255–256.
81. Merlino G, Serafini A, Dolso P, et al. Association of body rolling, leg rolling, and rhythmic feet movements in a young adult: a video-polysomnographic study performed before and after one night of clonazepam. Mov Disord 2008; 23(4):602–607.
82. Jankovic SM, Sokic DV, Vojvodic NM, et al. Multiple rhythmic movement disorders in a teenage boy with excellent response to clonazepam. Mov Disord 2008; 23:767–768.
83. Vogel W, Stein DJ. Citalopram for head-banging. J Am Acad Child Adolesc Psychiatry 2000; 39:544–545.
84. Gagliano A, Germano E, Pustorino G, et al. Risperidone treatment of children with autistic disorder: effectiveness, tolerability, and pharmacokinetic implications. J Child Adolesc Psychopharmacol 2004; 14:39–47.
85. Lavigne GJ, Khoury S, Abe S, et al. Bruxism physiology and pathology: an overview for clinicians. J Oral Rehabil 2008; 35:476–494.
86. Micheli F, Fernandez Pardal M, Gatto M, et al. Bruxism secondary to chronic antidopaminergic drug exposure. Clin Neuropharmacol 1993; 16:315–323.
87. Amir I, Hermesh H, Gavish A. Bruxism secondary to antipsychotic drug exposure: a positive response to propranolol. Clin Neuropharmacol 1997; 20:86–89.
88. Gerber PE, Lynd LD. Selective serotonin-reuptake inhibitor-induced movement disorders. Ann Pharmacother 1998; 32:692–698.
89. Winocur E, Gavish A, Voikovitch M, et al. Drugs and bruxism: a critical review. J Orofac Pain 2003; 17:99–111.
90. Lavigne GL, Lobbezoo F, Rompre PH, et al. Cigarette smoking as a risk factor or an exacerbating factor for restless legs syndrome and sleep bruxism. Sleep 1997; 20:290–293.
91. Lavigne GJ, Kato T, Kolta A, et al. Neurobiological mechanisms involved in sleep bruxism. Crit Rev Oral Biol Med 2003; 14:30–46.
92. Lavigne GJ, Huynh N, Kato T, et al. Genesis of sleep bruxism: motor and autonomic-cardiac interactions. Arch Oral Biol 2007; 52:381–384.
93. Kato T, Montplaisir JY, Blanchet PJ, et al. Idiopathic myoclonus in the oromandibular region during sleep: a possible source of confusion in sleep bruxism diagnosis. Mov Disord 1999; 14:865–871.
94. Vetrugno R, Provini F, Plazzi G, et al. Familial nocturnal facio-mandibular myoclonus mimicking sleep bruxism. Neurology 2002; 58:644–647.
95. Dubé C, Rompré PH, Manzini C, et al. Quantitative polygraphic controlled study on efficacy and safety of oral splint devices in tooth-grinding subjects. J Dent Res 2004; 83:398–403.
96. Ommerborn MA, Schneider C, Giraki M, et al. Effects of an occlusal splint compared with cognitive-behavioral treatment on sleep bruxism activity. Eur J Oral Sci 2007; 115:7–14.
97. Pierce CJ, Gale EN. A comparison of different treatments for nocturnal bruxism. J Dent Res 1988; 67:597–601.
98. Kato T, Thie N, Montplaisir J, et al. Bruxism and orofacial movements during sleep. Dent Clin North Am 2001; 45:657–684.
99. Lobbezoo F, Soucy JP, Montplaisir JY, et al. Striatal D2 receptor binding in sleep bruxism: a controlled study with iodine-123-iodobenzamide and single-photon-emission computed tomography. J Dent Res 1996; 75:1804–1810.
100. Lavigne GL, Soucy JP, Lobbezoo F, et al. Double-blind, crossover, placebo-controlled trial of bromocriptine in patients with sleep bruxism. Clin Neuropharmacol 2001; 24:145–149.
101. Lobbezoo F, Lavigne GJ, Tanguay R, et al. The effect of catecholamine precursor L-dopa on sleep bruxism: a controlled clinical trial. Mov Disord 1997; 12:73–78.
102. Raigrodski AJ, Christensen LV, Mohamed SE, et al. The effect of four week administration of amitriptyline on sleep bruxism. A double-blind crossover clinical study. Cranio 2001; 19:21–25.

103. Sjoholm TT, Lehtinen I, Piha SJ. The effect of propranolol on sleep bruxism: hypothetical considerations based on a case study. Clin Auton Res 1996; 6:37–40.

104. Bostwick JM, Jaffee MS. Buspirone as an antidote to SSRI-induced bruxism in 4 cases. J Clin Psychiatry 1999; 60:857–860.

105. Brown ES, Hong SC. Antidepressant-induced bruxism successfully treated with gabapentin. J Am Dent Assoc 1999; 130:1467–1469.

106. Saletu A, Parapatics S, Saletu B, et al. On the pharmacotherapy of sleep bruxism: placebo-controlled polysomnographic and psychometric studies with clonazepam. Neuropsychobiology 2005; 51: 214–225.

107. Montgomery MT, Nishioka GJ, Rugh JD, et al. Effect of diazepam on nocturnal masticatory muscle activity. J Dent Res 1986; 65:1980.

108. Huynh N, Lavigne GJ, Lanfranchi PA, et al. The effect of 2 sympatholytic medications—propranolol and clonidine—on sleep bruxism: experimental randomized controlled studies. Sleep 2006; 29:307–316.

109. Ivanhoe CB, Lai JM, Francisco GE. Bruxism after brain injury: successful treatment with botulinum toxin-A. Arch Phys Med Rehabil 1997; 78:1272–1273.

110. Tan EK, Jankovic J. Treating severe bruxism with botulinum toxin. J Am Dent Assoc 2000; 131:211–216.

111. Huynh NT, Rompre PH, Montplaisir JY, et al. Comparison of various treatments for sleep bruxism using determinants of number needed to treat and effect size. Int J Prosthodont 2006; 19:435–441.

112. Huynh N, Manzini C, Rompre PH, et al. Weighing the potential effectiveness of various treatments for sleep bruxism. J Can Dent Assoc 2007; 73:727–730.

113. Jagger R. The effectiveness of occlusal splints for sleep bruxism. Evid Based Dent 2008; 9:23.

114. Jacobsen JH, Rosenberg RS, Huttenlocher PR, et al. Familial nocturnal cramping. Sleep 1986; 9:54–60.

115. Coppin RJ, Wicke DM, Little PS. Managing nocturnal leg cramps—calf-stretching exercises and cessation of quinine treatment: a factorial randomised controlled trial. Br J Gen Pract 2005; 55:186–191.

116. Butler JV, Mulkerrin EC, O'Keeffe ST. Nocturnal leg cramps in older people. Postgrad Med J 2002; 78: 596–598.

117. Connolly PS, Shirley EA, Wasson JH, et al. Treatment of nocturnal leg cramps: a crossover trial of quinine vs vitamin E. Arch Intern Med 1992; 152:1877–1880.

118. Man-Son-Hing M, Wells G, Lau A. Quinine for nocturnal leg cramps: a meta-analysis including unpublished data. J Gen Intern Med 1998; 13:600–606.

119. Diener HC, Dethlefsen U, Dethlefsen-Gruber S, et al. Effectiveness of quinine in treating muscle cramps: a double-blind, placebo-controlled, parallel-group, multicentre trial. Int J Clin Pract 2002; 56:243–246.

120. Woodfield R, Goodyear-Smith F, Arroll B. N-of-1 trials of quinine efficacy in skeletal muscle cramps of the leg. Br J Gen Pract 2005; 55:181–185.

121. Sidorov J. Quinine sulfate for leg cramps: does it work? J Am Geriatr Soc 1993; 41:498–500.

122. Seligmann H, Podoshin L, Ben-David J, et al. Drug-induced tinnitus and other hearing disorders. Drug Saf 1996; 14:198–212.

123. Beyens MN, Guy C, Ollagnier M. [Adverse effects of quinine in the treatment of leg cramps]. Therapie 1999; 54:59–62.

124. Townend BS, Sturm JW, Whyte S. Quinine associated blindness. Aust Fam Physician 2004; 33: 627–628.

125. Khajehdehi P, Mojerleu M, Behzadi S, et al. A randomized, double blind, placebo-controlled trial of supplementary vitamins E, C and their combination for treatment of haemodialysis cramps. Nephrol Dial Transplant 2001; 16:1448–1451.

126. Bertolasi L, Priori A, Tomelleri G, et al. Botulinum toxin treatment of muscle cramps: a clinical and neurophysiological study. Ann Neurol 1997; 41:181–186.

127. Barone P, Amboni M, Vitale C, et al. Treatment of nocturnal disturbances and excessive daytime sleepiness in Parkinson's disease. Neurology 2004; 63(8 suppl 3):S35–S38.

128. Roffe C, Sills S, Crome P, et al. Randomised, cross-over, placebo controlled trial of magnesium citrate in the treatment of chronic persistent leg cramps. Med Sci Monit 2002; 8:CR326–CR330.

129. Young GL, Jewell D. Interventions for leg cramps in pregnancy. Cochrane Database Syst Rev 2002; (1):CD000121.

130. Broughton R. Pathological fragmentary myoclonus, intensified hypnic jerks and hypnagogic foot tremor: three unusual sleep-related movement disorders. In: Koella WP, Obàl F, Shulz H, et al., eds. Sleep '86. Stuttgart: G Fischer Verlag, 1988:240–242.

131. Chervin RD, Consens FB, Kutluay E. Alternating leg muscle activation during sleep and arousals: a new sleep-related motor phenomenon?. Mov Disord 2003; 18:551–559.

132. Wichniak A, Tracik F, Geisler P, et al. Rhythmic feet movements while falling asleep. Mov Disord 2001; 16:1164–1170.

133. Vetrugno R, Provini F, Plazzi G, et al. Propriospinal myoclonus: a motor phenomenon found in restless legs syndrome different from periodic limb movements during sleep. Mov Disord 2005; 20:1323–1329.

134. Cosentino FI, Iero I, Lanuzza B, et al. The neurophysiology of the alternating leg muscle activation (ALMA) during sleep: study of one patient before and after treatment with pramipexole. Sleep Med 2006; 7:63–71.

135. Allen RP, Picchietti D, Hening WA, et al. Restless legs syndrome: diagnostic criteria, special considerations, and epidemiology. A report from the restless legs syndrome diagnosis and epidemiology workshop at the National Institutes of Health. Sleep Med 2003; 4:101–119.

136. Walters A, LeBrocq C, Dhar A, et al., and The International Restless Legs Syndrome Study Group, Writing and central data collection and data analysis committee. Validation of the International Restless Legs Syndrome Study Group Rating Scale for restless legs syndrome. Sleep Med 2003; 4: 121–132.

137. Hening WA. Subjective and objective criteria in the diagnosis of the restless legs syndrome. Sleep Med 2004; 5:285–292.

138. Fulda S, Wetter TC. Where dopamine meets opioids: a meta-analysis of the placebo effect in RLS treatment studies. Brain 2008; 131(pt 4):902–917 [Epub October 11, 2007].

139. Hornyak M, Hundemer HP, Quail D, et al. Relationship of periodic leg movements and severity of restless legs syndrome: a study in unmedicated and medicated patients. Clin Neurophysiol 2007; 118:1532–1537.

140. Earley CJ, Yaffee JB, Allen RP. Randomized, double-blind, placebo-controlled trial of pergolide in restless legs syndrome. Neurology 1998; 51:1599–1602.

141. Michaud M. Is the suggested immobilization test the "gold standard" to assess restless legs syndrome? Sleep Med 2006; 7:541–543.

142. Allen RP. Improving RLS diagnosis and severity assessment: polysomnography, actigraphy and RLS-sleep log. Sleep Med 2007; 8:S13–S18.

143. Silber MH, Girish M, Izurieta R. Pramipexole in the management of restless legs syndrome: an extended study. Sleep 2003; 26:819–821.

144. Winkelman JW, Johnston L. Augmentation and tolerance with long-term pramipexole treatment of restless legs syndrome (RLS). Sleep Med 2004; 5:9–14.

145. Stefansson H, Rye DB, Hicks A, et al. A genetic risk factor for periodic limb movements in sleep. N Engl J Med 2007; 357:639–647.

146. Winkelmann J, Schormair B, Lichtner P, et al. Genome-wide association study of restless legs syndrome identifies common variants in three genomic regions. Nat Genet 2007; 39:1000–1006.

147. Mignot E. A step forward for restless legs syndrome. Nat Genet 2007; 39:938–939.

148. Winkelman JW. Periodic limb movements in sleep—endophenotype for restless legs syndrome? N Engl J Med 2007; 357:703–705.

149. Diagnostic Classification Steering Committee of the American Sleep Disorders Association. The International Classification of Sleep Disorders: Diagnostic and Coding Manual. –2nd ed. Chicago, Illinois: American Association of Sleep Medicine, 2005.

150. Lee HB, Hening WA, Allen RP, et al. Restless legs syndrome is associated with DSM-IV major depressive disorder and panic disorder in the community. J Neuropsychiatry Clin Neurosci 2008; 20:101–105.

151. Winkelman JW, Finn L, Young T. Prevalence and correlates of restless legs syndrome symptoms in the Wisconsin Sleep Cohort. Sleep Med 2006; 7(7):545–552.

152. Winkelman JW, Shahar E, Sharief I, et al. Association of restless legs syndrome and cardiovascular disease in the Sleep Heart Health Study. Neurology 2008; 70:35–42.

153. Siddiqui F, Strus J, Ming X, et al. Rise of blood pressure with periodic limb movements in sleep and wakefulness. Clin Neurophysiol 2007; 118(9):1923–1930.

154. Macedo CR, Silva AB, Machado MA, et al. Occlusal splints for treating sleep bruxism (tooth grinding). Cochrane Database Syst Rev 2007; CD005514.

| # Special Considerations for Treatment of Sleep-Related Movement Disorders

Birgit Högl

Department of Neurology, Innsbruck Medical University, Innsbruck, Austria

INTRODUCTION

This chapter will discuss special considerations for treatment of sleep-related movement disorders (SRMD).
These include specifically

- Side effects of treatment
- Age and gender effects of treatment
- Driving risks and medicolegal aspects

Because SRMD comprise such a heterogeneous group of disorders, special considerations will be discussed separately for each of the disorders.

RESTLESS LEGS SYNDROME

Side Effects of Dopaminergic Treatments
The treatment of restless legs syndrome (RLS) has been discussed in chapter 48. Dopaminergic agents (dopamine agonists and levodopa) are usually considered first-line therapy in RLS.

Common side effects of dopamine agonists include nausea, dizziness, orthostatic hypotension, and headache (refer to Chapter 48). A very slow dose titration will help minimize side effects.

Hallucinations are another common side effects of dopaminergic therapy in Parkinson's disease (PD), but have not been reported in RLS up to now. In fact, hallucinations may not be a problem in RLS patients who do not have dopaminergic cell loss and are usually treated with very low doses.

Of specific interest for dopamine agonists is *daytime sleepiness* as a side effect. Falling asleep at the wheel has been reported first in PD patients taking pramipexole and ropinirole (4), but later it became obvious that involuntary and even unnoticed napping and/or "sudden onset of sleep" (SOS) were quite common in Parkinsonian patients, and dopamine agonist treatment was only one of several possible causes (5–11).

It has been argued that daytime sleepiness in RLS is not a problem because of the very low doses used. However, unpublished data from our group and from others indicate that sleepiness as a side effect of dopaminergic therapy may also occur in a few patients with RLS, and this was even proven in one patient by polysomnography (PSG) in a double-blind design (12). Bassetti and coworkers reported the occurrence of daytime sleepiness in an RLS patient during reduction of pergolide and discussed this as a potential consequence of wake-promoting effects of higher doses of pergolide (13). Nevertheless, it seems that—apart from a few individual exceptions—for the average of RLS patients, dopaminergic treatment seems to be protective regarding SOS, and not a risk: Möller and coworkers investigated the frequency of SOS in 156 patients with RLS and 126 controls (14). A slightly higher frequency of SOS in RLS (33%) versus controls (20%) was found. The Epworth Sleepiness Scale score predicted SOS, and patients on dopaminergic therapy had a lower risk of SOS than untreated controls, which is in contrast to the findings in PD (14).

Another specific side effect of dopaminergic therapy is *cardiac valvulopathy*. This has been reported as a long-term side effect of treatment in PD, specifically with pergolide and cabergoline. Multivalvular insufficiency has been described in (ergot) bromocriptine (15), pergolide (15,16), and cabergoline (15). On the basis of this, a class effect of ergot-like dopamine agonists has been suggested (15). The pathogenesis of multivalvular heart disease is suspected to involve serotonin-mediated abnormal fibrogenesis by means of 5-HT2B receptors (15). In this context, it has been discussed that the 5-HT2B receptor agonist effect is responsible for cardiac valvulopathies, not the ergoline structure (17). In fact, it has been argued that no such side effects would occur with the isoergot derivatives, lisuride and terguride (17). A database and literature search comprising 360,000 patient years reported by a company on lisuride, a dopamine receptor agonist with 5-HT2B receptor antagonist properties, did not reveal a case of fibrotic cardiac valvulopathy and a very low incidence of any other fibrosis (18). In any case, it is important to remember that lack of reports do not mean nonexistence of a certain side effect (19).

In addition, Chaudhuri mentioned a fibrotic reaction in seven cases treated with ropinirole reported by the World Health Organization (WHO), and one case with pramipexole (20).

An echocardiographic study showed an increase of grade 2 or higher valvular regurgitation in 31% of pergolide-treated patients and 47% of cabergoline-treated patients, and a frequency in the normative range for patients treated with nonergot compounds (21).

On the basis of these data, pergolide is no longer considered first-line treatment for RLS (22) and, if other treatments fail, at least echocardiography before onset and every 6 to 12 months during treatment is warranted for patients on pergolide (22), possibly also on cabergoline treatment.

Because a cumulative dose-dependent risk for the occurrence of cardiac valvulopathies has been reported, this side effect might, as many others, again be less problematic in RLS, but the precautions should be maintained (regular echocardiograms).

Lastly, RLS patients prescribed dopaminergic agents should be warned of the development of *compulsive behavior*, including pathologic gambling and hypersexuality, which occurs infrequently in patients taking these medications.

Augmentation and Rebound

Augmentation is the most serious and specific side effect of dopaminergic treatment in RLS. According to original criteria, augmentation requires a two-hour advance in the time of symptom onset during the day, or at least two of the following: an overall worsening of symptoms despite increasing dose and an overall improvement of symptoms when dose is decreased, an expansion of RLS symptoms from legs to arms, a shorter latency to symptoms at rest, or a shorter duration of treatment effect (23). Augmentation has been reported with greatly varying frequencies between absent and higher than 80%, but the definitions of augmentation have not been uniform, and most studies have been retrospective, hampering a reliable comparison of frequencies. Nevertheless, the highest frequencies of augmentation have been reported with levodopa (24). Augmentation was reported in 48% of patients on different dopamine agonists, namely, ropinirole, pramipexole, and pergolide (25) or 8% to 32% of cases with pramipexole, but in the latter study, quite mild worsening covered by a slight dosage increase was also defined as augmentation (26,27). Even with cabergoline, a dopamine agonist with a 65-hour plasma half-life (28), a 9% frequency of augmentation was reported (29). Of course, reported frequencies of augmentation depend very much on the fact, if this phenomenon has been recognized at all and/or systematically assessed.

Several risk factors for augmentation have been identified, namely, a high levodopa dose (24), previous augmentation or tolerance, albeit controversial (27,30), lack of neuropathy, familial RLS (25), and secondary RLS in another study (26).

A novel hypothesis, well based on experimental data, suggests that augmentation results from a treatment-induced imbalance between decreased analgesic D2 receptor activation and increased pain-enhancing D1 receptor activation (31), and that the clue to avoiding augmentation lies in administering very low doses of dopamine agonists to RLS patients (31). Once augmentation has occurred, it is necessary to withdraw the patients from the causative agent (e.g., levodopa) and to switch to a dopamine agonist, opiate, or a combination of both; frequently it will be necessary to hospitalize the patient for a few days (32).

Similar symptoms like augmentation may be caused by tolerance, which has been viewed as a first step toward augmentation by several authors. However, tolerance should not necessarily include a time advance of symptoms, and symptoms should not be worse than baseline (27).

Frequently, a slight dose increase will sufficiently cover tolerance, but patients should be monitored closely in order not to miss the conversion into frank augmentation.

Rebound, specifically early morning rebound, is another related symptom. It refers to the reoccurrence of symptoms in the second half of the night or in the early morning and is a result of short-acting levodopa (33). In this case, one would consider adding a sustained release levodopa formulation (33) or middle-of-night or morning dose, or switching to dopaminergic agonists.

The knowledge about augmentation and its risk factors will certainly increase when the new uniform criteria are used in prospective studies, and new instruments to assess the presence [Structured Interview for Diagnosis of Augmentation (SIDA)] (34) or severity of augmentation [Augmentation Severity Rating Scale (ASRS)] (35) are incorporated into clinical studies and routine practice. It might also occur that novel ways of drug delivery in RLS, for example, transdermal systems, may change the appearance of augmentation. On the basis of experience gathered in the past few years since the publication of the first uniform criteria for augmentation in 2003 (23), a new version with some slight adaptation and modification is currently being prepared.

Side Effects of Nondopaminergic Treatments

Nondopaminergic treatments in RLS include opiates and some antiepileptics, for example, gabapentin (36,37). Constipation is among the most relevant side effects of opiates and may definitely be prohibitive for treatment specifically in elderly patients with comorbid diseases impairing bowel function (e.g., Parkinson's disease) or a history of diverticulitis. Gabapentin has been used in high doses in RLS (38), but side effects like sleepiness may limit its use. It has to be taken into account that gabapentin can only be used in very low doses (200–300 mg per day) in patients on dialysis (39).

Side Effects of Iron Treatment

Iron treatment is now being proposed not only in patients with iron deficiency but also in patients with low normal serum ferritin levels (40,41).

Oral iron is well known for its limited tolerability (nausea, diarrhea). Its absorption is good only from an empty stomach and an acidic environment. It may cause severe esophageal inflammation and focal erosion (42).

Intravenous (i.v.) iron may have severe, local, and generalized side effects, such as local tissue necrosis in case of paravascular injection, and anaphylactic and/or anaphylactoid reactions. Anaphylactic reactions have been described with various i.v. iron injections. They are observed more frequently with iron dextran (43).

A significant 0.6% rate of life-threatening complications has been reported with i.v. iron dextran treatment in 481 hemodialysis patients (44).

One hundred and ninety-six cases were published in the literature from 1976 to 1997 (43). The incidence of complications was lower with iron saccharates between 1.5 and 6 permille (e.g., iron III saccharose complex), and between 1976 and 1997, 74 cases were published (43).

In addition, in contrast to dextrans (31 deaths), with iron saccharates no deaths were observed (45) On the basis of the possibility of anaphylactic or anaphylactoid reactions, it has been recommended to use oral iron whenever possible and implement i.v. applications only when necessary (43,46).

Another iron preparation is sodium ferric gluconate complex, which is considered to be the safest option. However, an anaphylactoid or anaphylactic reaction to sodium gluconate complex administered in a pregnant woman has been reported (44). In another four-year study with repeated i.v. iron administration, iron sucrose and sodium ferric gluconate in 57 patients, no cases of anaphylactic reactions, two cases of flushing, and one hypotension case were reported (46).

Despite the impressive benefits of i.v. iron dextran reported in the past few years (40,41), these side effects will have to be carefully weighed against the risks mentioned above, and the least harmful preparation and administration method selected.

Age and Gender Effects of Treatment

It is well known that the frequency of RLS is related to gender (47). In addition, the comorbidities of RLS have been reported to be different in men and women, for example, higher rates of coexistent hypothyroidism were reported in women with RLS (48). Women also had a higher frequency of multisymptomatic sleep disturbance from RLS (48).

An increasing frequency of RLS has been noted across decades in many studies, but it may be in the highest age group that a decline in prevalence is observed (47,49). However, RLS may still be widely unrecognized in cognitively impaired persons, for example, demented elderly. New criteria for recognizing RLS in this patient group have been defined, which include observation of behavior (e.g., rubbing the legs, moaning while holding the legs) (23).

Specifically in these patient groups, interactions of RLS exacerbations and RLS treatment, concomitant medications (e.g., neuroleptics), or aggravation by comorbid conditions (e.g., untreated anemia) may be far more frequent than expected.

Possibly, dopamine agonists can be used safely for the treatment of RLS in the highest age group, but no specific study is available to prove this possibility.

In contrast, treatment of RLS in children has completely different caveats, for example, impaired osteogenesis by benserazide given together with levodopa in some preparations.

In an epidemiological study of RLS, subtle, albeit nonsignificant, differences were found for the concentration of soluble transferrin receptors (sTfR) in plasma, which was elevated in individuals with RLS ($p < 0.001$) compared with a nonaffected population. The association was particularly strong in men and somewhat less pronounced in women, even though from a statistical viewpoint gender was not a significant effect modifier. In men, high sTR was found in 22.7% of patients with RLS and in 3.8% of nonaffected individuals, and in women, high sTR was found in 13.5% of patients with RLS and in 8.3% of the nonaffected group (47).

In periadolescent rats, it has been reported that gender affects locomotor response to quinpirole (50).

Kompoliti and coworkers reported a greater bioavailability of levodopa in postmenopausal women compared to men, but an equivalent pharmacokinetics of pramipexole (51). Craig and coworkers investigated growth hormone response to subcutaneous apomorphine in postmenopausal women with and without estrogen therapy. The area under the curve was greater in estrogen-treated women, suggesting that estrogen therapy enhances dopaminergic responsivity in postmenopausal women (52). Gender has been reported to have no effect on the pharmacokinetics of ropinirole (53), but clearance was slower in women taking hormone replacement therapy compared to those without therapy (53).

Pregnancy is another gender-related condition very relevant for treatment of RLS. Controlled studies are lacking. Many RLS medications imply potential harm to the unborn (e. g., impairment of osteogenesis in levodopa-benserazide, inhibition of lactation in dopamine agonists) and controlled studies are lacking (54). Therefore, in pregnancy, most authors recommend to carefully weigh the need for treatment, and if possible, get along with iron supplementation, magnesium or physical measures such as cold showering, massages, etc. Folate supplementation might also be helpful, albeit the available evidence is not high (55). If pharmacological treatment cannot be avoided, opiates are considered to be least harmful by some (www.rls.org).

Driving Risks and Medicolegal Aspects
Although, as discussed above, levodopa or dopamine agonist–induced sleepiness may be infrequent in RLS treatment, all patients should be clearly warned when a new RLS medication is started, that sleepiness may occur in the beginning of (or during stable) treatment. Patients should also be educated on how to recognize sleepiness, and that chronic sleepiness may sometimes lead to habituation and misperception (10). It is important that patients understand how their driving abilities may be impaired by sleepiness (56). On the other hand, one should take into account that untreated RLS may also severely disturb sleep and cause sleep deprivation–induced daytime sleepiness.

PERIODIC LIMB MOVEMENT DISORDER

Classically, the occurrence of any periodic limb movements (PLMs) during sleep was sometimes considered synonymous with periodic limb movement disorder (PLMD), and this was supported by the previous *International Classification of Sleep Disorders* (*ICSD-1*), where bed partner observed leg movements that were sufficient to complete diagnostic criteria.

The new *ICSD-2* makes a more definite statement: PLMD can only be diagnosed in patients with PSG-confirmed PLMs and additional clinical sleep disturbance or daytime fatigue.

In the authors' opinion, the occurrence of PLMD always requires that symptomatic PLMs due to another sleep disorder must be carefully ruled out. Specifically, it is important to check again for RLS in patients with unexpected PLMs during PSG. Walters and colleagues have reported unsuspected but clinically significant RLS in a large proportion (specify) of patients undergoing PSG for suspected sleep apnea (57). PLMs may also be prominent in narcolepsy or rapid eye movement (REM) sleep behavior disorder (RBD) (58). Therefore, one should never simply diagnose PLMD if a patient complains of daytime sleepiness and exhibits PLMs in the PSG, but in all cases, one should first rule out other reasons. Another caveat refers to the increasing use of actigraphs. What is classified as "PLMs" in actigraphy may be due to undiagnosed sleep apnea.

Usually, dopaminergic agents are considered the first choice for treatment of PLMD (58), but data are limited. Moreover, the first ever occurrence of RLS after the start of dopaminergic treatment of PLMD has been reported previously (59) and confirmed by others (60). Maybe dopaminergic treatment triggers RLS, and this further supports the hypothesis that PLMD is a forme fruste of RLS (61).

One study on the basis of one single night also proposed benzodiazepines (62), but effects were nonspecific, and the risk of worsening of sleep-disordered breathing (63) must be taken into consideration.

Age and Gender Effects for Treatment of PLMD

There are too little data to discuss specific age and gender effects for treatment of PLMD. PLM indices higher than 15 per hour of sleep are generally considered indicative of the disorder in adults; however, in children, a much lower cutoff of 5 per hour applies (*ICSD-2*). Given the uncertain clinical significance of PLMs alone, treatment is usually considered only in cases where a connection between the PLMs and the patient's complaints of insomnia or daytime fatigue seems probable, and other causes have been ruled out. Nevertheless, an increasing number of studies deal with autonomic activation during PLMs (arousal, blood pressure, and heart rate increases) and a possible risk for hypertension induced by PLMs, including all its pathophysiologic consequences, namely, increased risk for cardiovascular disease (64–66).

Driving Risks

PLMD per se may go along with daytime sleepiness and reduced capacity of driving. More than treatment-induced driving impairment, the primary underlying sleep disorder (e.g., narcolepsy, sleep apnea syndromes) may pose a person at risk for involuntarily falling asleep. In cases of doubt, full PSG and a multiple sleep latency test have to be performed.

SLEEP-RELATED LEG CRAMPS

Leg cramps have been associated with many different medications. For example, leg cramps have been reported to be a side effect of donepezil (67) and numerous other medications such as raloxifene (68), dihydroergotamine mesylate for intractable headache (69,70), and analgesics (71).

Compared to men, women have a higher predisposition for cramps (71). Quinine sulfate is used for treatment of leg cramps. Side effects include cardiac arrhythmias. A study of patients on long-term repeat prescriptions has demonstrated that trying to stop quinine temporarily will allow a significant number to be able to stop use of this medication (72).

SLEEP-RELATED BRUXISM

The prevalence, symptomatology, clinical implication, and suspected pathophysiology of bruxism have been discussed in chapters 43 to 45.

Dental splints are among the most often prescribed treatments for bruxism. A splint will help reduce damage to the teeth, possibly also the temporomandibular joints, but may worsen bruxism or sleep apnea (73). A marked aggravation of respiratory disturbances as evidenced by a more than 50% increase of the apnea-hypopnea index in 50% of the patients was observed in 10 patients with snoring and sleep apnea by the use of an oral (occlusal) splint (73). Moreover, excess salivation occurring with any intraoral device may be a significant problem, not just at the beginning of treatment. Botulinum toxin has been proposed for the treatment of bruxism for years, but good evidence, specifically controlled studies, are still lacking. In botulinum toxin treatment, swallowing difficulties and masticatory muscle weakness are among the side effects to be expected.

Dopaminergic medications have also been studied for bruxism, but results were negative (74). On the other side, bruxism itself or worsening of bruxism may be side effects of antidepressant treatment (75,76), neuroleptics (77), and amphetamines (78). Bruxism and other intraoral manifestations may even be a first hint for the physician regarding methamphetamine or other stimulant use in dental patients (79).

β-Blockers are among the alternative treatment options, their side effects include bradycardia, hypotension, sleep disorders, and even a case of exacerbation of REM sleep behavior disorder has been reported (80).

More recently, tiagabine has been proposed as an off-label, second-line treatment for bruxism of grinding and clenching. Based solely on reports by bed partners, a beneficial effect on bruxism and associated temporomandibular joint pain was observed in four out of five patients of a case series treated with tiagabine for psychiatric indications (bipolar depression and anxiety) (81). Somnolence, depression, emotional lability, tremor, etc. are among the many side effects that have been observed with tiagabine treatment, and several interactions (e.g., with antiepileptics and rifampicin) must be taken into account.

Age and Gender Effects of Treatment of Bruxism

In children, bruxism is so frequent that it is often considered a developmental phenomenon (*ICSD-2*). Rhythmic masticatory activity during sleep without bruxism must be differentiated from bruxism; it is present in normals and possibly necessary for airway lubrication and patency (82).

Medicolegal Aspects of Bruxism

On the basis of the fact that bruxism is a side effect of stimulants such as amphetamines and other amphetamine-based drugs (e.g., "speed" and "ecstacy") (83,84), and a high prevalence of bruxism and temporomandibular disorders is present in heavy drug addicts compared to a normal control population (85), it is important to note that the presence of bruxism and related disorders may point to drug or stimulant abuse. Thus, patients should be questioned for illicit drugs used if signs of bruxism are seen.

There are also some differential diagnoses to sleep bruxism, which are also a side effect of treatment, for example, dopaminergic-induced jaw dystonia and decreased lateral jaw excursion in PD (86).

SLEEP-RELATED RHYTHMIC MOVEMENT DISORDER

The clinical features of rhythmic movement disorder (RMD) have been described in chapters 43 and 45, and treatment approaches have been discussed in chapter 48.

Age and Gender Effects of Treatment

Sleep-related rhythmic movements have a very high prevalence in newborns and very young children, which then continuously declines with advancing age (60% at 9 months, 22% at 2 years, and 5% at 5 years) (87).

The new *ICSD-2* requires a significant sleep disruption, daytime impairment, or potential injury in association with the rhythmic movements during sleep onset or within sleep to classify them as RMD (*ICSD-2*), analogous to PLMs versus PLMD. RMD can persist into adulthood, but it is then very rare.

In toddlers and infants, the very high prevalence of rhythmic movements has generated discussions about the possible biologic function of RMD, for example, vestibular stimulation for maturation of the vestibular system, tranquilizing effect, etc. The latter is also supported by the persistence of RMD in mentally incapacitated children and adults. It is unknown if RMD recur in the cognitively impaired elderly but stereotypic movements are frequent in cognitively impaired patients [e.g., frontotemporal lobar degeneration (88), mental retardation (89)], and these movements might in some cases resemble RMD.

The differential diagnosis of RMD includes other treatment side effects, for example, neuroleptic induced akathisia or rabbit syndrome (90).

RMD has also been described as an adverse reaction to specific foods in a few patients (91).

Treatment Side Effects

While SRMD as a developmental phenomenon in infants and toddlers is usually considered not to require treatment, individuals exhibiting violent episodes should be treated. If treatment is not initiated, severe consequences may result from RMD, for example, alterations in the parietal and occipital bone structure as a consequence of violent head banging (92); in very rare cases even subdural hematomas and carotid dissection (93), and other injuries, specifically in mentally retarded children, have been reported (94).

Benzodiazepines are most frequently mentioned as a possible treatment for RMD (87), but worsening of sleep apnea in predisposed individuals (63) and nocturnal falls as well as "hangovers" must be taken into account as possible treatment-induced side effects.

Behavioral treatments for RMD have often been suggested (87) but not effectively studied (95). A small actigraphy-controlled treatment case series of sleep restriction together with hypnotic administration for the treatment of RMD has been published. A three-week transitory one-hour sleep restriction and concomitant administration of choral hydrate for one week produced a very favorable long-term resolution or marked improvement in six children with RMD (96). However, one has to keep in mind that sleep restriction can easily result in partial sleep deprivation, and the enormously negative outcomes of long-term partial sleep deprivation on cognitive function (97), attention, accident risk, as well as immune and metabolic function (98) have been extensively studied and reviewed.

CONCLUSIONS

In conclusion, special considerations for treatment of sleep-related movement disorders will have to take into account age and gender effects, as well as specific side effects. Medicolegal aspects and driving risks in sleep-related movement disorders mostly derive not only from concomitant sleep restriction but also from drug-induced sleepiness.

REFERENCES

1. Stiasny-Kolster K, Kohnen R, Schollmayer E, et al. Patch application of the dopamine agonist rotigotine to patients with moderate to advanced stages of restless legs syndrome: a double-blind, placebo-controlled pilot study. Mov Disord 2004; 19(12):1432–1438.
2. Trenkwalder C, Hundemer HP, Lledo A, et al. Efficacy of pergolide in treatment of restless legs syndrome: the PEARLS study. Neurology 2004; 62(8):1391–1397.
3. Trenkwalder C, Garcia-Borreguero D, Montagna P, et al. Ropinirole in the treatment of restless legs syndrome: results from the TREAT RLS 1 study, a 12 week, randomised, placebo controlled study in 10 European countries. J Neurol Neurosurg Psychiatry 2004; 75(1):92–97.
4. Frucht S, Rogers JD, Greene PE, et al. Falling asleep at the wheel: motor vehicle mishaps in persons taking pramipexole and ropinirole. Neurology 1999; 52(9):1908–1910.
5. Hobson DE, Lang AE, Martin WR, et al. Excessive daytime sleepiness and sudden-onset sleep in Parkinson's disease: a survey by the Canadian Movement Disorders Group. JAMA 2002; 287(4):455–463.
6. Ferreira JJ, Desboeuf K, Galistzky M, et al. Sleep disruption, daytime somnolence and sleep attacks in Parkinson's disease: a clinical survey in PD patients and age-matched healthy volunteers. Eur J Neurol 2006; 13(3):209–214.
7. Rye DB. Excessive daytime sleepiness and unintended sleep in Parkinson's disease. Curr Neurol Neurosci Rep 2006; 6(2):169–176.
8. Paus S, Brecht HM, Koster J, et al. Sleep attacks, daytime sleepiness, and dopamine agonists in Parkinson's disease. Mov Disord 2003; 18(6):659–667.
9. Högl B, Poewe W. Disorders of sleep and wakefulness in Parkinson's disease. Swiss Arch Neurol 2003; 154:374–383.

10. Merino-Andreu M, Arnulf I, Konofal E, et al. Unawareness of naps in Parkinson's disease and in disorders with excessive daytime sleepiness. Neurology 2003; 60(9):1553–1554.
11. Parkinson's disease: a questionnaire survey. Mov Disord 2003; 18(3):319–323.
12. Frauscher B, Kunz K, Brandauer E, et al. Ropinirole associated induction of sleepiness in a patient with restless legs syndrome: a polygraphic, double-blind, placebo-controlled, crossover study. Proc Austrian Neurol Soc 2005.
13. Bassetti C, Clavadetscher S, Gugger M, et al. Pergolide-associated sleep attacks in a patient with restless legs syndrome. Sleep Med 2002; 3(3):275–277.
14. Möller JC, Körner Y, Cassel W, et al. Sudden onset of sleep and dopaminergic therapy in patients with restless legs syndrome. Sleep Med 2006; 7:333–339.
15. Horvath J, Fross RD, Kleiner-Fisman G, et al. Severe multivalvular heart disease: a new complication of the ergot derivate dopamine agonists. Mov Disord 2004; 19(6):656–662.
16. Scozzafava J, Takahashi J, Johnston W, et al. Valvular heart disease in pergolide-treated Parkinson's disease. Can J Neurol Sci 2006; 33(1):111–113.
17. Horowski R, Jähnichen S, Pertz HH. Fibrotic valvular heart disease is not related to chemical class but to biological function: 5-HT2B receptor activation plays crucial role. Mov Disord 2004; 19(12):1523–1524.
18. Hofmann C, Penner U, Dorow R, et al. Lisuride, a dopamine receptor agonist with 5-HT2B receptor antagonist properties: absence of cardiac valvulopathy adverse drug reaction reports supports the concept of a crucial role for 5-HT2B receptor agonism in cardiac valvular fibrosis. Clin Neuropharmacol 2006; 29(2):80–86.
19. Rascol O, Pathak A, Bagheri H, et al. Dopaminagonists and fibrotic valvular heart disease: further considerations. Mov Disord 2004; 19(12):1524–1525.
20. Chaudhuri KR, Dhawan V. Valvular heart disease and fibrotic reactions may be related to ergot dopamine agonists, but non-ergot agonists may also not be spared. Mov Disord 2004; 19:1522–1525.
21. Peralta C, Wolf E, Alber H, et al. Valvular heart disease in Parkinson's disease vs. controls: an echocardiographic study. Mov Disord 2006; 21(8):1109–1113.
22. Corvol JC, Schüpbach M, Bonnet AM. Valvulopathies sous pergolide: revue critique de la littérature et conduite á tenir an pratique. Rev Neurol 2005; 161:637–643.
23. Allen RP, Picchietti D, Hening WA, et al. Restless legs syndrome: diagnostic criteria, special considerations, and epidemiology. A report from the restless legs syndrome diagnosis and epidemiology workshop at the National Institutes of Health. Sleep Med 2003; 4(2):101–119.
24. Allen RP, Earley CJ. Augmentation of the restless legs syndrome with carbidopa/levodopa. Sleep 1996; 19(3):205–213.
25. Ondo W, Romanshyn J, Vuong KD, et al. Long-term treatment of restless legs syndrome with dopamine agonists. Arch Neurol 2004; 61(9):1393–1397.
26. Ferini-Strambi L. Restless legs syndrome augmentation and pramipexole treatment. Sleep Med 2002; (suppl 2):S23–S25.
27. Winkelman JW, Johnston L. Augmentation and tolerance with long-term pramipexole treatment of restless legs syndrome (RLS). Sleep Med 2004; 5(1):9–14.
28. Hogl B, Rothdach A, Wetter TC, et al. The effect of cabergoline on sleep, periodic leg movements in sleep, and early morning motor function in patients with Parkinson's disease. Neuropsychopharmacology 2003; 28(10):1866–1870.
29. Stiasny-Kolster K, Benes H, Peglau I, et al. Effective cabergoline treatment in idiopathic restless legs syndrome. Neurology 2004; 63(12):2272–2279.
30. Silber MH, Girish M, Izurieta R. Pramipexole in the management of restless legs syndrome: an extended study. Sleep 2003; 26(7):819–821.
31. Paulus W, Trenkwalder C. Less is more: therapy-related augmentation of symptoms in restless legs syndrome caused by dopaminergic overstimulation. Lancet Neurol 2006; 5(10):878–886.
32. Trenkwalder C, Canelo M. Management of augmentation in patients with restless legs syndrome. Mov Disord 2005; 20:S10, P151.
33. Collado-Seidel V, Kazenwadel J, Wetter TC, et al. A controlled study of additional sr-L-dopa in L-dopa-responsive restless legs syndrome with late-night symptoms. Neurology 1999; 52(2):285–290.
34. Högl B, Garcia-Borreguero D, Gschliesser V, et al. On the development of the "structured interview for diagnosis of augmentation during RLS treatment" (RLS-SIDA): first experiences. Sleep Med 2005; 5(S2):S158.
35. Garcia-Borreguero D, Högl B. Validation of the augmentation severity rating scale (ASRS): first results from a study of the European Research RLS Group (EU-RLSG). Sleep Med 2005; 6(S2):S67.
36. Lesage S, Hening WA. The restless legs syndrome and periodic limb movement disorder: a review of management. Semin Neurol 2004; 24:249–259.
37. Hogl B, Poewe W. Restless legs syndrome. Curr Opin Neurol 2005; 18(4):405–410.
38. Garcia-Borreguero D, Lardosa O, de la Llave Y, et al. Treatment of restless legs syndrome with gabapentin: a double-blind, crossover study. Neurology 2002; 59(10):1573–1579.

39. Thorp ML, Morris CD, Bagby SP. A crossover study of gabapentin in treatment of restless legs syndrome among hemodialysis patients. Am J Kidney Dis 2001; 38(1):104–108.
40. Earley CJ, Heckler D, Allen RP. The treatment of restless legs syndrome with intravenous iron dextran. Sleep Med 2004; 5(3):231–235.
41. Earley CJ, Heckler D, Allen RP. Repeated IV doses of iron provide effective supplemental treatment of restless legs syndrome. Sleep Med 2005; 6(4):301–305.
42. Nordt SP, Williams SR, Behling C, et al. Comparison of the toxicities of two iron formulations in a swine model. Acad Amerg Med 1999; 6(11):1104–1108.
43. Fiechter R, Batschwaroff M, Conen D. Anaphylaktische Reaktion nach intravenöser Fe-Injektion. Praxis 2005; 94:209–212.
44. Cuciti C, Mayer DC, Arnette R, et al. Anaphylactoid reaction to intravenous sodium feric gluconate complex during pregnancy. Int J Obstet Anesth 2005; 14:362–364.
45. Faich G, Strobos J. Sodium ferric gluconate complex in sucrose: safer intravenous iron therapy than iron dextrans. Am J Kidney Dis 1999; 33(3):464–470.
46. Maslovsky I. Intravenous iron in a primary-care clinic. Am J Hematol 2005; 78:261–264.
47. Hogl B, Kiechl S, Willeit J, et al. Restless legs syndrome: a community-based study of prevalence, severity, and risk factors. Neurology 2005; 64(11):1920–1924.
48. Bentley AJ, Rosman KD, Mitchell D. Gender differences in the presentation of subjects with restless legs syndrome. Sleep Med 2006; 7(1):37–41.
49. Rothdach AJ, Trenkwalder C, Haberstock J, et al. Prevalence and risk factors of RLS in an elderly population: the MEMO study. Memory and morbidity in Augsburg elderly. Neurology 2000; 54 (5):1064–1068.
50. Frantz KJ, Van Hartesveldt C. The locomotor effects of quinpirole in rats depend on age and gender. Pharmacol Biochem Behav 1999; 64(4):821–826.
51. Kompoliti K, Adler CH, Raman R, et al. Gender and pramipexole effects on levodopa pharmacokinetics and pharmacodynamics. Neurology 2002; 58(9):1418–1422.
52. Craig MC, Cutter WJ, Wickham H, et al. Effect of long-term estrogen therapy on dopaminergic responsivity in postmenopausal women—a preliminary study. Psychoneuroendocrinology 2004; 29(10): 1309–1316.
53. Kaye CM, Nicholls B. Clinical pharmacokinetics of ropinirole. Clin Pharmacokinet 2000; 39(4): 243–254.
54. Littner MR, Kushida C, Anderson WM, et al. Practice parameters for the dopaminergic treatment of restless legs syndrome and periodic leg movement disorder. Sleep 2004; 27(3):557–559.
55. Manconi M, Govoni V, De Vito A, et al. Pregnancy as a risk factor for restless legs syndrome. Sleep Med 2004; 5(3):305–308.
56. Zesiewicz TA, Hauser RA. Sleep attacks and dopamine agonists for Parkinson's disease: what is currently known? CNS Drugs 2003; 17(8):593–600.
57. Lakshminarayanan S, Paramasivan KD, Walters AS, et al. Clinically significant but unsuspected restless legs syndrome in patients with sleep apnea. Mov Disord 2005; 20(4):501–503.
58. Montplaisir J, Michaud M, Lavigne G. Periodic limb movements in sleep. In: Chokroverty S, Hening W, Walters A, eds. Sleep and Movement Disorders. 1st ed. Philadelphia: Butterworth Heinemann, 2003:300–309.
59. Santamaria J, Pranzo A, Tolosa E. Development of restless legs syndrome after dopaminergic treatment in a patient with periodic leg movements in sleep. Sleep Med 2003; 4:153–155.
60. Högl B, Paulus W, Clarenbach P, et al. RLS: Diagnostic assessment and the advantages and risks of dopaminergic treatment. J Neurol 2006; 253(suppl IV):22–28.
61. Bonati MT, Ferini-Strambi L, Aridon P, et al. Autosomal dominant restless legs syndrome maps on chromosome 14q. Brain 2003; 126(6):1485–1492.
62. Saletu M, Anderer P, Saletu-Zyhlarz G, et al. Restless legs syndrome (RLS) and periodic limb movement disorder (PLMD): acute placebo-controlled sleep laboratory studies with clonazepam. Eur Neuropsychopharmacol 2001; 11(2):153–161.
63. Schuld A, Kraus T, Haack M, et al. Obstructive sleep apnea syndrome induced by clonazepam in a narcoleptic patient with REM-sleep-behavior disorder. J Sleep Res 1999; 8(4):321–322.
64. Pennestri M, Montplaisir J, Richard M, et al. Differential rise of blood pressure in periodic leg movements associated or not with micro-arousals in patients with restless legs syndrome. Sleep 2006; 29:A290–A291.
65. Winkelman JW. The evoked heart rate response to periodic leg movements of sleep. Sleep 1999; 22 (5):575–580.
66. Ali NJ, Davies RJ, Fleetham JA, et al. Periodic movements of the legs during sleep associated with rises in systemic blood pressure. Sleep 1991; 14(2):163–165.
67. Birks J, Filcker L. Donepezil for mild cognitive impairment. Cochrane Database Syst Rev 2006; 3: CD006104.
68. Morii H. Safety profile of raloxifene. Clin Calcium 2004; 14(10):100–104.

69. Ford RG, Ford KT. Continuous intravenous dihydroergotamine in the treatment of intractable headache. Headache 1997; 37(3):129–136.
70. Queiroz LP, Weeks RE, Rapaport AM, et al. Early and transient side effects of repetitive intravenous dihydroergotamine. Headache 1996; 36(5):291–294.
71. Abdulla AJ, Jones PW, Pearce VR. Leg cramps in the elderly: prevalence, drug and disease associations. Int J Clin Pract 1999; 53(7):494–496.
72. Coppin RJ, Wicke DM, Little PS. Managing nocturnal leg cramps—calf-stretching exercises and cessation of quinine treatment: a factorial randomised controlled trial. Br J Gen Pract 2005; 55(512): 186–191.
73. Gagnon Y, Mayer P, Morisson F, et al. Aggravation of respiratory disturbances by the use of an occlusal splint in apneic patients: a pilot study. Int J Prosthodont 2004; 17:447–453.
74. Lavigne GJ, Soucy JP, Lobbezoo F, et al. Double-blind, crossover, placebo-controlled trial of bromocriptine in patients with sleep bruxism. Clin Neuropharmacol 2001; 24(3):145–149.
75. Bostwick JM, Jaffee MS. Buspirone as an antidote to SSRI-induced bruxism in 4 cases. J Clin Psychiatry 1999; 60(12):857–860.
76. Romanelli F, Adler DA, Bungay KM. Possible paroxetine-induced bruxism. Ann Pharmacother 1996; 30(11):1246–1248.
77. Amir I, Hermesh H, Gavish A. Bruxism secondary to antipsychotic drug exposure: a positive response to propranolol. Clin Neuropharmacol 1997; 20(1):86–89.
78. See SJ, Tan EK. Severe amphetamine-induced bruxism: treatment with botulinum toxin. Acta Neurol Scand 2003; 107(2):161–163.
79. Rhodus NL, Little JW. Methamphetamine abuse and "meth mouth". Northwest Dent 2005; 84(5):29, 31, 33–37.
80. Iranzo A, Santamaria J. Bisoprolol-induced rapid eye movement sleep behavior disorder. Am J Med 1999; 107(4):390–392.
81. Kast RE. Tiagabine may reduce bruxism and associated temporomandibular joint pain. Anesth Prog 2005; 52:102–104.
82. Lavigne GJ, Kato T, Kolta A, et al. Neurobiological mechanisms involved in sleep bruxism. Crit Rev Oral Biol Med 2003; 14(1):30–46.
83. Kraner JC, McCoy DJ, Evans MA, et al. Fatalities caused by the MDMA-related drug para-methoxyamphetamine (PMA). J Anal Toxicol 2001; 25(7):645–648.
84. McGrath C, Chan B. Oral health sensations associated with illicit drug abuse. Br Dent J 2005; 198 (3):159–162.
85. Winocur E, Gavish A, Volfin G, et al. Oral motor parafunctions among heavy drug addicts and their effects on signs and symptoms of temporomandibular disorders. J Orofac Pain 2001; 15(1):56–63.
86. Robertson LT, Hammerstad JP. Jaw movement dysfunction related to Parkinson's disease and partially modified by levodopa. J Neurol Neurosurg Psychiatry 1996; 60(1):41–50.
87. Mahowald W. In: Ferber R, Kryger M, eds. Principles and Practice of Sleep Medicine in the Child. Philadelphia: WB Saunders, 1995:115–123.
88. Shigenobu K, Ikeda M, Fukuhara R, et al. The stereotypy rating inventory for frontotemporal lobar degeneration. Psychiatry Res 2002; 110(2):175–187.
89. Applegate H, Matson JL, Cherry KE. An evaluation of functional variables affecting severe problem behaviours in adults with mental retardation by using the questions about behavioral function scale (QABF). Res Dev Disabil 1999; 20(3):229–237.
90. Levin T, Heresco-Levy U. Risperidone-induced rabbit syndrome: an unusual movement disorder caused by an atypical antipsychotic. Eur Neuropsychopharmacol 1999; 9(1–2):137–139.
91. Gerrard JW, Richardson JS, Donat J. Neuropharmacological evaluation of movement disorders that are adverse reactions to specific foods. Int J Neurosci 1994; 76(1–2):61–69.
92. Carlock KS, Williams JP, Graves GC. MRI findings in headbangers. Clin Imaging 1997; 21(6):411–413.
93. Aldrich M. Sleep medicine. Parasomnias. New York: Oxford University Press, 1999:267–268.
94. Thorpy MJ. Rhythmic movement disorder. In: Thorpy MJ, ed. Handbook of Sleep Disorders. New York: Marcel Dekker, 1990:609–629.
95. Kuhn BR, Elliott AJ. Treatment efficacy in behavioral pediatric sleep medicine. J Psychosom Res 2003; 54(6):587–597.
96. Etzioni T, Katz N, Hering E, et al. Controlled sleep restriction for rhythmic movement disorder. J Pediatr 2005; 147(3):393–395.
97. Durmer JS, Dinges DF. Neurocognitive consequences of sleep deprivation. Semin Neurol 2005; 25 (1):117–129.
98. Copinschi G. Metabolic and endocrine effects of sleep deprivation. Essent Psychopharmacol 2005; 6(6): 341–347.

50 | Medical Disorders

Scott M. Leibowitz

The Sleep Disorders Center of the Piedmont Heart Institute, Atlanta, Georgia, U.S.A.

INTRODUCTION

Sleep complaints are a common finding amongst patients with acute and chronic medical conditions. Many medical conditions are directly interrelated to sleep. As a result of this relationship, an exacerbation of a chronic disease frequently parallels worsening sleep quality. Additionally, some sleep disorders may directly exacerbate or even cause a chronic disease state [i.e., obstructive sleep apnea (OSA) and hypertension], which is an important consideration in the diagnostic evaluation of a variety of disease states. Many major medical conditions in fact occur at significantly higher rates in individuals with severe insomnia as compared with those without insomnia. These conditions include hypertension, congestive heart failure (CHF), clinical and subclinical depression, diabetes, and acute myocardial infarction (1). This chapter explores the relationship between medical disorders and sleep and important clinical considerations when evaluating patients with sleep complaints and chronic medical conditions.

MEDICAL CONDITIONS

Cardiovascular Disease

Much attention has been garnered about the association of cardiovascular disease and sleep disorders, in particular, OSA. It appears that the autonomic nervous system (ANS) seems to be the common thread linking these two processes together. Sleep under normal circumstances is a state of marked variability in the activity of the ANS. As a part of normal phasic rapid eye movement (REM) sleep, significant sympathetic nervous system bursts occur while during non–rapid eye movement sleep (NREM) sleep, a predominance of parasympathetic nervous system activity is seen. A perturbation of the normal sleep process may significantly impact and alter this autonomic variability and potentially create a physiologic landscape for a variety of disease states.

In no disease state is this phenomena better demonstrated than in OSA. This condition is characterized by cyclical or repetitive obstructive respiratory events that occur during sleep with microarousals occurring at the termination of a respiratory event (2,3). Associated with these events are frequent desaturations, hypercapnea, and autonomic arousals, all of which significantly elevate the outflow of the sympathetic nervous system and simultaneously cause withdrawal of vagal activity (4,5). This abnormal modulation of the ANS causes significant hemodynamic changes, including increased heart rate, blood pressure (2), decreased cerebral blood flow (3), and increased myocardial oxygen demands, to name a few. In turn, patients with untreated OSA have elevated levels of ANS activity not only during the discrete events but during wakefulness (Fig. 1) (4,6).

This process, as well as oxidative stress (7), hypercoagulability (8), and endothelial dysfunction (9) are all implicated in the development of comorbid cardiovascular consequences in patients with untreated OSA.

Treatment with continuous positive airway pressure (CPAP) has been shown to reverse these processes (10–13). CPAP acts as a "pneumatic splint" to brace open the airway via a nasal or nasal-oral interface, providing continuous positive pressure to the upper airway while sleeping. By stabilizing the airway walls, the tendency for the upper airway to collapse is alleviated, breathing disturbances are ameliorated, autonomic and electroencephalographic (EEG) arousals are eliminated, and sleep continues much less interrupted.

AWAKE

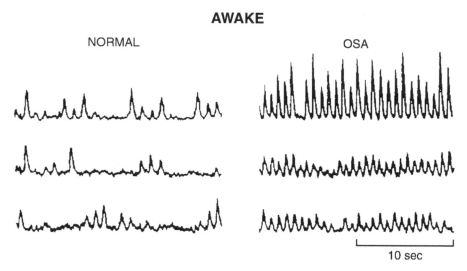

Figure 1   Recordings of sympathetic nerve activity (SNA) during wakefulness in patients with obstructive sleep apnea and matched controls showing high levels of SNA in patients with sleep apnea. *Source*: From Ref. 4.

Hypertension

A strong link between OSA and hypertension has been found in multiple longitudinal studies. The seminal Sleep Heart Health Study found that mean systolic and diastolic blood pressure and prevalence of hypertension increased significantly with increasing severity of sleep-disordered breathing (SDB) including apnea-hypopnea indices (AHI) and percentage of sleep time below 90% oxygen saturation (14). Additionally, the odds ratio for developing hypertension in the presence of severe (AHI > 30) untreated OSA in this study was 1.37. In a separate cross-sectional study of 1069 subjects, even patients with mild SDB (AHI < 5) had 42% greater odds of developing hypertension than individuals who had an AHI = 0. This study also found that there was a linear relationship between severity of OSA and risk for hypertension, and that at the four-year follow-up period, patients with an AHI ≥ 15 had a 2.89-fold increased risk for developing new hypertension over patients with an AHI = 0 (15). Due to the accumulating data on the causal relationship of OSA and hypertension, the Joint National Commission (JNC) guidelines for the diagnosis and management of hypertension has recognized OSA as the number one treatable cause of hypertension (16).

Fortunately, the use of nasal CPAP improves blood pressure control. Studies have varied on the impact of CPAP on blood pressure, but decreases between 2.5 mmHg and 10 mmHg have been seen in placebo-controlled CPAP trials (17,18). One notable study in patients with refractory hypertension found that an astounding 82% of patients had OSA and after two months of treatment with CPAP, an improvement in the 24-hour mean systolic blood pressure of 11 mmHg was observed (19).

Congestive Heart Failure

Patients with severe CHF have consistently been found to have highly fragmented sleep, with frequent arousals and sleep changes (20). A recent study has shown that at least 21% of patients with CHF complained of excessive daytime somnolence (EDS) and 48% of patients complained of being awake more than 30 minutes during the course of the night (21). Additionally, studies indicate that upward of 30% to 60% of patients with heart failure suffer from sleep-related breathing disorders, which further causes significant sleep disturbance (22). These numbers include both OSA and Cheyne–Stokes respiration with central sleep apnea (CSR-CSA). This pattern of respiration is characterized by a crescendo-decrescendo respiratory pattern, with periods of hyperventilation followed by periods of central apneas (Fig. 2). This respiratory pattern is thought to represent breathing instability. It also appears to correlate with CHF severity, and has been shown to increase mortality risk in CHF (24–26). In about 30% of heart failure populations, the prevalence of OSA is approximately 30% (35% in patients with

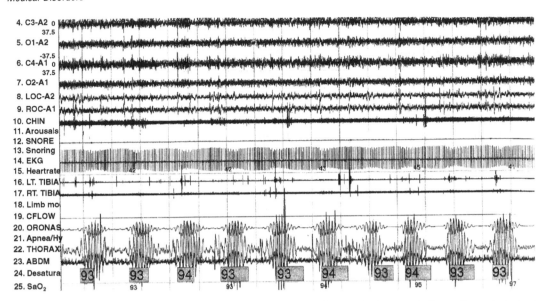

Figure 2 Respiration pattern in obstructive sleep apnea and Cheyne-Stokes respiration with central sleep apnea. Note the crescendo-decrescendo respiratory pattern in the abdominal, thoracic, and oronasal airflow channels. *Abbreviations*: C3 and C4, central electroencephalographic (EEG) electrodes; O1 and O2, occipital EEG electrodes; A1 and A2, reference electrodes; LOC and ROC, left and right outer canthi electrodes, respectively; CHIN, chin electromyographic (EMG) electrodes; TIBIA, tibialis EMG electrodes; ORONAS, oronasal airflow sensor; THORAX and ABDM, thoracic and abdominal wall movement; SaO_2, oxygen saturation. *Source*: From Ref. 23.

diastolic dysfunction) (27,28) while CSR-CSA has been estimated to be 40% to 60% (24,27,28). Importantly, in the Sleep Heart Health Study, the presence of OSA was associated with a 2.38 greater risk for coexistent CHF, independent of other recognized risk factors (29).

Benefits of CPAP therapy in patients with CHF and OSA have shown a marked improvement in left ventricular ejection fraction and functional class after initiation of CPAP therapy, with improvements of up to 12% in ejection fraction after treatment was initiated. Studies to date looking at the benefits of CPAP in these patients, however, have been limited by small sample size (30,31).

The optimal treatment for CSR-CSA is still unclear. Patients with CHF and CSR-CSA seem to improve with optimization of cardiac function; however, this approach only improves the breathing disorder in a minority of patients (32). While CPAP has been shown to improve cardiac function when used chronically (33), a recent study of CPAP and CSR in CHF patients failed to show any significant improvement in number of hospitalizations, quality of life, or significant difference in death and heart transplantation in the CPAP-treated group (34). Other modalities including supplemental nocturnal oxygen (35), acetazolamide (36), and other medications (37) have not proven to be consistently effective for treatment in these patients. A recent new treatment using an adaptive servo-ventilator (AutoSet CS, ResMed, Sydney, Australia) has shown great promise in more effectively treating CSR-CSA than other previous therapies, and importantly, has been found to be better tolerated than traditional positive airway therapy (38,39).

Stroke

Stroke is another cardiovascular disease that has been found to be strongly associated with OSA. Approximately 60% to 70% of stroke patients have OSA, as defined by an AHI $\geq$ 10 events/hr (40). After an acute cerebrovascular event, both OSA and CSR-CSA are not uncommon (41,42). A 2005 study showed that OSA showed a significant association with stroke and death [adjusted hazard ratio, 1.97; CI, 1.12–3.48; $p = 0.01$] (43). The effectiveness of treatment has not been well established, perhaps in part due to patient intolerance of CPAP (44); however, the benefits of CPAP on blood pressure and on the normalization of ANS activity would imply a significant benefit in cardiovascular morbidity and mortality related to stroke patients.

Patients who have suffered a stroke may also have difficulties with EDS (45), insomnia (46), and REM behavior disorder (47), depending on the site of the stroke. The latter condition is a condition where the normal atonia of REM sleep is lost and individuals may act out their dreams.

Cardiac Arrhythmias

A relationship between OSA and cardiac arrhythmias has also been found in a number of cross-sectional epidemiologic and case-control studies. Some of these studies have found that OSA increases the risk of developing atrial fibrillation and increases the risk of recurrent atrial fibrillation after cardioversion (21,26,48–50). Other studies have shown an increased frequency of nonsustained ventricular tachycardia in patients with CHF and CSA (50,52). A 2005 study showed a relative risk increase of 2.57 (95% CI, 1.87–3.52) for patients with OSA of sudden cardiac death during sleep as compared to individuals without OSA (51). Treatment with CPAP has been shown to prevent OSA-associated bradyarrhythmias (52,53), decrease recurrence of atrial fibrillation after cardioversion (54), and abolish ventricular arrhythmias (55,56), but definitive conclusions about the impact of treatment on arrhythmias from these studies are also limited due to their sample size.

Coronary Artery Disease

It does appear that a relationship between OSA and coronary artery disease exists; but again, this relationship is still under great scrutiny due to limitations of the studies performed to date. In spite of these limitations, there is compelling epidemiologic evidence to further reinforce this relationship. These connections are logical in light of the associations between cellular mechanisms of atherosclerosis, the ANS, and OSA. The Sleep Heart Health Study showed an increased odds ratio of 1.42 (95% CI, 1.13–1.78) for patients with severe OSA to develop at least one manifestation of cardiovascular disease (myocardial infarction, angina, coronary revascularization procedure, heart failure, or stroke) (28). A Swedish study found that over a seven-year period, cardiovascular disease developed in 36% of subjects who had OSA, as compared to 6% of subjects who did not have OSA (57). An earlier study found that during a seven-year follow-up period, the relative risk of developing new vascular problems in patients with OSA was 2.3 times greater in patients who were advised to lose weight (conservative therapy) as opposed to those who underwent tracheostomy (58). A 10-year observational study from Spain showed that untreated severe OSA significantly increased the risk of fatal (odds ratio, 2.87; 95% CI, 1.17–7.51) and nonfatal (3.17, 1.12–7.51) cardiovascular events compared to subjects without OSA (59).

Pulmonary Hypertension

OSA is also an important consideration when evaluating patients with pulmonary hypertension. In 1998, the World Health Organization conference on pulmonary hypertension recognized SDB as a secondary cause of pulmonary arterial hypertension (PAH) (60). While severe OSA and severe hypoxemia are more commonly associated with PAH, mild PAH is also common in patients with OSA (61–63).

Respiratory Disease
Asthma

Mild nocturnal bronchoconstriction occurs in normal individuals due to a circadian variation in airway caliber. It appears that this process is exacerbated in asthmatics, as evidenced by frequent patient reports of nighttime exacerbations of asthma (64,65). A 15% decrement in peak expiratory flow rate between bedtime and morning is objective evidence of nocturnal worsening of asthma. Nocturnal asthma may be a separate but related entity to asthma, or it may be a poorly controlled variant of typical reactive airway disease. There are many factors that may be involved with nocturnal asthma any of which may control, in part, the normal circadian variation of airway caliber. These include airway inflammation, circadian changes in vagal tone, circadian variation of cortisol and epinephrine, allergens and airway cooling, gastroesophogeal reflux, and changes in mucociliary clearance (66). The end result of these processes is bronchial hyperactivity.

Another potential mechanism of nocturnal worsening of asthma is the presence of a sleep-related breathing disorder. Several studies have shown patients with asthma and coexisting OSA have shown improvement of nocturnal worsening of asthma with initiation of CPAP to treat the OSA (67–69).

It is important to recognize that, as previously stated, nocturnal worsening of asthma may be a marker of overall asthma severity. Therefore, aggressive standard treatment following the recommended clinical guidelines should be followed. These include the use of inhaled corticosteroids, short- and long-acting inhaled β-adrenergic agents, and leukotriene inhibitors. There are some data to suggest that sustained-release theophylline may have utility in nocturnal worsening of asthma; however, long-acting β-adrenergic agents appear to have less central nervous system and gastrointestinal effects and therefore should be used before addition of theophylline (70,71).

Chronic Obstructive Pulmonary Disease

Chronic obstructive pulmonary disease (COPD) is recognized as one of our country's most rapidly growing health problems, with over 14 million adult Americans having this disease. These patients have frequent complaints of disrupted sleep, insomnia, and daytime sleepiness. These symptoms increase directly with the severity of disease (72). Patients with COPD tend to have a high degree of nocturnal hypoxemia, in particular, during REM sleep; however, treatment of hypoxemia does not necessarily guarantee improved sleep efficiency, as evidenced by a 1982 study by Calverly et al. (73).

There are no data to suggest that OSA occurs with greater frequency in patients with COPD. While patients with COPD have a significant degree of nocturnal hypoxemia, in patients without OSA, there is nothing to suggest that this nocturnal hypoxemia occurs due to airway obstruction. It appears rather to be caused by a combination of hypoventilation (74), ventilation-perfusion mismatch (75), and a decrease in functional residual capacity (FRC). Sleep-related hypoxemia appears to be more common in the "blue bloaters" variant of COPD, as compared to the "pink puffers" variant. "Blue bloaters" tend to have lower baseline arterial oxygen saturation, and accordingly, larger drops in oxygen saturation and more frequent desaturation events (76).

An overlap syndrome of COPD and OSA does exist and treatment with CPAP is indicated in these patients, though bilevel ventilation may be better tolerated (77). The routine use of positive airway pressure (PAP) therapy in these patients in the absence of OSA has not been proven. Noninvasive positive pressure ventilation (NIPPV) has been found to reduce intubations, complications, and mortality rate in patients with acute hypercapnea due to a COPD exacerbation (78); however, it is still unclear whether patients with chronic, severe hypercapnea will derive significant survival benefit from prolonged NIPPV (79).

Restrictive Lung Disease

Restrictive lung disease is another category of pulmonary disorders that may have exacerbation of its usual disease state during sleep and resultant sleep disturbance. Patients with any one of these diseases may require nocturnal PAP therapy. Lung restriction is most commonly seen in obesity, kyphoscoliosis, neuromuscular disease, interstitial lung disease (ILD), and pregnancy. PAP therapy should be used unequivocally in these patients if they have coexisting OSA. However, in the absence of OSA, PAP therapy must be considered on a case by case manner, depending on the disease process being considered.

Interstitial lung disease. ILD is a broad group of restrictive pulmonary disorders of over 100 different etiologies. Patients with ILD tend to complain of disrupted sleep. Decreased sleep efficiency, frequent nighttime awakenings, increased stage N1 sleep, and decreased REM sleep frequently lead to the complaints of daytime fatigue and sleepiness, even in the absence of OSA (80,81). Patients with ILD often manifest disordered sleep due to difficulties with nocturnal breathing, especially in patients with baseline SaO_2 < 90% (80). Additionally, nocturnal hypoxemia is fairly common in this group of patients and is likely due to episodic or persistent hypoventilation relative to waking ventilation, and may be more severe in REM sleep (82). PAP therapy is only indicated in patients with coexisting OSA and although no definitive clinical trials have validated its use, nocturnal oxygen in appropriate individuals is likely the treatment of choice (83).

Obesity. Obese individuals have compromised respiratory function while awake and upright due to decreased compliance of the thoracic cage as a result of fat accumulation in and around the ribs, abdomen and diaphragm (84). This restriction is exacerbated by the supine position and then even more so once in the sleep state. The supine position causes a decrease in the FRC, which is further exacerbated by the weight of the diaphragm and the abdomen being applied to the lungs. Not all obese patients have OSA, though there is a subset of patients, with and without OSA, that suffers either nocturnal hypoventilation or day and night hypoventilation, termed the obesity-hypoventilation syndrome (OHS). Criteria for the diagnosis of OHS include a diagnostic polysomnography that documents an increase in PCO_2 of ≥ 10 mmHg, or oxygen desaturations not explained by apnea or hypopnea. Additionally, it is common to find other features of chronic hypoventilation including cor pulmonale, pulmonary hypertension, erythrocytosis, daytime sleepiness, and/or awake hypercapnea (85).

Obese patients with and without OSA and OHS may benefit from nocturnal PAP therapy: CPAP, bilevel PAP, or volume-cycled NIPPV. Bilevel PAP or volume-cycled NIPPV allow for increased ventilatory assistance than PAP therapy with CPAP. Initiation of PAP therapy should be performed in an attended setting as these patients may, at times, be medically unstable, and/or require supplemental oxygen in addition to positive pressure therapy; however, oxygen therapy alone is insufficient in these patients. NIPPV has been shown to improve long-term outcomes in patients with OHS (86).

Kyphoscoliosis. Kyphoscoliosis involves a deformity of the spine that characteristically consists of an anteroposterior angulation of the spine, a lateral displacement of the spine, a curvature of the spine, or both (87). This deformity may compromise respiratory function to the point of respiratory failure due to decreased lung and chest wall compliance, increased elastic load on the respiratory muscles, and a resultant increased work of breathing (88). Patients with kyphoscoliosis should be considered for PAP therapy in the absence of OSA if there are complaints of daytime sleepiness or sleep disruption and/or evidence of hypoventilation, CSRs, or central apneas, all of which may be seen in these patients (88,89). Acute respiratory failure due to PAP therapy may occur in these patients with its initiation due to the increased work of breathing, which may result from an increased FRC coupled with extreme chest wall stiffness. Once evidence of hypoventilation is observed, bilevel PAP or volume-cycled NIPPV will be required to adequately ventilate these patients at night and may stave off invasive ventilation for some time (90–92).

Neuromuscular disorders. Patients with progressive neuromuscular disorders will manifest the beginnings of chronic respiratory failure with nocturnal hypoventilation. In these cases, NIPPV should appropriately be started at night with a formal, supervised titration. Stable neuromuscular disorders with partial ventilatory function, including sequelae of poliomyelitis, tuberculosis, Duchenne's muscular dystrophy (DMD), or high-level spinal cord injuries, may successfully be ventilated at night, which may, in turn, improve clinical and physiologic daytime function and may, like patients with respiratory failure due to kyphoscoliosis, stave off continuous NIPPV and/or invasive ventilation (93,94).

Pregnancy. The latter part of pregnancy is a time where many women complain of sleep difficulties. Seventy-nine percent of women surveyed in a 1998 National Sleep Foundation poll reported sleep was disturbed and 59% reported less refreshing sleep (95). The discomfort of carrying a growing fetus, especially during the third trimester, makes this finding not unexpected. While snoring does become more common as pregnancy progresses, the development of frank OSA in a patient without OSA prior to pregnancy is unlikely (96). Many of the components of lung restriction that exist in the obese individual also exist in the pregnant individual; however, it is uncommon to find significant oxygen desaturations in an otherwise healthy pregnant woman (97). This finding is likely in large part due to the respiratory stimulant properties of progesterone whose production is greatly stimulated in the pregnant woman (98). There has been some evidence to suggest that a relationship between preeclampsia and untreated OSA exists; however, more studies are needed to clarify this connection (99).

Gastrointestinal Disease

Gastroesophogeal Reflux

The lower esophageal sphincter (LES) is the primary barrier to prevent reflux of stomach acid contents into the esophagus. Normally, the LES relaxes with swallowing during wakefulness. During sleep, LES tone is decreased transiently with arousals, so that nocturnal gastro-esophogeal reflux (GER) occurs primarily during arousals from sleep (100). Esophageal clearance of acid is prolonged during sleep and also requires an arousal (101). Saliva secretion, which neutralizes acid, is virtually absent during sleep as is swallowing (102). The combination of all of these mechanisms increases the likelihood of symptomatic GER during sleep. Accordingly, it is not surprising that nocturnal GER is common. A 2003 Gallup poll reported that 79% of all heartburn patients had symptoms at night, and approximately 75% reported that heartburn impaired their sleep (103). Another 2001 survey found a prevalence of 10% of the general population with nighttime complaints of reflux (104).

Symptoms of sleep-related GER are similar to that of diurnal GER, including chest discomfort, indigestion, substernal burning, and sour taste. However, because nocturnal GER occurs during sleep, an added consequence is disturbed sleep, and because of the supine position, reflux can be more significant with frequent tracheal aspiration resulting in a nocturnal cough, or even choking. Additionally, sleep-related GER can potentially exacerbate nocturnal asthma and occurs in up to 50% of asthmatics (105,106). Any condition that may cause frequent nocturnal arousals also increases the risk of episodes of GER. One study showed that prior to treatment, 68% of patients with OSA had episodes of sleep-related GER, which improved to 48% after treatment with CPAP (107).

GER has also been implicated in nocturnal laryngospasm. This condition is characterized by abrupt awakenings from sleep with an intense feeling of suffocation, often accompanied by stridor and choking. One small study found that 9 of 10 patients with sleep-related laryngospasm had GER as documented by esophageal pH testing (108).

Nocturnal GER is best confirmed via an esophageal pH probe, placed 5 cm above the LES, either in an ambulatory manner or during diagnostic polysomnography. Episodes of reflux are characterized by a pH of less than 4. Treatment is usually the use of H2 receptor antagonists or proton pump inhibitors for preventative therapy or antacids for acute symptom control. Prokinetic agents have been used successfully for the treatment of sleep-related GER; however, central nervous system (CNS) side effects may limit its use. Positional therapy can be helpful in milder cases. Antireflux surgery can be highly effective but should be reserved for refractory cases. Finally, CPAP can be useful in patients who have exclusively nocturnal GER and coexisting OSA (105).

Irritable Bowel Syndrome

Sleep disturbances are frequently reported in patients with functional bowel disorders. Recurrent nighttime awakenings and nonrestorative sleep were the most common complaints, and abdominal pain was the primary reason reported for nighttime awakenings (109). While one study showed no measurable differences in sleep architecture in patients with irritable bowel syndrome (IBS), a different study showed increased amount of REM sleep in these patients, in conjunction with very low activity of the small bowel during the day, leading to the speculation that there is a CNS component to IBS (110,111).

Renal Disease

The patients with renal disease who have been most studied with regard to sleep disorders is primarily those with end-stage renal disease (ESRD), on and off chronic hemodialysis or peritoneal dialysis. These studies have consistently reported a high prevalence of sleep complaints in these patients in the form of nighttime awakenings, early morning awakenings, periodic limb movements, and EDS (112). Studies vary in terms of the order of common complaints. Holly et al. found that early morning awakenings were reported in 80% of chronic hemodialysis and ambulatory peritoneal dialysis patients, while 72% reported restless legs syndrome (RLS), 83% reported "leg jerking," 67% reported nighttime awakenings, and 28% reported daytime sleepiness (113). Other studies have shown a higher prevalence of EDS and RLS (114,115). It is clear, however, that RLS, periodic limb movement disorder (PLMD) and OSA occurs much more commonly in dialysis patients than in the general population (116,117).

RLS is a clinical syndrome characterized by an unpleasant or uncomfortable sensation in the legs, occurring more commonly at night, which causes an almost irresistible urge to move the legs. Symptoms of RLS may often result in delayed sleep onset and disrupted sleep (118). Approximately 80% of patients with RLS also have PLMD, a seemingly separate but related condition from RLS characterized by episodic limb movements that are often associated with nocturnal awakenings and disrupted sleep. RLS has been reported in up to 80% of dialysis patients, while PLMD has been reported in up to 70% (113–115,119). The pathophysiologic mechanism of RLS and PLMD in patients with ESRD have not been entirely elucidated; but it is clear that central nervous system dopaminergic dysfunction plays a major role in the etiology RLS and PLMD, and that CNS iron deficiency likely plays a role as well (120–123). Iron is a cofactor in the rate-limiting step in dopamine production (124). It is probable that alterations of dopamine synthesis and metabolism are in large part responsible for the prevalence of RLS and PLMD in ESRD patients as total brain content of tyrosine, the amino acid precursor for dopamine, has been reported in patients with uremia (125). Treatment with dopamine agonists is the mainstay of treatment while trying to identify and treat any secondary causes (126,127).

OSA occurs in patients with ESRD with a significantly higher prevalence than the general population, with a prevalence rate reported to be between 30% and 80% (116,128,129). It is not clear why this disorder is higher in ESRD patients but there are a number of proposed theories. Accumulation of uremic toxins affecting airway muscle tone, instability of respiratory control, and/or discoordination of diaphragm and upper airway muscle activity are a few proposed mechanisms that may play a role in these patients (130). Additionally, fluid overload may make upper airway collapse more common (131). Finally, it may be in part that the prevalence of SDB increases with increasing age and patients with ESRD tend to be an older population.

Endocrine Disease

Endocrine disorders comprise another chronic disease group wherein patients may complain of EDS. It has long been observed that sleepiness is a symptom of hypothyroidism. Additionally, there are considerable data to show that hypothyroidism is a risk factor for the development of OSA (132). It is not clear whether the sleepiness that hypothyroid patients experience is due to a direct effect of the hypothyroid state on sleep or to coexisting sleep-related breathing disorders (SRBD).

Patients with Cushing's disease have frequent sleep complaints, perhaps in large part due to the increased prevalence of OSA (32%). However, patients who have Cushing's disease without OSA still have been found to have fragmented sleep (133).

Patients with acromegaly have also been shown to have an increased prevalence of sleep apnea, with rates between 39% and 58.8% in various studies (134,135). Additionally, CSA has been noted in these patients, which may indicate a central ventilatory control issue, creating a landscape fertile for the development of SDB (136). On the other hand, patients with growth hormone deficiency consistently report a reduced level of energy, fatigue, and impaired sleep quality (137).

Rheumatologic Disease

Patients with fibromyalgia frequently characterize their sleep as being restless, light, and unrefreshing (138). These patients often have a characteristic EEG finding during sleep of alpha-frequency activity intrusion during delta-frequency activity or "alpha-delta" sleep (139). Alpha activity is characteristic of the EEG pattern seen during quiet wakefulness with the eyes closed and does not typically occur during deep sleep (wherein delta activity occurs) in normal controls. This EEG finding has been reported to also occur in rheumatoid arthritis and chronic fatigue syndrome (82,140,141). Researchers have found a positive correlation between the frequency of alpha-delta sleep and severity of overnight pain in patients with fibromyalgia and an inverse correlation between frequency of alpha-delta sleep and subjective sleep depth and refreshing sleep (142,143).

Patients with chronic pain, of rheumatologic origin or otherwise, consistently report sleep disturbances. Studies have shown that 50% to 70% of patients with chronic pain report sleep impairment, with sleep disturbances correlating with higher pain intensity. Likely related to this finding is that 40% of patients with chronic pain report depression (144).

Cancer and Sleep

Patients with cancer also have increased reports of EDS. Prevalence rates of 54% to 68% for "feeling drowsy" and 21% to 40% for being "overly sleepy" have been found in studies of this population (145,146). Causes of EDS reported in this population may be related to increased risk of primary sleep disorders due to age alone (average age of onset of cancer is 55 years); insufficient sleep due to insomnia, depression, or pain; disruption or erratic hormone secretion due to the malignancy or chemotherapy, with subsequent sleep disruption or shortened sleep periods; effects of cytokines and inflammatory mediators induced by cancer cells, biotherapy, or radiotherapy; and/or side effects from chemotherapy or other adjunctive medications (147).

Evaluation of Medical Patients With Sleep Complaints

Patients with sleep complaints need to be evaluated in a systematic fashion. Understanding the nature of the complaint, the duration, frequency, and timing of the problem are essential components in the evaluation process to fully comprehend the factors at play causing the disturbance. As with any medical evaluation, of key importance in evaluating the patient complaining of a sleep disturbance is a detailed history and physical exam. Obtaining a detailed sleep history in addition to a medical history is essential. Documentation of total daily 24 hour sleep time and daily sleep pattern, number of nocturnal awakenings, prolonged sleep latencies, snoring, witnessed apneas, symptoms of restless legs syndrome, periodic limb movements, and restless sleep are highlights of the sleep history that should be covered at minimum. Alcohol or drug abuse can be a significant contributor to sleep disturbances and if suspected, appropriate evaluation should ensue. Special note should be made of chronic sedating medications or stimulating medications taken at night.

The sleep history should be supplemented with questionnaires evaluating degree of sleepiness and impact on daily living. These questionnaires include, but are not limited to, the Epworth Sleepiness Scale (ESS) (148), the Stanford Sleepiness Scale (149), and the Sleep-Wake Activity Inventory (150). The ESS is the most commonly used questionnaire due to its ease of use and small, but statistically significant, correlation with sleepiness measured by an objective test of sleepiness known as the multiple sleep latency test (MSLT) (151,152). While a normal value of the ESS is considered to be less than 10, this test is neither highly specific nor sensitive for the existence of pathologic sleepiness and these values are not entirely representative of true level of sleepiness; however, the ESS serves as a useful screen for those who are severely sleepy (153). With the ease of use of the ESS and the high prevalence of sleepiness in the general public, we advocate the administration of this tool to all adult patients in any clinical practice. To further characterize a patient's sleep, nightly sleep logs can be helpful in establishing circadian tendencies and patterns of sleep. If the patient is unable to give a reliable history or nightly sleep times are in question, several days of actigraphy monitoring, a device that registers movement by the patient, may be a useful tool in evaluating patterns of waking and sleep.

Once a thorough history and physical examination are performed, if a physical sleep problem is considered, the primary diagnostic tool available is the nocturnal polysomnogram (PSG). The PSG is used to evaluate sleep disturbances leading to sleep fragmentation, including sleep-related breathing disorder (SRBD), periodic limb movements of sleep (PLMS), REM sleep behavior disorder, and/or, more rarely seen, nocturnal seizures.

To objectively evaluate the degree of sleepiness of an individual, the MSLT can be used. The MSLT consists of four or five 20 minute polysomnographically monitored daytime nap opportunities separated by two-hour intervals wherein the patient is placed in a sleep laboratory bed in a dark room with instructions to fall asleep. The primary assessments made by the MSLT are the rapidity of sleep onset, which correlates to degree of sleepiness, and to establish the presence of REM sleep, if sleep occurs during the nap opportunity. REM sleep episodes (a period of sleep during which dreams occur) at or close to sleep onset are known as sleep-onset REM periods (SOREMPs).

Typical sleep latencies in the normal adult are between 10 and 20 minutes while pathologic sleepiness is manifested by a latency of less than 5 or 6 minutes (154). The MSLT should be performed immediately following a nocturnal polysomnogram to exclude other causes of EDS due to either sleep fragmentation or insufficient sleep. If the polysomnogram is positive for other causes of EDS, these conditions should be adequately treated before an evaluation of EDS with an MSLT is pursued.

The maintenance of wakefulness test (MWT) is another diagnostic test used in the sleep laboratory, but rather than evaluating the tendency to fall asleep, as the MSLT does, the MWT assesses the capacity to maintain wakefulness in a sedentary setting during the patient's regular waking hours. This test is often used to evaluate impact of treatment for OSA-related EDS in heavy equipment operators and/or airline pilots.

TREATMENT

Treatment of patients with chronic medical conditions and sleep complaints can prove to be challenging. In the case of patients who have sleep complaints due to exacerbations of their primary illness, optimizing therapy for that disease process is crucial. In cases of transient sleep difficulties due to acute disease state exacerbations, the judicious use of short to intermediate half-life benzodiazepines, non-benzodiazepine hypnotics [benzodiazepine receptor agonists (BZRAs)] or melatonin receptor agonists (i.e., ramelteon) may be appropriate and efficacious; however, treating the primary disease will likely yield positive and long-term results (155,156). Any sedating hypnotic medication runs the risk of side effects and the use of BZRAs do carry important side effect profiles that must be taken into consideration before prescribing. However, in one of the largest longitudinal database analyses for insomnia to be completed to date, the presence of untreated insomnia alone was found to be a larger risk factor for hip fracture in nursing home patients than was the use of these medications (157). Appropriate patient selection is critical when prescribing these medications as well as understanding the etiology of the sleep problem. In the setting of chronic insomnia, these drugs have proven to be effective and useful for short-term use and in some cases, long-term use; however, cognitive-behavioral therapy for insomnia appears to be at least equally effective, with seemingly longer sustained results, without the risk of adverse events that accompany the benzodiazepine agonists (156,158–160). Based on the results of the 2005 National Institutes of Health consensus conference regarding the management of chronic insomnia, the use of sedating antidepressants and sedating antihistamines are not recommended for the short-term or long-term treatment of insomnia due to lack of efficacy and outcomes data supporting their use (159).

As stated earlier, the use of CPAP for the treatment of SDB is the current recommended first-line strategy. Dopamine agonists, and in patients with iron deficiency, iron supplementation, are the recommended treatment of RLS/PLMD. Patients with complaints of hypersomnolence require a comprehensive evaluation before considering the use of stimulants and should be referred to a sleep specialist for this evaluation.

CONCLUSIONS

Patients with chronic medical conditions are a patient population at great risk for the development of sleep complaints. Understanding the relationship between chronic disease and sleep disorders is essential for all clinicians as many patients with chronic disease, at some point in time will invariably complain of sleep difficulties. Initial assessment and treatment should be predicated upon the nature of the complaint as well as comorbidities that may predispose patients to a particular sleep disorder. Addressing the sleep complaint in an effective and comprehensive manner will ultimately improve both the care of the patient as well as the patient's quality of life.

REFERENCES

1. Katz DA, McHorney CA. The relationship between insomnia and health-related quality of life in patients with chronic illness. J Fam Pract 2002; 51:229–235.
2. Guilleminault C, Tilkian A, Dement WC. The sleep apnea syndromes. Annu Rev Med 1976; 27: 465–484.
3. Bassiri AG, Guilleminault C. Clinical features of evaluation of obstructive sleep apnea-hypopnea syndrome. In: Kryger MH, Roth T, Dement WC, eds. Principles and Practices of Sleep Medicine, 3rd ed. Philadelphia, PA: Saunders, 2000:868–878.
4. Somers VK, Dyken ME, Clary MP, et al. Sympathetic neural mechanisms in obstructive sleep apnea. J Clin Invest 1995; 96:1897–1904.
5. Mancia G. Autonomic modulation of the cardiovascular system during sleep. N Engl J Med 1993; 328:347–349.
6. Narkiewicz K, van de Borne PJ, Cooley RL, et al. Sympathetic activity in obese subjects with and without obstructive sleep apnea. Circulation 1998; 98:772–776.
7. Lavie L, Vishnevsky A, Lavie P. Evidence for lipid peroxidation in obstructive sleep apnea. Sleep 2004; 27:123–128.
8. Von Kanel R, Dimsdale JE. Hemostatic alterations in patients with obstructive sleep apnea and the implications for cardiovascular disease. Chest 2003; 124:1956–1967.
9. Ip MS, Tse HF, Lam B, et al. Endothelial function in obstructive sleep apnea and response to treatment. Am J Respir Crit Care Med 2004; 169:348–353.
10. Narkiewicz K, Kato M, Phillips BG, et al. Nocturnal continuous positive airway pressure decreases daytime sympathetic traffic in obstructive sleep apnea. Circulation 1999; 100:2332–2335.
11. Phillips BG, Narkiewicz K, Pesek CA, et al. Effects of obstructive sleep apnea on endothelin-1 and blood pressure. J Hypertens 1999; 17:61–66.
12. Chin K, Ohi M, Kita H, et al. Effects of NCPAP therapy on fibrinogen levels in obstructive sleep apnea syndrome. Am J Respir Crit Care Med 1996; 153:1972–1976.
13. Bokinsky G, Miller M, Ault K, et al. Spontaneous platelet activation and aggregation during obstructive sleep apnea and its response to therapy with nasal continuous positive airway pressure: a preliminary investigation. Chest 1995; 108:625–630.
14. Nieto FJ, Young TB, Lind BK, et al. Association of sleep-disordered breathing, sleep apnea, and hypertension in a large community-based study. Sleep Heart Health Study. JAMA 2000; 283(14): 1829–1836.
15. Peppard PE, Young T, Palta M, Skatrud J. Prospective study of the association between sleep-disordered breathing and hypertension. N Engl J Med 2000; 342:1378–1384.
16. Joint National Committee on Prevention, Detection, Evaluation, and Treatment of High Blood Pressure. The seventh report of the Joint National Committee on Prevention, Detection, Evaluation and Treatment of High Blood Pressure. JAMA 2003; 289:2560–2572.
17. Becker HF, Jerrentrup A, Ploch T, et al. Effect of nasal continuous positive airway pressure treatment on blood pressure in patients with obstructive sleep apnea. Circulation 2003; 107:68–73.
18. Pepperell JC, Ramdassingh-Dow S, Crosthwaite N, et al. Ambulatory blood pressure after therapeutic and subtherapeutic nasal continuous positive airway pressure for obstructive sleep apnoea: a randomized parallel trial. Lancet 2002; 359:204–210.
19. Logan AG, Tkacova R, Perlikowski SM, et al. Refractory hypertension and sleep apnoea: effect of CPAP on blood pressure and baroreflex. Eur Respir J 2003; 21:241–247.
20. Yamashiro Y, Kryger MH. Sleep in heart failure. Sleep 1993; 16:513–523.
21. Brostrom A, Stromber A, Dahlsrom U, Fridland B. Sleep difficulties, daytime sleepiness, and health-related quality of life in patients with chronic heart failure. J Cardiovasc Nurs 2004; 19:232–242.
22. Javaheri S, Parker TJ, Liming JD, et al. Sleep apnea in 81 ambulatory male patients with stable heart failure: types and their prevalences, consequences, and presentations. Circulation 1998; 97: 2154–2159.
23. Chokroverty S, Thomas RJ, Bhatt M. Atlas of Sleep Medicine. Philadelphia: Elsevier, 2005.
24. Lanfranchi PA, Braghiroli A, Bosimini E, et al. Prognostic value of nocturnal Cheyne-Stokes respiration in chronic heart failure. Circulation 1999; 99:1435–1440.
25. Findley LJ, Zwillich CW, Ancoli-Israel S, et al. Cheyne-Stokes breathing during sleep in patients with left ventricular heart failure. South Med J 1985; 78:11–15.
26. Hanly PJ, Zuberi-Khokhar NS. Increased mortality associated with Cheyne-Stokes respiration in patients with congestive heart failure. Am J Respir Crit Care Med 1996; 153:272–276.
27. Sin DD, Fitzgerald F, Parker JD, et al. Risk factors for central and obstructive sleep apnea in 450 men and women with congestive heart failure. Am J Respir Crit Care Med 1999; 160:1101–1106.
28. Solin P, Bergin P, Richardson M, et al. Influence of pulmonary capillary wedge pressure on central apnea in heart failure. Circulation 1999; 99:1574–1579.

29. Shahar E, Whitney CW, Redline S, et al. Sleep-disordered breathing and cardiovascular disease: cross-sectional results of the Sleep Heart Health Study. Am J Respir Crit Care Med 2001; 163:19–25.

30. Malone S, Liu PP, Holloway R, et al. Obstructive sleep apnoea in patients with dilated cardiomyopathy: effects of continuous positive airway pressure. Lancet 1991; 338:1480–1484.

31. Kaneko Y, Floras JS, Usui K, et al. Cardiovascular effects of continuous positive airway pressure in patients with heart failure and obstructive sleep apnea. N Engl J Med 2003; 348:1233–1241.

32. Tremel F, Pepin J, Veale D, et al. High prevalence and persistence of sleep apnoea in patients referred for acute left ventricular failure and medically treated over 2 months. Eur Heart J 1999; 20:1201–1209.

33. Naughton MT, Lie PP, Bernard DC et al. Treatment of congestive heart failure and Cheyne-Stokes respiration during sleep by continuous positive airway pressure. Am J Respir Crit Care Med 1995; 151:92–97.

34. Bradley TD, Logan AG, Kimoff RJ, et al. Continuous positive airway pressure for central sleep apnea and heart failure. N Engl J Med 2005; 353:2025–2033.

35. McNicholas W, Carter J, Rutherford R, et al. Beneficial effect of oxygen in primary alveolar hypoventialion with central sleep apnea. Am Rev Respir Dis 1982; 125:773–775.

36. White D, Zwillich C, Pickett C, et al. Central sleep apnea: improvement with acetazolamide therapy. Arch Intern Med 1982; 142:1816–1819.

37. Guilleminault C, van den Hoed J, Mitler M. Clinical overview of the sleep apnea syndromes. In: Guilleminault C, Dement W, eds. Sleep Apnea Syndromes. New York: Alan R Liss, 1978:1–11.

38. Teschler H, Dohring J, Wang YM, Berthon-Jones M. Adaptive pressure support servo-ventilation: a novel treatment for Cheyne-Stokes respiration in heart failure. Am J Respir Crit Care Med 1999; 160:1124–1129.

39. Pepperell JC, Maskell NA, Hones DR, et al. A randomized controlled trial of adaptive ventilation for Cheyne-Stokes breathing in heart failure. Am J Respir Crit Care Med 2003; 168:1109–1114.

40. Turkington PM, Bamford CR, Wanklyn P, et al. Prevalence of upper airway obstruction in the first 24 hours after acute stroke. Stroke 2002; 33:2037–2042.

41. Parra O, Arboix A, Bechich S. Time course of sleep-related breathing disorders in first-ever stroke or transient ischemic attack. Am J Respir Crit Care Med 2000; 161:375–380.

42. Iranzo A, Santamaria J, Berenguer J, et al. Prevalence and clinical importance of sleep apnea in the first night after cerebral infarction. Neurology 2002; 58:911–916.

43. Yaggi HK, Concato J, Kernan WN, et al. Obstructive sleep apnea as a risk factor for stroke and death. N Engl J Med 2005; 353:2034–2041.

44. Palombini L, Guilleminault C. Stroke and treatment with nasal CPAP. Eur J Neurol 2006; 13:198–200.

45. Scammell TE, Nishino S, Mignot E, et al. Narcolepsy and low CSF orexin (hypocretin) concentration after stroke. Neurology 2001; 56:1751–1753.

46. Leppävuori A, Pohjasvaara T, Bataja R, et al. Insomnia in ischemic stroke patients. Cerebrovasc Dis 2002; 14:90–97.

47. Kimura K, Tachibana N, Kohyama J, et al. A discrete pontine ischemic lesion could cause REM sleep behavior disorder. Neurology 2000; 55:894–895.

48. Blackshear JL, Kaplan J, Thompson RC, et al. Nocturnal dyspnea and atrial fibrillation predict Cheyne-Stokes respirations in patients with congestive heart failure. Arch Intern Med 1995; 155:1297–1302.

49. Mooe T, Gullsby S, Rabben T, et al. Sleep-disordered breathing: a novel predictor of atrial fibrillation after coronary artery bypass surgery. Coronary Artery Dis 1996; 7:475–478.

50. Lanfranchi PA, Somers VK, Braghiroli A, et al. Central sleep apnea in left ventricular dysfunction: prevalence and implications for arrhythmic risk. Circulation 2003; 107:727–732.

51. Gami AS, Howard DE, Olson EJ, et al. Day-night pattern of sudden death in obstructive sleep apnea. N Engl J Med 2005; 352:1206–1214.

52. Becker H, Brandenburg U, Peter JH, et al. Reversal of sinus arrest and atrioventricular conduction block in patients with sleep apnea during nasal continuous positive airway pressure. Am J Respir Crit Care Med 1995; 151:2215–218.

53. Stegman SS, Burroughs JM, Henthorn RW. Asymptomatic bradyarrhythmias as a marker for sleep apnea: appropriate recognition and treatment may reduce the need for pacemaker therapy. Pacing Clin Electrophysiol 1996; 19:899–904.

54. Kanagala R, Murali NS, Friedman PA, et al. Obstructive sleep apnea and the recurrence of atrial fibrillation. Circulation 2003; 107:2589–2594.

55. Harbison J, O'Reilly P, McNicholas WT. Cardiac rhythm disturbances in the obstructive sleep apnea syndrome: effects of nasal continuous positive airway pressure therapy. Chest 2000; 118:591–595.

56. Javaheri S. Effects of continuous positive airway pressure on sleep apnea and ventricular irritability in patients with heart failure. Circulation 2000; 169:156–162.

57. Peker Y, Hedner J, Norum J, et al. Increased incidence of cardiovascular disease in middle-aged men with obstructive sleep apnea: a 7-year follow-up. Am J Respir Crit Care Med 2002; 166:159–165.

58. Partinen M, Guilleminault C. Daytime sleepiness and vascular morbidity at seven-year follow-up in obstructive sleep apnea patients. Chest 1990; 97:27–32.

59. Marin JM, Carrizo SJ, Vicente E, et al. Long-term cardiovascular outcomes in men with obstructive sleep apnoea-hypopnoea with or without treatment with continuous positive airway pressure: an observational study. Lancet 2005; 365:1046–1053.

60. Rich S, ed. Primary Pulmonary Hypertension: Executive Summary from the World Symposium on Primary Pulmonary Hypertension. Geneva: World Health Organization, 1998.

61. Sanner BM, Doberauer C, Konermann M, et al. Pulmonary hypertension in patients with obstructive sleep apnea syndrome. Arch Intern Med 1997; 157:2483–2487.

62. Chaouat A, Weitzenblum E, Krieger J, et al. Pulmonary hemodynamics in the obstructive sleep apnea syndrome. Chest 1996; 109:380–386.

63. Laks L, Lehrhaft B, Grunstein RR, et al. Pulmonary hypertension in obstructive sleep apnea. Eur Respir J 1995; 8:537–541.

64. Bellia V, Pistelli R, Fillippazzo G, et al. Prevalence of nocturnal asthma in a general population sample: determinants and effect of aging. J Asthma 2000; 37:595–602.

65. Turner-Warwick M. Epidemiology of nocturnal asthma. Am J Med 1988; 85:6–8.

66. Martin RJ. Nocturnal asthma: circadian rhythms and therapeutic interventions. Am Rev Respir Dis 1993; 147:S25–S28.

67. Chan CS, Wookcock AJ, Sullivan CE. Nocturnal asthma: role of snoring and obstructive sleep apnea. Am Rev Respir Dis 1998; 97:2154–2159.

68. Guilleminault C, Quera-Salva MA, Powell N, et al. Nocturnal asthma: snoring, small pharynx and nasal CPAP. Eur Respir J 1988; 1:902–907.

69. Yigla M, Tov N, Solomonov A, et al. Difficult-to-control asthma and obstructive sleep apnea. J Asthma 2003; 40:865–871.

70. Wiegand L, Mende CN, Zaidel G, et al. Salmeterol vs theophylline: sleep and efficacy outcomes in patients with nocturnal asthma. Chest 1999; 115:1525–1532.

71. Shah L, Wilson AJ, Gibson PG, et al. Long acting beta-agonists versus theophylline for maintenance treatment of asthma. Cochrane Database Syst Rev 2003; CD001281.

72. Klink ME, Dodge R, Quan SF. The relation of sleep complaints to respiratory symptoms in a general population. Chest 1994; 105:151–154.

73. Calverley PM, Brerzinova V, Douglas NJ, et al. The effect of oxygenation on sleep quality in chronic bronchitis and emphysema. Am Rev Respir Dis 1982; 126:206–210.

74. Catterall JR, Douglas NJ, Calverley PM, et al. Transient hypoxemia during sleep in chronic obstructive pulmonary disease is not a sleep apnea syndrome. Am Rev Respir Dis 1983; 128:24–29.

75. Catterall JR, Calverley PM, MacNee W, et al. Mechanism of transient nocturnal hypoxemia in hypoxic chronic bronchitis and emphysema. J Appl Physiol 1985; 59:1698–1703.

76. DeMarco FJ Jr., Wynee JW, Block AJ, et al. Oxygen desaturation during sleep as a determinant of the "blue and bloated" syndrome. Chest 1981; 79:621–625.

77. Resta O, Guido P, Picca V, et al. Prescription of nCPAP and nBIPAP in obstructive sleep apnea syndrome: Italian experience in 105 subjects. A prospective two centre study. Respir Med 1998; 92:820–827.

78. Lighttowler JV, Wedzicha JA, Elliot MW, et al. Non-invasive pressure ventilation to treat respiratory failure from exacerbations of chronic obstructive pulmonary disease: Cochrane systematic review and meta-analysis. Br Med J 2003; 326:185–187.

79. Meecham Jones DJ, Paul EA, Jones PW, et al. Nasal pressure support ventilation plus oxygen compared with oxygen therapy alone in hypercapnic COPD. Am J Respir Crit Care Med 1995; 152:538–544.

80. Clark M, Cooper B, Singh S, et al. A survey of nocturnal hypoxemia and health-related quality of life in patients with cryptogenic fibrosing alveolitis. Thorax 2001; 52:482–486.

81. Perez-Padilla R, West P, Lerzman M, et al. Breathing during sleep in patients with interstitial lung disease. Am Rev Respir Dis 1985; 132:224–229.

82. Tatsumi K, Kimuar H, Kunitomo F, et al. Arterial oxygen desaturation during sleep in interstitial pulmonary disease: correlation with chemical control of breathing during wakefulness. Chest 1989; 95:962–967.

83. Crockett AJ, Cranston JM, Antic N. Domiciliary oxygen for interstitial lung disease. Cochrane Database Syst Rev 2001; (3):CD002883.

84. Naimark A, Cherniack RM. Compliance of the respiratory system and its components in health and obesity. J Appl Physiol 1960; 15:377–382.

85. American Academy of Sleep Medicine, . Sleep-related breathing disorders in adults: recommendations for syndrome definition and measurement techniques in clinical research. Sleep 1999; 22:667–689.

86. Perez de Llano LA, Golpe R, Ortiz Piquer M, et al. Short-term and long-term effects of nasal intermittent positive pressure ventilation in patients with obesity-hypoventilation syndrome. Chest 2005; 128:587–594.

87. Bach JR. Update and perspective on noninvasive respiratory muscle aids-Part 2, the expiratory aides. Chest 1994; 105:1538–1544.

88. Mezon BL, West P, Israels J, et al. Sleep breathing abnormalities in kyphoscoliosis. Am Rev Respir Dis 1980; 122:617.

89. Guilleminault C, Kurland G, Winkle R, et al. Severe kyphoscoliosis, breathing, and sleep: the "Quasimodo" syndrome during sleep. Chest 1981; 79:6.

90. Hill NS, Eveloff SE, Carlisle CC, et al. Efficacy of nocturnal nasal ventilation in patients with restrictive thoracic disease. Am Rev Respir Dis 1992; 145:365–371.

91. Buyse B, Meersseman W, Demedts M. Treatment of chronic respiratory failure in kyphoscoliosis: oxygen or ventilation? Eur Respir J 2003; 22:525–528.

92. Masa JF. Noninvasive positive pressure ventilation and not oxygen may prevent overt ventilatory failure in patients with chest wall disease. Chest 1997; 112:201–213.

93. Ward S, Chatwin M, Heather S, et al. Randomised controlled trial of non-invasive ventilation (NIV) for nocturnal hypoventilation in neuromuscular and chest wall disease patients with daytime normocapnia. Thorax 2005; 60:1019–1024.

94. Konagaya M, Sakai M, Wakayama T, et al. Effect of intermittent positive pressure ventilation on lifespan and causes of death in Duchenne muscular dystrophy. Rinsho Shinkeigaku 2005; 45: 643–646.

95. Johnson ED, ed. 1998 Women and Sleep Poll. Datastat 199. Ann Arbor, MI: National Sleep Foundation, 1998:1–122.

96. Loube DI, Poceta JS, Morales MC, et al. Self-reported snoring in pregnancy. Association with fetal outcome. Chest 1996; 109:885–889.

97. Nikkola E, Ekblad UU, Ekholm EM, et al. Sleep in multiple pregnancy: breathing patterns, oxygenation and periodic leg movements. Am J Obstet Gynecol 1996; 174:1622–1625.

98. Lyons HA. Centrally acting hormone and respiration. Pharmacol Ther 1976; 2:743–751.

99. Roush SF, Bell L. Obstrucitve sleep apnea in pregnancy. J Am Board Fam Pract 2004; 17:292–294.

100. Freidin N, Fisher MJ, Taylor W, et al. Sleep and nocturnal acid reflux in normal subjects and patients with reflux oesophagitis. Gut 1991; 32:1275–1279.

101. Orr WC, Johnson LF. Responses to different levels of esophageal acidification during waking and sleep. Dig Dis Sci 1998; 43:241–245.

102. Schneyer LH, Pigman W, Hanahan L, et al. Rate of flow of human parotid, sublingual, and submaxillary secretion during sleep. J Dental Res 1956; 35:109–114.

103. Shaker R, Castell DO, Schoenfeld PS, et al. Nighttime heartburn is an under-appreciated clinical problem that impacts sleep and daytime function: the results of a Gallup survey conducted on behalf of the American Gastroenterological Association. Am J Gastroenterol 2003; 98:1487–1493.

104. Farup C, Kleinman L, Sloan S, et al. The impact of nocturnal symptoms associated with gastroesophageal reflux disease on health-related quality of life. Arch Intern Med 2001; 161:45–70.

105. Harding SM. Gastroesophogeal reflux and asthma: insight into the association. J Allergy Clin Immunol 1999; 104:251–259.

106. Gislason T, Janson C, Vermeire P, et al. Respiratory symptoms and nocturnal gastroeophageal reflux. A population-based study of young adults in three European countries. Chest 2002; 121: 158–163.

107. Green BT, Broughton WA, O'Connor JB. Marked improvement in nocturnal gastroesophageal reflux in a large cohort of patients with obstructive sleep apnea treated with continuous positive airway pressure. Arch Intern Med 2003; 163:41–45.

108. Thurnheer R, Henz S, Knoblauch A. Sleep-related laryngospasm. Eur Respir J 1997; 10:2084–2086.

109. Fass R, Fullerton S, Tung S, et al. Sleep disturbances in clinic patients with functional bowel disorders. Am J Gastroenterol 1999; 94:2447–2452.

110. Elsenbruch S, Harnish MJ, Orr WC. Subjective and objective sleep quality in irritable bowel syndrome. Am J Gastroenterol 1999; 94:2447–2452.

111. Kumar D, Thompson PD, Wingate DL, et al. Abnormal REM sleep in the irritable bowel syndrome. Gastroenterology 1992; 103:12–17.

112. Parker KP. Sleep disturbances in dialysis patients. Sleep Med Rev 2003; 7:131–143.

113. Holley JL, Nespor S, Rault R. Characterizing sleep disorders in chronic hemodialysis patients. ASAIO Trans 1991; 37:M456–M457.

114. Walker S, Fine A, Kryger MH. Sleep complaints are common in the dialysis unit. Am J Kidney Dis 1995; 26:751–756.

115. Hui DS, Wong TY, Ko FW, et al. Prevalence of sleep disturbances in Chinese patients with end-stage renal failure on continuous ambulatory peritoneal dialysis. Am J Kidney Dis 2000; 36:783–788.

116. Pressman MR, Benz RL. High incidence of sleep disorders in end stage renal disease. Sleep Res 1995; 24:417.

117. Mendelson WB, Wadhwa NK, Greenberg HE, et al. Effects of hemodialysis on sleep apnea syndrome in end-stage renal disease. Clin Nephrol 1990; 33:247–251.

118. ASDA. The International Classification of Sleep Disorders. Rochester, MN: American Sleep Disorders Association; 1997.
119. Holley JL, Nespor S, Rault R. A comparison of reported sleep disorders in patients on chronic hemodialysis and continuous peritoneal dialysis. Am J Kidney Dis 1992; 19:156–161.
120. Staedt J, Stoppe G, Kogler A, et al. Dopamine D2 receptor alteration in patients with periodic limb movements in sleep (nocturnal myoclonus). J Neural Transm 1993; 93:71–74.
121. Trenkwalder C, Walters AS, Hening WA, et al. Positron emission tomographic studies in restless legs syndrome. Mov Disord 1999; 14:141–145.
122. Turjanski N, Lees AJ, Brooks DJ. Striatal dopaminergic function in restless legs syndrome: 18F-dopa and 11C-raclopride PET studies. Neurology 1999; 52:932–937.
123. Ruottinen HM, Partinen M, Hublin C, et al. An FDOPA PET study in patients with periodic limb movement disorder and restless legs syndrome. Neurology 2000; 54:502–504.
124. Allen RP, Earley CJ. Restless legs syndrome: a review of clinical and pathophysiologic features. J Clin Neurophysiol 2001; 18(2):128–147.
125. Furst P. Amino acid metabolism in uremia. J Am Coll Nutr 1989; 8:310–323.
126. Allen R, Becker PM, Bogan P, et al. Ropinirole decreases periodic leg movements and improves sleep parameters in patients with restless legs syndrome. Sleep 2004; 27:907–914.
127. Trenwalder C, Garcia-Borreguero D, Montagna P, et al. Ropinirole in the treatment of restless legs syndrome: results form the TREAT RLS 1 study, a 12 week, randomized, placebo controlled study in 10 European countries. J Neurol Neurosurg Psychiatry 2004; 75:92–97.
128. Hallett MD, Burden S, Stewart D, et al. Sleep apnea in ESRD patients on HD and CAPD. Perit Dial Int 1996; 16(suppl 1):S429–S433.
129. Wadhwa NK, Mendelson WB. A comparison of sleep-disordered respiration in ESRD patients receiving hemodialysis and peritoneal dialysis. Adv Perit Dial 1992; 8:195–198.
130. Fein AM, Niederman MS, Imbriano L, et al. Reversal of sleep apnea in uremia by dialysis. Arch Intern Med 1987; 147:1355–1356.
131. Hanly PJ, Perratos A. Improvement of sleep apnea in patients with chronic renal failure who undergo nocturnal hemodialysis. N Engl J Med 2001; 344:102–107.
132. Resta O, Paanacciulli N, Di Gioia G, et al. High prevalence of previously unknown subclinical hypothyroidism in obese patients referred to a sleep clinic for sleep disordered breathing. Nutr Metab Cardiovasc Dis 2004; 14:248–253.
133. Shipley JE, Schteingart De, Randon R, et al. Sleep architecture and sleep apnea in patients with Cushing's disease. Sleep 1992; 15:514–518.
134. Blanco Perez JJ, Blanco-Ramos MA, Zamarron Sanz C, et al. Acromegaly and sleep apnea. Arch Bronconeumol 2004; 40:355–359.
135. Rosenow F, Reuter S, Deuss U, et al. Sleep apnoea in treated acromegaly: relative frequency and predisposing factors. Clin Endocrinol (Oxf) 1996; 45:563–569.
136. Grunstein RR, Ho KY, Sullivan CE. Sleep apnea in acromegaly. Ann Intern Med 1991; 115:527–532.
137. Bjork S, Jonsson B, Westphal O, et al. Quality of life of adults with growth hormone deficiency: a controlled study. Acta Paediatr Scand Suppl 1989; 356:55–59.
138. Campbell SM, Clark S, Tindall EA, et al. Clinical characteristics of fibrositis, I: a "blinded" controlled study of symptoms and tender points. Arthritis Rheum 1983; 26:817–825.
139. Hyyppa MT, Kronhom E. Nocturnal motor activity in fibromyalgia patients with poor sleep quality. J Psychosom Res 1995; 39:85–91.
140. Modolfsky H, Saskin P, Lue FA. Sleep and symptoms in fibrositis syndrome after a febrile illness. J Rheumatol 1988; 15:1701–1704.
141. Moldolfsky H, Lue FA, Smythe H. Alpha EEG sleep and morning symptoms of rheumatoid arthritis. J Rheumatol 1983; 10:373–379.
142. Perlis ML, Giles DE, Bootzin RR, et al. Alpha sleep and information processing, perception of sleep, pain, and arousability in fibromyalgia. Int J Neurosci 1997; 89:265–280.
143. Moldolfsky H, Lue FA. The relationship of alpha delta EEG frequencies to pain and mood in "fibrositis" patients with chlorpromazine and L-tryptophan. Electroencephalogr Clin Neurophysiol 1980; 50:71–80.
144. Morin CM, Gibson D, Wade J. Self-reported sleep and mood disturbance in chronic pain patients. Clin J Pain 1998; 14:311–314.
145. Davidson JR, MacLean AW, Brundage MD, et al. Sleep disturbance in cancer patients. Soc Sci Med 2002; 54:1309–1321.
146. Portenoy RK, Tahler HT, Kombilth AB, et al. Symptom prevalence, characteristics and distress in a cancer population. Qual Life Res 1994; 3:183–189.
147. Vena C, Parker K, Cunningham M, et al. Sleep-wake disturbances in people with cancer part I: an overview of sleep, sleep regulation, and effects of disease and treatment. Oncol Nurs Forum 2004; 31:735–746.
148. Johns MW. A new method of measuring sleepiness: the Epworth sleepiness scale. Sleep 1991; 14:540–545.

149. Hoddes E, Zarcone V, Smythe H, et al. Quantification of sleepiness: a new approach. Psychophysiology 1973; 10:431–436.

150. Rosenthal L, Roehr TA, Roth T. The sleep-wake activity inventory: a self-report measure of daytime sleepiness. Biol Psychiatry 1993; 34:810–820.

151. Chua, LWY, Yu NC, Golish JA, et al. Epworth sleepiness scale and the multiple sleep latency test: dilemma of the elusive link. Sleep 1998; 21(suppl):184.

152. U.S. Modafinil in Narcolepsy Multicenter Study Group. Randomized trial of modafinil for the treatment of pathological somnolence in narcolepsy. Ann Neurol 1998; 43:88–97.

153. Johns MW, Hocking B. Daytime sleepiness and sleep habits of Australian workers. Sleep 1997; 20:844–849.

154. Carskadon MA, Dement WC. Cumulative effects of sleep restriction on daytime sleepiness. Psychophysiology 1981; 18:107–113.

155. Roth T, Seiden D, Sainati S, et al. Effects of ramelteon on patient-reported sleep latency in older adults with chronic insomnia. Sleep Med 2006; 7:312–318.

156. Morin CM, Hauri PJ. Espie CA, et al. Non-pharmacologic treatment of chronic insomnia: an American Academy of Sleep Medicine review. Sleep 1999; 22:1134–1156.

157. Avidan AY, Fries BE, James ML, et al. Insomnia and hypnotic use, recorded in the minimum data set, as predictors of falls and hip fractures in Michigan nursing homes. J Am Geriatr Soc 2005; 53:955–962.

158. Jacobs GD, Pace-Schott EF, Stickgold R, et al. Cognitive behavior therapy and pharmacotherapy for insomnia. Arch Intern Med 2004; 164:1888–1896.

159. NIH State-of-the-Science Conference Statement on Manifestations and Management of Chronic Insomnia in Adults. June 13-15, 2005. Available at: http://consensus.nih.gov/2005/2005InsomniaSOS026html.htm

160. Siversten B, Omvik S, Pallesen S, et al. Cognitive behavioral therapy vs zopiclone for treatment of chronic primary insomnia in adults: a randomized controlled trial. JAMA 2006; 295:2851–2858.

51 | Neurologic Disorders

Theresa M. Buckley and Christian Guilleminault
Sleep Disorders Center, Stanford University School of Medicine, Stanford, California, U.S.A.

INTRODUCTION

Neurologic disorders can affect sleep on multiple levels, depending on the location of the lesion or dysfunction. Many classifications can be used, such as classifications related to the location of the lesion or classifications related to the clinical presentations. The latter have the advantage of enticing the practitioner to systematically evaluate specific sleep disorders. Such classifications include neurodegenerative disorders, neuromuscular disorders, movement disorders, auto-immune disorders, cerebrovascular diseases, seizures, and headaches. The manifestations in terms of their impact on sleep often depend, of course, on the location of the lesion. Some neurologic diseases involve the sleep-wake system. For example, dementing disorders may affect diffuse neural pathways that impact the strength of the circadian rhythm, but also instability of sleep and sleep states. In contrast, other disorders secondarily impact sleep and its quality. As an example, neuromuscular disorders can impact control of swallowing and the airway, which can increase susceptibility to obstructive sleep apnea (OSA).

Below, key disorders within each classification will be described. For each class, an approach to their evaluation from a sleep medicine perspective is given. Attention to specific aspects for each disorder within a class is given, when relevant. Though a complete summary of all neurologic disorders and their associated sleep complaints is not feasible within the limited scope of this chapter, a similar approach to evaluation and treatment from a sleep perspective can be applied. It is assumed that the clinician will have completed the appropriate neurologic workup and treatment.

Before proceeding with a discussion of key disorders, Table 1 can help provide a framework for this approach. See also Ref. 1 for more details on sleep and brain lesions. In the first column, we list the location of the nervous system affected. In the second column, we list potential resulting sleep disorders to consider. In the third column, we list sample neurologic disorders that could cause the lesions in the area listed. The clinician should decide on a case-by-case basis what information is relevant to his or her patient in light of the neurologic syndrome and regions affected in the specific patient's case.

NEURODEGENERATIVE DISORDERS

Typical dementing disorders include Alzheimer's type dementia, Lewy body disease, Jacob–Creutzfeld disease, and fatal familial insomnia (FFI). Because of the impact on diffuse neuronal pathways in many cases, the dementing illnesses can impact regulation of the sleep-wake system, including transmission of the suprachiasmatic nucleus time signal to other parts of the brain.

Description
Alzheimer's type dementia is an insidious onset disorder characterized by deposition of extracellular plaques (β-amyloid protein) and intraneuronal tangles (hyperphosphorylated τ protein), most prominently in the hippocampus and later, in other areas as well. There is loss of cholinergic neurons in the nucleus basalis of Meynert. Loss of neurons in the suprachiasmatic nucleus of the hypothalamus may also occur. Early clinical symptoms include difficulty with short-term memory and relative preservation of long-term memory. As the disease progresses, more pervasive cognitive deficits ensue. Typical sleep disturbances and

Table 1 Sample Sleep Disorders and Location of Neurologic Deficit

Region affected	Potential sleep disorders	Potential neurologic syndromes (that may cause lesions in aforementioned region)
Anterior and dorsomedial thalamic nuclei	Insomnia	Fatal familial insomnia
Nucleus of the solitary tract	Insomnia	Stroke, tumor, encephalitis
Posterior hypothalamus (Tuberomammillary nucleus)	Hypersomnia	Stroke, tumor, encephalitis
Anterior hypothalamus (VLPO)	Insomnia	Stroke, tumor, encephalitis
Lateral hypothalamus (prefornical)	Hypersomnia	Stroke, tumor, encephalitis
Bilateral cerebral hemispheres	Cheyne–Stokes breathing	Stroke, encephalitis
Brainstem	Central sleep apnea, hypoventilation, OSA, insomnia, RBD	PD, OPCD, MSA, Lewy body disease, AD, pontine infarcts, ALS, MS
CNS white matter	Narcolepsy, excessive daytime sleepiness, insomnia, RLS, PLMD, OSA, RBD	MS, encephalitis
Cervical spinal cord	PLMD, Dysregulated circadian rhythm	Cervical spinal stenosis, MS, syringomyelia, Arnold–Chiari malformation
Lumbar cord	Muscle cramps	Lumbar spinal stenosis, MS
Lumbosacral plexus	RLS, PLMD	Pelvic tumor
Peripheral nerve	RLS, PLMD	Neuropathy
Retinohypothalamic tract	Insomnia, circadian dysregulation	Blindness (noncortical), craniopharyngioma, MS
Frontal lobe		Nocturnal paroxysmal dystonia
Multiple	OSA and others (depends on location of lesion)	Stroke, tumor, encephalitis

Abbreviations: VLPO, ventrolateral preoptic region; RBD, REM behavior disorder; REM, rapid eye movement; OPCD, Olivopontocerebellar degeneration; MSA, multiple system atrophy; ALS, amyotrophic lateral sclerosis; MS, multiple sclerosis; RLS, restless legs syndrome; PLMD, periodic limb movement disorder.

behaviors include insomnia, excess daytime napping, and sundowning behaviors. Disruption of the circadian sleep-wake system contributes to many of these symptoms. Sleep complaints appear correlated to cognitive decline.

Sundowning behaviors encompass wandering, vocalizations, aggression, and agitation (2). Most commonly, subjects cannot maintain sleep. The presence of darkness enhances disorientation and confabulation. Nocturnal wandering with uncontrolled behavior will occur. Polysomnographic findings include increased wake after sleep onset, decreased total sleep time (TST), decreased sleep efficiency, decreased rapid eye movement (REM) sleep, and increased latency to REM (2). REM changes may be secondary to decreased acetylcholine (3). OSA is more frequent in Alzheimer's disease (present in 33–53%), compared with the healthy population. No change in periodic limb movement disorder (PLMD) is reported.

Dementia with Lewy bodies results from deposition of Lewy bodies throughout the brain, involving both cortical and subcortical structures (4). Clinical symptoms include cognitive, neuropsychiatric, motor, sleep, and autonomic changes. In the cognitive domain, executive function, visiospatial memory, and attention/concentration are most affected (5). Complex visual hallucinations may be present during the day (6) and hallucinations may also disrupt sleep at night (7). In addition to insomnia and neuropsychiatric changes such as seen in Alzheimer's disease, Lewy body dementia is associated with increased movement disorders, especially REM behavior disorder (RBD) (6). RBD is characterized by loss of atonia during REM and "acting out of dreams" (8). This can manifest as vocalizations, limb movements, and so on and can result in injury to the bed partner. Violence to the bed partner or oneself is common, with the risk of serious injuries. The abnormal sleep behavior may precede the wake manifestations of the neurologic syndrome by 20 to 30 years.

Two prion diseases (9) associated with sleep disturbances include *Jacob–Creutzfeld disease* and *FFI*. These two disorders are now associated due to their linkage to prion disease. They were initially separated due to their clinical presentations.

Jacob–Creutzfeld disease is characterized by neuronal destruction and subsequent vacuolization of brain tissue, creating a spongiform appearance to the brain tissues. Clinical symptoms include fatigue, disordered sleep, cognitive changes, cerebellar ataxia, and myoclonus (4). In time, progressive myoclonus and dementia predominate (9). Disruption of REM sleep is reported (10). Triphasic sharp waves by electroencephalography (EEG) and 14-3-3 protein in the cerebrospinal fluid (CSF) are characteristic (4).

FFI is an autosomal dominant progressive insomnia that results from a genetically transmitted prion disease. Destruction of brain tissue is initially localized to the thalamus and inferior olivary nucleus (11). Clinical features include severe insomnia, autonomic disturbance (e.g., pyrexia, excess salivation), and myoclonus (11). Additionally, there is cardiac and respiratory dysfunction and progressive worsening of autonomic nervous system symptoms. Neuronal loss without spongiosis occurs in this form (11). EEG shows a dissociated REM characterized by bursts of generalized theta rhythm, loss of sleep spindles, and absent slow wave sleep. With progression, the EEG progressively flattens (8). The neurologic workup includes EEG and CSF analysis. Unfortunately, FFI is rapidly progressive and fatal, with time to death of 8 to 72 months (12).

Parkinson's disease (PD) results from destruction of dopamine containing neurons in the basal ganglia and thalamus, key pathways involved in control of movement. Clinical features include bradykinesia, rest tremor, masked facies, and cogwheel rigidity. When severe, dysphagia may occur, increasing susceptibility to aspiration. PD is associated with increased incidence of a myriad of sleep disorders (13). These include insomnia (32%), OSA, and RBD (15–47%), restless legs syndrome (RLS) (20.8%) and nightmares (32%) (13). Obstruction of the airway and restriction is highly prevalent (13). Hallucinations are common with RBD (13). In addition, other features of the disorder and its treatment can lead to disrupted sleep and excessive daytime sleepiness (EDS). Though the tremor usually goes away in sleep, if severe enough, it may persist. Hypertonia is more often disruptive. Foot pain is common (13). Sleepiness and/or insomnia may occur secondary to dopaminergic agents used to treat the disorder.

RBD can be a harbinger of PD (5,14), when other symptoms are absent. Increased nocturnal hallucinosis and nightmares may also disrupt sleep (15). Though dopaminergic agents can increase visual hallucinations, a dysregulation of REM sleep may contribute as well. Dopaminergic agents can contribute to insomnia, but can also cause excess sleepiness in some patients. There is an increased incidence of sleep attacks in PD compared with the normal population, and this is thought secondary to dopaminergic agents (16). Nocturia may disrupt sleep. Autonomic disturbances from the disorder may induce nocturnal sweating as well as dysregulation of the circadian sleep-wake system (13). Additionally, disability, poor sleep hygiene, and other environmental factors may also impair strength of the sleep-wake system.

Multiple system atrophy (MSA) is a neurodegenerative movement disorder that includes parkinsonism as well as cerebellar dysfunction and dysautonomia. Three forms include MSA with olivopontocerebellar degeneration, MSA with dysautonomia, and MSA with striatonigral degeneration (4). In MSA with olivopontocerebellar degeneration, ataxia is a key feature, especially of gait. There is dysmetria of upper arm movement and cerebellar dysarthria. Dementia and personality changes may also coincide. Magnetic resonance imaging (MRI) may show atrophy of both the brainstem and cerebellum. MSA with dysautonomia may include orthostatic hypotension, incontinence, and impotence. There may be distal muscle wasting with distal dysmetria. In MSA with striatonigral degeneration, the tremor of PD is absent, but rigidity is prominent. Patients may experience axial rigidity, bradykinesia, and falls. MRI may show bilateral putamen gliosis. RBD and nocturnal stridor is common, with the latter secondary to vocal cord abductor weakness (17).

Progressive supranuclear palsy (PSP) shares the rigidity and bradykinesia of PD but lacks the tremor (4). Gait is slow. Additional features include difficulty with eye movements, especially on down gaze. Thus, falls can occur frequently. Blepharospasm may be present as well. Cognitive changes include slowing as well as depression and difficulties with regulation of emotions. A recent study reports that RBD is as frequent in PSP as it is in PD (18). Insomnia is worse than in PD and AD, possibly secondary to greater brainstem involvement (17).

Huntington's disease is an autosomal dominant neurodegenerative disorder (4). The caudate and putamen are affected. Clinical characteristics include choreiform movements as well as cognitive decline (subcortical dementia). Movements may progress to Parkinsonian features such as dystonia, postural instability, and bradykinesia. Psychiatric manifestations include hallucinations, depression, and mania (4). There can be disintegration of the sleep-wake cycle due to circadian disruption (19).

Leigh's disease, a neurodegenerative disorder of the brainstem, will lead to more sleep-related breathing disorders (SBDs) initially.

Evaluation

In general, sleep complaints may be categorized as those of insomnia, EDS, or parasomnia with or without violence. Once categorized, the workup of sleep disturbance is directed toward the complaint. A sleep diary (kept by either the patient or the caregiver) and daytime activity log may offer a glimpse of circadian rhythm sleep disturbances and sleep habits.

If insomnia with new onset nocturnal agitation is present in a patient with dementia, the workup should be directed first to rule out medical causes, including infection (acute urinary tract infection), metabolic (hyperammonemia) and toxic causes. Nocturnal agitation may also represent RBD. If RBD is suspected, it is diagnosed with a polysomnogram to discern for the characteristic electromyographic (EMG) augmentation during REM sleep seen in this disorder (8). A polysomnogram is also useful to evaluate for OSA and PLMD (as a cause of EDS and confusional arousals) (20).

Figure 1 illustrates an approach to evaluation and workup of sleep complaints. A similar approach can be used for the other neurologic disorders described herein.

Step 1: Neurologic diagnosis.
Step 2: Identify areas of central nervous system (CNS) and peripheral nervous system (PNS) affected and hypothesize index of suspicion for potential sleep disorders (e.g., bilateral cerebral hemispheres—Cheyne–Stokes; brainstem—respiratory control and bulbar function, etc.).
Step 3: Take complete sleep and health history (include daytime activity).
Step 4: Classify complaint (EDS, insomnia or sleep-wake disruption, parasomnia or extra activity).
Step 5: Proceed with workup (diary, activity log, polysomnogram) to establish *International Classification of Sleep Disorders* (ICSD-2) sleep diagnosis.

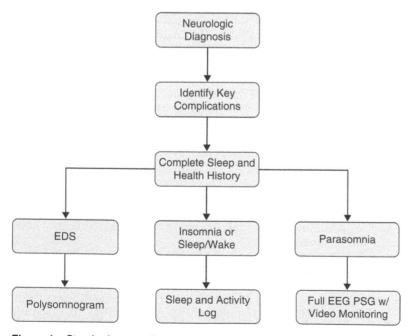

Figure 1   Standard approach to sleep disorders in neurologic patients.

Treatment

Nonpharmacologic treatments in the case of dementia and disability include means to reenforce a weakened circadian rhythm. These include regular activity and meals during the day, exposure to bright light during the day, (21) and limited exposure to light at night. A controlled trial of 2500 lux bright light in the morning (9:30 a.m. for 2 hours) shows benefit in improving sleep and circadian activity rhythms and in reducing agitation. Limiting sleeping and lying in the supine position during the day may also improve sleep at night. Despite the diagnosis of Alzheimer's disease, education and implementation of the behavioral techniques of sleep hygiene education, daily walking, and increased light exposure improve sleep in this population (22).

If sleep apnea is present, a trial of continuous positive airway pressure (CPAP) may be beneficial and has been shown to reduce daytime sleepiness in this population (23), though the equipment may not be well tolerated in more advanced cases. In the case of neuromuscular disorders, sleep-related hypoventilation and desaturations are best treated with bilevel positive airway pressure (BPAP) and, if needed, O_2.

Pharmacologic treatments directed to the treatment of insomnia are best used by keeping the following techniques in mind (24). The lowest dose that is effective is ideal. Intermittent use (2 to 4 times per week) is preferable over nightly use. If used nightly, limit the duration of treatment to three to four weeks. Discontinue medications gradually to avoid rebound insomnia. Consider agents with a shorter half-life in order to limit residual morning and daytime sedation.

Agents include the traditional benzodiazepines as well as the newer nonbenzodiazepine hypnotics. In a meta-analysis (24) of 23 trials of treatment of chronic insomnia in the elderly, short-term efficacy for triazolam, temazepam, flurazepam. quazepam, and zolpidem was found. Newer nonbenzodiazepines hypnotics include zaleplon, zopiclone, and eszopiclone. Ramelteon, a melatonin receptor agonist (at the MT1 and MT2 receptors), has been approved by the U.S. Food and Drug Administration (FDA) for treatment of chronic insomnia in the elderly.

Other off-label treatments of insomnia have included trazodone as well as the atypical antipsychotics. Both have cardiac side effects. Though quite effective for their calming and sedating properties in assisting with both insomnia and agitation, cardiac and metabolic side effects suggest caution when antipsychotics are used. In fact, increased mortality has been observed in elderly patients given atypical antipsychotics, and this is not recommended for psychosis and agitation in this population. If used for sleep purposes in the younger population only, smaller doses than the typical antipsychotic dose are usually adequate. For example, there are anecdotal clinical reports of 25 mg of seroquel as effective.

Although the first-line agents for PLMD and RLS are dopamine agonists (25), these agents may be activating as well as contribute to insomnia in elderly patients. Doses up to a maximum of 1 to 1.5 mg are usually effective. It is best to start with very small doses, 0.125 mg, and gradually increase to minimize side effects. As with hypnotics, stopping at the minimum effective dose is ideal. Other agents besides the dopamine agonists include anticonvulsants (e.g., gabapentin, carbamazepine, etc.) and benzodiazepines (e.g., clonazepam) (26). As any benzodiazepine can exacerbate sleep apnea (due to the muscle relaxant properties of drugs), underlying sleep apnea should be treated before implementing such medications.

Since patients with Lewy body dementia are extremely sensitive to neuroleptics, these agents should be avoided in this population (27). The major problems are the nocturnal wanderings with abnormal behaviors. Drugs, including clonazepam and haloperidol, the most commonly used drugs, have not demonstrated clear efficacy, but when tried, clonazepam should be the first drug to be considered.

NEUROMUSCULAR DISORDERS

Neuromuscular disorders are those that affect the nervous system beginning at the level of the nerve root and extend distally. Some disorders affect the CNS as well, such as amyotrophic lateral sclerosis (ALS). They may affect the sensory loop, the motor loop, or the integrative centers. Neuromuscular disorders may affect sleep in many ways. For example, subjects may have difficulties moving in bed and may wake up due to overall discomfort, with difficulties in changing positions. Lung expansion is worse during sleep, and urinary difficulties as well as abnormal bowel movements may also fragment sleep. Poor control of oropharyngeal musculature may lead to increased incidence of sleep apnea. Thus, neuromuscular disorders may affect sleep in many ways.

Description

A classic neuromuscular disorder not described elsewhere in this text is ALS. ALS is a neurodegenerative disease with progressive neuronal loss involving both upper and lower motor neurons. Survival ranges from three to four years (28). Generalized weakness, including both bulbar and respiratory muscles, leads to progressive disability. Respiratory deficits include daytime hypoventilation leading to hypercapnea.

Clinical symptoms at various stages of progression include fasciculations, difficulties with control of the or pharyngeal musculature, poor transmission of neural signals to the diaphragm to control breathing, and deficits in accessory respiratory muscle activity (4). ALS is associated with increased incidence of sleep apnea, though not as marked as would be expected for the degree of bulbar weakness (29). One hypothesis is that there is insufficient respiratory muscle activity to overcome the oropharynx closing pressure, thereby causing less obstruction (29). Nocturnal hypoventilation, however, is evident (30).

Interestingly, ALS is associated with decreased REM sleep in some cases (28). Since OSA and hypoventilation may worsen during REM due to atonia of accessory respiratory muscles and there is less REM sleep in some ALS patients, a partial compensation may occur. Other causes for poor sleep in ALS may include insomnia from hypercapnea.

Lumbar spinal stenosis may complicate sleep secondary to pain, calf muscle cramps, and paresthesias (31). *Cervical spinal stenosis* may complicate sleep secondary to pain as well. If sufficiently severe, bulbar weakness may predispose to OSA. Spinal cord pathology is associated with increased incidence of RLS and PLMD. Cervical spinal cord injury can reduce nighttime melatonin secretion and contribute to insomnia (32). Unilateral RLS should prompt consideration of a pelvic tumor causing a *lumbosacral plexopathy* in the differential diagnosis. Likewise, a plexopathy should prompt consideration of the RLS and PLMD in the differential as well. Finally, *neuropathies* are associated with increased incidence of RLS and PLMD.

Evaluation

Once the neurologic workup and treatment is complete, evaluation should begin with a diagnostic workup directed to the primary sleep symptom. For example, EDS may be secondary to OSA, central sleep apnea, hypoventilation, pain, RLS, and PLMD. Even without a presenting complaint of EDS, respiratory disorders are intimately linked with diseases such as ALS, in that a polysomnogram to evaluate for a SBD, including hypoventilation, is warranted. A similar approach as described in Figure 1 is applied, with an index of suspicion raised for certain sleep disorders, based on the above descriptions. For example, a neurologic diagnosis of cervical spinal stenosis may increase the index of suspicion for both SBD and PLMD.

Treatment

Nonpharmacologic treatment begins with evaluating current medications. In those disorders wherein oropharyngeal musculature or respiratory muscle involvement is expected, any medications that induce respiratory relaxation or central neural suppression should be avoided, given the comorbid breathing difficulties that occur during the day with exacerbation at night. When hypoventilation is found, BPAP is the preferred treatment (compared with CPAP).

Pharmacologic treatments, in addition to any pharmacologic interventions for the neurologic disorder itself, should be according to the current practice parameters for the sleep disorder identified. In some cases, certain medications may be useful for treatment of both the neurologic disorder and the sleep disorder. An example is the use of gabapentin in peripheral neuropathy. It may be effective for both pain and treatment of PLMD.

AUTOIMMUNE DISORDERS

Description

Sleep disorders and EDS are common in *multiple sclerosis* (MS), an autoimmune disorder that causes white matter plaques in affected areas of the brain. The most common sleep complaints include EDS and insomnia (33). Approximately 40% of patients with MS have insomnia. Other sleep complaints include RLS and PLMD (36%) and OSA and RBD. There is increased incidence of narcolepsy as well. Depression is a common comorbid condition in MS and some of the symptoms of fatigue, daytime sleepiness, and insomnia may be further complicated by depression. Finally, chronic pain (present in 50%) can exacerbate insomnia and both pain (34) and insomnia (35) increase susceptibility to depression. Nocturia and urinary incontinence can also contribute to fragmented sleep.

The syndrome of fatigue commonly reported in MS may or may not be related to abnormal nocturnal sleep. The differential diagnosis is difficult and a polysomnogram may be needed.

Evaluation
As in other disorders described in this chapter, the evaluation is the same. The neurologic disorder is treated first. A sleep evaluation is performed as in Figure 1, while maintaining a higher index of suspicion for certain disorders based on the descriptions above and location of lesions in the particular patient.

Treatment
Pharmacologic treatment should be directed as described elsewhere to treat the identified sleep disorder. As fatigue is common in MS, addition of modafinil may be helpful. The smallest effective dose, up to 400 mg per day, is appropriate. If insomnia occurs, limiting afternoon dosing should help. Modafinil may not be helpful if symptoms of fatigue are not related to abnormal sleep. If benzodiazepines or other respiratory depressing medications are used, sleep apnea should be evaluated and treated first.

Nonpharmacologic treatment should be directed as described elsewhere to treat the identified sleep disorder.

CEREBROVASCULAR DISEASES

Stroke can contribute to sleep disorders in a number of ways (36). Stroke can disrupt neural pathways responsible for proper control of the sleep and wake system. This can induce insomnia, hypersomnia, and dysregulation of the circadian cycle of sleep and wake across the 24-hour period. Alternatively, stroke may cause secondary sequelae, and these sequelae may also contribute to poor sleep quality (e.g., pain, rigidity, spasticity, hypertonia, urinary and bowel movement impairment).

Description
Key brain regions responsible for regulation of the sleep and wake system include the preoptic nucleus (sleep active neurons), the tuberomammillary nucleus of the hypothalamus (wake active neurons), the lateral hypothalamus (hypocretin neurons important for strengthening the wake signal and the circadian system), the reticular activating system (alertness), as well as other diffuse pathways.

Multiple opportunities for disruption of the sleep-wake system thus exist, depending on the pathways impacted. A summary of reported stroke syndromes [condensed from (36–38)] and associated sleep disruption is given in Table 2, demonstrating the diverse sleep changes that may occur, even with similar locations of lesions.

There is increased prevalence of OSA in patients who have suffered a stroke (36–39). Cheyne–Stokes breathing and central apneas are also of greater incidence (36). Conversely, sleep apnea is a risk factor for stroke (37), so its evaluation and treatment is important in patients who have already suffered a stroke to decrease risk of recurrence. The independent role of sleep-disordered breathing as a causal factor in stroke has recently been demonstrated. As important is the demonstration of the significant increase of recurrent stroke, impairment of rehabilitation, and secondary death with untreated sleep disordered breathing after the initial stroke.

In contrast to direct effects on the neuronal regulation of sleep-wake cycles, stroke can contribute to secondary sequelae that disrupt sleep quality. For example, sleep apnea is common in stroke patients and not only impacts quality of sleep and daytime function, but

Table 2 Stroke Syndromes

Stroke location	Sleep-related changes
Subcortical hemispheric and thalamic stroke	Presleep behaviors (yawn, stretch, eyes closed, sleep postures) and EDS
Subcortical, thalamic, mesencephalic, pons	Insomnia; can include inversion of sleep-wake cycle
Pontine tegmentum	RBD
Pontine tegmentum, mesencephalic, thalamic	Lhermitte's peduncular hallucinosis with visual hallucinations at sleep onset
Thalamic, temporal, parietal, occipital	Increased dreams, nightmares
Occipital, deep frontal, thalamic, parietal lesions	Decreased or absence of dreaming
Lateral medullary stroke	Insomnia and loss of dreaming
Hemispheric strokes	Decreased sleep spindles and slow wave sleep
Hemispheric strokes	Decreased saw tooth waves
Paramedian thalamic strokes	Decreased spindles, K-complexes, slow-wave sleep
Pons	Reduced REM sleep, loss of sleep spindles, K-complexes, vertex waves

Abbreviations: EDS, excessive daytime sleepiness; RBD, REM behavior disorder; REM, rapid eye movement.

also increases risk of subsequent stroke. OSA is associated with lack of the normal nocturnal dip in blood pressure during sleep. Persistent elevated blood pressure may increase the risk of hypertensive stroke and may also negatively impact recovery in the acute setting (39).

When stroke occurs in the brainstem pontine pathways, RBD may result. Finally, stroke may cause significant changes in daytime routine, due to secondary disability. Less activity and more time in bed during the day may decrease strength of the circadian rhythm and sleep drive at night, thereby contributing to insomnia.

Evaluation

As in other disorders described in this chapter, the evaluation is the same. The neurologic disorder is treated first. A sleep evaluation is performed as in Figure 1, while maintaining a higher index of suspicion for certain disorders based on the descriptions above.

Though guidelines exist for cerebrovascular and cardiovascular workup in the post-stroke setting, no endorsed guidelines exist for workup of sleep disorders for the post-stroke patient. Given the increased incidence of sleep apnea in stroke patients and the risk of stroke in sleep apnea patients, polysomnography would be a prudent study to perform in all stroke patients, once stabilized. The role of sleep disordered breathing in occurrence of a second stroke is today well demonstrated. Although in-house polysomnography is the gold standard (20), this may be prohibitive given the level of disability. In this case, portable monitoring may be helpful to accelerate evaluation and treatment. When subjects complain of sleep disturbances, a sleep diary and careful history may be helpful in better discerning the etiology.

Treatment

Nonpharmacologic treatment should be directed as described elsewhere to treat the identified sleep disorder.

Pharmacologic treatment should be directed as described elsewhere to treat the identified sleep disorder.

SEIZURES

There is both increased association of seizures with sleep deprivation as well as increased incidence of seizures during non–rapid eye movement (NREM) sleep. In fact, 7.5% to 45% of patients with seizures have events confined to the sleep period (36). Sleep disturbances in patients with epilepsy are a key predictor of quality of life in these patients (40). A brief description of seizures and clues from their sleep that may contribute to their diagnosis is given (4,8,40). Those reviewed by age of peak onset (40) include continuous spike and slow wave discharges during sleep, Lennox–Gastaut syndrome, absence epilepsy, juvenile myoclonic epilepsy, epilepsy with generalized tonic-clonic seizures (GTCS) on awakening, benign childhood epilepsy with centrotemporal spikes, frontal lobe epilepsy, and temporal lobe epilepsy. Nocturnal paroxysmal dystonia is considered a form of frontal lobe epilepsy and will be described as well.

Continuous spike and slow wave discharges during sleep (CSWS) is characterized by continuous slow spike-and-wave complexes on the EEG throughout at least 85% NREM sleep (8). It is formerly known as electrical status epilepticus of sleep. Movement does not occur. During wake and REM sleep, epileptiform activity is more focal and noncontinuous. It may be associated with progressive intellectual decline (41).

Lennox–Gastaut syndrome is a severe epilepsy syndrome with onset in childhood (peak onset 3–5 years). Cognitive and neurologic deficits are present (41). Seizure types range from axial tonic seizures that occur during sleep (in particular NREM) to tonic-clonic seizures, atypical absence, and myoclonic and atonic seizures. Interictal EEG reveals 2 to 2.5 Hz spike-and-wave complexes.

Juvenile myoclonic epilepsy (peak onset 14 years) is characterized by myoclonic jerks, tonic-clonic seizures, and absence seizures (4,41). Events commonly occur within a few hours of awakening. EEG reveals 3.5 to 6 Hz spike-and-wave discharges worsened with photic stimuli.

Absence seizures are generalized seizures with peak onset at age six to seven years. The duration is brief (5–10 seconds), with disruption of ongoing activity and a blank stare, then return to activity. Eye blinking and lip smacking may be present. EEG shows a characteristic three-second spike-and-wave discharge. Such patterns and behavior should lead to systematic sleep investigations despite absence of clinical manifestations during sleep. Sleep activates seizures, which are most prominent during NREM sleep and the first sleep cycle (41).

Epilepsy with GTCS on awakening is another generalized epilepsy, with peak age of onset at age 11 to 15 years. A genetic basis is probable. Seizures occur almost predominately upon awakening or during evening drowsiness.

Benign childhood epilepsy with centrotemporal spikes peaks at age 9 to 10 years and is characterized by perioral numbness, guttural sounds, excess salivation, and focal facial twitching (4,41). Clonic jerks of the arm and leg may also occur. Events most often occur during sleep and drowsiness. They resolve by adulthood. EEG shows centrotemporal sharp waves in the region of origination (4).

Nocturnal frontal lobe epilepsy (NFLE) can present with both motor and cognitive changes and may be difficult to detect on the EEG, depending on depth of focus (42). It may present with partial arousal from sleep with behaviors that mimic parasomnia, as nocturnal paroxysmal dystonia, and as unexplained arousals or stereotyped behavior (8). EEG may show a focal epileptiform abnormality that is, by definition, localized to the frontal lobe.

Nocturnal mesiotemporal seizures may also underlie abnormal stereotyped behavior out of NREM sleep, mimicking sleepwalking in a manner similar to mesiofrontal seizures.

Evaluation

In general, when seizure is expected, evaluation should begin with a careful history and neurologic workup directed to any daytime symptoms. Sleep-deprived EEG evaluation for characteristic EEG features is diagnostic in many cases, though up to three EEGs may be required to increase sensitivity. When symptoms are confined mostly to the sleep period, nocturnal video-polysomnography is indicated. This is the case when NFLE is suspected (43). If seizure disorder is already known, diagnostic workup is directed to the primary sleep symptom. For example, EDS may be secondary to OSA, central sleep apnea, hypoventilation, RLS, and PLMD. Since sleep disturbances can impact quality of life, a high index of suspicion for their evaluation and treatment is important. Improvement of seizure frequency is reported following CPAP in patients with sleep apnea and epilepsy (26,44)

Treatment

Nonpharmacologic treatment should be directed as described elsewhere to treat the identified sleep disorder. Given the increased incidence of seizure with sleep deprivation, educating the patient regarding keeping a regular sleep-wake cycle is important.

Pharmacologic treatment should be directed as described elsewhere to treat the identified sleep disorder.

HEADACHES

Several types of headaches are unique to sleep and its disorders (8,45,46). Thus, evaluation of headache should also include temporal information during the 24-hour cycle, which may offer clues to the diagnosis. Key headaches that are classically associated with sleep include cluster headaches, migraines, chronic paroxysmal hemicrania, and hypnic headaches. Additionally, sleep apnea can help trigger headaches, in particular (45).

Description

Cluster headaches are characterized by unilateral severe headache of rapid onset (5–15 minutes) and short duration (30–45 minutes) with autonomic changes in 97% of the cases (4). Autonomic changes are attributed to involvement of the carotid sympathetic plexus in the cavernous sinus. Symptoms include a unilateral Horner's syndrome, lacrimation, and injection of the conjunctiva of one eye. A link to REM sleep is considered characteristic (43). More recent studies suggest a link to OSA and hypoxemia (47,48) and raise the possibility that the sleep disordered breathing, which is often worse during REM sleep, may be the etiology of the association with REM sleep (rather than REM sleep itself).

More recent studies suggest a link to OSA and hypoxemia (47,48) and raise the possibility that the sleep disordered breathing, which is often worse during REM, may be the etiology of the association with REM sleep (rather than REM itself).

Migraine headaches are neurovascular headaches that may result from inflammation of the trigeminovascular system with secondary vasodilatation and throbbing pain (4). Headaches are more often unilateral than bilateral. Nausea and photophobia is common. Aura occurs in 20% and, when present, results from a slow march of neurologic symptoms across the affected region due to vasodilatation and secondary vasoconstriction. Common triggers include stress, sleep deprivation, excess sleep, menses, weather changes, chocolate, and alcohol. Exercise is exacerbating. Fifty percent occur during sleep, from 4 a.m. to 9 a.m. (8) An association with REM and stage NREM N3 (stages 3 and 4) sleep is reported (8). One must be careful to check for the presence of sleep-disordered breathing as the initial cause as OSA may lead to "pseudo sleep-related migraine" that becomes repetitive due to inappropriate prescription of an antimigraneous treatment.

Chronic paroxysmal hemicrania is rare and more common in females than males. Similar to cluster headaches, pain is unilateral and can be stabbing, pulsatile, or throbbing in nature (4). Autonomic symptoms such as lacrimation, ptosis, conjunctival injection, and nasal congestion are common. Headaches are more frequent than in cluster headaches, occurring from 1 to 40 times per day with duration on the order of minutes to two hours. A strong association with REM sleep is evident (8).

Hypnic headaches are strictly related to sleep and cause awakening at the same time each night. Pain is more often bilateral than unilateral. The duration is typically 5 to 15 minutes, and the frequency is at least 15 times in one month (8). They tend to occur during REM sleep.

Headaches associated with OSA commonly occur in the morning on awakening and are distinct from migraine headaches. Some debate exists on whether or not the actual association is to disrupted sleep, rather than sleep apnea itself [reviewed in (46)]. Assuming the latter association, mechanisms proposed for headache in OSA include vasodilatation secondary to hypoxemia and hypercapneic vasodilatation, autonomic and blood pressure surges, and increased intracranial pressure during the apneas (see above for issues with migraine).

Evaluation

Evaluation should begin with a neurologic diagnosis of the headache syndrome. Once diagnosed, standard neurologic interventions are implemented according to the latest clinical guidelines for the type of headache. A sleep and headache diary may be helpful if the above headache disorders are suspected. Once one of the above types of headaches is diagnosed, given the increased association with sleep apnea, a polysomnogram is warranted.

Treatment

Nonpharmacologic treatments include standard methods to treat any underlying sleep disorder determined on polysomnogram. If the sleep diary and headache logs reveal a pattern associated with excess sleep or sleep deprivation, modifying the patient's sleep schedule may be used to decrease occurrence. If sleep apnea is present, a headache diary and sleep may be helpful to monitor response to treatment and enable reduction of medications. If certain foods or beverages are triggers in an individual patient, they should be avoided as well. Withdrawal from inappropriate headache treatment may be needed.

Pharmacologic treatments are directed to the standard treatments currently available for each type of headache (4). In this regard, cluster headaches respond well to oxygen, triptans, dihydroergotamine (DHE), lidocaine, and butorphanol (4), acutely. Prophylactic treatments include verapamil, methysergide, divalproex sodium, lithium, topiramate, and baclofen. Migraines are treated with preventive as well as abortive agents. Abortive treatments include aspirin, acetaminophen, aspirin plus caffeine, non-steroidal anti-inflammatory drugs (NSAIDS), triptans, DHE, opioid nasal sprays and ergotamine. Prophylactic agents include tricyclic antidepressants, β-blockers, and anticonvulsants. Chronic paroxysmal hemicrania is very responsive to indomethacin. Alternative treatments may include aspirin, verapamil, steroids, and naproxen. Treatments for hypnic headaches include caffeine, lithium, indomethacin, atenolol, cyclobenzaprine, melatonin, prednisone, and flunarizine.

HEAD TRAUMA

Sleep disorders are common in the acute phase of head trauma (e.g., the first 3 months post head trauma or concussion). They include nocturnal disrupted sleep, sleep onset and sleep maintenance insomnia, early-morning awakenings, nocturnal headaches of all types, snoring and sleep-disordered breathing, daytime sleepiness and tiredness, and circadian rhythm disorders (particularly sleep phase delay syndrome).

A relationship between the importance of head trauma and the presence and absence of initial loss of consciousness and severity of sleep complaints has been shown. Whiplash without loss of consciousness has been shown to induce some degree of diaphragmatic and upper airway muscle dyscoordination leading to sleep disordered breathing and abnormalities of sleep.

These disorders may persist after the acute phase and regression of other symptoms associated with the head trauma. If they are still seen after 18 months post injury, one may need to consider the changes to be permanent sequelae. OSA, daytime NREM sleep, hypersomnia, and nocturnal awakening with or without headache are the most common permanent sequelae. Their presence leads to difficult medicolegal problems, including determination of severity of disability and compensation.

The most devastating is the permanent hypersomnia that may also be associated with intellectual decline and other neurologic sequelae. Such conditions respond poorly to modafinil. Stimulants of the amphetamine family are more effective. Often in severe cases, stimulants may only be partially effective; thus permanent disability may result.

CNS MALFORMATIONS AND SPINAL CORD TRAUMA

Many CNS malformations involving hydrocephalus (with or without pressure change), syringomyelia, syringobulbia, Arnold–Chiari type I and type II (49,50), spinal cord malformation, spinal cord trauma (51), and craniovertebral (52) and vertebral malformations will lead to different types of sleep complaints and syndromes, depending on the location affected.

Nocturnal sleep disruption, daytime sleepiness, abnormal breathing during sleep, and abnormal movements during sleep will be commonly associated with these malformations. Sometimes neurosurgical treatment of the problem, such as posterior cervical fusion, will be responsible for the problem (53). In some cases, neurosurgical treatment can improve breathing, such as in the case of Arnold–Chiari syndrome (54).

CONCLUSIONS

Neurologic disorders often affect sleep and the sleep-wake system. Neurodegenerative disorders such as Alzheimer's type dementia, Lewy body disease, Jacob–Creutzfeld disease, FFI, PD, MSA, PSP, Huntington's disease, and Leigh's disease can result in sleep complaints, such as insomnia, EDS, and parasomnias with or without violence. Treatment options include specific pharmacologic agents, as well as nonpharmacologic treatments such as improved sleep hygiene and CPAP for sleep apnea. Neuromuscular and nervous system disorders such as ALS, lumbar or cervical spinal stenosis, lumbosacral plexopathy, and neuropathies may affect sleep and/or daytime alertness, and improved sleep hygiene and specific medications, such as gabapentin, may be indicated. Autoimmune disorders such as MS may result in EDS and insomnia, and stimulants such as modafinil to combat the fatigue that is also associated with this condition may be helpful. Cerebrovascular disease may result in insomnia, hypersomnia, OSA, and dysregulation of the sleep-wake cycle, and treatment options include improvement in sleep hygiene and treatment with CPAP. Seizures can also disrupt sleep, and treatment of the underlying abnormality as well as good sleep hygiene and avoidance of sleep deprivation is often helpful. Headaches that affect sleep are managed by standard neurologic interventions, and if the headaches are associated with sleep apnea, treatment of this SBD may improve the headaches. Head trauma can severely affect sleep, particularly in the acute phase, and this trauma may result in a permanent hypersomnia that may or may not respond to stimulants. CNS malformations and spinal cord trauma may result in sleep disruption, daytime sleepiness, and abnormal breathing or movements during sleep, and neurosurgical treatment may improve these sleep-related symptoms.

REFERENCES

1. Autret A, Lucas B, Mondon K, et al. Sleep and brain lesions: a critical review of the literature and additional new cases. Neurophysiol Clin 2001; 31:356–375.
2. Bliwise DL. Sleep disorders in Alzheimer's disease and other dementias. Clin Cornerstone 2004; 6 (suppl 1A):S16–S28.
3. Chokroverty S. Sleep and degenerative neurologic disorders. Neurol Clin 1996; 14:807–826.
4. Evans RW. Saunders Manual of Neurologic Practice. Philadelphia: WB Saunders, 2003.
5. Boeve BF, Saper CB. REM sleep behavior disorder: a possible early marker for synucleinopathies. Neurology 2006; 66:796–797.
6. McKeith IG, Dickson DW, Lowe J, et al. Diagnosis and management of dementia with Lewy bodies: third report of the DLB Consortium. Neurology 2005; 65:1863–1872.
7. Provini F, Lombardi C, Lugaresi E. Insomnia in neurological diseases. Semin Neurol 2005; 25:81–89.
8. Sateia M. The International Classification of Sleep Disorders. Westchester, IL: American Academy of Sleep Medicine, 2006.
9. Johnson RT. Prion diseases. Lancet Neurol 2005; 4:635–642.
10. Gourmelon P, Amyx HL, Baron H, et al. Sleep abnormalities with REM disorder in experimental Creutzfeldt–Jakob disease in cats: a new pathological feature. Brain Res 1987; 411:391–396.
11. Taratuto AL, Piccardo P, Reich EG, et al. Insomnia associated with thalamic involvement in E200K Creutzfeldt–Jakob disease. Neurology 2002; 58:362–367.
12. Surhbier D. Diencephalic and brainstem sleep disorders. In: Carney P, Berry, R., Geyer, J, ed. Clinical Sleep Disorders. Philadelphia: Lippincott, 2005:347–359.
13. Thorpy MJ, Adler CH. Parkinson's disease and sleep. Neurol Clin 2005; 23:1187–1208.
14. Postuma RB, Lang AE, Massicotte-Marquez J, et al. Potential early markers of Parkinson's disease in idiopathic REM sleep behavior disorder. Neurology 2006; 66:845–851.
15. Kulisevsky J, Roldan E. Hallucinations and sleep disturbances in Parkinson's disease. Neurology 2004; 63:S28–S30.
16. Tan EK, Lum SY, Fook-Chong SM, et al. Evaluation of somnolence in Parkinson's disease: comparison with age- and sex-matched controls. Neurology 2002; 58:465–468.
17. Bhatt MH, Podder N, Chokroverty S. Sleep and neurodegenerative diseases. Semin Neurol 2005; 25: 39–51.
18. Arnulf I, Merino-Andreu M, Bloch F, et al. REM sleep behavior disorder and REM sleep without atonia in patients with progressive supranuclear palsy. Sleep 2005; 28:349–354.
19. Morton AJ, Wood NI, Hastings MH, et al. Disintegration of the sleep-wake cycle and circadian timing in Huntington's disease. J Neurosci 2005; 25:157–163.
20. Kushida CA, Littner MR, Morgenthaler T, et al. Practice parameters for the indications for polysomnography and related procedures: an update for 2005. Sleep 2005; 28:499–521.
21. Fetveit A, Bjorvatn B. Bright-light treatment reduces actigraphic-measured daytime sleep in nursing home patients with dementia: a pilot study. Am J Geriatr Psychiatry 2005; 13:420–423.
22. McCurry SM, Gibbons LE, Logsdon RG, et al. Nighttime insomnia treatment and education for Alzheimer's disease: a randomized, controlled trial. J Am Geriatr Soc 2005; 53:793–802.

23. Chong MS, Ayalon L, Marler M, et al. Continuous positive airway pressure reduces subjective daytime sleepiness in patients with mild to moderate Alzheimer's disease with sleep disordered breathing. J Am Geriatr Soc 2006; 54:777–781.

24. Kupfer DJ, Reynolds CF III Management of insomnia. N Engl J Med 1997; 336:341–346.

25. Littner MR, Kushida C, Anderson WM, et al. Practice parameters for the dopaminergic treatment of restless legs syndrome and periodic limb movement disorder. Sleep 2004; 27:557–559.

26. Lesage S, Hening WA. The restless legs syndrome and periodic limb movement disorder: a review of management. Semin Neurol 2004; 24:249–259.

27. Henriksen AL, St Dennis C, Setter SM, et al. Dementia with Lewy bodies: therapeutic opportunities and pitfalls. Consult Pharm 2006; 21:561–575.

28. Arnulf I, Similowski T, Salachas F, et al. Sleep disorders and diaphragmatic function in patients with amyotrophic lateral sclerosis. Am J Respir Crit Care Med 2000; 161:849–856.

29. Ferguson KA, Strong MJ, Ahmad D, et al. Sleep and breathing in amyotrophic lateral sclerosis. Sleep 1995; 18:514.

30. Gay PC, Westbrook PR, Daube JR, et al. Effects of alterations in pulmonary function and sleep variables on survival in patients with amyotrophic lateral sclerosis. Mayo Clin Proc 1991; 66:686–694.

31. LaBan MM, Viola SL, Femminineo AF, et al. Restless legs syndrome associated with diminished cardiopulmonary compliance and lumbar spinal stenosis—a motor concomitant of "Vesper's curse". Arch Phys Med Rehabil 1990; 71:384–388.

32. Scheer FA, Zeitzer JM, Ayas NT, et al. Reduced sleep efficiency in cervical spinal cord injury; association with abolished night time melatonin secretion. Spinal Cord 2006; 44:78–81.

33. Fleming WE, Pollak CP. Sleep disorders in multiple sclerosis. Semin Neurol 2005; 25:64–68.

34. Ohayon MM, Schatzberg AF. Using chronic pain to predict depressive morbidity in the general population. Arch Gen Psychiatry 2003; 60:39–47.

35. Lustberg L, Reynolds CF. Depression and insomnia: questions of cause and effect. Sleep Med Rev 2000; 4:253–262.

36. Bassetti CL. Sleep and stroke. Semin Neurol 2005; 25:19–32.

37. Yaggi H, Mohsenin V. Obstructive sleep apnoea and stroke. Lancet Neurol 2004; 3:333–342.

38. Neau JP, Paquereau J, Meurice JC, et al. Stroke and sleep apnoea: cause or consequence? Sleep Med Rev 2002; 6:457–469.

39. Turkington PM, Elliott MW. Sleep disordered breathing following stroke. Monaldi Arch Chest Dis 2004; 61:157–161.

40. Alanis-Guevara I, Pena E, Corona T, et al. Sleep disturbances, socioeconomic status, and seizure control as main predictors of quality of life in epilepsy. Epilepsy Behav 2005; 7:481–485.

41. Malow BA. Sleep and epilepsy. Neurol Clin 2005; 23:1127–1147.

42. Derry CP, Davey M, Johns M, et al. Distinguishing sleep disorders from seizures: diagnosing bumps in the night. Arch Neurol 2006; 63:705–709.

43. Dexter JD, Weitzman ED. The relationship of nocturnal headaches to sleep stage patterns. Neurology 1970; 20:513–518.

44. Hollinger P, Khatami R, Gugger M, et al. Epilepsy and obstructive sleep apnea. Eur Neurol 2006; 55: 74–79.

45. Poceta JS. Sleep-related headache syndromes. Curr Pain Headache Rep 2003; 7:281–287.

46. Rains JC, Poceta JS. Sleep-related headache syndromes. Semin Neurol 2005; 25:69–80.

47. Graff-Radford SB, Newman A. Obstructive sleep apnea and cluster headache. Headache 2004; 44: 607–610.

48. Chervin RD, Zallek SN, Lin X, et al. Sleep-disordered breathing in patients with cluster headache. Neurology 2000; 54:2302–2306.

49. Botelho RV, Bittencourt LR, Rotta JM, et al. Adult Chiari malformation and sleep apnoea. Neurosurg Rev 2005; 28:169–176.

50. Botelho RV, Bittencourt LR, Rotta JM, et al. Polysomnographic respiratory findings in patients with Arnold–Chiari type I malformation and basilar invagination, with or without syringomyelia: preliminary report of a series of cases. Neurosurg Rev 2000; 23:151–155.

51. Guilleminault C, Yuen KM, Gulevich MG, et al. Hypersomnia after head-neck trauma: a medicolegal dilemma. Neurology 2000; 54:653–659.

52. Botelho RV, Bittencourt LR, Rotta JM, et al. A prospective controlled study of sleep respiratory events in patients with craniovertebral junction malformation. J Neurosurg 2003; 99:1004–1009.

53. Guilleminault C, Li KK, Philip P, et al. Anterior cervical spine fusion and sleep-disordered breathing. Neurology 2003; 61:97–99.

54. Gagnadoux F, Meslier N, Svab I, et al. Sleep-disordered breathing in patients with Chiari malformation: improvement after surgery. Neurology 2006; 66:136–138.

INTRODUCTION

Psychiatric disorders are amongst the most frequent disorders encountered in clinical practice. A majority of patients with psychiatric disorders also present with prominent sleep disturbances. The full diagnostic criteria of the different disorders can be found in *Diagnostic and Statistical Manual of Mental Disorders (DSM-IV)* (1).

MOOD DISORDERS

Major Depression

Major depression is probably the most studied psychiatric disorder from the perspective of sleep issues, as insomnia and/or hypersomnia are integrated in the diagnostic criteria published in the *DSM-IV* (1) Women are twice as likely as men to be affected by depression, as the overall lifetime prevalence reaches up to 25% in women and 12% in men (1). Pathophysiology of depression has generated many hypotheses, some of them directly related to sleep physiology. Imbalance of cholinergic and monoaminergic systems (2), deficiency of homeostatic sleep drive (process S) (3), and dysregulation of the hypothalamo-pituitary axis (4) have all been postulated as possible explanations for generation of sleep dysregulation in major depressive disease. Insomnia is clearly the key sleep symptom, as it may precede and persist beyond resolution of the depressive episode. This has led many investigators to actually consider insomnia as a potential causative factor of depression and not merely as another symptom (5). This issue obviously has not been resolved yet. Clinical manifestations of sleep disturbances in depression include difficulty initiating sleep, sleep maintenance issues leading to fragmented sleep, frequent arousals and decreased total sleep time, as well as terminal insomnia (6). Available polysomnographic (PSG) data, although sometimes equivocal, shows definite trends toward certain patterns that correlate with the stated sleep symptoms. We can divide the data in sleep quantity, which encompasses duration, fragmentation and arousal issues, non–rapid eye movement (NREM) sleep distribution, and rapid eye movement (REM) sleep quality. Insomnia being the chief complaint of a majority of patients, it is not surprising to find PSG evidence of increased sleep latency, increased arousals leading to fragmented sleep episode, and increased wake after sleep onset (WASO). Sleep efficiency, as would be expected, is decreased. Studies have shown that NREM slow-wave activity can be diminished, especially in the first sleep cycle, as spectral analysis can substantiate a reduction of delta power compared with the other sleep cycles.

REM sleep analysis is probably the aspect of sleep that has generated the most interest. PSG findings consistently demonstrate reduction in the first REM episode latency combined with its prolonged duration, increased REM density (number of eye movements per REM time), and sometimes increased REM percentage in the night's hypnogram (7). The changes in REM sleep activity account for the hypothesis of dysregulation of the monoaminergic/cholinergic balance as a causal factor of major depression. Cholinergic hypersensitivity has been proposed. It has also been proposed that the REM sleep abnormalities might reflect a certain biologic trait indicating susceptibility to depression, as they can persist in the absence of current depression in the same individual and can also be found in family members of these index cases (8).

Treatment of depression involves classical pharmacotherapy with all classes of antidepressant drugs. Most share REM suppressant qualities, although bupropion, which is known to increase REM sleep in some patients, is also effective in treating depression. Special consideration should be taken in selecting pharmacologic therapy for the patient in whom insomnia is a prominent symptom. The more sedating antidepressants, such as mirtazapine and trazodone might be considered, as some selective serotonin reuptake inhibitors (SSRIs) might exacerbate the sleep problems. If insomnia persists after resolution of the acute depressive episode, cognitive behavior therapy (CBT) is a proven tool in helping to resolve chronic insomnia and should be considered in the ensuing management (9).

Bipolar Disorder

Bipolar disorder is characterized by recurrent episodes of depression alternating with mania. Interestingly, although insomnia is still the most common sleep disturbance in the depressed cyclothymic patients, a significant number of them exhibit hypersomnia, such as an increased total sleep time, difficulty arousing in the morning, and excessive daytime sleepiness. Insomnia or decreased need for sleep is also a cardinal symptom of mania (1). PSG data is scarce in mania as compared with depression, but the overall findings are quite comparable to the ones found in unipolar depression in terms of sleep disruption, slow-wave sleep decrease, and a REM sleep increase (10). Pharmacologic treatment with mood stabilizers (lithium, antiepileptic drugs) and, if necessary, with antidepressants should achieve control of the problem. Advantage of the sedating effects of antiepileptic drugs might be taken into consideration in the insomniac patient (9).

SCHIZOPHRENIA

Schizophrenia prevalence is 1% of the population. Sleep complaints are common, especially in the form of disruption of sleep. Insomnia, in particular, can be a prodromic symptom. Reversal of circadian pattern can also be present (sleeping during the day, awake during night) (1). Polysomnogram data reveals prolonged sleep onset latency, decreased total sleep time, and increased WASO (11). Sleep architecture has also been found to be disturbed in some patients, much like in patients with depression, with decreased slow-wave activity, and with shortened initial REM sleep latency (12). Successful treatment of schizophrenia with available neuroleptics will usually reverse the sleep disturbance but chronicity can ensue in some, especially with insomnia, that may need specific therapy (9).

ANXIETY DISORDERS

Panic Disorders

The prevalence of panic disorders is higher in females than males, as it varies between 2% and 3% in females and around 1% in males, with prevalence decreasing with age. Patients presenting with panic attacks have a higher prevalence of insomnia (1). Panic attacks can occur during sleep, as the patient will typically awaken in transitional NREM stages 2 and 3 with the classic symptoms. Other polysomnograms show that total sleep time and sleep efficiency are commonly decreased, although these findings are not universal (13). One also has to take into consideration the presence of comorbidities, particularly depression, as a confounding factor in the interpretation of the sleep data (14). Treatment includes avoiding stimulants (e.g., coffee, etc.), using SSRIs, benzodiazepines, as well as CBT (9).

Generalized Anxiety Disorder

Prevalence data taken from population surveys have given a 3% prevalence rate. Sleep disturbances, in the form of either initial insomnia, difficulty maintaining sleep, or non-refreshing sleep, are actually part of the *DSM-IV* diagnostic criteria (1). Polysomnogram findings have been unremarkable, unless insomnia is present (15). However, patients with generalized anxiety disorder frequently have associated depression (16), as this may alter sleep architecture, especially REM sleep. Treatment is accomplished with benzodiazepines, SSRIs, or CBT (9).

Social Phobia

In laymen terms, social phobia can be described as an unreasonable fear of a certain situation that leads to either avoidance of that situation or extreme discomfort while confronted with it (1). Sleep disturbances are generally not present but insomnia may be seen as an expected event gets closer. Polysomnogram recordings are typically normal (17). Treatment includes pharmacotherapy [benzodiazepines, SSRIs, norepinephrine serotonin reuptake inhibitors (NSRIs), monoamine oxidase inhibitors (MAOIs), β-blockers, and CBT (9)].

Obsessive-Compulsive Disorder

Lifetime prevalence data of obsessive-compulsive disorder (OCD) is in the range of 3%. Normally, sleep disturbances are not a prominent feature of this disorder, unless the obsession and/or compulsion involve a sleep-related activity (e.g., getting up from bed to check if the door is locked, etc.) (1). Polysomnograms show normal sleep architecture (18). Pharmacotherapy with SSRIs, tricyclic antidepressants (TCAs), and/or CBT have been advocated to help resolve this problem (9).

Posttraumatic Stress Disorder

Lifetime prevalence of posttraumatic stress disorder (PTSD) is about 7% to 8%. Sleep complaints constitute a major part of the symptoms, as vivid, recurrent nightmares and insomnia, either sleep initiation or sleep maintenance type, is frequently present. These features are included in the diagnostic criteria (1). Sleep studies have focused on disturbances of REM sleep. Studies of postwar veterans have shown fragmented REM sleep (i.e., frequent arousals from REM sleep), higher frequency of muscle twitches, thought to represent heightened autonomic activity (19,20). However, recent data collected from a large study population and compared with a control group did not show any convincing evidence of differences in sleep architecture of both groups. So, even though the sleep symptoms can be prominent, polysomnogram results can be unremarkable (21). The presence of sleep-related symptoms is often the most distressing feature for the patient and proper management is of great importance. Treatment for PTSD includes pharmacotherapy with SSRIs, TCAs, MAOIs, α-1 adrenergic receptor antagonists, antiepileptic drugs, and atypical neuroleptics. Psychotherapy might be particularly helpful for sleep disturbances (9).

EATING DISORDERS

Anorexia nervosa and bulimia nervosa are the prototypical primary eating disorders. Meta-analysis of PSG data failed to reveal clear differences between patients with eating disorders and normal controls (7). Claims of shortened REM sleep latency should be taken with caution, especially since comorbidity with mood disorders is common (22).

SUBSTANCE ABUSE

Probably the two most commonly legally used substances that affect sleep are alcohol and caffeine. Alcohol might be the most widely used nonprescribed "hypnotic," and caffeine is the stimulant of choice all over the world.

Alcohol

In normal subjects, alcohol has a short-term effect, as it decreases sleep latency, increases NREM sleep, and reduces REM sleep. After a few hours, blood levels drop, which results in autonomic activation, fragmented sleep, and an increase in REM sleep (23). Overall, alcohol has a disruptive effect on sleep quality. Also, alcohol intake increases the risk of developing or unmasking sleep-disordered breathing, as it decreases muscle tone and increases airway resistance (24). Periodic limb movements of sleep can also be exacerbated by alcohol consumption (25). PSG data on true alcoholic patients show prolonged sleep latency, poor sleep efficiency, and decreases in total sleep time, REM sleep, and NREM sleep (7). Daytime hypersomnia can also be present as part of a disrupted circadian rhythm. Abstinent former alcoholics still can have a disturbed sleeping pattern, as evidenced by PSG findings, many years after cessation (26). The presence of insomnia is a negative predictor of abstinence (27). Treatment of the sleep disturbances must take into account the consumption of alcohol, as compliance is difficult to obtain in an intoxicated patient.

Caffeine

Caffeine is the prototypical legal stimulant. It promotes wakefulness by blocking adenosine receptors in the brain. Regular caffeine intake leads to tolerance, and mild withdrawal symptoms can occur with abrupt cessation. Besides enhancing vigilance, caffeine also produces sympathetic activation (28). It is important to recognize coffee intake as a possible cause of insomnia and increased anxiety, and a potential precipitator of panic attacks (9,29).

CONCLUSIONS

Psychiatric disorders have been associated with sleep disturbances and sleep disorders. Major depression has a profound impact on sleep, with insomnia as a key sleep symptom of this disorder and a reduction in the first REM episode latency prominently observed during polysomnography. Hypersomnia as well as insomnia can be seen in patients with bipolar disorder, which manifests as an increased total sleep time, difficulty arousing in the morning, and excessive daytime sleepiness. Insomnia and reversal of circadian pattern coupled with the PSG findings of prolonged sleep onset latency, decreased total sleep time, and increased WASO can be found in patients with schizophrenia. Panic disorders are associated with insomnia, with fragmented sleep, and sometimes with decrements in total sleep time and sleep efficiency. Patients with generalized anxiety disorder frequently have insomnia and non-refreshing sleep. For patients with posttraumatic sleep disorder, insomnia and vivid, recurrent nightmares are characteristic of this condition. Sleep complaints or abnormal sleep studies are not typically identified in patients with social phobia, OCD, and eating disorders. Lastly, alcohol has a disruptive effect on sleep quality and regular caffeine use may lead to tolerance as well as insomnia, increased anxiety, and possibly panic attacks.

REFERENCES

1. American Psychiatric Association. Diagnostic and Statistical Manual for Psychiatric Disorders IV. Text Revision. Washington, D.C.: American Psychiatric Press, 2000.
2. Janowsky DS, Davis JM, El-Yousef MK, et al. A cholinergic-adrenergic hypothesis of mania and depression. Lancet 1972; 2:632–635.
3. Borbély AA, Wirz-Justice A. Sleep, sleep deprivation and depression: a hypothesis derived from a model of sleep regulation. Hum Neurobiol 1982; 1:205–221.
4. Nestler EJ, Barrot M, DiLeone RJ, et al. Neurobiology of depression. Neuron 2002; 34:13–25.
5. Ohayon MM, Roth T. Place of chronic insomnia in the course of depressive and anxiety disorders. J Psychiatr Res 2003; 37:9–15.
6. Riemann D. Insomnia and comorbid psychiatric disorders. Sleep Med 2007; 8(suppl 4):S15–S20.
7. Benca RM, Obermeyer WH, Thisted RA, et al. Sleep and psychiatric disorders: a meta-analysis. Arch Gen Psychiatry 1992; 49:651–668.
8. Lauer CJ, Schreiber W, Holsboer F, et al. In quest of identifying vulnerability markers for psychiatric disorders by all-night polysomnography. Arch Gen Psychiatry 1995; 52:145–153.
9. Kryger MH, Roth T, Dement WC. Principles and Practice of Sleep Medicine. 4th ed. Philadelphia: Elsevier, 2006:1297–1358.
10. Hudson JL, Lipinski JF, Keck PE, et al. Polysomnographic characteristics of young manic patients. Comparison with unipolar depressed patients and normal control subjects. Arch Gen Psychiatry 1992; 49:378–383.
11. Chouinard S, Poulin J, Stip E, et al. Sleep in untreated patients with schizophrenia: a meta-analysis. Schizophr Bull 2004; 30(4):957–967.
12. Poulin J, Daoust AM, Forest G, et al. Sleep architecture and its clinical correlates in first episode and neuroleptic-naive patients with schizophrenia. Schizophr Res 2003; 62(1–2):147–153.
13. Mellman TA, Uhde TW. Electroencephalographic sleep in panic disorder: a focus on sleep-related panic attacks. Arch Gen Psychiatry 1989; 46:178–184.
14. Roy-Byrne PP, Stang P, Wittchen HU, et al. Lifetime panic-depression comorbidity in the National Comorbidity Survey: association with symptoms, impairment, course and help-seeking. Br J Psychiatry 2000; 176:229–223.
15. Monti JM, Monti D. Sleep disturbance in generalized anxiety disorder and its treatment. Sleep Med Rev 2000; 4:263–276.

16. Wittchen HU, Zhao S, Kessler RC, et al. DSM-III-R generalized anxiety disorder in the National Comorbidity Survey. Arch Gen Psychiatry 1994; 51:355–364.

17. Brown TM, Black B, Uhde TW. The sleep architecture of social phobia. Biol Psychiatry 1994; 35:420–421.

18. Robinson D, Walsleben J, Pollack S, et al. Nocturnal polysomnography in obsessive-compulsive disorder. Psychiatry Res 1998; 80:257–263.

19. Mellman TA, Kulick-Bell R, Ashlock LE, et al. Sleep events among veterans with combat-related posttraumatic stress disorder. Am J Psychiatry 1995; 152:110–115.

20. Ross RJ, Ball WA, Dinges DF, et al. Rapid eye movement sleep disturbance in posttraumatic stress disorder. Biol Psychiatry 1994; 35:195–202.

21. Breslau N, Roth T, Burduvali E, et al. Sleep in lifetime posttraumatic stress disorder: a community-based polysomnographic study. Arch Gen Psychiatry 2004; 61:508–516.

22. Levy AB, Dixon KN, Stern SL. How are depression and bulimia related? Am J Psychiatry 1989; 146:162–169.

23. Lobo LL, Tufik S. Effects of alcohol on sleep parameters of sleep-deprived healthy volunteers. Sleep 1997; 20:52–59.

24. Dawson A, Bigby BG, Poceta JS, et al. Effect of bedtime alcohol on inspiratory resistance and respiratory drive in snoring and non-snoring men. Alcohol Clin Exp Res 1997; 21:183–190.

25. Aldrich MS, Shipley JE. Alcohol use and periodic limb movements of sleep. Alcohol Clin Exp Res 1993; 17:192–196.

26. Drummond SPA, Gillin JC, Smith TL, et al. The sleep of abstinent pure primary alcoholic patients: natural course and relationship to relapse. Alcohol Clin Exp Res 1998; 22:1796–1802.

27. Brower KJ, Aldrich MS, Robinson EA, et al. Insomnia, self-medication, and relapse to alcoholism. Am J Psychiatry 2001; 158:399–404.

28. Zwyghuizen-Doorenbos A, Roehrs T, Lipschutz L, et al. Effects of caffeine on alertness. Psychopharmacology (Berl) 1990; 100:36–39.

29. Hughes JR, Higgins ST, Bickel WK, et al. Caffeine self administration, withdrawal, and adverse effects among coffee drinkers. Arch Gen Psychiatry 1991; 48:611–617.

Index

Milton Keynes UK
Ingram Content Group UK Ltd.
UKHW051901071024
449327UK00025B/2043